A MANUAL

OF

MEDICAL JURISPRUDENCE

A MANUAL

OF

MEDICAL JURISPRUDENCE

FOR

INDIA,

INCLUDING THE OUTLINE OF A HISTORY OF CRIME AGAINST
THE PERSON IN INDIA.

NORMAN CHEVERS, M. D.

GYAN

Published by

Gyan Publishing House
5, Ansari Road
Daryaganj, New Delhi-110002
Phone: 011-47034999, 9811692060
E-mail: books@gyanbooks.com

Distribution Network
gyanbooks.com
India, USA, Canada, UK, Australia, France

ISBN: 978-81-212-8378-6 (PB)
First Published, 1870

2nd Impression 2023

Printed at: Gyan Press, Delhi.

A MANUAL OF MEDICAL JURISPRUDENCE
Author: NORMAN CHEVERS

MEDICAL JURISPRUDENCE IN INDIA.

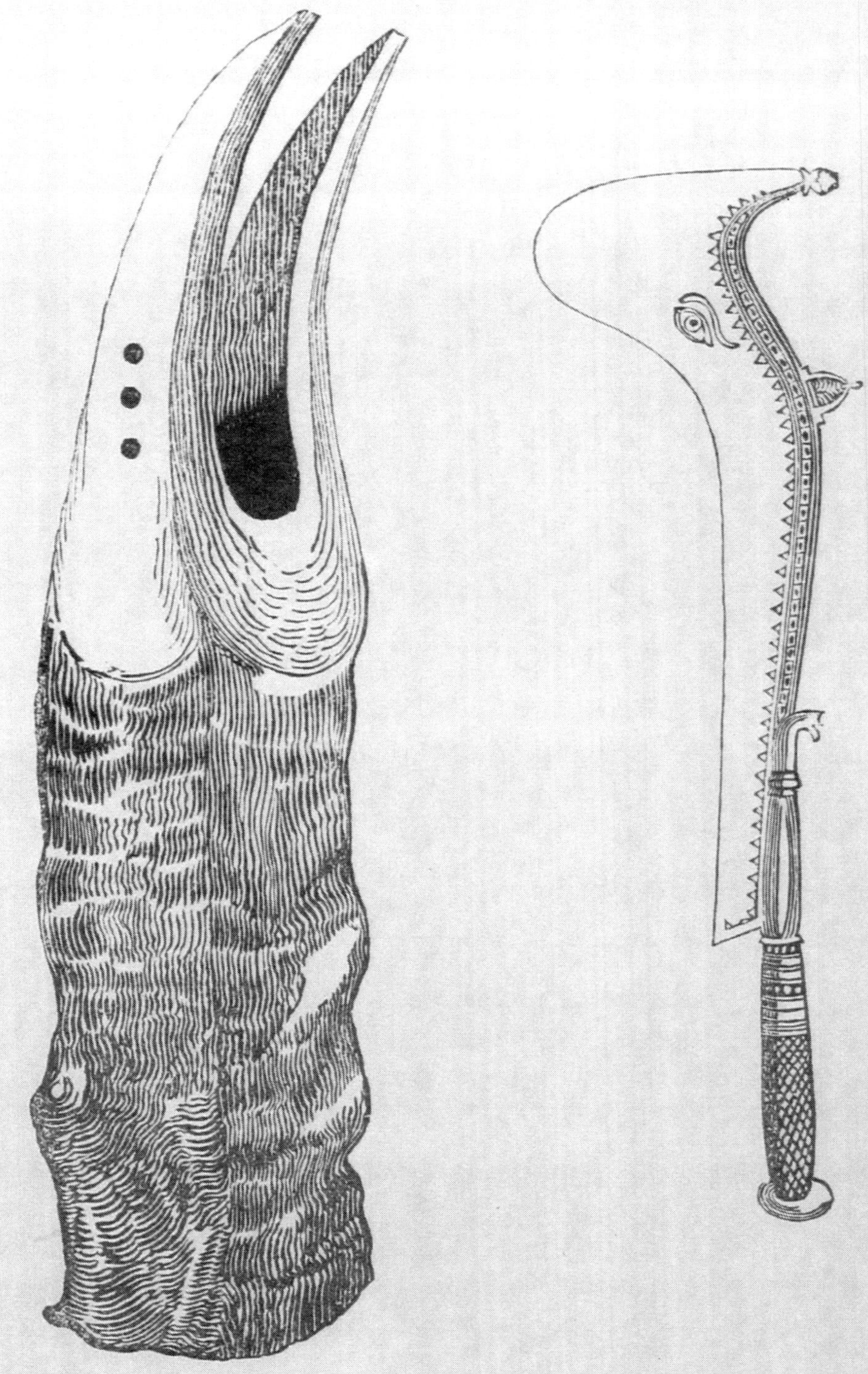

Sacrificial Instruments used in the murder of a child in a temple at Jessore, vide p. 413.

DR. KENNETH MCLEOD, DEL.

A MANUAL

OF

MEDICAL JURISPRUDENCE

FOR

INDIA,

INCLUDING THE OUTLINE OF A HISTORY OF CRIME AGAINST THE PERSON IN INDIA.

BY

NORMAN CHEVERS, M.D.,

SURGEON-MAJOR, H. M. BENGAL ARMY;
PRINCIPAL OF THE CALCUTTA MEDICAL COLLEGE, PROFESSOR OF MEDICINE, AND SENIOR PHYSICIAN IN THE COLLEGE HOSPITAL;
PRESIDENT OF THE BENGAL SOCIAL SCIENCE ASSOCIATION.

"As a hunter traces the lair of a wounded beast by the drops of blood, thus let a king investigate the true point of justice by deliberate arguments."—MENU.

CALCUTTA:

THACKER, SPINK & CO., PUBLISHERS TO THE UNIVERSITY.

BOMBAY: THACKER, VINING & Co. LONDON: W. THACKER & Co.

1870.

To

THE PEOPLE OF INDIA

This Work,

WHICH BENEFITS THEM

BY PROTECTING THEM AGAINST

THEIR ONLY POWERFUL OPPRESSORS,

THEIR CRIMINAL CLASSES,

IS DEDICATED,

BY THEIR FRIEND,

THE AUTHOR.

PREFACE TO THE THIRD EDITION.

THE previous (second) edition of this work appeared in January 1856, by the command of the Most Noble the Marquis of Dalhousie, Governor-General of India, conveyed in the letter of which a copy is subjoined:

No. 1342.

FROM

C. ALLEN, ESQ.,
Offg. Secretary to the Government of India,

To

NORMAN CHEVERS, ESQ., M.D.

Dated the 15th December 1854.

Home Department.

SIR,

I am directed to inform you that the Most Noble the Governor-General in Council has read, with the greatest interest, your able and valuable Report on Medical Jurisprudence published in the Indian Annals of Medical Science.

2. His Lordship in Council is of opinion that the distribution of this Report, among the Magistrates and Political Officers in India, would be a most useful measure; and, with reference to your two letters dated respectively the 4th and 5th instant, is pleased to subscribe for 500 copies, of which 100 copies will be placed at your disposal, and 400 copies distributed to Judicial Officers.

3. His Lordship in Council accepts your offer to correct the press and to make such alterations and additions to the Report as may be necessary. When you have done this, you will be good enough to have the 500 copies subscribed for, printed at the expense of the Government, and 400 of them forwarded to this office.

I have the honor to be,

Sir,

Your most obedient Servant,

C. ALLEN,
Offg. Secy. to the Government of India.

Gratifying as this arrangement, which was carried out in strict obedience, was to myself, it tended considerably to limit the publicity of my work, copies of which are only to be found in Magistrates' and Judges' Offices, and in a few Indian Libraries. In fact, the second edition of the work was never *published*, in the booksellers' sense of the term; and it is now so rare that I have been obliged to spoil my only remaining copy in printing the present edition.

This is not an elementary treatise on Medical Jurisprudence. It is a system for India intended to be used by those who have already mastered the science of Legal Medicine as it stands, well-nigh complete for Europe, in the works of Taylor, Casper, and Guy.

The work, as it is now offered, has been re-arranged, and, in a great measure, re-written. Not only have the contents of the book been doubled, nearly every subject having received fresh illustration, but the scope of the work has been greatly enlarged, and the view of the whole subject presented to the reader is very much clearer and more extensive than that which was disclosed in the previous edition.

I venture to believe that the amount of information which I have been able to obtain regarding the crimes which prevail in the two sister Presidencies, is calculated to render this volume as useful in the Courts of Madras and Bombay as in those of Bengal.

Four years subsequently to the appearance of the last edition, the introduction, throughout the Judicial Courts of India, of the Indian Penal Code (Act XLV of 1860) and of the Code of Criminal Procedure (Act XXV of 1861, and Act VIII of 1869), completely changed, at least in form, the Criminal Law of this country.

I trust that I have succeeded in adapting my work to the existing Law; at the same time, full references to older Laws have been retained, generally in the form of foot-notes.

In the present edition, the Table of Contents has been rendered as full as possible, and a copious Index has been added.

The History of Crime against the Person in India, contained in this book, is, even now, a mere outline; still the body of facts brought together for the illustration of this subject has become so considerable as to deserve the attention, not only of the Legislator and the Medical Jurist, but also of the Sociologist. Carefully read, this work will be found to throw considerable light upon the true origin, nature, and distribution of crime in India; and, by defining with fair clearness the classes among whom crime prevails, and by discovering the traditions upon which these criminals act, its facts do justice to the people at large, who, it is true, have certain illegal national practices of great antiquity not unlike our own duelling and boxing, and who suffer grievously from the persecution of their criminal classes,—the Dacoits, Thugs or Road-Poisoners, Wall-Piercers, &c., &c.,—but whom it would be as unjust to stigmatize generally as Phansigars and Lattials, as it would be to characterize the English as a nation of Garotters and Prize-Fighters.

The most facile, and the most fatal, error into which delineators of national character have fallen, in all ages, is that of representing prevalent crimes as national customs.

Nearly every page of this volume bears evidence of my indebtedness for valuable facts to my Brother-Officers and Friends; among whom The Hon'ble Elphinstone Jackson, Baboo Kanny Lall Dey, Additional Chemical Examiner to Government, and Teacher of Chemistry and Medical Jurisprudence in the Medical College, Dr. Robert Faure Hutchinson, and Moulvie Tumeez Khan, Khan Bahadur, Teacher of Medicine, have my best acknowledgments.

I shall feel greatly obliged to those gentlemen who may supply me with additional facts illustrative of questions of medico-legal importance in this country, especially in the Bombay and Madras Presidencies.

THE MEDICAL COLLEGE, CALCUTTA,

11*th October* 1870.

PREFACE TO THE SECOND EDITION.

THE remarks embodied in this volume first appeared as a "Report on Medical Jurisprudence in the Bengal Presidency," published in the Indian Annals of Medical Science, for October 1854. They are now reprinted, by direction of the Government of India. In the present edition, however, the original article has received so many and such extensive additions and alterations, that it may be said to have been almost entirely re-written. The chief of these additions consists in the insertion of a great number of important facts and cases, chiefly derived from the printed Reports of the Court of Nizamut Adawlut of the North-Western Provinces: these quotations have, for greater facility of reference, been marked in the notes by distinctive letters.*

It is hoped that these additions will render the work equally useful to Judicial and Medical Officers in Bengal and the North-Western Provinces.

It should be clearly understood that this Manual is not professed to embody even an outline of the well-known principles of Medical Jurisprudence,—the writer's object has merely been to bring together those facts, bearing upon medico-legal questions of frequent occurrence in this country, which are not to be found in the works of our standard authority on the subject—Dr. Alfred Taylor;—the "Manual of Medical Jurisprudence;" and the "Treatise on Poisons."

The author trusts that, without deviating from the main object of his work, he has succeeded in embodying in this volume some useful contributions towards *A History of Crime Against the*

* Thus: "Nizamut Adawlut Reports, N. W. P."

Person in India. A knowledge of the principal facts of which this outline is made up, while it is altogether indispensable to the Judicial Officer in the daily performance of his duty, is required by the Surgeon in the investigation of nearly every medico-legal question that can be brought before him in this country.

This sketch is, avowedly, a very slight and imperfect one; still it is believed that it is the first that has been attempted; and it is trusted that it will, at least, serve to demonstrate the importance which would attach to a thoroughly complete and elaborated HISTORY OF CRIME IN INDIA.

In performing this not uninteresting task, it has been found necessary to dwell somewhat at length upon many painful details; this, however, has been done unhesitatingly, under the conviction that, for the censor of morals and the dispenser of laws, the vices of society must be laid bare with a strong and untremulous hand:—knowing where the moral canker lies, it is a resolve neither of wisdom nor of delicacy to permit it to fester on in concealment.

The Legal Authorities referred to in this Manual are—

Taylor's Manual of Medical Jurisprudence, Fifth Edition.

Baynes's Notes on Medical Jurisprudence in India. (A carefully drawn-out abstract of the leading portions of Taylor's larger work, with notes from the Editor's own experience, especially intended for the use of Judicial Officers.)

The Institutes of Menu.

Mahomedan Law. Harington's Analysis of the Laws and Regulations, &c., Folio, 1809.

Beaufort's Digest of the Criminal Law.

Skipwith's Magistrate's Guide.

Macnaghten's Reports.

Reports of the Nizamut Adawlut of Bengal.

Ditto of the North-Western Provinces.

The Reports of the Superintendent of Police, Lower Provinces.

CALCUTTA, 10*th January* 1856.

GENERAL TABLE OF CONTENTS.

LIST OF ILLUSTRATIONS.

ERRATA ET CORRIGENDA.

Page 68, line 1, *omit* "the" at the beginning of the line.
,, 100, ,, 23, *for* "Benglee" *read* "Bengalee."
,, 107, ,, 3, *for* "vendor" *read* "vendors."
,, 114, ,, 5, *for* "dicease" *read* disease."
,, 125, ,, 12, *for* "ACETO-ARSENIC" *read* "ACETO-ARSENITE."
,, 137, ,, 5 from bottom, *for* "detatchment" *read* "detachment."
,, 143, ,, 3 ,, *for* "*kishnak*" *read* "*bishnak*."
,, 169, head line, *for* "INDIA" *read* "IN INDIA."
,, 220, line 18 from bottom, *for* "toxnological" *read* "toxicological."
,, 227, ,, 2 ,, *for* "onan" *read* "on an."
,, 234, ,, 16 ,, *for* "Malwas" *read* "Malwa."
,, 246, ,, 3 ,, *for* "angmentation" *read* "augmentation."
,, 254, ,, 20 ,, *omit* "the" at the beginning of the line.
,, 281, ,, 1, *insert* "of" *between* "Bengal" and "a."
,, 307, ,, 12, *insert* "all" *between* "it" and "over."
,, 315, ,, 21, *for* "confectionary" *read* "confectionery."
,, 318, ,, 16, *for* "Societies'" *read* "Society's."
,, 334, ,, 11, *for* "cresentic" *read* "crescentic."
,, 341, ,, 14 from bottom, *for* "*aconilum*" *read* "*aconitum*."
,, 357, ,, 12, *for* "daed" *read* "dead."
,, 360, ,, 10, *for* "itseltf.he" *read* "itself the."
,, 378, ,, 23, *for* "*itelf*" *read* "*itself*."
,, 380, ,, 15, *for* "relaity" *read* "reality."
,, 410, ,, 9 from bottom, *insert* "the" *between* "to" and "notice."
,, 423, ,, 22, *omit* the word "in" at the end of the line.
,, 429, ,, 4 from bottom, *for* "brothe 's" *read* "brother's."
,, 463, ,, 9 ,, *for* "expriments" *read* experiments."
,, 478, ,, 7 ,, *for* "Wyh" *read* "Why."
,, 545, ,, 8 ,, *fon* "Bukland" *read* "Buckland."
,, 621, ,, 11, *for* "of Raneegunge" *read* "at Raneegunge."
,, 627, ,, 3, *omit* the words "and drowned them."
,, ,, ,, 4 from bottom, *omit* the words "Only a few months since."
,, 635, ,, 2 of note, *for* "page 56" *read* "page 24."
,, 649, ,, 1 ,, *for* "1833" *read* "1853."
,, 651, ,, 13 from bottom, *for* "He" *read* "We."
,, 660, ,, 10, *omit* the word "he" before "resolved."
,, 662, ,, 15, *for* "honor" *read* "horror."
,, 679, ,, 2 from bottom, *for* "pp. 641-42" *read* "pp. 990 *et seq*."
,, ,, ,, 3 ,, *for* "p. 244" *read* "p. 996."
,, 682, ,, 15, *for* "struck" *read* "stuck."
,, 684, ,, 7, *for* "of submission" *read* "for submission."
,, 693, ,, 15, *for* "infracture" *read* "infraction."
,, 697, ,, 14 from bottom, *for* "and Nizamut," *read* "of Nizamut."
,, 704, ,, 14 ,, *for* "1864" *read* "1868."
,, 765, ,, 1, *for* "Ushru" *read* "Ushruff."
,, 771, ,, 1 of note, *after* "Taylor" *insert* "Fifth Edition."
,, 807, last line of note, *for* "Pschycological" *read* "Psychological."
,, 831, line 10 from bottom, *for* "Saxus Baccata" *read* "Taxus Baccata."

MANUAL OF MEDICAL JURISPRUDENCE

FOR

INDIA.

INTRODUCTORY REMARKS.

WHEN performing the duties of a Civil Surgeon, I was frequently struck with the remarkable singularity and intricacy of the medico-legal questions upon which my opinion was required by the Magistrates and Judges of the districts, and I, consequently, perceived that our Indian Medical Literature stood greatly in want of a treatise on Medical Jurisprudence, embodying clear and practical expositions of the various and peculiar modes by which the natives of this country are wont to effect crimes against the person, and to attempt their concealment; as well as full illustrations of the many difficult questions regarding Unsoundness of Mind, Identity, Suicide, Torture, &c., which frequently occur here, under circumstances entirely dissimilar to those which call for the like investigations in Europe.

Dr. Mouat informed me, in the year 1853, that, while occupying the Chair of Forensic Medicine in the Calcutta Medical College, he became so strongly convinced of the necessity of illustrating the leading principles of his subject by examples occurring in India, that he was, subsequently, led to apply to the Court of Nizamut Adawlut for copies of all depositions, made by Surgeons in the Zillah Courts within their jurisdiction, forwarded to the Judges subsequently to 1840, in which year the several Magistrates of Bengal were directed to take the depositions of Medical Officers in cases of murder or wounding. Full copies of nine years' reports were furnished by the Court. These Dr. Mouat very liberally made over to me, previous to his departure on furlough, for analysis in the *Indian Annals of Medical Science*.

I attentively went over the whole of these interesting documents. The principal facts which they contain are embodied in the following pages.

Although the formation of a judicial opinion upon the general merits of cases in which his medico-legal evidence may be required is, of course, altogether beyond the province of the Medical Jurist, it is generally necessary,—first, that he should possess a wide and intimate knowledge of the dispositions, customs, prejudices, and crimes of the people among whom his investigations are to be pursued; and, secondly, that he should be made acquainted, as fully as possible, with every ascertainable detail of the cases upon which his opinion is demanded.

The circumstances which generally lead to the perpetration of various crimes against the person, the descriptions of crimes usually committed, and the means commonly employed to effect and to conceal them, form an essential portion of the Medical Jurist's knowledge. A very few illustrations will sufficiently set forth this principle.

The body of a woman is discovered on the floor of a London garret. The evidences of want and sorrow are stamped upon her countenance, as deeply as the recent gashes and bruises which disfigure it. The surgeon and the policeman hold an undivided opinion upon this case;—it is not one of accident or robbery; life has been taken away by the hand sworn to protect it; and the criminal must be sought for with the fumes of liquor still in his brain, and with his victim's blood still upon his clothes and behind his nails.

A girl lies dead in a small room in Paris; the Medical Inspector, on entering, presses his handkerchief to his face, to exclude the suffocating atmosphere, glances at a charcoal pan beside the bed, tears out a caulking of rags from the crevices of the sash;—and the leading facts of the case are before him.*

In like manner, the body of a female is discovered beside a tank in Bengal, mutilated by a dozen wounds, each sufficient to cause almost instantaneous death. The skull is cloven, a hand has been lopped off, the shoulder is gashed through muscle and bone to the lungs. Whether the remains are those of a Hindu woman or of a Mussulmanee, the matter scarcely admits of a doubt;—the murder has been committed by her husband or paramour, in a fit of jealousy; search must be made for a *dhao*, or bill-hook, which will probably be discovered with the evidences of crime upon its blade.

Still again,—the body of a native of good condition would be found buried near a water-course, scored from head to heel with enormous gashes; these, however, would be entirely passed over in the examination, the evidences of strangulation by a Thug's girdle would alone be sought for.

Various as are the modes of effecting and of concealing crime in different countres, a large experience will always show that a really new crime is an unexampled event in the cirminal annals of any land.

As the hunter and the brute-tamer learn to approach and to subdue the cunningest and the strongest beasts and the most venomous reptiles,

* Happily the crime of suicide by charcoal fumes appears to be far less prevalent in Paris now than it was when the above was written, fifteen years ago.

the detective officer follows the criminal through all his feints and doublings towards escape ; while the Medical Jurist,—guided here by a scratch or a blood spirt, there by a dingy stain, or an almost invisible speck of powder, or a metallic film weighing the twentieth part of a grain,—tracks out and lays bare the evidences of his crime, almost with the certainty of an irresistible fate. To start fairly on the scent, however, it is necessary, as we have seen, that he should know something of the propensities and customs of the criminal, and be thoroughly practised in the unravelling of similar cases.*

A very large proportion of the experience and tact essential to the attainment of this end in India has yet to be gained ; somewhat, however, is known at present, and sufficient for all practical purposes may, doubtless, be acquired by the combined labours of several close observers, pursuing their investigations in various parts of the country, each noting the varieties in the modes of effecting and of concealing crime, according to the religious classes, habits, and races of the offenders.

---

* "As a hunter traces the lair of a wounded beast by the drops of blood; thus let a King investigate the true point of justice by deliberate arguments."—*Menu.*

It is told of Camille Desmoulins that, when urged to apprehend a body of royalist conspirators somewhat prematurely, he said—"A hen always lays in the same place. Wait till the eggs are all laid and then take them."

An Indian criminal's or escaped prisoner's movements almost always tend ultimately towards his own village, in the neighbourhood of which the police should maintain as long a watch as the importance of his apprehension may justify. Such watch was laid for the Nana at his birth-place, Narel, on the railway line to Poonah.

Previous to the introduction of the Approver System, the police frequently succeeded in apprehending dacoits by rendering the mistresses of the suspected ringleaders furiously jealous.

Who is *she?* was the well-known enquiry of an Eastern potentate whenever the cause of deep-laid mischief had to be brought to light.

Governor Holwell said :—"During five years that we presided in the Judicial Court in Calcutta, never any murders or other atrocious crimes came before us in which it was not proved that a Brahmin" [one of those who mingle in worldly pursuits] "was at the bottom of it."

A London detective, suspecting that one of a party of coal-heavers had just committed a sanguinary murder, would probably look for an individual with clean hands. A deeper insight into class habits was shown by the Judge of Rajshahye, when he enquired of a Hindu, who confessed that he had been one of a party who had committed a murder, whether, upon throwing down the body, he and his associates *bathed.*

The meaning of this will be rendered clear to the inexperienced reader by what came out at another trial before the same Judge. Certain Hindus, having strangled a woman and thrown the body into the Ganges, were asked, "if they did not mean to bathe;" they replied, "no; for if they did, they would be suspected." The person who asserted that he asked this question, was tried for the murder. The Judge remarked, "What convinces me that the prisoner lent a helping hand to remove the body, was the question he put to his associates about bathing. It is notorious that, when natives touch a corpse, they consider themselves defiled and impure *(asood)*, and invariably bathe, whatever hour it may be. Now, if the prisoner had been a mere looker on, the idea of bathing *at night* would never have suggested itself to him, nor would he have adverted to the fact in his confession."—*Nizamut Adawlut Reports*, Vol. V., Part 2 of 1855, p. 406.

CHARACTERISTICS OF THE CRIMINALS OF INDIA.

It would probably be impossible to point to any races of men whose great crimes more distinctly emanate from and illustrate their national character, than is the case with those various classes of natives who inhabit the British possessions in India. A thorough insight into the intimate peculiarities of the native character could only follow a life-long acquaintance with Hindus and Mussulmans of all classes, and has probably never yet been fully mastered by any European. Still, the strong broad features which stand prominently forth upon the surface of their national characters, and which are displayed with the greatest expression in the details of their crimes are, of course, open to every cautious observer, and especially demand the study of the Lawyer, the Physician, and the Medical Jurist.

I shall, therefore, make no apology for citing here the opinions formed of the moral characteristics of two foremost classes of the people in India as viewed by two great Lawyers,—verdicts evidently weighed on the judgment-seat with regards unrelentingly directed to the criminal aspects of the natures judged :—

" The *Rajpoots* are the representatives of Hinduism. In them are seen all the qualities of the Hindu race unmitigated by foreign mixture, exerted with their original energy, and displayed in the strongest light. They exhibit the genuine form of a Hindu community, formed of the most discordant materials, and combining the most extraordinary contrasts of moral nature ; unconquerable adherence to native opinions and usages, with servile submission to any foreign yoke ; an unbelieving priesthood, ready to suffer martyrdom for the most petty observance of their professed faith ; a superstition which inspires the resolution to inflict or to suffer the most atrocious barbarities, without cultivating any natural sentiment, or enforcing any social duty ; all the stages in the progress of society brought together in one nation, from some abject castes, more brutal than the savages of New Zealand, to the polish of manners and refinement of character conspicuous in the upper ranks ; attachment to kindred and to home, with no friendship, and no love of country ; good temper and gentle disposition ; little active cruelty, except when stimulated by superstition ; but little sensibi-

" The physical organization of the *Bengalee* is feeble even to effeminacy. He lives in a constant vapour-bath. His pursuits are sedentary, his limbs delicate, his movements languid. During many ages he has been trampled upon by men of bolder and more hardy breeds. Courage, independence, veracity, are qualities to which his constitution and his situation are equally unfavourable. His mind bears a singular analogy to his body. It is weak, even to helplessness, for purposes of manly resistance, but its suppleness and its tact move the children of sterner climates to admiration, not unmingled with contempt. All those arts which are the natural defence of the weak are more familiar to this subtle race than to the Ionian of the time of Juvenal, or to the Jew of the dark ages. What the horns are to the buffaloe, what the paw is to the tiger, what beauty, according to the old Greek song, is to woman, deceit is to the Bengalee. Large promises, smooth excuses, elaborate tissues of circumstantial falsehood, chicanery, perjury, forgery, are the weapons, offensive and defensive, of the people of the Lower Ganges. All those millions do not furnish one sepoy to the Armies

lity, little compassion, scarcely any disposition to relieve suffering, or relieve wrong done to themselves or others. Timidity, with its natural attendants, falsehood and meanness, in the ordinary relations of human life, joined with a capability of becoming excited to courage in the field, to military enthusiasm, to horoic self-devotion. Abstemiousness, in some respects more rigorous than that of a western hermit, in a life of intoxication. Austerities and self-tortures almost incredible, practised by those who, otherwise, wallow in gross sensuality; childish levity, bare-faced falsehood, no faith, no constancy, no shame, no belief in the existence of justice."

MACKINTOSH.

of the Company. But as usurers, as money-changers, as sharp legal practitioners, no class of human beings can bear a comparison with them. With all his softness, the Bengalee is by no means placable in his enmities or prone to pity. The pertinacity with which he adheres to his purposes, yieids only to the immediate pressure of fear. Nor does he lack a certain kind of courage, which is often wanting in his masters. To inevitable evils, he is sometimes found to oppose a passive fortitude, such as the stories attributed to their ideal sage. An European warrior, who rushes on a battery of cannon with a loud hurrah, will sometimes shriek under the Surgeon's knife, and fall into an agony of despair at the sentence of death. But the Bengalee, who would see his country over-run, his house laid in ashes, his children murdered or dishonoured, without having the spirit to strike one blow, has yet been known to endure torture with the firmness of Mucius, and to mount the scaffold with the steady step and even pulse of Algernon Sydney."

MACAULAY.

Eminently clear and graphic as these sketches of the native character are, it is self-evident that they have both been taken from the same standpoint,—the road which leads to the jail. Macaulay's picture is placed as a frontispiece to the history of the criminal Nundcomar.

Absolutely unfair to the people of India at large, these characters are highly valuable to us in our present enquiry.

Missionaries and Physicians do not write of the people as these two brilliant Lawyers did; still the readings of nature which they have left us were just and practical as far as they went, and no further.

Close observation of the "night-side" of London and a diligent study of the police reports and the Newgate Calendar would afford any quick-sighted foreigner an equally dark picture of the British character.

These sketches display to us, in keen but narrow glimpses, the native character just as it verges upon criminality.

After long opportunity of becoming acquainted with the people of India, we freely admit that these legal opinions upon their character are of infinite value *in court*—but nowhere else.

The operation of the great moral defects laid bare by these stern judicial critics in stamping a peculiar and distinctive character upon the crimes most frequently committed by the natives of India, is abundantly evidenced in every page of our criminal reports, in which Theft, Perjury,* Personation, Torture, Child-stealing,† the Murder of Women and of Aged Men, Assassination, Arson, the Butchery of Children for the sake of their ornaments, Drugging and Poisoning, Adultery, Rape, Unnatural Crime, the Procuration of Abortion, are among the leading villanies.

Faithfully graphic as the above delineations of the worst features of native character unquestionably are, they still afford but little insight into the deeper and darker recesses of the Bengali and Hindustani nature when warped to evil ; into those springs of action which develope the criminal characteristics of the people, without a knowledge of which it is impossible that we should acquire the power—so indispensable to the successful tracing or just weighing of any description of guilt—of regarding the natives' crimes from those points of view whence they themselves regard them. It is only by thoroughly knowing the people, and by fixing the mind sedulously upon the records of their crimes, that an European can learn how strange a combination of sensuality, jealousy, wild and ineradicable superstition, absolute untruthfulness, and ruthless disregard of the value of human life, lie below the placid, civil, timid, forbearing exterior of the Indian criminal.

When we recollect that all these qualities are ruled by the traditions of custom and of ancient sanguinary laws which, in the absence of what they regard as rightful authority, the people generally still hold to be just and absolute ; that the masses have over them a police constabulary drawn from their own lower ranks, and, therefore, marked with all the worst features of the national character ; that they are uneducated and borne down by all the temptations and degrading influences of extreme poverty ; that the women of the ruder classes are even more ignorant and brutalized than the men ; that the belief in woman's virtue or man's honesty does not exist amongst them ; that, cowardly as the common people are, they are all armed, and are often necessitated to act in self-defence ;—when we take together these and many other facts which experience will afford, we may gain some insight into the "Pathology" of crime in this country, and into the modes of analysing and of dealing with it.

---

* In his report for 1866, the Inspector-General of Police, Lower Provinces, states that, in this country, "Perjury is the rule and not the exception."

† "This crime is very common in Mahomedan towns, the children being mostly girls, stolen to be sold as slaves, or for purposes of prostitution."—*Mr. Dunbar's Police Report*, L. P., 1845.

Of late years, the Government have been most zealous in stamping out this wide-spread atrocity. The crime of enticing away married women is now more prevalent, especially in the Dacca and Backerguuge Districts.

According to William of Malmesbury, the mother of Godwin Earl of Kent was in the habit of purchasiug companies of slaves in England, and sending them to Denmark, more especially girls, whose beauty and youth rendered them more valuable, that she might accumulate money by this horrid traffic.

Between Hindus and Mussulmans the disparity is rather in the frequency than in the characters of the offences.* The only prevailing crimes that appear to be inconsistent with the habits of the people are the *Dacoitees* (gang robberies) and *Dungas* (faction fights) formerly so prevalent in Bengal. In these, however, the ringleaders were mostly robbers by birth and profession, forming what the police call "regular gangs," or in the word of the law, "professional dacoits systematically employed in carrying on their lawless pursuits in different parts of the country;" and Up-country men, or Bengalis of unusual daring, who calculated rather upon the weakness of their opponents than upon their own prowess.† To the eye of the experienced official, the distinctions may probably

* I have not succeeded in discovering any fully satisfactory data with regard to *the comparative frequency of crimes of magnitude among the Hindu and Mahomedan inhabitants of India.* It appears, from the Chief Magistrate's Report for 1852-53, that the number of Hindus committed to the Calcutta House of Correction in 1853, was 704, while that of Mahomedans was 718; showing a very large excess against the latter, when it is remembered that the proportion of Mahomedans to Hindus, in Calcutta, is reckoned as 4 to 10. These numbers, however, do not give a fair idea of the comparative frequency of the graver offences among the two classes—a comparison which is much needed.

Dr. Mouat has sought to obtain this information which is, in part, given in a series of district reports annexed to his annual report of the Jails of the Lower Provinces for 1868. On sifting the tables, I find that there are ten Jails in which the proportion of Hindu and Mussulman prisoners confined for Murder can be ascertained. These are Patna and Deegah, Shahabad, Rajshahye, Purneah, Furreedpore, Burdwan, Hooghly, Maunbhoom, and Calcutta.

Of 15,562 Hindus confined in these Jails, 298, or 1·91 per cent., were for Murder. Out of 6,344 Mussulman prisoners, 203, or 3·26 per cent., were for Murder.

Dr. Mair, of Madras, has compiled the following statistics showing the *comparative prevalence of Murder in the Bengal Presidency and in British Burmah* (Annals of Indian Administration in the year 1866-67, by George Smith, LL.D.). The detected Murders in Bengal were 257, or 1 in 145,937 of the population; in the North-Western Provinces, 319, or 1 in 87,158; in Oudh, 102, or 1 in 88,235; and in British Burmah 48, or 1 in 47,355. The average, in a population of 132 millions, is 1 in 92,557; in England, it is 1 in 91,210.

† I speak of the crime of Dacoitee as an offence of the past, because, although very serious dacoitees still are of almost constant occurrence, especially in Bengal, they appear to be now far less frequently committed by *professional* robbers, such as were the Budhuk or Bagree Dacoits, the Sanseea and other robbers by hereditary profession of India, whose atrocities and partial suppression are described in a report by Colonel Sleeman, published in 1849. The establishment of an Approver System has considerably checked the systematic gang Dacoitee which formerly had its centre in the districts of Hooghly and Baraset, but it would appear from the police reports, that, during the late famine, there was a tendency to reorganize the old bands in certain districts, such as Hooghly, Bancoorah, and Midnapore. I am informed that the heads of this system were a peculiar sect of Shikaree (hunter) Gipsey-like people, tall and of strong growth, with a language of their own; and that the *Shikarees* and *Prostitutes* obtained between 1750 and 1800, sunnuds, under which they became entitled to hold land rent-free in several parts of Bengal,—the prostitutes being confined to certain quarters of towns.

In the same manner the Abbe Dubois speaks of the Calla-bantru, a caste of thieves or sharpers by profession and right of birth, whom he described as holding a rather advantageous position in the Mussulman kingdoms of India, being secretly authorized by the Government, which granted them a license in consideration of receiving half the booty.

The people of the Rajwar Hills, a small tribe of heriditary gang robbers, on the border of Hazareebaugh and Behar, systematically plunder where they feel themselves strong enough to do so, in the vicinity of the Grand Trunk Road and the Shergotty and Gya roads.

appear sufficiently broad; but, to the ordinary observer, it would certainly seem to be almost impossible to detect any absolutely characteristic differences between the modes adopted by the Hindus and by the Mussulmans of Bengal Proper, in effecting and in concealing the majority of grave crimes against the person. Indeed, the lower grades of these two sects are so closely blended together—not only as regards means, social position, and the operation of surrounding circumstances generally, but even with respect to their origin, their habits, and their religious superstitions,—that they can scarcely be considered as separate races, adopting broadly distinctive trains of criminal action. It can merely be said, with regard to the crimes of both, that they are, for the most part, essentially "*Bengali*" in their characters. Certain descriptions of crime occur nearly alike throughout the whole of India. The chief of these are Dacoitee, Dunga, and Thuggee. Mussulmans and Hindus have combined to perpetrate each of these atrocities in innumerable instances; and—since the active measures of Government have nearly extinguished the profession of Thuggee by strangulation—the drugging of travellers, with a view to robbery and murder, has threatened to become an established practice among criminals of both sects in every part of the country. Several of the smaller tribes inhabiting our border districts, however, display very characteristic national traits, both in the motives which lead to crime and in the devices adopted in its perpetration and concealment.

The Kole, dwelling in the hills which lately formed the South-Western frontier of this Presidency, lays wait for the man whom he believes to have wronged or bewitched him, and effects his deadly purpose without any unnecessary exposure of himself. He shows no anxiety to reveal the crime, which by no means weighs heavily on his conscience; but, upon being distinctly charged with it, he admits his guilt at once without a shadow of equivocation.* His neighbour, the Khond, with a character full of rude and perverted courage, fidelity, and generosity, was wont, until a few years back, to indulge his rapacity and his vengeance to the uttermost, to purchase human victims for

---

The Report of the Police Administration of the N. W. Provinces, for 1869, furnishes a great deal of information regarding certain organized bands of professional thieves, burglars, dacoits, and druggers who traverse the country. The Bhowreas, Jogees, Beloochees or Rinds, and Sunoreahs caused, a few years ago, much trouble to the Police over the N. W. Provinces, their habits being like those of the Brinjarries of Central India, dispersing and robbing over the whole country, separating and combining at will.

The gang robbers still so prevalent in Bengal are mostly Budmashes, thieving vagabonds, nearly corresponding with the class formerly notorious in England as "masterless men." There are still many bands who prepare themselves for the night attack upon some wealthy zemindar's house by a devout performance of the Kalli Poojah, but there are few who can say, with a Dacoit mentioned in Hunter's *Annals of Rural Bengal*, "I have always followed the trade of my ancestors. My ancestors held this profession before me. We train boys in the same manner."

* See Lieutenant Tickell's Memoir on the Hodésan (improperly called Kolehan).—*Journal of the Asiatic Society*, Vol. IX., p. 79.

sacrifice to his deities, and to perpetrate female infanticide with all the systematic regularity of one who performs a grateful religious duty. Again, the Reaug, Cookie or Chuckma,* inhabiting the hills eastward of Tipperah and Chittagong, with apparently far less development of the nobler instincts, plunders and lays waste every undefended settlement that attracts his cupidity, employs poisoned weapons against those whom he fears, slaughters every opponent whom he is not desirous to steal, and pours out the blood of his human sacrifices before his gods, like water.† Until the advent of European power among them, the Jainteas and the Kasias of the hills east of Sylhet, practised human sacrifice and polyandry (which, of course, involved infanticide),—even now they use poisoned arrows in the chase. The Nagas come down from their hills, attack and plunder the villages of the plains, and scrupulously take home with them the heads and, if possible, also the hands and feet of both friends and enemies slain in action, he being accounted the noblest warrior who possesses the greatest number of foemen's skulls. Still, with all their distinctive traits of barbarity, the crimes of these several Mongolian tribes would alone be sufficient to stamp them as branches of one great aboriginal family, inhabiting the hill districts of Lower Bengal, who have always remained perfectly distinct from the people of the Delta; and as representatives of those primitive savages whom the author of the *Annals of Rural Bengal* shows to have been characterised in the Sanscrit as "The black-skinned, human-sacrificing, flesh-eating forest tribes."

Again, certain rather marked characteristics distinguish crime in several of the other districts of India. In his own country, the Ooriah criminal betrays but little craft in effecting his nefarious designs, and displays a singular propensity to confess. Many of the Hindustanee's greatest crimes are committed in moments of ungovernable rage; indeed the frenzy which reproachful language is apt to evoke in these people is so well understood, that the law has provided accordingly;‡—at the same time, it would appear that *the weak* are usually the victims of their fury. The murder of female infants, long the prevailing crime of Rajpootana, appears to have had its centre in Mairwharra. It has been equally prevalent in Mynpoory, in the Jullundur Doab, in Oude, and in the Benares district; and the Hon'ble Mr. Strachey has lately shown that, in some parts of the country, this atrocity is still perpetrated among the Mahomedans.

The Hindustanee usually strikes with the sword *(tulwar)* or iron-bound cudgel *(lohar ki latthee* or *lohbanda)*. The Bengali's readiest weapons are the *dhao* (bill-hook), the *kooralee* (axe), and the bamboo *(bans ki latthee)*. As would be expected in a rocky country like Chota-

* These tribes are now much divided, but have evidently sprung from a common stem.

† See the case of Joodhomonee and others.—*Nizamut Adawlut Reports*, Vol. II., Part 1 of 1852, p. 899.

‡ Macnaghten's Reports, Vol. I., page 53.

Nagpore, heavy stones are frequently used as instruments of destruction, just as opium-poisoning is most prevalent in opium districts. The *lotah* (a heavy brass vessel with a narrow neck, which may be conveniently slung to a waist-cloth) formerly afforded our prisoners a dangerous weapon. Within doors, the Bengali, moved by sudden homicidal rage, readily takes up the *dhao* (bill-hook), *bhuttee* (knife fixed in a stand at right angles for cutting fish and vegetables), or *peerah* (wooden stool). In the field, either a bamboo, a sickle (*hussooa* and *kachtya*), a *durmush* or *moogur* (hammer for breaking clods), or a hoe (*kodalee*) is generally at hand.

Class and local position, of course, have their effect in determining the comparative prevalence of various crimes. Sexual jealousy is probably the most frequent cause of homicide among Mussulmans; Criminal Abortion and Child Murder are rifest among the unhappy class of Hindu widows. Dungas and affrays on account of cattle trespass occurred principally in the great indigo districts, in spots where the estates of rival Zemindars were crowded together, and in situations where, the means of irrigating the land being defective, water-rights were mainly insisted upon. Fatal squabbles about fish traps (*ara*) are common in Bengal. Dacoits and other robbers, of course, infest those roads and rivers which are most frequented by natives, and those districts where the probabilities of resistance are least.*

Although the proportionate frequency of certain crimes varies much in the three states, I can find no very marked distinction in the characteristics of crime as practised in Bengal, in the North-West Provinces, and in the Punjaub. The same observation is applicable to the Bombay and Madras Presidencies.

Altogether it would certainly appear that, neither in the planning, nor the effecting, nor the concealment of great crimes, does any class of the natives of India display that remarkable subtlety, calmness and power of baffling investigation which might be expected on observation merely of the tact, duplicity, and *finesse* which characterize their minor rogueries of every-day occurrence. The timid nature cannot rise with the occasion; it fails under the terrific weight of enormous crime.

In India, as elsewhere, the intelligence of the criminal is generally found to be below the average—a very low type of cunning easily dealt with.

A deep and cautious investigation into the habits and opinions of the people of India, in their relation to crime, would afford to any judicial officer an almost untrodden path of research, leading to practical results which would abundantly repay the labour employed. Hitherto, the attention of Magistrates in India has been sufficiently occupied in the tasks of detecting crime and of carrying out the penal system.† The time long

* A great deal of curious information regarding the Prevailing Crimes in the several districts of the Lower Provinces will be found in the Appendix to Dr. Mouat's Jail Report for 1868, already cited.

† The administration of the jails throughout the Bengal Presidency is now entrusted to the Civil Surgeons.

ago arrived, at which the true nature or "Pathology" of Crime in India might be investigated with advantage both to the people and to their law-givers. The officially printed Police Reports, and the Reports of the Courts of Nizamut Adawlut of Bengal, the North-West Provinces, and Bombay, and those of the High Courts, afford abundant materials for a HISTORY OF CRIME IN INDIA. Such a work, ably and carefully compiled, and deeply reasoned out by one of truth-seeking, moderate and philosophic mind, and of long and extensive judicial experience in this country, while it would materially aid the daily investigations and decisions of every Judicial Officer in the land, would, probably, go further than any other book that has appeared since the commencement of the century in advancing the progress of civilization here, by enabling us to detect and grapple with those deeply-rooted errors in the native character which now, in eluding our notice, most effectually baffle all our best-laid schemes of improvement. For this noble task I am not fitted; but, with this view, I have ventured, in several of the following pages, to digress somewhat from the direct line of my subject, while endeavouring to show the Causes, Antiquity, and Prevalence of the criminal practices which are brought under consideration.

Every one who has spent even a month in India will have learned how strong an influence CUSTOM has over the conduct of natives of all classes, in all the opinions and actions of their lives.* This traditional "Custom"—throughout the details of which scholars may still detect the faint but indelible traces of ancient laws—is inextricably interwoven with the native's religion. He does not always pause to consider whether this act or that is right or wrong, or will be viewed in the same light by the English as by the Hindu or Mahomedan law;—he is satisfied to act precisely as his forefathers have acted for centuries.†

* In their Report of 1838, the Committee on Prison Discipline remark:—"The general morals of the people may possibly be bad enough, but an Indian criminal is probably a better man than any other criminal of the same sort. His general character certainly differs less from that of the mass of his countrymen than would be the case in more civilized and moral countries. A large proportion of the crimes in this country are committed by persons whose tribe have done the same time out of mind, and they are almost as naturally the result of birth as another man's honest trade. Many more are committed, as it were professionally, by the members of immense confederations, who are not much worse than other people in matters unconnected with their profession. Owing to feelings and principles which we can never" [?] "comprehend, there is little or no consciousness of moral guilt amongst these classes, on account of the exercise of what they regard as their proper business."

† Many years after the above was first written, the same observation presented itself, in his daily experience, to the mind of my friend, Mr. W. W. Hunter, who says, in the "Dissertation" which precedes his *Comparative Dictionary of the Non-Aryan Languages of India and High Asia*:—"As a magistrate I came in contact with prejudices and traditional convictions which, however unfounded they may seem to us, nevertheless amount to a sense of duty, and supply motives of action to millions of British subjects; prejudices an convictions for which English criminal justice makes no allowance, yet which, as I shall show, sometimes affect English Officers with a sense almost of sickness in administering the law."

Hence the antiquity of a crime must always be taken into account in legal investigations here; indeed the general practice of an atrocity, like the general prevalence of a superstition, has usually been received as mitigatory, as in the practices of Sati, Leper-Burying, Suicide, &c., until it has been found necessary to adopt extreme measures for its absolute extirpation.*

This CUSTOM has, from very primitive times, tyrannised over the men of all nations, forcing them into crime against their better instincts. In the Mahabharata, Yudhishthira tells Drupada—" The law, oh! King, is subtle; we do not know its way. We follow the path which has been trodden by our ancestors in succession."

Our own Sir Thomas Browne has precisely the same idea: " Men count it venial to err with their forefathers," apparently adopting it from the old law maxim—" *Vetustas pro lege semper habetur.*"

So also, as, a few years ago, two of the best men in England, " following the wicked old traditions of their order," were, at any moment, liable to be forced by an unexpected train of circumstances into fighting a duel, are the Bengalis and Rajpoots of the present day tempted to commit certain atrocities *more antiquorum.*

Out of this principle spring two facts of great practical importance to the Indian jurist:—(1) that an altogether new crime is probably never committed in India, every criminal act being founded upon recent practice or old tradition; hence the task of defining the characters of Indian crime is distinctly finite; I venture to hope that there are not many crimes against the person, prevalent in India, which are not described in this treatise:—and (2) that, as it has been lately well put, " there is but

---

* In 1802, five women were tried, at Patna, by a native tribunal, for sorcery; and, being found guilty, were put to death. The Governor General ordered the principal persons who conducted this affair to be tried for murder at the Circuit Court. The Court sentenced them to death. It appeared, however, that this custom had prevailed from time immemorial. Several of the witnesses remembered numerous instances of persons having been put to death by the Brahmins for sorcery; and one of them, in particular, proved that his own mother had been tried and executed as a witch. The Government, therefore, pardoned the offenders, but issued a proclamation declaring that any one forming a tribunal for the trial of persons charged with witchcraft, or aiding and encouraging in any act to deprive such persons of life, shall be deemed guilty of murder, and suffer the penalty attached to that offence.—*Asiatic Annual Register for* 1802.

In 1835, Putho Jora was tried at Ahmedabad (Bombay) for instantly killing a man whom he caught in the act of adultery with his wife, and for inflicting a wound on the woman's nose and face. The Sessions Judge sentenced him to death, but urged that " the offence, severely punishable as it is by the laws, is one which has always been viewed by native legislators in a far more lenient light, and no doubt the prisoner has grown up from his youth with sentiments conforming to the general feeling of his countrymen on these subjects." Urging the absence of vindictive premeditation, and the suddenness, severity, and irritating nature of the injury done to his feelings, the Judge warmly recommended the prisoner to mercy. He was acquitted.—*Bellasis's Reports of Criminal Cases determined in the Court of Sudder Foujdaree Adawlut of Bombay*, p. 95.

one step from the popular belief in the prevalence of any stated crime to the fact of its occasional perpetration among the people."

Deeply impressed with the principle that it is as essential to the medical jurist as to the judge of criminal cases to possess a full knowledge of the machinery by which guilt is wont to effect its ends, I long ago broached these important questions, in the hitherto unfulfilled but not yet abandoned hope that they will eventually find illustration from abler hands.

SEARCH FOR THE BODIES OF MISSING PERSONS.

In Bengal, a country abounding in jungles and patches of waste land, in ploughed fields, dirt heaps, sandy tracts, dry water-courses, tanks, swamps and muddy streams, and infested by multitudes of carrion-feeding animals, as well as by myriads of those insects which prey upon animal matter; where, further, human remains may be found thickly strewn on every river brink and upon the outskirts of every village,—the discovery and identification of the bodies of missing persons often becomes a task of no ordinary difficulty. Under these circumstances, error and fraud, doubtless, occur, and many bodies remain undiscovered. Still it is remarkable in how very large a proportion of cases such searches prove successful. Few police agents are so well fitted for these investigations as the burkundauze.* With all his energies stimulated into activity for the time being, by his immediate superior, the inquisitiveness, bustling importance, love of ransacking, and by no means inconsiderable cleverness and tact, which are leading features in his character, come fully into play. Where, as is usually the case, a large number of these men are scattered over the country, with every nook and corner of which they are familiar, their search is rarely baffled. It has been frequently asserted that the native police employ promises, menaces, and even torture in the detection of hidden crime; placing this question aside for the present, we have sufficient facts before us to show that, by the exercise of a fair amount of tact and acquaintance with the habits of criminals, the desired result may generally be obtained, without recourse to any measures so unjustifiable.

Apart from the ordinary difficulties attendant upon such a search, and from the means of concealment adopted by the criminal parties, the selfish timidity of the natives frequently delays and even counteracts the discovery of homicide. Experience certainly tends to show that the generality of natives, on witnessing a murderous attack, unhesitatingly prefer flight to rescue.†

* I have less personal experience of the modern police constable. His acumen is probably as great.

† This is the rule, but the reports contain a few highly honorable exceptions—here the courageous acts have generally been performed by Up-Country men. The concealment of crime by those who are unwilling to incur the trouble or risk of a police investigation is probably an almost daily occurrence. In a trial for murder at Mirzapore in 1853, three

The dread of a judicial inquiry, or the fear of offending a powerful criminal, very frequently induces the zemindars and others, in whose land the bodies of murdered persons are found, to conceal the remains.*

I find among my papers the following memorandum, on the *Causes which prevent murder from coming to the knowledge of the police*, which must

---

men deposed that, on a certain day, their attention was called to a well 25 cubits deep, from which the sound of a voice proceeded. Upon looking down, they saw a woman lying in the shallow water, who exclaimed that one Jokhoo Singh had wounded and thrown her down. A severed hand was lying on the side of the well, and blood was sprinkled about three or four cubits around the well. "*On seeing the hand and blood, they were going to run off*," when they met a fourth neighbour, with whom they returned to the place. The woman implored them to take her out; but, not having a rope, the fourth man went to Ishree Singh *karinda* for one, and the other three went to gather grass for thatching. Upon the man's arrival at the nearest village, which was two miles off, several people were despatched with a rope to the well: two ghurries elapsed before they got there; they looked in and saw the woman lying on her back; on getting no reply, they believed that she was dead, and all returned home. Ishree Singh agreed with them, that it would be better to leave her where she was, in order that she might be taken out in the presence of the police.—*Nizamut Adawlut Reports, N. W. P.*, 27th August 1853.

* In a case tried at Furruckabad in 1852, where there could scarcely be a doubt that a man had murdered his wife and had thrown her body into a well, but had afterwards disposed of it otherwise by the aid of accomplices, two brothers testified that they were ploughing together, when one of them observed what seemed to be a dead body in the well, and called the other. From fear, one of them told no one what he had seen. The other said that, next day, he met the woman's husband with his accomplices, whom he asked where they had since removed the body to. They replied that, if he said a word, they would kill him. Witness, therefore, remained silent.—*Nizamut Adawlut Reports, N. W. P.*, October 30th, 1852.

The following is from the Bengal Police Report for 1866 :—"This murder was committed (in the Gowalpara district) four years ago. The deceased was generally detested by his neighbours on account of being supposed to practise sorcery. The head of the village conspired with seven persons of his caste to kill him at night, and did so, and buried the body the following morning. Some other villagers observed blood and palpable marks of violence on the corpse previous to burial, but were deterred, through fear of the head-man, from either reporting or saying anything of what they had seen. About four years afterwards, the deceased's wife having become intimate with a constable of the adjacent police station, informed him of these occurrences, and the latter reported them at once to the District Superintendent, who proceeded to the spot himself, and, after a little trouble, succeeded not only in procuring reliable evidence against the criminal, but also in recovering the skeleton which had unmistakeable marks of violence upon it. Six of the criminals were arrested. All were convicted."

In 1852, one Gungadeen was murdered by two of his servants and another person in the Government Bungalow of a village called Sohagee. The deceased's father received information from a Brahmin of the place of his son's death, and of his body having been thrown into a well. Upon reaching the place, he found that the body had been discovered about 14 days previously; and, being in a state of extreme putridity, had been thrown outside the village; he found nothing but the skull and some bones; but, upon the skeleton, were portions of a necklace of beads, which he identified as having been worn by his son.—*Nizamut Adawlut Reports, N. W. P.*, 12th February 1853.

In a case of murder tried at Bareilly in the same year, two gardeners swore that, early in the morning, on their way to their work in their fields, they saw the body of the deceased lying close to their field. There were fourteen sword cuts on it. From fear, they took up the body and threw it into the dâka jungle near at hand.—*Ibid*, February 15th, 1853.

A thug, who was tried at Meerut in 1852, in confessing various crimes, mentioned that, having strangled a man, he threw the body into a well. Five or six days afterwards, he heard that the zemindars had taken the body out of the well and burnt it.—*Ibid*, 11th June 1852.

have been written for me by a native friend about twelve years ago. I regret that it does not bear any signature :

"1. From the apathy of the relatives and neighbours to appear before the magistrate and give deposition on oath and suffer the lingering proceedings of the criminal law, and partly from regard to the honor of the parties concerned.

"2. Through the corruption of the police officers in the mofussil ; because, in many cases, it has been discovered that the dead bodies of the murdered have been concealed or thrown into small rivers even with the knowledge of the police officers, until, later, some family dissensions among the parties have brought the fact to the knowledge of the magistrate. But, here, in the absence of the dead bodies and of other corroborative evidence, the cases often prove unsuccessful.

"3. The state of the mofussil witnesses is so miserable" (*i. e.*, they are so poor and abject) "that a very small expense on the part of the accused is sufficient to overturn the facts of the case ; so, until the character of the people and state of the mofussil police be perfectly reformed, there is no opportunity for the criminal authorities to execute those excellent laws which have been enacted by our benevolent Government for the protection of native society in India."

"Murder is committed by persons at night, and the police are so corrupt that their myrmidons, the chowkeedars, voluntarily take upon themselves to despatch the dead bodies from one jurisdiction to another for fear of their being held responsible by the authorities. So it occurs that dead bodies are sometimes carried away for some 12 or 16 miles, in the course of the night, and are thrown into rivers."

The Reports contain many cases in which village chowkeedars have aided in the concealment of murder.*

"There is another kind of murder which generally takes place in passenger boats. The boatmen are the murderers, they conceal their arms in the bottoms of the boats, and throw the dead into the river."

In 1844, three individuals, Hindus "of the better class," were tried for conspiracy at Dhaolia (Bombay Presidency), and convicted of having, when empanelled as members of an inquest held upon the body of one "who, they had ample reason to believe, and moreover were fully con-

* As in the following instance : "The prisoner belongs to the village police and, having heard that a woman had come to a violent death, he persuaded her father-in-law, if he wished to escape any enquiry, to give him a bribe of 20 rupees and some grain. He then sent information to the regular Police that the woman had been drowned."—*Remarks of the Nizamut Adawlut*, N. A. R., Vol. V., Part 2, for 1855, p. 724. What these men now are in the N. W. P. may be judged of by an extract from the Report for 1867 of the Inspector-General of Police, page 33 : "To show how utterly worthless the village Chowkeedar is,—out of the twelve cases of burglary above mentioned, not one was reported at the police station, which was only two miles distant." Again (p. 32), "thirty chowkeedars were punished (in the Cawnpore District) and only one rewarded." In the Allyghur Report (p. 6), it is stated that "fifty-nine chowkeedars were punished, and not one rewarded."

vinced," had been murdered, purposely returned a false verdict, stating that the deceased had committed suicide by hanging himself. Before the magistrate they stated that the contents of the Inquest Report were false; that it had been drawn up by the order of the mamlutdar (since dead); and that, although they believed Tejah had been murdered, they certified, at the instigation of the mamlutdar, that he had committed suicide.*

The Report on the State of the Police in the Lower Provinces for the first six months of 1842 contains reference to a case in which suspicion of some foul play fell on certain persons in consequence of their having, without any reason, filled up a well which they had just dug for the irrigation of their fields, and the police officers were sent with orders to dig out the well, *which they reported as giving no cause for suspicion.* The mohurir, however, having gone on the same day, to a village near, learnt that a woman who appeared to be travelling, had stopped for the night at the prisoners' cattle-shed, and that they had murdered her for the sake of her ornaments, and thrown the corpse into the well, which they had then filled up. He immediately proceeded to the spot, and had the well dug out to the bottom. The effluvia left no doubt as to a corpse having been deposited there, and a quantity of long hair was also found; but the body had been removed, and no trace of it could be discovered, nor could all the subsequent endeavours of the magistrate procure any clue to the identity of the woman.

There are even instances where the timidity, imbecility, or venality of natives has led them to conceal the murder of their near kindred. In 1854 a wretch, whose nephew had been murdered for the sake of his ornaments, stated at the trial,—"I went and saw he was lying thrown down in the *khet;* the ornaments he used to wear were not present on his person. He had been strangled with the stalks of the *urhur*, and the gold rings in his ears were also gone. Cashee, my nephew, was with me: *we both took up the body and threw it in the river* and came home in the evening and remained without sense" (*behosh*). "On Friday" (three days subsequently) "Daveela *putwaree* came to the village, and I told him, and was lamenting, when he said, 'Go in the morning, to Bugool *lohar*, and you will get the jewels, &c.'"†

Again, in 1856, a man at Bareilly, whose child, four years and-a-half old, had also been strangled for its ornaments—"was in such a state of mind as to yield to the selfish suggestion of his neighbours to adopt, or to report to the police, the conclusion that a wolf had carried him off, there being known similar facts in most parts of the country of the daring attacks of those animals when pressed by hunger."‡

A case occurred, some years since, in Tirhoot, where a man was sentenced to 18 months' imprisonment for concealing his father's murder,

* Bellasis's Rep., S. F. A. of Bombay, p. 203.

† Nizamut Adawlut Reports, N. W. P., 9th May 1854.

‡ *Ibid*, 5th March 1855.

which had been committed under circumstances of great atrocity by the servant of a rich zemindar. Here the money and influence of his powerful neighbour were, doubtless, operative.*

The following appears in the Report of the Police of the Lower Provinces for 1866: "The mother of the deceased informed the police that her son had committed suicide by hanging himself. The police found that he had been murdered by Sreekant and others. Deceased is said to have had an intrigue with Sreekant's wife. Sreekant and three others came at night and killed him, and instructed his mother to lodge information that her son had committed suicide. The four defendants were arrested, committed, and sentenced to transportation for life." Doubtless, the poor mother yielded in sheer terror.

The whole of this miserable system is summed up in a few words recorded by the Nizamut Adawlut in 1856. "Instances of persons consenting to forego the prosecution of those who have committed the most serious injuries on their persons or properties are within the common experience of every magistrate in this country."†

It has already been mentioned that murdered bodies are not unfrequently removed to a considerable distance from the scene of the crime, often to the environs of a neighbouring village.

In 1842, it appeared in a trial at Ahmedabad (Bombay), that two coolies were accompanying a wedding party at about 4 o'clock one morning, when they met three Gosaens leaving a village with a mare and a colt. On the back of the mare they saw a man lying wrapped up in a quilt. The posture of this man attracted their attention and induced them to enquire why he was lying in such a position. The Gosaens replied that the man was suffering from fever, and was unable to sit up. The Gosaens then proceeded on their way. On talking over the matter, the coolies were of opinion that the man was dead; they, therefore, turned back in pursuit. After proceeding about half a mile, they overtook the Gosaens, but no longer saw the body of the man lying on the back of the mare. The coolies apprehended two of them, and described a spot where the body, murdered by stabbing, was found buried in a water-course. The prisoners were condemned to death.‡

In 1856, three men in the Midnapore district were so remorselessly beaten and otherwise ill-used that they died. Each of the bodies was tied to a bamboo and carried to a maidan (plain) about two-and-a-half miles from the village where the crime was committed.§

In a case of dacoity with murder in the Hooghly Zillah in 1855, it was shown that it was not until three days after the crime was committed

* Mr. Dunbar's Police Reports, L. P., 1849, p. 8. The law no longer binds zemindars to give notice of suspicious deaths.

† Nizamut Adawlut Reports, Vol. VI., for 1856, p. 801.

‡ Bellasis's Bombay Reports, p. 147.

§ Nizamut Adawlut Reports, Vol. VI. (1856), p. 481.

that the darogah succeeded in finding the corpse on the plain adjoining a village nine or ten miles distant from the scene of the murder.*

The same practice appears to exist in the North-Western Provinces. In 1867, a body was found in a well in the south of the Hameerpore district. It was bound all over with ropes in such a way as to bend the head down towards the knees. This was evidently done to make it occupy a smaller space, and probably, too, for facility of transport (this is a rather frequent practice in Bengal). The Deputy Inspector-General of Police remarked that murders of this kind are not uncommon in Bundelkund. He has had before him several cases where the murderers, after despatching their victim, carried the body at night and threw it down a well several miles distant from the scene of the crime.†

In 1852, the native police of Kumaon discovered the body of a murdered person by an ingenious deception which would almost appear to have been devised with a knowledge of the case of Eugene Aram. A man named Mungloo having been missing for some days, one Moosa, with whom Mungloo's wife was living in adultery, was suspected of making away with him. The body, however, could not be found, although a reward of rupees 200 was offered for its discovery. Nine months afterwards, the body was brought in. It then appeared that the local police had entrapped Moosa into the discovery of the corpse, by digging up and showing him another corpse, when he denied the identity of the body, and said that one Kitroo would point out the place of Mungloo's burial. Kitroo was then seized, and immediately took the police to a spot near his own house, and caused the body to be dug up from a considerable depth. At the same time Moosa, the accused, showed great anxiety to be recognized as the first pointer-out of the grave; and, in fact, claimed the reward for its discovery. The corpse was immediately recognized, by competent witnesses, as that of Mungloo. Kitroo at once accused Moosa and three others of the murder, naming himself as an eye-witness, and acknowledging his *forced* privity. Moosa confessed that he had killed the deceased. The trial, which developed several remarkable circumstances, resulted in the sentencing of Moosa to imprisonment for life in transportation.‡

In India, as elsewhere, homicidal crime is not unfrequently discovered by *Traces of Blood*, by the *Tracks of Footsteps*,§ and by *Marks left on the Ground over which a corpse has been dragged.*

---

* Nizamut Adawlut Reports, Vol. V., for 1855, p. 726.

† Report on the Administration of the Police of the N. W. P., for 1867, p. 109.

‡ Nizamut Adawlut Reports, N. W. P., 12th June 1852, p. 537.

§ At Dacca, in 1856, two witnesses stated that, owing to a malformation in the prisoner's foot, they were able to identify his foot-marks in the clayey mud where the body of his alleged victim was found. The Judge remarked that he "should have considered such proof perfectly satisfactory, had it been tendered by the darogah, on his arrival at the spot. There is nothing on record about the recognition of foot-steps till the date of the prisoner's con-

TRACES OF BLOOD.—Considerable ingenuity is occasionally displayed by criminals in the obliteration of blood-marks. In 1854, the kotwal of cantonments at Furruckabad was sent to make enquiries regarding a person who was believed to have been made away with at a village called Mozadeenpore. Upon his arrival, he gave notice to the chowkeedar and zemindars of the village. The chowkeedar named all the villagers but two ; one of these persons, on being apprehended, took the kotwal to a field, where some of the earth had been lately smoothed down, which he said was the spot of the murder, adding that the chowkeedar had told him to smooth the earth in order to conceal the marks of blood. The chowkeedar had allowed the other murderer to abscond.*

In 1853, one of the accomplices in a murder at Kumaon confessed that, three days subsequently, one of the perpetrators "killed a calf at the site of the murder with his *halce*, in order to falsify the former blood-marks."†

In the trial of a man who was sentenced for the murder of a girl for the sake of her ornaments, it was shown that the prisoner endeavoured, with some ingenuity, to make it appear that the child had been devoured by a wolf ; and that, in the course of the original search, *he made his gums bleed and spat blood* to give a colour to his indication of the place where the child's torn apparel was found, and where he asserted that she had been killed by some wild animal. He afterwards pointed out the body in a hole where he had buried it.‡

FOOTMARKS.—In a trial at Midnapore in 1853, it appeared that a man, having been struck a fatal blow on the head, was carried to a nullah by three persons and thrown into the water. On the return of these men, they were apprehended, when they admitted that deceased had been murdered. In the Judge's Court two of the men pleaded not guilty, and set up an *alibi.* In the mofussil and before the magistrate, one of these men had confessed to having proceeded a part of the way only towards the nullah with the body and then returned ; the sooruthal, however, stated that there were footmarks of *three* persons on the banks of the nullah in which the body was found, and the witnesses swore that the clothes of the three prisoners were wet when they returned home at night.§

The *Forms of Natives' Feet* is a matter worthy of study alike by the ethnologist and the medical jurist. In climbing and in executing many

fession. This destroys the weight of that evidence. It is not credible that, with such strong proof at hand of the prisoner's guilt, the darogah should continue daily to report that he was acting only on suspicion."—*Nizamut Adawlut Reports*, Vol. VI. of 1856, p. 533.

* Nizamut Adawlut Reports, N. W. P., 16th May 1854, p. 542 ; also *Ibid*, 3rd January 1854, p. 9.

† Nizamut Adawlut Reports, N. W. P., 30th August 1853, p. 1048.

‡ *Ibid*, 8th September 1854, p. 332.

§ Nizamut Adawlut Reports, Vol. VI., Part 2, p. 645.

kinds of what is, in Europe, exclusively "handiwork," various classes of natives use the foot with great precision and power as a prehensile organ. Hill-men generally have the great toe so much developed and set so widely apart from the others, that we could surely fail to distinguish their footsteps from those of men inhabiting the plains.

The marks of DRAGGING SOME HEAVY BODY ALONG THE GROUND are frequently alluded to in the Reports as having assisted the police in the discovery of corpses. These are, of course, most likely to be found in cases where the murderer has been single-handed; where there are several accomplices, the body is, as I have already stated, often fastened to a bamboo, or tied up in a cloth, and so carried to a distance.

In 1853 one Mooloo, a person in the habit of plucking corn and stealing from fields, went out to visit his field, and did not return. A search was instituted next morning. In the field of his neighbour Mohun, some human ordure and the cap of the deceased, partly hidden in the ground, were discovered, the earth around was also trodden down, and some *bajra* stalks were lying about. Marks of dragging extended to a well in the field; drags were procured, and the body of Mooloo was extracted; a cloth was tied round the throat, and had evidently caused strangulation, and the hands were also bound with the same; the well had eight *haths* of water in it. Mohun was sentenced to seven years' imprisonment.*

In the same year, certain persons entered a house at night with intention to steal. A conflict ensued, in which one of the thieves was wounded on the leg. The prosecutor recognized one of the thieves. Two chowkeedars came almost immediately and lighted a torch. They observed that something bleeding had been dragged a certain distance; and, the next morning, they tracked footsteps from the spot where the body had been lifted up, to a village, in which Dabeea, one of the accused, lived. On entering his house, they saw spots of blood on his clothes and person; and, on asking for his brother Seeta, they were told that he was absent. Subsequently, the mother of Seeta pointed out where her son's body had been buried the previous night, in a cow-shed. Over the grave a buffaloe was tied. The body was exhumed, and a severe wound was found behind the knee. The prisoners confessed their crime, and were sentenced accordingly.†

What would, at first sight, appear to be a very trifling circumstance, has frequently been found to throw considerable light upon obscure cases of homicide in this country. Native women of the poorer classes generally adorn their arms with bracelets. The cheapest and commonest ornaments of this kind, in Bengal, are made of shell-lac and sand. When fixed on the arm, these *choorees* are heated and joined in such a manner as

---

* Nizamut Adawlut Reports, N. W. P., 3rd February 1854, p. 116.

† Nizamut Adawlut Reports, N. W. P., 30th March 1854, p. 346.

to surround the limb in continuous circles ; other *choorees* are of thin glass. They appear to wear well, with care ; but can scarcely fail to be broken during any violent struggle. I find several instances in which the discovery of broken *choorees* assisted in the detection of crime. In 1853, a woman, believed by her relatives to be unchaste, disappeared ; a careful search was instituted in a field belonging to certain suspected parties ; and there, about the middle of the field, were found portions of broken *choorees ;* the ground was here dug up, and the corpse of the missing woman disinterred.*

Again, in the same year, a woman was murdered by a person with whom she had carried on an illicit connexion. Upon her disappearance, search was made, and on the bank of a nuddee were found a shoe, recognized as belonging to the prisoner, two metal ankle ornaments worn by females, and pieces of glass arm-rings, identified as belonging to the missing woman. Search was made for the prisoner, who was apprehended with blood on his clothes. Under his guidance, the body was found sunk in the bottom of the nuddee, frightfully gashed.†

A man was heard to exclaim in the night that Gungajulee (his kept mistress) had wounded him and was making off. He had been wounded in the throat, and died almost immediately. His son, a very intelligent boy of nine, stated that he saw the woman struggling with and stabbing his father. Some pieces of broken bangle were found on the bed, which were proved to be her property. She admitted that these fragments belonged to her, but asserted that she was attracted by the outcry ; and, going to see what was the matter, fell over the bedstead, and so broke her bangle. Plausible as this statement might appear to be, the Court held that it was of no avail against the evidence upon which her crime was established. They therefore upheld the sentence of death.‡

A young woman was seen at noon to throw a boy, aged ten years, into an unenclosed dry well, 20 feet deep, by a man, who ran to the village, and informed the boy's father of what had taken place.§ The father went immediately to the spot, but the corpse was not taken out until the *evening !* Some fragments of ***kanch choories*** were picked up at the well, corresponding with those the accused was in the habit of wearing ; and were found to be similar to those she wore at the time of her arrest. The joint magistrate, who investigated the case with extreme care, did

---

* Nizamut Adawlut Reports, 17th January 1853, p. 63.

† Nizamut Adawlut Reports, N. W. P., 1st April 1853, p. 487.

‡ Nizamut Adawlut Reports, Vol. VI., Part 2, p. 728. See also a case in which a man identified certain broken *choorees*, which were found with some blood and hair near a well, as those of his daughter, who had been made away with.—*Nizamut Adawlut Reports, N. W. P.*, 30th October 1852, p. 1269.

§ His excuse for not rendering more efficient aid was that he could not pursue and overtake the murderess, as he had a boil on his foot, and a load of fuel on his head, which, moreover, he did not throw down to be enabled to pursue her !

not attach much weight to this last circumstance, as the fragments of glass bangle were not discovered until the following morning ; and as it appeared that, on the evening before, the boy's mother (who lived next door to the accused, was of the same caste, and *might probably* wear bangles of the same pattern,) went to the well accompanied by other women. She, it was held, might have broken one of her bangles in the excess of grief, or the ornament may have been lost by one of her companions. Sentence of death was, however, awarded.*

In 1856, it appeared in the trial of a Nuddea man (Hindu) for killing a woman with whom he had intrigued, by striking her violently and breaking her ribs, that an armlet belonging to him was found in the clothes of the corpse.†

The materials available are scarcely sufficient to allow of a numerical comparison, and it is doubtful whether such statistics, if collected, could be rendered practically useful ; it, however, appears that the most frequent modes of disposing of the bodies of murdered persons in this country are as follow :—By concealment in *Jungles* and *Mango Topes*, in *Standing Crops*, in *Wells*, *Rivers*, *Tanks*, in *Dung-Holes*, in *Fallow Fields*, in *the Sand of Water-Courses*, in *Houses*, and in *Porcupine's Holes.*

The concealment of bodies in the dense recesses of JUNGLES where, in a very short time, birds of prey, jackals, dogs, and insects reduce them to skeletons, is, probably, the most frequent practice of those criminals who live at a distance from any deep and rapid river. I was assured, upon authority which I cannot doubt, that, shortly before 1865, upon clearing a certain jungle, which had long been regarded as a covert for suspicious persons, no less than seven skeletons and one recent body were discovered !

The following passage from the report of a trial at Luckimpore, Assam, in 1856, affords some slight idea of the nature of these searches :—" The darogah asked Bancha to tell where the body was, and not to give unnecessary trouble, but he would not tell. Next morning, however, he led the way to a tank in the jungle, six miles off, and showed where the body had been put, but it could not be found. He then said that it must have been taken away by a tiger, and shewed pieces of bamboo with which the body had been pinned down. Search was made, but no body found. The prisoner then said he would show something belonging to the deceased, and produced from the mud the *towa*, old cloth, and shoe, saying they belonged to the deceased. The jungle was set on fire, but nothing was found ; next day, the search was renewed, when the prisoner (No. 2) took the darogah to a place where human bones were found."‡

Where the remains of a human body, not admitting of special identification, are discovered in a jungle, the circumstance, standing alone, can

* Nizamut Adawlut Reports, N. W. P., September 1st, 1853, p. 1068.

† Nizamut Adawlut Reports, Vol. VI., of 1856, p. 273.

‡ Nizamut Adawlut Reports, Vol. VI. of 1856, p. 50.

scarcely be regarded with much suspicion. Pilgrims, fukeers, and others may die unnoticed in these remote spots: lunatics, sick, or intoxicated persons may be lost in the jungles, and there be attacked and devoured by the smaller wild animals—(*On this point consult the chapter on* INJURIES INFLICTED BY WILD ANIMALS)—and it is to be feared that, when strangers arrive at villages in a dying state, they are not unfrequently thus exposed, even before life has departed.* Under a strict observance of the Hindu Law, the bodies of suicides, and of those who died a violent death, were cast into the jungles without any funeral rites. The law and the practice, however, appear to be alike unknown to those high caste natives of Bengal of whom I have made enquiry.

The practice of sinking bodies in TANKS by means of large earthen vessels, or by bricks, sand-bags, or other weights, is very common in Bengal. The following instances may be cited from many:—In August 1865, the body of a Mussulman old woman was found floating on the surface of a tank in a village near Patna. Six gurras were fastened to it, two round the neck, two to the waist, and two to the knees. It appeared that her husband and two accomplices had strangled her, and had sunk her body in the tank in the manner described. It was proved that some of the gurras had been in the house of one of the accomplices, and the string with which the gurras were tied was shown to have belonged to the husband.†

In 1855, certain Hindoos were capitally sentenced at Tirhoot for the murder of a Mussulman. The deceased having beén missing for eight

---

* "I beheld," says Dr. Buchanan, in his Christian Researches, speaking of Juggurnauth, "another distressing scene this morning, at the place of sculls, a poor woman lying dead, or nearly dead, and her two children by her, looking at the dogs and vultures which were near. The people passed by without noticing the children. I asked them where was their home. They said, 'they had no home but where their mother was.'" The author of "Fifteen Years in India" (1822) says, at page 211,—" I have beheld the dead bodies of natives, not yet cold, who had expired under the trees in the vicinity of Calcutta, mangled and torn by adjutants, while crowds of Hindoos were passing to bathe in the Ganges; and, when the corpses were pointed out to their countrymen, the cold answer was, 'hum janta ne Saheb,' (I know him not, Sir). Ah, but remove the body and burn it—'Mera dustoore ne, Saheb,' (it is contrary to custom), answered they. Hence it may be inferred that it is the lot of no Hindoo to meet with a good Samaritan."

Cases of this kind sometimes come before the police authorities. In 1846, six persons were tried at Purneah on a charge of having made away with a sick traveller. This unfortunate, in passing through a village, became too ill to proceed, and lay down opposite a shop. The owner, seeing that he was very ill, and fearing that he and others would be exposed to much trouble and expense from the enquiries of the police, if he died there, had him conveyed to a tope of trees which was about a mile distant, and left him exposed to the rain during the night. In the morning he died, having mentioned what had occurred to other persons passing that way. Mr. Dampier remarks—he fears that this is a very common practice, at least he has heard it frequently mentioned, and the lives of many poor travellers and pilgrims are sacrificed to the fear of incovenience to the villagers, should they be allowed to remain and perhaps die in their town. It is, from the nature of the case, almost impossible to procure sufficient evidence to secure the punishment of the parties.—*Police Report, L. P., for* 1846, p. 21.

† Bengal Police Report, for 1865, p. 124.

days, a man, who was gathering lotus leaves in a tank, felt a corpse touch his leg under water. On the thannadar's proceeding to the tank, it was found that a gurra had been tied round the waist on each side, in order that, when the gurras filled, the corpse might remain under water. It appeared that the deceased had been strangled.*

In Northern Bengal and in the N. W. Provinces, the numerous WELLS scattered over the country are commonly made receptacles of the bodies of murdered persons. Forbes states that, during 1808 and 1809, no less than 67 bodies were taken out of wells in the single district of Etawah. They had probably been deposited there by thugs. It sometimes happens that criminals adopt the unsafe expedient of filling up the wells in which the bodies of their victims have been deposited.†

Dr. Edward Goodeve informed me that, in some observations which he made upon the comparative rapidity of animal decomposition in various media, he found that, under ordinary circumstances, bodies submerged in wells up-country decompose more rapidly than they would do if exposed to the air. It appears probable, however, that this must depend much upon the depth and condition of the water. In a body immersed in a well plentifully supplied with spring water, the progress of decomposition would, doubtless, be considerably retarded ; but, in shallow stagnant water, which had merely drained into the receptacle, and had been evaporating for several months, the remains would, of course, decompose rapidly, as in a macerating tub.—Further remarks on the discovery of bodies in Wells, Tanks, and Rivers will be found in the chapter on DROWNING.

The burial of corpses and of plundered property in the sands of DRY WATER-COURSES is a frequent practice among criminals in Bengal and the N. W. Provinces ; the sand is easily dug out, and all traces of the burial are speedily obliterated. This was a common mode of disposing of the victims of thuggee by strangulation.

Both in Bengal and in the N. W. Provinces, bodies are often buried in the MUD FLOORS OF HOUSES. As there is no solid foundation, the grave may be dug to any depth (although it is generally shallow), and the extra

* Nizamut Adawlut Reports, July 1855, p. 11 :—It appeared, in a trial at Chota-Nagpore, in 1855, that it having become known to certain villagers that the corpse of a murdered woman had been thrown into a tank, they, with characteristic apathy, *waited till the body rose.* The "marine telescope," as it is called, might frequently be used with advantage in the search for sunken bodies. It is a cask with a plate of strong glass at the bottom. A man plunges the closed end a few inches below the surface, and looks down. The glare and confused reflections and refractions from and through the rippled surface of the water, are thus entirely shut out ; and, unless the water be foul and turbid in the extreme, all that lies below is rendered visible.

† See an instance already cited. Police Report, L. P., for 1844 :—In 1852, a youth of 15 or 16, having been persuaded to rob his father by two persons with whom he decamped, was thrown into a well by them. They then cast heaps of earth down at him. The water was very deep, but he contrived to support himself on a projection; and, after about three hours, he managed to climb up the sides and got out.—*Nizamut Adawlut Reports, N. W. P.*, 14th September 1852, p. 990.

earth can be disposed of in raising the level of the floor which, when leeped over with a mixture of water and cow-dung, presents no traces of disturbance. It is probable that, in most cases, this mode of sepulture is only intended to be temporary. It is frequently resorted to in cases of infanticide, and where children are decoyed into the houses of criminals and murdered for the sake of their ornaments.

N. B.—In Madras (not in Bengal) it is usual to bury first-born Hindu infants of some castes, temporarily, within the precincts of their houses.

In 1853, a woman was sentenced at Jounpoor for murdering her illegitimate child ; she confessed that she had pressed the infant's neck and strangled him. She had placed the corpse in an earthen vessel, which she had buried in a corner of her house.*

In 1852, a girl, seven years old, was decoyed into the house of one Bhickna, and murdered by him for her ornaments, worth only a few rupees. The criminal's son made disclosures which led to the discovery of the body buried at about four fingers' depth below the floor. The neck bore marks of strangulation, both legs were cut off near the ankles, and were found apart from the trunk, and there were marks of the jaw having been stoven in by a brickbat.†

Still again, in Tirhoot, the body of a female child, aged six years, was found buried under the floor of the prisoner's house. He had murdered her for the sake of her ornaments, valued at about three rupees.‡

Adult bodies are also sometimes disposed of in this manner :—In 1853, a man was sentenced at Cawnpore as an accessory to the murder of his own sister.§ He confessed that the deceased's son and another relative had beaten her to death, and had absconded with her property, and that he afterwards witnessed the partial burial of her body in one of the apartments of the building in which they all resided as a joint family. He had deceived the neighbours as to the cause of the unpleasant effluvium which proceeded from his house, by attributing it to the death of a snake in one of the drains. The body was found, several days after the murder, in the condition of a skeleton, imperfectly buried in a locked room, the key of which was in the prisoner's possession.||

In 1854, a boy was missing at Futtehpore ; suspicion fell upon a woman of disreputable character, named Mendeea, who had been in the habit of giving the child sweetmeats. Her house was searched, and there the body of the child was found, buried in the ground, with the throat cut

* Nizamut Adawlut Reports, N. W. P., 30th July 1853, p. 937.

† *Ibid*, 29th October 1852, p. 1254.

‡ Report of the Superintendent of Police, L. P., for the second six months of 1838, p. 14.

§ Cases of atrocity parallel to this are, unhappily, not rare in India. A perfectly well ascertained instance occurred up-country some years since, in which a wretch, tempted by avarice, strangled his own grand-daughter for the sake of her gold ornaments, and buried her body in a corner of his house.

|| Nizamut Adawlut Reports, N. W. P., 11th June 1853, p. 765.

and with other wounds. On the following day, search was made for the knife with which the crime was committed ; when, upon taking a number of earthen pots out of the house, and digging into the floor, the bone of a leg appeared, and then an entire skeleton. This, Mendeea confessed, was the body of a Brahminee widow, named Duryaee, who had disappeared nine months previously, and had been killed with a sword. Mendeea was sentenced to death.*

Both in the N. W. Provinces and in Bengal, THE COOKING PLACE is, not unfrequently, that chosen as the securest spot for the concealment of a body.

In 1854, a woman in Bundlekund decoyed a girl four years old into her house and murdered her ; and, after pretending to assist in the search for the child, locked her house and absconded. Upon being apprehended, she refused to deliver the key. The door was then forced by the police ; and in an interior room, which formed the prisoner's cooking place, and in a hollow close to her *choolha,* the child's body was found buried in the ground, but with her hand and foot protruding. Over the body was found a massive stone, three or four seers in weight, smeared with blood. The face and nose were somewhat flattened and defaced, one foot had disappeared, having been cut off at the ankle joint. A cord was found tightly fastened round the neck, so as to cause strangulation. The ornaments, valued at rupees 13 or 14, were found on the person of the murderess. On being questioned regarding the motive, she used a word *(ukus)* which was interpreted as envy or jealousy. She was childless, and the word used expresses a feeling very common amongst the native women towards those who are more fortunate than themselves. She was condemned to death.†

Four brothers were found guilty, at Delhi, in 1852, of the murder of Peerdan, of the village of Bhinee Bhirroo, who, there was every reason to believe, had seduced their sister, and caused her to procure abortion. Having enticed him into their house to smoke, they strangled him, and buried him deeply under the *aharah* (fire-place) in their compound. Upon searching their house in vain, a pitchfork was struck into the ground over the *aharah,* from which a stench immediately issued. One of the prisoners, then in custody, was desired to point out where the body was ; he said that the corpse would be found there, buried with his clothes and shoes on ; on digging, the body was found in the state described.‡

The following account of a similar search contains some useful particulars. Upon the disappearance of a young child, a burkundauze was deputed to the village of Sarunpore. He reported that, upon his arrival there, he assembled the four chowkeedars, four moquddums, and Shady

* Nizamut Adawlut Reports, N. W. P., 9th September 1854, p. 345.

† *Ibid*, 18th September 1854, p. 404.

‡ *Ibid*, 19th August 1852, p. 830.

Khan tanet. They searched the jungle, and the wells, and some heaps of *bhoosa.* Having placed watches round the village, the next day they searched again till noon ; but, finding no trace of the child, they made further enquiries, and desired the moquddums to search all through the village *mohullas* by turning over the heaps of manure and rubbish. On coming to the premises of Rambuksh, there was some appearance of the rubbish having been removed to a distance. He sent for four *Chumars,* and, after digging three times in the dirt and manure heap, discovered the body of the child concealed underneath. The wife of Rambuksh accused her husband and another of having brought in the child smothered up in their clothes, and then of cutting his throat with *khoorpas,* which would be found in the *choollees* (earthen receptacles under the flooring of the house). He searched, and perceived an odour, and that the earth had been moistened with blood. Scraping up the earth, a *khoorpa* was found. The woman said that, on killing the child, they had, in the first instance, buried the body near the *choola* (or cooking place), but that Rambuksh had the following day taken up the body, at noon, and buried it in the rubbish heap. The child's ornaments were found buried in the *choollees,* or earthen receptacles, underneath the *palehnda,* or place for water-vessels.* See also a very remarkable case in which the body of a child, murdered for the sake of its ornaments, was buried in a recently-made *tengrah,* or earthen mound used for placing cooking utensils on. The attention of the police was called to the spot *by observing that ants were travelling in and out of a hole in the newly-raised heap.*†

The bodies of murdered persons are occasionally found concealed in the houses of individuals wholly innocent of all participation in the crime.‡

A very remarkable case of this kind was tried at Bundelkund, a few years since :—A Bunnea having missed his child, about six years of age, was informed that one Chitooa, a man of notoriously bad character, had decoyed the boy away by a promise to get him a young *bulbul.* Chitooa denied all knowledge of the child. His and other houses were searched, but in vain, until they came to the house of one Thakoor. Finding the door locked, suspicion was excited, but they patiently awaited the man's return. On being required to do so, he immediately opened the door. The house was very dark within, and they were obliged to light a *chiragh* to enable them to search it. They found one part of the earthen floor of the inner room soft to the touch, as though it had been recently dug up, and then beaten down again. They discovered, at the depth of four

---

* Nizamut Adawlut Reports, N. W. P., 8th September 1853, p. 1127.

† Nizamut Adawlut Reports, Vol. III., Part 1, of 1853, p. 228.

‡ See an instance of this kind in which a wretch, having strangled his own nephew, placed the body in an out-house belonging to a neighbour ; and, upon the first enquiry, discovered it to the child's father,—his brother, and to the police.—*Nizamut Adawlut Reports, N. W. P.,* 17th February 1854, p. 204.

or five fingers, the corpse of the child, with the head nearly cut off, but with all its ornaments on. Upon repairing to Chittooa's house, under a large heap of *kundahs,* was found the *ghurasa,* with which the murder was committed, covered with fresh blood ; this was recognised by two *lohars* as having been made by them for the prisoner. Chittooa said that he and Doorja, an accomplice, called the child, when Doorja, having opened the lock of Thakoor's house with a stick, took the boy in, and, having gagged his mouth with a cloth, cut his throat with the *ghurasa.* The padlock was produced in Court. It was the commonest description of native lock, and was easily opened before the Judge with a small piece of bamboo. Chittooa was sentenced to death.*

In a trial of certain persons, Hindus and Mussulmans, for the murder of a Hindu and his mistress, in Zillah Dinagepore, in 1856, two of the Hindu prisoners are stated to have confessed that it was originally plotted that "*the woman's body should be buried in some Mussulman grave,* and that the man's should be left in his house, that it might appear that he had been murdered by his concubine. It, however, appears that it was decided to sink the woman's body in the river.†

Many instances will be found in the Criminal Records of the N. W. Provinces (where wheat is plentiful) in which dead bodies have been concealed in dwellings and out-houses under HEAPS OF BRAN OR CHAFF *(Bhoosa).*‡

In that part of the country also, the HOLES OF PORCUPINES afford ready places of concealment for the corpses of murdered persons.§

"Wheresoever the body is, there will the eagles be gathered together"—is a fact, which has daily illustration in India, and which has often been turned to good account in searches for the remains of missing individuals. Cases in which attention was called to a murdered body by the noise of crows hovering over it :—Nizamut Adawlut Reports, N. W. P., 30th January 1852. Crows and Vultures, *Ibid,* 17th September of the same year. Jackals and Vultures, *Ibid,* 29th April 1853, p. 618. Vultures, *Ibid,* 3rd June of the same year, p. 743. Kites and Vultures, *Ibid,* 30th August of the same year. Nizamut Adawlut

---

* Nizamut Adawlut Reports, N. W. P., 2nd October 1852, p. 1121.

† Nizamut Adawlut Reports, Vol. VI., of 1856, p. 856.

‡ Nizamut Adawlut Reports, N. W. P., 20th July 1853, p. 880 ; 20th March 1854, p. 324 ; 12th May 1854, p. 514 ; 2nd September 1854, p. 310 ; 23rd October of same year, p. 602 ; 3rd March 1855, p. 297. It is worthy of notice that, in all of these six cases, the bodies were those of children murdered for the sake of their ornaments ; and that, in all but one (in which it does not appear that the body was actually buried in the chaff), death had been caused by strangulation.

§ For instances of this mode of concealment, *see* Nizamut Adawlut Reports, N. W. P., 30th September 1852, p. 1095, a boy aged 12. *Ibid,* 27th January 1853, p. 112, body of a man. *Ibid,* 6th May 1854, p. 485, body of an adult female. Also 10th October of same, year, p. 512, of a boy aged 14 years.

Reports, Vol. II., Part 1, of 1852, p. 685, by the howling of a Jackal, *Ibid*, Vol. VI. of 1853, p. 660. A remarkable instance in which the friends of a murdered child, searching for his body with torches at night, were directed to the spot where it lay by the noise of Jackals quarrelling and snarling over it, *Ibid*, Vol. VII. of 1853, p. 72. We are told that, in this way, the sacrilegious slaying of a cow, which led to the Battle of Pundooa in 1340, was brought to light. Vultures flying over a tank by which a body lay. Corpse of a murdered woman discovered by Jackals and Dogs tearing away the earth with which it was covered, Police Reports, L. P., 1840, p. 5. There is a case narrated in the Bengal Police Report for 1866, p. 221, in which it would appear, as far as can be gathered from the by no means clear narrative, that a murderer, having first buried his victim, placing a quantity of stones over it, found that the body had been unearthed by wild animals, and therefore threw the corpse into a nullah.

I have long thought that the common pariah dog of the country, and, very possibly the vulture also, could be trained for the discovery of missing bodies. The dog would, probably, be found tolerably manageable, but could rarely be useful in cases where the corpse lay at a considerable distance. The keener sense and wider visual range of the vulture would tell far more advantageously ; and, although this bird appears to be absolutely untameable, small supplies of food will generally induce it to resort to a particular locality, where its movements can nearly always be under observation.* Indeed, a tree resorted to by vultures will be found in the neighbourhood of every station ; and a look-out for the direction in which the birds left or returned thither, might often assist a search. The subject certainly deserves the attention of Surgeons and Magistrates in the Mofussil.

RULES FOR THE TRANSMISSION AND EXAMINATION OF WOUNDED PERSONS AND DEAD BODIES.

It is, of course, a matter of paramount importance that, upon entering upon any medico-legal enquiry, *the surgeon should be made acquainted by the police and others, with every ascertainable detail of the cases upon which his opinion is required.*

The rules which obtain in British India for conducting and reporting inquests, and for sending wounded persons and the bodies of those who

* The best kept burial-grounds in India are resorted to by Adjutant Birds and Vultures. Here there are no open graves to satisfy their rapacity, neither can the small fragments burrowed for by Jackals tempt creatures of such large size and rapid digestion. They, doubtless, batten upon the rats and other vermin which infest those places.

have died under suspicious circumstances, with all necessary information, to the civil surgeons, are as follow :*

"161. It shall be the duty of the officer in charge of a police station, on receiving notice or information of the unnatural or sudden death of any person,

---

* Since the second edition of this work appeared, in 1856, the Law has undergone great change, especially in the promulgation, throughout British India, of the Indian Penal Code (Act XLV. of 1860), of the Code of Criminal Procedure (Act XXV. of 1861), and of the new Police Rules. Citing the existing law and practice in the text, I have thought it right to give those previously in force in the Bengal Presidency as foot-notes.

Rules in force previous to 1860.

"505.—On receiving information of suspicious or unnatural deaths, the darogah, or some responsible person deputed by him, shall proceed to the spot and examine the wounds or other corporal injuries ; but he shall not probe them, and he shall record the length, breadth and apparent depth of each, and the weapon with which the wounds appear to have been given, and whether the body appeared to have been brought and laid there. He should also ascertain, if possible, the name of the deceased, and whether any one can recognise him or her.—*Regulation XX. of* 1817, *Section XIV., Clause* 6; *Circular Order No.* 9, *August* 10*th*, 1847.

"508.—After the inquest, the body or bodies shall be given up to the relations, or be buried or burnt, and shall not be sent to the magistrate except in cases of poison or doubt ; and then only if the weather or distance will allow of their being sent without the risk of putrefaction ; and the notice of the sessions judge shall be directed, on the trial, to the observance, or otherwise, of these rules.—*Regulation XX. of* 1817, *Section XII.; Circular Order No.* 17, *April* 19*th*, 1789 (*a*).

"510.—In sending the bodies to the civil surgeon for examination, the magistrate shall furnish him with all available information, as to the cause of death.—*Circular Order No.* 152, *November* 24*th*, 1843.

"1134.—All enquiries held by the police relative to unnatural deaths or woundings, as well as to dacoity and other heinous offences, shall be attested by the police officer holding the enquiry, and a sufficient number of creditable persons present at the investigation.—*Regulation XX. of* 1817, *Sections XIV., XV.*

"1127.—The sooruthals required by Sections XIV. and XV., Regulation XX. of 1817, in cases of deaths, robberies, &c., shall be sent to the magistrate, in place of a report, the moment they are drawn up.—*Circular Order No.* 138, *June* 16*th*, *Para.* 2, *Section III.*

"In cases of murder, homicide, or unnatural death, accompanied with suspicious circumstances, as also in cases of severe wounding, the corpse or wounded person will be forwarded by the police, as soon as the customary 'sooruthal' has been recorded, to the officer in charge of the sub-division, should his station be in the direct line between the place where the

---

(*a*). In 1853, the Officiating Sessions Judge of Bundlekund recorded his opinion that,—"In all cases where there has been severe wounding, and death subsequently ensues, *the corpse should be sent into the station without leaving the police any discretion in the matter*." There was a proceeding, dated 3rd June 1845, however, by a former joint magistrate of that district, to the purport, "that when people are killed by wounds of sword or spears, and there is no doubt but that they have died from such wounds, their corpses should not be sent to the station." Although this order is conformable to the letter of the law, Regulation XX. of 1817, Section XIV., Clause 12, yet it seemed to him that, in almost all cases of death ensuing a few days after the infliction of wounds, there is doubt whether unskilful treatment or other causes may not have operated, and that nothing can be imagined more injudicious than the above order, the only certainty which we have in this country of the actual cause of death arising from the *post-mortem* examination of the surgeon.—*Nizamut Adawlut Reports, N. W. P.*, March 24th, 1853.

Experience would certainly tend to show that this is, by far, the safer view of the case.

immediately to give information to the nearest magistrate, and to proceed to the place where the body of such deceased person is; and there, in the presence of two or more respectable inhabitants of the neighbourhood, to make enquiry, and report the apparent cause of death, describing any mark of violence which may be found on the body, and stating in what manner, or by what weapon or instrument, such mark appears to have been inflicted. The report shall be signed by such police officer and other person, or so many of them as shall concur therein, and shall be forthwith forwarded to the magistrate. When there may be any doubt regarding the cause of death, such police officer shall forward the body, with a view to its being examined by the civil surgeon, if the state of the weather and distance will admit of its being so forwarded without risk of putrefaction on the road. In the Presidencies of Madras and Bombay, it shall be the duty of the head of the village, in like manner, to make the enquiry, and report as aforesaid."—*Code of Criminal Procedure.*

The Government have further ordered—

"1*st.*—That, when the death occurs in the sudder sub-division, the body should, in suspicious cases, be forwarded to the civil surgeon.

"2*nd.*—When the death occurs in a sub-division, and there is a sub-assistant surgeon or European medical officer attached to it, he should hold the *post-mortem.*

"3*rd.*—In a sub-division where there is only a native doctor, whenever the state of the dead body, the distance, the weather, or the state of the roads renders it improbable that the body will reach the sudder station in such a condition as to enable the civil surgeon satisfactorily to hold a *post-mortem*, the body must be sent to the sub-divisional medical officer. A copy of the report of such officer will, however, be submitted to the civil surgeon, who will make any remarks he may think proper in the margin of the report, for the information of the sub-divisional officer. When the body bears external marks of violence, the sub-divisional officer should, if possible, view the body in the presence of the native doctor.

"When, on the other hand, circumstances permit, the body should be sent to the sudder station for examination by the civil surgeon, and at such examination the native doctor or sub-assistant surgeon at the sudder station should be present, so that he may be able to attend, if required, at the sub-divisional court, and give evidence as to the cause of death, in cases in which the absence of the surgeon on duty would be attended with inconvenience to those under his medical charge."—*B. G. Cir. O., No.* 4970, 1863, *and O'Kinealy's Ed. of the Code of Criminal Procedure*, 1868, *p.* 85.

"Magistrates should be careful that, in every case of suspected death, the body is taken *direct* to the civil surgeon by the police, who should lose no time in despatching it, with such information as to the history of case, symptoms, &c., as can be procured without the occurrence of delay. After the civil surgeon,

---

investigation is going on and the sudder station of the magistrate. The deputy or assistant, after inspecting the corpse, or wounded person, as the case may be, will lose no time in sending the same on to the sudder station for examination by the civil surgeon.—Rule 4 of Rules for the Guidance of Deputy Magistrates and Assistants in charge of Sub-divisions, Government Circular Order, February 18th, 1846.—*Skipwith's Magistrate's Guide*, 3*rd ed.*, 4*to.*, 1849.

*

on completion of the *post-mortem* examination, and preparation of the subjects for despatch to the chemical examiner, has communicated the necessity for such despatch to the magistrate, the latter will prepare the report of the circumstances attending the death as they can be ascertained. The magistrates should instruct the police, that, after the despatch of the body with the requisite information to the civil surgeon, they are to abstain from further communication with that officer, except through the magistrate."—*Agra Sudder Court Circular* 11, 1866.

The Judicial Commissioner, Punjab [10th January 1862], instructed the police to hold enquiries in all cases of unnatural or sudden death; but, if the homicide did not appear to have been culpable [s. 299, Penal Code,] he directed them not to interfere or mulct the perpetrator.—*Prinsep's Code of Criminal Procedure*, *2nd ed.*, *p.* 73.

In 1865, the Principal Inspector-General of the Medical Department in Bengal having brought to notice that, owing to the very meagre information collected, and to the imperfect manner in which, in cases of poisoning* or death, the first investigations are frequently conducted, much important medico-legal evidence is often lost,—the following hints drawn up by Dr. Hutchinson, the Civil Surgeon of Patna, were circulated to the police, for general information :—

In cases of Hanging or Strangulation.

1. Note, if possible, before cutting down the body, or removing the strangulating medium, any lividity of face, especially of lips and eyelids; any projection of the eyes; the state of the tongue, whether enlarged and protruded, or compressed within the lips; the escape of any fluid from mouth and nostrils, and direction of its flow.
2. On cutting down the body, or removing the strangulating medium, note particularly the state of the neck, whether bruised along the line of strangulation.
3. Note the direction of the mark, whether circular or oblique.
4. Note the state of the thumbs, whether crossed over the palm.
5. If possible, bring away the materials by which the hanging or strangulation has been effected.

On finding a Body in a Tank or Well.

1. Note any marks of blood about the mouth, or on the sides of the well or tank.
2. On removing the body, carefully examine for and note any external marks of injury, especially about head and neck.
3. Note state of skin, whether smooth or rough.
4. Examine the hands, and carefully remove anything they may hold.

In the case of a Body found murdered in an Open Field.

1. Note the number, character, and appearances of any injuries.
2. Should a weapon be found, cover with paper, and seal any marks of blood, and especially note and preserve any adherent hairs.

---

* *The Rules to be observed in cases of suspected Poisoning will be found in the Chapter on Poisons.*

3. In the case of an exposed infant, note the state of the cord, especially if tied, and any marks of violence.

In a case of presumed Murder and Burial of the Remains.

1. Examine for and note any marks of violence, about the skull especially.
2. Note carefully any indications of sex; especially bring away a jaw and the bones of the pelvis.
3. If any suspicions of poisoning, bring away (sealed) the earth where the stomach would have been.
4. If the body, presumed to have been murdered, has been burned, collect and bring in any fragments of bones which may be found among the ashes.

In Rape or Unnatural Offences.

Send in the lower garments worn by the persons when assaulted.

It is held to be the duty of medical officers to examine all bodies sent in by the police, as soon as practicable after their arrival at the sudder station.

In Bengal, police officers are supplied with the form of printed letter, a copy of which is given below, which is forwarded to the civil surgeon, not only in cases of assault, &c., but also in those where an explanation of the cause of death is required :

BENGAL POLICE FORM, No. 27.

No.

FROM

THE DISTRICT SUPERINTENDENT OF POLICE,

To

THE CIVIL SURGEON OF

SIR,

I HAVE to request the favor of your examining sent to the hospital on the

Be so good as to fill up the columns on the reverse of this letter, and return it to me with such remarks as you may consider necessary, to show clearly your opinion of the cause of

2. All that is at present known of the case is as follows :—

I have the honor to be,
Sir,
Your most obedient servant,

District Superintendent.

DISTRICT SUPERINTENDENT'S OFFICE,

The 18

1	2	3	4	5	6
Nature of injury, *i. e.*, whether a cut, a bruise, or a burn, &c., &c.	Size of each injury in inches, *i. e.*, length, breadth, and depth.	On what part of the body inflicted.	Slight, severe, or dangerous.	By what kind of weapon inflicted.	REMARKS.

HOSPITAL,

The *of* 18

Civil Surgeon.

At the end of this letter, police officers usually insert a few words indicative of the alleged cause of death ; such as—" Reported to have died with symptoms of poisoning ;" or—" Stated to have been severely beaten." Indeed the form, being printed rather widely on one side of a half sheet of foolscap paper, does not admit of the insertion of many explanatory remarks.

I stated in 1855 that it by no means unfrequently occurred that, either from delay on the part of the darogah in transmitting the sooruthal (*sooret-hal*, narrative or report of inquest), or from some other cause, the medical officer finds himself called upon to examine and to report upon the cause of death in a case regarding which he has not been furnished with a single guiding fact.

Upon this *My Commentator* remarked : " The sooruthal has nothing to do with the sending in of the body." [It had in Bengal, as will be seen on reference to the rules then in force—Note to page 30.] "It is *the abstract of the case* which is made up after the *completion of the thannah enquiry :* this may occupy two, three, or more days. If every corpse were kept in the thannah till the completion of the sooruthal, the position of a civil surgeon would be trying indeed ; the sooruthal, however, has nothing to do with the medical investigation, the information for which is forwarded in a small *nuksha* with the body. This information is generally meagre, often incorrect, and not unfrequently downright false. It does not follow, however, that the thannahdar is to blame. He is not omniscient, and he can only give what information he may have obtained from others ; nor is it always possible to punish the fabricator of false information, for his identity is as difficult of discovery as the identity of a seven days' corpse. The thannahdar trusts to the chowkeedar, who says that he was told by the zemindar, who heard it from some one else who turns out to be the father of the accused man himself. Perhaps the information given, although apparently false, may be substantially true. We will relate a case in point. A gentleman beat his punkah coolie with a slipper for going to sleep ; some hours after, the man was taken seriously ill. He became giddy and partially comatose. In this condition he was immediately taken before the doctor. He was made to vomit, and brought up a quantity of dhatoora seeds, which he had taken in a fit of passion after a love quarrel. Now, if this circumstance had occurred away from the station, and the man had died, the body would have been sent in with the remark 'said to have died from the effects of beating.' The medical examination would have established death from the effects of *dhatoora ;* or, in default of *a thorough examination,* 'no apparent traces of injury.'

" A consideration of these circumstances will show how difficult it is to furnish the civil surgeon with really trustworthy information, by which his researches may be guided. The sooruthal, which gives an abstract of the whole case, contains this information ; but it can never be ready in time for transmission with the body. As to the suggestions which Dr. Chevers gives about obtaining an accurate description of the position of the body, &c.,* there is not a magistrate who does not try to obtain this desideratum, but natives *will not be accurate.*" [They will, in time, if those who teach them are sufficiently persistent in selecting men who have fair powers of observation and in training them into habits of accuracy, and then make it worth their while to be accurate ; a man is generally accurate in his observation of that which tends to his own personal interest.] "A darogah considers that he has performed a feat of accuracy, when he has measured the length of a wound, and distinguished a graze or a hatchet blow from the stroke of a tulwar. He cannot expect accurate descriptions from men who are not accurate observers ; and to tell a darogah to observe accurately is to tell him to change his nature."

It is certainly difficult to make a man change his nature, but it is observed that the hope of Κυδος and of promotion often modifies and improves human nature considerably. No doubt there is a great deal of truth in the above commentary, still it is evidently the duty of civil surgeons to insist inflexibly upon the fullest *possible* reports—and a good deal of guiding information is, in most cases, immediately procurable.

A very experienced civil surgeon in this neighbourhood writes me—"Very little information, as a rule, is sent with the request to examine, and my impression is that the inquest held by native inspectors is generally very superficial." Another old officer, in medical charge of a very important district, tells me that, until very lately, he used to receive with the bodies nothing but the short vernacular *chellans.* When the brevity of these came to the point of "*the body of —— sent for examination,*" he urged and obtained a reform.

The following letter, from the Sessions Judge of Bhaugulpore to the Magistrate of the district, points out the action which ought to be taken by civil surgeons in noticing important irregularities or omissions in reports of mofussil police inquests :

"In the within trial before this court, the police inquest, 17th March 1857, No. 3, on the murdered boy Ram Sein, though describing death generally to have been caused by strangulation, was utterly wanting in the following particulars deposed to by Dr. Farncombe,—'and from the protrusion of the eyes and tongue, I think it very likely that strangulation was the cause of death.' Neither inquest, nor the attesting witnesses thereto, observe anything of the kind. Such grave discrepancy ought to be cleared up at the time by the magisterial authorities, as it is vain to expect it when brought up at a distant period before the sessions court.

"It is the practice, in other districts, for a copy of the mofussil inquest to accompany the body. This copy is handed to the medical officer for his information, simultaneously with his examination of the body, and he

* See page 43 of this volume.

countersigns it in acknowledgment of his having done so, when it should be duly filed with the record. It will then, of course, be the duty of the medical officer to bring to your notice any important irregularities or omissions in the mofussil inquest which may seem to call for emergent enquiry ; and in that case, of course, timely enquiry will duly follow, and the matter be cleared up before it comes before the sessions court. I would, therefore, suggest your duly instructing your subordinates and the medical officer on the subject." *

A curious glimpse of the Crowner's 'Quest Law of the Madras Village Punchayets in 1862, is given by Native Surgeon Ruthnum Moodelly :†

He tells us that the members of the punchayets are often men from the dregs of society, picked up indiscriminately without the slightest regard to their discretion and respectability. They perform their temporary duty very reluctantly, pay no attention to the proceedings at the inquest, and are glad to get rid of a vexatious task by finding any verdict they please. "Never differ" is their motto—and they, on every occasion, concur in the same opinion. "Who is to know that these worthies are not themselves privy to the base and sordid underhand dealings of some village moonsiff ?" But, if a medical opinion on the case before them is thought necessary, the depositions are not completed until the doctor arrives and gives a certificate on the results of his *post-mortem* examination ; and, on his retiring, the arbitrators change their opinion, if they had formed one, and the record is made to tally with the views of the medical officer. A little extortion from both the innocent and the guilty concludes the proceedings. He adds that he has attended a great number of inquests, and that his description is by no means exaggerated. On the contrary, he is fully convinced that the monstrous evils complained of are but poorly represented, inasmuch as they interfere with the medical evidence which they sometimes supplant. We can readily agree with N. S. Moodelly that "the institution of the punchayet is a complete failure," and also assent to the argument of one who has recently advocated the substitution of the punchayet system for the village police in Bengal that "the utility of the institution will be contingent on the possibility of finding honest and intelligent men to work it."

When, as generally happens, death has taken place several days previously, and decomposition of the body has advanced to a horrible extent, the task placed before the surgeon, who is really desirous to throw some light upon a case which he doubts not involves questions of vital moment, is a very trying and difficult one. The order forbidding the police to send in bodies for examination whenever it is probable that, on account of the weather or of the distance, they will reach the sudder station in a state

---

* Nizamut Adawlut Reports, June 27th, 1857, p. 796. It is directed, in Bengal Police Circular, No. 19 of the 17th September 1869, that the final order in every case shall be communicated to the Civil Surgeon—see Chapter on *Medical Evidence.*

† Madras Quarterly Journal of Med. S., for October 1862, p. 311.

of advanced putrefaction, is not always attended to ; and account is not generally taken of the rapidity with which decomposition advances in a body wrapped in a sheet of matting, hurried along some thirty or forty miles through a burning atmosphere, at from two to ten days after death. Judging by my own experience at different stations, a body can seldom be sent in, from a remote part of the district, within less than two or three days after death. Under these circumstances, its very appearance, when freed from its swathings, is almost appalling, even to the initiated :—bloated in every part, almost to bursting, with its limbs widely separated by sheer gaseous distention ; the eyes dissolving and forced from their sockets ; the tongue enormously swollen and protruded between the teeth, through which the gases of putrefaction bubble with loud crepitations ; the skin everywhere separated, displaying the *white* surface beneath, marbled with gangrenous blotches and veinings, and preyed upon by gigantic ants and beetles of sinister aspect, and by maggots which roll forth in measures-full when the cloths are unloosed. A body of this kind offers no very safe or encouraging field for the morbid anatomist's researches.

It is true that, in all such cases, the civil surgeon is at liberty to decline to make an internal examination ; still, if furnished with a distinct clue, he would very often be able to throw a light upon the cause of death, sufficient for the purposes of justice, even when decomposition had advanced considerably. Too great stress needs not be laid upon the rule of avoiding to send in bodies, when it is even certain that they will reach the sudder station in an extremely putrid condition, as it will frequently happen that even a single glance at the most decomposed corpse will reveal much to the experienced eye. For instance, a body was sent to my hospital at Chittagong in a very advanced state of putrefaction ; the history was not furnished. I was about to desire that it might be buried, when I was struck with something unusual in the position of the head. Upon further examination, I found a fracture of the vertebræ of the neck. A person was stated by the police to have died in consequence of a severe beating ; the accused declared that death had resulted from cholera. The body was so offensive as to be scarcely approachable. No wound or fracture could be perceived,—the presence of solid fæces in the mats, however, enabled me to declare that the case had not been one of cholera. When at Howrah, I viewed the body of a pregnant female, in which the work of decomposition had fully revealed the history of her death. After it had been placed in the dead-house, accumulation of gas in the intestines had caused the contents of the uterus to be expelled,—there lay a much-decomposed fœtus of about four months, and with it a portion of the intensely acrid root of the *Plumbago Rosea,* seven inches and a half in length, thickly coated with inflammatory mucous deposit. An almost precisely similar case occurred to Dr. Clementson in the Dispensary at Berhampore (Madras Presidency) in 1866.* Again, in a case of alleged death by hanging, where any idea of dissection was quite out of the question, a close examination of the skin of the neck revealed perfectly convincing traces of the pressure which the rope had occasioned. In the Court of Criminal Referred Jurisdiction, January 17th, 1868, Mr. Justice Elphinstone Jackson suggested,—in the case of Beebun Aurut, who had been sentenced to death by the Officiating Sessions Judge of Moorshedabad, on a charge of murdering her niece, aged three years, by throwing her into a small water-hole,—that, although the civil surgeon did not examine the brain as the body was too far advanced in decomposition, such an examination might have proved that the child had suffered injury to the brain by a fall upon its head (the prisoner having alleged before the magistrate that the deceased running after her, she had given it a push which caused it to fall down senseless), and that the death was not caused by drowning. The extremely decomposed state of a body cannot afford any grounds for overlooking anything remarkable in its outward condition. Thus, in a certain trial of a man for cutting his wife's throat, the medical officer testified that the wound was two inches deep and extended from the back to the front of the neck on the left side; and that such a wound would cause death. But the corpse was in so decomposed a state, when it reached him, that he could not positively state whether the wound was inflicted before or immediately after death. The state of the body need not have prevented examination of the hands, the sound or wounded condition of which forms so leading a criterion in cases of cut-throat. Many other similar instances might be enumerated. They, however, merely tend to confirm and strengthen the necessity of the principle that the police should furnish ample information for the guidance of the medical officer in every case; and, most especially, in those instances where it is evident that the task of unravelling the truth will be one of exceeding difficulty. I believe that, in nearly all cases, police officers and magistrates are perfectly willing to afford the medical officer every information and assistance in their power; still it appears probable that there exists a very prevalent idea that it is merely necessary to place a body, however decomposed, before a medical man, to enable him to reveal fully the causes of death. It is certainly a truth, which the criminal histories of every year show forth with almost supernatural distinctness, that—

> "Murder hath speech, and will declare itself
> With most miraculous organ"†——

Still, a very close devotion of thirty-five years to the study of morbid anatomy has convinced me, that this is one of the most unfair and most

---

* Madras Quarterly Journal of Medical Science, Vol. X., p. 181.

† A belief in the maxim that "Murder will out" is general among the Natives of India. "*Sin is never hidden*" is a Bengali proverb, for which I am indebted to the kindness of the Rev. James Long.

unsafe questions that can be put to a medical man. In England,—where such investigations are, of course, made with very much greater facility than in India,—a difficulty of this kind exceedingly rarely comes before those who are most engaged in *post-mortem* examinations. There, in at least ninety-nine cases out of every hundred, the operator is enabled to obtain, beforehand, some kind of clue which may guide him in his obscure inquiry. Except in cases where it is found absolutely impossible to obtain information, no surgeon can be fairly expected to unravel every tissue of a body from which life may have been expelled by any one of a hundred causes,—such as by the softening of part of a nervous centre, by a stroke of lightning, by a snake-bite, by exposure to a poisonous gas, by a blow over the stomach, by a bodkin thrust into some vital organ, from hydrophobia or idiopathic tetanus, by the effects of a few drops of prussic acid, or of a few grains of strychnia,—the detection of every one of which would become an undertaking of greater and greater difficulty with every hour that elapsed after the departure of vital heat. When the process of decomposition has fully commenced, the surgeon cannot fairly be expected to succeed in throwing any light upon the cause of death,—or even to undertake the examination,—unless he can be enabled to judge with precision in what direction his search must be pursued, as, for instance, where it is known that a blow has been inflicted over a certain vital part, or it is believed that a mineral poison has been swallowed. In the absence of the necessary information regarding the circumstances preceding death, the best surgeon is frequently liable to deduce a partial, and therefore erroneous, opinion from his examination of the bodies even of the recently dead. Two or three probable instances will suffice in illustration. A person suffering from cholera has his end hastened by a (let us say homœopathic) dose of arsenic; or a plague-stricken wretch is strangled ; or an unfortunate, in this country, is attacked and suffocated :—are the surgeons to blame if, on discovering the ordinary vestiges of destructive intestinal disease, the deadly carbuncles, and that cerebral congestion which may so sufficiently represent the effects of heat apoplexy,* they form their decisions, and record their evidence upon these, overlooking entirely the few scattered grains of impalpable powder, the finger-marks upon the swollen neck, and the evidences of asphyxia, wherein the truth lay hidden ?

Although the Regulation guiding the police in sending bodies with sufficiently explanatory details to the medical officers for examination is, as we have seen, very frequently overlooked, it rules in a perfectly clear and unequivocal manner that the civil surgeon is to be held as a party

* It is well known that heat apoplexy (or, more properly speaking, death from extreme heat) may occur quite out of the influence of the sun's rays. In India, many cases occur at night. As in nearly all cases involving a severe shock to the nervous system, the first effect of the destructive influence is to arrest the supply of blood to the cerebral system. With reaction, however, we have all the evidences of intense congestion of the brain.

in the judicial inquiry ; that no attempt is to be made to keep him in the dark ; and that all possible aid and information are to be afforded him in his task of unravelling the medico-legal difficulties of the case. The Circular Order, No. 152 of November 24th, 1843, directed that—

"*In sending the bodies to the civil surgeon for examination, the magistrate shall furnish him with all available information as to the cause of death.*"

This rule, however, does not appear to have been formerly adhered to with strictness in the North-West Provinces. In a case of child murder, tried at Cawnpore in 1852, the civil surgeon stated that the infant *probably* died from concussion of the brain, but that he did not make an examination of the head or brain ; that, not having any idea of the circumstances under which the examination was required, and the infant being newly born, he, not perceiving any appearance of a blow, satisfied himself with examining the bowels and viscera, where disease or appearance of poisoning would, most probably, be detected. He had become aware that this was omission on his part, which he assured the judge would not occur again. He desired, in future, to have an outline of the circumstances under which bodies for report might be sent to him, in order that he might have some guide to the organs most requiring scientific examination. "*This,*" however, the judge thought, "*would interfere with a principle of criminal justice, and would be analogous to putting leading questions, the answers to which would not be evidence*, nor would it be fair to the prisoner ; for, though a severe sword-cut might be reported on, the presence of a diseased lung or spleen might pass unnoticed, though the actual cause of death." In their remarks upon this case, the superior Court decided that "the communication which had passed between the sessions judge and the civil surgeon was altogether irregular and objectionable."* As, however, the animadversion of the Court does not appear to have been particularly directed to the above opinion, and as there is reason to believe that a similar view of the question may be entertained by other judicial officers, this point still appears to demand an authoritative decision.

It would, of course, be presumptuous to attempt to discuss the question here, except in its medical bearings. Still many able jurists, among whom those of France may be especially mentioned, disapprove of that strict avoidance of leading questions which so strongly marks all judicial proceedings in England.†

---

* Nizamut Adawlut Reports, N. W. P., December 21st, 1852.

† "The Scottish lawyers regard with a sacred and scrupulous horror every question so shaped by the counsel examining as to convey to a witness the least intimation of the nature of the answer which is desired of him. These scruples, though founded on an excellent principle, are sometimes carried to an absurd pitch of nicety, especially as it is generally easy for a lawyer, who has his wits about him, to elude the objection."—Sir W. Scott.

The position of the medical witness in a criminal question, is, however, altogether different from that of an ordinary witness to matters of fact. When consulted by the police in a case of assault, wounding, or poisoning, he is not, in the first place, a *Witness;* he is, like the police themselves, *an active Agent in the inquiry.* Can it be that each of the parties concerned in this inquiry is under obligation to pursue the search throughout, guided only by his own light, keeping all the others sedulously in the dark? When, later in the inquest, the evidence of the medical witness is called for, it is evident that, in nearly nine cases out of ten, he has to be questioned, not upon plain facts, but upon obscure points of opinion and judgment. He can have no motive for collusion; it is a Decision rather than an Evidence which the law demands of him; he is, in fact, the arbitrator of a most essential portion of the case: with him alone lies the determination of those leading portions of the inquiry which are set before him,—upon these he stands in judgment; and all attainable light must be thrown upon every point of difficulty which he may be called upon to weigh.

In short, medical jurists cannot be too conversant with the details of the judicial inquiries in which their opinions are called for; and all reserve in furnishing them with the information which they require involves an infraction of the law as established both in England and in India.

About two years ago, the Judicial Commissioner, N. W. Provinces, ordered that every report of a *post-mortem* examination, in a judicial case, should comprehend the *whole appearances* discovered on full inspection of the body. Mr. George Barnard demurred at this, admitting that the fullest possible examination should invariably be made, but holding, with Casper, that extraneous facts only tend to confuse the judicial mind when introduced in such reports.

The true principle of action is that,—while the civil surgeon's official statement of the cause of death, as revealed in the autopsy, cannot well be too concise, if fully to the point,—the examination of the body should be *thorough,* and the surgeon's own notes (preserved for reference) of the appearances discovered should be as minute as possible. The plan of making partial autopsies is altogether wrong.

It has occurred, in cases where the surgeons' reports have shown merely that (1) death was caused by injury to the head, and (2) that a woman had died by strangulation; that it subsequently appeared that, in the first case, the ribs were also crushed in; and that, in the second, rape had been committed. Here thorough examinations and full notes would have furthered the ends of justice, and would have protected the medical officers from a charge of carelessness.

At the request of the late Mr. Ward, when magistrate of Howrah, I, in 1854, suggested the following *Rules to be observed by darogahs in sending dead bodies to the sudder station for examination.* It must, however, be premised that, in this country, the approach and progress of decomposition can be only in some degree retarded, whatever means we may adopt. Still, it is within our power to preserve the remains against attacks of insects and vermin, and to provide that the advance of putrefaction shall not be unnecessarily accelerated :

"I would recommend that supplies of strong acetic acid, or of the solution of the chloride of zinc* be sent to each thannah in the station. The free application of either of these fluids over a body will tend to delay somewhat the progress of decomposition externally, and will be very effectual in protecting the corpse against the destructive attacks of insects and small animals. I find that the cost of either of these fluids will be three rupees per quart. Rather more than a pint of the acetic acid would be required for each body. The chloride of zinc would go considerably farther, but is somewhat objectionable, as it would soon destroy the cloths used for enveloping the bodies.

"I would, therefore, beg to recommend that, immediately upon the discovery or disinterment of a body, the darogah [*now Police Officer*] having carefully observed and made notes of its position, the state of its garments, the marks of injury, any appearances of blood, &c., on the ground, floor, walls, or furniture, &c., &c., should have it placed on a clean rattan-bottomed charpoy (one of which might be supplied for that purpose, at small expense, to each police station), and covered with a clean sheet.

"Care should be taken not to remove any traces of blood and mud which may be found on the body. Any cord, &c., on the neck or limbs, or any grass or weed grasped in the hands, should be allowed to remain untouched, as should also be the case with any weapon left sticking in the body. Should delay be likely to attend the first investigation, the body should be despatched at once, with a memorandum to the magistrate of the cause of death *assigned*, as well as of that which is *suspected* by the police,—such as, 'Alleged to have been drowned ; but supposed to have been beaten with latthees.' The regular sooruthal should follow as speedily as possible.

"When considerable delay is quite unavoidable, it will be necessary to envelope the corpse carefully in a sheet saturated with the acetic acid. Some of the acid should also be poured into the mouth, and a cloth soaked in it should be placed carefully over any wound that may be present.

"Where it is possible to send the body to the medical officer within twelve hours after death, it should merely be enveloped in a dry sheet and despatched at once.

"As the present mode of sending bodies enveloped in mats and slung on a bamboo is, in many respects, objectionable, I would recommend that a wooden shell, with a closely fitting cover, protected above and at the sides and ends with thick sheets of sola† and furnished with poles for the bearers, should be kept at every thannah. For each shell should be supplied two sheets of very strong cotton cloth or thin canvas, and a quantity of charcoal, broken up into small pieces, could always be kept in the shell.

---

* It is now generally considered that *Carbolic Acid* should be supplied for this purpose, and that it will prove most useful.

† The spongy wood of the *Æschynomene Paludosa*,—a great non-conductor of heat, from which "rice paper" is manufactured.

"I would also recommend that, if possible, four *dome* bearers should be encouraged to live in the neighbourhood of every thannah for the speedy conveyance of bodies. Upon repairing to the spot at which a suspicious death had occurred, the darogah could be accompanied by these men with the shell, charcoal, cloths, and a bottle of acid.

"Before placing the body in the shell, the charcoal should be emptied out upon one of the sheets spread on the floor. The other sheet should then be placed at the bottom of the shell, with its ends hanging out evenly over the edge. Upon this sheet, the body, enveloped in its winding sheet saturated with acetic acid, should be placed within the shell. The other sheet, with a portion of the charcoal still upon it, should then be placed evenly over the body with its ends also hanging over the edge of the shell. The shell should then be filled to the edge with charcoal, and the lid fitted on.

"By this arrangement, we should be enabled to lift off the whole of the charcoal in the upper sheet, finding the body unsoiled beneath it. The body could then be lifted from the shell, for inspection, by grasping the corners of the lower sheet.

"The charcoal need not be used again, but it should be the duty of the *domes* to clean the shell, and to wash the sheets before taking them back to the thannah.

"If possible, the bodies should be brought from thannah to thannah, or along tracks where additional bearers may be obtained. The above plan, although it would be attended with some outlay at first, would not, in all probability, be more expensive, ultimately, than the use of bamboos and mats, which are never employed a second time.

"Should it be found impossible to abandon the present plan of conveying bodies, the corpse should be enveloped, 1st, in the sheet saturated with acid, as already directed; 2ndly, in a mat of close texture; 3rdly, it should be placed on a coarse mat spread with a thick layer of charcoal, broken small. The coarse mat should then be closed over, the space between the mats being first closely packed with charcoal, and the whole carefully bound round with split rattans."

Less than two years ago, it was still the practice, in the neighbourhood of Calcutta, to send in bodies for examination wrapped in matting and slung from bamboos. I learnt at the same time, in a communication from a civil surgeon, that, in Behar "the bodies are sent on *charpaies* fully exposed to the sun and rain, no attempt at protection or preservation with any antiseptic being made."

The need for good Dead-houses has been much felt in most stations in this Presidency. Not only is it absolutely necessary that a building should be provided sufficiently well built to protect bodies from being eaten by jackals or gnawed by rats, but it is also of the greatest importance that the civil surgeon should conduct his *post-mortem* examinations (which in some stations are very numerous) in a cool, well-lighted room, furnished with all needful appliances,—punkah, water-supply, tables, &c. Probably, the best dead-house ever devised for a tropical climate was one erected by Dr. Payne in the grounds of the Dullunda Lunatic Asylum, Calcutta, a few years since. As regards plinth and roof, it resembled an ordinary bungalow, but its walls and door were made of a thick iron gauze so close-meshed as to exclude flying insects. The arrangement, which was literally that of a large meat-safe, was so accurate that, while the bodies were completely protected, the medical officer did his work within, perfectly free from all avoidable inconvenience.

I feel confident that the general introduction of such dead-houses would prove a valid aid to pathological and medico-legal research in India.

IDENTITY OF DEAD BODIES.

The identification of dead bodies is among the most difficult of the tasks which fall within the province of the Medical Jurist. When such cases as that which occurred two years ago at Hackney almost defy solution in England, where the course of judicial enquiry is generally so clear, it must not cause surprise that, in India, where the truth almost always lies deeply concealed, our means of detection should often falter.

As the Hackney case has not appeared in any work on Medical Jurisprudence, a brief abstract may be given with advantage. On the 8th April 1868, the dead body of a man was discovered in an unfinished house. It appeared that he had been dead two or three months. The hair, moustache, and beard were mottled with blood, the eyes had been completely destroyed. The body was identified by Dr. Ellis, of St. Luke's Lunatic Asylum, as that of a patient named Heasman, who escaped from the institution on the night of the 1st of February. The brother of the patient corroborated this statement. A Mrs. Banks, however, most positively identified the deceased as her husband with whom she had lived for thirteen years, and who had been missing three years. She had minutely examined the remains on two occasions, and she had not the least doubt that they were those of her husband. She knew this to be the case from the fact of there being a mark on the forefinger of the right hand, which was caused by a cut when he was very young, and round which the flesh had never grown since. She mentioned the mark to the police before she saw the body, and the constable who accompanied her to the mortuary found it upon the body. Mr. E. Heasman deposed that he identified the body as that of his brother Benjamin Heasman, who had been a clerk in the same office as himself up to the early part of 1866. Witness last saw him alive at St. Luke's during the winter of 1867. The delusion he entertained was that he had been poisoned, and was a dead man. He had a suicidal tendency. The witness was enabled to identify the body by the squareness of the forehead, the high cheek-bones, and the general contour of the features. He was aware that, five years since, the deceased injured one of his fingers by doing something with the slates on the roof of his house, but the witness had never observed the mark. It appeared that no insurance money was likely to fall due upon proof of the death of either Banks or Heasman. The stockings found upon the body were marked with the name "Heasman," in the handwriting of his wife. The wife had viewed the body, and, looking at the face, was quite sure that it was that of her husband. She had been married to him fifteen years, and saw him last on the 9th of January this year. She had never noticed any scar on his finger from the accident alluded to by his brother. She was pecuniarily a sufferer by his death. She recognised the handwriting on the underclothing of the deceased as being her own, and also stated that the trowsers found upon the body were machine-made and of her own working. Dr. Ellis showed that, in escaping, Heasman took with him some articles of clothing belonging to other patients. The boot found by the side of the deceased, and marked "Harnett," belonged to a patient of that name. In the left jaw of the patient named Heasman, a tooth was missing, and this was also the case in the body in question. The dress found upon it was also identical in every respect by that worn by Heasman. A sister of Mrs. Banks thought the lower part of the body was exceedingly like her sister's husband, but she could not say positively that it was he. She had not seen him for seven or eight years, and had no remembrance of the scar her sister had referred to.

It is singular that, in the reports which I have seen, nothing appears to have been said by Dr. Gant, who made the *post-mortem* examination, regarding the scar on the finger. Dr. Ellis had not observed it.

It was, subsequently, found that deceased had died from swallowing a large quantity of opium. At the close of the first sitting of the Court, Mrs. Banks admitted that she was thoroughly satisfied that the body was that of Mr. Heasman and not that of her husband.

When the above case was under discussion, two other instances were also brought forward,* which are valuable in their resemblance to cases which have occurred in India.

In the number of the *Times* which appeared on the 24th of March 1866, there is a curious case recorded of a body found drowned and much decomposed, which was claimed by two young men as that of their father—a Mr. Etherington—and which they buried under that name. Some months after his burial, however, this Mr. Etherington walks into his daughter's house alive and well. Of course, under these circumstances, it becomes necessary to find out, since the body which had been interred was not that of Etherington, whose it really was; and then it comes out that a certain William Turner—who when last seen had been in a very wretched condition, covered with boils and sores, and suffering from ague, and who had told some one that he could never go back to live where he had previously been residing—had also been missing lately, and so it gradually got to be suspected that the body which had been found must

* In *Once a Week.*

really have been his. This suspicion soon became converted into an absolute certainty, when a portion of the neckerchief which had been found on the deceased was discovered in an odd corner of the very last lodging which William Turner had occupied.

This story is very like one authenticated by the coroner of Burton-upon-Trent, and communicated by him not long afterwards to the *Times*. Only in this latter case the body identified is that of the brother, and not the father, of the persons claiming it ; and moreover, when this last comes forward, still in the flesh, the question as to whose, after all, were the remains which were found in the Trent, is left unanswered.

Another story, something akin to both of these, is quoted from the *Annual Register*, by a correspondent of the *Times*, on the 15th of April 1868. It was a woman this time whose body was discovered in the water (with marks of violence on it), and it was her own father who identified it. It was his daughter's body, he said, and so said the neighbours also, and she had been murdered, he was sure, by her husband, who always used her ill. His evidence was so convincing that, at last, this bad husband was sent for by the police, in order that he might be duly examined by the authorities. They came back after a while, unsuccessful as to the main object of their mission, but not unsuccessful altogether either. They had not been able to find the man, they said, but that mattered the less as they had found his wife—the old man's *murdered* daughter—alive and well, and had brought her back with them.

In August 1869 the body of a woman was discovered in a canal. Death, it was considered, had been caused by violence, and not by suicide. A young woman named Kate Macdonald having disappeared, her parents identified the body as that of their daughter. It, however, subsequently appeared that Macdonald had, since her disappearance, been living at Rochdale, where she was discovered by a police inspector. The girl seems to have heard of the rumours of her death, but stated that she kept out of the way because she did not wish her relatives to know where she was.

Here then are cases in which both parents, and again a father, were wrong as to the identity of their own daughters, just as we have seen before two sons mistaken as to that of their father, brethren as to that of a brother, and a wife in reference to her husband.

The following case occurred within my own Indian experience. A. was a patient in my European ward,—a portly Scotchman, of rather striking appearance, approaching middle age. Some few weeks subsequent to his discharge, a tall, stout man was brought to the hospital, one evening, dying from the united effects of alcoholism and insolation. B., having an interest in A., heard that his body was lying in the dead-house. She went the next morning, saw the body, cried over it, and covered it with a sheet which she provided for the purpose. Some one now suggested that the body might not be that of A. after all ; and B. was advised to write a note of enquiry to A.'s address. He immediately replied that he was quite well,—and I trust that he is still living. Here, most probably, the error arose mainly from the fact that, in the Calcutta hot season, the bodies of fat men certainly do become very much alike after decomposition has fully set in.

Again, an unrecognised body may be identified for some fraudulent purpose. This appears to have happened in London in January 1870. The body of a young woman was found in the bed-room of a waiter in a hotel near Finsbury Square. The head and face had been so completely disfigured by blows as to render identification nearly impossible. A girl of eighteen, however, came forward, and identified the deceased as her sister Cecilia Aldridge. Upon enquiry, the girl's mother was found by the police, and her evidence proved that the whole story told by her daughter was false from beginning to end. It was also discovered that she was the same girl who, when the Clerkenwell explosion occurred, told a melancholy tale of the loss of her father and mother, and received a considerable sum from kind-hearted sympathisers.

The whole question of the *corpus delicti*, in cases of homicide, is surrounded with peculiar difficulties in India.

There is no place in the world where it is so needful that the body should be (1) *produced* and (2) *fully identified* as in India.

At the same time no criminals have greater facilities than those of India in availing themselves of a relaxation of the rule demanding the actual proof of the *corpus delicti*, in the placing aside of which Bentham argued : " A murderer, to secure himself with impunity, would have no " more to do but to consume or decompose the body by fire, by lime, or by " any other of the known chemical *menstrua*, or to sink it in an un- " fathomable part of the sea."*

Goodeve holds that, " according to Indian law, as administered by the Nizamut Adawlut, the finding of the body is not *indispensably* necessary to warrant even a capital sentence ; but, in such cases, an irrevocable sentence is not usually passed."† Goodeve here cites the case of Kealal *v.* Chundwa, 2 Nizamut Adawlut Reports, 82—bones were found, but these not being identified, the court withheld the capital sentence, notwithstanding a confession ; and, in one of Haubil *v.* Nuzeer Khan, 3 Nizamut Adawlut Reports, 122, the result was the same notwithstanding the recognition of the skull by a peculiarity in the jaw-bone.

I shall cite the two following instances of a crime, by no means rare in India, as being merely introductory to our argument of the special necessity which exists for establishing the *corpus delicti* in this country. The first is abridged from Allen's Asiatic Journal.

---

* 3 Judicial Evidence, 234, as cited by Goodeve.—*The Law of Evidence as administered in England applied to India*, p. 300.

† Beaufort's Digest, 1857, Homicide and Murder, Index C., section 3980.

At the time when ships only came up the Hooghly as far as Diamond Harbour, a passenger hired a dinghee to convey him to Calcutta. Being unacquainted with the language of the native boatmen, and becoming greatly exasperated by their apparent inertness, he laid about him with a stick so vigorously that three of the boatmen threw themselves overboard, and were immediately lost to view. The drowning, as it appeared, of these men brought him to his senses ; his alarm became manifest, and the rest of the crew, weeping and wailing, exerted themselves to convey him to his destination. Immediately on their arrival, they gave him in charge, the case was heard before a magistrate, and the stranger was immediately committed to jail. A true bill was found against him by the grand jury. At the trial the charge was clearly proved on the deposition of the survivors, and a verdict of guilty was brought in without the slightest hesitation. His counsel, however, brought forward a point of law which was to be argued before the judges, and sentence was, therefore, deferred. In the meantime, the unhappy man was visited in person by one who spoke very fluent English, and who gave him to understand that, upon the payment of a certain sum, he would be able to get him off by producing the identical parties supposed to have been long ago the food of fishes. He produced all the cash that he could command, and, accordingly, the missing men presented themselves on the following day, and, their identity being satisfactorily proved, the accused was discharged. These fellows were expert divers, who, immediately upon jumping out of the boat, sank; and, coming up again at some distance, swam to the shore. Their comrades knowing very well how to avail themselves of the circumstance, and acting in concert, the fugitives remained concealed until it was their interest to come forward. No conspiracy could be proved against them, as they declared they knew nothing of the proceeding, and had concealed themselves in alarm at having been forced overboard ; and, though no credit was given to this declaration, it could not easily be gainsaid, while the party who negociated the business took care to be out of the way. The stranger was too glad to escape to be anxious to pursue the matter further.

My *Commentator* gives the following similar case, which appears to have occurred in Calcutta about forty years ago. A ship's captain was tried for the manslaughter of a native by knocking him overboard. He did not deny the blow, and crowds of witnesses saw the man fall overboard and disappear. During the progress of the case, the rascal was recognised in the bazar by a jemadar in the service of a family with whom the accused was intimate. He had dived after his immersion, and, having risen up among a crowd of bathers unnoticed, he went quietly to his home, and remained in fond anticipation of seeing the *sahib* hanged. An acquittal followed the identification of this man in court.

A very prevalent crime amongst the Natives of Bengal is that of causing a person to disappear, and of charging some obnoxious individual with his murder. Here the culprits either offer a probable explanation of the disappearance of the body, or a putrid corpse, readily procured from the river and disfigured with wounds, is brought forward as that of the missing individual.

Upon examination of this body, the medical officer can probably do little more than report that the remains are those of a male or female, young or old, upon which he observes certain wounds, regarding which he cannot venture any opinion as to whether they were inflicted before or after death. Here the safety of the accused is, of course, imperilled ; unless, as has not unfrequently happened, his alleged victim be speedily produced in full life and vigour. A fairly characteristic example of the first kind is recorded in the Nizamut Adawlut Reports, Part I., of 1853, p. 259, in which " certain of the prisoners were convicted, on their own confessions of perjury, in having falsely deposed to the fact of a murder and to the burial of the corpse, in a trial, at the conclusion of which the alleged deceased made his appearance in court." "It would be impossible," writes the sessions judge in his report of this trial, " to imagine a case more completely satisfactory, as regards at least the guilt of Abdool Kurrem" [the unfortunate accused,] " than this became when the darogah's report was completed, and as in fact it remained, until the appearance of Pertaubnarain" [the *murdered* man] " brought to light its real character. The prosecutrix was the mother of the missing man ; the principal witnesses were his wife, Shurasattee, and his cousin Kanaram, while the prisoner's own servants detailed at length the circumstances attending the burial of the body. There were no inconsistencies and no contradictions in the evidence, which, from first to last, gave the hearers the impression that a heinous crime had indeed at last been brought to light, in spite of a powerful combination to conceal it."

In the Annual Report of the Bengal Police for 1863, it is noted (p. 84), that the detective police had succeeded in the production of a man said to have been murdered at Kishnagur.*

---

* My late esteemed friend, Dr. Kenneth MacKinnon, gave me the following notes, from memory, on a very remarkable case of this description: " When I was at Cawnpore, a case occurred strongly illustrative of the desirableness of producing the bodies of persons supposed to have been murdered. Two boys set out on a journey from Bundlekund, and, while bathing together, one, for the object of appropriating his property, threw the other into deep water, where he was supposed to have been drowned, as he disappeared for a long time. The supposed murderer returned to Cawnpore and, after a time, I think confessed his crime. At any rate, he was tried by Mr. Spiers, one of the most conscientious and cautious men that ever sat on the Bench, and condemned to death. While the proceedings were before the Agra Sudder, the lad supposed to have been drowned returned to his home."

It appears that Dr. MacKinnon's recollection of this case involved one or two inaccuracies. My *Commentator* remarks,—" The boy *was not condemned to death* ; he was sentenced to transportation for life, *as the body had not been found.* Substantially, the confession was correct, for the recovery of the victim was a perfect marvel. He was found insensible by a

I shall quote another case from the paper on *Native Society in India*, in Allen's Asiatic Journal, because in it we find *the accused confessing to the murder of a living person*, and obtain an important hint for our guidance in question of Identity in India. *Parents deny the identity of their daughter, of whom they have lost sight only for three years.*

In 1809, Nubia, the daughter of a respectable Hindu named Dhur, living in a village in the Doab, become attached to one Kulian. Her family being adverse, she eloped with the young man, taking her valuables to a considerable amount. The father went to Cawnpore, where he found Kulian, but without the girl, and had him apprehended as his daughter's murderer. Kulian readily acknowledged that he had taken Nubia from the village; and, while under examination, he informed a friend that he had buried the greater portion of her clothes and ornaments which she had carried away in the house which he then inhabited, pointing out the precise place, and requesting that they might be given up to her father. He at first preserved a mysterious silence respecting the fate of the owner, but, the property being found, he was taken to the thannah. Here he admitted that he had killed the girl, stating that he had thrown her body into a nullah, and offering to show the police officers the spot. Upon their arrival, they searched in vain for the usual indications; no remains of a body could be found, nor any signs of the perpetration of a murder. He then said that, being apprehensive of ill-usage at the thannah, he had pleaded guilty. He also asserted that he had left his companion alive and well in the neighbourhood of the camp at Cawnpore, but knew not what had become of her afterwards. At the trial, the police positively declared that neither threats nor violence had been employed to induce him to confess. He readily admitted that he had eloped with the girl, and also acknowledged that he had confessed the murder imputed to him, but declared that he had been beaten and menaced by the police, and had, therefore, confessed through fear. He declared his perfect ignorance of Nubia's fate, saying that, when they neared the cantonments, they being afraid of being seen together, it was determined that he should go into the city and procure a house, and she entrusted her bundles to him. Leaving her beside a well, until his return, they parted early in the morning; on his return, at mid-day, she had disappeared. He was sentenced to thirty lashes and to imprisonment for fourteen years, the proof being considered insufficient to warrant capital punishment. About three years subsequently, Medaree, Kulian's brother, brought forward one whom he alleged to be Nubia. She made oath that she was. The father and mother, however, denied her identity. Consequently,

---

worthy Brahmin who took him home and nursed him. He did not, however, come forward till the sentence had been passed.

See an extraordinary case, apparently of this kind, in Nizamut Adawlut Reports, N. W. P., Sept. 18th, 1854, p. 381; and another in the Police Report, L. P., for 1844, p. 37.

Medaree and the girl were sued for perjury. The father, mother, and an intimate friend of the family, who had been acquainted with Nubia from infancy, positively denied that she was Nubia. On the other hand, four witnesses were found who had known Nubia from her childhood, who as positively testified to her identity. The family disgrace and the loss of caste which she had incurred created a suspicion in the mind of the Court that Hindus of respectability might be unwilling to admit that a person, known to have misconducted herself for years, really belonged to them. She stated that, being tired of waiting at the well for Kulian, she set forward in search of him, and, while thus fruitlessly employed, met with a soldier belonging to one of the regiments stationed there, and, after considerable persuasion, was induced to place herself under his protection, and accompany him home. The regiment being shortly afterwards ordered away, she had quitted Cawnpore, and had only lately returned, when meeting Kulian's brother, she had come forward in his justification. No evidence was adduced in support of this statement, and the whole question rested entirely upon the probability of the parents denying their daughter, in consequence of motives which, under the circumstances, were very likely to influence them. The Court also perceived a resemblance between the mother and the alleged daughter, and, the testimony of the person calling herself Nubia being the individual whose identity she claimed appearing to preponderate, she and Medaree were acquitted. The sentence of Kulian now required revision ; he was only amenable to punishment for the abduction of an unmarried female, and for carrying off property of considerable value ; but, as he had voluntarily returned the greater portion, and moreover had suffered nearly four years' imprisonment, the punishment undergone was deemed quite adequate to the offence. He was discharged.

In the case of Pertaubnarain [page 50], as well as in three similar instances of which I possess notes, *no body was produced.* It was stated that the corpse of the murdered man had been dug up, and thrown into the sea for greater security.* Still, in cases of this complexion, it merely requires a little more audacity in the criminals to produce, if necessary, a wounded body as that of the murdered person, trusting to its disfigurement and to the medical officer's inexperience ; and such instances have occurred.

Some thirty years ago, the Collector of Chittagong, having been charged with the duty of carrying out a new and very unpopular system of assessment, made enemies ; and, on waking one morning, was astonished to find in his verandah two maugled dead bodies, which it was, doubtless, intended should be regarded by the public as the victims of his cruelty.

In his report for 1866,† the Inspector-General of Police, L. P., states

---

* An admirably graphic description of a doubtless true case of this kind will be found in the *Revelations of an Orderly*, p. 13.

† Page 47.

that a head constable at Rungpore induced a woman to say that a certain corpse found floating on a river was that of her adopted father. He further instigated her to charge five men with the murder. At this juncture a sub-inspector took up the case, and the five men were arrested and kept for the night in the custody of these constables; these men maltreated their prisoners, and thereby induced them to confess that they had committed the murder. When the trial was going on, the missing man came into court. The police officers concerned in the enquiry were sentenced to five years' rigorous imprisonment, with the exception of the sub-inspector, who was acquitted. *(For a full detail of this case, see p. 69).*

In 1855, Ali Jamin Sheikh was convicted at East Burdwan of conspiracy and perjury, and sentenced to seven years' imprisonment under the following circumstances. Disputes were going on between a tolookdar and some of his ryots. A jemadar was sent to the village to prevent a breach of the peace. He saw the body of Umbicachurn, brother of one of the ryots engaged in the dispute, wrapped in a bloody cloth. The thatch of the roof was burning. The dead man's brother told him that the talookdar had come to his house with an armed force, and, the deceased having annoyed him, the man was, by his order, struck on the head with a bamboo, and died in consequence, and the house was set fire. The body was examined by the civil assistant surgeon, who found that it was much emaciated; that a bad form of diarrhœa was the cause of death; and that there were two parallel cuts on the head, which had probably been made after death, and which could not possibly have been the cause of death. There was evidence that the prisoners had consulted together and agreed to accuse the talookdar. Ali Jamin Sheikh stated that he saw ten or fifteen men, with lattees, running off; and that he saw deceased "lying murdered in his house, and blood issuing from his head, where there were two wounds made by lattees, and that his skull was fractured." "He must have been aware," the sessions judge observed, "that deceased died from natural causes, and there is no reason to suppose that he was really deceived as to the true cause of the man's death."*

In the previous year certain prisoners at Tirhoot were convicted by the sessions judge of "conspiracy for the purpose of proving a false and malicious charge of murder against Sookhlall Rai; and, for that purpose, fabricating wounds on a dead body, in order to induce the belief that deceased had died from violence." Many witnesses testified that deceased died a natural death, and the medical officer reported that, in his opinion, the wound had been fabricated after death, deceased having died from natural causes. The statement of the late Dr. Simpson (a most able officer) is as follows: "The body was that of an old man much emaciated, the head was almost separated from the trunk between the 3rd and 4th verte-

* Nizamut Adawlut Reports, October 30th, 1856, page 834.

bræ of the neck, the cut through the integuments in front was a clean, unjagged cut, as if made at one incision with a sharp cutting weapon. There was also a deep cut at the back of the neck near the trunk, wounding the spine. Along the top of the left shoulder, there was a deep cut, wounding the shoulder joints, collar bone, and shoulder blade. There was also a deep cut in front of the right shoulder-joint, wounding the arm-bone, collar-bone, and shoulder-blade. There were also two slight cuts on the back ; there was no material effusion of blood, nor extravasation of blood into the surrounding parts, or retraction of the muscles, *showing that all these injuries had been inflicted after death ; of this there cannot be a possibility of a doubt.* "The right lung was completely disorganised by disease, being in a state of suppuration from long-standing tubercular disease. The left lung was also affected, but to a less extent. This was the cause of death. The body was undecomposed, and in a fit state for medical examination, so as to leave no doubt as to the above points."

In consequence of certain irregularities in the manner in which the depositions were taken, the conviction was not upheld by the court of appeal.*

The following is from Allen's Asiatic Journal :—

A wealthy mahajun had a young and handsome wife, of whom he was known to be exceedingly jealous. They had no family, and, in the event of his death, his property would go to a relative, with whom he was at variance. This person, named Khan Beg, an idle, dissipated fellow, glanced a longing eye upon the inheritance, and cast about for the means by which he might succeed to it. Reduced to poverty by his extravagance, he knew that it would be vain to ask assistance from a kinsman whom he had justly incensed by repeated transgressions ; and, finding a ready accomplice in a domestic in the merchant's establishment, he set a scheme on foot, which promised to be successful. It appeared that Ibrahim Beg had, in a fit of jealousy, sold, discharged, and otherwise got rid of his wife's female attendants, and that she had nobody to wait upon her but a slave girl, so stupid, as to be incapable of being very observant respecting what was going on in the house. Hitherto, the husband had treated his wife with kindness, but, being irritated by suspicions instilled into his mind in the most Iago-like manner by Emamee, the servant, he lifted his hand against her, and the poor girl, frightened and in pain, screamed dreadfully. The next morning she was not to be found, and information was given at the nearest thannah that the woman had been murdered. The officers of justice immediately came, and Emamee deposed to the quarrel, but said that his master had sent him away on a message after it had occurred, and that he knew nothing more of the matter. Search was made throughout the premises ; some of the

* Nizamut Adawlut Reports, July 31st, 1855, page 180.

earth in the court-yard appearing to have been removed ; on looking farther, the body of a woman was discovered, but the head was nowhere to be found. Ibrahim Beg was of course apprehended, and carried to prison ; it was in vain he protested his innocence, declaring that, immediately after the unfortunate quarrel with his wife, either exhausted by the violence of his emotions, or stupefied by some drug administered to him in his drink, he had fallen fast asleep, and remained unconscious of everything that had occurred until a late hour in the morning. The absence of Emamee upon his master's business was satisfactorily proved by some of his confederates ; he identified a bangle found upon the arm of the corpse as one belonging to his mistress, which he got mended for her ; while the slave-girl, who said that she had run away and hidden herself when his master beat his wife, and had found the door of the apartment locked upon her when she desired to leave it, expressed her conviction that the body was that of Chumbelee, her mistress. Nothing, in fact, could be more conclusive, the head alone being wanted to complete the chain of evidence. Ibrahim Beg's jealousy of his wife was notorious, and her screams were heard by all the neighbours on the fatal evening. At trial, notwithstanding the opinion of the native law-officer, who stickled for the production of the head, the case was referred to the Nizamut Adawlut, and not a doubt was entertained of the murder. Ibrahim Beg had some friends, and the greater number endeavoured, by every means in their power, to induce him to confess the crime with which he had been charged. Generally speaking, natives of India are very willing, after apprehension, and more especially after condemnation, to acknowledge their guilt, and to state all the circumstances connected with it. In many instances, the confession of the prisoner forms the principal evidence against him, and a relation of the whole particulars in a case of murder is seldom wanted for the satisfaction of the inquirers, who hear the whole account from the perpetrator himself. Ibrahim Beg, however, continued stoutly to deny all participation in his wife's disappearance, and as peremptorily to declare that the body produced was not that of Chumbelee. Unfortunately for him, he had kept her too strictly secluded for many persons to be able to question the identity, and his asseverations went for nothing. Time passed away ; the evidence against the prisoner was deemed conclusive by the superior court, and a day was appointed for his execution. Khan Beg's spirits rose at the prospect of immediate possession ; already he gave himself the airs of a man of great wealth, and it was observed that Emamee had entirely deserted his old master, and become attached to his heir and successor : circumstances which raised some indignation against the faithless domestic, who had so long eaten the prisoner's salt, but did not create any suspicion of treasonable acts towards him. At length, the very day before that on which the sentence was to be carried into effect, the assistant to the judge and magistrate received intimation that Chumbelee was in existence, and living not above twenty miles from the scene of her alleged murder. Though scarcely crediting the intelligence, yet, a life being at stake, he determined to ascertain the fact in person, and, having despatched horses and bearers to the place, rode over himself in the evening. The woman, it appeared, had been placed in the custody of a gang of fakeers, who had established themselves in a tomb; and, as these fellows were expert in all sorts of devices, it would be necessary to take them by surprise. Accordingly, the village police were summoned cautiously, the tomb surrounded, and search being made, Chumbelee was found in a subterranean apartment. She was immediately placed in a *doolee* prepared for her, and conveyed to the city. Emamee and Khan Beg were apprehended. The former, on perceiving that the whole plan had failed, gave the necessary explanation. He stated, in the first instance, that an unfortunate propensity to gambling had put him into the power of Khan Beg, who assailed his integrity with temptations too strong to be resisted; that the affair had been projected for a long time, and was executed the moment a body could be procured which might pass for that of Chumbelee; that, at length, a not very disconsolate widower was found, who was very willing to part with the corpse of his wife for a consideration, but, being afraid to produce the head, they cut it off, and contented themselves with the trunk; that Emamee inflamed the mind of his master by a fabricated account of his wife's misconduct, and, when she had wept and moaned herself to sleep, and Ibrahim had become insensible from the effects of a drug, the slave-girl being locked up in the room in which she had hidden herself, he enveloped Chumbelee in a dark blanket, and, giving her into the custody of the fakeers of the tomb, who were in waiting to receive her, proceeded to dispose of the corpse; that, in this undertaking, he was assisted by Khan Beg, and having managed everything, as they thought, very dexterously, they repaired to the abode of the former, and he (Emamee) went to sleep; that, in the morning, he returned to the house of his master, pretending that he had executed a commission with which he had charged himself on the preceding night; that, soon afterwards, Chumbelee was missed, and Ibrahim, concluding that she had fled with a paramour, abandoned himself at first to grief and resentment; that he (Emamee) took care to report the circumstance, and the neighbours, recollecting the screams they had heard, were easily induced, by a few hints and surmises, to suspect foul play; the confederates, therefore, soon had the satisfaction of seeing Ibrahim in the gripe of the law. A trifling matter about a few rupees, it appears, ruined this hopeful scheme. Khan Beg refused to pay one of the subordinates employed in this affair, who had contrived to get deeper into the secret than the principals were aware of, and this man it was who acquainted the young English civilian with the circumstance of Chumbelee's existence. Khan Beg and Emamee were tried for the abduction and conspiracy, and sentenced to work upon the roads for life.

To carry out fully a deception of this kind, it would be necessary that the body produced should, in nearly all respects, correspond with that of the missing person ; and to compass this would certainly be regarded as no safe or easy undertaking, where it was understood that the medical officer could distinguish, in any body that might be brought to him, not only the age, constitutional state, and cause of death of the deceased, but also his caste and condition in life, and a great variety of other distinctive particulars. Strongly impressed with the necessity that medical men in India should possess this discriminative power, I have been at considerable pains to collect accurate information upon the subject.* Attention to the following rules will be sufficient to establish the *Religion* of the deceased under all ordinary circumstances :

MALES.—The body of a *Mussulman* male, above the age of 11 years, always presents the marks of circumcision.

A (born) *Mussulman* never has the lobes of *both* ears pierced.

Every *Hindu*, above the age of 11 years, has had the lobes of *both* ears pierced for earrings. Where a necklace of beads is worn, the wearer is a *Hindu*.†

FEMALES.—Where a mark of tattooing is found between the eyes, the female may generally be known as a (born) *Hindu*.‡

The *Hindu* female wears her saree *single*, that of the *Mussulmanee* is always *double*.

When an iron kharoo, or bracelet, is worn on the left wrist, the wearer is a *Hindu* woman whose husband is living.

The *Hindu* women pierce the ears irregularly through the fossa innominata above, in one or two places ; through the lobe also, in one or two places ; and, perhaps, at one spot through the concha.

When the openings are numerous, and are found extending in a line completely along the helix, and where the rings worn are *silver*, the female is certainly a *Mussulmanee*.

With the exception of the first, these tests fail us when *headless and entirely denuded bodies* have to be reported upon.

* I was indebted to Baboo Grish Chunder Ghose, then Deputy Magistrate of Howrah, and to Baboo Peary Lall Banerjea, now Moonsiff of Sylhet, for a very large mass of interesting facts bearing upon this point. The details would, however, occupy too much space in a practical work.

† In a trial at Rajshahye, the Judge remarked : "These bead *mallas* are worn both by males and females, and this makes it very doubtful if any person could identify the *malla*.—*Nizamut Adawlut Reports*, September 18, 1855, p. 406.

‡ Moulvie Tumeez Khan Bahadur informs me that no Mahomedan lady of the upper or middle class tattoos ; but that, in the Eastern districts of Bengal, Patna, Jessore, and Dacca, as well as in Midnapore, Hooghly, Burdwan, and other parts of the country where the manners of the Mahomedans retain many characteristics of Hinduism, very low class women, as Dhoomeeas or Jolahas, use tattooing between the eyes (*oolkee*) and elsewhere.

Upon this very difficult question of the identification of the *Religion*, where headless bodies are discovered, I have consulted two, Hindu and Mahomedan, medical men of great learning and experience. I obtain the following results from the very careful notes made for me by Moulvie Tumeez Khan Bahadur and Baboo Kanye Lall Dey.

Mussulman Males.

The marks of circumcision.

Those who wear the chupkan or myrzaee, without under garment, have a narrow line, about an inch broad and five or six inches long, on the *left* side of the chest, tanned by exposure to the sun.

In the Hindu accustomed to wear a similar dress, this mark is to be looked for on the *right* side.

On the bodies of devout Mahomedans, certain callosities, with discoloration of the skin, are produced by the various attitudes in which they pray. These spots or corns (Ghutta—in Arabic Mujool) are most conspicuous over (1) the centre of the forehead. This is most observable in the Sheeahs, less in the Sonnees, and is caused by pressing and rubbing the forehead strongly over the prayer-carpet ; (2) the tip of the external malleolus of the left ankle ; (3) one midway between the last and the tendon of the *tibialis anticus,* as it passes under the annular ligament ; (4) one a little below and to the outer side of the last, just over the junction of the os calcis with the cuboid bone ; (5) two or three smaller spots over the metatarso-phalangeal joints on their dorsal aspect, that over the *third* toe being most marked ; (6) another is sometimes found over the tarso metatarsal joint of the *fourth* toe ; (7) a deep and dark callosity is invariably found below the apex of the patella, and over the tuberosity of the left tibia. No such marks are to be found on the right foot or leg. In consequence of their mode of sitting, both Mahomedans and Hindus have thickening and discoloration of the skin over the outer malleolus of either ankle and over the base of the metatarsal bone of the fifth toe only.

Occasionally a Mahomedan man will have the palm of his left hand and tip of the little finger stained with *henna.* No Hindu male ever does this.

Hindu Males

Are distinguished by the absence of the above marks.

Mussulman Females.

Mahomedan *ladies* of the upper and middle classes invariably wear shoes. Hence greater fairness of the protected skin up to the middle of the metatarsal bones, and frequently corns and bunnions. *Ladies* never tattoo.

In *ladies,* just under the level of the mammæ, a darkish, slightly furrowed line surrounds the chest. It is most conspicuous laterally, and is caused by the pressure of the tightly laced *urigeea* or boddice. The *kachoolee,* worn by Hindu females in the Deccan and Rajpootana, is not so tightly laced, and is, therefore, less liable to produce this mark.

Every Mahomedan female wears an under *coorthee*, which is so cut that, just over the upper part of the sternum, and on either side of it, a cordate portion of skin is left exposed. This and the skin of the arms, below the insertions of the deltoid muscles, become darker from exposure.

The palms of the hands, fingers, finger nails, soles of the feet and toes are tinted with *henna*.

Hindu Females.

There are no signs of the feet having been compressed by shoes. They preserve their natural form. The toes being wide spread and apart.

In Bengal, the mark of the *Saree* surrounds the body above the navel. In the North-Western Provinces, it is about two inches below the navel, and has an obliquity downwards. When there is tattooing on the inside of the wrist, near the pisiform bone, the woman must be a Hindu. The hands and feet are painted with the *carmine*-red, *aultha*, which may be readily distinguished from the *brown*-red *henna* or *mehndee* used by Mahomedans.

Hindu women of bad character may have *henna;* and, similarly, *low* Mahomedan women *aultha*.

If anything be left on the body, it will probably be the iron ring on the left wrist, which is positive proof that the wearer is a Hindu woman whose husband is living.

When, in either male or female, the nail of the left little finger is extremely long, the probability is that the individual is a Hindu.

In every case of suspicious death, the police should be expected to give, in their sooruthal, accurate descriptions of all marks of tattooing, scars, &c., on the bodies sent in, as well as of the clothes, ornaments, and amulets worn. The apparent age should also be stated.

In India, as elsewhere, judicial and medical officers may often gain valuable knowledge by close observation of minute varieties in the dress and physical characteristics of the people. Many points of distinction, almost as marked as those between the appearance of the hands of the blacksmith or seaman and those of the gentleman or penman, may thus be elicited. Ali Beg, the traveller, was recognised as an European at Morocco by his *Corns.* A very able officer in the Cossya Hills has occasionally formed a tolerably just estimate of a woman's character by noticing the size of her *Calves.* The Cossya women generally gain their living by constantly toiling up and down the hills with extremely heavy loads ; consequently, their legs rival those of ballet dancers in muscularity. One in whom this respectable development does not exist, probably lives by prostitution. Upon differences in the *Feet* of Hill and Plain-men, *vide supra*, p. 19.

Here, as everywhere else, the *Teeth* frequently prove an important clue to identity. One of the latest examples of this was the aid which the presence of a small pointed supernumerary tooth, between the middle incisors of the upper jaw, afforded in discovering the identity of the body of Rose Brown, in Calcutta, in 1868. This, however, is not a very rare abnormality. I have, without any search, observed it in three other instances within the last two years. Dr. Shortt has published* a very suggestive narrative of the examination of the bones of a child at Chingleput (Madras Presidency), in which he decided that the age was between 12 and 13 years, in part, because the second permanent molar *Teeth* were ready to come through the gum. As the presence of *False Teeth* led to the identification of Dr. Parkman's ashes and of the skeleton of Patrick O'Connor, the Mannings' victim, so the body of the Prince of Benares, who was slain in battle by Cuttub, in A. D. 589, of the Higera, was recognised among the heaps of slain, by its *Artificial Teeth,* which were fixed in by golden wedges and wires.†

The following, from Bellasis's Bombay Reports, p. 199, affords a fair idea of the information which may occasionally be obtained, even by a native jury of inquest, from a careful examination of the skeleton. "The Inquest Report stated that a jury had been assembled, on the 23rd April 1844, to examine the remains of a dead body discovered in a nullah in the field of Ekinshah Fukeer ; that the jury had found a number of human bones, and among others a skull, which was very perfect with the exception of the front teeth, which were wanting in the upper jaw ; that the skull and part of the neck were separated from the body ; that one of the vertebral bones had been cut, as with a sword or other sharp instrument, for it was not divided at a joint ; there were some marks of dried blood on the sides of the nullah, and a cholna, an iron bracelet, and a silk kurgota were lying scattered about near the spot, and that they were identified as having been the property of Wittoo Wullud Chrishna. The jury stated that they had probably known Wittoo, and, from the peculiarity of his *Teeth,* which were very small and wide apart, and from the other circumstances which had come to their knowledge during the examination and enquiry, they are of opinion that the remains discovered were those of Wittoo, whom they further believed to have been murdered about 10 or 12 days previously.

In a case which was tried in 1830, all that was discovered of a murdered man was portion of scalp, with *a tuft of Hair,* which formed a very important evidence of identity. My *Commentator* relates it as follows. Richard Amies, commonly known as Dick Sahib, and one Gong, were head assistants in rival indigo factories in the Nuddea district. They had frequent altercations. One evening, as Dick was sitting in his verandah with his family, he was seized by a band of armed men, said to have been

* Madras Quar. Jour. of Med. Science, January 1st, 1862, p. 227.

† Dow's Hindoostan, Vol. I., p. 145.

headed by Gong, and carried off forcibly towards the factory of the latter. The unfortunate man was never seen again except by witnesses who deposed to seeing him die under Gong's hands. Information of the outrage was given on the following morning to Dick's employer, by his native mistress. Owing to that gentleman's apathy, apparently four days were allowed to elapse before any active enquiries were instituted, and, consequently, Dick's body was not discovered ; but, in Gong's cow-house, some human hair was found, which, when shown to her, the prosecutrix, identified as the hair of Dick's head. The deposition of the nazir who conducted the search is as follows, and it does not appear from the printed record to have been disputed.

Mohummud Suleem, nazir of the Nuddea Fouzdary Court, stated that he was directed by the magistrate to investigate the affair of Dick's disappearance. About three russuns north-east of Gong's tent, observed a spot which appeared recently disturbed, dug that and discovered the carcase of a dead horse. Afterwards went into the cow-house of the Katlamaree (Gong's) factory, and probed about with a spear, observed the ground in one place uneven, and covered with cow-dung ; dug there ; after they had dug a cubit and a half, a putrid smell issued from the hole, which increased as they continued to dig. At length, about two cubits below the surface, they found some human hair of a reddish colour, with a piece of the skin of the head attached to it. Izzutoolah and Dhun Mullick, who were present, and well acquainted with Dick, recognised it as his hair. Found nothing else. The earth was very soft to the depth of 3½ cubits, 2 cubits in width, and 4½ cubits in length. Put the hair which had been dug up in a pot, and showed it to prosecutrix. She said that it was Dick's hair, and that Dhan Mullick and Ramdhun Nyee could identify it ; afterwards saw the hair in the Supreme Court. It was then comparatively dry ; when dug up, it was moist.

My *Commentator* goes on to say that there can be little doubt that the hair thus found with the skin attached to it was Dick's hair ; for red hair is not a common deposit in Bengali ground. No one, reading the nazir's evidence (which there appears no reason for disbelieving) can doubt that Dick was buried in Gong's cow-house, and that the body was hurriedly removed upon information of the nazir's approach. *Perhaps, if the carcase of the dead horse had been closely examined, the murdered man might have been discovered within.* Be this as it may, Dick was proved by witnesses to have died under the cruel treatment of Gong and his accomplices. This discovery in the cow-house established the credit of the witnesses. In spite of direct and circumstantial evidence, Gong was acquitted by the Supreme Court, where, as an European British subject, he was tried. The evidence which did not satisfy the Supreme Court did, however, satisfy the Sudder. The three principals, Peer Allee, Nemye Nundun, and Sartuk Biswas were imprisoned for life. Their accomplices were sentenced to terms of 14 and 7 years' imprisonment. He adds, "A consideration of the facilities of escape offered to crime by too rigidly insisting on identification will, therefore, cause some relaxation of this rule. This is no fault of the legislature or of the bench, but an unfortunate consequence of the circumstances peculiar to this country. If a mass of bones can pass in an English court of law, we see no reason why a tuft of red hair should not be accepted in Bengal. The irrevocable sentence of death need not be pronounced, but, when direct evidence and a mass of concurrent circumstances render us virtually certain of a man's guilt, it is mere weakness to let him go wholly unpunished, because the proof is incomplete. What earthly investigation can be complete? Some men can be made to doubt their own senses; and we know that, in this country, a bullying counsel force a native witness to admit anything. We must try, therefore, to administer justice with the means at our disposal, and not attempt to attain an unattainable perfection."

I remarked, in 1856, that an accurate comparison of the *Skulls* of the various races inhabiting India is a great desideratum in ethnology, and would prove a considerable aid to medico-legal inquiry. The small compact cranium of the Bengalee—"good if there were but enough of it;"—the spreading retreating forehead and projecting malar bones of the Chuckma, Mugh, Burman, and Chinese, each receding from the Caucasian and approaching the Mongolian type nearly in the above order; the nobly Caucasian heads of the educated Brahmin and the Rajpoot; and the high, ovoid, and essentially Jewish cranium of the Affghan,—all present distinctive peculiarities which, thoroughly studied, would afford many valuable clues to identity.

During the fourteen years which have elapsed since the above remark was recorded, great advances have been made in our knowledge of the comparative forms of the skulls of the various races of men, especially by Dr. Barnard Davis, the learned author of the *Thesaurus Craniorum.* Still, apart from the fact that a complete collection of skulls representing the various races which inhabit India has never yet been made, a small and handy work displaying the forms, and giving the measurements of those skulls (authenticated as being of pure race), which have already been catalogued, is much needed for use in India.

It will frequently happen that the medical officer's opinion will be required upon *Skeletons or detached Bones.* The smallness and delicate formation of the skeleton of the Bengalee may often lead to considerable doubt regarding the age and sex of the deceased, unless the pelvis or a femur be produced.*

* The following case (N. A. R., Vol. VI., of 1856, p. 999) illustrates very forcibly the necessity of minute accuracy in conducting these investigations. It also shows how little importance is attached, in India, to the production of "probable" bones. In a trial at Backergunge the Sessions Judge observed:—"On the 31st of December 1855, the prisoner, Boodhagi, denied

In this country, as elsewhere, it is of course needful that no suspicious *Bone* should be decided to be human, except upon the testimony of an anatomist. This is particularly to be attended to, as, no use being made of the bones of the lower animals in India, they generally lie about in profusion wherever there is population. Some years ago, walking through the Park Street Cemetery of this city, a friend expressed to me great disgust at the fact that the paths were literally covered with fragments of bones. I explained to him that not one of these was human. The place being seldom visited, the birds which resort to the trees carry thither bones from the whole neighbourhood, and especially from the adjacent native shambles. But for my explanation, my friend would have had fair presumptive evidence, that he had seen in the cemetery large quantities of the bones most likely to abound there.

It will be noticed that, in his *Hints for the Police*, *supra* p. 32, Dr. Hutchinson has very judiciously insisted that, when the body of a person,

---

the charge" (of murder and concealment of the body) "before the Police. On the 3rd of January 1856, he, it is alleged, made an elaborate confession, and is said to have pointed out bones and a piece of cloth as belonging to the deceased. These bones and piece of cloth were found at a considerable distance (six *gurrees*) from the houses of the prisoner and the missing man.

"The medical officer in the magistrate's court deposed to the bones being those 'of an adult male lately deceased.' With all due deference to the opinion of Dr. ———, I may be permitted to doubt whether such opinion must necessarily carry conviction with it. It is an admitted fact that it is extremely difficult to pronounce an opinion as to the age or sex of a deceased party on the mere inspection of one or two bones. Dr. Chevers, in his work on Medical Jurisprudence in India, remarks, that 'the smallness and delicate formation of the skeleton of the Bengalee may often lead to doubt regarding the age and sex of the deceased.' The magistrate, it appears, did not deem it necessary to question the medical officer to elicit on what grounds he arrived at the opinion so deliberately given, and I was unable to examine Dr. ——— in my Court, as the bones were not produced in it in a regular manner. But, even admitting the bones to be those of an 'adult man lately deceased,' it by no means follows that they are the bones of the missing man Moonar. Bones, it must be well known to the Court, are procurable in any number, of any age and sex, on the banks of any river. Further, two witnesses in this Court state that the prisoner was on board the boat of the darogah when these bones were found, and that, though adduced as witnesses to the prisoner having pointed out the bones to the police, they did not see him do so. So much for the bones.

"The rag produced in my Court, said to be a portion of the *gamcha* of the deceased, and which some witnesses identify as such, is torn and dirty. I can distinguish no mark or peculiarity in the rag admitting of its easy and certain identification, and, with my experience of the too ready way in which natives identify any article, I hesitate not in rejecting this link in the chain of circumstantial evidence, looking upon it, as I do, as a part of the machinery of the case, which has been got up against the prisoner."

With much deference I do not consider that anything appears above to shake the civil surgeon's positive assertion that "the bones were those of an adult male lately deceased." It is, however, much to be regretted that the bones upon which this opinion was given are not named. If Dr. ——— reported upon a pelvis, his statement was unanswerable. It would, I think, only be when a medical witness declared that a humerus or tibia was that of a female, that the above quotation from this work could be urged against him.

To render such cases intelligible, the names of the bones should always be stated in the record.

suspected to have died by violence, has been burnt, any portions of *Bone* which may remain unconsumed should be carefully preserved and examined. Bodies of murdered Hindus are occasionally got rid of by burning in the regular way, but this would, of course, generally be avoided, as likely to excite suspicion, where the condition of the deceased was not such as to render his cremation a matter of course. Few criminals in India attempt to dispose of bodies as a wretch in the Bood-Bood Division (Burdwan) is stated (in the Bengal Police Report for 1866, p. 172) to have done. She having murdered a child for the sake of its ornaments, which were worth less than six rupees, the child's body was found burning on her (chula) fire-place. She confessed and suffered capital punishment.*

---

* NOTE ON THE INCINERATION OF HUMAN BODIES.—As it is very difficult, so also the complete destruction of a body by fire is rather expensive. The Medical College Hospital pays the Municipality of Calcutta Rs. 1-9-6—the price of firewood being from 3 to 3½ maunds (of 80 lbs. each) per rupee—each, for burning the Hindu dead with wood. We read, in Strype's Life of Cranmer, that three loads of wood fagots at 12*s*., and one load of furs (furze?) fagots, at 3*s*. 4*d*., were charged for in the burning of Ridley and Latimer; and 100 of wood at 6*s*., and 150 furze fagots at 3*s*. 4*d*., for burning Cranmer.

In most of the incremations in England, during Queen Mary's reign, a bag of gunpowder appears to have been hanged around the neck or body of each martyr. This not only abridged suffering, but must also have much assisted the destructive action of fire, when, in exploding, it tore open the great cavities of the body. Under ordinary circumstances, it is usually found that portions of the solid viscera long resist the action of the fire. Germannus says that Joan of Arc's heart was found unconsumed. M. Tardieu found, in the remains of persons who perished in a conflagration in Paris, that the soft parts exhibited great diminution of volume. This was more especially observed upon the viscera, which had been more or less protected from the immediate action of the fire. Some of these were mummified. The blood in the heart, aorta, and other large vessels presented an extraordinary appearance, resembling wax or fatty matter of most beautiful carmine colour. The cerebral substance was contracted to half its bulk, and in consistence resembled a half-dressed sweetbread.

These appearances of partial destruction represent the effects of slack, irregular, insufficient accidental heat upon the structures of the human body. In India, those whose business it is to burn the dead to ashes, effect this within a few hours, with great completeness, and with a moderate consumption of fuel,—*i. e.*, about 400 pounds of wood.

Dr. Hutchinson, of Patna, an active observer of all that can throw light upon our knowledge of Medical Jurisprudence in India, took an opportunity to ascertain exactly the amount of wood which would be necessary to destroy entirely an adult healthy body, and the time that would be necessary for its complete cremation. The pyre was composed of ten maunds of wood, but an equal amount of jala straw was necessary, as also two bottles of oil. The pile was lighted at 6-30 p. m.; and at 3 a. m. next morning, the consumption of the body was declared to be complete. When he visited the spot, he found, in the centre of the ashes, the heads of two femora entire, but competely calcined, and a mass of incinerated matter, as large as two fists, said to be the remains of the liver. Thus 20 maunds, or 1,600 pounds, of wood and straw, and two bottles of oil were required to consume a healthy body, and 8½ hours were required for the operation which, even then, was virtually incomplete. Here, however, five times the needful quantity of fuel was consumed.

Baboo Ram Lall Chuckerbutty, of the Medical College Hospital, and my pupil Baboo Rajendranath Mullick, have been at some pains to ascertain for me what the practice at the Nimtollah Burning Ghaut, Calcutta, is. The attendants there say that *five* maunds of fuel (wood and

I am indebted to Dr. E. Goodeve for a very useful hint with regard to the importance of *preserving the cut ends of the Bones* in cases where—for example, as not unfrequently occurs—a headless body, or a detached limb, is brought in for examination. Unless this precaution be taken, it may often be impossible to judge, with certainty, whether parts sent for examination subsequently belong to the same or to another body. This precaution was attended to in matching the scattered remains of the woman Brown, who was murdered and cut to pieces by Greenacre.

In a trial which took place at Bancoorah, in December 1833, a question arose relative to the identity of certain human *Bones*, which involved more than one important medico-legal point. Mr. Belts was accused of the murder of Meah Khan. Two witnesses deposed that *a few hours* before his death, defendant had beaten the man, striking him several blows on the cheek, and had broken his rib—the only bone purporting to have been that of the accused produced in Court. This had been broken, and, as it had an osseous callus formed upon and around the fractured ends, Mr. Cheek, the civil surgeon, was of opinion that the fracture must have occurred several days, at least seven or eight, before death. This fact having sufficed to upset the charge, the question of the identity of the bones as those of Meah Khan does not appear to have been fully gone into. Still the question was one of interest. The skeleton was pointed out by one of those who asserted that he had buried Meah Khan. After some search they were found on the verge of the bank of the river Damoodah. The body, it seems, was buried pretty deep in the land above the common water-mark, at a distance of sixty or eighty yards from the proper bed of the river, at a place which the waters had never reached, or could only reach on extraordinary occasions. The bones were uncovered, but not removed until five days afterwards. It does not appear to have been clearly shown whether other bodies were ever interred on that spot. Twelve of the vertebræ, six of the ribs, and the sacrum were wanting. The whole of the bones were found clean and free from periosteum, ligament, and cartilage. Mr. Cheek never heard of an instance of bones being cleared of soft parts and ligaments by natural decomposition in

---

dry stalks) with about a chittack (two fluid ounces) of ghee are sufficient in ordinary cremations. I saw what remained after two of these cremations,—chiefly the heads of large bones, bodies of vertebræ and portions of skull. Doubtless, much tact and skill, with a view to expedition and economy of fuel, are employed, and, latterly, the incandescent remains are frequently stirred together with poles.

In this manner, it is said, fat bodies may be consumed in 2 or 3 hours; emaciated ones in 4 or 5. Nothing can be more complete than the destruction of parts; for, although portions of bone retain their shape, pressure between the fingers reduces them to dust. This result is unexpected, seeing that many dead bodies weigh more than two hundred pounds. In the cremation of the bodies of wealthy men, 8 to 10 or more maunds of fuel (much of which is sandal-wood) with from one to twenty seers (each a quart) of ghee are expended,—but all fuel in excess of five maunds is waste.

three months. He considered it extremely improbable that those were the bones of Meah Khan, or of a person who died in the preceding June.

Considerable weight was given to the circumstance of the separation of the sacrum, which was wanting. It was then considered, and is now held by Dr. Taylor, that "it may readily be conceived that the entire separation of this bone by decomposition would require, even in a hot climate, an extremely long period in a body in the ground—probably from three to ten years. Now, when we consider that the deceased had not been buried above three months, it is clear, both from the entire destruction of the soft parts, and the separation of the sacrum, that the bones discovered on the bank of the river could not have been belonged to the deceased, but must have been part of the skeleton of a person whose body had been buried in the spot many years before. There was, therefore, a complete failure of identity, and the accused was discharged."

This is, undoubtedly, true and cogent reasoning from experience of the manner in which bodies decay in northern climates. It also has great weight as being the view held by one so acute and so well acquainted with the locality as my friend the late Mr. Cheek. Still I have seen the banks of the Damoodah in the neighbourhood of Bancoorah, and I have doubts as to whether the denudation of the bones of all soft parts did not occur during the five days subsequent to their discovery, throughout which period they appear to have been left exposed to a great variety of influences tending to the destruction of the soft parts. It is not stated that Mr. Cheek was present at the disinterment, or in what state the skeleton was when first disinterred. The loss of the sacrum, many of the vertebræ, and some of the ribs, may be taken as strong presumptive evidence that the missing parts were removed to be mumbled at a distance by jackals and dogs. Placed thus, on the sandy banks of the Damoodah, multitudes of ants and insects would attack the bones and rapidly clear them of all soft parts. In a similar case, the *cleanness* of the bones would not be so much a turning point in evidence as their *freshness*. In specific gravity, in appearance, and in odour, the condition of a recent bone, thus rapidly cleaned by insects, would, in no way, resemble that of one which had gradually undergone denudation underground.*

An instructive case, involving an unusual amount of doubt as to the identity of certain human bones, was tried at Meerut, in May and June 1852. One Kulloo, a native policeman, was generally known in his village to have a criminal intimacy with a married woman, Mussamut Gowra. The age of this woman is stated to have been 28 years ; she had a girl four or five years old, born previous to her last marriage. On the 13th of March, the woman's husband being absent, Kulloo was seen

* This case is cited by Dr. Taylor, Ed. of 1865, p. 111. I have also used Dr. Taylor's authority, the Indian Journal of Medical Science, Vol. I, p. 69.

by several neighbours leaving the village followed by the woman with her child in her arms. He was absent from his duties on that night; on returning the following day, he was questioned regarding his absence and the disappearance of the woman, whom he promised to bring back forthwith, and went away ostensibly for that purpose. He did not return; but, several days afterwards, he was apprehended selling ornaments, which were proved to be hers, in a distant bazar. He attempted this sale clandestinely; and, when discovered, offered rupees 15 to two *bunneeas*, and afterwards a share to the police jemadar. Upon being examined by the joint magistrate, he accused other parties of the murder (altogether falsifying the statements which he had made at the thannah), and especially implicating one Dilsookh. On the 24th March, eleven days after the disappearance of the woman and child, the prisoner was sent with the jail darogah to point out the remains of the woman, which he said had been thrown by the murderers into a well. Nothing was found in the well. He then took the police to search the house of Dilsookh: some property was found, but this was afterwards ascertained to be Dilsookh's own. On the following day, he was again taken to the well, which was searched in vain by a diver. The prisoner now pointed in a direction in which he said he perceived a smell, and led the police to a raised spot, about 100 paces from the well, where, among stacks of wheat which had evidently been trampled down by the feet of birds and wild animals, certain human bones were found—*viz.* two pieces of a small skull, ten small ribs, two pieces of a larger skull, the lower jaw with the teeth, half the upper jaw, with the teeth, part of the nasal bone, and six other bones not described. The police stated that no smell was perceptible from the bones when close to them; they were dry, and bore the appearance of the remains of a person who had been dead ten or fifteen days; the weather was hot, the bones had been dismembered, as if torn to pieces by dogs or jackals. Near these were a *ghagree* and *nougree*, recognised as those worn by the child Luchmee, and a small child's *chooree* in three pieces, also recognised. He then said that he had forgotten the day before where the wearing-apparel of Gowra had been concealed in the house of Dilsookh, and took the police to an out-house where they were found in a *mutka*, where he had, some days previously, stated before the joint magistrate that they had been concealed. Upon the bones being sent to the civil assistant surgeon, however, this officer certified as follows:—"I examined, about a week ago, sundry bones forming portions of the bodies of two children: one I should suppose to have been about eight years old, the other about as many months; not one of the bones I saw formed any portion of an adult skeleton." Upon this report, the joint magistrate, considering that it afforded conclusive proof that the bones were not those of the murdered woman, without examining the civil surgeon, or calling for his attendance, found the prisoner guilty of the

the theft only, and sentenced him to three years' imprisonment. The matter was, however, taken up by superior authority, and re-investigated. The trial at the Sessions Court was held 14 months subsequently. The civil surgeon stated that he examined skeletons of two chidren, one belonging to a child eight years old. What these bones were, was not mentioned; no anatomical examination was made, nor record kept of them; they were simply stated to be bones assumed, from their size, to be those of a child eight years old. The judge remarked that Fonblanque shows that the size of bones varies so greatly in individuals that it forms no certain criterion of age; the bones of the female are said to differ from those of a male from their being generally smaller and more delicate, and from the muscular impressions and asperities being less distinctly marked; it, therefore, appeared to him by no means improbable that the bones of a small adult young woman should have been mistaken, at a hasty examination, for those of a boy eight years old. The *sooruthal*, continued the judge, recorded among the bones an entire upper jaw and half a lower jaw* with the teeth attached, but the medical officer did not remember to have seen anything of the kind, nor did his unsatisfactory report, recorded at the time, allude to them, though these, it was held, would have afforded a much more certain criterion of the person's age. The evidence of the civil surgeon, regarding the smaller bones, was viewed as equally unsatisfactory; a small skull in two pieces [" two pieces of a small skull"?] was stated in the *sooruthal* to have been found, and the sutures would have enabled an anatomist to state, with something approaching to certainty, whether it belonged to a child of eight months or four years; but the civil surgeon, without knowing whether or not there was a skull, and judging merely from the size of the [other] bones, of which the ribs are alone mentioned in the *sooruthal*, states most decidedly that they belong to a child of eight months. The chemical composition of the bones is said by Fonblanque to vary, in relation to their phosphate of lime and gelatine, at different ages; but the difference in those proportions in an infant and an adult appears to be only ascertainable with certainty by chemical analysis; but the civil surgeon states most decidedly that he could, from the mere appearance of the bones, determine whether they belonged to a child of eight months or four years: so slight, however, was his recollection of the bones, that he does not remember whether they were connected or dismembered. On these grounds, the judge did not attach any weight to the civil surgeon's evidence, as refuting the assertion of the prisoner that the bones produced were those of Mussumat Gowra and her female child. This view of the case was upheld by the judge of

* In the printed report it is stated, " the lower jaw and half the upper jaw"—but this discrepancy is immaterial.

the superior court who desired that a copy of the sessions judge's remarks on the subject of his hasty and unsatisfactery report upon the bones sent to him should be communicated to the medical officer. The prisoner was convicted ; but—following what appears to have been the more general practice of the Courts, in cases of this nature, where the body is not forthcoming, or circumstances may prevent its recognition—the prisoner was sentenced to imprisonment in transportation with hard labour in irons for life.*

On the discovery of a nameless murdered body in India, its identification may sometimes be accomplished with greater facility than accuracy. Thus my *Commentator* relates a case which occurred in the Mirzapore District, in which, the headless body of a woman having been found in a well, suspicion attached to some Rajpoots, whose sister, a widow, was known to be unchaste. Suspicion became conviction when it was found that their sister was missing. Upon enquiry, the men confessed and gave a circumstantial account of their sister's death. Their confessions were repeated before the magistrate and sessions judge, and, as circumstances were strong against them, they were convicted of wilful murder. When the case was pending before the Sudder, the *Dea ex machinâ* appeared in the *missing woman herself!* She had eloped with a paramour, and, hearing by chance that her brothers were charged with killing her, she voluntarily came forward to clear them. At first, the woman was disbelieved, as the whole thing appeared to be a *ruse*. As she persisted in her story, she was placed among chance crowd in Court, and the prisoners were filed in, as if to hear their sentence. Directly their eyes fell upon their sister, they raised a glad cry of recognition, and with tears of joy praised God, after their own fashion, that they were saved. The woman was identified, and the defendants' further statements were taken. They had confessed because, finding facts—and that thing more terrible than fact, *rumour*—against them, they thought that it was hopeless to plead innocence. The unexpected sight of their sister, of whose fate they were as ignorant as their accusers, appeared to them like a miracle. They immediately retracted their confession, and the strong case against them vanished into thin air.

Thus the partial truth came out, though the original mystery remained as dark as ever ; who the "good woman" in the well really was, never became known.

The following very important case, in which *the police, discovering a murdered body, determined to create a murderer*, appears at p. 290 of the Bengal Police Report for 1866. A corpse, bearing marks of violence, having been found floating in the Teesta River, it was supposed that a

* Nizamut Adawlut Reports, N. W. P., July 22nd, 1852.

murder had been committed. Head constable Banee Madhub Roy, of Rungpore, who received the first information report, proceeded to investigate, and, reaching the neighbourhood of the place where the corpse had been discovered, ascertained from Cheepoo, a prostitute that her "dhurumbap" (father by adoption) Ootum, by name, was missing, having left his house some days before. On being shown the corpse, Cheepoo at once professed her inability to identify the body as that of Ootum, and adhered to her statement for several hours, until noon of the next day, when, having, in the interval, passed the night with the head constable, she consented to make a false identification of the corpse, and declared it to be that of Ootum. This, however, was by no means all that the head constable required, and his next step was to force others to corroborate Cheepoo's false statement. This he did by means of threats and ill-treatment, and then induced Cheepoo to name one Bocha and four others as the murderers of Ootum. At this stage of the "enquiry," Sub-Inspector Juggut Chunder Sein appeared on the scene, and relieved his subordinate, the head constable, of charge of the case. It was then evening, too late in the day for further proceedings, and the five persons named by Cheepoo as the murderers of Ootum were taken for the night to a certain house, where they were kept till next morning in the custody of three constables. It was proved at their trial that during that night, the constables maltreated three prisoners to such an extent as constituted the crime of "causing hurt," the result being that, when brought before the sub-inspector next morning, they one and all made a false admission of having murdered Ootum, and they were, on that admission, and on the false evidence extracted from Cheepoo, forwarded for trial. While the magistrate of the district was actually engaged in holding the preliminary enquiry into the charge of murder, Ootum, the man said to have been murdered, appeared. His appearance anywhere else would, probably, have been followed by his final disappearance, and thus the case would have been quite complete.

The true history of the case was elicited, and the three constables put upon their trial. They were committed to the sessions charged with "causing hurt to extort confession;" the sub-inspector and the head constable being convicted for abetment of the same, and all were, on conviction by the judge, sentenced to five years' rigorous imprisonment. This sentence was upheld by the High Court on appeal, except as regards the sub-inspector, who was acquitted and released. He, subsequently, appealed for reinstatement in the police, on the ground of his acquittal by the High Court, but his conduct in the enquiry, after it came into his hands, showed that he had been guilty of such utter carelessness and neglect that his restoration was refused.

Regarding all the circumstances, under which the confessions of murder were made in this case, and in several others given above, they appear to suggest some exception to a ruling of the Calcutta High Court in 1865 to the effect that—

"When prisoners confess, in the most circumstantial manner, to having committed a murder, the finding of the body is not absolutely essential to a conviction."*

Goodeve holds that "it has been doubted, and still remains unsettled, whether even a *confession* of the crime, not being a judicial one, would be sufficient to dispense with the proof of the *corpus delicti*. In India, in the Courts of the Nizamut Adawlut, it is apprehended, however, that no confession, unsupported by other evidence, would avail, it not being regular to commit a prisoner solely on his own confession.—Beaufort's Digest, 1857, p. 126.†

In this country, dead bodies are generally available when needed. We have seen that the practice of laying a corpse, wounded after death, at an enemy's door, is by no means unfrequent, and the atrocity of committing a murder (usually upon some very young, aged, feeble, crippled, or idiotic victim) with the design of bringing an adversary to ruin, is almost equally common.

One of the latest instances of this kind is cited in the Bengal Police Report for 1866, p. 128. Ill-will having, for some months, existed between the Ticcadar of Sheodabad (Patna) and his ryots, the latter resolved to bring him into trouble. With this view they murdered Chummna Gowalah, an unfortunate cripple, and then laid his death at the door of the Ticcadar. Ten persons were tried, of whom two were hanged.

Under nearly similar circumstances, certain persons were tried at Tirhoot in 1856. The body of an unfortunate deaf and dumb beggar having been discovered frightfully hacked before the house of one, against whom it was alleged the accused had a grudge. The sessions judge convicted four persons on this charge, but they were acquitted by the higher Court.‡

Three years previously "the servants of a zemindar in the Midnapore district, deliberately decoyed an old woman into a house, and then murdered her for the sole purpose of throwing the crime upon a neighbouring zemindar."§

Probably the most atrocious case of the kind on record is that of a woman in the Patna District, who poisoned *her own* little daughter, and having concealed her body on the premises of a neighbour with whom she was at enmity, accused him of having murdered her.‖

---

* Sutherland's Weekly Reporter, Appellate High Court, Vol. IV., Crim. Rulings, p. 19.

† Op. Cit., p. 802.

‡ Nizamut Adawlut Reports, Vol., VI., for 1856, p. 810.

§ Bengal Police Report, for 1863, p. 25.

‖ Police Report, L. P., for 1868, p. 139. This case appears to give confirmation to a statement, which has been by some regarded as untrue, made by Father Martin, in 1709:—"Not long since, at a little distance from the Church whence I write, two of these barbarians happening to quarrel, one of them ran to his own house, snatched up one of his children (about four years

Indian criminals, not unfrequently, disfigure the dead bodies of their victims that they may not be easily recognized. The custom of the Garrows and Nagas of cutting off and carrying away the heads and hands of both friends and enemies slain in their raids has already been alluded to. This, however, is rather a usage than a criminal device.*

Dacoits have been known to cut off the heads of their dead, and even of their severely wounded, when in fear of pursuit. In the Euterpe of Herodotus, an Egyptian thief being caught in a trap, when in the act of robbing the royal treasury, entreats his brother to cut off his head that his body may not be recognized. A similar practice has been observed in Japan. Captain Osborne states, in his Japanese Fragments, that, at Yedo, a hostile prince directed his retainers to cut off one who was regent to the young Taikoon. They failed, although they wounded the regent. The assailants fled, followed by the imperial forces. A few only escaped, as when any one of the retreating party fell through wounds or fatigue, their comrades decapitated them, in order that no evidence should be forthcoming to inculpate their chief.

In his remarks upon a fatal affray, the leaders of which were tried at Rajshahye in 1858, the sessions judge observed that the party having failed in their object of taking the cutcherry, were yet strong enough to carry away their dead and wounded. As, however, "Lalkhan was a well-known sirdar, it was necessary for their purpose to prevent recognition of his body, which they sought to do by cutting off his head. The head was buried and found many days afterwards by the police."†

---

old) and, coming in sight of his enemy, beat out his child's head between two stones. The other, without discovering any emotion, took up a daughter of his, who was but nine years old, and plunged his dagger in her breast. Your child, said he afterwards, was but four years old, and my daughter was nine; give me, therefore, a victim equal to mine. 'That I will,' replied the other; when, spying at his side his eldest son, whom he was about to dispose of in marriage, he gave him four or five stabs with his dagger; and, not contented with having spilt the blood of his two sons, he also killed his wife, that his enemy might be forced to murder his wife also. This tragical scene ended with the murder of a little girl, and a child sucking at the breast; so that, in one day, seven persons were sacrificed to the vengeance of two men, who thirsted after human blood, and were more cruel than the fiercest beasts."

The murder of their wives and children, under circumstances of disappointment, has been attributed to the Bhauts of Guzerat. The *Motive* is explained by Forbes.—Oriental Memoirs, Vol. I., pp. 493–96.

* The remains of their own dead are burnt to ashes by the Garrows, lest on any account the skull of a Garrow should be passed off for that of a Bengalee. Their enemies' skulls are suspended as trophies in the houses of the victors. We are told that the skulls are valued in proportion to the rank of the persons to whom they belonged. In 1815, the skull of a Hindoo zemindar was valued at one thousand rupees; that of a talookdar at five hundred; while a mere peasant's skull would not pass for more than ten or twelve rupees.

When Nagas do not find it convenient to take away their enemies' heads, they cut off the hair, and bury the bodies.—*Vide* N. A. R., Vol. VI., for 1856, p. 264. A warrior ranks low until he can adorn his spear with such a spoil of his own winning. I have two Naga spears thus decorated.

† Nizamut Adawlut Report, Vol. VIII., for 1858, p. 168.

A very characteristic instance of this mode of concealing crime came to light in a trial in the Court of the 24-Pergunnahs. In 1855, certain dacoits having attacked a house were beaten off, and had to make a precipitate retreat with one of their gang badly wounded near the groin. No one was recognised ; but the disappearance of a noted dacoit by name Gopal, taken with the above facts, led to a report among the country people that the wounded man had been murdered by the dacoits to prevent detection. Certain suspected parties having been apprehended, pointed out a shallow nullah, where the headless body of Gopal was disinterred ; the persons confessed to having cut off their companion's head after he was dead. The Nizamut Adawlut held that there was not "a particle of proof that the wounded dacoit was murdered." The wound, as described by the witnesses for the *sooruthal*, "was not one which killed him on the spot." It is to be regretted that it was not examined by a medical man.*

In August 1869, it was reported in the public prints that a very daring dacoity had, a short time previously, been committed at the village of Hasalong in Lohardugga, upon which the zemindar gave chase to the gang and, in a fight, succeeded in wounding two of the gang so badly that their heads were cut off by their comrades to prevent their being recognised or giving any information.

In 1857, the remains of one Nokoor Chandra Chuckerbutty were found in the bed of a river at a distance of about half a mile from his house. The legs, arms, and head had been severed from the body. The prosecutor recognised the body as that of his uncle owing to its having a hump on the back. The head and right arm were found in the bed of the river at a distance of 40 yards from the spot where the trunk had been discovered. It appeared that the deceased was strangled in his house, and that the prisoners carried his body to the river bank, and there dismembered it with a sword.†

In 1866, one Maroop Mundul being missing from his village in the Moorshedabad district, it was suspected that he had been waylaid and murdered. After some delay, it was discovered that his head had been severed from his body, and the head and body thrown into a beel. The beel was carefully drained, and the skeleton of a headless body discovered. Seven men confessed being implicated in the murder.‡

Considering that the regular mode of disposing of a Hindu pauper body is to hold burning straw or a torch to its face, and then to throw it into the river, such disfigurement may prevent the recognition or identity without conveying any suspicion of crime. I, however, do not know of any instance in which this point has come forward in Court in Lower Bengal,

---

* Nizamut Adawlut Reports, Vol. V., Part I., for 1855, p. 824.

† *Ibid*, Vol. VII., for 1857, p. 292.

‡ Bengal Police Report, for 1866, p. 202.

and, as a general rule, the faces of the Hindu bodies brought to the dissecting room of this College are very little, if at all, disfigured by fire.

In the North-West Provinces, however, Thugs, when obliged to abandon a body without burial, used to drag it to some secret spot, and deface the features with fire.*

I remarked, in the Edition of 1856, that there could scarcely be a doubt that PHOTOGRAPHY would, before many years elapsed, be employed throughout India as a means of identifying bodies, anticipating the disfigurement of rapid decay, and enabling the magistrate and the civil surgeon to examine, in their offices, every detail of a scene of bloodshed, as it appeared when first disclosed to the police, in a place perhaps sixty miles from the sudder station, which no activity on the part of the police or themselves could enable them to visit in time. This process had then been employed, with advantage, by the police at home, in the identification of old offenders ; and I expressed my confidence that no measure would afford more aid to police inquiries in India, or impress more vividly, even upon the minds of the ignorant and superstitious common people, a conviction of the difficulty of eluding our vigilance and of our accuracy in the detection of crime. Although many uneducated Natives are scarcely able to comprehend the meaning of ordinary pictures, we have yet to judge of the effect which would be produced upon the conscience of a hardened savage, obstinate in the denial of guilt, by placing before him, in the stereoscope, the actual scene of his atrocity—the familiar walls, the charpoy, the ghastly faces—as they last appeared to his reeling vision—the sight which has haunted his brain every hour since the act was done—while he believed to certainty, that its reality could never come before his eyes again.

Every magistrate and surgeon will perceive under how many circumstances photography could be made available. It would be especially useful in showing the actual position of the body in cases of hanging, strangulation, &c. The experiment certainly deserves a portion of the time and consideration of judicial and medical officers ; and a few successful trials would recommend it to the attention of Government. Although the difficulties of rendering such a system general would, of course, be numerous, there is every reason to believe that the expectation of reward would encourage many young and intelligent darogahs to master the art of taking sun pictures, which is already easy, and which will, doubtless, be further simplified in the hands of the many who now give it their attention. Photography has occasionally been employed as an aid to police and medico-legal investigation in India. I am indebted to Mr. John Blessington Roberts, Coroner of Calcutta, for photographs by which alone

* Remarks of the Deputy Inspector-General of Police, North-Western Provinces, Annual Report for 1867, p. 109.

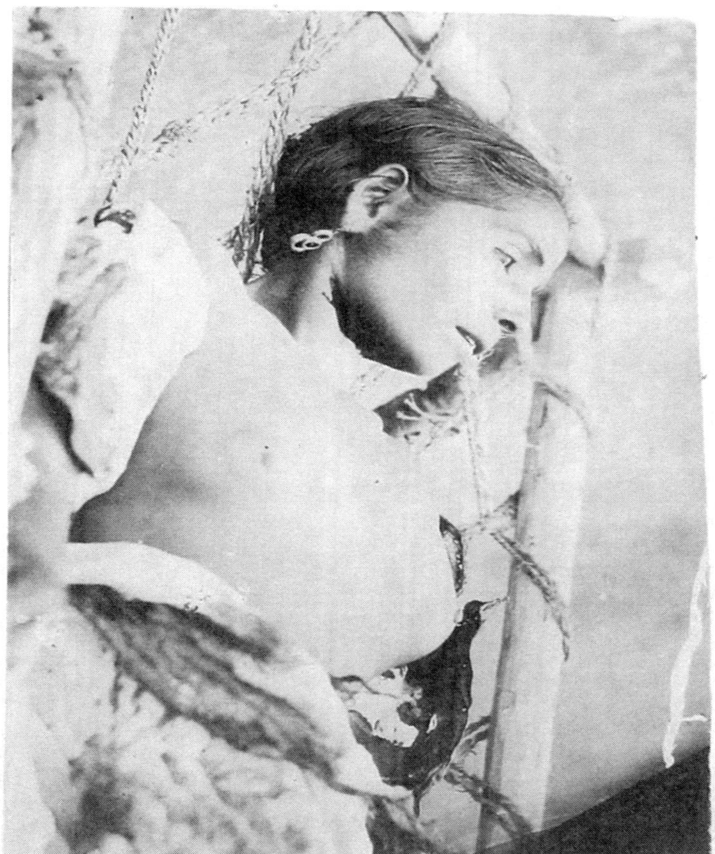

Photograph by means of which the victim of the "Amherst Street Murder" was identified.
See also p. 424.

the remains of Rose Brown, whose dead body was found in a Calcutta street with the throat cut in 1868, were identified.

UNCERTAINTY OF GENERAL EVIDENCE IN INDIA.

Supposing all attainable information to have been furnished by the police, the Medical Jurist, in this country, has to contend with a cause of embarrassment which is almost unknown at home. In England, it may be taken, as a general rule, that all the information, contributed in aid of a medico-legal enquiry, contains nothing that can be regarded as a wilful misrepresentation, unless emanating from a prosecutor, whose anger or vindictiveness has got the better of his judgment or honesty, or from the criminal, or his direct abettors. There, men all combine, with earnest purpose and sharpened faculties, to reveal the hidden guilt. In India, however, the deceit inherent in the character of the lower class of Natives surrounds all judicial investigations with an atmosphere of obscurity. Whenever the case has involved loss of life, the friends of the deceased are not, unnaturally, prone to give, to say the least, an exaggerated coloring to their statements. Other witnesses, less personally concerned in the issue, either speak under intimidation or for a price, or do not hesitate to endeavour to gain credit by asserting more than they know. The neighbours, if not personally affected by the occurrence, are either quite indifferent, or more or less adverse to the police and to their enquiry.

The extortion of confession by intimidation, and even by torture, is a practice often attributed to the police of this Presidency, and occasionally brought home to them in extreme cases ;* and, in certain instances, darogahs and their subordinates have been under strong suspicion of fabricating cases, and of suborning witnesses.†

The above moderate remark was sufficient allusion to that which I positively had proof of regarding the "Old" Police fourteen years ago. Subsequently, however, the evidences of their great untrustworthiness rapidly increased, until a new, and it is to be hoped a more valid, organization was established. The records show that, as the evidences of the necessity for this reform became glaringly apparent, the distrust displayed by judicial officers, and especially by the Court of Appeal, of all *thannah* evidence, whenever it was not supported by the most tangible proof, was extreme. Thus, in 1855, we find the Officiating Sessions Judge of Patna observing, in a case of stabbing : "I do not credit the evidence of the eye-witnesses as to the place where, and the mode in which, the wound was inflicted. I am

---

* Decisions of the Nizamut Adwalut, N. W. P., Vol. IV., p. 54.—" A tehseeldar and two chuprassees convicted of cruel torture" (with a view apparently of obtaining information regarding a robbery) " and sentenced to imprisonment for four and two years respectively, January 21st, 1854." See also Nizamut Adawlut Reports, Vol. IV., p. 508, April 1854, &c.

† See Reports of Nizamut Adwalut, Vol. III., Part 1, of 1853, p. 259 ; and Part 2, p. 130. Report on the State of the Police in the Lower Provinces, for 1845, p. 64 ; for 1846, p. 35.

of opinion that there was no reason why prisoner should follow his brother out of the shop ; that the blow was struck with a bread-knife inside the shop, and in the sight of no one ; that the deceased staggered out of the shop and died on the spot without saying a word ; and that the eye-testimony of the knife and the blow on the road was an after-thought of the police to make the case more complete (*muzboot*) according to their infamous custom in these parts."*

Again we find the same judge remarking, nearly at the same time : "If retribution for the murder of Chumars, and such like, depended on the consistent and concordant evidence to the fact of the witnesses of the same or of like castes, after it has passed through the police darogah's hands (who never will leave a case alone, but must always prepare it, and patch it up, by teaching the witnesses to learn their evidence off by heart beforehand, and to say more than they know), every Chumar and Dosadh in the country could be beaten to death or murdered without any one receiving punishment."† A short time previous to this, we find the Judges of the Nizamut Adawlut, in a case appealed from Tipperah, observing : "The mode in which the woman is said to have met her death seems most improbable ; nor is it clear whether the witnesses attribute it to the beating or to the suspension. We doubt whether they even saw what they relate, and we are led to suspect that the whole of this part of the case has been got up by the police." . . . "The confessions, in our opinion, are not calculated to remove the impressions that the police have got up the evidence in this case ; and, with nothing before us to justify reliance on any part of it, even as to the death of the woman, we must acquit all the prisoners of the charge, and direct their release."‡ In a case from Mymensingh, the Nizamut Adawlut Judges recorded the following : "No proofs whatever of burglary, such as the court could accept, are to be found on the record, and yet the prisoners, with the exception of one, plead more or less guilty to that charge ; and, if we convict the prisoners at all, we must convict them as having been actuated by motives which are not, in our opinion, in any way established by the evidence before us. There is, in our judgment, such " [much?] " strong reason to believe that the whole story has been got up with the view to screen others, at the cost of the prisoners ; but we cannot convict them on their admissions even before the magistrate, which, it is to be remarked, in some instances, vary materially from their mofussil confessions. Upon a careful consideration of all the circumstances on record, we come to the conclusion that there is not a single fact upon which we can with confi-

---

* Nizamut Adawlut Reports, Vol. V., Part 2, for 1855, p. 812.

† *Ibid*, p. 360.

‡ *Ibid*, Vol. V., Part I, of 1855, p. 18.

dence rely."* In a case from Tipperah, where the prisoners, in their capacity of witnesses, positively denied, in the judge's court, the evidence which they had given at the thannah and before the magistrate, stating that they had been tutored under threats and ill-treatment by the *kotwalli* darogah, the sessions judge observed : "I must admit my belief that the prisoners' story" (imputing illegal pressure to the darogah) "is true, and that the darogah, acting on an unhappy impression that an officer of his high character for efficiency (he has twice been honored by *khellauts* by Government) must support, and might add to it by being successful, where two other darogahs had failed, resorted to most unjustifiable means to extort confessions and create evidence to prove that murder, and not suicide, had been committed." Upon this the Nizamut Adawlut remark : "The Officiating Sessions Judge should not have ordered the commitment of the prisoners for perjury, as he was convinced that they had been subjected to ill-treatment to cause them to depose as they did before the magistrate. We, therefore, acquit them, and direct their release."†

In fact, Napoleon's saying—"The Police invents more than it discovers"—was scarcely an exaggeration of the general opinion in Bengal.

I find it alleged, in more than one instance, that *prisoners have been drugged by the police.* Thus, at Midnapore, in 1856, a prisoner named Nazur Mundul, asserted that he was forced to confess, but could not remember what was written ; and, after coming to the station, the darogah, early in the morning, gave him a hookah to smoke, which took away his senses, and when, before the joint magistrate, he was asked whether he had committed the dacoity, he denied and remained silent, and the mohurrir copied what had been written by the darogah.‡ Again, Tojoomoodeen and two others, when under trial for dacoity at Backergunge, in 1858, declared, that they were under the influence of some intoxicating liquor or drug when they were brought before the magistrate, and are unable to recollect what they may have said on that occasion,—in short they retract their confession. This plea of being under intoxication was, the sessions judge remarked, then resorted to in that court by every confessing prisoner who thought fit to retract his confession. The confessions of the three persons were recorded in the magistrate's house in his immediate presence. There was nothing to distract the magistrate's attention, and it was quite impossible to believe that, had the prisoners been under the influence of liquor or of any intoxicating drug then, the fact would have escaped the magistrate's notice.§

---

* Nizamut Adawlut Reports, Vol. V., Part I., p. 327.

† *Ibid*, p. 400.

‡ *Ibid*, 19th November 1856, p. 951.

§ *Ibid*, 11th August 1858, p. 332.

At a trial of several men, Hindus and Mahomedans, for dacoity, at Jessore, in 1856, all the prisoners ignored, in the judge's court, the recorded confessions taken by the police and the magistrate. One prisoner pleaded that the case was maliciously got up against him by a burkundaz, who must have drugged him previous to his going before the magistrate. The sessions judge remarked that the confessions were attested by respectable witnesses, who asserted that the confessions were voluntary, and that no kind of compulsion or persuasion or intimidation was exercised; and that the prisoners who confessed were, at the time, in the full possession of their faculties, and not in any way under the influence of any drug or intoxciating liquor.*

Distinct traces of some traditional knowledge of the Mahomedan Law appear in the plea made by these dacoits. It was held possible that wine might be administered to a person by force or menace, and was ruled that "*a confession, made during a fit of intoxication, is invalid.*"†

I do not find on record any positive proof that the police have ever practised the drugging of prisoners with a view to eliciting confession; but we have only too abundant evidence of the fact that the police authorities have always experienced difficulty in preventing their subordinates from practising torture. Several illustrations of this fact will be found in the Chapter on Torture, and in other parts of this work.

The modes of torture adopted, formerly and of late, by the police have generally been those which leave no discoverable bruise, or other trace of injury.

In 1855, a darogah and a party of burkundazes were convicted in the Court of the 24-Pergunnahs of having tortured a man into confession by tying his hands behind him with a cloth, and then by hoisting him up to a beam in the roof by a rope attached to the cloth. In this position he was beaten.‡ A very similar conviction was made in the same Court in the following year.§ In 1857, a darogah was convicted at the Sessions Court of Behar of torturing a prisoner. It was stated that the man's hands and feet were bound together with a cloth, that a stick was introduced between them, and that a party of chowkeedars, holding the ends of the stick, dashed him against the door of the thannah, and beat him with a shoe on the hinder part.‖ In 1866, it was proved that an inspector and sub-inspector of police in the Nuddea Division ill-treated four suspected persons by trussing them up to the roof of the house, keeping them without food, beating them with slippers, and practising other indignities upon them.¶

---

* Nizamut Adawlut Reports, September 23rd, 1856, p. 575.

† Harington's Analysis of the Laws and Regulations of Bengal, Part 2, p. 296.

‡ Nizamut Adawlut Reports, January 23rd, 1855, p. 103.

§ *Ibid*, February 25th, 1856, p. 501.

‖ *Ibid*, April 24th, 1857, p. 530.

¶ Report of the Police of the Lower Provinces, for 1866, p. 283.

Torture *by Cold* is sometimes had recourse to by the police. In 1855, a darogah and some of his people were convicted at Dacca upon a charge of having caused the death of a weakly, but not diseased, man, by placing him over the side of a boat, and leaving him in water not sufficiently deep to drown him, for many minutes.* In 1866, a sub-inspector of police in the Dinagepore Division was transported for life on proof of having beaten and ill-treated a man, suspected of docoity, until he died. It appeared that, when beating with a whip was found to have no effect, the unfortunate was tortured, in a cold February night, by pouring water on, and then fanning his naked body.†

The practice of the Indian Courts was, we repeat, for many years, full of evidences of distrust of *thannah* confessions. We find magistrates required to take special care that persons, upon being apprehended, are not made to suffer corporal punishment, or to be otherwise ill-treated under the pretence of compelling them to answer truly to questions that may be put to them, or under any other pretext whatever. In repeated decisions, the Court of Nizamut Adwalut held that a thannah confession must be borne out by other evidence, and is alone insufficient for conviction ; and that, even though acknowledged and confirmed by the prisoner, it requires corroboration by other evidence ; but, if proved to have been freely and voluntarily made, and if supported by other evidence, it is sufficient.‡ The existing practice, as prescribed in the Code of Criminal Procedure, is far more definite.

"148. No confession or admission of guilt made to a police officer shall be used as evidence against a person accused of any offence. It is now ordered that, in sending up cases for trial, police officers should not send in witnesses to prove confessions made before them."

"149. No confession or admission of guilt made by any person whilst he is in the custody of a police officer, unless it be made in the immediate presence of a magistrate, shall be used as evidence against such person."

The following rules are now in force in the Bengal Police :

Note to section 146 *of the Code of Criminal Procedure.*—"Extorting a confession by torture is punishable under sections 330, 331, 348, Penal

* Niźamut Adawlut Reports, January 12th, 1855, p. 49.

† Report of the Police of the L. P., for 1866, p. 239. In the reign of Henry the First, Ascelin de Goel, having taken William of Breteuil prisoner, and desiring to extort money from him, tormented him for three months, exposing him in his shirt all the morning in the north windows of his castle, after having thrown over him some buckets of cold water which froze one after the other over his body.—*Bell's Historical Sketches of Feudalism*, p. 189.

" *Cold Burning, Bottling.*—This punishment is thus inflicted. The offender is set against the wall with the arm which is to be *burned* tied as high above his head as possible. The executioner then ascends a stool, and having a bottle of cold water, pours it slowly down the sleeve of the delinquent, patting him, and leading the water gently down his body till it runs out at his feet. This is repeated to the other arm if he is sentenced to be burned in both. Bottling was at one time much in use in the cavalry branch of the service.—*Henry Marshall's Military Miscellany*, p. 156.

‡ Beaufort's Digest of the Criminal Law of the Presidency of Fort William, 1860, paras. 644 and 661.

Code. Extorting or attempting to extort a confession by criminal intimidation, is punishable under section 506, Penal Code."

"In all cases where the police are accused of extorting confessions or maltreating persons arrested, the district superintendent will immediately proceed to the spot, and thoroughly investigate the matter, reporting the circumstances fully not only to the district-magistrate, but to the inspector-general of police and the deputy inspector-general of the circle. Should it appear that there is any foundation for the charges, the deputy inspector-general will lose no time in proceeding to the district in which the occurrence has taken place, and reporting the action to the superior officers of the police in the matter."

Note to section 149.—"When an accused person makes a confession, or offers to do so, he is at once to be sent to the magistrate, and not to be detained by the police until they can hunt up corroborative evidence. Any omission to do this tends to make such confession valueless."

These restrictions are thus explained by Norton : "In this country, the quality of confessions made before the police is proverbial, and the Indian Law Reform Commissioners propose, in their report, to forbid the taking of confessions by the police in any case whatever, perhaps as the surest and shortest mode of putting an end to the evil."*

It was probably hoped that this action of the law, in reducing to a minimum the value of *thannah* confessions, would have put an end to the practice of torture and intimidation by the police.

Reform in this respect has, doubtless, been in progress for several years past, but it appears to have been much retarded by the retention in the force of men obstinately attached to the old system.

In his report for 1866, Colonel Pughe observes that, "as certain condemnatory reports have been made by the High Court, with reference to the many cases of torture by the police, which have lately come before it, and in which the judges suggested that, if the higher officers of the police did their duty, such cases could not occur, I have deemed it due to the department to go through every case which has been reported during the past year." He then gives memoranda of twelve cases, in which the police had been accused of torturing or ill-treating prisoners. In five of these the accused were acquitted. Most of the others were serious cases.

Colonel Pughe adds that, "it is to be presumed that the practice of flogging to induce confession was not uncommon in days gone by, for, shortly after the new police was introduced into the Hooghly district, a case occurred, in the year 1864, in which a sub-inspector of old standing, in open day, in the middle of a large bazar, not four miles from the sudder station, ordered a chowkeedar to be tied up and flogged, in order to

---

* Norton on Evidence, p. 108.

extort confession from him; and, so little was the occurrence thought of, that no complaint whatever was made by the chowkeedar, and it was by the merest accident that the circumstance came to notice. Cases of this kind still occur, now and then, without doubt; but no one who has the slightest acquaintance with a district will venture to say that such cases are anything nearly so frequent as they were a few years ago. Again, with regard to the getting up of false charges by police officers, it has been found that, in nearly every instance, the delinquents were men who had been for years in the old police. The inference is but fair that the men thus convicted have been in the habit of indulging in these practices, but that now only have their deeds been found out."* Elsewhere, in this report, we read of a sub-inspector in the Sonthal Pergunnahs, who, with six of his constables, was found guilty of torturing a man for the purpose of extorting confession. It turned out that he "had been frequently in the habit, when in the old police, of torturing his prisoners to extort confession.†" It would appear that—like the Byrajee who, after long confinement to a couch studded with spike nails, could not repose easily upon any softer bed—the people of Bengal have become somewhat attached to this ancient iniquity. In his report for 1865, the inspector-general writes: When ill-treated, the people now seldom fail to complain. There are two authorities to whom they can always appeal, and they know full well that they are immediately listened to, and their complaints investigated. To give an idea of native opinion on this subject, it may be observed that, in a late newspaper, the editor mourns over the loss of the old police, "because, under the new system, the constables are severely punished for the ill-treatment, however slight, of guilty parties; their hands are thereby tied, and offenders escape, because, not having descended from heaven, they will not confess." "A pretty clear hint," Colonel Pughe adds, "that, in the opinion of the writer, torture should be reverted to."‡

The public mind in Bengal is, at least, well inured to the idea of police pressure. Writing as lately as March 1870, the editor of the *Indian Mirror* says—"The first thing which a *pahara-wallah* is known to do, after catching a supposed delinquent, is to flog him soundly, and this system has gone on for such a length of time with utter impunity, that it is thought" (*sic*) "by the native community as a matter of course, any exception to it being a subject of much surprise."

Undoubtedly, matters have improved in this respect considerably of late. In the last published police report, for 1868, Col. Paterson shows that "whilst no less than fourteen charges of torture were preferred

---

* Report of the Police of the Lower Provinces of the Bengal Presidency, for the year 1866, pp. 46-9.

† *Ibid*, p. 111.

‡ *Ibid*, p. 7.

against the police, only three were proved, and one of these is pending final judgment."*

In the Garrow Hills, a head constable was sent to direct the Luskurs to assist the Mymensing police in capturing the murderers of one Neamut Sheikh, who was supposed to have taken refuge in the Garrow Hills. The head constable and one Gungia Luskur arrested a man on suspicion; and, at the instigation of the head constable, Gungia tortured him so severely to extort a confession that, in the course of three or four days, death resulted from the injuries he had received. The head constable and his accomplices were tried, and the former was sentenced to ten years' rigorous imprisonment.† The suspicion of the district superintendent of police at Bogra was aroused by the marks of wounds on the corpse of a reported suicide, and was directed against his own subordinates, whom he believed guilty of homicide in attempting to extort confession. He pressed the case, and obtained the conviction of an acting sub-inspector and three constables, under sections 330 and 114, Indian Penal Code.‡ At the Criminal Sessions of the Calcutta High Court, in March 1870, the following incident occurred:§ During the progress of a trial, one of the witnesses for the prosecution having related that he had accompanied the police constable who had arrested the prisoner, was asked whether the prisoner had made any statement. The following dialogue ensued:

Witness.—"At first he denied the charge, but afterwards when the *jemadar* scolded him and thereatened to beat him ———"

The Court.—"Threatened to beat him! did he say that he threatened to beat him?"

On the question being repeated, the witness denied that the *jemadar* had beaten the prisoner, and, to a succession of questions, affirmed that he did not recollect anything more than that the *jemadar* had scolded the prisoner in a loud and angry tone. On being asked who the *jemadar* was, he named one Mofeezoodeen, and then, being confronted with the man, who, unknown to him, had been standing close behind him whilst he gave his evidence, denied that it was Mofeezoodeen who had scolded the prisoner, but said that it was some constable in plain clothes whose name he did not know. Mofeezoodeen was next called, and having said that he did not beat or scold the prisoner, and that his statement was purely voluntary, was asked by the Court: "If the witness who has just given evidence has said that you scolded the prisoner, and threatened to beat him, has he committed perjury?" He replied promptly, "yes." At the close of the trial Mr. Justice Phear, addressing the superintendent

* Report of the Police of the Lower Provinces of the Bengal Presidency, for the year 1868, p. 41.

† *Ibid*, p. 40.

‡ *Ibid*.

§ As reported in the *Englishman*.

of police, directed that the matter might be brought to the attention of the commissioner of police.

Shortly after this, it was stated in the public prints, that a native who was lately sentenced to death, by the sessions judge of the Nundidroog division, for murder, has had his sentence reversed, and has been discharged by the judicial commissioner, on the ground that the confession made by him before the magistrate was vitiated by the mistaken zeal of the police in inducing him to make it. The sub-magistrate also appears to have been too anxious to induce the prisoner to confess, as he three times told him to tell the truth, adding that, "if he told the truth, justice would follow; but, if he told a lie, he would be punished." This was clearly holding out hopes to the prisoner that he would be leniently dealt with if he confessed, and yet he was sentenced to death on his own confession.

The prevalence of these abuses will diminish, if the exertions of a large body of able European officers, upheld by the full authority of Government, can avail in extirpating this ancient and deeply-rooted evil. For the present, however, those engaged in medico-legal investigations here cannot well exercise too much caution in distinguishing between EVIDENCE and FACT. Indeed, we must feel that this caution can never be relaxed, seeing that—could it be ordained to-day that, henceforward, police testimony throughout the land should become unusllied truth,—the same deceit which we now battle with would continue ingrained in the vulgar popular mind, and would still demand our unceasing vigilance.

"If," writes Goodeve, "in the system of Police Administration which exists in India, the barbarous usage of torture, as it may be feared it does, still holds its ground there, in spite of all the efforts of the Government to put it down, it may be safely asserted that India is the only portion of Her Majesty's dominions which has not yet been freed from the stain; and that it has there survived so long is attributable rather to the character of the people than to any oppressive tendencies on the part of their rulers."*

Cases frequently come to light in which the people and the police are equally in fault. It was reported in May 1869, that six wealthly zemindars of Serampore, near Calcutta, were charged before Mr. Ryland, the magistrate, with oppression towards a small landowner and ryot in their village, named Halimudin Shaik. The ryot had a small piece of land to sell in another village, and the chief zemindar wish to buy it. But he spoke too late—it was already sold; and then the zemindar determined to seize it without further parley. He and his labourers went to the ryot's huts, bound one of his relatives to a tree outside as a caution to the neighbours not to interfere, and at once proceeded to carry off every-

* Op. Citat., p. 94.

thing the poor man possessed. The cattle were driven off, the brass pots and other indispensable articles of the native kitchen taken away. Some money and papers were also stolen. All this was openly done, and two of the zemindars were present on the scene, while the others looked on from their houses hard by. Mr. Ryland committed the defendants on a charge of dacoity, and they were brought to trial. But the native police did all in their power to suppress or mutilate the evidence, and the jury acquitted the defendants, although the judge summed up for a conviction. Mr. Ryland said in his memorandum: "The difficulty of getting any independent evidence at all in such a case can only be appreciated by those who have experience of the terror exercised by an unscrupulous landlord in the mofussil, and upon which, together with a corrupt police, the offenders in this case doubtless trusted for impunity."

Let us take one or two examples of the manner in which evidence is got up without the tutorage of the police.

In 1855, the naib of the talookdars of a village in the Hooghly district, having made himself detested by the villagers, was dragged out of his home in the middle of a winter night, and beaten to death by an infuriated crowd. Upon the evidence of certain witnesses, the sessions judge remarked: "It is not impossible that different witnesses might, even in a dark night, recognise, out of a body of twenty men, two or three different persons with whose appearance and voices they were each familiar; but it is not probable that the same six witnesses could, under the circumstances supposed, identify the same eight persons. A recognition of eight persons out of twenty, all huddled together in a dark night, is an improbable thing, but the recognition of the same eight persons by the same six witnesses is altogether beyond the pale of probability. I, therefore, cannot yield that belief to the evidence of recognition to find the prisoners guilty upon it; not that I would have it supposed that, because of this improbability, I would reject the evidence *in toto*; far from it, for it is natural to suppose that different witnesses did recognise some of the persons; some recognised some, and some others, and, native-like, they communicated the names one to another; and each witness, under the circumstances, thought he might safely adopt as his own the borrowed recognition of his fellow eye-witnesses. Though, individually, their evidence is open to objection, I have not myself much doubt that the evidence *in the main*, as to recognition, has indicated the right parties."*

It has been proved repeatedly that, throughout the rural districts of India, men are willing to swear in Court that they have actually *seen* that which it turns out they have only *heard* of from one on their own side. Probably, the Hindu law was somewhat in fault here. Goodeve remarks: "If

---

* Nizamut Adawlut Reports, Vol. V., Part 1, of 1855, p. 725.

Sir W. Macnaghten correctly represent the text of Menu, that ancient sage of the Hindus, declares that,—'Evidence of *what has been seen or of what has been heard* is admissible ;' And Sir W. Macnaghten, on the authority of the passage, says,—A witness may be either from *seeing* or *hearing*, as has been declared by Menu (*Macnaghten's Hindu Law*, 239). Possibly this may merely mean to enunciate that evidence derived through the perception of *either* sense, seeing or hearing, is admissible ; and to restrict evidence generally to what is derived from *one of these two* sources. If it intend the indiscriminate adoption of what is ordinarily termed 'hearsay,' the Code of Menu is very much at variance with the Codes of most civilised nations" (page 416). Observing what the common practice is, it is but charitable to believe that a tradition of this latter reading of the law has come down to the common people, and somewhat justifies their action.

Let us take one more illustration. In 1837, Luxiah bin Budiah, a Bheel, was tried for perjury at Khandesh. It appeared that, in a trial for highway robbery, a witness for the prosecution was called, when the prisoner answered, personating Kalliah bin Dowjee. The prisoner deposed that his name was Kalliah bin Dowjee; that on a certain date he had followed up the foot-prints of certain robbers, &c. On being cross-questioned, respecting various particulars he had not come prepared to answer, he admitted that his name was not Kalliah bin Dowjee but Luxiah bin Budiah, and further that he was not present when the robbers were traced. The prisoner urged that his friend Kalliah was sick, and unable to attend the Court, and that, therefore, he came to depose for him ; that the facts to which he had deposed were perfectly true ; and, although he was not himself an eye-witness, yet they were notorious to all the people of his village. He was sentenced to one year's imprisonment with labor, and to receive twenty-five stripes in the bazar.* On reference to Goodeve we read that "Mahomedan law, in certain prescribed cases, allowed the singular expedient of giving evidence *by proxy*. In the event of the death of the principal witness, the *absence of the witness on a three days' journey*, or his *sickness*, and in a certain class of cases where the judgment was not barred by doubt, a witness or the person who would have been such was permitted *to supply a proxy*, substituting another person to detail facts or opinions for him."†

"*What is truth?*"

In more than one recent decision of the Privy Council, the untrustworthiness of native evidence in India is taken as a received fact. Thus, in Bunwarree Lall *v.* Hetnarain Sing, "the general fallibility of native

---

* Bellasis's Bombay Reports, p. 116.

† Beaufort, section 635 ; Goodeve, p. 116.

evidence in India" is spoken of; and, in the case of Modhoosoodun Sundeal *v.* Surroop Chandra Sircar Chowdhry, reference is made to "the lamentable disregard of truth prevailing amongst the natives of India." *(Cowell)*.

Then we have the expressions of the Inspector-General of Police, Lower Provinces, that this is "a country where perjury is the rule and not the exception, where no man will tell the whole truth or the simple truth, and where exaggeration is perfectly natural;"—and also "where false witnessess can be bought for a few annas."*

The painful patience with which Indian Judges winnow the evidence before them for any grain of truth which it may contain, is shown in a late ruling of the Calcutta High Court: Wise and others *v.* Sundul-oonissa Chowdranee and others.† "A native case is not necessarily false and dishonest, because it rests on a false foundation, and is supported in part by false evidence."

In a recent report upon the criminal classes of Cachar,‡ we are told that "perjury and false charges are common offences enough, but the false charge is generally an extrmely exaggerated version of something that really happened, and the perjury is not often of a very aggravated character. The false witness, for the most part, believes that the facts to which he swears are true in the main, and that, if he had been luckier, he might have seen the things he says he has seen, or heard the things he says he has heard. I think too that the Cachar Bengali generally would prefer to tell the truth if he were quite sure that it would not hurt himself or his friends. The Munipoorie, on the other hand, never tells the truth if he can possibly tell a lie. He has been gifted by nature with a very pretty turn for perjury, and he has done his utmost to cultivate the talent."

As we are not writing a work on evidence, but merely desire to show reason for cautioning medical jurists in India not to be too easily satisfied with specious evidence, we shall be satisfied with choosing for illustration, out of many, one kind of *benowed* or prepared evidence, which Goodeve designates *The too perfect;* and of which he cites the following instance from the judgment of the Court in a case furnished by the records of the Sudder Dewanny Adawlut of the Presidency of Bengal, which is not only valuable as a case of actual occurrence, but as a specimen of a very ordinary Indian trial. "Now it is clear," says the judge, "that the memories of these witnesses must be either wonderfully retentive, or that their recollections must have been recently *refreshed*, to enable them to speak of *details with such remarkable precision and accuracy;* their testimony could scarcely be more perfect than it is in every minute coincidence. But evidence, I apprehend, may be *too perfect;* and, after such lapse

---

* Annual Report for 1866, pp. 10 & 53.

† Cowell, p. 269.

‡ Appendixes to Report on the Bengal Jails, for 1868, p. 234.

of time, naturally creates suspicion ; for, without very recent *refreshing*, this concordance in regard to *dates in different eras*, the *number of bags*, the *amount in each*, even the *number of sheets of stamped paper* on which the bond was engrossed, and the *conversation* which took place, seems almost impossible ; the only inference to be drawn is that the witnesses must have been *tutored*."*

Mr. Baynes† speaks of the "*incredible* minuteness with which in our" [Indian] "Courts the prosecutor and his witnesses almost invariably detail the particulars of an assault or affray,—*e. g.* '*The first prisoner, standing to the south, struck me one blow on the arm with a stick two cubits long and two fingers thick ;* the second prisoner kicked me with his right foot on my left leg,' &c. Here, however, apart from embellishing details, the assault may have been a fact."

The above examples are sufficient to prove that the District Superintendent of Police, the Magistrate, and the Civil Surgeon have frequently little but their own knowledge and acumen to guide them in the discovery of crime. In fact, the latter often obtains no truth from any but that silent witness who never lies—the Corpse.

For valuable notes upon the circumstance under which "*False Testimony*" became admissible under the Hindu law, and *Equivocation* in testimony was permitted by the Mahomedan law, *vide* Goodeve, pp. 114-16.

The following case strongly illustrates the character of the uncertainties which may present themselves to the medical jurist in this country, when in quest of reliable evidence. In the cold season of 1850, I received a small fragment of recent bone with an official letter from the magistrate of the Chittagong district. The bone was evidently a portion of the shaft of the humerus or femur of a young child ; it was nearly two inches long, and weighed about three drachms. It had formed less than half of the circumference of the shaft, and had evidently been broken out by a jackal, the dent of a small canine tooth being impressed distinctly on its edge. I was informed that a little native girl, about four years old, had been taken away from her home, by one Tofan Alee, who was some time afterwards seized by the police, in attempting to cross the river. The child's silver ornaments were found upon him ; he at once confessed that he had strangled the infant, and pointed out the spot where he had buried the body. Upon close search, however, nothing could be found there except the fragment of bone described, and the *ghoonsee*, or waist-string, which the child had worn. A place near a tank was also pointed out by the prisoner, in which the child's jacket was found concealed. After confessing to the police, and repeating

* Goodeve, p. 95; Sudder Dewanny Report, 1853, p. 25.

† Points on Medical Jurisprudence for British India, p. 20.

every circumstance of his crime before the magistrate, the prisoner retracted his avowal; and, in the absence of any evidence beyond that afforded by the splinter of bone (which might have been brought by dogs or jackals from a distance), it appeared questionable whether the prisoner might not have committed the not by any means unfrequent crime of stealing the child, and selling her, after having stripped her of her clothes and ornaments in the place indicated.

After examining the splinter of bone, I expressed my belief that the body had been devoured by wild animals; but told the darogah that diligent search must still be made for the skull, which would, doubtless, be discovered. I was convinced that small animals, like jackals, could do no more than gnaw the perfectly ossified skull of a child of that age, and roll it from place to place. The darogah failing to make any further discovery, I accompanied the magistrate to the scene of the alleged crime, a very distant solitary spot, on the bank of a narrow, but deep and rapid marsh stream, by which any fragments of the body might have been carried down towards the river. As, however, it appeared unlikely that the jackals would resign any portion of their prey, I still maintained confidently that the skull must be found, probably among the thickets of wild pine-apple with which the ground was covered. Shortly after this, the skull of a child was brought to me by the police; it was recent, corresponded with the age of the missing child, and had, evidently, been gnawed by small wild animals, the marks of whose teeth traversed the calvarium in every direction. Still, again, this prompt discovery of the skull, upon my reiterated assertion that it must be forthcoming, after the ground had been searched again and again for nearly a week by the whole *posse comitatus*, was somewhat startling; and the suspicion obtruded itself—have the police been so much impressed with the confidence of my assertion, that some burkundauze, failing to discover the head, and feeling himself unpleasantly responsible to the darogah, has endeavoured to resolve the difficulty by borrowing a credible head from one of the many bodies daily floating down the adjacent river? The skull was shown to the child's father, who asserted that he could identify it by the shape of the front teeth; but still it was questionable whether, in his anxiety to convict the man who was known to have kidnapped his child, he would have hesitated to identify any skull that might have been produced.* When tried, the prisoner recalled his confession, and pleaded "not guilty." The sessions judge, however, sentenced him to death, and the judges of the superior court confirmed the decision, recording their opinion that "the

* This recognition of the skull appears not to have been admitted at the sessions court as the judge's report says, "there is no satisfactory recognition of the corpse."

Upon this my *Commentator* remarks, "Natives will swear to anything,—to bajra stalks, ears of grain, and lotas stolen ten years ago: much more would a father swear to the teeth of a skull to obtain vengeance for his stolen, murdered child."

corpus delicti being proved, non-recognition should not absolutely and invariably be ruled to bar capital punishment. Each case should be tried with reference to the circumstances, and to the facts established." The prisoner suffered the last penalty of the law.

SIMULATED DEATH.

The *Lash* (corpse) having been brought in for examination, it is needful to be certain, in the first place, that it is, in reality, dead. India is probably the only country in the world where a person, wishing to prefer a false charge against his enemy, would venture to simulate death and allow himself to be brought to a medical man for examination. I have heard of more than one case of the kind. We begin to comprehend this when we occasionally find natives carrying animosity to such a length as to destroy themselves in the hope of bringing down present and eternal punishment upon their enemies,—*see* the Chapter on Suicide.

The late Dr. Kenneth Mackinnon informed me that the body of a man, alleged to have been murdered, was brought to him many years since. Finding that the deceased had a very tolerable pulse, he adopted means which assisted the corpse in making off with great rapidity. In another case, an offer to save the deceased's friends the expense of burning his remains was attended with the best results.

In his "First Impressions of Hindustan," Captain Bacon mentions having seen a squalid-looking corpse brought to the house of a civilian, with two or three wounds on the chest, and with many marks of violence on other parts of the person. Believing the dead man to be a simulator, the magistrate approached to examine the body, but was assailed with a thousand importunities not to pollute the corpse before the rites of sepulture had been performed. He, therefore, refrained from touching the body with his hand; but stuck the sharp end of his billiard cue, which he had in his hand, into the side of the supposed corpse. This did not produce any effect beyond disconcerting the throng. The blow was repeated with such force that the sharp point of the cue penetrated the flesh between the ribs. A very slight quiver of the muscles and an almost imperceptible movement of the head discovered the cheat. The people were then told that they had better take the body to the hospital, for that life was not yet extinct. The reply was, "The man has been dead since cock-crow!" A kettle of hot water was then brought and, notwithstanding the entreaties of the friends that the body might be spared, a small quantity was poured upon his foot,—when he "bounced from the charpai and fled like a spirit."

"When some officers in India were breakfasting in the commander's tent, the body of a native, said to have been murdered by the sepoys, was brought in and laid down. The crime could not be brought home to any one of them, yet there was the body. A suspicion, however, crossed the adjutant's mind and, having the kettle in his hand, the thought struck him that he would pour a little boiling water on the body. He did so; on which the murdered remains started up and scampered off."*

Baboo Kanny Lall Dey informed me in 1868, that he had, a short time previously, been called to see one who, wishing to terrify his master, simulated death rather cleverly for many hours. When an attempt was made to open one of his eyes the orbicularis acted. A call for a red-hot iron had a surprisingly restorative effect.

When practising, many years ago, in an out-of-the-way station, among dull people, I was, more than once, called upon to satisfy friends of the reality of a death. I did so by the use of boiling water. The best test, in cases of doubt, however, is that recently brought to notice by Dr. Martenot, principal physician of the Hospital de Lyon. Produce a blister on one digit of the hand or the foot, by the flame of a candle left in contact with it for some seconds, till the vesicle forms, which it always does. If the vesicle contain serous fluid, it is an evident sign of life. If it contain only vapour, it is a proof of death. In other words, a dry vesicle—*death*; a liquid vesicle—*life*. No possibility of error.†

DYING DECLARATIONS.

In cases of very severe wounding, &c., the letter sent to the civil surgeon with the injured person generally also conveys a request that, should the case be likely to terminate fatally, timely intimation may be given that the patient's deposition may be taken in writing.

In India, the rule, as laid down in para. 371 of the Code of Civil Procedure, is that "The declaration of a deceased person, whether it be made in the presence of the accused person, or not, may be given in evidence if the deceased person, at the time of making such declaration, believed himself to be in danger of approaching death, although he entertained at the time of making it hopes of recovery."‡

By the English law, as expounded by Guy,§ "Death-bed declarations are admitted on evidence in cases of homicide, where the death of

---

* Family Library No. 63, Sketches of Imposture, &c., E. 9, p. 139, cited by Best and Goodeve.

† The British Medical Journal, April 25th, 1868.

‡ The action of the *Police* in these cases is as follows :—"Where a police officer, making an enquiry in any case, has reason to believe that a person whose statement may have an important bearing on the case is in a dangerous state, and likely to die before the completion of the proceedings, or before the deposition of such person can be taken on oath in the presence of the accused before a magistrate, he should be most careful first to ascertain in the presence of respectable witnesses the apparently dying person's own impression of his condition, and then to take down his statement *verbatim*. Should there be reason to believe that the statement as recorded by the police officer is not *word for word* as it was uttered by the deceased, it may seriously damage the case on trial, and district superintendents should carefully impress on their subordinates the great importance of bearing the above instructions in mind when enquiring into cases of the nature noted."

§ Principles of Forensic Medicine, 3rd edition, p. 26.

the deceased is the object of the charge, and the circumstances of the fatal injury the subject of the declaration. It is assumed that the declarant, having lost all hope of recovery, is induced to speak the truth by considerations as powerful as an oath administered in a court of justice. It is not necessary, however, that he should express his conviction. It may be inferred from the nature of the injury, or from other circumstances of the case. But, if any hope whatever be entertained, or may be inferred to exist, whether it be spontaneous, or on the suggestion of others, death-bed declarations cannot be received in evidence."

Goodeve remarks (p. 491) : "The distinction between the English and the Indian law, it will be noticed, is that, to render the declaration admissible, the former requires a full apprehension of the danger ; while the latter admits the element of *a hope of recovery.* It may not always be very easy to draw the line between *apprehension* of danger and *hope* of recovery. *Practically,* the Act would only seem to *lower the scale or degree* of apprehension. According to English law, *any* hope of recovery would exclude."

In the absence of any intimation from the police to that effect, it is clearly incumbent upon the surgeon to communicate with them, whenever he may perceive that a case involving criminal charges is likely to terminate fatally. In the absence of the police, it is desirable that the civil surgeon, or indeed any trustworthy bystander, should take down the statement of the dying man. There does not, however, appear to be any rule rendering such a course incumbent upon medical officers.

The administrators of the law in this country have, in more than one case, wisely decided, that unless supported by collateral evidence, the dying declaration of a native cannot be received as conclusive.

In a trial for murder, it was held that the dying deposition of the deceased, taken by the police officers, should have been brought on the record of the trial ; and that evidence to its accuracy should be taken.* The dying declaration of a murdered person (taken down in writing by a *sezawul*) was considered alone insufficient for conviction.†

In a case tried at Bundelkund in 1852, the judge of the superior court held that the deceased, after receiving seventeen wounds (some of which were mortal, and from the effects of which he died shortly after), could scarcely have had sense or strength sufficient to make the statement attributed to him. The judge was not disposed to place much more faith in the dying declaration of the deceased (supposing such really to have been made), than he would in a statement delivered by him when in the enjoyment of complete bodily health, and in the full possession of his

---

* Nizamut Adawlut Reports, Vol. V., p. 9.

† Nizamut Adawlut Reports, Vol. IV, p. 31. *Ibid*, 402, 404. The doubt here probably applied rather to the Police than to the declarant.

mental faculties. Natives of this country are not sensible of the same impressions as Europeans on the point of dissolution ; and, in their dying moments, not unfrequently accuse any one whom they may only *suspect* of being the perpetrators of the attack on them. The accused was acquitted.*

In May 1868, some person or persons unknown entered the house of Rutton Bewa, a woman of bad character, in the Moorshedabad district, and inflicted upon her wounds, of which she died on the following morning. Before her death she accused one Parboo, the chowkeedar of the village, as being the man who had wounded her. He was arrested and tried ; but, as there was no further evidence against him, he was acquitted.†

Under these circumstances, the medical witness in India is not likely to be closely questioned with regard to the point, formerly so strongly insisted upon by English lawyers,‡ as to whether, at the time of making his declaration, the injured person was evidently convinced that he was about to die. While it may be questionable whether, even in the most enlightened mind, all hope of recovery can always be dispelled by the sense of immediately impending death ; and whether, in the surprise, the excitement, the agony, the confusion, and the failing consciousness which result from the infliction of a deadly injury, the judgment and the passions can be sufficiently calm for the delivery of a testimony which deserves to be received hereafter as absolutely and unimpeachably true,—especially when it may be doubted whether the wounded person is not utterly unprincipled and false by habit—it is fortunate that this ancient legal superstition has not been brought to bear upon a people who have, in repeated instances, committed murder and even suicide§ with the design of bringing down present and eternal punishment upon an enemy, who do not recognize veracity as a principle of morality, and who almost invariably answer as they believe that they are expected to answer ; who meet inevitable death with an apathy which has been mistaken for stoicism, but whose cry of —" I am dying, I am dying,—Death, Death" !—is almost daily evoked by ordinary circumstances of misfortune or pain.

" The person or persons," says Guy, " inculpated by the declarant's statement, are not precluded from giving evidence as to his state of mind and behaviour in

---

* Nizamut Adawlut Reports, N. W. P., for 8th May 1852. See also report of a case tried on the 23rd of the following July, in which scarcely any weight was given to the dying statement of the deceased.

† Bengal Police Report, for 1868, p. 239.

‡ Dr. Taylor has shown that it is no longer necessary, to render a declaration valid, that the person making it must entertain " no hopes of recovery." At the Special Commission in Ireland (Jany. 1848, *Reg. v. Butler*,) a declaration was admitted where the words were, that the deceased entertained " little or no hope" of recovery.—*Medical Jurisprudence*, Fifth edition, p. 899.

§ See the Chapters on Identity of Dead Bodies, p. 71 ; and Suicide.

his last moments. They may be allowed to show that the deceased was influenced by vindictive motives, or was not of a character to be impressed by a religious sense of his approaching dissolution."*

The great importance of medical evidence regarding the *State of Mind and Body* of the declarant, at the time at which he made his declaration, was very forcibly illustrated in the case of Finlayson tried in Calcutta in 1869. On the 7th May (a season at which, in Calcutta, to become intoxicated is to incur imminent risk of death by insolation) a European shut himself up in a room with his wife, and appears to have continued to drink spirits up to the evening of the 12th, when, upon an alarm, he was found bleeding from a wound on the back of the head. A police officer enquired "How did this happen ?" He replied, " She threw a glass at me." The wife said, "Don't say that ; you know I did not do it." She said that he had fallen out of bed on a cup. This was towards 8 o'clock. At about half-past eight, Dr. Charles Palmer saw him. He spoke incoherently ; his pulse was pretty strong, but his skin was cold. Dr. Palmer could not tell whether he was in liquor. He was brought to the Medical College Hospital soon after 9 o'clock,—drunk, and with oozing of blood from the scalp wound. He tossed about and abused the coolies, but never spoke rationally up to the time of his death, which occurred at about 11 o'clock. The appearances after death were by no means those of excessive hœmorrhage. There was intense congestion of the meninges and substance of the brain, with a sub-arachnoid extravasation of blood upon the upper surface of the left anterior lobe of the cerebrum, occupying rather more than an inch of surface. At its centre the clot was between two and three lines deep ; the brain was not torn ; the extravasation of blood was attributed to *contre-coup.* Portions of the enamel of a teacup (bloody fragments of which were found scattered about the room) were removed from the wound on his admission, and it was found that some minute flakes of the enamel had been driven under the pericranium. I reported that "Death might be attributed to the combined influence, in an intemperate and unhealthy man, of alcoholism in a very aggravated degree, of heat, and of congestion of the brain, with traumatic extravasation of blood." Here the universal medical opinion was that the wife's was the true statement ; and that, when the man accused her, he was not in a condition to know how the injury was inflicted. A fall upon a teacup would produce the appearances described, whereas the power of a woman's arm would be insufficient to throw a teacup with such strength as to force the enamel under the pericranium. The case, however, went to the sessions, where, the medical opinion being at once accepted, the wife was acquitted.

A case of great importance, as bearing upon the weight of dying declarations in India, was tried at Sholapore (Bombay Presidency) in July

---

* Forensic Medicine, 3rd Edition, p. xxvi.

1843.* Appa was charged with the wilful murder of Koondee, and Yadoo and Sheekoo as accessaries with aiding and abetting.

The conviction in this case rested entirely on the credit due to the dying declaration, taken on solemn affirmation, of the deceased Koondee. He affirmed that, on the morning after the Hoolee, *viz.*, on the 16th of March, he was awoke by the prisoners Yadoo and Sheekoo seizing him by the hands, and while these prisoners held him down, the prisoner Appa deliberately wounded him twice with a hatchet on the forehead ; that he was enabled to recognize the prisoners by the light of the moon. The declarant next described the nature and extent of the wounds he had received, and was about to enter into other particulars, when he became speechless, and shortly afterwards expired. In corroboration, it was proved by the evidence of Buckma, the deceased's wife, that she, at day-light on the morning of 16th of March, found the deceased, her husband, lying wounded near the village gate of Zowlgaum, and that he then accused the prisoners Yadoo and Sheekoo with holding, and Appa with wounding, him. Three other witnesses deposed to the same effect. The prisoner Sheekoo before the Police Amilder admitted that Appa was at enmity with the Mhars of Zowlgaum, and that he had three days before the Hoolee expressed his intention of killing the first Mhar he would find alone. Sheekoo, however, denied this statement before the magistrate and the sessions court.

On the trial, the prisoners disclaimed all knowledge of the murder, and called several of their relations to prove that they did not leave their homes on the night of the Hoolee. The sessions judge (W. Birdwood) was of opinion, that the testimony of the deceased was consistent throughout, and being sanctioned by an oath, was deserving of credit, and he thereon convicted the prisoners, and sentenced them severally to be transported for the terms of their natural lives, subject to the confirmation of the superior court.

By the Court of Sudder Foujdaree Adawlut, Mr. W. Simson :—"In this case the evidence of the deceased is entitled to the highest credit ; no imaginable reason is supposed or suggested why the deceased should have charged the prisoners falsely, and his statement is corroborated by concurrent circumstances, and by the deposition of one of the prisoners. The defence and the *alibis* set up are not, in my opinion, worthy of any belief. The evidence is certainly scanty, but it is sufficient to leave no moral doubt that the deceased met his death at the prisoners' hands very much as he states. On the whole, I would confirm the conviction and sentence." Mr. B. Hutt :—"This conviction rests solely on the statement of the deceased Koondee Mhar, who is represented by the persons who went to his assistance on his being discovered lying in a wounded state at the gate

* Bellasis's Reports, p. 174.

of the town, to have said that the prisoners wounded him, and on his deposition to the same effect before the police authorities, which is recorded; but there is no evidence to show that the deceased was sufficiently collected to know what he was saying, and this paper recorded as his deposition throws great doubt on this from the abrupt manner in which it breaks off, and which is stated to have occurred in consequence of his being unable to proceed, and this doubt is greatly strengthened by the nature aud position of the wound. It is to be regretted that so important a matter should have been neglected. Further, I see great reason to distrust the deposition said to have been made by the deceased, from its containing a description of the size and nature of the wound, which, being on the forehead, it is obvious he could know nothing whatever of. This must have been an addition by another, and if so, the whole becomes valueless, as it is impossible to say how much more may have been similarly added. Again, the crime is described as having been perpetrated at about 4 A.M. At this time of the morning, from the declining state of the moon, it would be extremely difficult to distinguish another person even near, and it seems most improbable that persons would go to commit such an act without some disguise, which makes it far from improbable that the deceased may have been deceived in the imagined recognition of the prisoners, even if the statement could be trusted. I would not then convict the prisoners on such evidence, even though one of the prisoners' statements seems to render it probable that they were concerned in the crime."

The Court being divided in opinion, the case was referred to a third Judge.

Minute recorded by F. Pynes, Esq., Puisne Judge :—"The declaration of the deceased, which was subsequently reduced to writing when he was on the point of death, before constituted authority, and under an oath, is, I am of opinion, deserving of every credit. On being visited immediately after the assault, and while he was lying on the spot where it took place, he, without hesitation, affirmed that the prisoner Appa struck the blow, and the other two prisoners were aiding. The day afterwards, before the Police Amildar, he confirms this statement and, while in the act of delivering his evidence, becomes speechless.

"There is no assignable cause why he should have made a wilful misrepresentation, or why, *in articulo mortis*, he should have persisted in the same; and, though the evidence of an accomplice cannot be adduced in support of the prosecution, the confession of the prisoner Sheekoo stamps the evidence with the mark of truth. There is no cause to doubt that the deceased had his faculties about him when he recognized the prisoners; and, as no motives are assigned or attempted to be assigned for his falsely charging them with his death, I am prepared to confirm the conviction and sentences."

The conviction and sentences were, accordingly, confirmed.

MEDICAL EVIDENCE.

Previous to the introduction of the Code of Criminal Procedure, the civil surgeon's written statement, in reply to the magistrate's letter of inquiry, was received as evidence in ordinary cases of assault. The Regulation, however, directed that,—

In cases of murder, or wounding, endangering life, when the body or wound may have been inspected by the civil surgeon, the deposition of the surgeon should be invariably taken on oath, whether before the magistrate or the sessions judge.—Circular Order, No 54, para. 7, 16th July 1830; Circular Order, No. 42, 1st May 1840.

Something farther was, however, necessary to render such depositions valid as evidence in the sessions courts.

In May 1853, a case of murder was tried at Mynpoorie, in which the sessions judge apprehended that, although the civil surgeon had left the station on leave for Europe before the trial, that officer's depositions having been taken on oath, before the magistrate, in accordance with Circular No. 42 of 1st May 1840, he was at liberty to refer to those depositions as evidence which, under any legal view whatever, it would be impossible to ignore. He, however, abstained from placing the examination of the civil surgeon before the magistrate on the record of his court. It was ruled by the superior court that,—although the Circular Order quoted by the sessions judge directs that the examinations of medical officers in the magistrates' courts shall be taken on oath, in order to their being available on the trial,—in the event of the unavoidable absence of the officers making them, it is necessary that such examinations should be proved, on the trial, in the usual manner, in conformity to the injunction contained in the Circular Orders of the 16th July 1830, otherwise, they cannot be accepted as proof against the accused. This precaution not having been observed in the present instance, the deposition of the medical officer was held by the court not to be, in its existing state, admissible as evidence against the prisoner.*

A similar ruling was adhered to by the Court in a case tried at Cawnpore, in 1852, where the sessions judge had placed on the record of his court an original letter from the civil surgeon, and other papers which, in their then form, were inadmissible as proof; and again, in a case tried at Bareilly in the same year, where the statement on oath of the civil

---

* Nizamut Adawlut Reports, N. W. P., of 31st May 1853. In a case tried at Bareilly, in January 1854, the court observed that the mere occupation of the civil surgeon on other duty, and his consequent non-attendance at the trial, by no means justified the procedure here adopted of placing his foujdaree deposition on the record of trial, after causing it to be attested by the subscribing witnesses; such a course is only allowed in the "*unavoidable absence*" of the Surgeon, under Circular Order, dated 1st May 1840 (N. W. P.), as explained by Construction No. 1280.—*Nizamut Adawlut Reports*, N. W. P., 30th January 1854.

surgeon, not having been duly attested and proved, was ignored by the higher court.*

The medical officer's evidence was to be taken in full and *de novo* in the sessions court. The superior court, N. W. P., ruled, in 1854, in a case where the sessions judge, in examining the civil surgeon, had not called on him to repeat *seriatim* his previous deposition in the magistrate's court, but had allowed him to read that document, and had asked him if the replies therein recorded contained the facts of the case,—that this was not the proper mode of conducting an examination. The civil surgeon should, like any other witness, have been directed to state, *de novo*, all the circumstances, to the best of his recollection, referring to any notes he might have to refresh his memory.†

Again—"The evidence of the civil surgeon should have been taken in detail; a mere attestation on oath of a written report, made on inspecting the corpse, is not sufficient, and would imply a want of proper attention on the part of the sessions judge to his duty of elucidating by questions the exact nature of the wounds causing death, and of the weapon with which they were apparently inflicted.‡

In cases which had come under the immediate notice only of a native doctor or sub-assistant surgeon, the civil surgeon may be called upon for an opinion upon the evidence of the subordinate medical officer.

At Moradabad, in 1854, the sessions judge was required by the superior court to obtain the evidence on trial of the civil assistant surgeon as to the cause of death. They directed that the evidence of the sub-assistant surgeon should be read over to the civil assistant surgeon, and such other questions put to the former as the latter might suggest, with a view to elicit more fully the symptoms apparent on the *post-mortem* examination; the opinion of the civil assistant surgeon should then be taken on oath as to the cause of death to be inferred from the symptoms described; and the degree of confidence between mere suspicion and certainty with which the deponent's opinion on the subject might be formed, should be particularly noted. §

In commenting upon the record of a case tried at Bareilly, the judges of the higher court ruled that—"In taking the examination of the civil surgeon, the additional sessions judge should have shown him the cap and dhotee, on which he deposed to having observed spots of blood, and have obtained identification of the same; the omission must be noticed, and the additional sessions judge informed that the examination of the civil surgeon, in its present form, does not reach the prisoner.‖

---

* Nizamut Adawlut Reports of 23rd June and 29th November 1852.

† *Ibid*, 4th April 1854. Again, *Ibid*, 7th April 1854.

‡ Nizamut Adawlut Reports, N. W. P., 11th November 1854.

§ *Ibid*, 27th May 1854.

‖ *Ibid*, 30th October 1852, p. 1260.

The rule at present in operation is that—

"The Court shall receive as *primâ facie* evidence the examination of a civil surgeon or other medical witness taken and duly attested by the magistrate: Provided that it shall be competent to the court to summon such civil surgeon or the medical witness, if it shall see sufficient cause for doing so."—*Code of Criminal Procedure, para.* 368.

It has been ruled that "the substance of a report from a subordinate medical officer, with an expression of concurrence by his superior, cannot be received in evidence under section 368 of the Code of Criminal Procedure.

It is directed, in Bengal Police Circular, No. 19, dated the 17th September 1869, that—"With a view to facilitate the compilation and circulation, for general information, of complete medico-legal reports of the most important criminal cases,—

"1*st.* On receipt of the memorandum (Form No. 26) from the court officer, showing the result of a case in which a report has been asked for from the civil surgeon, the district superintendent will communicate the final order in the case to the civil surgeon in as few words as possible, with a reference to the report above mentioned. Ordinarily, it will be sufficient to note whether the accused has been convicted or accquitted; but in cases where the final order appears to be opposed to the medical evidence, the civil surgeon should be furnished with any remarks made in the decision regarding that evidence. These remarks will be communicated to the district superintendent by the court officer when reporting the result of the case.

"2*nd.* In sessions cases, the court inspector will obtain necessary information through the Government pleader (who will have access to the records) and will furnish it to the district superintendent in the same manner as in other cases."

In a trial at Furreedpore, in 1850, the sub-assistant surgeon gave conflicting testimony before the magistrate and the sessions judge, as to the cause of death. This, of course, led to the acquittal of the parties. The superintendent of police attributed this to his want of knowledge of medical jurisprudence, and to his not having been accustomed to give evidence in public, so that he became confused.*

I pay no undue compliment to my own Profession when I state that, having read carefully from every source whence my research has been able to draw them, all trials conducted in India bearing upon the subject of this work, I have met with very few and trivial instances in which the *Medical Evidence* has not been given with knowledge, caution, and precision.

The following evidence, in which a want of clearness and accuracy is apparent, is one of the very few to which judicial objection has been made.

It appeared that the accused was seen by certain witnesses to strike the deceased, with a *surkee* (or small spear), in the calf of the right leg, as he was running away. The judge remarked that certain

* Police Report, L. P., for 1851, p. 43.

witnesses proved the sooruthal, which stated that the deceased had four wounds on the calf of the right leg; but the civil surgeon deposed to there having been, in reality, only two wounds, both of which passed through the leg, and consequently left four marks, which would account for the witnesses (being ignorant natives) imagining these marks to be distinct wounds; and that these wounds had been caused by a sharp weapon like a spear, one of the blows having divided the artery; and that the death of the deceased resulted from the loss of blood occasioned by the wound. The judges of the higher court observed that "the whole of the eye-witnesses depose, in the most circumstantial manner, to what is clearly a deliberate falsehood. It appears that, when the body of the deceased was examined in the mofussil, the impression of the bystanders was that there were four distinct wounds in the leg. The prosecutor's witnesses have, accordingly, framed their story so as to meet this state of facts. They swear that Puddolochun first inflicted one wound, and that Ramanund followed, and inflicted *two* or *three*. When the body was examined by the civil surgeon, however, it turned out that, in reality, there were only *two* wounds. It is impossible, we think, for any one who reads the evidences, and observes the minuteness with which witness after witness details the circumstances attendant on the wounding of the deceased, to suppose that this could possibly have been a mistake. It is clearly intentional, and is fatal to the credibility of the evidence.

"We acquit the prisoners, and direct their release. We should have ordered the witnesses for the prosecution in this case to be committed for perjury, but that the evidence of the civil surgeon has been so carelessly given that it would be impossible to found a conviction upon it. In his letter to the magistrate, reporting the result of his examination of the body, he describes *one* wound, and says, 'I did not observe any other wound or mark of injury on the body.' In his evidence before the magistrate, he says: 'there was also another superficial wound on the same leg.' Before the judge he states that 'there was also, not far from it' (the principal wound) 'another wound, but this was merely superficial and of no consequence; but it passed superficially through the integuments of the leg, so that a native may have considered them four wounds, but, in reality, there were only two.' He states also that he 'cannot say from the appearances of the wound whether it was inflicted from before or behind, because it was probably inflicted by a weapon of about the same breadth throughout.' This is a very unsatisfactory answer, and we cannot comprehend why the judge did not question the civil surgeon further on this point, which was one of great importance. If the wound was given from behind, the orifice in front of the leg must, necessarily, have been considerably lower than that behind; and the reverse must have been the case if the wound was given in front; while, if the two orifices of the wound were on a level, the inference would be that the man must have been lying down when the wound was inflicted. The judge will be good enough to furnish the civil surgeon with a copy of these remarks ; and be more careful himself, in future, not to leave in doubt a point of so much importance to the elucidation of the case."

IDENTITY OF THE LIVING.

Some of the reviewers of my edition of 1856 were rather severe upon my disregard of this question. One of them observed : "This omission is extraordinary in a work on Medical Jurisprudence, for a country in which fraudulent personation is very common, and the difficulty of identifying criminals is very great."

The fact is, that there have not occurred, within my experience or reading, many Indian cases in which medical evidence could be brought to bear upon questions of Identity of the Living.

My *Commentator* remarked that : "The crime of fraudulent personation, like many other crimes, receives great facilities from the custom of *purdah nusheenee*. The object in view is generally the unlawful securing of an inheritance, or the prolongation of a lapsed pension. In the latter case, the fraud may continue for years undiscovered, as the only loser is Government ; but, in the former case, private interests being at stake, the opposition of the real heirs will generally elicit the truth. The audacity of some of these frauds is quite astounding. In a case, which was tried before the Supreme Court three years ago, an impostor had the face to pretend that he was identical with a Benglee gentleman whose death-consignment to the Ganges, some years before, was plainly proved. He allowed the latter fact, though he denied the former ; and declared that he had revived after being thrown into the river, and had since lived as a fakeer. In this case the medical evidence was of importance, as the body of the deceased had been eaten away by an incurable disease. The converse of this case is the denial of Identity of criminals who have for some time eluded justice. Men commit crime and disappear. They are at last apprehended at a distance from their homes, or in their own villages, where, after many years, they have returned and settled, saying, 'surely the bitterness of death is past.' In many cases their appearance is so altered by age or disease, that it is very difficult to identify them. We have seen a man apprehended, some ten or fifteen years after he absconded, in the last stage of atrophy. He absconded in consequence of having been concerned in an affray ; so the inference is that he had then some personal strength and activity. When captured, he had scarcely the strength to stand, and his frame was so emaciated, so shrunk, so utterly hapless and lifeless, that he looked more like a mummy than a man. Others conceal their identity by much simpler means. Shoobratee, who was hanged at Benares for murder, by poison, in 1853, returned to his own village at the time when the search was hottest for him, with no other disguise except a thick beard. He was so altered by this appendage that, for some time, his own friends did not know him. At last his own step-father, or father-in-law, recognized him, and gave him up to justice. The greatest difficulty of all is not when the witnesses cannot, but when they will not, identify a person to whose criminality they have previously sworn. Cases of this kind are not of unfrequent occurrence; they are quite heart-breaking to men who take an interest in bringing criminals to punishment instead of opening every loophole for their escape. Here is a case of the kind, and unfortunately it is founded upon" [?] "fact. Ramsuhai, son of Gunga Ram, of Loochapore, Zillah Moorshedabad, was concerned in a barbarous murder. The deed was committed before a crowd of witnesses, who all swore to Ramsuhai as one of the perpetrators and gave an accurate description of his person. Ramsuhai, being an accomplished ruffian, had, among other personal peculiarities, the scar of a sword-cut on his forehead, and a few other scars on difficrent parts of his person. All these were recorded at the time of his flight, with his parentage, caste, residence, and other particulars. A few years afterwards, Ramsuhai was apprehended, but lo! not a witness would identify him. Their depositions were read to them—yes; they allowed that the depositions were true, but 'THIS is not the Ramsuhai whom I saw commit the murder.' Name, father's name, residence, height, appearance, apparent age, and particular marks, all tallied with the recorded description; still the witnesses swore that 'this was not the Ramsuhai; they had never seen this man;'—and so the ruffian escaped."

The most remarkable Indian case in which medical evidence may yet be useful, in a great question of Personal Identity, is that of the most atrocious of unapprehended criminals. He, if still existing, bears upon his body marks of surgical treament which might be recognised with absolute certainty.

Several persons have been taken into custody in consequence of their personal resemblance to this miscreant. One of these was admitted in a dying state to the Medical College Hospital, and my curiosity has seldom been so highly excited as it was when I made search (of course in vain) for these damnatory *stigmata*.

The extreme difficulty which may attend questions of Personal Identity received such typical illustration in that which will be long known as the Cannon Street Murder of 1866, that I shall preserve the facts in the words of a contemporary writer.*

"Never did circumstances tell so terribly against an innocent man. A woman, known to have been subject to threats, was found murdered, and the man who threatened her was almost accidentally discovered. This man, when traced, proved to be a bad sort of scamp, not exactly of the

* The *Spectator*, June 16, 1866.

criminal class, but still bad enough to extort money from a poor woman, distrusted by his own relations, and associating with a very doubtful set of characters. He himself, moreover, not only admitted that he had extorted money from the murdered woman, Sarah Millsom, but that he had expected the police to arrest him on that charge—an admission the police probably thought extremely unlikely if the expectation had been genuine, while the device of confessing a minor offence to conceal a capital one is exceedingly frequent. Then spots were found on his coat believed to be blood-stains, though they were only stains from some material used in his trade, which might very well have been blood-stains if Smith had cut himself in shaving or accidentally touched a newly-killed animal. Further, it seemed that he was long enough away from his home at Eton to have been in London at the time of the murder, about ten p. m. on May 11. It was proved that he said he was going to London about seven o'clock on that night, and that the remark excited some surprise. It was also deposed by a lamplighter and another witness that they had seen William Smith going at half-past seven on the 11th towards the Slough station, that they had spoken to him, and that he had on a tall hat and a dark coat. It was proved by a constable that he was in the High Street of Eton about a quarter to twelve, and it was shown by satisfactory evidence that there was one train from Slough at 7-43, by which he might have gone to London, and another by which he might have returned before the constable saw him. Finally, a respectable person, housekeeper in a neighbouring house in the City, swore that she saw him leave Messrs. Bevingtons' house just at the time when the murderer must have left it. There was no reason whatever for suspecting this woman of improper motive of any kind, and she firmly believed the accused to be the man she said, singled him out among fourteen people, and swore most positively to a high hat and dark clothes. It would be almost impossible for circumstantial evidence to be more perfect. Here was a man of bad character who acknowledged himself guilty of a crime towards Sarah Millsom, who was shown to have said he was going to London, shown to have been seen going to a station which a London train would pass, and recognized by an honest witness as having left the house in which the murder was committed at a time which tallied exactly with its commission. Nothing but a motive was wanting, and, in the face of undoubted facts, the law does not always require that motive should be proved.

"And yet there cannot be a doubt, if evidence is worth anything at all, if in fact the very basis of every system of trial is not rotten, that William Smith was totally innocent of the murder. The circumstances had lied against him almost as if they had been sentient. There was but one train from Slough that evening by which Smith could by possibility have reached London in time to commit the crime, and that train left Slough at 7-43. By that train the prisoner, though he did walk towards Slough 'to meet a woman,' as he told one witness, certainly did not go. Henry Harris, a hatter, met him in Eton Square at 20 minutes past 6, and did not leave him till 10-10, still in a beershop in Eton. Henry Coster, photographer, confirmed this statement in detail. So did John Starling, a brazier, so did Henry Holderness, a gardener, so did G. Dodner, a boot-maker, so did John Mathews, a photographic printer, so in fact did ten or twelve men, all of whom stated circumstances which induced them to recollect the day, and all of whom must have combined to perjure themselves if the accused was not in Eton while the murder was being committed in London. The theory of such combination is too absurd for consideration. In the first place, they had no motive for such a crime; in the second, average English scamps abhor murder just as much as English respectables, drawing a distinct line between it and every other crime; and, in the third, they were supported by a very remarkable bit of moral evidence and an equally remarkable bit of physical testimony. The accused from the first said he had never left Eton that night, this point being fully admitted by the police. Now, we take it to be almost a certainty that, had Smith committed the crime, he would not have denied going to London, but have invented some story to account for his going, sure that the mere fact of his journey would be traced. The physical evidence was merely that, as Smith certainly was in Eton at 7-30, he must have run the whole way to the Slough station, while the Windsor station was quite close, and the same train stopped there. Nobody, aware how a man like Smith detests exertion, would believe any assertion of the kind, unless supported by positive evidence, instead of being denied by a cloud of independent witnesses. The evidence for the defence is unanswerable, so perfect that no one who reads it will doubt that Baron Bramwell, in declaring Smith 'not only acquitted, but innocent,' was right."

Of late, the art of Photography has been used, in Bengal, with considerable success, as a means of identifying criminals,—their portraits being taken bearded and shaved. I showed, three years ago, in *Notes and Queries*, that this custom is a revival of one which prevailed in England in the time of Elizabeth. The "*Ugly Pictures*" of some notorious impostors and malefactors of that period are still preserved.

POISONS.

The abundance in which a large variety of deadly plants spring up in the hot and moist atmosphere of Bengal, and the unrestricted freedom with which nearly all the most potent kinds of mineral and vegetable poisons can be purchased in every Indian bazar, added to the familiarity with the action of narcotics which has arisen from their daily habits of opium-eating and hemp-smoking, sufficiently account for the prevalence of the crime of secret poisoning among a timid people, who, except when wrought up to a state of frantic excitement, always prefer treachery to violence in the execution of their crimes.

It cannot be doubted that, under the Mussulman dynasty, assassination by poison became, if not the most prevalent, undoubtedly one of the most prominent of court atrocities. As the closing act of a great political contest, as a means of removing a stubborn minister or an intriguing kinsman, the Datoorah, with its power of gradually drowning the astutest intellect in a state of drivelling fatuity; and the Arsenic, certain to destroy existence in a night, with symptoms which the most learned hakeems could not distinguish from those of cholera (even then one of the most prevalent diseases of India), wrought as effectually, and, as the assassins doubtless consoled themselves, far less noisily and unseemly than the wheel at the Grêve and the axe on Tower Hill.

According to Strabo, the custom of burning Indian widows was introduced as a check to the women's practice of poisoning their husbands. Captain Hamilton, who traded in India between 1688 and 1723, reports this legend, apparently from oral tradition :—" In Canara there are several customs peculiar to itself, and many of them are spread abroad to remote countries. Here it was that the custom of wives burning on the same pile with their deceased husbands had its beginning. It is reported that, before the Brahmins invented this law, poison was so well known and practised, that the least quarrel that happened between a married couple cost the husband his life, and this law put a great stop to it ; and now custom so far prevails that, if any faint-hearted lady has not courage enough to accompany her spouse to the other world, she is forthwith shaved and degraded, and obliged to serve all her husband's family in all kinds of drudgery."

So also Purchas quotes Plericus to the effect that " the cause of burning the wives is by some ascribed to their wonted poisonings of their husbands before this law. He also cites the narrative of W. Methold :— " It is, amongst these Indians, a received history that there was a time when wives were generally so luxurious that, to make way for their friends, they would poison their husbands, which to prevent, a law was made that, the husbands dead, the wives should accompany them in the same fire."

Several poisons and some harmless substances are not unfrequently employed in India as philtres or as aphrodisiacs. In 1864, a woman, who was tried at Kurrachee for administering stupefying drugs to her husband, pleaded that it was a love-charm for the purpose of regaining his affections, which had become weak. In 1863 a woman in the Midnapore District caused her hushand's death by mixing what she was led to believe was a love-potion in his food. She was acquitted of criminal intention by the Magistrate.*

The author of an article on witchcraft in the Central Provinces affords us† a very interesting glimpse of this mode of poisoning as it prevailed in

* Second Annual Report of the Inspector General of Police, Lower Provinces, 1863, p. 23.
† Once in a Way,—a Jubbulpore Miscellany.

that part of India so recently as 1866. He tells us that the art of preparing philtres, love-potions, and other potent mixtures for producing magical effects on mind or body, flourishes now in India as widely as ever it did among the Greeks and Romans, or in Europe, where it cannot yet be said to be quite extinct. "It is," he says, "mostly practised here as everywhere else, by jealous women, or desperate lovers of either sex, for the purpose of captivating affection, of infatuating and enthralling the object of desire. But it is also used for baneful purposes, to cause disease, death, or some strange aberration ; and whether employed by love or by hate, it has certainly always been intimately connected with some real knowledge of medicine, and has veiled a great deal of downright poisoning. Many months ago a man was tried before one of the courts of these provinces for giving to a woman a poisonous mixture which she administered to her husband, and from which the husband died. His defence was that the wife asked for a love-potion, and that he supplied nothing else ; but there was clear evidence of an intrigue, and he was convicted of abetting the murder. The ingredients of which these philtres are ordinarily compounded, are, to this day, not a whit less disgusting than the contents of the witch's chauldron in 'Macbeth' ; and perhaps Shakespeare got from the East the idea of adding a tiger's chauldron (entrails), and a baboon's blood."* For further information on this point see next chapter—*Employment of Arsenic as an Aphrodisiac.*

I was, some years since, consulted by a judicial officer in Bengal upon the question whether a person could be rendered impotent by eating owl's flesh. Upon this we are told, at p. 15 of the *Taleef Shareef* (the work of a Delhi Hakeem), that "those who eat of owl's flesh may expect to be deprived of all reasoning faculties with loss of memory." "The women of India give it to their husbands, that, by the mental weakness it produces, they may obtain more liberty of conduct than might otherwise be agreeable."

We are told in the same work, that—"If the flowers of the Black Dhatura be bruised, and a little of your own blood added, and this used as a *tilak* or ornament on the forehead, betwixt the eyes, whoever sees it will become your slave, be it man or woman. If a wife uses it her husband will never forsake her." †

It would appear from the remarks on poisons in the Shastras, that this crime was by no means unfrequent among the Hindus at an early period, and the story of the Indian king who sent to Alexander the Great a fair woman fed with aconites, is at least evidence that there was great affectation of subtlety in the professors of this crime. We read,

* See Herklots's Customs of the Mussulmans of India, p. 341, "*Concerning the method of establishing Friendship between two persons.*" Also Forbes, who says (*Orient. Mem.*, Vol. 2, p. 266), "The instances brought to light in Court" (in the Bombay Presidency) "were generally more intended for destruction by poison than for the creation or renewal of love."

† Page 82.

in Wise's translation, that—"It is necessary for the practitioner to have a knowledge of the symptoms of the different poisons, and their antidotes; as the enemies of the Raja, bad women, and ungrateful servants sometimes mix poison with food. On this account, the cook should be of a good family, virtuous, faithful, and not covetous, not subject to anger, pride, or laziness. He should also be cleanly, and skilful in his business. The practitioners should have like qualities, with an intimate knowledge of poisons; and should examine the food to be eaten by a Raja in the cooking room. This should be large, airy, light, and surrounded with faithful servants, and no one should be allowed to enter unless he is first examined. In the *Mitakshara* Shastra there are copious directions regarding the manner of detecting a person who gives poison—he does not answer questions, or give evasive answers; he speaks nonsense; rubs the great toe along the ground, and shivers; his face is discolored; he rubs the roots of the hair with his fingers; and he tries by every means to leave the house. The food which is suspected should be first given to certain animals, and, if they die, it is to be avoided."*

As rarely fails to happen when crime of any kind is the lesson taught, the common people of this country were in no way behind their masters in the practice of empoisonment; and it is probable that various modes of assassination by drugs, first made known by the hukeems of Aleppo and Bagdad, and freely employed by Shah Jehan and Aurungzebe, are still practised in the jungle villages of Hindustan and Bengal.

A complete and accurate list of all the vegetable poisons obtainable in Indian bazars, especially of those which are known to have been employed in the destruction of human life, together with full details of the operation of those the effects of which upon the system are least known, is still a great desideratum.

Impressed with this fact, Dr. Mouat, in 1843, addresssd the Government of India, reporting that the greater number of cases of poisoning which

---

* Tavernier, in describing his visit to Gwalior, the great state prison of the Mahomedan sovereigns, says—"When Aurungzebe sends any great lord to this place, at the end of nine or ten days he orders him to be poisoned; and this he does, that the people may not exclaim against him for a bloody prince."

It can scarcely be doubted that Hyder Ali dealt in this manner with some of his English prisoners. James Bristow states, in the narrative of his captivity, that "the month of September 1793 was distinguished by the inhuman murder of General Matthews, who was certainly poisoned in a very barbarous manner, being starved until he had consented to eat of the food which he had discovered contained poison. He refused for several days to taste nourishment, but hunger surmounted at last the desire of protracting a miserable existence, and he swallowed a plentiful portion of the victuals prepared for him, and in a few hours after expired in violent convulsions."

Again, "Captain Rumley, when he found that he would be constrained to swallow poison, put an end to his own existence." "Lieutenant Frazer had poison forced down his throat, of which he soon after died." There is confirmation of this statement in the memoirs of Captain Philip Melville and in Forbes's Oriental Memoirs.

he was called upon to examine, in his capacity of Chemical Examiner to Government, were those in which vegetable substances were used, from its having become generally known, among native hukeems and vendor of drugs, that mineral poisons can invariably be discovered, even when existing in extremely minute quantities; but that most vegetable matters cannot be distinguished by any processes of analysis known to, or practised by, European chemists. With a view, if possible, to prevent this, and to put a stop to the large amount of crime which can thus be committed with impunity throughout the country, he suggested that he might be furnished with the means of carrying out an extended series of experimental inquiries on the subject. For this purpose, he recommended that a circular letter should be addressed to the various magistrates in this presidency, requesting them to procure from the bazars, native druggists, and other sources from which such substances are likely to be obtained in their several districts, samples of the various vegetable poisons known to be usually resorted to for criminal purposes, with their names, the modes in which they are prepared and administered, the properties ascribed to them by the natives, and, in fact, every information which could be elicited on the subject, and which would be likely to serve hereafter as a guide to the judicial and chemical investigation of such cases. He observed that the substances should, if possible, be procured in such quantities as to enable the examiner to perform a series of trials, so as to modify them in the many ways that would be necessary in endeavouring to arrive at any determinate result in a comparatively untrodden field of observation.* The Government, considering that the magistrates were not the proper authorities to be called upon for the information sought by Dr. Mouat, requested that the Medical Board would consult the civil surgeons at the different stations, whether samples of the various vegetable poisons, known to be usually employed for criminal purposes, could be procured by them for Dr. Mouat's examination; requesting them, at the same time, to furnish such information as might be useful to Dr. Mouat in his proposed experiments. A circular to that effect was accordingly issued by the Board. This appears, by the filed reports, to have been responded to by only twelve medical officers,† who sent in the names of about thirty-six vegetable substances stated to be used as poisons and procurable in their stations. These articles have been embodied in the "*List of Vegetable and Mineral Poisons procurable in the Bazars of India.*"—Appendix A.

Many of the vegetable substances described,—as the Datoorah, Gunjah, Aconite, Kurrearee, Gunch, Lall Chitra, Kuchila (*Nux Vomica*) with its

---

* Letter No. 57, of May 18th, 1853.

† Messrs. Dickens of Balasore; Morton, Banda; Cumberland, Pooree; Macnab, Ghazeepore; Pitt, Backergunge; Shaw, Agra; J. McRae, Muttra; Lightfoot, Bolundshuhur; Barber; Griffith, Jubbulpore; Greig, Seetapore; J. Macrae, Monghyr.

Viscum, Kakmari (*Cocculus Indicus*), and Kurrubee (*Oleander*) are poisons, and are employed by the natives as such. Others, as the Mishmee Bish, &c., &c., are somewhat doubtful, both with regard to their botanical characters, and to most of the circumstances under which they are employed, and deserve a very careful investigation. A third set, among which are the Isamel or Esser Mhool (*Aristolochia Indica*), and probably several others, are to be considered as powerfully medicinal rather than poisonous.* Several of the reports bear strong evidence of the great unwillingness and suspicion which are nearly always displayed by uneducated natives when called upon to afford aid in the elucidation of questions of this kind. Still, the result of the inquiry was sufficiently encouraging to render its repetition highly advisable.

Of late years, the increase in the number of dispensaries and the importation of chemicals into India have occasionally led to poisoning by such agents as the Sulphate of Zinc, Burnett's Solution, Prussic Acid, Strychnine, Cyanide of Potassium, Chloride of Cadmium, Belladonna, Chlorodyne, &c.; but these must still be regarded in the light of extraordinary accidents.

Great as is the obscurity which envelopes the history of many of the poisonous substances used in India, the present inquiry leads me to feel convinced that the number of poisons which are used freely by the natives of the three Presidencies, is very limited indeed. The chief of these are comprised in the following table :—

I. The Preparations of Arsenic Aconite ... ... Nux Vomica ... ... Opium ... ... Lall Chitra ... ... Oleander	For Assassination and Suicide.		
II. Datoorah ... ... Gunjah	With a view to producing intoxication, insensibility or fatuity, but not perhaps with intent to kill, although death frequently results from their use.		
III. Lall Chitra	For Abortion.		
IV. Sulphate of Copper ...	... ...	Given as medicines in poisonous doses.	
Arsenic ... ... Snake Poison, &c.	In the *Bish Baree.*		

Doubtless, further experience may call for additions to this list, and especially to the 3rd and 4th classes; but it must be repeated that the number of poisons commonly employed with criminal intent in India

* The *Aristolochia* was, however, ranked by the ancients among the weak poisons.

probably does not much exceed that given in the 1st and 2nd classes of the above list.

A few notes on the employment of these poisons in India may usefully supply the deficiencies in the English standard works on Medical Jurisprudence.*

For the earlier editions of this work, I carefully perused and made use of the records of the office of the Chemical Examiner to Government, which (together with a published report by Sir William O'Shaughnessy Brooke) comprise details of all the chemical examinations made in cases of poisoning, &c., by Dr. O'Shaughnessy, Dr. Mouat, Mr. Siddons, and Dr. Francis Macnamara, from 1840 to 1844, from January 1849 to January 1851, and from May 1852 up to June 1854.

For an abstract of the most important facts which have been elicited in the Calcutta Chemical Examiner's Office, subsequently to 1854, by Dr. Macnamara and Baboo Kanny Lall Dey, Additional Chemical Examiner, I am indebted to the courtesy and able diligence of the latter officer.

ARSENICAL POISONING.

Arsenious Acid, and the Yellow and Red Sulphides of Arsenic are imported into this presidency in remarkably large quantities. I have ascertained that the principal supplies of White Arsenic are brought to Calcutta from the Gulf, in Arab ships. Some also is brought from Europe. The bazar value of Arsenious Acid was, 14 years ago, about twenty-five rupees per maund (of eighty pounds). The Yellow Arsenic comes from Oude; that of a superior quality brought from eighty rupees to ninety rupees per maund. Another cheaper and coarser description of the Yellow Sulphide is imported in greater quantities from Rangoon, where its value was then about thirty rupees per maund; this latter appears to pass largely into the interior of the country. Red Arsenic also comes from the territories of Oude; and it is found native in China. Its value was then from thirty rupees to forty rupees per maund, according to its quality. The prices are now considerably higher than they were fourteen years ago, that of White Arsenic being rupees 30 per maund; Red, rupees 50; Yellow (from Rangoon), rupees 50; and Yellow (from Oude), rupees 100.

It has long appeared to me a matter of great practical importance that the Arsenic trade in India should be strictly and authoritatively watched.

In a table given by Horace Hayman Wilson, in his *Review of the Exter-*

---

* I have, with much reluctance, refrained from adopting the usual scientific mode of classifying the poisons spoken of in the following pages; but, upon full consideration, I think it most convenient to adhere to my old arrangement, in which the foremost places are given to those poisons which are most used in India.

nal Commerce of Bengal, from 1813-14 to 1827-28, I find that there were 4 out of the 15 years in which White Arsenic was imported to Calcutta from Pegu, at the value per annum of from rupees 5,467 to rupees 28,818. Yellow Arsenic was imported from the same source in 6 of the 15 years, to the value annually of from rupees 2,220 to rupees 15,988. At rupees 30 per maund; this would give a (rarely occurring) maximum annual importation of 533 maunds. In 1850-51, 422 maunds and upwards passed the Custom House. In the following year it was only 83 maunds. In 1852-53 it was 260, and in the two following years it was only 6 and 13 maunds respectively. Mr. J. A. Crawford, Collector of Customs in Calcutta, has most kindly furnished me with a table showing the total quantities of Arsenic (of all kinds) which were imported through the Custom House every year from 1854-55 to 1868-69 inclusive. The quantities imported in each of these 15 years were as follow,—in hundred-weights :—2,501 ; 1,342 ; 1,020 ; 304 ; 407 ; 674 ; 1,162 ; 830 ; 551 ; 464 ; 11,813 ; 758 ; 2,234 ; 378 ; 2,035 ; and 502 in January and the first 26 days of February 1870.

The following are among *the* (legitimate) *Uses to which White Arsenic is put* in India. Large quantities are thrown into the holds of vessels,—an imperfect, and of course dangerous, mode of cyanising the timber, and of checking putrefaction and the generation of animal life.

In the same manner, when piles are used in filling up tanks in the loose moist soil of Bengal, with a view to building on the sites thus obtained, large quantities of Arsenic are sometimes thrown in, on, and around the wood.

There is a considerable consumption of White Arsenic in wall-washes and about the ends of roof-beams as a protection against white ants, bugs, and other insects. It is also used in the preparation of the thicker kinds of leather by harness-makers, &c. The Arsenic trade seems to be almost entirely in the hands of natives.

ARSENIC.—*Arsenious Acid*; *White Oxide of Arsenic.*—*Sumool-Khar,* H. *Sanchya,* S. (Fleming) *Phenáshmabhasma,* S. (Wise), *Suffed Súmbhul,* Ind. and Cash. (Honigberger)—May be bought freely, at a very low price, in nearly all Indian bazars.* Dr. Honigberger says that, in former times, and probably at the present day, any one could purchase Arsenic at Lahore from the druggists, on simply stating that he was in the habit of eating it or *that he wanted it for the destruction of rats.*

This ancient and almost universal pretext for buying the strongest of all poisons, and most useless of all chemical substances, likewise prevails in Bombay, and also in Madras. This is the common plea upon which

* In 1868, Dr. Mair, Deputy Coroner of Madras, wrote—" Reported cases of murder by poi-son are exceedingly rare, and yet perhaps in no other part of the world do there exist greater

criminals purchase the drug from the only too facile bunneahs Up-Country. The wife of a man who had died by poison declared that she had administered to her husband a powder, given her by her paramour, to cure him of impotency! The bunneah from whom the Arsenic was bought, stated that the male prisoner had purchased two pice-worth of arsenic (about one and a half masha weight) *to kill rats.** A prisoner at Seharunpore asserted, in his foujdaree confession, that he had purchased Arsenic for the purpose of *destroying rats*, and that his wife had taken it by mistake. It was proved, however, that he had purchased arsenic, mercury, and sulphur, with the object, as he stated, of curing itch.† In 1854, one Bijyee, Brahmin, of Bareilly, confessed that his widowed sister having been seduced and thrown upon him for support while pregnant, he determined to kill her. Telling her that he would take her back to her late husband's relatives, he, while on the road, poisoned her with Arsenic, with which he had provided himself on pretence of *poisoning rats.*‡

Again, at Tipperah, upwards of 700 miles from the scene of the above tragedy, we find a prisoner giving his mistress a fatal dose of poison, with a view, as he said, of procuring abortion, although he must have been well aware of its effects, as he had previously used it *to kill rats.*§

I, many years ago, published the first draft of the subjoined statement, which displays at a glance the steady and almost systematic manner in which the lives of men have been sacrificed to this particular mode of vermin-killing, from Chaucer's day up to the present time.

---

facilities for procuring poison than in the bazars and gardens of India. Arsenic and its various compounds, corrosive sublimate, opium, stramonium, and other deadly poisons are openly sold in the bazars in any quantity, and unrestrained by any license; while many other equally deadly poisons are to be found in gardens. With such facilities for procuring poison, there is little doubt that advantage is taken of them to commit murders which are never recorded as such, and when some suspicious circumstance does ooze out afterwards, all attempts to prove the crime are rendered abortive by the absence of the best of all evidence, *viz.*, the dead body, which has been burned within a few hours after death."

Two interesting cases of poisoning by Arsenic in *Bombay* are recorded by Mr. Heddle in the first volume of the *Bombay Medical and Physical Transactions.* See also two others in Bellasis' *Bombay S. F. A. Reports*, Vol. 1, pp. 37 and 178.

Several, occurring in *Madras*, are narrated by Native Surgeon Moodelly in the *Madras Quarterly Journal of Medical Science* for October 1862.

* Nizamut Adawlut Reports, N. W. P., 8th March 1852, p. 1607.

† *Ibid*, 9th April 1853, p. 522.

‡ *Ibid*, 13th October 1854, p. 551.

§ Police Report, Lower Provinces, for 1848, p. 37.

XIV. CENTURY.

" And forth he goth, no longer wold he tary,
Into the town unto a potiocary.
And praied him that he him wolde sell,
Some poison that *he might his ratouns kill;*
And eke there wal a polcat in his heme.
And fayn he wolde him wreken if he might,
Of vermine that destroied him at night."

(Chaucer's Pardonour's Tale.)

XVI. CENTURY.

" Thou art accused of giving eight shillings money to William McGillivirie's dame, to pass to Elgin, for buying *rateoun poison*, who wared thereof but sixteen pennies; and brayed the said poison, and put it in one piece leather, and delivered it to thee in June," &c.—*Indictment of the Lady Fowlis for Witchcraft and Poisoning*, 1590.*

XVIII. CENTURY.

" Lieutenant Oglivie told him that he wanted to buy some arsenic in order to *destroy some dogs* which spoiled the game."—*Medical Evidence in a Trial for Poisoning in* 1765.

It appeared at the trial of Donellan for the poisoning of Sir T. Broughton, 1781, that the deceased was in the habit of keeping large quantities of Arsenic in his room, and that he used it, with very little caution, *to poison fish*.

"She" (Eleanor Johnson) "purchased three penny-worth of white mercury at an apothecary's, under pretence of its being *to kill rats.—Report of an Inquest in the Literary Magazine* for 1789, p. 315.

XIX. CENTURY.

" She purchased one penny-worth of Arsenious Acid, 'for the purpose,' she said, '*of destroying rats.*' "

" He swallowed half an ounce of Arsenious Acid (purchased) upon the usual pretext of *killing rats*."—*Northern Jour. of Medicine*, Novr., 1845.

" She stated that she had procured poison twice for the purpose" (of poisoning her mother, her four brothers, and two other persons). " She had procured it on both occasions by saying that she *wanted it for the destruction of rats*."—*Med. Gazette*, June, 1846.

" She was proved to have gone to one shop to buy poison under the pretence of *destroying rats;* and, at another, where she succeeded in procuring an ounce, she stated that it was for destroying bugs."—*Ibid*, August 1847.

" She said that, knowing where her master kept Arsenic *for the destruction of rats*, she had taken and put it into the milk."—*Report of a Trial at Nemours*, in July, 1851.

" He added that it was he who had furnished Arsenic to Paris (the murderer) who said *he wanted it to poison rats.* This witness kept arsenic by him, using it occasionally for diseases of his sheep."—*Report of a Trial at Aube*, August, 1851.

* Burton's Narratives of Criminal Trials in Scotland.

Strange, that so weak a lie should be traceable as having passed current in all Europe, as a cloak for homicide, since the fourteenth century; and that it should be equally valid throughout all India at the present moment!

"The *Rat*," said my *Commentator*, "is usually a Husband."

Still again, fourteen years later, on the 28th of October 1869, we find the following verdict delivered in the Calcutta Coroner's Court:—"The deceased died from the effects of Arsenic, having eaten some sweetmeat which had been mixed with arsenic by his master *for the purpose of poisoning rats*."

I am indebted to a native medical officer of considerable experience in Upper India for the following note on *some of the Diseases in which Arsenic is used by native practitioners*.

Arsenic has long been used among the natives of Asia in the following diseases:—

(a).—In intermittent fevers, the White Arsenic of commerce and its Sesquisulphuret (Orpiment) are both used by the native physicians, who generally prefer the ashes in prescribing this poison instead of the raw mineral.

(b).—In remittent, the common continued, and typhus fevers, Arsenic is also used by the native physicians; in fact, it is indiscriminately used by them in all classes and types of fever.

2. Arsenic is also used as an aphrodisiac, in cases of recent, as well as in long-standing impotence. The up-country fakeers, who are generally considered to be a very skilful class of *hakeems* for this complaint, suppose that it has a wonderful effect in invigorating and in exciting the virile powers.

3. Opium-eaters in India are sometimes known to have recourse to Arsenic in lieu of their favourite drug, and they generally suffer very little in gradually accustoming the system to the use of the new drug, and in abstaining themselves from the use of the old one. Sub-Assistant Surgeon Meer Ashruff Ally has seen this done at Agra.

4. It is moreover used, as an alterative, in rheumatism, gout, and in secondary syphilis.

5. Lastly, Arsenic is likewise an useful external remedy among the native hakeems, who generally use it as a wash, made up with milk or some such bland liquid, in various skin diseases, especially the scaly varieties, such as, lepra, eczema, psoriasis, &c., &c.

Arsenic is, I believe, rather largely employed in itch and other skin diseases in India. A few remarks on this subject have been recorded* by Sub-Assistant Surgeon Ockhoy Coomar Dey of Urmitsur. One of my own students systematically took Arsenic for itch. In the case of one Kisto Moochee, who was tried at East Burdwan for poisoning a child

---

* Indian Medical Gazette, November 1, 1866, p. 327.

with White Arsenic,* the prisoner is stated to have asserted at different times that "some rats had bitten and dropped some poison," he did not say what poison, from the roof on to the floor of the house, and that the child had eaten it ; and again, that one Gobordhun Moochee was suffering from a dicease called *goorgooree,* and that he had been about to apply some arsenic to him externally, and had put some out to-day for that purpose in the sun, when the child took it up and ate it. White Arsenic is given by the Bengal koberajes in the Bish Baree and in some other preparations. For further information regarding the employment of Arsenic in native medicine, see the *Chapter on the Employment of Poisons by Native Practitioners,* and the *Taleef Shereef,* page 99 (*Soombool Khur*).

The records of the Chemical Examiner's office, during the periods already referred to, contain reports of the discovery of White Arsenic, either in food, &c., known to have been given with a felonious intention, or in the stomachs, &c., of persons dying under suspicious circumstances in *twenty-three instances.*

I am indebted to Baboo Kanny Lall Dey for a table which shows that, between the years 1855-56 and 1870 (up to the 25th of March), there have been brought before the Calcutta Chemical Examiner *two hundred and eleven* cases in which White Arsenic was used to poison man. In the 15 years the number of cases ranged from 6 to 20 annually.† Guy says that, in the two years 1837-38, Arsenious Acid was the ascertained cause of 185 deaths ; according to the *Times,* the number of deaths from Arsenical poisoning in England and Wales, in the five years 1863-67, was 83.

In some few of these Indian cases, the quantity detected amounted to a mere trace ; but in many, it was noticed as being sufficient to destroy eight or ten persons. In a large proportion of cases of poisoning by White Arsenic, up-country, the drug is administered in enormous quantities. The late Dr. Kenneth Mackinnon informed me that, in some of these cases, he has known vomiting occur so rapidly, and with such great activity, as to free the stomach before the poison could enter the circulation.

In one case, a woman confessed that she had administered three doses of White Arsenic to her son-in-law. The man appears to have been ill three or four days and received native medical treatment.‡

In another case, where a small quantity of arsenic was discovered in the stomach, the individual survived four days.§ In Europe, the speediest

---

* Nizamut Adawlut Reports, 9th September 1859, p. 245.

† It will be observed that these statistics of the Calcutta Office do not represent at all fully the extent to which poisoning by this and other drugs exists in the Bengal Presidency, as for some years past Chemical Examiners to the Governments of the Punjaub and the N. W. Provinces have been established at Lahore and Allahabad.

‡ Nizamut Adawlut Reports, N. W. P., 6th February 1852, p. 105.

§ *Ibid,* 2nd September 1852, p. 960.

death observed was in twenty minutes (with tetanic symptoms). Some cases have proved fatal as late as the second or third week; and, from secondary symptoms, in two or three years (Guy).

Many years ago, Mr. Macleod Wylie related to me the following case, as an illustration of the difficulty which is often experienced in fathoming crime in India.

Two Bengalees, say T. and S., were always quarrelling and getting up law-suits against each other. S. was sent to jail. It was then given out that peace had been concluded between them. T. visits S., at his request, in jail, and brings him a present of sweetmeats from Kali Ghat. S. gives the alarm that he has been poisoned, is seen vomiting into a vessel, the contents of which are sent to Dr. O'Shaughnessy, the Chemical Examiner, who reports that the vessel contained enough White Arsenic to poison a horse. On further investigation, the Chemical Examiner said that it was by no means certain that the poison had ever been in the stomach of S.*

In the generality of cases of poisoning by Arsenic, the criminals state that their victims died of *Cholera*. See Nizamut Adawlut Reports, N. W. P., 9th April 1853, p. 522; *Ibid*, 31st May 1854, p. 596, &c. Dr. Morehead (Vol. I., p. 377) cites a report of one of the Bengal Charitable Dispensaries, in which it is stated that advantage is sometimes taken of the prevalence of Cholera for the perpetration of acts of criminal poisoning, in consequence of the lessened chance of detection which exists under such circumstances of the public health. Dr. Morehead says—"I concur in the justness of this remark, for I am sure, from my own observations in Bombay, that criminal poisoning, chiefly by Arsenic, is not rare, and that the great collapse which speedily comes on after a large quantity of the poison has been taken, sufficiently resembles that of Cholera to render the mistake, in Cholera seasons, when suspicion has not been aroused, by no means an improbable one. If we have the opportunity of examining the vomited and dejected matters during life, there can be little difficulty in determining the question. The florid tongue and tender epigastrium of gastritis will also assist in the diagnosis; but if, in fatal cases, doubt still remains, a *post-mortem* examination will at once remove it."

---

* This mode of destroying an enemy, by placing him in the light of a criminal, is well understood in India. At the beginning of the present year, one Syed Abdoolla was convicted at the Bombay Criminal Sessions on a charge of fabricating false evidence against one Mahomed Bucksh, with a view to procuring his conviction as a forger of Government promissory notes. He caused a box, containing some false notes, and all the necessary implements for forgery, to be placed in his enemy's house, and then led the police to its discovery. He was sentenced to three years' rigorous imprisonment.

Not many years ago, the implements of coining were discovered in a Bengal jail. The circumstance was, at first sight, a very astonishing one, but it is probable that they were introduced with the intention of still further implicating a prisoner.

The circumstances under which the poison was administered are frequently left altogether unexplained ; in many cases, however, it was evidently given with intent to kill or disable. In my second edition, I stated that I found three instances in which it was employed with a view to procure abortion. Baboo Kanny Lall Dey has recently mentioned to me a similar case which occurred at Hooghly. It terminated fatally. Another case occurred at Barrackpore. It appeared at a trial at Tipperah, in 1857, that the first means adopted for the purpose of making a girl abort was to administer a mixture of chitta root and some Arsenic. This failing, other still more violent measures were resorted to.

As most of the cases of poisoning by White Arsenic reported in the Chemical Examiner's Records do not present any peculiar features which distinguish them from similar instances occurring in Europe, I shall only cite one of them as an example of the utterly reckless manner in which the thugs and other robbers of this country —whose criminal practices will presently be described—employ poisons with a view to disable their victims. In January 1854, two travellers were attacked at eight o'clock in the evening with vomiting and purging soon after having taken food in the neighbourhood of Allahabad. They died about day-break next morning. Upon examination, the medical officer found a bright redness in the stomachs and upper part of the small intestines of both, leading to the opinion that a poison had been administered, although no irritant was detectable by the naked eye. The stomachs, with their contents, were forwarded for analysis, together with a powder found on the person of the suspected party (one Bhowaneedeen—doubtless a thug poisoner by profession), described by him as cough medicine, and some of the flour with which their bread was made. Dr. Macnamara discovered considerable quantities of Arsenic in both stomachs ; this poison was also detected in the powder and in the flour.

The powder containing the Arsenic was described as being of a *black* colour. In a case also, where a young woman, at the instigation of her paramour, administered Arsenic (as was afterwards proved on *post-mortem* examination) to her husband's parents, the prisoner declared that the poison was a *black* powder.* In this case it was proved that the Arsenic, when purchased, was white—the man who bought it also spoke of it as white ; but the woman, who asserted that he gave it to her to administer to her husband for the cure of his impotence, always described it as black. It is, however, probable that, in these cases, the colour of the poison is disguised, perhaps with ground spices, before it is administered. In this trial, the Judge questioned a native druggist, who stated that a preparation made from Arsenic, by a slow and expensive process of refinement, is sometimes

* Nizamut Adawlut Reports, N. W. P., 18th January 1854, p. 49. *Ibid*, 8th March 1852, p. 160.

given as medicine for impotency ; this substance he called "Kooshtah," and said that it is white. He added that ignorant persons might, by subjecting Arsenic to the process of burning, make it black, and administer it for medicine, without any of its deadly properties being refined out of it.*

Use of Arsenic as an Aphrodisiac. At page 110 allusion has already been made to the practice of *Arsenic-eating* in India. This is by no means unfrequent in the Punjab, where (except when it is made an alternative of opium-eating) it is, I believe, generally employed as an aphrodisiac agent. The avidity with which medicaments of this class are sought for in Upper India may be judged by any one who casts his eye down the pages of the *Taleef Shereef*, the *Ulfaz Udwiyeh*, and Percival Lord's papers in the first and fourth numbers of the *Bombay Medical and Physical Transactions*.†

Mr. Bowser, Purveyor to the Medical College Hospital, informs me that, when at Rawal Pindee many years ago, he used frequently to speak to a Fakeer, who avowed that he ate White Arsenic largely as an aphrodisiac. This man was found one morning dead in his hut—perhaps from an over-dose of the poison.‡ He also knew a wood-carver who used Yellow Arsenic in colouring his work. Enquiring once of this man how he could venture to handle a deadly poison so freely, he put some of the flakes into his mouth, and said that he would not mind eating a lump of Hurtal. [Yellow Arsenic is given rather freely to horses in this country. It is said to make them froth at the mouth when champing the bit, and to improve the smoothness and glossiness of the skin. I understand that, in Calcutta, this coarse preparation has now given way to Fowler's Solution, —one or two drachms being given twice a day in low condition, dry skin, eczema, &c.]

---

* According to Baboo Issurchunder Gangooly, Arsenic, as well as several other powerful drugs used in native medicine, is made to undergo certain preliminary processes, called "*Sodhana*," by which it is supposed that their medicinal qualities are enhanced, and their deleterious ones modified, or redered mild in the required degree. Two plans are practised near Midnapore. In the first, the Arsenic is pounded and macerated in cow's urine for 36 hours. In the other, it is introduced into a portion of the green trunk of the munsasij (*euphorbia ligularia*), and, being covered with the bark of the same plant, the whole is exposed to a good fire until the external parts of the wood are completely charred. The Arsenic is then fit for use. This may possibly explain the black appearance of the Arsenic.

Native Surgeon Moodelly says that, in Madras, Arsenic, as well as all powerful native medicines, is subjected to a series of boilings in milk, cow-dung, urine, the juices of leaves, &c., and is then said to be purified. He considers that this purification renders Arsenic, in medicinal doses, more easily tolerated by the system.

For much information regarding the various forms of Arsenic, and the manner in which they are prepared, see the *Taleef Shereef*, pp. 99 and 173.

† No. I, page 276, and No. IV., page 115.

‡ I find the following note among my papers ; but I have lost the clue, probably in consequence of my never having had an opportunity of making enquiry of Dr. Macrae before his unexpected death :—

"Dr. James Macrae,—(Byragees' bags seized, and found to contain *Arsenic.*") Arsenic used as an Aphrodisiac by Fakeers, *vide supra* p. 113.

Several allusions to the use of Arsenic in Impotence have been made in the preceding pages (111, 113, 116).

The Jubbulpore case (*supra* page 105), in which a husband was killed by some drug administered as a philtre, was singularly repeated, many hundred miles off, at Raneegunge in 1868. A woman confessed, on being apprehended, that she had obtained a drug from an old woman who told her that, if she could get her husband to eat one of the pills, he would love her ever after and not ill-treat her again. On the old woman's house being searched, several pills of the kind the deceased had given her husband were found, and the Chemical Examiner reported that each of them contained a large quantity of Arsenic. The accused afterwards declined to confess. Two witnesses proved that she gave her husband some *goor* and *choorah*, on eating which he complained of a burning sensation in the throat, commenced vomiting, and died shortly after. The accused was committed to the Sessions, but acquitted by the Judge. The Judges of the High Court, however, expressed it as their opinion that there was sufficient evidence for conviction.*

Here the question will naturally occur—granted that the Jubbulpore man had a sinister motive in supplying the poison—what could have induced the old woman at Raneegunge to incur the great peril of dispensing the Arsenical pills ? The reply is that, as in native medicine Arsenic is one of the most powerful of all aphrodisiacs, it is within the bounds of possibility that both of these poor creatures gave this poison without any desire to kill. The author of the *Taleef Shereef* tells us that, on account of the danger which attends the use in medicine of the six kinds of Arsenic, he seldom gave these remedies internally, and adds—"I usually confine my use of them to external application, *and as Aphrodisiacs, which I prescribe to a few friends who may have derived no benefit from Yunani prescriptions.* It is better, however, to use as few of them as possible."†

The author of this work states that White Arsenic is used by alchemists in the transmutation of metals.

In a note to the index of this book, it is stated that a few articles contained in the original work, *viz., medicines principally used in Sorcery and Incantation,* have been omitted. This is rather to be regretted.

Arsenic given in poisonous doses as an Anti-Syphilitic, vide supra page 113.—Dr. Beatson alludes‡ to a case of death from poisoning in which the defence set up was—administered medicinally for the cure of a venereal affection. Arsenic amounting to twenty times a medicinal dose was, how-

---

* Bengal Police Report for 1868, p. 214.

† Page 99.

‡ Precis of Medico-Legal *Post-Mortem* Examinations made in Dacca during the year 1865.—*Indian Medical Gazette,* Vol. 1, p. 82.

ever, discovered in the contents of the stomach by the Chemical Examiner; therefore, there must have been, on the part of the administrator, either murderous intent, or gross ignorance of the nature of the drug.

In another case, it appeared that the deceased had sought the advice of one Bhanoo Bebee, who was believed to be possessed of a sovereign remedy for venereal disease. The remedy, it is said, was effectual, though violent. Several persons had been subjected to it, and the effect had always been pain in the stomach, vomiting and purging, which, passing away in a day or two, left the patient thoroughly cured. The accused Bhanoo admitted that she had administered some pills with the intention of curing the deceased. They were composed, she said, of "*Darmooch*" and a white substance, a quantity of which had been left her by her late husband. What it was she did not know, and she had none left. Dr. Beatson adds,—"The substance *Darmooch* is said to be a poisonous wood." I do not find mention of such a wood by Watson, Balfour, or elsewhere. In the *Taleef Shereef, Darma* is one of the six kinds of White Arsenic; in my own list of poisons procurable in India, we find—"*Darmooz*, preparation of arsenic?" and in a MS. list of poisons used in Bengal obtained by my friend the late Mr. Joseph R. Bedford, *Darmooz* is also given as a preparation of Arsenic.

At a trial at Midnapore in 1857, it appeared that Ramakant Pandah, being desirous to remove Binodram Nund, sent for a Hindu having several *aliases* who (Bindoram being a sufferer from syphilis, and desiring to restore his virility) administered to the unfortunate man a mixture of White Arsenic and *mera shingah* (aconite), which caused his death the following afternoon.*

The diabolical crime of *Poisoning Well or Tank-Water*, upon a probably false suspicion of which multitudes of Jews were executed during the prevalence of the Black Death in Europe, is, unhappily, not unknown in India. It is mentioned† that, in the winter of 1815, the army in Guzerat, on reaching their camping ground near a respectable town called Cheekansir, learned that the enemy's cavalry had been there, and had poisoned all the tanks and wells with wheat impregnated with Arsenic, a plan which, it was supposed, would prevent the mineral from sinking and losing its deadly properties. The water in the wells was highly poisonous, and orders were given not to draw any from them. Some of the followers, however, suffered before this was known; but the body of water in the tanks was too great to be affected by the quantity of Arsenic thrown in.

In January 1868, Dr. Thomas of Kyouk Phyoo sent to the Calcutta Chemical Examiner, a bottle containing a blackish looking matter (decomposed vegetable matter) mixed with a substance of clay-like appearance in

* Nizamut Adawlut Reports, July 21, 1857, p. 90.

† Fifteen Years in India, p. 355.

a semi-solid state. It was obtained from a well in the station of Kyouk Phyoo, the water of which, when used, " produced vomiting, giddiness, and irritation over the surface of the body." Baboo Kanye Lall Dey subjected the clay-like substance to Reinsch's test, and discovered Arsenic in considerable quantity. R. Fitch, who visited this part of India early in the seventeenth century, says, that he went from Bengala to the country of Couche (Cooch Behar), where " in time of warre they poyson all the waters." The remark has been volunteered to me by one well acquainted with the country, that this practice is by no means unknown in peaceful Bengal. For notes on poisoning tank water in Nipal and Burmah, see the Chapter on *Aconite*.

The late Mr. Henry Piddington, Coroner of Calcutta, sent me two cases, in which unmistakable and very violent symptoms of irritant poisoning distinctly arose from eating the *salted ox tongues* commonly sold in the bazars of Calcutta. It is certainly also remarkable that I was, two years ago, consulted in the fatal case of an European lady in this city, who was attacked with cholera shortly after having eaten some cold slices of such a tongue at breakfast. I should have considered that the poison here was an animal one, except that Mr. Piddington notes—" I have heard from several persons that, in hot weather, *Arsenic* is used to make the meat take the salt, a portion being mixed with the salt." Thus used, it would, doubtless, also assist to prevent the meat from becoming tainted. It is remarkable that, in one of Mr. Piddington's cases, where several of a family were poisoned, a dog, which it was believed had eaten of the tongue, was also sick. It appears that, in Europe (Taylor, M. J., p. 277), dogs and cats are not affected by eating diseased or tained meat which produces symptoms of irritant poisoning in man.

Mr. Bowser, Purveyor to the Medical College Hospital, tells me that a married soldier of H. M.'s 44th Regiment, at Kurnaul, obtained from the mess khansamah some stale salt beef, of which the whole family, consisting of five persons, ate at breakfast. Shortly afterwards all were seized with symptoms of cholera, severe purging, incessant vomiting, and very great prostration. The extremities were cold, but there was no lividity or shrivelling of the fingers, as in cholera. The youngest, a child of three, died ; the rest recovered. Some thought this was copper poisoning, but the copper cooking vessels were surveyed, and were found to be properly tinned. This may have been either animal or mineral poisoning.

State of the Heart in Deaths from Arsenical Poisoinng.—In 1866, Dr. Bonavia, of Lucknow, stated* that, in several cases of Arsenical poisoning, he had invariably found livid patches in the inner lining of the heart, more especially that of the left ventricle, about the *columnæ carneæ*, so much so that, in cases of suspected poisoning, he always examines the heart first, and, if he discovers these patches, he invariably finds Arsenic in the stomach. The greater or less size and depth of colour of the

* Indian Medical Gazette, Vol. I., p. 252.

patches appears to bear some proportion to the more or less extent and intensity of redness in the mucous membrane of the stomach.

He refers to an observation by Andral that Arsenic is one of the causes of *endocarditis*, and gives the following quotation from Pereira:—"The heart is mostly flabby, and it is asserted that, on its inner surface (especially the *carneæ columnæ and valves*, particularly on the left side) is observed redness, sometimes diffused, sometimes in the form of spots, which penetrate a line in depth into the substance of the heart."

He, however, notices that Dr. Taylor, in his work on Poisons, rejects the idea that there are any heart changes which indicate Arsenical poisoning. Dr. Bonavia suggests that—"when the natives use Arsenic for poisoning they do it thoroughly;" and suggests that, where death is caused by comparatively small doses, this cardiac lesion may not be produced. Dr. Bonavia's observation has since been confirmed by several Indian authorities.

Dr. Kenneth McLeod, then of Jessore, gives the case of a young man, of good caste, and well educated, who, having contracted syphilis, took the disgrace so much to heart, that he killed himself by swallowing half a tolah (90 grains) of Arsenious acid.

On *post-mortem* examination four hours after death, the left ventricle of the heart was found empty, *lining membrane of a dark livid colour;* this tint was deeper on the *columnæ carneæ* than between them, and was well marked over the whole surface of the cavity. The deep colour extended about an eighth of an inch into the substance of the heart, and seemed to be owing to a layer of blood extravasated beneath the lining membrane, which was quite smooth; otherwise the heart was not in any way affected by the poison.

Mr. McReddie found, in a Mussulman of Hurdui,—"patches, which might be termed *sub endocardinal ecchymosis* in the left ventricle, about the *carneæ columnæ*, not in them. These patches extended about a line in depth. They were not numerous, but were well marked." The Chemical Examiner for Oudh found "unequivocal proofs of Arsenic in the stomach."* Dr. Harris, of Shahjehanpore, narrates† the case of a young Mussulman, who committed suicide by swallowing White Arsenic. The following were among the more important *post-mortem* appearances:—pia matral vessels immensely congested; extensive sub-arachnoid effusion of serum; a little extravasation of black blood on the upper surface of the left hemisphere. The left ventricle of the heart contained a little fluid blood, and its lining membrane was deeply stained in vertical patches of an inch in length, penetrating to the depth of a line or two into the substance of the heart; no Arsenic in the stomach; mucous membrane not highly congested. The small intestines contained lumps of White Arsenic of the

* Ind. Med. Gaz., March 1, 1867, p. 75; see also a similar case by Mr. M., *Ibid*, April 1, 1868, p. 84.

† *Ibid*, May 1st, 1867.

size of a pea. The large intestines were filled with fluid fœces deeply tinged with bile, and the mucous membrane was covered, in one or two places, with what looked like a little dab of yellow paint. Dr. Harris's remarks on these appearances are very suggestive :—

"It has been said that the size of the patches in the heart appears to bear some relation to the extent of those met with in the stomach; I think, however, it should rather be said that they both are related to the greater or less amount of the poison taken. As some small doses of Arsenic cause congestion of all the internal organs, it does not require a great stretch of the imagination to conceive that a larger dose may produce a stage of disease in advance of this, in the form of effusion from the already congested vessels of these organs, constituting, in the brain, serous or sanguinous effusion into the meshes of the arachnoid ; and, in the heart, sanguinous effusion into the endocardium. The last, perhaps, immediately due to the bruising of the congested capillaries of the endocardium, by the powerful muscular action of the left side of the heart. It will be very interesting in future to observe the stethoscopic sounds in these cases during life. With reference to the *post-mortem* symptoms of serous apoplexy in this case, I may mention that I have met with this state of the brain before. I find entered in my case book, on 29th August last, in a *post mortem* on a case of undoubted Arsenic poisoning, the following :— 'Much effusion of blood and serum upon the brain.' This state of the brain is worthy of remark, as Taylor does not mention it in the 6th edition of his Medical Jurisprudence. The patches of yellow paint-like substances found in the large intestine in this case, have been before observed by me in suspected poisoning by *White* Arsenic, and they give one the idea that the drug used was Orpiment, though really the colour is due to the presence of bile."

My friend and colleague, Dr. Woodford, Police Surgeon of Calcutta, lately gave me what appeared to be a few minute *Gall-Stones.* He found about half a salt-spoonful of these loose in the stomach of one who hanged himself (probably when suffering from belly-ache, *vide* Chapter on Suicide). The stomach presented patches of inflammation nearly resembling those of arsenic poisoning. Dr. O'Shaughnessy also had a similar case of *Gall-Stone* in the stomach, with similar inflammation of the mucous lining of that organ. *Vitiated Bile* a powerful irritant—Paris, M. J., Vol. II, p. 159.

Yellow Sulphide of Arsenic.—*Orpiment.*—*Hartal,* H ; *Haritala,* S. (Fleming). In Calcutta, the kind imported from Oudh is called *Basputtee.* This is probably the preparation of Arsenic most frequently employed as an internal medicine, as a depilatory, and as a pigment in India. All the bright yellow colour which Hindus apply to their foreheads, and which they use in painting their Doorgas, &c., is prepared from the Yellow Sulphide. In this Presidency, very large quantities of Orpiment are consumed in the manufacture of shell lac, chiefly at Mirzapore, Beerbhoom, Bancoòrah, and Calcutta. Hartal is extensively used in the Bengal Presidency in making paper which, thus prepared, is secure against the attacks of white ants and all other insects. The story of the king who was poisoned in the turning over the leaves of a manuscript has been used as an argument that the *Alf Lailah wa Lailat,* or Thousand and One Nights, is of Indian origin, because it was only in India that such paper was known in ancient times. Formerly, Yellow Arsenic was much used by rich Calcutta natives in colouring the walls of their rooms. According to Dr. Percival Lord, the natives inhabiting the borders of the Indus sometimes employ the *Zurd Sunkiah,* or Yellow Sulphide* in small doses (they said *half a ruttee,—three quarters of a grain*) for obstinate cases of intermittent fever. A similar practice prevails among the Bengalee doctors, and is sometimes followed by calamitous results. I understand that a case occurred some years since, in which a respectable native, enraged with a kobiraj who had administered a fatal dose of Arsenic to his child, seized a weapon and struck the unfortunate practitioner dead.

For some of the uses of *Hartal* in native Medicine, see page 173 of the *Taleef Shereef.* Hartal as a horse-medicine, *vide supra,* p. 117.

The Chemical Examiner's Records (anterior to 1856) contain *eight* instances in which this poison was discovered, either in very suspicious compositions, or in the stomachs of persons dying with symptoms of irritant poisoning. The subsequent records, from 1856, inclusive, give a further total of *fifteen* cases.

Baboo Kanny Lall Dey has obliged me with notes of the following case. A sepoy at Ballygunge (a suburb of Calcutta) attempted to poison his comrade by mixing Yellow Arsenic with the cooked dal kept ready for his dinner when he was away on duty. Although the bright yellow colour of the dal disguised that of the poison, the discovery of a large lump of the Hartal created suspicion. *A handful* of Yellow Arsenic was found mixed with the dal.

The following case is abridged from Dr. O'Shaughnessy's printed report :—

On the 21st October 1840, Dr. O'Shaughnessy received the remains of a rice pudding on the copper plate in which it had been cooked. It was stated that this pudding had been served, the evening before, at Major H——n's table ; that Mrs. H., her European servant, and metranee had eaten of it ; that Major H. had tasted it ; and that all had been immediately taken ill. A bitter taste was observed by the parties, and the pudding was said to be discoloured. Upon analysis, it was found that it was the

* Mr. Campbell, C. S., when at Azimghur, stated that the natives of that country describe as " Yellow Arsenic " a variety of the White Arsenic which has a yellowish tinge, but which is quite different from Orpiment.

Sulphuret of Arsenic which had been used, and that impregnation of the pudding with copper was not the cause of the illness of the sufferers. Dr. O'Shaughnessy was inclined to believe that the substance introduced was one of the compound native poisons, of which Orpiment is an ingredient, and not the pure arsenical poison alone. The bitterness of taste, the proportionately small quantity of Arsenic present, and the symptoms of giddiness and intoxication experienced in two of the cases, were his chief reasons for entertaining this opinion.

This report also records a case of murder by (Yellow ?) Arsenic, and detection of the poison in the remains of two individuals after *ten months'* interment without coffins.—A most interesting and instructive detail.*

Dr. Burton Brown also notices† that, when much Arsenic is present, the stomach often remains, even in the hottest weather in India, firm, hard, and with a peculiar smell, and the tissue is so little altered that the condition of inflammation can be easily recognized. This, however, he adds, is not always the case ; sometimes the tissues are dried up or partly converted into adipocire.

He cites the case of a native of Mozuffergurh, who ate a small chupattee cooked separately, while his companions shared a large one between them. Almost immediately afterwards he complained of great pain and became violently sick, and died two hours afterwards. He was buried without a coffin. A month afterwards suspicion was excited, and the body was dug up. It was very much decomposed with the exception of the stomach, which was evidently much inflamed and contained the remains of a chupattee, and a large quantity of Yellow Sulphuret of Arsenic.

RED SULPHIDE OF ARSENIC—*Realgar,*—*Mansil,* H.,—*Manah Sila,* S. (Fleming).—This was detected in a suspicious powder sent for examination from Hooghly in March 1841. It only appears twice in the Calcutta Chemical Examiner's records since June 1855. It is sold in all the bazars. I am informed that it is also used by the hakeems and kobirajira. I have found it among a bunneah's stock forwarded by the police. It appears to be employed for the removal of superfluous hair, &c.‡

Dr. Burton Brown refers in his work to two cases of poisoning by ARSENIATE OF POTASH AND LIME, probably made by heating common White Arsenic with impure nitre, "shora." It was employed in both cases for poisoning cattle. In animals this drug produces symptoms similar to those excited by Arsenious Acid—diarrhœa especially being very severe.§

In the Calcutta *Englishman* of the 19th November 1867, Baboo Kanye Lall Dey states that a medical friend at Agra had recently sent him for

---

* Bengal Dispensatory, pp. 721-28-29.

† A Description of the Poisons used in the Punjab.

‡ For descriptions of several preparations of Arsenic used medicinally by the Byeds, kobirajira, and hakeems of Bengal, *see* papers by Baboo I. C. Gangooly,—*Bengal Hurkaru* Medical Column, for Feb. 7, and Dec. 11 and 18, 1852.

§ Op. Cit., pp. 45 & 56.

analysis a powder which he said was largely used in the Upper Provinces for dyeing native sweetmeats. The powder was *Magenta* (roseine), an aniline colour, and preparation of Arsenic. The proportion of poison it contained appeared to him so great, that he was of opinion that the use of it in confectionery would have a most injurious effect on the health of those eating such sweetmeats. He learnt from another medical friend in Calcutta, that certain wealthy Mahomedans were in the habit of tinging their pilaus with red Magenta. He noticed that it was also much used by native women and children in painting the lips, hands, and feet. He has since seen a child endangered by swallowing a small portion of it while painting the lips.

Chronic Poisoning by ACETO-ARSENIC OF COPPER.—Two cases of *slow poisoning, caused by sleeping in rooms papered with Arsenical Green,* have been reported in India.

Dr. Shortt relates* that, during the extreme heat of July 1862, a gentleman at Chingliput (Madras Presidency) slept in one of two papered rooms which communicated by an open arch. He soon found that, although he slept well, he awoke unrefreshed with a feeling of malaise, nausea, loss of appetite, diarrhœa, and sometimes syncope, thoroughly unfitting him for his work ; but, towards evening, this feeling gradually passed away, and he felt better. These symptoms continuing for a few days, suspecting that there was something wrong in the room, his medical adviser directed him not to sleep there. No sooner was this room given up, than the patient felt better, and the most prominent symptoms disappeared. The diarrhœa and tendency to syncope, continuing to be persistent, called for tonics and astringents. The paper in the room had an apple-green ground, on which are large green flock leaves, the dust of which can be easily rubbed off by the finger ; and that these symptoms arose from Arsenical poisoning, there can be no doubt, for, on scraping off a small quantity of the dust, and submitting it to Reinch's test, a large proportion of Arsenic was found to exist. The assistant to the Chemical Professor, Madras, detected "Arsenic in pretty good quantity" in this paper.

Dr. Shortt pointed out the evils likely to ensue when the house had been papered some four or five years previously.

Dr. Horace Day reports† the case of Mr. ——— of the Civil Service, who came under his care at Malwar, S. Conean (Madras Presidency), with symptoms to a certain extent resembling those of dysentery. This disease being rare in the station, Dr. Day sought another cause for the symptoms, which soon became patent. Mr. ——— had been using as a bed-room a room which had lately been re-coloured. This colour proved to

* Madras Quarterly Jour. of Medical Science, October 1862, p. 460.

† Indian Medical Gazette, Aug. 1, 1866, p. 219.

be ***Arsenite of Copper*** put on very loosely with size, ***a colour much used for decorating rooms in that part of India.*** The case proved to be, beyond any doubt, one of chronic poisoning by Arsenic. But besides the symptoms of poisoning by Arsenic, a periodic headache, lasting about six hours, came on every other day. It appeared that he had formerly suffered from Guzerat fever. Here then was a cause for the headache which lasted after the other symptoms had abated ; removal from the bed-room having removed those, quinine soon cured the headache. Attention is drawn to the fact that the Arsenic and the fever poison were simultaneously at work. Dr. Day suggests that, but for the Arsenic, tertian fever might have occurred instead of mere headache.

The men (habitual workers in this green colour) engaged in scraping the Arsenic off the walls appeared not to suffer in any way, although the room was closed while this was being done, to prevent the poison-laden atmosphere from getting about the house.

Paralysis from Arsenic Poisoning.—Dr. Morehead gives* the case of a Mussulman of Bombay, 17 years of age, who was brought to hospital on the 20th of April, suffering from symptoms of acute Arsenical poisoning. He had become affected the preceding night after having eaten curds. It appeared in evidence that the milkman (from whom the curds were obtained ?) had purchased Arsenic, he said, at the boy's request ***for killing rats.*** It was, however, held, in the subsequent trial, that the lad took the Arsenic with suicidal intent. He was discharged on the 30th of April, and re-admitted on the 7th of the following month. He had then pneumonia ; but, besides this, he had become considerably emaciated, and there was partial paralysis of both upper and lower extremities. The hands drooped from the wrists, and the fingers were bent somewhat backwards, and the hands were closed feebly and with difficulty. He was able to bend the knee-joints but imperfectly, and he lay stretched with the feet extending, and the toes pointing downward. The pulse was 100 and feeble, skin cool, the tongue whitish in the centre, not florid at the edges, but there was tendency to diarrhœa and evacuations were passed in bed. He complained at times of pain in the arms and legs ; and there was a good deal of desquamation of the cuticle of the hands and about the shoulders. He was discharged on the 4th September. The paralysis, though less, still existed in considerable degree. He was unable to walk. The emaciation was less, but still considerable. There had been no return of diarrhœa.

I have (unfortunately) only a slight note of the case of a Cavalry Officer, who came before the Medical Board in Calcutta, about ten years ago, in a state of considerable emaciation and cachexia, and with paralysis

* Clinical Researches on the Diseases of India, Vol. II., p. 618.

of the fore-arms almost as complete as I have ever seen in painters. This was clearly traced (I think by Dr. Clifford) to Arsenical poisoning.

Mr. Jayakar,* admitted one Foola Mona to hospital at Ahmedabad (Bombay Presidency) with Carter's Disease of the foot, in an advanced stage. The leg was amputated, and, except that there was an attack of secondary hœmorrhage, the stump did well ; but anœsthesia of both hands, which had been complained of on admission, continued to increase. The hands were partially paralysed, and the flexors of the fingers were strongly contracted. It was discovered that, two months before his admission, he had a poultice applied for about a week by a hakeem, which contained nearly three ounces of Arsenic, and an incredible quantity of cayenne pepper (seven pounds). This having given rise to constant vomiting and purging, the Arsenic was omitted after the second (?) application. It was followed by a burning sensation throughout the body, which, after the operation, continued to be present in the extremities, the stump not excepted. The symptoms in the hands made their first appearance a fortnight after the last application. He gradually improved under peroxide of potassium and tincture of belladonna, until he was discharged cured in about nine weeks. These cases of Arsenical Paralysis may be advantageously collated with others mentioned by Pfeffer (*Taylor on Poison*, p. 316) and Guy (3rd edition), p. 453.

In the *Quarterly Journal of the Calcutta Medical and Physical Society*, for July 1838, Dr. Duncan Stewart published some observations showing the *injurious effects of the Yellow Sulphuret of Arsenic employed in the manufacture of shell lac.* He showed that the employment of Hartal in this manufacture produced upon the bodies of the work-people "an eruption of a miliary, dry, and popular character."

See Taylor on Arsenical Eczema, *Medical Jurisprudence*, p. 197, and Guy on the eruption produced by Aceto Arsenite of Copper in makers of paper-hangings, p. 453.

Native Surgeon Ruthnum Moodelly says that the village quacks in Madras occasionally use sulphate of copper as an antidote (emetic) in Arsenical poisoning. A lump of the salt, of unknown weight, is rubbed on a cut-lime, which is then squeezed into the mouth to be swallowed. An acquaintance of his assured him that a sister of his died from the effects of this poison when given as an ordinary emetic.

He adds that the froth of the soap-nut is extensively used as an errhine and emetic, but that it is very disagreeable, irritant, and uncertain in its action on the stomach.† Baboo Ka ıye Lall Dey informs me that the washings of stinking fish, and human ordure, are used by the natives of Bengal as emetics in cases of poisoning. In a case of Arsenical poisoning, which

* Indian Medical Gazette, September 1, 1869.

† Madras Quarterly Journal of Medical Science, October 1862, p. 312.

occurred lately at Tipperah, we are told that the "symptoms were not relieved until the man swallowed some human fœces!"

The Baboo tells me that human ordure is also much trusted in Bengal as an antidote in the bites of snakes and go-samps—(the innocuous guana, *varunus flavescens*, much feared in India).

CATTLE POISONING.

The Hindus in ancient times appear to have been prepared against the villanies of Cattle Poisoners. It is ordained in the institutes of Menu that, when cattle die, the herdsman shall carry to his master their ears, their hides, their tails, the skin below their navels, their tendons, and the liquor exuding from their foreheads (?) He was also directed to point out their limbs (VIII., 234).

It is a very remarkable fact that the English Gypsies (whose affinity to the chumars and moochees, who are the most active cattle poisoners in India, has been frequently argued by philologists and historians) are notorious for this practice. Borrow says*—"The accusation of producing disease and death amongst cattle is far from groundless. Indeed, however strange and incredible it may sound in the present day to those who are unacquainted with this caste, and the peculiar habits of the Romanees, the practice is still occasionally pursued in England, and in many other countries where they are found. From this practice, when they are not detected, they derive considerable advantage. Poisoning cattle is exercised by them in two ways; by one they merely cause disease in the animals, with the view of receiving money for curing them upon offering their services. The poison is generally administered by powders cast at night into the mangers of the animals. This way is only practised upon the larger cattle, such as the horses and cows. By the other, which they practise chiefly on swine, speedy death is almost invariably produced, the drug administered being of a highly intoxicating nature, and affecting the brain. They then apply at the house or farm where the disaster has occurred for the carcase of the animal, which is generally given them without suspicion, and then they feast on the flesh, which is not injured by the poison, which only affects the head." So the Miris and other Assamese Hill-tribes eat animals killed with poisoned arrows.

The following case shows that the crime of poisoning the cattle for the sake of their hides has long been prevalent in the Bombay Presidency. In 1846, one Pandoo Wullud Bappoo was tried at Sholapore upon an accusation of having administered to a bullock and a buffalo balls composed of a white substance sewn up in kurbee leaves. The animals died on the same day. The Sessions Judge considered the evidence conclusive of the prisoner's guilt; and, taking into consideration the numerous instances in

* The Zincali, 4th ed., p. 12.

which *mhars* had been detected in poisoning cattle for the sake of their carcases, which by custom are their perquisites, he sentenced the prisoner to be imprisoned.*

Lieut. Bacon, who came to India in 1831, gives a striking account of the practice of poisoning horses, which was long well known to officers, especially to those in the Horse Artillery, as prevailing wherever there were Chumar (skinner) villages along the Grand Trunk Road. He says†—"In the hope of obtaining a horse's skin, which they could sell in the Cawnpore market for one rupee, they would wantonly poison the finest animals, without regard to their value or their blood. Strict attention was necessary to keep all strangers from the neighbourhood of the horses, or otherwise there was little hope of the creatures' preservation. For many years the method of poisoning the horses was a mystery, and it was generally supposed that the edges of the wells or tanks were besmeared with some poisonous matter, in expectation that one horse out of the many might happen to partake of it. It was, however, remarked that the fattest and sleekest horses invariably fell victims, and at last the secret was discovered. The poison was administered in the form of a small pill cast into the horse's hay while feeding.

It appears that the drug was sometimes thrown into the grass before it was brought into camp, possibly by some insinuating villager, who would find an opportunity while standing to talk with the grass-cutters. The plan of cutting the hides to pieces was very generally adopted, and with great success. The moment travellers were seen to be over-secure, they were sure to suffer, especially when they arrived from the Lower Provinces, as they were supposed to be ignorant of the system. Cawnpore is the largest leather mart in all India, hence the inducement to practice this infamous trade.

The Calcutta Chemical Examiners' records contain much interesting correspondence relative to the very prevalent crime of poisoning horses, cattle and elephants. The animals are generally destroyed by the administration of balls, one of the principal and commoner constituents of which appears to be the root of the *Aconitum Ferox*, which is doubtless also the substance most in use among the hill tribes for poisoning spears and arrows. The following details will afford sufficient illustration of this subject.

In September, 1852, the Sub-Assistant Commissary General, in charge of the Government elephants at Dacca, forwarded a portion of the contents of the stomach of an elephant which had died with symptoms of irritant poisoning, together with a portion of meetha bish (*aconitum ferox*)—the poison supposed to have been administered. Mr. Siddons failed to procure even a trace of aconitine from the contents of the

* Bellasis's Reps. of the Bombay S. F. A., Vol. I., p. 261.

† First Impression in Hindustan, Vol. I., p. 356.

animal's stomach. He, however, testified to the poisonous character of the root sent, and gave it as his opinion that about three ounces of root, as fresh as that sent, would be sufficient to destroy the life of a half-grown elephant. It is, however, very difficult to prejudge with accuracy the effects of any vegetable poison upon one of the lower animals. A somewhat similar, but very questionable, case was investigated in the following August, without any satisfactory result. In the preceding May, the Magistrate of the 24-Pergunnahs forwarded a ball which a person had been charged with giving (?) to an elephant with intent to poison it. This was found to be of the size of a small orange. In its interior were found imbedded, without any attempt at intermixture, a small piece of *fresh aconite root* weighing about 20 grains, and a portion of *sulphuret of mercury* nearly a drachm in weight. In August of the same year, the Joint Magistrate of Pubna was informed that the Chumars of a certain village had been for some months in the habit of killing cattle in the neighbourhood, for the sake of their skins, by thrusting into the rectum certain poisonous balls. Some of the prisoners confessed and produced several balls, two of which were sent to the Chemical Examiner. They also produced a pointed stick, at the end of which the ball, it was understood, was fixed, and so thrust into the body. When the stick was withdrawn, the ball remained; the consequences were, that the belly swelled, in some cases a small quantity of blood was passed, and the animal died in about 12 hours in great pain. The balls were found to be perforated with an aperture for the pointed stick, and contained a resinous matter, kept in form by being mixed with a large quantity of hair rolled up somewhat like a silk-worm's cocoon with one end cut off. The nature of the resinous matter could not be decided by analysis. In 1851, four Chumars of Sarun were sentenced by the Nizamut for poisoning cattle with intent to steal their hides. There could not be a doubt that the cows had been killed by inflicting a punctured wound into which poison ('*mahoor*'—Aconite) was inserted. (Returns for 1851, p. 1102.) Balls said to be extensively used for poisoning cattle in Jessore were sent for examination in November 1853. Their poisonous ingredients could not be detected.

When at Lahore, Dr. Honigberger received from the English cantonment, for analysation, a vegetable compound which had been discovered in the form of a ball in the artillery department, where it had probably been deposited for the purpose of destroying the cattle. He ascertained the presence of aconite root in that mass. The coarse pieces were white, having the texture and pungency of the root.

Mr. H. Alexander obliged me with the following interesting note:—
" The principal crime committed in the district of Beerbhoom is poisoning cattle for the sake of their hides. This crime is committed by the hill-men, who invariably confess. The manner in which it is effected is

this. These men lurk amongst a large herd of cattle; and, when they observe one that looks sickly, they puncture the hide near the hip joint with iron needles which have been soaked in some vegetable poison: their arrows are poisoned in a similar manner. The animal lingers for about two or more days, and seldom leaves the spot where it once lies down. Several of these hill-men have been brought to me with the instruments and poison upon them. If I remember right, I sent some of the poison to Dr. W. B. O'Shaughnessy to be analyzed, but I forget the result." (It was, doubtless, a preparation of aconite root.) "The skins are sold to the Chumars."

The Punjabees not infrequently poison their neighbours' cattle (generally with large doses of arsenic) out of revenge, and it is said that in the very north of India, horse dealers sometimes have their horses poisoned.

A surprisingly extensive system of cattle poisoning was discovered, late in 1854, by Mr. G. Campbell, then the Magistrate of Azimghur. The following perfectly trustworthy account is from the *Friend of India*:— "A child was detected administering poison to a cow. Inquiries were made as to his motive, and his replies furnished a clue, which was vigilantly followed, and at last revealed the existence of a widely-organized conspiracy. A few men, perhaps not more than two, had adroïtly availed themselves of the village organization, and turned it into a source of vast pecuniary profit. Every village in the North-West numbers among its officers a Chumar. These men, of the very lowest caste, perform all offices too repulsive for the more respectable inhabitants. As a reward, they obtain the skins of all dead animals. They have, therefore, a direct interest in such deaths; and a leather dealer, aware of this fact, resolved to induce them to increase the number by artificial means. In concert with a native merchant, he procured vast quantities of arsenic, which was distributed, by agents sworn to secresy, to other subordinates. From their hands, it reached the Chumars, who administered it to the cattle, usually in the shape of a ball of flour. The cattle died, and the skins were sold by the Chumar to the poison-distributor at two-thirds of the ordinary price. The agent, in his turn, obtained a commission on the skins, and the bunneah an exorbitant price for his arsenic, while the leather dealer was contented to find skins plentiful and cheap. With such inducements, the practice rapidly increased. Whole classes became initiated into the use of a fearful agent of destruction, and the wealth of the cultivator was swept away, without either detection or remedy."

In the course of this inquiry, Mr. Campbell found that the wholesale arsenic merchants principally resided in the city of Patna, and got their supplies direct from Calcutta. These men all held that the traffic in arsenic was not prohibited by law, and acknowledged that they carried it on actively, not knowing that the arsenic was used for illegal purposes.

They all stated that this traffic had enormously increased within the previous two or three years, and especially within the last year, and that the drug had, of late, been much reduced in price. They knew of no legitimate use to which it was ever applied, except in the composition of medicines, and to mix with the white-wash of English gentlemen's houses to keep off insects. The Patna merchants, their books, and the white arsenic found in their shops, were brought before Mr. Campbell. One man admitted that he had received from Calcutta during last year no less than one hundred maunds, or nearly four tons of the poison, of which his books showed the sale of upwards of eighty-eight maunds, and upwards of eleven maunds were seized in his shop. In the shops of seven dealers in Patna, the total quantity of white arsenic seized amounted to upwards of twenty maunds. It would seem that arsenic had been accumulating in Calcutta for some years previous to the discovery of this system, as the quantity imported had diminished greatly during the preceding five years,—*viz.*, as we have already shown, in 1850-51, 422 maunds and upwards passed the Custom House ; in the following year the quantity was reduced to 83 maunds ; in 1852-53, it rose to 260 ; and in the succeeding years, it fell to 6 and 13 maunds respectively. At the same time, it appeared that, during the nine years ending 1848-49, the average exports of hides and skin of sorts to Great Britain was 14 lakhs of pieces. In 1853, the exports to that quarter of hides alone amounted to 23½ lakhs of pieces. The aggregate of exports, during 1853, of hides to Great Britain, North America and France (the three principal destinations) amounted to 3,209,483 pieces.

It is to be feared that, during the fourteen years which have elapsed since the publication of the above details (in which I consider that I was the first who brought this important subject fully to public notice in all its leading particulars), the crime of cattle-poisoning has not received any permanent check.

The table prepared for me by Baboo Kanye Lall Dey shows that, from the year 1855, a total of *sixty-two* cases of cattle-poisoning, by white arsenic alone, appear in the records of the Calcutta Chemical Examiner. *Twenty-one* of these cases were recorded in 1869, and *six* in the first three months of 1870.

In 1863, Dr. S. E. Burton Brown, Chemical Examiner for the Punjab, reported,* that arsenic is not unfrequently used to destroy cattle in the Punjab in order to obtain their skins, which, in many parts, are the perquisites of the Chumars. Many such cases have been referred from the Peshawur district. In some of these, the poison, in the form of white arsenic, has been simply mixed with attah, and made into a ball of an

* At page 48 of his valuable *Description of the Symptoms and Treatment of Poisons principally used in the Punjab.*

oval shape, about $1\frac{1}{2}$ inches long, which, in one case, contained 19 grains of white arsenic in 1,000 grains. Sometimes grass is mixed up with the ball, to make it more attractive to cattle. In two cases, pieces of grass were moistened with a solution of *arseniate* of *potash*, probably made by fusing white arsenic with nitre, and these were left about for the cattle to eat.

Aconite is, Dr. Brown adds, sometimes used for this purpose, the root being made up into a ball with flour. It usually causes vomiting, great weakness, sometimes purging and foaming at the mouth, and, at last, death.

Native Surgeon R. Moodelly states* that, in Nellore (Madras Presidency), *Chucklers* make it their profession to poison cattle by causing the animals to swallow the poison (often arsenic) in balls of fat or similar bland vehicles. Horses, belonging either to the residents or to travellers passing through the districts, are often sacrificed in this way. Indeed, it has been officially reported by the Collector that the crime is notorious in that province.

In 1856, a man was tried at Sarun for poisoning a bullock, for the sake of its skin. It appeared that the prisoner, in company with three other Chumars, threw down a small bundle of grass in front of the bullock, on eating which it began to bellow, whereupon the owner ran to the spot and took the grass out of the bullock's mouth, and found that some white arsenic was mixed with the grass. In the grass sent for his inspection, the Civil Surgeon found fifty-three grains of white arsenic.

It was discovered that the defendants made a trade of selling skins, and it was shown by the prisoner's own deposition that he had, on a previous occasion, been punished for cattle-poisoning.

The Sessions Judge remarked that thousands of bullocks had been in this way destroyed in a neighbouring district, and many in Sarun.

The crime, he added, was one punishable under the Mahomedan law.

He was sentenced to imprisonment with labor and irons for seven years.†

In the appendix to the Bengal Jail Report for 1868, it is stated that in Jeindah (sub-division of Jessore), the Moochees, it is believed, poison a great number of the cattle for the sake of the hides, but they do it in a manner which renders it difficult to find them out, and, consequently, very few of them are ever brought to trial. Their practice, it would seem, is to put some of the poison in a piece of plantain-leaf, and, in passing through a herd of cattle in the fields, to drop it on the ground. Some one of the cattle is sure to pick it up and eat it. The poison used is a very strong one, and causes death in a very few hours.

Early in 1869, it was discovered that an organized system of cattle-poisoning on a large scale existed at Mymensingh.

---

* Madras Quarterly Journal of Medicine, October 1, 1862.

† Nizamut Adawlut Reports, February 1, 1856, page 313.

*

It is stated in the *Indian Daily News*, that a number of men were observed by some villagers feeding the cattle with plantain and other leaves smeared with a white substance, which the Civil Surgeon ascertained to be arsenic. The criminals had also arranged to give a Mahomedan butcher four rupees for every score of cattle poisoned. Being unsuspected, he was able to lay the poison about among the herds—giving notice, when it was consumed, to the *Moochees*, who then went and skinned the dead cattle. The destruction of cattle in the neighbourhood has been very great, one man alone having lost a hundred head—all he possessed. Arsenic was found in the houses of the accused, and enquiry showed that considerable quantities of the poison had been sold in the bazar. The names of the purchasers, however, did not appear in the shopkeepers' books, and the trade was to a great extent kept secret.

In June 1869, Captain Hedayet Ally forwarded to the Cantonment Magistrate of Dinapore a letter descriptive of this system, as he is of opinion that it is at present in operation. This document is of so much interest that I have given it in the *Appendix B.*

It has been stated in the public prints that, not long ago, the Stud suffered considerably, until the old precaution of cutting the hide in such a manner as to render it useless to traders was had recourse to.

In August 1869, First Class Veterinary Surgeon Hulse addressed a letter to the Government of India, in the Military Department, in which he unhesitatingly affirmed that "the so-called cattle plague or murrain in cattle," then prevalent, was wholly caused by "vegetable poison." I do not think that other observers have confirmed this conclusion. Doubtless the Chumars and Bungies are never more active in the employment of poison than at times when murrain is prevalent.

I was informed a few months ago by Sub-Assistant Surgeon L. N. Bose, in charge of the Chitpore Dispensary, near Calcutta, that, a short time previously, a shoemaker swallowed, in fear of detection, portion of an arsenical (?) ball prepared for poisoning cattle. A merchant in the Calcutta bazar informed Sub-Assistant Surgeon Meer Ashraff Ally that the cattle-poisoners select *Arsenic* with the idea that it gives to the hides of the poisoned animals a good and sleek appearance!

An officer of considerable local experience, now deceased, informed me that, along the Trunk Road, there is, particularly at about the time of the Sonepore Fair, a trick, much practised by up-country horse-dealers, of attempting to sell, as perfectly quiet animals, unbreakable brutes which have been drugged into temporary good behaviour.

In April 1870, Baboo Kanye Loll Dey showed me some babool pods, the seed of which had been removed, and the hollows filled with a white substance, consisting chiefly of arsenic.

These pods had been given to cows at Serampore.

It certainly appears to be a matter of great importance that the importation, or at least the sale, of Arsenic in India should be regulated by a stringent legislative enactment.

ACONITE.

Aconitum Ferox;—Bish, Bikh, Meetha Teelia, Meetha Zuher, Ati Singeea Bish, Singia Jur, S. Khar, Beechnak (the Taleef Shereef) Bishnak,* (O'Shaughnessy).—*Butsnab-bide,* Beng. *Mahoor,* Hind. *Butchnab,* By. *Ativassa,* Tel. (Birdwood). The Dakra, or Nepaul poison, is also considered to be the root of the Aconite; Dr. Bidie of Madras says that the root sold in most bazars called *Bish, Bikh Nabee,* or *Uasah Nabee,* which has generally been supposed to be that of *Aconitum Ferox,* is, according to Hooker and Thomson, derived from the *A. Napellus Ferox, palmatum* and *luridum,* which are indiscriminately called *Bikh.* N. S. Ruthnam Moodelly says, that *Nabi* plays a most important part in the Hindu Materia Medica in Madras. *Nirbisi* is, according to Royle, *Aconitum Ferox.* Dr. Birdwood explains (p. 2) that *Nirbisi* signifies "the antidote to *Bikh;*" still, as we have seen, the name is popularly applied to the poison itself both in Madras and in Northern India. Baboo Kanye Loll Dey says, that *Kalkoot* is the root of a species of Aconite differing from *Napellus* and *Ferox* by its peculiar smell, and is much used in native medicine. It has virulent properties similar to that of *Aconitum Ferox.* In an MS. note of poisons used in Bengal which I have, I find "*Kalkoot,* root from the hill districts." It is added that 30 grains kill a man. Baboo Kanye Loll Dey tells me that, in a strong cat, two grains of *Kalkoot* made into a paste with water, and placed on the tongue, caused all the symptoms of Aconite poisoning for two days; but the cat recovered.

In the last edition of this work, I mentioned that the late Sub-Assistant Surgeon Issur Chunder Gangooly described a root having a black bark, covering a white substance within. He observed, that these roots are indigenous to the mountainous tracts of Tirhoot, and are much employed by the native hunters in poisoning the points of their arrows: a few of which were placed at the Baboo's disposal by a former Magistrate of Midnapore, for the purpose of ascertaining the effects of the poison upon inferior animals. From the terrible character of the spasms pervading the whole body, which preceded the death of a couple of dogs experimented upon, he concluded that *Kalkoot* belongs to the family which produces the Strychnia. It appears nearly certain, however,

* In Nizamut Adawlut Reports, N. W. P., for 26th October 1854, p. 618, will be found a case of poisoning, in which Meetha Teelia is stated to have been used. Dhatoora, however, appears to have been the poison employed. "*Methel*" is one of the names of Dhatoora. Aconite-root appears to be best known, near Calcutta, as *Kath-Bish;* in Behar as *Dakra;* in the neighbourhood of Dacca as *Meetha-Bish;* and in the North-West Provinces as *Meetha Teelia.*

that the poison is Aconite. Baboo Issur Chunder Gangooly also held that the Aconite forms the basis of the Bish Baree.

Professor Hirtz finds that the cultivated Aconite does not contain any active principle (hence probably the fact mentioned by Linnæus that at a post-house in Lapland, large quantities of the *Aconitum Lycoctonum* were boiled for use at the table like cabbage), and that, in the wild plant, the root alone contains the active principle.

A portion of Dakra sent me by Dr. Chuckerbutty was evidently Aconite root. The tubers, which are used in several formulæ by the native practitioners, and also with a view to destroy life, are two or three, fasciculate, fusiform, two to four inches long, blackish externally, pale inside. They are brittle, *break with a resinous fracture*, and are readily reduced to a coarse powder; in this state they are destitute of smell, slightly bitter to the taste, the tongue being benumbed wherever touched on. The roots are sold in every bazar in India, and may be purchased in large quantities for about two rupees a pound.

A preparation of the root is much used in all the hill districts of India to poison arrows for the destruction of wild beasts.

In a tank of water destined for part of the British Army, on a halt in pursuit of the retreating Burmese, the water had been poisoned by the *Aconitum Ferox*, bruised and thrown in by the enemy, before they evacuated the place ; undoubtedly fatal consequences would have ensued, had not Dr. Wallich discovered it.*

Dr. Wallich says of the *Vishavish*, or *Bish*, that the Gorkhalese pretend that it is one of their principal securities against invasion from the low countries. See an early notice of this practice in Cooch Behar, *supra*, p. 120.

In medicine, the Bish is chiefly employed by the Natives in the treatment of leprosy, fever, cholera, and rheumatism.† A Lepcha described the root to Captain Walter Sherwill as being "useful to sportsmen for destroying elephants and tigers ; useful to the rich for putting troublesome relations out of the way; and useful to jealous husbands for the purpose of destroying faithless wives." For an account of its numerous uses in native medicine, from the casting out of devils to the cure of offensive breath, see the *Taleef Shereef*, p. 107. According to Dr. Honigberger, the natives report that, in its natural state, the root is white, and that,

---

* Beck, 7th Ed., p. 1042. "Howqua has sent notice to foreign merchants in Canton to be careful whence they procure their water for domestic purposes, there being reason to believe that the wells whence their servants are in the habit of procuring it have been poisoned."—*Allen's Asiatic Journal*, November 1842, p. 295.

† O'Shaughnessy. It appears, from the Dacca Dispensary Report, April and September 1854, that Sub-Asst. Surgeon Omeshchunder Dutt employed the Aconite root (called by the Natives of that place *Meetha Bish*) in chronic rheumatism and neuralgia, seemingly with some success. The doses are not mentioned.

when immersed in the urine of cows, it becomes black.* As it is met with in the bazars, it is lustrous when broken.

Many years since considerable attention appears to have been paid by some of the members of the Medical and Physical Society of Calcutta, in enquiring into the nature of a poison, used in Assam by hunters, called *Mismee Bish.* The fact does not appear to have been absolutely demonstrated, but there seems to be every reason to believe that this is the root of the *Aconitum Ferox.* Dr. Griffith sent some specimens down to the Society in February 1837. He stated that, as far as he could learn from the native accounts, the Assam poison resembles closely the Nepaul plant (Aconite). He believed it to be a very powerful drug, and attributed the failure of the experiments made with Dr. Wallich's specimens (brought down the previous year) to the age of the roots, which speedily become inert by keeping.

He stated that the apparatus employed for destroying animals with this poison consists of a short arrow, the head of which is plentifully smeared with the powdered root made up into a paste, by the help of the *Allengo juice*, as described by Dr. Wallich. This arrow is inserted into the barrel of a musket, the head projecting externally, and the gun is discharged in the ordinary way. It is said by the Mishmees that an elephant, wounded in the *shoulder* by this empoisoned weapon, dies in a few minutes; but, when struck in the hinder parts of the body, he lives till next day. This is evidently the poison alluded to by Dr. McCosh, in his Topography of Assam, published during the same year. He describes it as being grown only by the Abors, a mountain tribe inhabiting the banks of the Sampoo. Its cultivation is kept a great secret, and they carry their precaution so far as to boil it before leaving their country so as to destroy all vegetation (we have already seen that, in Bengal, the root of the *Aconitum Ferox* is generally made to undergo some soaking or *sodhana* process). It is brought into Suddia by the Abors, tied up in little bundles, and has the appearance of a small fibrous root. It is prepared for use by pounding the roots to powder, and mixing this into a paste with the juice of a tree called *Alengh*, so as to give it tenacity, and make it adhere to the arrow-head. So fatal are its effects that even a scratch from an arrow so poisoned is followed by almost instant death. This is the poison used by all tiger-killers for poisoning their arrows.

Dr. White, now of Debroghur, on his first appointment, went in medical charge of a detatchment of the Assam Light Infantry Battalion, on service against the Abors. Several of his men having been wounded with poisoned arrows, it is said that, with noble self-devotion, he sucked

---

* According to Baboo Issur Chunder Gangooly, the "Sodhana" process for *Bucknag* or *Butsnabh* (Aconite) is maceration in the juice of amrool, or three-leaved sorrel.

the wounds, and suffered in a marked degree from that numbness of the lips and tongue which characterises aconite poisoning.*

Captain Walter Sherwill mentions, in his Notes upon a Tour in the Sikkim Himalaya Mountains, that the poisonous effect of the *Bick* is so great that a Lepcha died at Darjeeling, having, while crossing the hot valleys, allowed the root, which was carried across his shoulder in an open cane basket, to rub against his moist naked body. Sufficient poison was thus absorbed to cause his death.

Baboo Kanye Loll Dey informs me that thirty-six cases of aconite poisoning came under the notice of the Calcutta Chemical Examiner in the ten years, 1860 to 1869.

This root, named emphatically BISH—*Poison*, but having an almost infinite variety of designations, is evidently the best known and the most frequently employed of all the stronger vegetable poisons in India.

In 1834, Mr. Burnard reported† that about seventy men, who had been drinking the intoxicating liquor prepared from the Mowah flower *(Bassia latifolia)* at a native spirit shop in Benares, were attacked with symptoms of poisoning. Forty-three were brought to hospital, and eighteen died outside. The symptoms were those of irritant poisoning, the brain being little affected, and the *pupils natural*.‡ There was a sense of constriction and burning at the upper part of the œsophagus, twisting of the tongue, in some instances protrusion of it, and cramps in the legs and arms; pulse, small and weak, and in none exceeding 65; in some it was imperceptible at the wrist. The treatment mainly consisted in removing the poison from the stomach and in giving ammonia to those who were collapsed. All who came under treatment were sufficiently well to be discharged on the following day. One of the servants of the liquor

---

* The author of *Notes on North Cachar* says that the deadly poison used by the Kookies is stated to be extracted from a tree, which does not grow in those parts. The article is brought to them for sale by tribes inhabiting the border of Manipur. The substance is of a dark blue or black colour, of about the consistence of common resin. To make it serviceable, it is ground down with capsicum seeds and tobacco juice, so as to form a pulp with which the weapons are smeared, cotton soaked in the mixture being also tied to the iron under the barb. He says that the *Panjies* (fine sharp splinters of bamboo planted obliquely in the ground in such a manner as to wound the feet of an attacking party) employed by the Kookies in the defence of villages, used to be poisoned when the feuds between the tribes were very fierce. The poison here alluded to was probably aconite.

Regarding the use of *Panjies* by the Eastern hill tribes of India, see '*the Chapter on Wounds.*' The Nagas use them as a defence against the attacks of both men and wild beasts under the name of Kumanchees, but do not usually poison them. In an attack made on an Angami Naga village in February 1868, by Lieutenant Gregory and Mr. James, three police constables were reported as wounded by *Panjies*, but nothing is said about poisoning.

† The India Journal of Medical Science, Vol. I., p. 286.

‡ This is no evidence against the conclusion that the poison used was Aconite. It will be seen, when we consider the physiological action of this poison, that it is only in very severe cases that it produces dilatation of the pupil.

shop, who had disappeared immediately after having served out the noxious liquor, confessed that he had put Singhera into the pots in which the mowah flowers, &c., were steeped.

I have taken a few of the many recorded cases of Aconite poisoning as presenting marked characteristics in regard to symptoms, &c. The following interesting cases of *supposed* poisoning by Aconite have been selected from the reports of the Chemical Examiners :

In October 1840, the Coroner of Calcutta ordered the examination of a liquid obtained from the stomach of one of three persons who had suffered from severe and peculiar symptoms, soon after their morning meal ; one died in *eleven hours,* the others recovered. Analysis gave no indication of the presence of any poisonous material. But, from the following circumstances, Dr. O'Shaughnessy felt himself warranted in giving it as his opinion, in evidence, that the deceased had been poisoned, and that the poison given was, in all probability, the *Bish,*—the root of the *Aconitum Ferox.* All these persons suffered almost immediately after taking food. The symptoms, in all, were burning in the throat, numbness of the extremities, transient loss of sight, and giddiness. To this succeeded collapse, sinking of the pulse, and, in one case, death in eleven hours. The food eaten was a prawn curry. Cholera was not epidemic at the time. Whilst the symptoms were different from those of all ordinary diseases, they coincided closely with those which the Doctor had witnessed as the effects of Aconite, when given medicinally to man or as a poison to animals. This Aconite, moreover, was one of the best known of the native poisons, and procurable in every bazar.

In April 1841, the Magistrate of Behar reported that three men, on their way from Bengal to the North-Western Provinces, were joined on the road by a fourth individual, who accompanied them about two stages, and took an opportunity of mixing poison of some description with some suttoo and goor (parched grain and treacle), which he gave them to eat. One of the men became insensible almost immediately, and *died in about four hours.* The other two, who had taken less, became also, after a short interval, insensible ; but recovered under treatment during the night, about 12 hours after taking the poison. The man who died lay down almost immediately after taking the poison, and never again betrayed any symptoms of animation beyond slight respiration. The others described their sensations as those of great heat and burning internally, accompanied with the most violent contortion of their limbs, and a feeling as if they were struggling with an exceedingly heavy load upon their shoulders. On examining the body of the deceased traveller, Mr. Dickson found a considerable degree of general inflammation of the intestines, the stomach contained a quantity of undigested suttoo, its lining membrane was in a very highly inflamed state. There was also some bloody fluid effused into the cavity of the abdomen. Having preserved the contents of the stomach, he, next day, gave a small portion to a chicken, which had the effect of making it apparently very uneasy during the day, and it died the next morning, about 20 hours after eating the suttoo. Dr. O'Shaughnessy analysed the contents of the stomach, which contained no metallic poison: owing to their putrefaction and state of admixture, no vegetable poison could be detected. He, however, inferred, from the symptoms described, that the Dakra, or root of the *Aconitum Ferox*, together with the seeds of the *Stramonium*, were the poisons employed.

A very demonstrative case of poisoning by Aconite was tried in Zillah Behar in 1820. A man who had embezzled a sum of money gave himself up as a slave to the defrauded party; he, however (as he afterwards confessed), mixed Dakra with his master's food. After having eaten some of the food, the unfortunate man remarked that it had a bitter taste. Having finished eating, he lay down, but soon complained of being unwell, and sent for one of the police, on whose arrival he said that he suspected his servant had poisoned him; emetics were administered by a native doctor, but without effect, for he died in a few hours; and a cat, which had eaten some of the flesh left by the deceased, died also before the next morning. The Judge of Circuit, in convicting the prisoner, remarked that the Dakra, which is brought from the Nepaul Hills, is well known to the Natives in general to be a most deadly poison, whether taken into the stomach or introduced into the circulation by a wound, and is commonly used to poison arrows for the destruction of wild beasts.*

In 1854, one Anundchunder Roy, having incurred the censure of his family by his dissipated and extravagant mode of life, conceived the idea of murdering them all. For this purpose, he purchased about an ounce of Aconite root. He was seen pounding some of the root on a brick, and was proved to have deposited the powder in a utensil, containing a vegetable broth, at his brother's house. The brother and three women partook of the broth. The man ate first, and probably got the largest share both of it and the poison. He was taken ill almost immediately, complaining of a burning sensation in his throat and stomach, vomited once, and expired during the night. The three women were seized with the like symptoms, and soon fell into a state of insensibility, but recovered after a lapse of several hours, the quantity of poisonous matter swallowed by them having proved insufficient to destroy life. The prisoner at first ascribed these events to Cholera. Having been upbraided and, as he asserted, beaten by Dwarkanath Roy and others, friends of the deceased, he laid a criminal information against those persons, charging them with having beaten the man to death. A child, the deceased's son, however,

* Macnaghten's Reports, Vol. II., p. 19.

stated that he had seen the prisoner enter the kitchen, and put something into the cooking vessel. Mr. F. P. Strong, the Civil Surgeon, examined the body, and stated that he was "unable to account for the death on any supposition other than that the deceased had swallowed some vegetable poison, as for instance Aconite." The prisoner was sentenced to death.*

Dr. William Palmer has given the two following cases in his valuable monograph on Datura and Aconite poisoning. A police constable at Brahmabaria, in Zillah Tipperah, was suddenly taken ill with burning pain in the epigastrium, frothing at the mouth, great restlessness, and inability to speak freely; his limbs soon became cold, and his pulse is reported to have been very weak. No mention was made in the report of the existence or non-existence of paralysis. The patient said somebody had administered poison with his pan,† when asked to account for his illness. He died in about four hours. On examining his body after death, a piece of root was found in the stomach, which was pronounced to be Aconite root, on the spot. It was, however, forwarded to Calcutta, where it was further examined in the following manner: After being cut into small pieces, it was macerated in spirit for twenty-four hours; a few drops of this tincture were next administered to a kitten with the following results. After half an hour her pupils were slightly dilated, though they became smaller when she was held towards the light to be examined. At this time, also, she made violent efforts to vomit, but only small portions of the contents of the stomach were ejected. After this she became very restless, walked about the room, seeking means to escape; not finding any, however, she returned to her original corner, where she sat staring vacantly with head erect, and pupils more widely dilated.

---

* Nizamut Adawlut Reports, Vol. IV., 1854, p. 560. See notes of cases of poisoning by Dakra, in sweetmeat, at Monghyr and Behar. Reports of State of Police, Lower Provinces, for 1846, p. 14, and 1848, p. 15. Also an instance, at Bijnore, in which particles of the *Meetha Teelia (or Aconitum Ferox)* were found in a portion of the dhall reported to have been given to certain persons, who were rendered insensible after eating, when one, the principal, was robbed of her jewels; the effects, however, were only temporary insensibility, and they recovered without remedies being administered to them.—*Nizamut Adawlut Reports, N. W. P.*, 27th November 1854, p. 766.

Several cases of Aconite poisoning are related by Dr. Burton Brown (Op. Citat. pp. 73 *et seq.*) Baboo Kanye Loll Dey has given me the case of a man treated in the Medical College Hospital, Calcutta, who was poisoned by a lump of Aconite among some dates; he recovered. In April 1870, I saw a boatman, in the ward of my colleague Dr. Chuckerbutty, who had marked symptoms from eating a small lump of the root as a remedy for rheumatic pains. See a case of *Meeta Bish* poisoning by Dr. Herbert Baillie.—*Indian Annals of Medical Science* for 1857, Vol. IV., p. 298. In February 1868, the Assistant Magistrate, Sealdah, sent to the Chemical Examiner some goor (country treacle) and chutto, after eating some of which a man was attacked with vomiting and insensibility. Aconite was found in the mess.

† Baboo Kanye Loll Dey informs me that *Aconite Root, in bits, is often mixed with prepared betel (pan) for poisoning purposes.*

After a few minutes she moved again about the room, not showing any marked signs of loss of power over her limbs. When her tail or foot was pinched with a pair of forceps, the limb was suddenly drawn up ; but when the skin of the back was similarly seized and forcibly twisted, she neither showed any sign of pain, nor made any effort to move away ; the feelers could even be pulled without exciting any appearance of displeasure. After the lapse of forty-five minutes, she was more inclined to sit still, or lie as if sleeping ; when called, however, she always opened her eyes and looked, showing at the same time her dilated pupils. After an hour and-a-half all these symptoms gradually began to disappear. A little of the same tincture, which was applied to the lip of the experimenter, caused numbness, which continued more or less for twenty-four hours.

The above signs and symptoms were considered sufficiently characteristic to confirm the suspicion that the root was Aconite.

At Ranchee, a man was suddenly seized with severe illness, after drinking some rice-spirit, and died the same day. No symptoms appear to have been recorded, but there was a suspicion of poisoning, and the stomach, with its contents, was forwarded to Calcutta for examination.

They were first examined for mineral poison by Reinsch's and the Magnesium tests. None being found, the contents were next submitted to a careful physical examination, but no known poisonous substance was detected by this means ; the whole stomach and contents were, therefore, subjected to a modification of Stas's process. The resulting extract was divided into two equal parts, one of which was injected into the stomach of a puppy at 10 A.M. His pupils became dilated in a few minutes ; he also began to froth in the mouth, and to lose power over his hind legs. He continued conscious, always looking up when called ; his pupils were generally dilated, but close and continued observation revealed much variation in their size ; they were often contracted to about their normal size, for a moment or two, but never absolutely small. At one o'clock he was brought out of his corner and placed in the middle of the room ; he then attempted to walk back again, but walked with a tottering gait ; his hind legs springing up again, in a state of great irritability, as soon as the feet touched the ground. When one hind foot was pinched with a pair of forceps, such violent reflex actions were produced that he immediately fell heavily to the ground towards the pinched side. His pupils were still dilated. No expression of pain was made when he was pinched severely on any part of his face or body. At 2 P.M. he lay apparently asleep, but raised his head and looked up the moment he was called. From this time he gradually recovered, and by the next morning was quite well. A little of the remaining portion was rubbed on the experimenter's lip at noon ; by 3 P.M., the part had become so benumbed that the point of a needle was not felt when applied. The peculiar action on the pupil, together with the insensibility to pain, caused by the suspected substance in the above case, were considered, in the absence of other signs, sufficiently characteristic to justify the opinion that Aconite, or some nearly allied poison, existed in the suspected stomach.

At 11 P. M. of the 8th of August 1865, one Choonee Ghazee, a resident of Tipperah, became very ill immediately after eating his evening meal. He is reported to have felt numbness over his whole body, and to have lost all strength, to have vomited frequently up to nine o'clock on the following morning, and to have died at noon on that day. At the *post-mortem* examination, the stomach was found congested, but quite empty; it was put into a bottle with some spirit, and forwarded to Calcutta for examination. One spirituous fluid was prepared as above described by repeated evaporations, solution, filtration, and re-evaporation, and the resulting extract, or essence, was divided into two unequal parts; the larger of these was injected into the stomach of a small cat; much, however, was lost by the struggling of the animal, and more was vomited within two minutes from the time it was given. After a lapse of five minutes, the following symptoms were seen: her pupils began to dilate, her breathing to be laboured, and her hind legs became so paralysed that she could scarcely walk, her hips falling to the ground from side to side as she attempted to do so. A little later she could not support the weight of her hips, but squatted down and pushed herself about by the fore-legs. Violent efforts to vomit were made from time to time, but only a little frothing matter was ejected. When pinched with tweezers in different parts of the body, no signs of pain were made. She appeared restless and distressed, staring wildly about, the pupils being more dilated. In half an hour from the time of administration, she began to lose power over her fore-legs also, and after an hour she had become quite still and motionless, and perfectly insensible to pain. At this time her pupils varied much in size; towards one o'clock, or two hours from the commencement, they were contracted rather than dilated. From this time she began to recover her normal condition. The smaller portion of the extract was applied to the lip of the experimenter without inducing any decided numbness: it was also tested chemically. The results were not considered sufficiently satisfactory at the time to justify a confident opinion that Aconite was contained in the stomach; when, however, the symptoms of the patient are considered in conjunction with those reproduced in the cat, it is scarcely possible to doubt that Aconite was the cause of death.

Mr. Peet, of Bombay, has recorded* the case of a Hindu priest, aged 50, who stated that, for twenty-four days, he had been taking daily *fifteen grains* of a native drug called *kishnak* (root of the *Aconitum Ferox*) as a remedy for leprosy. Until the morning of the day of his admission, he had

---

* Transactions of the Medical and Physical Society of Bombay, for 1853 and 1854, p. 309.

been using the ***black*** variety of the drug (probably altered and weakened by keeping, or by some ***sodahna*** process), but, at the recommendation of a friend, he substituted the ***white*** variety (doubtless a fresher kind), in the expectation that it would be more effective than the former, which did not appear to have much influence either upon the system or the disease. The dose was ***fifteen grains***, and was taken in the morning about 10 o'clock. He soon afterwards began to feel uneasy, had a disagreeable burning sensation in the mouth and fauces, a sense of formication, and some confusion of mind. A friend recommended milk, of which he drank a large quantity ; soon afterwards he vomited freely, and about an hour after the vomiting came on, and about four hours from the time of taking the drug, he was brought to the hospital. He was then sensible, had a stupid expression of face, and walked with an unsteady gait, like a drunken person ; he complained of heat and burning in the throat, some confusion of mind, and of a sense of formication over the surface generally. There was almost constant vomiting. Pulse feeble and rapid ; skin coldish, and covered with moisture ; pupils natural. A sinapism was applied to the epigastrium, and stimulants of ammonia were administered. The vomiting continued till 12 o'clock at night, after which he fell asleep. On the following morning, the skin had regained its warmth, and the pulse was better. The sense of heat about the throat had subsided, but he still walked with much difficulty. There was no return of vomiting. He was urgent for his discharge, and went home in the course of the day.

The following case, narrated* by my late assistant Baboo Taraprosunno Roy, sets forth very clearly the ordinary symptoms of Aconite poisoning. Phussee, a Mahomedan boatman, aged thirty-five, was admitted into the Medical College Hospital on the 29th November 1866, 2-45 P.M. He had taken with his *pan*, about half an hour before, a small portion of Aconite root, mistaking it for "Coorel," a dried root used by the Natives to relieve muscular pain. Immediately after chewing it, he felt a sweetish taste, which was soon followed by tingling of the lips and tongue, numbness of the face and severe vomiting. On his way to the Hospital, the symptoms gradually became aggravated, so that at the time of admission he was extremely restless, tossing his limbs about in all directions, constantly changing his position. He complained of a burning sensation in the stomach, and a tingling and numbness all over the body, excepting his legs. The tingling was specially marked in the face and tongue,—so much so, that he was constantly moving the latter to and fro, in order to scratch it against the teeth. Retching and vomiting occurred almost incessantly, and he constantly placed his hand over the cardiac region. His face was anxious, the eyes suffused, the lips pale and exsauguine,

* Indian Medical Gazette, Vol. II., p. 82.

the eye-lids swollen, pupils moderately dilated, and insensible to the stimulus of light. Respiration laboured 64 in a minute. Pulse small and feeble, 66. Unable to walk, owing to loss of volitional power over the muscles; mental faculties unimpaired, and consciousness perfectly clear. The contents of the stomach were washed out by the stomach pump, and white of eggs and milk freely administered. 6½ P. M.—The symptoms continue to increase in severity, lips more exsauguine. Eyes more suffused, tongue redder and more swollen. Pulse intermittent, feebler, and less frequent. Tingling and numbness extending to the legs. Retching and vomiting incessant ; mental faculties clear ; answers questions rationally. On examining the condition of the external sensibility of the patient with a pair of scissors, it was found that, on fully separating the blades and bringing the points in contact with the skin over the arms and forearms, he felt them as one, although they were four inches apart. But the sensibility of the thighs and legs was less obtuse, for he could feel the two points distinctly, when they were four inches apart, and he continued to do so until the distance between the points fell short of two inches and three quarters. He was ordered an ounce of rum mixture every hour. 11½ P.M.—Was now quieter. Pulse 56. Pupils contracting. Tingling and numbness less. Vomiting not so frequent as before. Since his admission he has not made any water, nor passed a stool, although a dose of castor oil has been administered. 30th—7½ A.M.—Pulse 84, regular, though small and feeble. Pupils contracted to the normal size, still paralysed. Numbness and tingling much less than before. Sensibility perfect in the forearms and legs ; has greater control over the muscles, so that he can move about his hands and legs without any trembling. He spits constantly, and vomits bilious fluid, but not so frequently as before. The burning sensation in the stomach is no more complained of. Calomel with opium substituted for rum mixture, as the latter seemed to keep up the vomiting. 4 P.M.—Much improved. No tingling in any part. Slight numbness of the arms and thighs only. On trial with a pair of scissors as before, the sensibility of the thighs and arms was found considerably increased. No more vomiting and retching. The patient gradually recovered, although he suffered from slight diarrhœa for a day or two afterwards. He was quite well, and was discharged on the 6th December.

The Baboo observes that the above case is a very fair illustration of poisoning by Aconite. The peculiar action of the poison, belonging as it does to the narcotico-acrids, was fully exhibited by this patient ; the acridity was manifested by the obstinate retching and vomiting, constant spitting of saliva, and burning sensation in the pit of the stomach. The depressant influence of the poison rendered the pulse small, slow, weak, and intermittent, and gave rise to the hurried laborious breathing, and the sense of void within the cardiac region. The narcotic action of Aconite was illustrated by the immediate impairment of sensibility, characterised by the tingling and numbness of the lips and tongue, almost coincidently with the chewing of the root, at first acting locally upon the peripheral distribution of the nerves ; but it subsequently affected the central ganglia, as proved by the tingling and numbness becoming universal, and the inability of the patient to stand on his legs. The great peculiarity of the poison was that it left the mental faculties perfectly clear, even during the height of the symptoms. We have seen how the patient was quite unable to walk or stand, owing to the paralysis of the lower extremities, whilst he could move his arms about without any difficulty, aud could steady them in any position at will. The disordered sensibility came on immediately after chewing the root, and continued more or less till the other symptoms of poisoning subsided, while the patient was perfectly rational throughout. The pupils dilated up to a certain degree only, and never reached that extreme dilatation which is characteristic of the solanaccous plants. They were totally paralysed without affording any sign of that irritability of the nerves of the iris indicated by alternate dilatation and contraction.

The question of *An Antidote* for Aconite, raised in the following case, from one of the Reports of the Superintendent of Police, Lower Provinces,* deserves investigation. There had been a dispute in the Bhaugulpore district, about a tauree tree, and a punchayet was held to settle it. When all was concluded, one of the parties said, who is for drink ? and the rest proceeded to his house to have some tauree. Poison was mixed with this, and the defendants, three in number, came provided with antidotes, known to the Hillmen, which they took : of the others, three died, and the remaining three, having procured antidotes, recovered. The antidotes were the roots and barks of trees, aud the poison administered was said to be "Dakra." If that was really the case, Mr. Dampier adds, the knowledge of the existence of such antidotes would be a matter of much medical interest. Unfortunately, however, no additional facts have since been adduced.

In a report (I think to the Agri-Horticultural Society of Calcutta) made by Colonel Lowther, when he was in Assam, it was stated that the Hill people there profess to have an antidote for Aconite. When I met Colonel Lowther some years afterwards, he told me that he had not obtained any definite information on this point.

At page 49, Vol. I of Royle's Botany of the Himalayas, will be found a learned enquiry with a view to identify the true *Nirbisi*, (*Nir* privative, and *Bis* poison). This point is also discussed by Birdwood, page 2 ; but an antidote to Aconite has still to be discovered.

---

* For 1844, p. 19.

The poison called *Jhur* (root) described by Mr. Brett, when serving with the Bhaugulpore Hill Rangers,* as commonly employed by the Hill-men to effect suicide, and in preparing the points of their arrows when hunting the wild boar, is evidently Aconite.

In the case related by Mr. Brett, a sipahi had taken a drachm twelve hours previously. He was sufficiently sensible to explain what had occurred. He suffered excruciating agony, and a sensation of burning heat in the stomach and within his body in every direction ; he complained also of pain in the head : pupils *contracted*,† pulse quick and small, countenance depicting alarm and horror. The stomach-pump and emetics failed to give relief, and he expired in about an hour and-a-half ;—extreme collapse of the features, *dilatation* of the pupils, coldness of the extremities, and feebleness of pulse having supervened an hour previously.

Mr. Brett introduced about half a drachm of *Jhur* into an incision, an inch long, over the glutæus maximus of a dog, and in a few minutes, the same quantity was placed in an old wound. Nothing apparently occurred during the first hour and-a-half ; after which the animal was seized with violent spasmodic action of the stomach, ejecting nearly its entire contents. It appeared to suffer great agony in its abdominal viscera, twisting its body in every direction, and foaming at the mouth ; pupils *contracted*, pulse quick and small ; expired after a collapse of fifteen minutes. The liver was found highly inflamed (?), as was also the cardiac half of the internal membrane of the stomach, and the peritoneum covering the liver, stomach, and large and small omenta.

Dr. Mouat published, in 1845,‡ the cases of two privates of H. M. 55th Regiment, at Chinhae, who suffered (in one of the cases fatally) from strongly marked symptoms of Aconite poisoning after swallowing a spirit called *samshoo*, supplied to them at a Chinese drinking-shop.

In his case of Aconite poisoning, given at the commencement of this Chapter (p. 138), Mr. Burnard says, that a servant of the liquor shop confessed that he had put Singhera, in coarse powder, into the pot in which the mowah flowers and other ingredients of the liquor were steeped. How much of the powder was used could not be ascertained, but a Buniya was found who stated that he had sold a quantity of Singhera to this man. Mr. Burnard learnt that different articles are said to be mixed with the ingredients for the purpose of rendering the liquor stronger, and that both Singhera and Buch-nag are thus employed. It is said that half a chittack of

* Transactions of the Medical and Physical Society of Calcutta, Vol. IV., p. 424.

† In this respect, the action of the poison differed from that of Aconite, which is liable to produce dilatation of the pupils, with more or less loss of sight. It will be seen, however, that the pupils were observed to be dilated before death.

‡ India Journal of Medical and Physical Science, N. S.

Singhera (an ounce) will double the strength of 16 quarts of mowah liquor. These additions are always made clandestinely, and the drinkers do not appear to be aware that they are made.

For full accounts of the Symptoms and Post-Mortem Appearances in cases of poisoning with Aconite,—See Taylor on Poisons and O'Shaughnessy's Bengal Dispensatory. For curious information regarding Aconite—See Wallich, Plant. Asiat. Rar., Vol. I., p. 35; *and Wight, Illustrations of Ind. Botany.*

THUGGEE BY POISON.

Writing in 1856, I observed that, while the whole system of organization of the bands of Phansigars who, a few years previously, overran India, had been thoroughly laid bare; and while an equally clear light had been thrown upon the practice of dacoity in Bengal, very little appeared to have been done towards revealing and placing a check upon the mysterious operations of those gangs of Poisoners by Profession who still infest every main road, and lurk in the purlieus of every large town throughout the country. I urged that the subject is one that especially calls for the closest judicial investigation. I had been able to collect but little definite information regarding it, beyond a few scattered remarks in the Reports of the Superintendent of Police, Lower Provinces, and some cases in the Reports of the two Courts of Nizamut Adawlut; still, the facts which these embody sufficiently proved that a system of Thuggee by Poison has spread itself over every portion of the Bengal Presidency. I added that it appeared certain that the crime was equally prevalent throughout Bombay and Madras.

The following table, compiled from Mr. Dampier's Reports, will give some idea of the *comparative* prevalence of this crime in the several districts of the Lower Provinces, during a period of nine years. It affords no guide, however, to the actual prevalence of the crime, as it is considered probable that very many instances escape discovery. Indeed Mr. Dampier more than once insisted upon the fact, that this is a crime in which the detection of the culprits is but seldom made.* Further, it would appear that this table merely comprises the discovered instances of the lesser offence of Theft by Drugging, the cases in which death by poison was occasioned being omitted.

* Report for 1846, p. 5, and for 1850, p. 1.

Cases of Theft by the Administration of Drugs—Lower Provinces.

	1843	1844	1845	1846	1847	1848	1849	1850	1851	Total.
Shahabad	1	2	5	5	3	1	4	2	4	27
Sarun	1	1	...	2	1	...	...	...	...	5
Champarun	...	...	...	...	...	...	...	...	...	...
Tirhoot	...	...	...	...	...	...	...	...	...	...
Patna	1	...	2	1	1	...	...	...	...	5
Behar	1	...	...	3	4	...	10	5	1	24
Monghyr	...	...	...	...	...	...	...	...	...	...
Bhaugulpore	...	...	...	...	...	...	...	...	...	...
Purneah	1	...	...	...	...	...	...	...	...	1
Dinagepore	...	...	...	...	...	...	2	...	...	2
Maldah	...	...	...	1	...	...	...	...	...	1
Rajshahye	...	...	...	...	...	...	...	...	...	...
Pubnah	...	...	...	...	...	...	...	1	...	1
Rungpore	...	...	...	...	...	...	...	1	...	1
Bograh	...	...	...	...	...	...	...	...	...	...
Mymensing	...	...	...	...	...	...	...	...	...	...
Sylhet	...	...	...	...	...	...	...	...	...	...
Tipperah	...	...	...	...	...	...	...	Not re- ported.		...
Noacolly	...	...	...	...	...	...	...			...
Chittagong	...	...	...	...	...	...	...			...
Dacca	...	...	..	...	...	5	...	...	...	5
Furreedpore	...	...	...	...	...	...	...	...	...	...
Backergunge	...	...	...	...	...	...	...	...	...	...
Jessore	...	...	...	...	...	...	...	...	...	...
Nuddea	1	...	...	1	...	...	...	...	...	2
Moorshedabad	...	...	...	...	..	...	...	...	...	...
Beerbhoom	...	...	...	1	...	3	...	1	1	6
Bancoorah	...	...	...	...	...	...	3	...	4	7
Burdwan	1	...	...	2	2	...	2	...	1	8
Midnapore	1	...	...	...	...	...	3	...	...	4
Hooghly	...	...	...	2	3	...	...	1	1	7
Howrah	1	1	...	...	...	...	2	...	1	5
24-Pergunnahs... ...	1	...	...	1	...	...	...	1	6	9
Baraset	...	...	...	...	...	...	...	...	...	...
	10	4	7	19	14	9	26	12	19	120

I argued that the first step in the investigation of this direful practice should be the discovery of *the precise Classes* to which the Professional Poisoners of India belong. Several of the deadliest poisons are so easily procurable, and are so well known in every part of the country, that it is not surprising that they should be employed by any unprincipled native in the furtherance of his criminal designs. Still, with due caution, no instance of drugging or poisoning, by any ordinary criminal, ought to be mistaken for an example of systematic Thuggee.

The individuals who might be expected to have the largest concern with poisons, and to be best acquainted with them, are the Druggists, the Bunneahs (who, although dealing in other articles, have, in many instances, collections of drugs by them), and the native Doctors. It is only too evident that the native dealers part with their poisonous wares with the most reckless indifference. It is well known that, a few years since, many Thugs assumed the characters of shop-keepers, as a means of facilitating their iniquitous designs; and I have, myself, met with one case, at Chittagong, in which a Bunneah was under very strong suspicion of having been concerned in drugging two travellers. Still I have not been able to meet with any instance in the criminal records, in which a Drug-seller, or a Bunneah, was tried as a principal in any case of poisoning; nor can I discover any fact which would lead to the belief that the byeds, kobirajira,* or hukeems of this Presidency afford the aid of their knowledge to criminal purposes. There is, in nearly every village throughout the country, a hag of low caste and evil repute, half *dai*, half *dain*, suspected as a witch, professedly a midwife; equally ready, at all times, to practise as a doctress, a sorceress, or a bawd; and carrying on a systematic trade in the procuration of abortion by the use of the most deadly poisons. It is the belief of persons well acquainted with the habits of the natives that these women are professional poisoners. Except, however, as regards the particular crime above mentioned, it is by no means certain that the suspicion rests upon valid grounds.†

---

* For a solitary exceptional case, see Nizamut Adawlut Report, January 9, 1856, p. 42.

† It appeared, in a trial at Bareilly in 1854, that a female having a daughter twenty years of age, who was blind, and therefore remained unmarried, went to consult a woman, named Musst. Goolshun, who pretended to work miraculous cures by aid of familiar spirits. They made a large offering of valuable property to the sorceress, who, however, dismissed them with their gifts, saying, this must not be done in presence of others; but if you come alone with trinkets and cash, your business will be done; the spirits will put on your trinkets, and will dance and be glad, and your eyes will recover sight. The woman collected rupees 200 worth of trinkets, and rupees 86 cash; and going to the house of the sorceress, were never seen again alive. The shoe of one of them was found, next morning, on the bank of the *nuddee*, distant from the prisoner's house four or five hundred paces; and upon search being made, their bodies were found in the *nuddee*; their mouths stuffed with cloth, as if they had been gagged before they were thrown into the water. Three days subsequently, information was given that the deceased persons had gone to the woman's house. The place was then searched, and a *ghoongroo* (toe ring), which was recognised by the father of the murdered girl as belonging to one of his children, was found concealed among *bhoosa* in a corner; and, in a recess of the inside wall, was found a piece of white arsenic. Upon being apprehended, the woman gave up rupees 17 and a pair of gold ear-rings which were identified as having been borrowed by the deceased. Upon a second search, money and jewels were found concealed; the latter, however, were not claimed. A cracked rupee found upon the prisoner was identified as having been lent to the deceased. The sorceress and her husband were found guilty of murder and sentenced to death by the sessions judge. This sentence, however, was annulled by the Superior Court.—*Nizamut Adawlut Reports, N. W. P.*, 2nd January 1854, p. 3. It may be worthy of remark that, nearly at the very time at which this crime was perpetrated in a remote part of India, a similar fraud was being transacted in Devonshire. The following is from *Notes and Queries* for October 21, 1854:—"Some gipsies having encamped in the neighbourhood of Northland, one of the female members of the tribe ascertained from the wife of a farm labourer, that she had a daughter in the last stage of

Again, there is a class of thieves, notorious ***budmashes,*** who eke out their other atrocities by occasional recourse to drugging or poisoning. It appears to be very difficult to ascertain whether these men practise their villanies alone and quite independently of others, or whether they are detached members of the Thug Association. Mr. Henry Alexander, of the Civil Service, showed me a collection of drugs (chiefly mineral and poisonous) which were taken, some years since, from a suspicious charac-

---

consumption. The gipsey represented that the child had been 'bewitched,' and that she could rule the spell which would effect a cure for two sovereigns. The mother cheerfully paid the money; but, the next day, the wily gipsey returned it, and said it was not sufficient, but 20*l.* more in gold would do it. The cottager's wife, in her native simplicity, went and borrowed 10*l.* from a neighbour; and, with another 10 sovereigns she had in the house saved from her husband's earnings, added the 20*l.* to the 2*l.* already in the gipsey's hands. As soon as the money was paid, the affrighted woman was bound over to secresy by the gipsey, who mumbled out a few disjoined texts of scripture and left, with the promise that the child would be cured on the following Friday, when an angel would appear and return the money. Since that time, however, it is needless to add, neither gipsey nor money has turned up."

"At the police-court in Merthyr Tydfill, the other day, a singular case of obtaining money under pretence of telling fortunes and 'ruling the planets' was investigated. The prisoner, a young gipsey woman of the Lovell tribe, was charged by Mrs. Thomas, a young, educated, and good-looking lady, the wife of an assistant surgeon in good circumstances, with having obtained from her £80 and 2*s.* 6*d.*, by false pretences. The prisoner, who had been in the habit of visiting Mrs. Thomas's house selling clothes' pegs, &c., took an opportunity of informing that lady that she possessed the power of ruling the planets, and for this trifling service only required half-a-crown. Having succeeded so far, she seems to have understood the character of the lady she had to deal with, and resolved to work upon her disposition for her own advantage. She paid her several visits, talking a good deal about working the circles, raising the spirits, &c., and at length induced Mrs. Thomas to hand her over £40, as there were four circles, and she was bound to put £10 on each. She promised to return the money, and singularly enough did so, but only for the purpose of increasing the amount, as the event proved. By playing on Mrs. Thomas's nervousness and superstition she induced her to deposit with her £80, promising as before to return it in a short time, when the 'circles' had been propitiated. This appointment the gipsey failed to keep, and it was only through the intermediancy of the police that Mrs. Thomas secured the next interview. In the meantime the £80 had disappeared, and has not since been heard of. The magistrates convicted the prisoner, and sentenced her to six months' hard labour. She left the dock with her baby in her arms, winking to some one she recognised in court, considering, no doubt, that on the whole she had not done a bad stroke of business."—*(Herald).*

"At the Newbury Petty Sessions on February 11, Maria Giles, a midwife, who has for many years borne the *soubriquet* of 'the Cunning Woman,' and William Tranter, a labourer with whom she cohabited, were charged with obtaining various sums of money from Issac Rivers by means of false pretences. The prosecutor is a respectable-looking countryman living in the village of Hampstead Norris, a few miles from Newbury. It appeared from his evidence that in December last he lost his watch—how he did not know—and hearing of the 'Cunning Woman' at Newbury, he consulted her with reference to his loss. She promised to get the watch back for him, and asked first for 12*s.*, but he only gave her 2*s.* 6*d.*, on which she showed him, in a sort of looking-glass, the face of the man who had the watch, but he could only see something in the form of a man's whiskers. There was no face. Two days later she got 9*s.* 6*d.* of him 'to get something from the chemists.' On a third occasion she got 9*s.* 6*d.* more of him, and on a fourth visit he gave her 25*s.* on an absolute promise to get his watch back between 12 and 1 o'clock the same night. Of course he neither got his watch nor his money. The prisoners were remanded."—*Home News, February* 1868.

ter of this kind at Beerbhoom. Among them were considerable quantities of white and yellow arsenic, and a slag of copper ore coated with verdigris.

In conversations which I had with natives when I first began to investigate this subject, and especially with Baboo Joykissen Mookerjea, of Ooturparah, an enlightened native gentleman of rank, thoroughly conversant with all matters relating to his own people, I learnt that they did not believe in any extensive confederacy among the Road Poisoners of Bengal, considering them to be merely *budmashes*, each of whom is willing to enter into any nefarious plan in association with others, or to practise any villany independently and on his own account;—to aid in a dacoity, to serve as a *lattial* in a zemindaree quarrel, to assist in a strangling or some other act of secret butchery, or to lurk upon the road with poison ready for the first unwary traveller. In the following cases, we gain some insight into the practices of men of this class, both in the North-West and in Bengal.

Petumber Doss, *alias* Dhowkul, was tried at Allyghur for the theft of Mohuna, a boy aged eight or nine years, for the purpose of selling him. The boy was seen following the prisoner and crying.* Upon his apprehension, the man confessed before the tehseeldar that he had stolen the child from his parents ; this the boy also asserted. Before the judge, Petumber Doss declared that the boy accompanied him voluntarily, as he was ill-used by his step-mother. In his confessions before the magistrate and at the thannah, he admitted having perpetrated at antecedent periods, several other atrocious crimes, for some of which he had undergone imprisonment ; but, for others, including several cases of robbery by the administration of *dhatoora*, it would appear that he had not been apprehended or punished. It could not be proved, however, that he had actually committed those crimes. Sentence—five years' hard labour in irons.†

One Purkhit Mytee was tried, at Midnapore, in 1853, and sentenced to imprisonment for life in transportation, for having administered the seeds of the *dhatoora* to three travellers on their way from Calcutta to Cuttack. The prisoner accosted them, and, saying that he was of their own caste, offered to share the expenses of the road. Putting up at a shop, the prisoner offered to cook rice for the party. After eating a portion, one of the party found some seeds sticking to his teeth ; and, on taking them out, and examining them by the light, it was agreed by all three that they were the seeds of the *dhatoora* plant. The prisoner, however, observed, that it was nothing but the seeds of *dhunia (coriandrum sativum)*, and encouraged them to finish their

* There are reasons for believing that intoxicating drugs are employed by child-stealers in this Presidency. It will presently be seen that they are commonly had recourse to by these criminals in Bombay, and a case, noticed in Dr. Esdaile's "Mesmerism in India," broaches the question whether Animal Magnetism may not sometimes be resorted to for this purpose.

† Nizamut Adawlut Reports, N. W. P., 7th January 1853, p. 35.

meal, although he declined eating any himself, saying that warm rice disagreed with him. Two of the people became insensible immediately after ; the other, suspecting that the rice was poisoned, had refrained from eating any, and gave the alarm. The intoxicated persons remained two days and-a-half before they recovered from the effects of the poison. On the prisoner's person was found a scrip or purse containing several pockets, in one of which were seventeen seeds of the *dhatoora* plant ; and, in the remains of the food, the darogah discovered some seeds of the same plant. The prisoner had been in jail no less than four different times, *viz.*, 1837, theft, one year ; April 1839, one year in default of security ; May 1844, accused of administering drugs, charge not proved, one year's imprisonment in default of security. February 1850, arrested on charge of poisoning travellers, not proved ; in default of security, three years' imprisonment. February 1853, released ; was again arrested, on a charge of administering drugs to travellers, but made his escape from custody of a burkundauze, 23rd March 1853.*

There appears to be, in the North-West Provinces, a class of miscreants who drug their victims by employing young persons—upon whose credulity or spirit of mischief they find no difficulty in acting—as cat's-paws, in effecting the crime of drugging. In 1852, one Goolma, a lad not more than thirteen years of age, was tried at Bundelkund for administering some drug mixed up with *goor* to a child younger than himself, almost in the presence of its father. Upon his child becoming excited and intoxicated, the father went to Goolma and taxed him with the fact, which he acknowledged, saying that he committed the act in consequence of the boy's mother being afflicted with fits, and his expecting to get a goat from her. The prisoner confessed, both at the thannah and before the deputy magistrate, that he had given two and half seeds [pods ?] of *dhatoora* to the boy at the instigation of Putchcowree, the boy's uncle, who wished to play a joke upon the mother. There was no proof of this Putchcowree having instigated the act ; but there appears to be strong reason for believing that the crime was devised by some wretch who had designs upon the child's ornaments, or who wished to revenge himself upon its parents.†

Two years later, a lad named Kalloo, sixteen years of age, was tried at Moradabad for drugging a man. He confessed, at the thannah, and before the magistrate, that one Ilahya had given him some *dhatoora*, and had desired him to administer it to the man, as it would make him intoxicated, and the sight would be amusing—a promise of one or two annas appears to have sealed the contract. The prisoner asked the man to dine with him, and mixed the powder in some sugar which was eaten, and

* Nizamut Adawlut Reports, Vol. VI. of 1853, p. 721.

† *Ibid*, N. W. P., 14th April 1852, p. 304.

rendered the victim insensible. The robbery, however, was prevented. Kalloo was sentenced to four years' imprisonment.*

In the following month, Nujeeb, a lad about fifteen years old, small and boyish in appearance, was tried for administering poison mixed with food, and stealing property while the owner was in a state of insensibility. At the same time, the above-mentioned Ilahya was charged with instigating the lad to administer the poison with intent to rob. It appeared doubtful what poison was administered. Nujeeb pleaded that the other prisoner called it *dhatoora*, but a portion of *dhall* sent to the Civil Assistant Surgeon of Moradabad, was found to contain particles of *Meetha Teelia (or Aconitum Ferox)*. The *dhall*, however, was not duly identified as a portion of that partaken of, and the symptoms of intoxication and the insensibility produced were but transient. Ilahya was sentenced to five, and Nujeeb to three years' imprisonment.† The name of Ilahya will be alluded to presently in another case of hocussing—page 167.

In 1854 a party of thieves, at Monghyr, entered the house of a Mohajun, living in the main bazar, and plundered the place : having first, through the instrumentality of Etwaree, his servant, a lad of fifteen or sixteen, nephew to one of the burglars, drugged the man and his wife with some strong narcotic (a yellow powder), in their usual evening draught of boiled milk.‡

It has been very clearly shown by Mr. Dampier, in his Police Reports, that there is a class of robbers whose occupation lies in *Administering Drugs to Women of the Town*, and then robbing them of their ornaments, brass plates, &c., in which these women generally invest all they gain. The parties, usually two or three combined together, find out what prostitute possesses a good portion of ornaments, and then visit her, one as master, and the other as his servant. After some acquaintance, a drinking bout is proposed, to which these women never object. As she becomes intoxicated, the drug is administered with liquor; and whilst she is insensible, all her property is carried off. Sometimes the parties make sure of their victims by strangling, or otherwise making away with them, whilst in a state of insensibility. Mr. Dampier seems to consider that this practice has only become prevalent of late years.§

This crime appears to be nearly as common in the North-West as in the Lower Provinces.

A few illustrative examples will suffice.

One Ramessur Bholah was tried at Beerbhoom in 1855, for theft. The prosecutrix, a prostitute, stated that, on the night of the occurrence, she

* Nizamut Adawlut Reports, N. W. P., 26th October 1854, p. 618.
† *Ibid*, 27th November 1854, p. 766.
‡ *Ibid*, 1854, p. 730.
§ Police Reports, L. P., 1849, p. 71, and 1851, p. 59.

was seated at the door of her house, when the prisoner came and asked for water. After some conversation, he offered her some sweetmeats, and proposed to remain with her during the night, promising to give her eight annas. She ate some of the sweetmeats, as did also the prisoner. About twenty-five minutes afterwards she felt giddy, and became senseless. Next day, at about 3 P.M., she recovered ; and, at the thannah, she saw the prisoner, and also the ornaments which had been taken from her person during her insensibility. A yellow powder was found upon the prisoner ; this and the remains of the sweetmeats, on being examined by the medical officer and the chemical examiner, were declared [?] not to contain any deleterious or poisonous ingredients [detectible on chemical analysis ?]. The sessions judge convicted the man of theft, but threw out the charge of administering some deleterious or intoxicating drug, believing that the woman was merely intoxicated by liquor. The prisoner was sentenced to imprisonment for one year, with labour and irons.* It would appear, from the police reports, that cases of this simple description are of frequent occurrence in Calcutta.

Again, in 1852, a prostitute at Meerut declared, that one Joogul came to her house at night, conducted by second prisoner, Pertab. The former agreed to pass the night with her. He paid her eight annas in advance, and, going away, returned presently with sweetmeats, part of which he gave her. Shortly after eating them, she began to vomit, and being alarmed, went to the door, where she found a chowkeedar, to whom she imparted her impression that Joogul had given her something to cause intoxication. She closed the door, and afterwards became insensible, remaining so for two days. The chowkeedar kept watch on the outside ; and, in the morning, sent for the police, when Joogul was seized in the house, and Pearee was found insensible. The man was searched, and on him were found several suspicious articles, including *a rope supposed to be used for strangling*, and a box containing pills of different colours. Joogul attempted to throw the criminality upon Pertab, who related that Joogul mixed the ground seeds of *dhatoora* with the sweetmeats. It was proved that Joogul was a notoriously bad character ; and, at the sessions court, both prisoners made a full confession of their having agreed that Joogul, being a stranger, should give the woman sweetmeats, in which *dhatoora* had been mixed, in order that they might rob the house while she was insensible. The superior court held that the charge was fully proved against the prisoner Joogul, and that the charge of "aiding and abetting" in the offence was clearly established against the prisoner Pertab. In consideration of the facts that consequences endangering life did not ensue from the *dhatoora* administered, and that the intention appeared to have been to cause insensibility, and not death, the

* Ñizamut Adawlut Reports, Vol. V. of 1855, p. 367.

court mitigated the penalty prescribed by law, under the authority conveyed in Clause 4, Section 8, Regulation XVII. of 1817, and sentenced both the prisoners to seven years' imprisonment, with labour in irons.*

A prostitute of Meerut, named Ucphal, was employed with some other persons to attend, as dancers, at the wedding of a palkee-bearer's nephew. Before setting out, she employed one Khoda Buksh, as cook, at one rupee. On reaching their destination, they got *ottah* and *dhall* from the bride's family, which food the cook brought and prepared. The woman and six other persons ate of this separately. It tasted bitter, and the prisoner said some *neem* berries had fallen into it, so the woman continued to eat. Afterwards, her head grew giddy, and he then brought her a *hooka:* she then became insensible ; whilst she was in that state, the cook took her gold ear-rings from her, and other property from the others, and went away. She recovered her senses in ten or eleven hours. The man was apprehended by the Thuggee Superintendent, before whom he admitted that he had given *dhatoora*. Sentence, fourteen years' imprisonment in banishment.†

In many cases, however, the criminals are not satisfied with "hocussing" their victims, but murder them, while in a state of insensibility. Thus,—

Two instances occurred near Calcutta, in 1849. In one, the culprits drugged a prostitute with whom they were drinking, and then completed their work by strangling her. The result was that three persons were sentenced to imprisonment in transportation for life. In the other case, the woman was first intoxicated and then robbed of her ornaments and stabbed. She died in consequence.‡

In the following year, the case of a woman of this class was reported. She was found in her house, in the town of Bancoorah, strangled and denuded of all her ornaments. There was no appearance of any struggle, and not the slightest noise was heard by the neighbours, who lived within four feet of her dwelling. The Superintendent of Police offered a reward for the discovery of the murderer, but without success.§ A rather mysterious case of this kind occurred at Benares in 1854. Two men, Gunput and Boochnoo, were tried for the wilful murder of two women of indifferent character, and for robbing them of their ornaments and clothes. The women, mother and daughter, who were described as next thing to common prostitutes, were found, one morning, lying dead in their house. The Civil Surgeon, on examining their bodies, could scarcely form an

* Nizamut Adawlut Reports, N. W. P., for 17th April 1852, p. 328.

† Nizamut Adawlut Reports, 8th July 1853, p. 834. See also a case in which one Juggobundoo Bose was convicted of having drugged two prostitutes of Dacca in their own house and of then robbing them of property valued at upwards of two hundred rupees.—*Nizamut Adawlut Reports*, Vol. IV., of 1854, p. 304.

‡ Police Report, L. P., for 1850, p. 62.

§ Nizamut Adawlut Reports for 1851, p. 59.

opinion as to the manner in which they met with their deaths; for, though there were some suspicious-looking marks on the neck of one of the women, still these marks did not extend to the cellular tissue below. From the general placidity of the features exhibited by both bodies, and other circumstances, he came to the conclusion that "*Burking*" must have been practised on these females. "He was led to this conclusion from the livid placidity shown by the features of the deceased." He was of opinion that they could not possibly have died of intoxication; that their stomachs contained, in the one some digested food, smelling of bazar liquor; in the other some *dhall* and meat. The evidence regarding the parties to the crime involved some uncertainties. There could be no doubt, however, that at least two men were in the house on the night of the murder, one of whom was the elder woman's nephew. The clothes which were stolen were found in his possession; the women's silver ornaments were found in the house of the other man. It was proved that these two men purchased liquor in the early part of the night on which the women were murdered. It appears that the prisoners made confessions, both to the police and before the deputy magistrate, in considerable detail, relating with minuteness the incidents accompanying the violent death of the two females by "smothering" after first intoxicating them. The printed report does not contain the full particulars of these confessions; it is mentioned, however, that, at the thannah, one of the prisoners asserted that the women had been throttled by pressing a stick across their throats (a very common practice). This statement he retracted in the magistrate's court, where both prisoners asserted that they had suffocated the women by compression with the hand. With reference, apparently, to the first mode of destruction alluded to, the medical officer decided that the account given by the prisoners must be false; as, had death been inflicted in this manner (by throttling with a stick), the features would have been distorted [?] and marks would have been left on the cellular tissue. The judge of the superior court held that, on the other hand, the *post-mortem* appearances seemed to be quite consistent with the fact of homicidal suffocation by compression with the hand. Dr. Taylor observes, respecting the evidences of death by suffocation, that there rarely exist appearances indicative of violence, or other than natural extinction of life, unless circumstances arouse suspicion, and direct the inquiry to such a result. Unless such a result be clearly referrible to the accident, it would not, he remarks, be attempted on healthy adult persons, unless they were in a state of intoxication, and thereby rendered defenceless. Most persons, unless thus rendered powerless, would be able to offer so much resistance as would leave on their bodies indubitable evidence of murderous violence. The incidents of the present case, it was held, exhibit a close correspondence to the above statement. The women must have been able to offer a vigorous resistance, if they had not been overpowered by spirits. Indeed, one of the prisoners particularly mentioned that "they died easy, being senseless from intoxication." Death was awarded.*

Thuggee of Travellers by Poison.

In 1856 I urged that a thorough and successful investigation of this atrocity would certainly prove an undertaking of national importance in India. At that time we had only to deal with scattered facts. These, however, sufficiently demonstrated :—

1. That the crime (which appears to have become more prevalent since the check given to Thuggee by Strangulation) is common throughout the three Presidencies of India.
2. That it is pursued systematically, as a trade, not being merely the device of a stray criminal here and there; and that, in great probability, those who practise it are Thugs in the commonly received acceptation of the term.

Lower Provinces.

The Table at the head of this chapter will show how generally this crime is practised in the *Lower Provinces of the Bengal Presidency.* It must not, however, be supposed that certain instances of its commission do not occur in the districts against which numbers are not found. In Chittagong, for example, the crime was, within my own knowledge, by no means very uncommon; although up to that time, cases may not have been fully detected and brought to trial.

Upper India.

In a brief tabular statement by Dr. Esdaile, upon the cases reported upon to the Magistrate of Azimghur, during the year 1834-35,† we have the following entries which afford strong evidence of the prevalence of road-poisoning in that district, and also throughout *Upper India:*

"Fifteen persons poisoned on the road for their property and recovered by timely vomiting."

"Eight travellers poisoned for their goods, by *dhatoora* probably."

"Four putrid bodies, probably poisoned, the bodies being stript, as is usual in these cases."

Madras Presidency.

A narrative given by Surgeon H. W. Porteous of the Civil Dispensary, Coimbatore, affords evidence of the great prevalence of this atrocity in the *Madras Presidency,* in 1851.‡ Dr. Porteous states that he had treated six victims to the nefarious practices of a gang of thieves who made use of the *dhatoora* to effect their purpose. The police authorities were put on the alert, and succeeded in apprehending the gang, who were brought to trial, when it appeared that, in one of their tours, they had administered

* Nizamut Adawlut Reports, N. W. P., 4th December 1854, p. 797.
† The India Journal of Medical Science, V. II., p. 262.
‡ Medical Reports selected by the Madras Medical Board, 1855, p. 334.

the drug to eleven persons. To one of these it proved fatal. In every case they succeeded in their object of robbing. Their method was to mix a portion of the pounded seeds in either the rice, curry, or pepper-water,—of which they invited travellers to partake. The charge was proved against them, and they were sentenced accordingly.

Dr. Porteous said that eight grains, or 48 seeds, are sufficient to produce the full effects of *dhatoora* poisoning in from two to three hours in a strong able-bodied man.

Bombay Presidency.

We find it reported* that at the Sessions of July 1838, at *Bombay*, one Luximon Balloo was convicted of murder, by administering *dhatoora* to a blanket-seller, and executed. The night before his execution, he made an ample confession of his guilt, stating also that two individuals named Jumsal and Hoosain Essoof, with a Fakeer, who generally sat under a tree near the bazar gate, were in the habit of entrapping the unwary to take *dhatoora* for the purpose of robbing them of any trifling articles that they might possess. The police were long upon the alert to apprehend these three, but were, until lately, unsuccessful. They were then, however, in the jail upon a charge of giving this drug to a cooly who, after being taken to the General Hospital, recovered sufficiently to identify them.

It appears from the reports of Captain C. Hervey, the Assistant General Superintendent for the Suppression of Dacoity, that, in *Bombay*, poisoning is a regular profession, the victims being generally children. In an interesting account of *dhatoora* poisoning published by Dr. Giraud in the Transactions of the Medical and Physical Society of Bombay for 1849, it is remarked that "viewing the most prevalent motive to *dhatoora* poisoning, it would seem as if some regularly organized band of thieves had, within the previous year, invaded that island." From 1837 and 1838, when a few cases of poisoning, supposed to be from *dhatoora*, were noticed by Drs. Bell and McLellan in the several reports on the Native General Hospital,—up to 1848, only from six to ten such cases had been annually recorded ; but, during 1849, *fifty-one cases* had come under hospital treatment ! Dr. Giraud also alludes to the practice of drugging children with sweetmeats containing the powdered seeds, that their ornaments may be more easily removed.

The *Sindian* of 17th May 1856 reported that "Poisoning seems to have become a profession in Sind, and in some cases a lucrative one. In another part of our paper will be found a few lines from Kotree on the subject. We have just received a communication from Shikarpore, which gives us the outlines of a diabolical system that has been carried on in Upper Sind for the last few years. A gang of notorious characters have just been unkennelled in that Collectorate, who have been

* Allen's Asiatic Journal for March 1839.

in the habit of disguising themselves as Fakeers, and administering poison to people possessed of wealth, which they appropriated to themselves, after they had succeeded in putting them to death. Their plan of operations was very simple, and from that fact they were the better able to delude their victims. About this time of the year the laboring population employed upon the canals are accustomed to return home with the earnings they have saved during the working season. These people were generally selected by this nefarious gang for destruction. They offered them, in God's name, food which was impregnated with some deadly poison, and, as soon as it had the desired effect, they plundered the dead bodies of any property found on them. Our correspondent informs us that last year no less than nine persons were sacrificed in this manner, and, within the last month, seven, out of twelve who were poisoned, died. Some time back, he tells us, Government offered a reward of one thousand rupees for the discovery of the guilty party, and this seems to have had the wished-for result, as the whole gang have been apprehended, and a minute enquiry into the extent of their murderous practices was promised."

In the investigation of the sources of this crime, it is of the first importance to bear in mind that old writers describe the use of Poison as an essential part of the Thug system. "*Deleterious drugs,*" says Forbes, "*are stated to be used only by novices in the business, the more experienced Thugs trusting rather to the certain effects of the knife or cord than to the doubtful operation of poison.*" Still, it is conceivable that, observing the attention of the police employed in their suppression to be mainly directed to the practice of Strangling, the Thugs should have, in a great measure, abandoned the use of the *roomal*, and have devoted all their craft to the easier and safer practice of Drugging.

At the same time, it does not appear that any absolutely demonstrative evidence has been adduced identifying either the *Meetawallas* of Bengal or the Up-country *Dhatooreeas* with the true Thugs.

Mr. Dampier, whose judgment in the matter is unimpeachable, alludes, in his Reports for the 1st and 2nd half years of 1840, to circumstances which, at about that time, brought to light the existence of a system of administering poisonous drugs to travellers which, "since the suppression of Thuggee, had increased along the lines of general communication and in other parts of the country." He, however, appears to have considered that this practice was not carried on by Thugs.

In 1842, the Police Superintendent of Bengal stated in his report that a line of professional poisoners (called *meetawallas*, the poison being contained in sweetmeats) had been discovered on the Sasseram road. This is not a new trait in the annals of crime in India. The *Hurkaru* says: "From Nobutpoor to Bancoorah, a line of poisoners had flourished for some time. In 1835, an old woman was seized in Jehanabad, fourteen miles west of Sasseram, and upon her were found credentials from the poisoning community at large, as also special recommendations to the good services of different police officers on the whole line of road."*

Colonel Sleeman wrote, in 1844, that the impunity with which this crime is everywhere perpetrated, and its consequent increase in every part of India, were among the greatest evils with which the country was, at that time, afflicted. These poisoners were then as numerous over the Bombay and Madras Presidencies as over that of Bengal. There was no road free from them ; and he believed that, throughout India, there must be many hundreds who gained their subsistence by that trade alone.†

Just at this time, we find this practice systematically practised in the Lower Provinces by the *Meetawallas* (the designation given by Mr. Dampier to this class of robbers). In 1854, two persons were reported as having been drugged to death in Behar by a party of professional poisoners on the Great Road. No traces could be found of the offenders, and the survivors of the party drugged could not give a clear description of them. The superintendent remarked upon the extraordinary fact that, although travellers were fully warned of the acts of these men, and notices to that effect were put up at the Serais and Chuttees, they constantly fell victims to the robbers.‡ Again, in his report of the following year, upon the state of crime in the district of Shahabad—(a portion of the country fearfully notorious in the history of the old Thuggee system ; and, as the table will show, still the most rife of all the districts in Bengal in cases of Thuggee by Poison)—Mr. Dampier mentions that all the thefts by administering drugs occurred to travellers passing along the road who, in spite of the continued precautions put up in all the Chuttees and given to them by the deputy magistrates and police officers on the Trunk Road to prevent strangers from joining their parties,§ continued to drink and receive tobacco and dry food from the hands of such persons, thus affording them opportunities of acquiring their confidence and administering drugs at a place favorable for the escape of the poisoners, who were constantly on the watch for their victims. In two of the cases which occurred that year, death ensued ; in two, no trace of the *meetawallas* could be discovered ; and, in the last, one party was convicted. He considered that the reason for more offences of this kind occurring in the Shahabad and the Behar districts, is that the victims have generally come near the end of their journey, and would separate from the poisoners if they delayed administering the poison ; and also that there are greater opportunities of escape through bye-roads into other jurisdictions, whilst

* Allen's Asiatic Journal, 1842, Vol. 39.

† Rambles and Recollections of an Indian Official, Vol. I., p. 114.

‡ Report for 1845, p. 13.

§ Similar warnings to Sepoys going on leave to their homes have appeared, from time to time, in General Orders.

the person drugged is in a state of insensibility. Again, in 1849, we find Mr. Dampier reporting the continued prevalence of this crime on the Grand Trunk and other roads; and, while annexing a statement showing the number of persons arrested, punished, and acquitted upon charges of the kind,* remarking that, unfortunately, the chances of detection are but few. The poison, generally the seeds of the *dhatoora*, is to be found on the road side; and, reduced to powder, is nearly tasteless, when mixed with tobacco or food; while, if the victims do recover, they are for so long a time in a state of stupefaction, and unable to give any account of the transaction, that there is every opportunity afforded for the escape of the criminals. In commenting upon his statement showing the charges of poisoning which came before the assistant general superintendent for the suppression of Thuggee at Patna in 1850, Mr. Dampier again insists that this document does not give the slightest idea of the prevalence of the crime, particularly along the Grand Trunk Road, where the want of caution on the part of travellers, and the easy avoidance of detection on that of the criminals, render its occurrence frequent; added to which, from Bukhtiarnugger or Munglepore, in Bancoorah, to Sasseram in Shahabad, there was then not a single officer posted along that line of road, and the police arrangements throughout for the protection of travellers were very deficient.

Mr. Dampier considered that a combination existed along the lines of road frequented by travellers, pilgrims, &c., for robbery by this atrocious method; and that the dawk bearers, petty muddees at the halting-places, bhuteearas, and common thieves, were in it.†

Colonel Sleeman describes the professional road-poisoners, or *Dhatooreeas*, as commonly employing the *dhatoora* which they sometimes give in the hookah to be smoked, and at others in food. Their intention, he considers, is almost always to destroy life, as "dead men tell no tales;" but the poisoned people sometimes recover, and lead to the detection of the poisoners. The cases in which they recovered were rare (when Colonel Sleeman wrote); and of those who recovered and traced the criminals, very few would ever undertake to prosecute them through the magistrates and the sessions courts. These people put on all manner of disguises to suit their purpose; and, as they prey chiefly upon the

* The statements of cases of professional poisoners before the assistant superintendent for the suppression of Thuggee for the Patna Division, of this and the following year, show that thirty-seven persons were apprehended during that period, upon charges of this kind—eight were found guilty and sentenced, four were noted as having been transferred to other jurisdictions, or as under trial, and the remainder were acquitted.

† Beaufort's Digest of the Criminal Law—para. 3117.

poorer sort of travellers, they require to destroy the greater number of lives to make up their incomes.*

A party of two or three poisoners have very often succeeded in destroying another of eight or ten travellers with whom they have journeyed for some days, by pretending to give them a feast on the celebration of the anniversary of some family event. Sometimes an old woman or man will manage the thing alone, by gaining the confidence of travellers, and getting near the cooking pots while they go aside ; or when employed to bring the flour for the meal from the bazar. The poison is put into the flour as opportunity offers. People of all castes and callings take to this trade, some casually, others for life, and others derive it from their parents or teachers ; and the habit of cooking, eating, and sleeping on the side of the road, and the custom of smoking with strangers of seemingly the same caste, greatly facilitate their designs. The small parties are, this authority believes, unconnected with each other, and two parties never unite in the same expedition. The members of one party may be sometimes convicted and punished, but their detection is accidental ; for the system, he considers, which has enabled us to put down the *Thug* associations cannot be applied, with any fair prospect of success, to the suppression of these pests of society, seeing that the Thugs went on their adventures in large gangs ; and two or more gangs were commonly united in the course of an expedition in the perpetration of many murders. Every man shared in the booty according to the rank he held in the gang, or the part he took in the murders ; and the rank of every man, and the part he took generally, or in any particular murder, were for the most part well known to all. From these gangs when arrested, the authorities elicited the first clue to the evidence required for their conviction. This thorough unravelment of the whole organization by the confession of a few parties implicated, or by what is called the *approver* system, is not to be expected when, as in the case of the poisoners, the gangs are small and wholly distinct from each other.

The following are abstracts of the principal cases of *Drugging on the Highway*, which appeared in the Reports of the N. W. and Lower Provinces, from 1852 to 1855. It will be seen that the always available poison,—the Datura Seeds,—was believed to have been used in all the cases of this class, and that, in two instances only, was it considered probable that other poisons (Nux Vomica and Gunjah) were added to the seeds.

I remarked in 1856 that it was to be borne in mind that, although it had evidently become much more frequent of late years than it was during the

* This author details the case of a poor old Fakeer (mendicant,) and his young son, who were beset, drugged, and plundered by a family of these miscreants for the sake of a blanket—their only property. The child died, the father recovered after three days' intoxication and stupor.

unrestrained prevalence of Thuggee by Strangulation, this crime is by no means of recent origin. A very marked instance, which occurred in 1809, is reported by Macnaughten* and will be cited in full under the head of Poisoning by Dhatoora. It appears, however, that the first law instituted for controlling this crime, was promulgated so late as the year 1817.

In 1852, two men—Bhowany,† and Bhola, his nephew, were tried at Meerut, on the accusation of a man who deposed that, when on his way to Lucknow, he met Bhowany at Umballah, who said he would travel in company with him. On their way, Bhowany took him to a bunneah's shop and purchased some *ottah* and *dhall;* after cooking it, deponent went, at Bhowany's request, for some water; returning, he ate the food and became insensible. Bhola, who had lately joined them, was present. Bhowany placed the man within a hut; they then robbed him, and pretended to the police that their party consisted only of two. The police found the prosecutor insensible and concealed in a corner of the hut. A bag of *dhatoora* seed was found on Bhowany, some of this had been ground to powder, also some *Churus*—concrete juice of the *Cannabis Indica.* The prisoners mutually accused each other.—Sentence, fourteen years' imprisonment.‡

The following case singularly closely resembles, in its main features, one already cited (at p. 156). The prisoners' names were the same, and both cases occurred near Meerut, but they were quite distinct.

A prostitute, named Durbarun, who gained her livelihood by singing, was proceeding from Meerut to Allyghur, accompanied by her mother and six other persons. They were met on the way by one Khodabuksh, who appears to have had some acquaintance with the party at Meerut. He said that he was in want of service, and was engaged by the woman as cook to the party. On arriving at Coel, they put up at a Serai, and the prisoner was given food to cook. This

---

* Vol. I. p. 216. In 1812 one Joolsee Tewaree drugged four fakeers in Shahabad. They all became insensible and one died—*Ibid*, p. 209. In 1820, Kulwa, disguised as a Chuprassee, joined two brothers travelling by Bandah. He offered them some sweetmeat called Peeran (a kind of consecrated food); each received about two pice weight. The thief forbade them to spit any out. The stuff had an unpleasant taste. In a short time both fell down senseless. Joolsee made off with their effects. One of the brothers speedily died; the other recovered his senses on the following day. It appeared, at the trial, that the accused was an infamous character, who had travelled about plundering by administering poisonous drugs to all whom he could entice into taking them. *Ibid*, Vol. II., p. 51.

This trick of giving poison in food said to be consecrated was practised upon a Modee (supposed to be rich) at Godie in 1865. Sunkur, a gang poisoner, and three of his party disguised themselves as a *Gosain*, or priest, and his *Chelas*, disciples. They sat themselves down before the shop. Sunkur began to act the priest, muttered munters, performed poojah, and passed on the *pershad*, or offering, to his pretended disciples, who kept it in their hands, as they knew it was drugged. They then proffered a portion of their offering to the unfortunate Modee, who, at first, refused to eat it, but being told it was *pershad*, he ate it, and became delirious, and then insensible. The neighbours becoming alarmed, the thieves had to decamp without booty.—*Rep. of I. G. Jails, L. P.*, for 1565, p. 33.

† Bhowany was a very favorite name among the organized Thugs.—See Index to names in Col. Sleeman's "Thug Gangs of Upper and Central India." See also the case of one Bhowaneedeen, convicted of an atrocity of the kind, at p. 116 of this Manual.

‡ Nizamut Adawlut Reports, N. W. P., June 19th, 1852, p. 568.

was eaten at about nine in the evening. At midnight, the chowkeedar of the *Serai* observed some of the party rolling about the ground; he went up, and found them all more or less affected by some intoxicating drug. The prisoner lay among them feigning sleep, and some gold and silver ornaments belonging to the prostitute were found on his person. Four of the men who were most intoxicated were sent to the Dispensary, and, by judicious treatment, recovered in three days. The three women, and the rest of the party, who had eaten less, recovered after having been given some medicine to make them vomit. The prisoner confessed before the magistrate that he procured the *dhatoora* from a neighbouring garden, which he pointed out, on pretence of requiring it for a sick bullock. The civil surgeon deposed that the four *meerasees* were brought to him in a state of muttering delirium, and he detailed the symptoms as peculiarly the effects of an overdose of *dhatoora.* He stated that this drug is poisonous, or merely intoxicating, in proportion to the quantity taken, in relation to the strength and constitution of the patient; and that, as the patients brought to him were all strong men, he thinks it probable that the effects would have gone off, without proving fatal, even if prompt measures had not been taken. There was reason to believe that this was not the first instance in which the prisoner had been guilty of the same offence.—Imprisonment for fourteen years.*

Two travellers were putting up at the new *Serai* at Mirzapore, when one Ramtuhul also came there and made acquaintance with them. One of the men, having been preparing his food, asked Ramtuhul, who was close by, to look after it while he went to fetch water at the well.

During his short absence the other took the opportunity of putting some *dhatoora* into the *dhall*, which rendered one of the travellers insensible a few hours afterwards; the other became so during the night. The prisoner confessed, at the kotwalee and in the foujdaree, that he had put some *dhatoora* in the *dhall*, and made no defence on trial. Imprisonment for life in transportation.†

---

* Nizamut Adawlut Reports, N. W. P., November 26th, 1852, p. 1389. The practice of hiring themselves out as *Cooks* is an old and rather frequent one among the Dhatooreeas. A case, which occurred in the beginning of this century, will be found in Macnaghten's Reports of the Nizamut Adawlut, Vol. I., p. 368. A woman had been employed by the complainant as a household servant. Her first act appears to have been to prepare the evening meal for the family. Of this her master partook. He was alarmed, on rising from his repast, to observe every individual in his house in a state of stupefaction; and, at the same time, became aware, from the dryness of his mouth and a giddiness with which he was seized, that he had swallowed some deleterious substance. Although scarcely conscious of what he did, he found means to call to his assistance two persons who resided near, by whose aid the proper remedies were administered to the whole family;—before this, however, the prisoner escaped with a pair of silver foot-ornaments and a necklace. In another instance, this prisoner was proved to have prepared cakes for four sepoys, who, shortly after eating, became so violently intoxicated, as to be utterly unconscious of what they said or did. Three other persons also partook of the same food with similar results. The prisoner, taking advantage of the confusion thus created, decamped with several articles. She alleged, in her defence, that the state of her health made a constant use of the *dhatoora* seeds necessary. She, consequently, carried a quantity about her, and that it was probable some might have fallen into the food without her knowledge. See other recent instances at p. 178.

I learn that a band of Road Poisoners was detected at Meerut about 1845. The Chiefs were a Bheestie and the Kansamah of the Station Mess.

† Nizamut Adawlut Reports, N. W. P., March 23rd, 1854, p. 306.

In the previous January, a man and his son, while journeying towards the Punjab, halted at a mosque in Paneeput. One Ullayar Khan fell into conversation with them; and at last offered them something to eat. The father went into the city to purchase food. On his return, he found bread moistened with *sherbut*, which his son told him had been brought by the person who promised them food. They partook of this, and, shortly afterwards, began to feel stupefied, in which state the prisoner came to them, and removed them to another mosque, where they became totally insensible. On recovery of their senses, after three or four days, they found that they had been robbed of their money. The native doctor deposed that the men were under his treatment for three or four days, suffering from the effects of violent stupefaction, induced, as he supposed from the symptoms, by *dhatoora*. The prisoner was a known bad character. Sentence, fourteen years' imprisonment.*

In April 1853 the thannahdar of Bohsha (Jounpoor) sent in two men, Sheogholam and Sheochurn, with a small quantity of *dhatoora* tied up in a piece of cloth, together with other articles belonging to them. He reported that, in the preceding months of October and December, two cases of administering poisonous drugs or *dhatoora* to three persons named had occurred at Mouzah Lukneepoor, and in another spot; both places being near the high road leading to Allahabad. A strict search had been instituted, but without success, until the two prisoners were seized. Their conversation and behaviour exciting the suspicion of a police jemadar, he searched a bundle, their joint property, and found in it a patlee of *dhatoora*. One of the prisoners escaped, but was recaptured. They both confessed that they had brought the *dhatoora* with them to mix either in the water or food prepared by travellers, whenever a fitting opportunity offered. *This, they said, was their business.* They denied being implicated in the former cases alluded to above, but their appearance corresponded with the description given by the sufferers of the persons who had given them intoxicating drugs in their food. The *dhatoora* was sent to the civil surgeon for examination. One Koosial stated that he was a grass-cutter in the service of an officer, and was returning to his home in Zillah Azimghur, having with him Rs. 29 in cash, &c. The prisoners and another man, who called himself a sepoy, joined him at Futtehpoor. After travelling together some days, one of the prisoners bought some *ottah*. They prepared bread, some of which was given to him: after eating it, he became insensible, when the three men plundered him and made off. A woman recollected to have seen the prisoners and the grass-cutter together. The judge of the superior court considered that there were the strongest grounds for believing that the prisoners were poisoners by profession, and belonged to a class who infest the high roads for the purpose of entrapping unwary travellers. He observed, from a proceeding from the Magistrate of Azimgurh appended to the record, and from police reports of the Jounpoor District, also filed in the case, that no less than four cases of poisoning with theft took place in the high roads, in the same vicinity, within the period of three months previous to the capture of the prisoners, in which eight persons were drugged and robbed; and which, in one of the instances,

* Nizamut Adawlut Reports, N. W. P., January 6th, 1854, p. 592.

ended fatally. He therefore confirmed the sentence of imprisonment for life in transportation passed on the prisoners.*

In January of the same year Kureemoollah, *bhutteearah*, was tried on the following charge. Three men, who were in the habit of coming to the cattle mart of Chundowsee with cattle for sale, deposed that they were there on a certain date. Early in the morning, they left their quarters in the *Serai* which belonged to the defendant, and went to the market. On their return, the prisoner said to them, "Some calamity will occur to-night; give me what money you have about you, and I will lock it up." They replied, "What! is not this place under the British rule?" and refused to give up the money. They then called for dinner. At this time a violent storm arose, which uprooted large trees, and did a great deal of damage throughout the country. During the storm, the prisoner called them to dinner. They commenced eating *dhall* and *chuppattees* which he had cooked. One of them observed that the *dhall* was very bitter. The prisoner insisted twice that he had merely put too much salt to it. Immediately after eating the *dhall*, the three men became insensible in the prisoner's house. The young son of one of them took a mouthful of the *dhall* which caused him to vomit—and he ate no more. Seeing his father and others insensible, he ran out, although the prisoner tried to prevent him, and called a chowkeedar posted hard by. The police found the three men insensible, but the prisoner was well and in his senses: they went off to the thannah, and, on their return, found the prisoner feigning insensibility. He and the others were carried to the thannah on charpoys. Shoobratee Muqbool and Hussun Jurrahs were called to prescribe for all four. They did so, and made the three travellers swallow some peera and milk, forcing it down their throats, and tickled their throats with a feather, which caused them to vomit. The prisoner drank the peera and milk himself, whence it was evident that he was sensible, and the feather was not put down his throat. He was quite well the next morning, whereas the three men did not recover until the third day. The civil surgeon detected *dhatoora* in the *dhall*, and the prisoner admitted its presence in the food. The prisoner was sentenced to seven years' imprisonment.†

It is worthy of remark that the prisoner stated in his defence that one Ilahya (Illaheea) came to his house several times during the storm; and that, perhaps, he threw something into it. At the trial he recalled his hints against Ilahya, and endeavoured to criminate others. This was probably the Ilahya who was convicted at that place two years later as a systematic poisoner—See page 154.

In the following case, it would appear that the robber administered the *dhatoora* so freely to his victim as to cause death. It is not certain, however, that other unfair means were not resorted to, while the unfortunate man lay insensible at the prisoner's mercy.

When on trial at Bundlekund in 1853, one Kashee confessed that he gave a portion of *chutnee* in which *dhatoora* seeds had been inserted, to five persons, but pleaded not guilty to the murder of Bunsroop, one of the five. It appeared

* Nizamut Adawlut Reports, N. W. P., July 25th, 1853, p. 910.

† *Ibid*, January 12th, 1853, p. 50.

from the united testimony of the four survivors that they, with the deceased, formed a travelling party, and were joined by the prisoner. On cooking their dinner, the prisoner, to improve its flavour, offered them some *chutnee*, which they accepted and mixed with their dish—of this all the travellers partook, and became intoxicated and temporarily frantic. While in this state, two of them were robbed. After the effects of the intoxication had gone off, Bunsroop was missing, and his body was discovered on the third day in a neighbouring nullah. The prisoner was seen in company with the travellers. Evidence of their intoxicated condition was adduced—the stolen property was found in the possession of the prisoner, and with it a large quantity of *chutnee*, which was also produced in Court. The poisonous and deleterious nature of the *chutnee* was proved by the evidence of Dr. Ransford and two native druggists, who deposed that the seed contained therein were those of the *dhatoora*. The druggists asserted that the administration of fifteen or twenty seeds would be fatal to life. Dr. Ransford alleged that the death of Bunsroop was to be ascribed to the administration of *dhatoora*, or *stramonium*, as the indications of congestion in the lungs, head, and brain were such as would be caused by that poison. The prisoner was sentenced to death.*

In the following cases, there appeared to be reason for believing that *mixed poisons* were administered by the robbers to their victims.

Thana and Kishnoo, of Moradabad (a district singularly rife in cases of this description), were tried in 1852, upon the accusation of one Dya, who deposed that he and his brother Munsookh went to Kant to sell wheat. While disposing of the grain at a disadvantage, Thana came to them, telling them that, if they would accompany him to his village, he would take their wheat off their hands. They agreed; while on the way, they ate some parched wheat. Thana said that he would give them sugar to eat with it. He took some out of a bundle containing about one-and-a-half seer, and gave them each about six chittacks [12 ounces] of it. They ate the whole of the sugar with their wheat! and had not got 200 yards when they became insensible. Dya's belly began to burn, and his throat became dry; he did not completely recover his senses until the second morning, when he had vomited. Munsookh died the next day at twelve o'clock. Their property had disappeared. Some of the stolen articles were subsequently found in the house of Kishnoo, Thana's father; Thana had disappeared, but was afterwards seized. A bundle of sugar was found in the house. Thana, who was a notorious *budmash*, confessed before the thannahdar that he gave the men sugar, and then plundered them. Many witnesses deposed that both prisoners, father and son, were bad characters; "they administered poison to travellers and then plundered them;" but, the elder being a chowkeedar, no one interfered with them. Thana withdrew his confession in the Sessions Court, and said that the police had extorted it by beating him with a *kora*. Dr. Stiven deposed that the sugar sent to him for examination in this case contained the powder of the seeds of *dhatoora* and *nux vomica*, and that the statement given by Dya was highly probable, *viz.*, that he and his brother had been poisoned by eating each about twelve ounces of such sugar. The younger prisoner was sentenced to imprisonment in banishment for life. The elder was acquitted.†

* Nizamut Adawlut Reports, N. W. P., February 22nd, 1853, p. 262.

† *Ibid*, August 21st, 1852, p. 853.

One Khoman was tried, at Cawnpore, in 1854, upon three charges of poisoning and robbery. In the first of these cases, it was shown that a conversation was overheard by one Nidha between the prisoner and his mother, in which the latter accused her son of spending the money which he obtained by robbery and violence in debauchery. Nidha, having heard of the death of three hackery men by poison, made inquiries as to the description of the person who had hired the hackeries ; this agreeing with that of the prisoner, he gave information to the police. On being apprehended, the prisoner admitted his concernment in the crime, but implicated others as accomplices. A young intelligent boy, named Chowdhree, was with the murdered men. He stated that the deceased's hackeries were hired by the prisoner, who said that he wished to have some sugar conveyed towards the Jumna. Setting out, they halted, at night-fall, at a small village, and the prisoner prepared a *sherbut* by pounding up *bhang* (Indian hemp), &c., and *ottah*, which he gave to the three men and also to the witness ; the latter took a very small quantity and escaped, but the other three fell into a state of insensibility, from which they never awoke. The magistrate, after investigating other charges against the prisoner, arrived at the conclusion that the "prisoner was a professional murderer and robber by administering poison." He was identified, while in jail, by the victims of two other cases, who at once pointed him out from a crowd of the prisoners, and whose previous description of the person who had robbed them exactly coincided with that of the prisoner. The plan resorted to in all the cases being, as in this, to hire the hackeries of men who, having just completed a contract, would probably have the profits derived from it on their persons. Proof was absent as to the nature of the poison used. The bodies of the deceased men were in too advanced a stage of decomposition to admit of examination. The contents of a bottle sent to the Chemical Examiner were not ascertained by analysis to be poisoned, "though the known difficulty in detecting vegetable poisons is acknowledged," and the presence of *dhatoora* (the most usual poison in such cases) is not readily detectible, even when the examination of the contents of the stomach is immediate. Hemp (*bhang*) is, however, itself a strong poison, and the administration of an inordinate dose, intentionally, in the prosecution of a felonious purpose, would be quite sufficient to justify a conviction for murder. In the present case, the mixture composed by the prisoner was, by his own statement, shown to have contained three parts of hemp, which, in addition to the powder or the infusion [?] of *dhatoora* would abundantly account for the destruction of human life which followed." After a careful trial of each of the three cases, all of which were clearly proved, the prisoner was sentenced to death.*

* Nizamut Adawlut Reports, N. W. P., October 3rd, 1854, p. 479. A very iniquitous case, involving the murder of a hackery driver by a systematic road poisoner, was tried at Benares in July and October 1853. It appeared that a very young country-born girl, named Victoria Adelaide Hassey, eloped from her mother's house in company with one Henry Halpin, Chumroo, and a lad named Kandhaee. On the arrival of the party, by boat, at Bhaugulpore, a quarrel arose between the girl and Halpin, who deposed that she herself mixed *dhatoora* and cooked the food with which he was drugged as well as the boatmen [?], so that they did not recover their senses for two or three days. The girl then decamped with the native Chumroo, and came to Monghyr, accompanied by one Shubrattee. Here they engaged a hackery, whose driver's name was said to be Sookhun. On their way to Dinapore, they are alleged to have drugged this driver, and to have made away with him, and to have sold the hackery and bul-

In the Chapter on Arsenical Poisoning, the details of a case have been given (p. 116) in which a road poisoner deliberately administered a fatal dose of Arsenious Acid to his victims. It would appear that this crime is of by no means very rare occurrence in the North-West Provinces. In his observations upon a case of Arsenical poisoning tried at Bareilly, Mr. G. D. Raikes, the additional sessions judge, mentioned that, in several cases of poisoning which had come to his knowledge in another district, the poison had been disguised as a sweetmeat of tempting quality; and being offered as a refreshment to a wayfaring man on the road, had frequently caused death to the unsuspicious partaker of it.*

In 1855, it appeared that one Madhoo Sahoo joined six men travelling from Calcutta to their homes in the Midnapore District. While they were cooking their dinner, it appeared that there was no *huldee* (turmeric). Madhoo said he had some, and immediately dropped some powder into the vegetables. He said that he had fever, and threw away his food. The travellers were all poisoned, and one died. A white powder, declared to be arsenic, was found on his person, but it is very doubtful whether this was given, as the sufferers "had scarcely swallowed the food when they were all thrown into convulsions," while those who recovered "were not restored to their senses until the second day." Sentence, death.

In 1853, one Sheo Bux waylaid two poor travellers on the parade ground at Cawnpore, and having induced them to partake of some *suttoo* and *goor*, after eating which they became insensible, robbed them of their little property. When found, one of the men was *in articulo*, the other was relieved by an emetic. A search was made in the prisoner's house, and a considerable quantity of poisonous minerals was found, consisting of White Arsenic, and also *Hartal*, or Orpiment. He accounted for the possession of these deadly poisons by saying that he practised chemical experiments, and that he had learnt the art of making silver from them, and was enabled to produce four annas worth of silver per diem.† This wretch had been a Hindu, a Mahomedan, and it was said, for some time, an avowed convert to Christianity, leading a vagabond life, with no fixed means

---

locks at Arrah (Shahabad). Hence they hired another hackery and bullocks, driven by one Jugroop. On nearing Sydpore, Chumroo and Shubrattee enticed the unfortunate driver into a nullah—desiring some boys whom they had met to drive the hackery on with the woman. The body of the driver was found in this nullah with three frightful hacks upon the head and neck. The murderers overtook the hackery at midnight, bringing with them the ring and other property of their victim. They were apprehended at Benares endeavouring to dispose of the cart and bullocks. Chumroo afterwards made his escape. The wretched girl said in her defence that the men had threatened to kill her, that they gave her poison, and that, since she left her mother's house, she had not been in her proper senses. It was, however, clearly proved that she claimed the hackery and bullocks as her own, and offered them for sale for Rs. 30, and also that she said the murdered man's earrings were hers, and asked a woman to sell them. She was sentenced to imprisonment for life with labour; Shubrattee to death.—*Nizamut Adawlut Reports, N. W. P.*, 28th July 1853, p. 1240.

* Nizamut Adawlut Reports, N. W. P., September 2nd, 1852, p. 960.

† Regarding the use of Arsenic by those who profess Alchemy in India, *vide supra*, page 118.

of subsistence. The native doctor who examined the body was satisfied that it contained Arsenic. The superior Court, however, observing that this opinion did not appear to have been derived from analysis, or from the symptoms exhibited by the deceased, and holding that the single fact of the finding Arsenic in the prisoner's house did not amount to proof of guilt, as "the natives not unfrequently keep Arsenic by them for other purposes," ordered the prisoner's release.*

In my edition of 1856, I remarked that, of late, these cases of Road Poisoning had, for the most part, been brought under the investigation of the assistant general superintendents for the suppression of Thuggee, and that much valuable information upon the subject might, doubtless, be collected from the records of those officers at Dacca and Patna and elsewhere. It would appear that the Approver system, employed with such valuable results in the detection of professional stranglers and dacoits, was adopted in some of these cases,† and I suggested that it might be worthy of re-consideration whether a judicious modification of that system might not afford the best prospect of furnishing the judicial authorities with an insight into the true nature of this daily extending crime.

For cases in which prisoners pleaded that the police had drugged them, and thus compelled them to confession, *vide supra*, Uncertainty of General Evidence, page 77.

Much light has been thrown upon this form of Thuggee since I gave the above history of it in 1856.

North-Western Provinces.

Dr. Irving, of Allahabad, has given‡ "*the Confessions of a Professional Poisoner*," from which it appears that Muan Khan was a member of a rather extensive body of systematic druggers, whose victims were mostly prostitutes. Some of their victims died, and some are said to have recovered. He said, "we buy our drugs of Hoorul Pensari (druggist) who lives in the Khaja Kulan, in Patna. He makes us pay five rupees for a pice worth. He was once seized in a Thuggee case, but got off." Most, if not all, of the names of the accomplices whom he mentioned were known to the police, or to the Thuggee Department, as having been implicated in poisoning cases. He was executed for the murder of a woman who, Dr. Irving considered, died of Datura poisoning. Just before Muan Khan was swung off, Mr. Court asked him with what poison he had killed his victim. He replied, tauntingly :—"Your Doctor Saheb

---

* Nizamut Adawlut Reports, N. W. P., August 27th, 1853, p. 1036.

† See Report on the State of the Police, L. P., for 1849, p. 83.

‡ Indian Annals of Medical Science, No. XV., for 1862, p. 46.

could not find it out." "Whilst standing on the drop with the rope round his neck, he was offered his life on condition of turning approver and revealing the nature of the poison. To this he made no reply, but swung himself on the rope by drawing up his legs. The officer who superintended the execution wrote—'this determined act was apparently to resist the temptation offered to him of sparing his own life by betraying his friends.'" Possibly, if he got his drugs from a *pensari*, he was ignorant of their precise nature, especially if they were compounds.

In 1864, Dr. Irving published another paper,* which ought to be consulted by every one engaged, judicially or medically, in dealing with road poisoners or their victims, it being a perfect mine of information on the subject.

Dr. Irving has been unable to obtain much reliable information as to the prevalence of the crime of poisoning in the North-Western Provinces beyond that contained in the Annual Reports of the Nizamut Adawlut on the "Administration of Criminal Justice," for 1852, and for three following years. In 1852, twenty-two cases of theft by the administration of poisonous or stupefying drugs were brought to trial in the various districts of the North-Western Provinces, of which seventeen persons were acquitted, and only five convicted. The same Report shows that thirty-four persons were tried for poisoning, of whom only one was found guilty. In 1853, there were thirty-six persons tried for theft by means of poison, of whom thirteen were convicted, and twenty-three acquitted; besides twenty-one tried for poisoning, of whom four were punished, and seventeen released after trial. In 1854, there were twenty-six cases of theft by poisoning tried, in which conviction followed in twelve and acquitted in fourteen. There were also thirty-one trials for poisoning, in which four convictions and twenty-seven acquittals took place. Of thirty-two tried for poisoning in the year 1855, only three were convicted and twenty-nine acquitted; and of five tried for theft by administering poisonous and stupefying drugs, only one was convicted and four acquitted."

Colonel Harvey often experienced great difficulty in distinguishing between cases of poisoning committed by professional and those perpetrated by casual criminals; omitting, however, instances in which it was evident that the deed was not that of class criminals, the number of reported poisoning cases between 1864 and 1868, was a hundred and twenty-two.

After having shown that, in former times, there existed a body of Thug poisoners spread over all India, he gives grounds for the belief that, in the gangs of the present day, there is a very considerable amount of organization, although, doubtless, it is not so perfect as the older asso-

* Cases of Food Poisoning in the North-Western Provinces of Bengal, with remarks on the professional poisoners of India and their practices, especially Dhatoora Poisoning.—*Indian Annals of Medical Science, No. XVII.*, 1864.

ciation of Thuggee, in which Thugs, from very distant parts of India, who had never met before and whose language differed, could recognise each other by signs known only to the initiated, and had also a slang language of their own. The poisoners about Benares and Cawnpore have no language of their own, and no signs, but there is a large number of people of different castes, associated for this particular purpose, and under leaders, male and female, of different ranks, who direct their movements. Colonel Harvey states that the crime of administering poisonous drugs to travellers and others is known in the department as *Dhatoora* Thuggee, and in Western India as "Mawa."

In 1851, this officer reported that he had made particular enquiries to ascertain, with a view to repression, whether there existed any secret associations for the purpose of robbery by poison, forming such a general and systematic combination as "Thuggee." The result led him to decide that there was not any such general confederacy of this class of criminals as would warrant him to proceed against them as professional Thugs, with any prospect of the evidence of approvers being as efficient for their convictions as the comprehensive nature of Thuggee and Dacoity admits of in courts of law.

In the above enquiry, Colonel, then Major, Harvey obtained information of twenty-three cases of robbery by means of poison in five years, in which a man named Khadir was a principal, and, according to his account, nineteen others were accomplices. Subsequent enquiries by Mr. Court, superintendent general of police, N. W. P., and Capt. Watson, district superintendent of Benares, "resulted in the discovery of a system of poisoning hitherto unknown" (the employment of women was a very ancient practice of the Thugs), "and which, in the main, consisted in the employment of courtezans as decoys. They are generally good-looking young women, well dressed and wearing jewels, who frequent the great highways, and allure unwary travellers to some house of ill-fame, or elsewhere, and who, waiting their opportunity, at last generally manage to poison their victims, or at all events to stupefy them, and then become possessed of their property."

Dhatoora appears to be the usual poison. It is given in various ways, one of the most common being to mix it in flour or to give it in the bread itself, and great address is often shown in the manner in which the poisoner manages this. Khoman (*vide supra*, p. 169) hired carts, the drivers of which he intended to drug (they having probably lately received pay). When they halted to cook, he pretended to go to the bazar in order to purchase flour, but came back saying that there was no buniah to be found, upon which one of the cartmen said, "We have plenty of flour, take some of ours;" and he gave him about a pound and-a-half. He took it away, as if to cook, but returned in a short time saying, "You have given me too much; I only require enough for two cakes—take back the rest." Saying which he threw down a quantity of flour adulterated with powdered Dhatoora. Of the drugged flour the cartmen made their bread, after eating which they became insensible, and were robbed of all the money and property they had. The same Khoman, on another occasion, hired some cartmen, whom he knew to have money about them. On the night of the first halt, he and one of the cartmen went to a neighbouring village to buy food. The cartmen bought chaff for the bullocks, and Khoman flour for the men. Just as the bread was baked, Khoman left on pretext of an assignation. The others ate their food, and shortly afterwards became insensible. When they recovered, they found that they had been robbed of everything, and that their friend was not to be found.

Dr. Irving speaks of many ways of giving the seeds as mixed whole with *brinjal* (*solanum melongena*) between the seeds of which and those of the drug the victim does not observe any difference, and pounded in flour, goor, dhall, rice, milk, infused in spirits and in tea, and made up in sweetmeats. The leaves are also given as *sag* (spinach). These miscreants also use Arsenic, Opium, Hemp (Bhang), Aconite, and Oleander (Kunere). A woman confessed that she had been taught by a female to poison with Arsenic, Dhatoora and Oleander, and stated that she did kill a Rajpoot Sepoy with bread in which these poisons had been blended together.

Dr. Irving gives a case,* in which violence was resorted to in order to cause the victim to swallow the poison which, from its effects, was most probably Dhatoora. On the 26th August 1856, it was reported at Roorkee Police Station, that Roshun, son of Beharee, a banker, aged sixteen or seventeen years, had disappeared the previous night, and that there were strong suspicions of foul play, as the lad had on ornaments of the value of sixty rupees. A blind pauper mentioned that Roshun had gone to the hut of Debeegir, a fakeer, the night before; and he, accordingly, was suspected by the boy's relatives. In the meantime, messengers were despatched to look for him, and two men who had been sent towards Hurdwar met him on the road. He was then in a confused state, as if he had been drugged, dressed as a fakeer, and smeared over with ashes. He stated that, the night before, he went by appointment to the hut of Debeegir, in order to get a cure for earache; that he was taken inside, where he found other four fakeers; that he was gagged and drugged, his ornaments taken off, and he himself removed, he knew not how, as the drug administered to him had completely intoxicated him. Debeegir and another were sentenced to imprisonment for three years.

This system is carried on by miscreants equally ready either to hocuss or murder their victims—perfectly indifferent whether their drugs stupefy

---

* Nizamut Adawlut Reports, 1856.

or kill; but they are rather Budmashes than Thugs. One of them is thus described by Colonel Harvey :—

"I suggested to magistrates to require the police to look out for men, in the garb of religious mendicants, who should put up at *Serais*, or other resting-places, and to search their persons, in view to the discovery of poison or other noxious substance, upon some at least of them. Upon this a *Byragee*, as he pretended to be, was arrested on his return to Cawnpore, who had, after a very short stay at the *Serai* at that place, been perceived to go over into Oudh across the adjacent Ganges, leaving behind him, however, a bundle composed seemingly of tattered clothes only, too miserable looking, he thought, to excite any suspicion. Called upon to account for some seeds of the *Dhatoora* found tied up in a corner of one of the old garments, he unhesitatingly declared *that he used the drug as medicine*, and at once raised his hand as if to eat some of it on the spot. In this he was prevented by the sitting magistrate, by whom he was thereupon sent over to my assistant, Major Chamberlain, at that time located at Lucknow, where, on his making the same proposal, he was, in view to put him to the test, even permitted to do what he had offered. Nothing daunted, *he forthwith swallowed some of the seeds*, to the dismay of the above officer. Insensibility had already partially set in before the usual antidotes could be applied. On his being restored to consciousness, however, the further to disconcert beholders, he at once remonstrated at the measures taken for reviving him, declaring, as the Hasheesh Eater we may suppose would do, that 'he was just getting into the glory of the thing!' Transferred eventually to myself, he disclosed to me a long list of acts of poisoning and of dacoity both on land and river, in which he had taken part, and revealed too, among other like barbarities, that he was one of the infuriated band by whom Mr. St. George Tucker, of the Bengal Civil Service, was beset, and finally murdered in his bungalow at Futtehpore on the outbreak of the Mutiny in 1857, and that he had even received a bullet in his leg from the seldom erring rifle of that brave man."

In the *Report on the Administration of the Police of the North-Western Provinces*, for 1867, it appears that there had been "*no Professional Poisoning*," throughout the Province, during that year.

In 1868, the *Police Gazette, N. W. P.*, published the confession of one Ramadheen, not quite twenty-one years of age, who, for the previous twenty months, has followed the calling of poisoner. A local writer says: "There is no nonsense about Ramadheen. He does not pretend to scruples or remorse of any kind. He calls his victims 'shikar' (game), and alleges no other excuse for his practices than that it was very dull at home in his village. So far as we can enumerate the persons he poisoned in the year and a half, they are about twenty-seven; but he is very cavalier and careless in figures, and talks of a family whom he may murder with a lordly negligence as to the number of its members. Ramadheen is not in the least superstitious. Most of his victims were either Brahmins or fakeers, and his favourite hunting grounds were what he calls 'holy places'—Bindachull near Mirzapore, and the Megh Mela here."*

Punjab.

In his Chapter on Datura Poisoning, Dr. Barton Brown gives several cases which prove that this crime is practised in the Punjab.

In March 1869, it was remarked in *Indian Public Opinion* that "poisoning for plunder seems to be on the increase in that province. There have been several cases in the Sealkote, Amritsar, and Jalandhar Districts, but it is hoped that the case which we will presently narrate may lead to the detection of a gang of poisoners. We hear that there is now a prisoner committed to the sessions at Lahore for poisoning three travellers, whom he met near Taran Tarun, in the Amritsar District. He accompanied them on the pretext of being engaged on the same pilgrimage to the Pind Dadan Khan shrine. The Thug administered Dhatoora to them in some sweetmeat which he had purchased, and, after robbing them of some of their valuables, left them, as he thought, dying, under a tree, near the Lahore city gates. A constable discovered them, and after calling in medical aid, the three men recovered, and were able to describe their poisoner, who has been traced and arrested at Atari, and has confessed his crime."

The same paper for January 12th, 1868, states that a "most frightful case of Thuggee by the administration of Dhatoora took place a few days ago between Lahore and Amritsar. Five men, natives, left this city (Lahore) a few days ago for Amritsar, with about rupees 300 in their possession. They were all found dead, evidently from poison, and without any money on them, in the vicinity of Amritsar."

Bombay.

In 1866 it was reported† that there had, of late, been a systematic poisoning of natives of Bochara and Cabul in Bombay. Within the preceding twenty days, there had been no less than eighteen admissions, for poisoning with Dhatoora, into the Jamsetjee Hospital. About four months previously ten or twelve blind fakeers were taken to the hospital suffering from the effects of the same poison. One of the first party, a Cabulee mendicant, died on the day of his admission.

Mr. Burns wrote in 1868‡ that "there is a report that certain persons, apparently Brahmins, are going about distributing poisonous sweetmeats gratis. It is stated that one man appeared at first in Ahmedabad plying

---

* The *Pioneer* and the Calcutta *Englishman*, 30th November 1868.

† *Times of India*, 20th December.

‡ Notes from Guzrat in June 1868.

his incomprehensible calling ; since then a number of them have sprung up and created quite a panic among the inhabitants. These poisoners have now overrun the country. Of those who partook of the sweetmeats some are said to have died, and others were taken to hospital.*

Madras.

A family of six drugged, with Datura, and robbed. *Madras Quart. Jour. of Medical Science*, January 1867, p. 167.

Lower Provinces.

In 1865, the Bengal Police took cognizance of the existence of certain bodies of men who make it their trade to stupefy and rob persons travelling on the high road between Bhaugulpore and Patna ; in some instances death had resulted. The head of the Detective Department, Mr. Reily, was deputed to investigate the matter ; many cases of poisoning which had occurred long previously were brought to light, and more than one gang of professional poisoners who had plied their trade for years without suspicion was completely broken up. There were twenty-three cases in which 643 persons were arrested, eleven made Queen's evidence, fifty-two were committed for trial, and five were capitally punished. I am much indebted to Mr. Reily for the papers in some of these cases. The report of his operations will be found at pp. 23 to 50 of Colonel Pughe's Annual Police Report for 1865. It was proved that this system of drugging was introduced into the Bhaugulpore and Patna Districts by Hurree Sonar and Bhyrub Sonar, who had learnt the art from some men who came from Oudh. Hurree Sonar was arrested; admitted that he was the *Oostad* or master of all the poisoners in the district ; was convicted and sentenced to ten years' transportation. These men killed those victims who gave them any trouble. When opportunity offered, they committed dacoity. The Hon. Mr. Eden afforded Mr. Reily a clue to the detection of a gang of *Ooriahs* who were professional poisoners in Calcutta. When the house of their leader, Madhub, was searched, it was found that he had seven hundred rupees in a box. His gang displayed considerable *finesse* in the accomplishment of these crimes. Their victims were chiefly prostitutes whom they drugged and robbed of their ornaments and money, and men of their own province—Orissa. Their chief drug appears to have been Datura,—the seeds were discovered upon one of them, and their victims said that they felt giddy and thirsty or "dry in the throat," and then became insensible. The Bhaugulpore druggers appear always to have used *booknee*, a prepared powder which produced the symptoms of narcotic poisoning. Both parties administered the drug in ordinary food and drink, such as *goor*, spice, *kitchree*, *suttoo*, *sukker*, milk, *shurbut*, native spirit, *taree*, and even in water. One of the

* *Englishman*, 14th July 1868.

prisoners said, "The powder we use is made of Opium, Bhang, and Dhatoora; this is what is kept in the bag. I have seen them prepare the powder." Another said that the poison used by his party was made of Opium and Dhatoora. The poison is only stated to have been given once in sweetmeats, *jelabees*. Mr. Reily informed me, at the time, that these road poisoners thoroughly infested the way from Calcutta to Juggernath, on the one side, and to Patna on the other. They occasionally availed themselves of the advantages of railway transit. He considered that the crime was generally diffused through Oudh. These poisoners used principally Dhatoora and Koochila *(nux vomica)*,* generally adding a little opium to the Dhatoora. All these people (like the Thugs and the Dacoits) worship Kallee.

In the Bengal Police Report for 1866, p. 123, it appears that a traveller, having been induced to smoke, became immediately insensible, and remained so until morning. In the same year a family at Patna were drugged in sweetmeats by a woman who had been living in the neighbourhood for some days.† In 1868, a family of Taylees, in the same city, became insensible after taking their supper, and remained insensible throughout the night. The Sub-Divisional Native Doctor detected Dhatoora in the vegetables served up by the servant Mussamut Boodhna, a woman leading a vagrant life, who had recently entered the Taylees' service.‡ In the same year, a pilgrim, going to Juggurnath, was met at Searsole, near Raneegunge, by a professional thief, who asked him to buy some silver armlets (this trick has been played in other cases). The armlets were produced and, while the bargain was going on, the pilgrim was asked to smoke ; he did so, and immediately after felt a choking sensation, and became gradually stupefied. While in this state the thief asked him for the price of the armlets, and, as he was paying, the thief fell upon him and ran off with all that he possessed. The pilgrim, not entirely overcome with the drug he had smoked, raised the cry of "Thief!" Two constables on the spot succeeded in capturing the thief with the plated articles and all the pilgrim's money. Sentence of seven years' transportation was passed.§

At pp. 367-73 of the Bengal Police Report for 1868, will be found a very important narrative of the detection of a gang of poisoners—seventeen strong—who infested the road from Raneegunge to Gya. An approver stated that Islam, Ruffee, and Suffee were the heads of the gang from whom the rest had learnt to prepare the poison, and to follow their present pro-

* In the possession of one Haree Behrah, who was condemned at Midnapore for having drugged a party of travellers, was found a seed of the *nux vomica*, but it was entire, and the symptoms produced by the drug which he gave (poisoned turmeric rubbed into fish) were intoxication and insensibility.

† Bengal Police Report for 1866, p. 129.

‡ Bengal Police Report for 1868, p. 140.

§ *Ibid*, p. 215.

fession. He also stated that the gang divided into parties of three or four, and proceeded to different parts of the country, drugging travellers and robbing them. Islam, it appears, had formerly been to Mauritius, as a cooly, where, it was stated, he first learnt the act of drugging. It is remarked that "a similar statement has been made by most of the poisoners prosecuted by this" [the Detective] "Department. They assert that the art of poisoning with *dhatoora* seeds originated with men who returned from the Mauritius." It is probable that coolies in the Mauritius, like prisoners in jail, learn many things in conversation, of which they would have remained ignorant had they remained at home. Islam was apprehended and transported for three years. Ruffee and Suffee were also caught; made full confession, and were executed.

The same Report (p. 373) gives the case of one Hossainee "a vendor of poisons in the city of Patna," and for some time under the strong suspicion of the Detective Police as belonging to the gang of poisoners who drugged a Syce travelling with a horse to Dinapore, in a powder proffered as a specific for fever. He was sentenced to ten years' transportation.

For many years past, the Judges of the Calcutta Supreme Court have been sedulous in endeavouring to put down the crime of drugging prostitutes for the purpose of robbing them of their ornaments and money, but it is to be feared that the crime has not yet been effectually stamped out.

Baboo Kanny Loll Dey received, about four years ago, from a judicial officer, Up-country, a box containing "samples of different preparations of Datura employed by the Professional Poisoners of Upper India, for the purpose of robbery.

1. Datura Seeds.
2. Powdered prepared Datura Seeds, parched, but not cleaned, or fit to mix with food to drug a victim.
3. Powdered prepared Datura, fit to mix with food; dose half a tolah.
4. Distilled Essence of Datura, used with tobacco, sugar, attah, &c.; dose ten drops in a chillum, or a quarter tea-spoonful in a meal of attah.
5. Attah drugged with Datura Flour.
6. Suttoo drugged with Datura Flour.

DATURA.

DATURA FASTUOSA—Purple Flowered.
,, ,, ALBA—White Flowered.
,, ,, FEROX.

Vernacular, Black Species,—*Doostoora, Krishna Dhatura,* Sans.; *Kala-dhatura, Lal-dhatura,* Hind., Beng.; *Umana, Nela-hummatu,* Mal.; *Karoo-oomattay,* Tam.; *Nulla-oomatie,* Tel.; *Kaloo attana,*

Antenna, Cey.; *Bunjdhestee*, Arab.; *Goorzgeeah*, Pers.; *Rotecubung*, Malay. White Species,—*Sada-dhatura*, Hind., Beng. ; *Hummatu*, Mal.; *Yellay-oomattay*, Tam. ; *Tella-oomatie*, *Datturamu*, Tel.; *Suda-attana*, Cey. Both in common,—*Dhatura*, India ; *Towz-mazil (Methel Seed)*, Arab.—BIRDWOOD.

Popular superstition among the Hindus represents their deity Siva as constantly under the intoxicating effects of *Dhatoora* and *Gunjah*. Datura was ranked among the weak poisons *(Apabisha)* in the Shasters. Its use, for nefarious purposes, is of very long standing in India.

Purchas says:* "They have an Herbe, called Durroa, which causeth distraction, without understanding any thing done in a man's presence ; sometimes it maketh a man sleepe, as if hee were dead, the space of foure and twentie houres, except his feet be washed with cold water, which restoreth him to himselfe ; and in much quantity it killeth. Iarric cals it Doturo, and sayth that Pinnerus the Jesuite and his family at Lahor were by meanes of this herbe (given them by a theevish servant) distracted and the goods then carried out of their house. The women give their husbands thereof, and then in their sights will prostitute their bodies to their lewder lovers, and will call them *corundos*, stroking them by the beard ; the husband sitting with his eyes open, grinning like a foole ; when he returneth to himselfe, knoweth nothing but that hee hath slept."

We read, in Burton's Anatomy of Melancholy:† "Garcias ab Horto (plant. hist. lib. 2, cap. 26) makes mention of an hearb called *datura, which if it be eaten, for* 24 *hours following, takes away all sense of grief, makes them incline to laughter and mirth :* and another called *bunge*, like in effect to opium, *which puts them for a time into a kinde of extasis*, and makes them gently laugh.

"In the kingdom of Malabar, and about Goa in the East Indies, the women are so subtile that, with a certain drink from the herb Datura, they give them to drive away cares, as they say, *they will make them sleep for twenty foure houres, or so intoxicate them, that they can remember naught of that they saw done, or heard, and by washing of their feet* (the efficacy of cold affusion in datura poisoning is well understood by natives) *restore them again, and so make their husbands cuckolds to their faces*."

A case, which was reported,‡ as lately as 1864, gives singular confirmation to these quaint legends collected by Garcias ab Horto and Linschoten:— "A woman was tried at the Kurrachee Criminal Sessions early in the month for the offence of 'administering stupefying drugs.' That she did administer poison to her husband in his food she admitted, but it was a love-charm for the purpose of regaining his affections, which had become

* Op. Citat., Vol. V., p. 568.

† Page 457.

‡ *Friend of India*, September 1st, 1864.

'weak.' This defence was not good, as it was proved that, on her husband's becoming insensible, she had gone off with another man, and only returned when captured by the police. The assessors found her guilty, and the Judge sentenced her to six months' imprisonment."

In works of last century, I meet with more than one allusion to *Poisoning by Coffee* in India. Forbes says* that, having narrowly escaped being taken prisoner by the Garcias of Guzerat in 1783, he reflected upon the various modes of destruction to which he would have been exposed while in the hands of this fierce people, who were known to have determined upon his death. Among these he mentions "*the poisoned Coffee.*" Another passage in Forbes's work (Vol. II, p. 458) explains this. It was rumoured that General Mathews and two other officers were killed, at Tippo's durbar, with cups of poisoned coffee. Girdlestone mentions that, when cholera raged epidemically in Madras, in 1782, it was unanimously judged by a meeting of the Faculty that the disease proceeded from "damps from the earth, the not using of capsicum, bad arrack, and *a coffee made of stramonium.*" These two ideas, occurring nearly at the same time in Bombay and Madras, appear to point to the then prevalence of a mode of datura poisoning which is happily now forgotten.

Dr. John Fryer, who visited India between the years 1672 and 1681, (reign of Aurungzebe), gives the following description of the manner in which state criminals were then treated : " Upon an offence, they are sent by the king's order, and committed to a place called the *Post* (from the punishment inflicted), when the master of the Post is acquainted with the heinousness of the crime ; which being understood, he heightens by a drink, which at first they refuse, made of *Bung* (the juice of the intoxicating sort of Hemp), and being mingled with *Datry* (the deadliest sort of *Solarium* or *Nightshade*) named *Post.* After a week's taking, they crave more than ever they nauseated. *Ad illorum vicem qui degustato Sardonum graminum succo feruntur in morte ridere;* making them foolishly mad. Then they are brought into the inner lodging of the house, in which folding-doors open upon delicious gardens, where apes and cats, dogs and monkeys, are their attendants, with whom they maintain their dialogues, exercising over them their humour of an assassin, usurper, miser, or what their *Genius* led them to whilst themselves. After this manner are they imprisoned during the king's pleasure, or he orders their cure, to restore them to their senses again ; which otherwise, after their spirits are tired by a restless appetite of doing, and in the meantime have not a suitable recruit, they linger by a lasting leanness into the shades, which alive they represented."

Post is not, however, the *Datura*, but the *Papaver Somniferum.* Strictly it is an infusion of the virgin poppy-head, still used in the Pun-

* Op. Cit., Vol. II., p. 355.

jaub to produce intoxication. Bernier's account of the practice is, doubtless, more correct than Fryer's. "This *Poust*," he writes, "is nothing else but poppy expressed and infused a night in water. And it is that potion which those that are kept at Gwalior are commonly made to drink. I mean those princes whose heads they think it fit not to cut off. This is the first thing that is brought to them in the morning, and they have nothing given them to eat till they have drank a great cupful of it; they would rather let them starve. This emaciates them exceedingly, and maketh them die insensibly, they losing little by little their understanding, and growing torpid and senseless. And by this very means it is said that Sipeher Shekoh, Moorad Buksh, and Sooleeman Shekoh were despatched."

It is recorded that Mahomed Sultan, the eldest son of Aurungzebe, was detained in the fortress of Gwalior, under the slow influence of Post, for fifteen years.

Fryer describes the friends of Hindu widows as giving them the "*Datry*," as a preparation for burning—"When half mad, she throws herself into the fire." Tavernier also says, in speaking of the preparation for the Sati, "Many of our Europeans are of opinion that to take away the fear of death, which naturally terrifies humanity, the priests do give her a certain beverage to stupefy and disorder the senses, which takes from her all apprehension of her preparation for death." Captain Hamilton also states that some of the victims took "somnific medicines," and stood by the pile until they fell on it while asleep.

Mr. Ives, Admiral Watson's surgeon, who visited India in 1754, says that "if the Indian women have possession of any secret poison, it is the seed of this plant."

In an account of Tranquebar, published from narrations of the Missionaries in 1744, it is mentioned that the Datura is used to stupefy people, in order to carry them to some unknown place to be made slaves.

The author of the "Bengal Dispensatory" remarks that, for the purpose of facilitating theft, and other criminal designs, the seeds are very commonly given in Bengal, with sweetmeats, to stupefy merely, but not with the intention of killing [?]; intoxication or delirium is seldom produced, the individual sinks into profound lethargy, resembling coma, with dilated pupils, but natural respiration. These symptoms have been known to continue even for two days, and still recovery take place; cold affusion and strong stimulant emetics constitute the most effectual treatment; the vision often continues obscured long after the general recovery takes place. If given while the stomach is empty, a much smaller dose may induce all the preceding symptoms, and prove fatal. This is well known to the Indian poisoners, who suit the time of administration according to the purpose they mean to serve.*

* O'Shaughnessy.

The white *Datura* is found growing luxuriantly beside nearly every peasant's hut in Lower Bengal. The goats feed upon it ; and it is, doubtless, often tended for worse purposes.

The purple-flowered species (*Kala Dhatoora*) is comparatively uncommon. It is considered, both by our own botanists and by the native hukeems, to be by far the most potent of the daturas.

Of the species commonest in *Madras*, Dr. Shortt, then of Chingleput, writes :* "Two varieties of Stramonium are found growing in every part of this district : the *Datura Fastuosa*, or purple-flowered, and the *Datura metel (Alba)*, or white-flowered. The purple-flowered variety is rather rare, but the white-flowered is seen on the dunghill of every village, in waste places, and by the road side. It makes its appearance soon after the monsoons, and thrives with great vigour, pushing forth its large, conspicuous, white, tubular corolla, and giving beauty to localities otherwise defaced by refuse and neglect."

The *Datura Ferox* is found on the Malabar Coast (Dr. W. Palmer). Dr. Birdwood says that the *Datura Fastuosa* and *Alba* are frequently used criminally in *Bombay*.

Baboo Kanny Lall Dey informs me that, between 1855 and May 1870 (exclusive of 1866), forty-seven cases of Datura poisoning have engaged the attention of the Calcutta Chemical Examiner.†

Botanical Characters of the Seeds of the Indian Species of Datura.—This is a subject of great importance, as there is a close outward resemblance between the seeds of the *Datura Alba*, which is most used as a poison in India, and those of the common Capsicum (*Capsicum fratescens*), an ordinary ingredient of native diet, and a plant which is, botanically, very nearly allied to the Daturas. Dr. Burton Brown (page 66) and Dr. William Palmer have been at great pains to describe the differences in the characters of these seeds. Dr. Palmer‡ gives a case, which

---

* Cases of Poisoning by Stramonium.—*Madras Quarterly Journal of Medical Science*, Vol. VI., p. 286.

† The drug was given in such food as Suth, Chapaties, Rice, Dal, Dohee (Curds), Milk, Goor, &c.

Two native prostitutes, with their *Dullal*, who were brought into the Medical College Hospital in May 1868, had been poisoned by datura in Wine. At about the same time, a woman named Sajnee was tried in Calcutta for having datura-drugged an old malee in *Pán Soopáree*. He became insensible in 20 minutes. Sentence, four years' rigorous imprisonment.

This poison is often used in large quantities. In February 1870 the Calcutta Chemical Examiner received from Bhaugulpore about four ounces of bread, which had been used in Road Poisoning. This fragment contained 53 entire and a great many powdered seeds. An extract of this killed a powerful cat in two minutes. An ethereal extract from the cat's stomach produced, in the eye of another cat, marked dilatation of the pupil, which lasted more than 24 hours.

‡ *Practical Observations on the means of detecting Dhatoora and Aconite administered with the intention of inducing stupefaction, intoxication, and death.* Reprinted from the *Indian Medical Gazette*, 1868.

will be presently cited, in which the seeds both of the Datura and the Capsicum were found in the stomach of a poisoned man. He shows that, when the seeds of white Datura, or Datura metel, are boiled with rice, they appear in the midst of the white mass as yellowish pea or kidney-shaped bodies, so nearly resembling Capsicum seeds, which are used in the rice as a condiment, that they excite little suspicion either by their appearance or taste, for they have very little flavor.

Dr. Palmer goes on to show that these two seeds, differing so greatly in their therapeutical effects, belong to two plants which are, botanically, very nearly allied ; they have therefore many characters in common, and are constantly mistaken the one for the other, not only by the poor victims of the poisoner, but also by many others who have not carefully studied and compared them. The one great distinguishing feature above all others is the form and shape of the embryo. If one of each of the seeds be divided by cutting parallel with the flattened sides, the embryo of the capsicum will be found curved like the figure 6, while the end of the curve in the dhatoora is "twisted" or re-curved, not towards the down-stroke of the 6, but away from it, or towards the right hand. There are, however, many minor differences of great importance when taken together ; these may be contrasted thus :—

Seeds of the Common or White Dhatoora.	*Seeds of the Common Capsicum.*
1. Almost kidney-shaped, but one end much smaller than the other.	1. Kidney-shaped.
2. Outline angular.	2. Outline rounded.
3. Size, rather more than a quarter of an inch long, and rather less in width.	3. A little shorter and wider than the dhatoora.
4. Colour greenish-brown when fresh, changing to yellow when dry.	4. Yellow.
5. Attached to the placenta by large white fleshy mass, which separates easily, leaving a deep furrow along half the length of the concave border of the seed.	5. Attached to the placenta by a thin cord from a prominence on the concave border of the seed.
6. Surface scabrous, almost reticulate, except on the two compressed sides, where it has became almost glaucous from pressure of the neighbouring seeds.	6. Uniformly scabrous, the sides being equally rough with the borders.

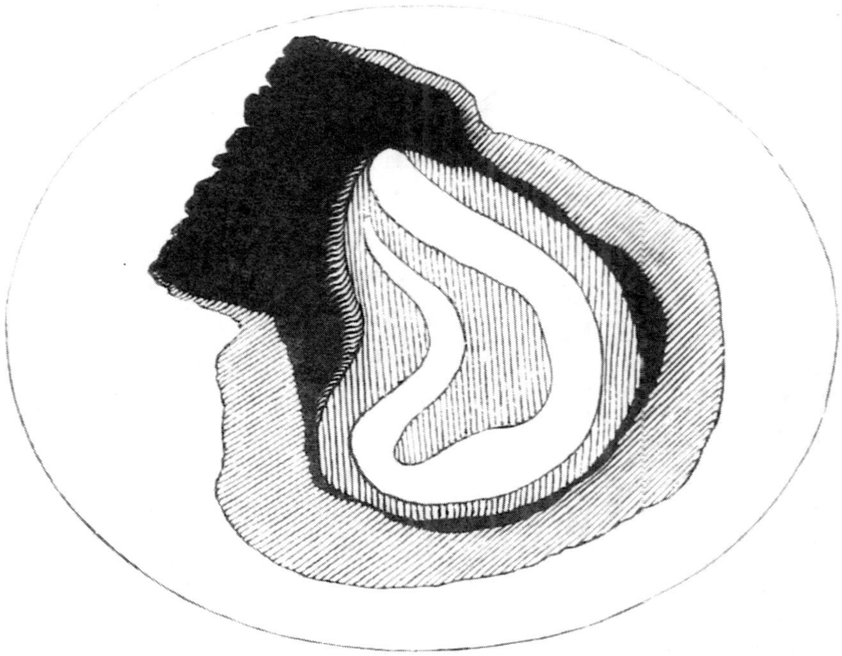

Embryo of Datura, × 13.

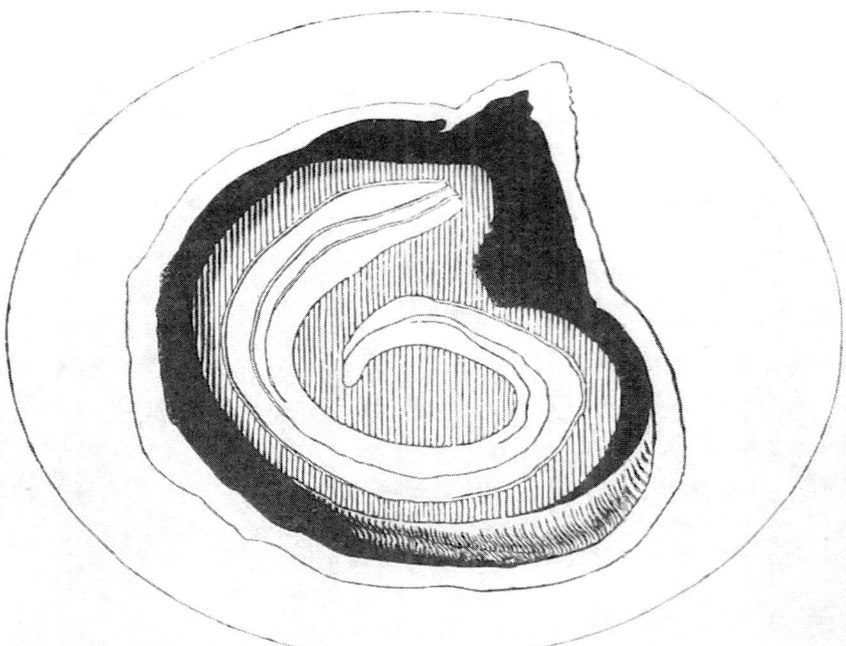

Embryo of Capsicum, × 13.

DR. D. D. CUNNINGHAM, DEL.

Seeds of the Common or White Dhatoora.	*Seeds of the Common Capsicum.*
7. Convex border thick and bulged, with a longitudinal depression between the bulgings caused by the compression of the two sides.	7. Convex border thickened, but uniformly rounded.
8. When divided into two, by cutting with a knife placed in the furrow on the convex border, the testa is seen irregular and angular in outline, the embryo is seen lying *curved* and *twisted* in a fleshy albumen.	8. When similarly divided, the testa is more uniform in outline, the embryo is seen lying in a fleshy albumen *curved,* but not twisted or re-curved.

Having separated the dhatoora from the capsicum seeds by the above physical examination, the following chemical and physiological tests may be applied for confirmation.

The seeds may be separated boiled in a little water and the decoction filtered through blotting paper. Both decoctions will appear a little turbid, and the dhatoora seeds will have become rather darker in colour by boiling, while the capsicum seeds either retain their bright yellow hue or become a little paler.

Chemical tests.	*Dhatoora decoction.*	*Capsicum decoction.*
1. Sol: Perchlor: Iron	No change ...	White cloud.
2. ,, Chloride Gold	Faint cloud ...	No change.
3. ,, Bichlor: Platinum ...	Faint cloud ...	No change.
4. ,, Ferrocyan: Potassium ...	Faint cloud ...	No change.

Physiological tests.	*Dhatoora decoction.*	*Capsicum decoction.*
1. Taste	Insipid	Pungent.
2. Dropped into the eye of man, cat, or dog.	Causes dilatation of pupil.	No change.

The above case is one of the simplest forms of dhatoora poisoning, in which only the simplest means of detection are required. Wherever seeds presenting the three following characters are detected, Dr. Palmer believes it may be positively stated they are dhatoora seeds, *viz.*:—

"1. *External form.*—From two to three lines long, and two lines broad, kidney-shaped, with one end much smaller than the other; or perhaps rather in shape like a flattened pear, with one border of the small end convex, the other concave. When the seed is fresh, an angular, white, fleshy *aril* is attached to the concave border ; when old and dry, this becomes broken off, its place of attachment being, however, still marked by a rough, rugged, triangular depression or furrow. The whole *testa* or covering of the seed has a scaly or scabrous appearance to the naked eye ; on the sides, however, which have been flattened by compression, this roughness is almost obliterated ; the same compression has bulged the convex border into two rounded shoulders with an intervening depression."

"2. *Internal structure.*—If the seed be equally divided by placing a knife in the above-named depression, and cutting parallel to the flattened surfaces, each cut surface will present a mass of white fleshy albumen, in the midst of which will be seen a *curved, twisted,* and *re-curved* embryo. This peculiar character of the embryo is characteristic of the genus dhatoora. The rudest diagram would perhaps convey a better notion of it than a mere verbal description ; some conception, however, may perhaps be formed of it by imagining a figure 6 to have been seized at its curved extremity, and twisted until its point became nearly parallel with the commencement of the down-stroke of the same figure, making it something like the neck of a swan in shape."

"3. *Physiological action.*—One drop of a decoction of the seed put into the eye of a cat causes well-marked dilatation of the pupil. All three of the above characters apply equally to the only forms of dhatoora commonly found in the plains of India,—*viz., datura metel, commonly called white* sada dhatoora, to distinguish it from the other common variety named *datura fastuosa,* commonly called black kala dhatoora, from its dark leaves. The two latter characters, as well as the peculiar structure of the *exosperm* which gives rise to the scabrous appearance of the surface, are, however, common to all the species of dhatoora, and, taken together, would be absolutely characteristic."

"The only other species of dhatoora found in India is the *datura ferox,* which has small, black, kidney-shaped, scabrous seeds. It is found on the Malabar coast. The ordinary medicinal plant—*viz.,* datura stramonium—has very similar small black seeds ; the surface of these is, however, quite *reticulate* as well as *scabrous.*"

"In the North-Western Provinces, the ordinary food of the people is wheat flour, made into unleavened cakes, called chupatties. Whole dhatoora seeds could not conveniently be clandestinely administered with these ; it is therefore common in those parts to find that the poisonous seeds have been ground before being used for drugging purposes. The testa of dhatoora seeds being tough rather than brittle, is not very easily reduced to fine powder ; when, therefore, it is mixed with flour, it appears as small brownish-yellow particles scattered through the white mass ; this appearance alone would give rise to suspicion in any country where sifted flour is ordinarily used; but in India, where the flour in common use is always mixed with bran, their appearance to the naked eye is not sufficiently dissimilar to excite any remark."

"The following case affords a good illustration of this class of dhatoora drugging or poisoning:—

"On the 24th January 1866, two patients were brought to the Chupra Dispensary suffering from the following symptoms:—chattering delirium, with a tendency to perform strange antics; they were stupid and unintelligible; their pupils were widely dilated; their skin was of a natural temperature; pulse quick and small; tongue white and moist. They both recovered under appropriate treatment. On subsequent inquiry, it was found that these curious symptoms supervened rapidly after eating chupatties made of flour, some of which was still found remaining.

"This flour was thus examined:—

"First, it *was sifted,* to separate all the coarser particles; these were then examined with the aid of a pocket lens. The grinding in this case had been so carelessly performed that whole kernels of dhatoora seeds were found, recognizable by the peculiar twisted and curved embryo above described; these kernels were scattered in a larger mass of broken seed-coverings (testæ) of both wheat and dhatoora; fortunately, these two are so utterly different in structure from each other that no difficulty is experienced in distinguishing and separating them. In each case the testa is composed of three distinct layers or coverings, but, for present purposes, our attention may be confined to the outer layer or exosperm. This, in the case of wheat, is a smooth, thin, dense, solid layer, of equal thickness throughout; it is made up of flattened cells placed horizontally, or parallel with the surface of the seed; while in the case of dhatoora it is made up of round open tubes, or pipes placed perpendicularly to the surface of the seed's surface. In the compressed portions these tubes are somewhat shortened, but in all the parts where their development has not been interfered with by pressure of the surrounding seeds they are long, wavy, and lie parallel to each other. It is the open mouths of these tubes which give the surface of the seeds its scabrous appearance; the exosperm of dhatoora further contrasts with that of wheat in being rough, thick, light, and friable, and of unequal thickness in its entire extent. It is scarcely possible for a person accustomed to examine ground dhatoora seeds with a lens to be unable to distinguish the peculiar characters of the dhatoora exosperm from any other known structure, unless it is ground very fine: fortunately, however, the physiological test above described is so easily applied for confirmation that dependence need never be placed on the physical characters alone."

"Cases, however, do occur where the dhatoora has been ground so carefully that the closest observation fails to detect the peculiar structure;

if in these cases the seeds or testæ have not been soaked long or boiled much, a decoction of them dropped in a cat's eye will afford all the additional evidence required for confirmation ; if, on the other hand, the seeds have been so macerated that most of their active principle is abstracted, a more minute chemical analysis will be required."

"In cases of suspected poisoning by dhatoora, where the most careful examination of the contents of the stomach by repeated washings and decantations fails to detect any portion of the seed sufficiently large to be recognized by the morphological examination above described, or where the portions so discovered have been already so long macerated that the active principle (daturia) has become generally diffused throughout the whole mass, so that a decoction of them fails, when applied, to dilate the pupil of a cat's eye, a more extended and elaborate process will be necessary."

Dr. Brown says that the kala dhatoora seeds *(datura fastuosa)* are of a black or reddish colour. Some, however, are of a fawn colour ; they are somewhat thicker but less broad than *capsicum* seeds ; 246 of the seeds of this *datura* are equal in weight to a two-anna piece, while only 107 of the seeds of *datura alba* and 286 of the *capsicum* equal that weight.

Detection of Datura by Chemical Means.—Dr. Palmer remarks that details of the process adopted in the following case afford a good illustration of what appears to be the best mode of procedure in the present state of our knowledge. Though this was a case of poisoning by the accidental eating of dhatoora leaves, no difference in the process now under consideration was required, the object being equally in both cases to present the alkaloid in a concentrated form, and separated as far as possible from all extraneous matter, for the application of physiological, chemical, and other tests.

"In March 1866, somewhere near Midnapore, father and mother, with their children, cooked and ate some 'greens' or *sag* which they had gathered, supposing it to be edible. The parents both died, but the children recovered, and afterwards pointed out where the supposed *sag* was gathered. It was then discovered they had eaten some young shoots of the dhatoora plant. The stomachs of the deceased, having been sent to Calcutta, were subjected to the following process :—The contents of the first being removed, the stomach itself was cut into small pieces ; these contents and pieces were then placed together in a bottle with some proof spirit acidulated with acetic acid, where they were allowed to macerate for three days, after which the fluid portion was separated from the solid by filtration, and the filtrate evaporated to dryness on a water-bath. The dry mass so obtained was next treated with rectified spirits of wine, in order to extract the active principles, and at the same time to coagulate the albuminoid, gummy, and other bulky substances ; these were separated by filtration, and the filtrate was again dried on a water-bath. This process of purification was twice repeated, the first time with rectified spirits, the second with absolute alcohol. In this way the bulk of the mass was very greatly reduced, and yet, at the same time, the whole, or almost the whole, of the alkaloids present in the original mass were extracted and gathered together in a concentrated form in the dried mass on the water-bath. This essence was now dissolved in a little water, and injected into the stomach of a puppy; vomiting unfortunately occurred almost immediately; enough, however, was retained to show the characteristic symptoms, as will be presently seen. In the meantime it should be remarked that, in order to avoid this inconvenient rejection of the matter given, very careful purification is necessary. Whenever this cannot be sufficiently done by repetitions of the process above described, the extract so obtained should be rendered alkaline by carbonate of soda, and the whole shaken frequently with three or four times its bulk of ether, for a period of thirty-six hours; by this operation most of the alkaloids, together with the fatty matter, will be extracted by the ether, and may be obtained by pouring off that fluid and allowing it to evaporate spontaneously. The presence of another similar stomach in reserve made it unnecessary to adopt this precaution in the present case.

"Very soon after the above-mentioned vomiting, the puppy performed a few antics, and fell over on his side into a deep sleep, from which tickling failed to rouse him; after ten minutes he got up, stared wildly about him, and appeared to see visions which he would scratch or snap at; finding, however, that they eluded him, he walked to his accustomed corner of the room, where he lay down and remained somewhat restlessly; at this time his pupils were much dilated; he did not again fall asleep, but moved constantly from one side to the other of his little corner; sometimes his eyes were closed, when he appeard to be in a restless slumber, disturbed by low moans. A little later he appeared more drowsy and sleepy, but he still opened his eyes when his name was called. The pupils continued widely dilated all this time. Half an hour later he was placed in the middle of the room, when he staggered towards his corner again, his feet and legs bending under him as he went, as if he had lost almost all power over them. When any part of his body was pinched with a pair of forceps, he screamed and turned his head towards the injured part. Half an hour later again, he, being still in his corner, looked very drunk, and performed such antics as a drunken beast might do. By evening—*i. e.*, after six hours—he had almost recovered, but the pupils were exceedingly dilated, and they continued more or less so the whole of the next day.

"The remaining stomach and its contents were treated in a manner precisely similar, including, however, the additional purification with ether, and the result was submitted to examination by chemical and microscopical tests; as, however, the above succession of symptoms, reproduced in the dog, were considered to afford satisfactory evidence that portions of some plant belonging to the natural order Atropaceæ were contained in the suspected stomach, it was desirable to defer the consideration of the chemical tests until the physiological evidence had been more carefully examined.

"In September 1866 another case occurred in the Midnapore District which is well worthy of attention. A sub-inspector of police was for some cause placed in custody, and died while he was in the lock-up. It was reported that he had taken opium, and the stomach was forwarded to Calcutta for examination; on its arrival, the whole contents were subjected to a careful physical and mechanical examination. No smell or appearance of opium could be detected, but particles were found which had the appearance of ground dhatoora seeds; a decoction of these particles, however, failing to dilate the pupil of a cat's eye when dropped into it. The examination was thus proceeded with :—A portion was examined in the usual way for opium, but none was found. Next, the absence of any metallic poison was ascertained by Reinsch's and the Magnesium tests; afterwards the whole remaining contents, as well as the the stomach itself, were submitted to the modification of Stas' process, described in the foregoing case. The resulting extract was equally divided, the first half being tested for narceine,* morphine, and meconic acid without any success, and the remaining half being given to a kitten at noon on the 27th September. The little cat soon began to breathe with difficulty, and to froth at the mouth; in ten minutes her pupils were dilated, and they continued to remain so, only to a still greater extent, the rest of the day, never for a moment being contracted, or even less dilated, when exposed to a strong sunlight. After 20 minutes she was placed in the middle of the room, and encouraged to walk, but she staggered and fell on attempting to do so. In half an hour from the time of administration, she was quite unconscious; up to this period she had felt pain when pinched with a forceps, but now a severe pinch only caused a slight movement of the limb, without any expression of pain. The respiration was still laboured; she continued to froth at the mouth, and the pupils remained very widely dilated. Consciousness began to return at two o'clock; she then got up, sat staring wildly, and commenced to perform a series of grotesque actions, uttering a low moan from time to time. When pinched, she felt pain, but not yet very acutely. She appeared very irritable, almost wild, but was neither vicious nor bad-tempered. At 3 p.m. the pupils were dilated extremely, the iris being a mere thread. By 4 p.m. she had recovered so far as to be able to come when called, and to feel acute pain when pinched, the pupils continuing as large as ever.

"* Narceine is very abundant in Indian Opium, and is readily indicated by the deep purple colour produced when treated with free mineral acids."

"A small portion of the same extract or essence was applied to the eye of another kitten; it caused the pupil to dilate in half an hour; another portion of the same was applied to the experimenter's lip, without producing any numbness.

"In reporting the result of this examination, it was stated that no opium could be detected, but that a portion of an extract, or essence, of the stomach and its contents, when given to a kitten, produced such a concatenation of symptoms as could only have resulted from the administration of one of the plants belonging to the natural order Atropaceæ, and that the particular one was probably a species of dhatoora."

According to Mr. James Taylor, the people of Dacca employ an intoxicating substance called *Bhauker* in the distillation of Arrack. This Bhauker is compounded of rice, opium, *Dhatoora*, and a number of other poisonous ingredients; it is imported from Tipperah, and sells at the rate of 1,000 balls (each weighing about 10 annas) for 2½ or 3 rupees. This is also frequently added to the Keitah (a fermented liquor) principally used by the Mussulmauns, but the low Hindus also indulge in this drugged compound during the feast of the Huli.*

I, some time since, had a specimen of this Bhauker, in the form of a light fawn-coloured powder. In other works,† I have spoken of the suspicion which has always existed that, occasionally, men are drugged in the bazar by liquor poisoned with narcotics, of which *Dhatoora* is probably one.

I then insisted that the failure to detect any poison in bazar liquor is no proof whatever that men are not thus poisoned, as it is stated that the lowest class of Native Christians have a mode of rendering *the bowl* intoxicating, by holding it over the smoke of burning Datura. Several Europeans, suffering from the effects of intoxication, have declared to me their belief that their liquor had been drugged. I have, however, met with several very far more suspicious cases in natives in Calcutta.—On the subject of *Poisoned Spirit*—vide *supra*, pp. 147 and 183 *note*.

In the highly valuable paper already cited, Dr. Giraud observes that the intoxicating properties of the indigenous species of the genus *Datura* have been known amongst Eastern nations from time immemorial. The botanical name of the genus has been adopted from the Sanscrit *Dhatoora*. They have also long been employed in China (where the *Datura Ferox* is used) and in the islands of the Indian Archipelago, to facilitate the commission of theft and other crimes. In Bombay, the cases of poisoning by the species of *Datura* are so frequent, that the natives usually recognise them by their characteristic symptoms. According to this authority, the motives which prompt the administration of the poison

---

* Topography and Statistics of Dacca, p. 280.

† On the Means of Preserving the Health of European Soldiers in India, and on the Preservation of the Health of Seamen.

are exremely various. Frequently, a shopkeeper is brought under the influence of the drug, that his articles of merchandise may be the more readily made off with : very often, a fortunate fakeer is made to yield up the contributions of the pious while thus intoxicated. Jealousy frequently appears to seek revenge in the use of *dhatoora.* During the preceding year, eight persons, a man, his wife, two children, and some friends were brought to the Jamsetjee Jeejehbhoy Hospital, all suffering from the effects of *dhatoora,* which it was supposed they took in a meal prepared by the man's other wife. In Dr. Giraud's own house, three horse-keepers were at one time drugged with *dhatoora,* which it was believed had been thrown into their meals by a fourth,—a man of different caste, and, at the time, on bad terms with the others. The fantastic antics that are exhibited under its action, sometimes tempt to the use of it as a practical joke —as in a case where a dog-boy gathered the seeds of *Datura Alba* in a garden, and threw them into a cook's rice.* Dr. Giraud is informed that the poison is, not unfrequently, had recourse to as a means of fortelling events—a person, while under its influence, being supposed to be possessed of faculties resembling those of the Pythian Priestess of old, or of the modern professors of clairvoyance. Notwithstanding the recent prevalence of *dhatoora* poisoning in Bombay, Dr. Giraud remarks that it has been only on the presumptive evidence of its characteristic symptoms that its action has been inferred. The poison is administered so stealthily, and the natives are so backward in aiding the cause of justice, that he has found it next to impossible to obtain positive evidence of the administration of the poison, or to trace it to the culprit ; although, from their familiarity with its nature, and the modes of its administration, it is, he thinks, evident that many of the lower orders of the people are acquainted with the adepts who employ it.

He finds that the *Seeds* are usually administered. They are powdered and thrown into rice, bajree, and other grains ; or mixed up with cakes and sweetmeats. Sometimes, however, an infusion or a decoction of the *Leaves* is prepared, and introduced into the vessels in which food is being cooked. In this Presidency also the seeds are usually administered

---

* Dr. Irving cites the case of Government *v.* Kulloo (Nizamut Adawlut Reports, N. W. P., for October 1854), in which the prisoner stated that Dhatoora was given to a man as it would make him intoxicated and the sight would be amusing. It, however, appears that in this case robbery was probably designed. He also quotes the case of Khooba *v.* Goomla (*Ibid,* for April 1852), in which the prisoner, who was only thirteen years of age, confessed that he had given another boy some drug mixed with *goor ;* this he said he had done at the instigation of the boy's uncle, who wished to play a practical joke upon the mother.

Dr. Ralph Moore told me that he was once sent for suddenly to his jail, and found the whole of the jail guards scattered about on the floor under the influence of Dhatoora. As there appears not to have been any attempt on the part of the prisoners to escape, this may also have been a practical joke.

in powder; they can rarely be detected *whole*, as in the cases noticed at pp. 152 and 168 and in the following instances.

The following case, which will be found at p. 6 of Dr. Palmer's Monograph, is of peculiar interest, inasmuch as *both Datura and Capsicum seeds were discovered in the stomach*:—

Early in the morning of the 3rd September, 1865, the bodies of two men were observed lying under a peepul tree, near Futtehpore, in Zillah Tirhoot. On examination, one was found to be dead, the other only in a state of insensibility. When, after a time, the latter became conscious, he stated that he, Beharee Mullah, and Jewlall, the deceased, had made the acquaintance of a Brahmin at Mozufferpore the day previous; that this same Brahmin met them again in the evening of the same day, while on their way home (eight miles from the town), and induced them to partake of some consecrated rice, or *prasadi* (*vide supra* p. 164); after eating this he and his friend Jewlall walked a short distance, when they felt their sight becoming confused and dim; they then became giddy, and sat down under a tree, when they groped about the ground until they became quite unconscious. Twelve hours after, he, Beharee, awoke, feeling as if he had been drunk, but neither he nor his friend had taken any spirits on the previous day; he then felt the body of his friend, Jewlall, and found it was quite cold, as if he had been dead some hours. The Civil Surgeon made a *post-mortem* examination of the body of Jewlall; a quantity of boiled rice was found in his stomach, which was forwarded to Calcutta for examination. On examining this partly digested rice, several roundish, flattened, kidney-shaped seeds, of a yellow colour, and measuring about a quarter of an inch in their long diameter, were found mixed with it. After careful examination, some of these were found to be seeds of the common *capsicum frutescens*, and others of the common or white dhatoora.

In September 1853, the Magistrate of the 24-Pergunnahs forwarded for examination a substance which was stated to have been picked out of some cooked *dhall*, the suspicions of the person eating it having been aroused by a bitter taste. After eating one handful of the *dhall*, in which the substance was found, this person vomited; and, within another half hour, became insensible from the same cause. Dr. Mouat replied that the substance in question consisted chiefly of the seeds of the *dhatoora*, which had evidently been boiled.

In 1854, one Mussamat Dhun Koour, being weary of leading a single life, had recourse to a barber useful in such exigencies, who procured her recommendation to a man named Kooraee, who, after an interview, approved of her appearance, and it was agreed that they should live together. It fell to her lot to prepare the meals for the family. On the fourth day, the man, his brother and mother, were discovered in a state of insensibility after eating their dinner. The female was missing, but upon being apprehended, confessed that, having taken offence, she had deliberately mixed some of the seed of the *dhatoora* in the food, but declared that she only wished to stupefy them, to enable her to make her escape. The civil surgeon found a large quantity of the *dhatoora* seed mixed with the food which he examined, "but could not say that the quantity was sufficient to cause death to persons freely partaking of the same." She was sentenced to fourteen years' imprisonment with labour.*

According to Professor Hirtz, the active principle of datura stramonium resides chiefly in the *seeds.* It cannot, however, be doubted that all parts of the Indian *datura* plants are full of daturine.

Leaves.

I am indebted to Dr. H. Cleghorn, of the Madras Medical Service, for the following interesting notes of a case of poisoning with the *Leaves* of the *dhatoora.*†

"A child aged two was brought in its last agonies; the fragments of three or four *leaves* were found in the stomach. This case is interesting, in as far as the poison was traced to its source, and I believe that, in all previously recorded cases, death resulted from eating the *fruits* or *seeds.*

"The mother of the child was reaping in a *raggy* field when it was discovered that her two children were eating the leaves of *dhatoora.* A leaf was found convulsively grasped in the hands of one of them. When I was afterwards taken to the spot, the plant was found to be the black *dhatoora (datura fastuosa),* which is esteemed a more virulent poison than the white-flowered species *(datura alba).* The elder child quickly recovered, as the sulphate of zinc which was given acted immediately; with the younger one, narcotism was so great that vomiting could not be produced."

In the paper already cited, Native Surgeon Moodelly gives two cases of poisoning by the *leaves.* In the first the woman took a quantity of the green leaves under the impression that they would cure a bowel-complaint. In the second a man drank, by the advice of a Fakir, a quantity of butter-milk, in which a handful of green *dhatoora* leaves had been soaked for twelve hours. In both cases the symptoms of *datura* poisoning were very marked. For a case of poisoning (fatal in the cases of two adults) by the leaves, *vide supra* p. 188.

Dr. Shortt gives‡ the case of a Brahmin of Chingleput, aged forty-one, apparently in the enjoyment of health, who, on returning from a visit to his rice-fields in the morning, grew giddy, and fell to the ground. He

---

* Nizamut Adawalut Reports, N. W. P., August 1854, p. 182.

† See also a case in which the leaves appear to have been used.—*Nizamut Adawlut Reports,* N. W. P., 22nd April 1854, p. 441.

‡ Madras Quar. Jour. of Medl. Science, Vol. VI, p. 286.

was able to say, on being questioned, that he had eaten "*Oomatum elai*" or stramonium leaves. He soon after grew violently delirious, and died comatose in about an hour. On *post-mortem* examination, on the following day, the only important appearances observed were dilatation of the pupils; heart empty and flaccid; mucous membrane of the stomach greatly congested throughout, more particularly along the great curvature; mucous membrane of the bowels congested throughout, but in a less degree than that of the stomach. Nearly two ounces of a green pultaceous mass were found in the stomach. On being washed, this was found to be made up of the *débris* of undigested leaves. The *duodenum* was empty. The *jejunum* contained a quantity of a pulpy mass of a green colour and peculiar musty odour.

In the middle of February 1869, I saw in Dr. Chuckerbutty's wards, in the Medical College Hospital, a family of four persons suffering severely, but not fatally, from the effects of eating datura leaves. Dr. Chuckerbutty has kindly permitted me to give the following details.

A policeman, when on guard at one in the morning, hearing a great noise of quarrelling in the house of a Mussalman labourer, entered and found the man and his wife, people about fifty years of age, and a boy and a girl, aged twelve and two, quarrelling and talking nonsense. They were brought to the hospital at about five in the morning. In the adults and in the boy the symptoms were, in a very marked degree, those of datura poisoning,—great excitement, rambling talk, and anger on being questioned, great and persistent dilatation of the pupils, which were at first insensible to the light. The infant was at first silent, with considerable dilatation of the pupils, and then fell asleep. They were all discharged well on the following day. On recovering her senses, the mother said that she had collected *sag* (wild spinach, as in Dr. Palmer's case), and made it with beans and peas into a curry, of which they all partook. She had no idea that the *sag* was datura.

A very well marked case of poisoning by a large quantity of the leaves in a muscular Rajpoot about fifty years of age, is given* by Mr. Hinder of the Calcutta Native Hospital. On admission, the patient lay quite unconscious, with severe spasmodic muscular twitchings and stertorous breathing, skin cool, pulse about 108, pupils dilated and insensible to light. By means of the stomach pump an enormous quantity of datura leaves mixed with boiled rice was evacuated. Next morning, about ten hours after admission, there was a slight subsidence of the muscular contractions (although during the night they had approached to tetanic rigidity), constant picking of the bed-clothes, spoke, but incoherently, articulation indistinct, pupils still dilated and insensible to light, pulse 108, firmer, skin cool, lips parched and dry. Towards afternoon, as the

* Ind. Med. Gaz. for Jan. 1, 1865, p. 10.

poisonous effects were passing off, he became wildly delirious, yelling and screeching striking out at and attempting to bite any one who approached, so that it was considered advisable to have him bound down to the bed. Head hot, and face flushed, lips parched and dry, skin warm. On the following day he wandered a little, but was not violent. From this time his recovery was rapid and complete.

He acknowledged that he took the leaves voluntarily. It is evident that, had he not been quickly relieved, he must have died.

Beck cites (p. 1032) the case of a soldier, in New Jersey, who, having dressed and eaten a quantity of leaves of *datura stramonium*, "was seized with genuine tetanus," and died.

We have thus five fatal cases of poisoning by the *leaves*, four in adults, and one in a child.

Capsules and Young Seeds.

Dr. Heude's Nagpore Dispensary Report, for the half year ending 31st March 1858, contains the case of a young man who died after taking two datura capsules. This appears to be a mode of taking the poison rather prevalent in Madras.

This, according to Linschoten, was the part of the plant employed by dishonest Portuguese women at Goa. He says,—"They have likewise an hearbe called Deutroa which beareth a seed, whereof, bruising out the sap, they put it into a cup and give it to their husbands."*

Dr. Shortt relates two cases in the paper already cited.

A girl aged fourteen, on admission, had a wild appearance, was stupid and unconscious of her state; when roused, she gave a foolish and vacant look around. Pupils widely dilated. A glairy fluid dribbling from the mouth. On recovery she stated that, having been beaten by her mother, she had plucked an *Oomatum Kai pinjee*, a young fruit of the stramonium, crushed it on a stone, and collected the young seeds, of which she ate about a third. On entering the house half an hour afterwards she staggered and fell; was able to state what she had done and remembered nothing afterwards. She was well the next day.

A girl aged eighteen, said to have been in good health, but subject to colicky pains, was observed early in the morning to be giddy and to stagger. When questioned, she hesitated for a time, and then replied that she had eaten *Oomatum Kai* which she had procured from a plant in the compound. In the course of an hour she became delirious, tossing about, picking her clothes, and talking incoherently. Convulsions then set in, and she died in few hours after taking the poison.

The brain had a dry firm appearance, the absence of moisture at once attracted attention. Some congestion of brain and meninges; the ventricles

* Part. 2, p. 175.

empty ; no fluid about the base of the skull ; pupils dilated ; heart small, empty, and flaccid ; stomach nearly empty ; and the mucous coat much congested, particularly along the great curvature. Several pieces of the spring capsule of the stramonium were found imbedded in the mucous membrane ; one or two of these were sufficiently large to be recognised at once as forming the prickly outer covering of the fruit of the thorn-apple. The duodenum contained 25 *stramonium seeds and also a good number of seeds of the common red chilly*, with portions of its [the pericarp of datura ?] skin mixed up into a greenish pultaceous mass, having a strong musty odour. The *jejunum* contained 35 *lumbrici* (hence probably the colicky pains ; and, according to Dr. Woodford's view, the tendency to Suicide—see Chapter on Suicide). In the *ilium* was some of the greenish mass with a few seeds of the stramonium.*

Dr. Giraud notices it, as a remarkable fact, that, although administered under such different circumstances and with such varied motives, *dhatoora* should so seldom prove fatal in Bombay, that not a single case in which the effects of *dhatoora* could be directly traced has terminated in death ; and that, of fifty-one cases which were treated in the Jamsetjee Jeejeebhoy Hospital, during the preceding year, only four presented very alarming symptoms. He considers it difficult to determine whether these comparatively mild results arise from a careful proportioning of the poison, or whether our Indian indigenous species of *Datura* are possessed of less virulent properties than those of the *Datura Stramonium*, of the fatal effects of which instances are not wanting.

As will be gathered, however, from cases already cited, the victims of *dhatoora* poisoning do not always escape with life. The following instances, in which death resulted from the practice, also deserve notice.

In August 1854, a woman was sentenced to death for having, upon her own confession, mixed a stupefying drug with the *attah*, which it was her duty to cook for the family. This was done at the instigation of her paramour. The result was, that a very aged man was taken ill with symptoms resembling those of *dhatoora* poisoning, and that three children died, after having been similarly attacked. Dr. Murray's inquiries led him to believe that the children died from taking *dhatoora* or some similar poison.†

---

* In both of these cases the girl took some *Eloopai poonak* (oil-cake from the seeds of the *Basssia longifolia*,) which is commonly used by the natives as an emetic. It failed to have this effect in the fatal case, but is considered by many to be generally efficient.

The girl who recovered was given some decoction of indigo leaves.

Dr. Shortt says that the indigo plant (*Indigofera tinctoria*) is considered by the natives to be an antidote in all cases of poisoning, more particularly in those by arsenic. The leaves are made into a decoction, and from 2 to 4 ounces are administered every two hours. The indigo itself is said to be an antidote to snake-bite.

† Nizamut Adawlut Reports, N. W. P., August 1854, p. 288.

In 1852, one Mussumat Jussodee, living with a widower, in the Hurdah District, as his mistress, destroyed her step-son, a healthy youth of fifteen or sixteen, by mixing the *dhatoora* seeds in his food, telling the man that his son had gone to his aunt's in another village. Six days afterwards, the man happening to go into a tobacco garden to the rear of his premises, his attention was drawn to a spot which a jackal was scratching up, and he perceived a human leg. Further investigation led to the exhumation of the corpse of his son, quite naked, much decomposed, but identifiable, the lower extremities only having been eaten by animals. The woman confessed her crime, and was apprehended. She acknowledged repeatedly, even in the Judge's court, that she gave the boy ten pods or heads of *dhatoora* seed in food, to kill him, as he was always quarrelling, and that he died in consequence. She adhered to this statement with great consistency. Eleven days after death, however, a *post-mortem* examination of the body was made by the medical officer at Hoshungabad (70 or 80 miles off). He gave it as his opinion that *rupture of the stomach* was the probable cause of death, adding that the organ was empty, showing no trace of digested food, nor any indication of the presence of *dhatoora* seed. (The woman said that she pounded the seed on a large stone, and then mixed it in one of two large *rotees*, which she baked for supper.) The Judge suggested that the state of the stomach might not improbably be dependent upon a natural *post-mortem* condition. The medical officer observed that the decomposition of the body had proceeded to such a degree that he was unable to pronounce an opinion as to the cause of rupture of the stomach ; indeed, under the condition in which the body was, he should have been doubtful as to the existence of the lesion of the stomach prior to the extinction of life, had not grumous blood been found contiguous to it. The Judge again inquired—Was it strange that digested food should, in the course of eleven days, have been absorbed, in the process of corruption, so as to be no longer traceable ? [It might, unquestionably, be very difficult to distinguish its presence.] The Judge then commented upon the seeming opposition between what the medical officer described as the first effect of poisoning by *dhatoora, viz.*, a condition of active maniacal excitement, and the woman's statement that, after his poisoned meal, her victim lay down to sleep, and she sat up watching him to see the effect of the poison ; that *he did not stir*, but passed from sleep to death ; and that, when about a *puhur* of night remained, she found he was dead. In the morning, she dug his grave. The Judge considered that, if the woman really did administer the quantity stated, it appeared to have been enough to kill ten men. As far as he could learn from the natives, any such dose would have thrown the person taking it into a stupor, followed by speedy death. It appears not improbable that the murderess may have inflicted violence upon her victim after he became insensible, or the rupture of the stomach may, possibly, have resulted from trampling the body down in a shallow grave, perhaps while life still lingered. The case should be referred to as an example of the care and discrimination in weighing every detail of evidence generally displayed by Judges in this country.*

It was proved on a trial at Agra, in the same year, that one Mussamat Rookma, having been superseded in certain village rights by a person named Thukoory, employed Cheetah, a youth living at a distance and having no concern in the matter, to mix pounded *dhatoora* with *bhang* (decoction of Indian hemp), which he gave to the unfortunate man, who drank it in the presence of three witnesses. Thukoory managed to reach the house of another witness, trembling and ill, and said that Cheetah and the woman had mixed poison in the *bhang* which they had given him. He soon after died. At the trial, the lad denied that he knew that what the woman gave him to mix was poison. The woman made no defence. They had made full confession of the crime at the thannah, as is usual. Cheetah was sentenced to death ; the woman, as an accessory before the fact, to imprisonment for life with labour.†

See three important cases of fatal poisoning by *datura*, at pp. 62, 63, of Dr. Burton Brown's work. In 1809, there occurred a fatal case of poisoning with *dhatoora*, which involved several important particulars. A woman, named Musst. Sookhao, while on her way from Benares, fell in with a very feeble man, nearly 80 years old, regarding whom she appears to have had previous knowledge. By his request, she gave him some flour of gram and barley mixed, which she had with her ; they then walked about a koss (two miles), when the deceased was suddenly taken ill, and told some people on the spot that he had taken some of the prisoner's *suttoo*, and was unwell, desiring them to secure her. He immediately after became senseless, rolling himself on the ground, tossing his legs in convulsive motions, foam issuing at the mouth. The man died *five days* afterwards. Two respectable Brahmins, whom the prisoner and the deceased met, when the latter was first seized with illness, also deposed that the prisoner then admitted that she had given the man *dhatoora* in the flour. She also appears to have confessed to the police that she had given the deceased one chedam's weight (less than a grain) of *dhatoora* among the flour ; that she had seen the deceased's son give him rupees 9 (which were found on the deceased) on parting, and that she had brought the *dhatoora* on purpose to give to the deceased. Before the magistrate, and on trial, she positively denied that she had given the deceased *dhatoora* or any other poisonous drug ; but acknowledged that she had upon her a small quantity of that vegetable, alleging that it was used by herself as a cure for certain disorders. She further

---

* Nizamut Adawlut Reports, N. W. P., January 22nd, 1852, p. 45.

† *Ibid*, 24th June, 1852, p. 580.

stated that the police had extorted her confession by maltreatment ; some flour, and about two chedams of pounded stuff, described by the prisoner as containing *dhatoora* and different kinds of spices, and used by her medicinally, were found on her person. The latter being mixed with some fresh flour was given to a dog, and the former to another ; but neither of the dogs was at all affected. The native docter stated that the deceased, having recovered his senses previously to his death, had told him that the prisoner had given him *dhatoora* among the flour. The Judge of Circuit, being informed that one Syud Sulamut Alee was a man skilled in the art of medicine, directed the following queries to be proposed to him :—*First,*—Whether *dhatoora* would cause death ; and, if so, what quantity was required to produce that effect ? *Secondly,*—Whether, if such quantity were mixed with $\frac{1}{2}$ or $\frac{1}{4}$ of a seer (a pound or half a pound) of flour, a person eating it would be sensible of the smell or taste ? *Thirdly,*—In what time death would ensue from a quantity sufficient to produce fatal effect ? Sulamut Alee replied, that there was one kind of *dhatoora* of which $4\frac{1}{2}$ mashas ($63\frac{3}{4}$ grains) would cause death in a man of middling strength ; but that none of the kinds produced in that part of the country caused death ; that, in small quantities, it was a useful remedy for several diseases ; but that, if more than two ruttees ($2\frac{14}{16}$ grs.) were taken, it would produce intoxication, insensibility, or madness; and that these effects usually lasted three days. The surgeon attached to the station also expressed his opinion that *dhatoora* would not produce death. There was read in evidence an extract from the records of a former trial, from which it appeared that twelve chedams of *dhatoora,* mixed in the juice of sugar (cane), had been given by some robbers to four travellers ; and that, from the action of the draught, these travellers had been deprived of their senses for three days, after which the effects had subsided. The law officers of the court of circuit declared the fact of the prisoner's having administered *dhatoora* to the deceased established ; but that it was uncertain whether his death had been occasioned thereby ; that, there being no prescribed penalty, under the Mahomedan law, for the offence of which she was convicted, she was punishable at the discretion of the ruling power. The judge of circuit declared his opinion that the prisoner gave the *dhatoora* (which he held to be a narcotic, not a poison,) to the deceased as a soporific, for the purpose of robbing him, without any intention of producing his death [it will, however, be noticed, that the point regarding the quantity of the poison administered only rested on the prisoner's statement] ; but that his death might have been occasioned by the effects of the dose on a person of his advanced years. The law officers of the Nizamut Adawlut declared in their *futwa,* that the *dhatoora* was a deleterious drug, and might, in the case of an infirm person, occasion death ; that the prisoner was convicted of having administered such drug to the deceased, to the effects of which alone his death could be attributed ; and that the offence of the prisoner not coming within the five-fold definition of culpable homicide, as laid down in the Mahomedan law, she was liable to discretionary punishment by *acoobut*. The Court of Nizamut Adalwlut, having no doubt of the prisoner's guilt in having occasioned the death of the deceased by an unlawful act committed in the prosecution of an intended theft, sentenced her, under the above *futwa*, to imprisonment for life.*

In 1823, a man was convicted and sentenced to ten years' imprisonment for having prepared *dhatoora* for the purpose of administering it to his rival. He, however, with some appearance of veracity, disclaimed an intention of killing, and maintained that *dhatoora* was not mortal.

Death resulted in several of the other cases of drugging for criminal purposes in India, published in the records of the Courts. It certainly was not *proved* that *dhatoora* was the poison employed in several of those instances; but any medical man who peruses their details will decide that this was, doubtless, the drug administered in nearly all.

The above cases must go far to explode the erroneous and dangerous opinion that *dhatoora* is to be considered as a narcotic and intoxicating drug; but not as a poison calculated, under ordinary circumstances, to destroy life—a belief which, forty years ago, was evidently prevalent both among Europeans and natives; and which is, doubtless, still held by the native public, and their Hukeems and Kobirajira.

There can be no doubt whatever that the *fresh seeds, cupsules,* and leaves of the Indian Daturas are very deadly, perhaps almost certainly so when taken in full dose, and when early measures are not taken for evacuating the poison by emetics and purgatives. Dr. Burton Brown states that, out of ninety-two cases, no less than twenty-one proved fatal; and it is probable that many other cases which result in death are never known (p. 57).

In my edition of 1856, I added that it is at the same time necessary to observe that, while there are many cases of fatal poisoning by the Indian species of *dhatoora* on record, and while the facts before us can scarcely leave a doubt that strong adults have perished from large doses of the plant, I had not succeeded in finding any unimpeachably proven case in which death was caused by the poison, *here,* in a healthy young adult. Children and aged persons have commonly been the sufferers, and the cases in which healthy men and women have died after being thus drugged, are open to the suspicion either of the *dhatoora* having been mixed with other and stronger poisons, or of other unfair means having been resorted to by the robbers after their victims became insensible. However, it is scarcely necessary to add that a poison which, when given in rather moderate doses, kills children and aged persons, will, if sufficiently largely administered, destroy persons of the strongest constitution.

* Macnaghten's Reports, Vol. I., p. 216.

Certain of the narratives given above lead me so far to modify the above opinion as to admit that there are about three cases (two by Dr. Palmer, and one by Dr. Shortt,) in which adults were killed with datura only.

It is, however, only positively stated that one of these three was healthy, and, in all these cases, the *fresh* plant was used.

Our highest authority in toxicology maintains that the "*Datura Stramonium* has decidedly the characters of a narcotico-irritant poison. All parts of the plant are poisonous."* He finds that, in Europe (where the *datura* certainly has not more virulent properties than it has in India), "several fatal cases are reported, one of which terminated in *six hours*." Among the fatal cases cited by Dr. Taylor are those :—(1.) Of a child aged two years, who swallowed 16 grains of the seeds and died in *twenty-four hours*, having been maniacally delirious, the symptoms resembling those of hydrophobia. (2.) Of a medical man's child, also two years old, who swallowed about 100 seeds of Stramonium weighing 16 grains: the usual symptoms were manifested in an hour; and although 20 seeds had been ejected by vomiting, and 80 by purging, the child died in *twenty-four hours*. (3.) A woman swallowed a decoction of the bruised seeds (about 120); she very soon became delirious, threw her arms about, and spoke incoherently: she *died in seven hours*. (4.) Three females swallowed an infusion of Stramonium leaves—all suffered most severely; stimulants were administered with success in two cases—the other proved fatal.

It must certainly be admitted that, although the *dhatoora* is employed for criminal purposes in the most reckless manner, it may, *possibly*, be true that it is not given with a decided intention to kill, and that there may still exist a popular opinion that its effects are not deadly, but merely intoxicating. The fact of its having been numbered among the "weak poisons" or active drugs in the Shastra, may explain the prevalence of this idea. This may, perhaps, still be considered to weigh in favour of prisoners convicted of the great and exceedingly prevalent crime in question. Still the evidence of medical witnesses, in such trials, cannot be otherwise than to the effect that *datura is a drug which is as certainly and as rapidly fatal in its effects as opium*; and that it is scarcely to be believed that any culprit can have long practised its administration, in a reckless manner, without discovering its destructive properties.

I observe that, in his valuable work on the Indigenous Drugs of India, published in 1867, Baboo Kanny Lall Dey appears to speak very distinctly upon this point, observing that the *dhatooras* "are very familiar to the Indian poisoners *who give them not with the intention of killing, but of stupefying their victims*† for the purpose of facilitating theft, and

* Dr. Taylor's Treatise on Poisons, p. 783.

† The italics are mine.

expediting other evil designs" (p. 48). This is a very important opinion, as coming from one of the most experienced of our Chemical Examiners. Still I think it a matter of importance that this question should be fully sifted. I am inclined to believe that the knowledge that *dhatoora*, especially *if given fresh*, and in sufficient quantity, is a deadly poison, is extensively spread among natives. Towards this opinion we have the following facts that Mussamut Jussodee (*vide supra*, p. 198) "acknowledged repeatedly, even in the Judge's court, that she gave the boy ten pods or heads of *dhatoora* seed in food to kill him, as he was always quarrelling, and that he died in consequence." Then we have Dr. Shortt's three Madras cases (*vide supra*, pp. 194 and 196). In the first of these a middle-aged brahmin returned as usual in the morning from his field, and fell, admitting, on being questioned by the women of the house, that he had eaten *dhatoora* leaves. Dr. Shortt says that, "in the absence of evidence to the contrary, it would be charitable to suppose that he committed suicide in a fit of temporary insanity." It appears never to have been doubted that the act was suicidal. Dr. Shortt believed that the suicide of this man was imitated by the two girls, who lived not far off, and who poisoned themselves with *dhatoora* while the sensation caused by his death prevailed. Still again we have Mr. Hinder's Calcutta case (p. 195) of a middle-aged Rajpoot, who very nearly killed herself with an enormous quantity of fresh *dhatoora* leaves avowedly swallowed with suicidal intent. It appears to me that, if these facts do not prove that it is generally known in India that *dhatoora* has power to kill, they at least call for re-consideration of this question.

The clear decision of this question was formerly a matter of the greatest moment, since the old law drew a marked difference between the crime of administering *poisonous* drugs to persons with a view to robbing them when in a state of insensibility, and that of administering drugs and substances of a merely *intoxicating* character, and not of a nature to endanger life, for the same purpose.* Upon this subject, Mr. Dampier recorded the following judicious remarks in commenting upon the practice of the *meetawallahs*:—† "The drugs administered are all stupefying; if the dose is large enough, it causes death; if small, stupefaction—not, in my opinion,

* Beaufort's Digest, para. 3118. Thus, in the case of Joogul, who gave a woman *datura* in sweetmeats which rendered her insensible for two days, punishment was diminished on the ground that the prisoner had only the intention of producing insensibility, and not of causing death.—*Nizamut Adawlut Reports*, N. W. P., for 1852, p. 329.

So also, in the case of Bhoboban Sahoo, the Judges of the Nizamut Adawlut decided: "There can be no doubt that *dhatoora* was the drug used on the present occasion; but, unless under very peculiar circumstances, it has only an intoxicating effect (see Chevers's Report on Medical Jurisprudence in the Bengal Presidency, pages 31, 2, 3). We therefore convict the prisoner of administering an intoxicating drug, with a view to theft, and of theft, and sentence him to seven years' imprisonment with labour in irons in banishment.—*Ibid*, July 27th, 1855, p. 1.

† Police Report for first six months of 1841, para. 123.

intoxication. The *meetawallah* mixes the drug by chance, and leaves his victim to recover or die as the chance may be; and I think a heavier punishment than six or seven years' imprisonment should always be given to this class of offenders; I would never give less than imprisonment for life, as such men should (like the Thugs) not be allowed again to be at large, to the injury of the community. That death does not ensue in every case is not the fault of the *meetawallahs* administering the drug in food or water; it arises from the mearest chances,—whether the stomach of the receiver is full or empty, the victim robust or weak, or the quantity of mixed food swallowed before the effect of the drug appears; and it is, I think, a mistake to charge this class of miscreants with administering *intoxicating* drugs when the parties recover, when they are always *poisonous* drugs dependent for their fatal effect on the quantity which the victim may swallow, or other circumstances,—not on any designed will of the administerer."

All subsequent experience has shown that every species of *datura* is a *poison,* in the strongest sense of the term; and it now seems to be generally so regarded by judicial officers in this country. Although, for the most part, reckless of consequences, it would certainly appear that some of the *dhatooreeas* and *meetawallahs* have acquired considerable skill in apportioning their doses; it is probable that the possession of such dexterity, as it must always be an evidence of long practice and numerous experiments, will not be regarded as mitigatory in the eye of the law.

The law now merely places in the same category "*any poison or any stupefying, intoxicating, or unwholesome drug.*"—Indian Penal Code, *Section* 328.

There existed, among Missionaries in this country, when this Manual was first published, a very strong conviction that *datura* is frequently administered by their relatives to natives who evince an inclination to embrace Christianity. In 1856, I was authorised to quote the following passage from a note lately written by an eminent and experienced Missionary, then residing in Calcutta, but now deceased, in reply to queries on this subject:—"I always understood that the drug administered in the cases referred to, was the *dhatoora* in small dose. The symptoms have been heavy dull eyes, with a prostration of mind, rendering the victim an idiot, and *looking* very much like one, with a listless heavy countenance, indicating that the brain has, somehow or other, been affected. I believe the victim can be for months in that listless, heavy, dreamy state; but, gradually, under a proper treatment and a change of scenery, I always heard recovery was possible. There is no mistaking the symptoms of the poison, as it transforms the victim in a *short time* into a *totally different being* from what he was in his normal state."*

* This very important subject will be recurred to in the Chapter on INSANITY, under the head of *Drugging with Datura.*

In 1838, the Rev. W. S. Mackay, of the Calcutta Church of Scotland Mission, stated, in a report of the case of a lad named Dwarkanauth Bose, that, "in their strong opposition to his determination to become a Christian, his father, having confined him, gave him a drug, with a view of gradually destroying his intellect."

The two following cases give us some insight into the operation of this fiendish process. They are the more remarkable because those whose destruction appears to have been attempted were Europeans.

It was reported in the *Bombay Gazette* in September 1865, that Mr. Uppham, an Inspector of the E. I. Railway at Jubbulpore, had charged three of his servants with poisoning him. The account goes on to relate :—"Mr. Uppham says that he saw (from a distance of ten paces) his servants pounding the *dhatoora* fruit, which one of them had got from a tree close by his house, and squeezing the juice through a towel into his stew. He called for the stew as if to partake of it, but after a little while told his kitmutgar that he was not hungry, and to keep the stew on the table for breakfast next morning, resolving to himself to make it over to the railway doctor next day. That night he wrote a letter to the doctor to be despatched the next day. Next morning, however, he called for 'chota hazree,' partook of tea and handcakes, and then mounted his horse, and rode towards the doctor's. He was obliged to halt at a bungalow on the line, as he felt his head affected. Mr. Augier, the occupant of the bungalow, took him in, and called in another person, but neither could make out what was the matter with Mr. Uppham, for he reeled to and fro like a drunken man, and yet was not drunk. They called in the doctor, but he was at a loss to discover the cause of indisposition ; the patient was talking incoherently, going reeling about the room, and every now and then squeezing and twisting his coat tail, and looking about the room as if to illustrate his meaning still further. After recovering from the stupor next day, Mr. Uppham left for home, and returned shortly after with a fruit from the same *dhatoora* tree ; the doctor then of course had no doubt on his mind that *dhatoora* had been administered to Mr. Uppham. Before the magistrate, who committed the prisoners to the Sessions, one confessed to having brought the fruit from the tree alluded to by Mr. Uppham, another confessed to its being pounded and made over to the kitmutgar, but he (the kitmutgar) says he did not give it to his master, but took it for ear-ache himself. The kitmutgar's own brother, who is Mr. Uppham's chupprassee, deposes that he never saw him using *dhatoora* for ear-ache."

Dr. David B. Smith gives* notes of the case of Mr. ——, aged forty-two, a European of very regular and temperate habits, residing at Mussoorie, the subject of "irritative" or "phosphatic dispepsia," but not otherwise diseased. On the morning of the 2nd November, Mr. —— was ill, and in a confused

* Ind. Med. Gaz., 2nd March 1868, p. 58.

state. On the 5th, the following notes were taken :—"Went to bed on evening of 1st November, perfectly well. Got up at usual hour in morning with a sensation of extraordinary giddiness, and a sense of rolling motion. In trying to reach his clothes, which were on a chair close by, felt a reeling sensation. In getting up to bathe, felt himself swaying from side to side. Lower limbs and arms felt perfectly powerless, and also the tongue. Could not speak properly. No pain in head or spine, no sickness of stomach. Could not see at all to write. Could see large objects, but not small ones, such as letters. Could not see to read. Any one approaching seemed to have a white muslin net over him. Face was puffy under the eyelids. Tongue moist-looking, but complains of dryness of mouth and throat." On the evening of the 6th, word was sent to Dr. Smith that Mr. —— was delirious (*behosh ho gya*). On visiting him, however, he was asleep. On being roused, his pulse was steady, and he answered some questions. His pupils were broadly dilated, and he was evidently drowsy. "Still," says Dr. Smith, "I had no suspicion of his having been unfairly dealt with." On the morning of the 7th, Dr. Smith received a note from Mr. ——. It appears that the beginning of it was steady, legible, and sensible, whilst the conclusion of it was rambling, confused, and almost illegible. Dr. Smith found him in a very peculiar state. Face somewhat purplish, eyes bright, the pupils greatly dilated and insensible to light. Pulse tolerably natural. He wandered about in a confused state, arching his eyebrows, rubbing his hands, and complaining of cold and numbness down the right side of his body. He went from room to room, and showed an inclination to wander outside. His daughter led him about, and prevented him from going out of doors.

He spoke incoherent nonsense. Looking out he suddenly exclaimed with a placid but startled expression, "See, doctor, there is *snow* on the ground." On being told "It is sunlight you see," he replied with an air of confusion and disappointment, "Oh ! sunlight is it ? I thought it was snow ;" and immediately he rambled incoherently about other matters. He then wandered into a room where Dr. Smith was writing a prescription ; came up to the writing-table and began touching various things without any definite object. He looked towards the pigeon-holes, where he had private papers tumbled in their direction, but took nothing out. His gait was peculiar, and he walked in a sort of stealthy manner, mumbling to himself. He appeared in a feeble and pitiable state. He was not the least violent.

Dr. Smith perceived that this condition was very peculiar. He apprehended a paralytic attack, but he did not yet suspect *foul play.*

On this day (7th), Dr. Smith heard that one of Mr. ———'s servants had expressed a suspicion that his master had been poisoned. Dr. Smith replied that, if so, the poison was probably *dhatoora.* On the 8th, he was found lying perfectly sensible, but weak, and still somewhat confused and unlike himself. On the 10th he wrote, still complaining of "dryness of the mouth and throat." On the 13th, he went to Dr. Smith's house, and talked the whole matter over. He then, for the first time, said that he felt convinced that he had been poisoned. He believed there were four occasions on which he had reason to suspect that poison had been administered to him. He could not recall dates. But, coupling his somewhat vague recollections of facts with notes in his own diary, Dr. Smith inferred that the first occasion was on the evening of the 1st of November, in his tea; the second on the evening of the 6th, in his soup; the third on the morning of the 7th, in his cocoa; and the fourth occasion he was not so certain about. On Sunday, the 10th, however, he still experienced dryness of the mouth and throat, and, otherwise, he felt peculiar sensations; but he stated that he could not be sure that, on that day, poison was administered to him. He said he thought it possible that his sensations then experienced were merely the after-effects of previous doses of poison. He said that the tea and cocoa which he drunk on the evening of the 1st and the morning of the 7th, had *a heavy muddy flavour like that of burnt milk*, and that he noticed and complained of this at the time. He said that the soup he took on the evening of the 6th *had a distinctly bitter taste*, and that he also remarked this, and complained of it at the time. Shortly after taking both the soup on the 6th, and the cocoa on the 7th, he lost all recollection of what happened around him. Meanwhile, however, he experienced a feeling of intoxication and giddiness, difficulty in swallowing, confusion of ideas, a coldness and numbness of the surface, a pricking sensation in the nose, and an irresistible inclination to rub the nose violently. He had also convulsive twitchings of the legs after taking the soup. He had no fever and no vomiting, but considerable drowsiness. In addition to the symptoms noticed above, there were observed frequent coughing; attempts to hawk and spit; haziness and confusion of objects, as if everything were badly focussed; a sensation as if smoke or fog were rising around him. The moment he touched any object, he went off in a purposeless manner to some other object at a distance. As he did this, he was led and supported by his daughter, and looked the picture of feeble nervous agitation. After recovering to a certain degree, he still evinced a partially incoherent mental state; his vision continued indistinct; the eyes were bright and glistering, and the pupils continued to be widely dilated. He also experienced a sense of very considerable exhaustion; walked about feebly; and was altogether sadly unlike himself.

Hence Dr. Smith concludes that he was powerfully under the influence of *dhatoora*. Mr. —— appears to have had considerable real causes of mental distress. Dr. Smith adds that, taking it for granted that an excessive quantity of *dhatoora* was administered in this case, it is not easy to determine with what specific object it was given, whether to kill at once, or to effect the same end by slow poisoning, or whether it was intended, by degrees, to stupefy and weaken the intellect. It is to be observed that the natives do believe in the possibility of rendering a person fatuous by such means. (Mr. —— is in possession of a good deal of valuable property.)

Reporting the case a year subsequently, Dr. Smith adds that his patient was then " perfectly well and happy."

It will be shown in the next Chapter that the use, as an intoxicant, of Indian hemp is an extremely frequent cause of acute mania in India. Whether *datura* has any similar power is a question which has yet to be settled, although native opinion answers it decidedly in the affirmative. In a table annexed to Baboo Kanny Loll Dey's valuable monograph on the *Uses of Narcotics and Stimulants, and their effects on the Human Constitution,** it is noted that, in the five years, 1863—67, three cases of mania, in which there was "*dhatoora* intoxication," were treated in the five Lunatic Asyla of Lower Bengal.

One of these, although not perfectly convincing, is very suggestive of the necessity for further enquiry into this question. In the Annual Report of the Lunatic Asylums in Bengal for 1867 (p. 91), Mr. W. D. Stewart, Superintendent of the Cuttack Asylum, reports the case of Mr. B ——, an European, who, as an inspector of irrigation works, had an extremely laborious duty, so that, at one time, he was doing the work of three men. His previous health had never been good ; he was subject to spasmodic asthma, for which his medical man ordered *dhatoora* smoking. He derived so much benefit from this, that he reverted to it whenever he was distressed. The leaves of the plant were chiefly employed. For six months he continued in this habit, on some occasions smoking two or three pipes a day. About this time he was heard to complain of pain and a sense of pressure on the head. Here, then, as Mr. Stewart observes, there were two exciting causes,—excessive mental and bodily occupation, and *dhatoora* smoking. The difficulties of the case were that, when relieved of some of his work, on giving over charge, he suddenly burst into a fit of craziness,† and declared he was poisoned, and surrounded by conspirators. For the first two months of his stay in the Asylum, he lost greatly in flesh, and was violently maniacal. For some days he was so morose that he refused all food, and had to be fed by the stomach pump.

He slowly improved, but had two or three relapses ; after that he steadily improved, but not sufficiently to justify his discharge. This case is of so much interest, that I enquired of Dr. Payne, Superintendent of

---

* Bengal Social Science Association's Transactions.

† This is characteristic of the over-worked brain; the crash comes *when the work ceases.* So it was that, as soon as the publication of the ——— Despatches was finished, the amiable editor of that most laborious undertaking cut his throat.

the Calcutta Asylum, to which Mr. —— was transferred. Dr. Payne writes :—"He had had an attack of acute mania, which may possibly have been occasioned by the drug; but I think it was not so, because his state was one which, if it arose from poisoning at all, would arise from long-continued and excessive use of the drug."

We have seen that the drug was smoked for six months, and that, on some occasions, two or three pipes were smoked daily. The case must stand, as a very suggestive one, for further illustration. Beck notices (p. 1033) that there is reason to believe that, in some cases, *datura*-smoking has proved injurious. Dr. Taylor notes (p. 367) that a death from this cause is recorded in the Return of the Registrar-General for April 1856.

Eleven clear cases of poisoning with *Datura* have come under my notice in twenty-two years' Indian experience. Mention may be made here of the first of these,—that of a rather elderly sepoy, who was found in his bed by the native doctor apparently in a state of collapse. When I was called to him, he appeared greatly depressed, with fixedly dilated pupils, cold surface, and a remarkably slow and feeble pulse. He recovered in a few hours, and then confessed that he had been drugging himself with *dhatoora*.* I cite this case on account of the marked tendency to *collapse*, which has been noticed in several other cases. As far as I have observed it, the coma of *dhatoora* poisoning differs from that of fever, apoplexy, alcoholic intoxication, and cerebral compression in the presence of marked collapse.

In some cases where the *dhatoora* is given, insensibility occurs almost immediately ; this probably happens when the poison is administered in solution, or in very fine powder. In a case tried in July 1852, the prosecutor declared that, while a person was handing him a *lota* of water, the prisoner snatched it away, on pretence of freeing the water from dirt

---

* Two cases, in which there was reason to believe that *dhatoora* had been given to travellers, have also occurred within my notice. In the first of these, two persons halted at a village, in the Chittagong District, where they obtained some food. After dining, they started together. One of them was afterwards found in a state of idiotcy, and many days elapsed before he was able to give any account of himself. He then stated that he had become insensible soon after leaving the village, and that he knew nothing of his companion's fate. A skeleton, supposed to be that of the missing traveller, was found in the jungle, and sent in for examination. I believe, however, that the crime was not distinctly brought home to any person. In the other case, a man who had been a native doctor was seized with symptoms of insanity after having partaken of a feast to which he was invited when on his way to Arrakan. This man was under my treatment for two or three days, during which he was apparently suffering from a very unusual kind of cerebral irritation ; he was exceedingly voluble and excited, speaking with a singular stutter, which evidently depended on a certain degree of local paralysis. His eyes were staring and bloodshot ; but there were no evidences of inflammatory action in the system. He was quite rational, and declared his conviction that he had been drugged with *dhatoora*.

or straws, and then gave it to him. After drinking only two mouthsful, and complaining of the bitter taste, he fell down insensible within forty yards of the spot where he had drank, and did not recover his senses until the third day after. In another case a man was struck down so suddenly that his feet were scalded by some hot water which he was carrying.

When the seeds are given, the symptoms continue as long as any of them remain in the intestinal canal; and, probably, in many cases, much longer.

This point, it must be insisted, is one of the greatest importance, not only to the physician, but also to the medical jurist. The very strong practical bearing of this principle was impressed on my mind in a conversation with Mr. Reilly, the head of the Detective Police in Bengal, who mentioned to me that, on one occasion, he failed to obtain a conviction, because the judge urged that the plaintiff had not been able to identify the accused *soon* after he recovered from *dhatoora* stupor. It is to be borne in mind that persons who have been thus drugged, *should have more than a week allowed them to recover their memory.* As long as seeds lurk in the bowels, memory is not to be depended upon.

There appear to be three sets or stages of symptoms observed in cases of poisoning with Datura—

1*st.*—Headache, dryness of the throat and fauces, urgent thirst, *faintness*, difficulty in walking, languor, and impairment of vision, the pupils being greatly dilated.* When the dose is considerable, insensibility rapidly supervenes.

2*nd.*—Maniacal delirium, flushed face, eyes glistening and in constant motion, the pupils being exceedingly dilated. There is no fever, but intense thirst, and violent perspiration from incessant motion, *the pulse remaining very slow.* All the symptoms are noticed as having a very remarkable resemblance to those occasioned by belladonna.†

3*rd.*—Those accompanying the fatuous condition already described.

In *fatal cases* of poisoning by the Indian Daturas, the person becomes giddy, staggers and falls, is then violently delirious with jactitation and subsultus, perhaps becomes convulsed and dies collapsed and comatose.

In a case, related by Dr. Aitchison, of a Chowdree, thirty-five years of age, poisoned by Datura‡ apparently in a mixture obtained from a hakeem,

---

* Cases by Messrs. Gould and Thurston, in which four persons partook of tea containing three table-spoonsful of stramonium seeds.—*Medical Times and Gazette*, Vol. IV, 1852, p. 197.

† Case by Dr. Schlesier, as quoted by Dr. Taylor.

‡ Probably the *Kala Dhatoora* was used in this case. The man had been ill for nearly six months with slight cough, and, now and then, vomiting; the dark-flowered plant is recommended in the Taleef Shereef as promoting appetite, and as being useful in disorders of phlegm.

there were epileptic fits. The man died from nervous exhaustion (having become quite sensible) five days after having taken the poison. There was considerable meningeal congestion with a trace of arachnitis, *i. e.* partial exudation of lymph.*

Dr. Burton Brown remarks that it would appear that a small dose of Datura only produces symptoms of intoxication or delirium, while, in almost all cases in which death occurred, insensibility coming on rapidly was the principal symptom. It is, therefore, his opinion that, when deep sleep and insensibility have been proved to have occurred early, the dose of the poison was so large as to render a fatal result most probable ; and that it may be fairly assumed, in such a case, that the prisoner gave such a dose as would produce death, unless he can prove the contrary. On the other hand, when delirium alone occurs, there is reason to suppose that the dose was too small to produce a fatal result, and that the prisoner only used the drug as an intoxicating agent. It is evident that, if the object was only to rob the individuals, and not also to prevent them from appearing against the poisoner hereafter, it would be quite sufficient to give a small dose, especially as the delirium is of such a nature that they generally throw off their clothes, rendering robbery easy, and as their state would prevent their evidence being taken with certainty for several days (p. 65).

There appears to be no drug known in the present day which represents, in its effects, so close an approach to the system of ***Slow Poisoning*** believed by many to have been practised in the Middle Ages as does the ***datura.***†

---

* Ind. Lancet, p. 227.

† Colonel Hugh mentions, in his "Proceedings in Military Law," that the natives of India have a mode of administering a substance which may be given insidiously, in small quantities, so as to cause death in a given period and in a manner which shall not cause the appearances on the body as in the case of poison. This, he adds, it would be unwise to publish.

The early writers on India appear to have communicated very nearly the above idea to the first Fellows of the Royal Society. We are told by Paris (M. J., Vol. II, p. 138), that "the power of so graduating the force of a poison as to enable it to operate at any given period, seems to have been considered possible by the earlier members of the Royal Society, for we learn, from Spratt's History of that learned body, that, very shortly after its institution, a series of questions were drawn up by the direction of the Fellows, for the purpose of being submitted to the Chinese and Indians, *viz.*, *Whether the Indians can so prepare that stupefying herb Datura, that they make it lie several days, months, years, according as they will have it, in a man's body, without doing him any hurt, and at the end kill him without missing half an hour's time.*"

I find that this idea was obtained from Linschoten, who, immediately after having spoken of the use of Datura, but not, apparently, with reference to that drug, says:—"There are many men poysoned by their wiues, if once they be moved; for they know how to make a certain poyson or venome, which shall kill the person that drinketh it, at what time or hour it pleaseth them; which poyson being prepared, they make it in such sort, that it will lie six years in a man's body, and never doe him hurt, and then kill him, without missing halfe an houre's time. They make it also for one, two, or three yeeres,

Dr. Giraud's observations on *Symptoms* and *Treatment* of poisoning by the Indian species of the plant being replete with practical value, I have cited them at length.—APPENDIX C.

We are indebted to Dr. Palmer* for a very elaborate review of *the Physiological Differences in the Signs of Poisoning by Aconite and by Datura.* He remarks that—

"On reviewing the several symptoms produced in the cat or dog by these two poisons, *viz., Dhatoora* and *Aconite,* it will be observed that some are constant, while others are variable; that some are common to both poisons, or so nearly resemble each other that they may be easily con-

---

moneths or dayes, as it pleaseth them best, as I have scene it in many, and there it is very common."—*Purchas, Part 2, p.* 1757.

It is now generally believed that the poisoners of the Middle Ages were never in possession of any chemical agent, the operation of which could be suspended and then manifest itself in the system after an indefinite interval (Taylor on Poisons, p. 38). The truth of the matter probably was that they could so accurately apportion their doses of some irritant (probably mercurial) poison as to cause their victims to be attacked with *Chronic Dysentery,*—then the most prevailing disease among all classes of persons, from the highest to the lowest, throughout Europe. It is very remarkable in how many instances it is left as a matter of historic doubt, whether persons of note died from the effects of Poison or of Dysentery. The cases of Geme or Zisimus, brother to Sultan Bajazet (a supposed victim of the Borgias, Anno 1494); Walter Devereux, Earl of Essex; Dudley Earl of Leicester (Queen Elizabeth's favourite); and Philip Earl of Arundel, who died in the Tower in 1595 (*vide* his Life by the Duke of Norfolk), may be instanced among others.

* Op. Cit., p. 27. The following are the principal conclusions of Dr. Van Praag upon a series of experiments upon the effects of Aconitine obtained from the blue variety of Aconite indigenous to Switzerland. Experiments were made upon mammalia, birds, and fishes. From his *post-mortem* examinations, he saw no reason to conclude that Aconitine produced gastro-enteritis; neither do his examinations lead him to place prominently forward, as Schroff has sought to do, a non-coagulable state of the blood as a symptom of poisoning by Aconitine. As to the physiological operation of Aconitine, the general conclusions drawn are, "that Aconitine exercises a retarding influence upon the respiration, a paralyzing operation on the voluntary muscular system, and a depressing influence upon the brain."

A retarding operation on the circulation was less marked than in the experiments of Schroff, and he concludes, "that Aconitine varies very greatly in the frequency with which it induces a reduction of the pulse." In general, it produces dilatation of the pupils. Schroff says that, at the commencement of the experiment, the pupil exhibits great variability, and from time to time even becomes contracted, but that this at length always terminates in dilatation. Salivation and increased excretion of urine must be regarded as amongst the less constant symptoms. Schroff describes, as occurring in the human subject, a peculiar contractile, compressing, even painful, sensation in the cheeks, over the jaws and forehead—in short, in the parts supplied by the trigeminus nerve. The only objective symptom observed by Van Praag that could be explained by such a sensation was licking of the mouth, which was noticed in two cases. Where death occurred suddenly, it was by asphyxia; but, in cases where it was deferred for some time, the animals died apparently from exhaustion. From one experiment made with the alcoholic extract of aconite, it was observed that, while for the most part its action agreed with that of the alkaloid, the symptoms referable to the stomach and bowels were more severe, and gastro-enteritis was moreover induced.

B. & F. Med. Chir. Rev., *January* 1856. *From Virchow's Archiv. fur Path. Anat., &c., Bd., VIII, heft.* 1.

founded ; while others are peculiar to, and characteristic of, one only. The more marked symptoms may now be examined in detail.

"1. *Dilatation of the Pupil.*—This symptom is common to both poisons ; there is, however, such a well-marked difference in the action of the two, that this one symptom alone, carefully observed, might suffice for a differential diagnosis. When *dhatoora* is taken, the pupil enlarges gradually and continuously until the iris is seen as a mere narrow band or thread ; it remains in this condition, without varying, for many hours, no exposure to light causing any contraction ; when, on the other hand, *aconite* has been taken, both the cervical sympathetic and the third nerve appear to be thrown into a state of excitement and irritability, the latter being the more paralyzed (or less excited, as the case may be) of the two ; for while the pupil is generally dilated to a certain extent, the dilatation is scarcely ever so extreme as in the case of *dhatoora ;* it manifests, moreover, a constant tendency to vary in size ; thus, while the animal is at a distance from the observer, it may be seen much dilated ; while, however, it is being watched, limited contractions will be seen to take place. If the animal is brought near, and its eye manipulated in a bright light for more minute inspection, these contractions may proceed to such an extent that it becomes doubtful whether there is any dilatation at all. Sometimes, as in Case II. (*vide supra*, p. 142), contraction to this extent, or even more, may take place without any manipulation or exposure to light.

"2. *General Paralysis* is also a symptom common to both, though generally less marked in the case of *dhatoora*. When complete, there is doubtless some difficulty in distinguishing between the two forms ; but in the less complete stages there are marked differences. In the case of *dhatoora* there is an absence of the co-ordinating power, together with inability to sustain any continued series of volitional efforts, which gives the animal a drunken appearance ; this appearance is greatly heightened by the curious antics which are played, which antics appear to be partly the result of spectral illusions, and partly of the awkward and misdirected efforts to attack the spectres. The paralysis of aconite is less constant in its mode of development. The hind legs appear to be attacked first in most cases, and the first sign appears to be an exaltation of the natural reflex actions ; if, at this time, the sole of the foot is pinched or irritated, the excitement produced in the reflex spinal centre appears to be so strong as to destroy, for the time, all volitional power, and the animal falls to the ground on the irritated side.

"3. *Insensibility to Pain*, when any portion of the skin is pinched with a forceps or pricked with a pin. This is the great characteristic symptom of *aconite* poisoning ; it is marked and decided, while the animal remains perfectly intelligent, and able to move about freely. It occurs also in poisoning by *dhatoora*, but not to any extent until the animal has lost all consciousness and power of motion.

"4. *Loss of Consciousness.*—This symptom occurs to a limited extent in all cases, however slight, of *dhatoora* poisoning, but it is only observed after *aconite*, when a large dose has been taken, or for a very short time, when the symptoms of a smaller dose are at their height.

"The other symptoms are less constant, and the distinction between those produced in the two cases less clearly defined. Difficulty of breathing is common to both. Frothing at the mouth also occurs in both ; but the free and abundant flow of saliva is more marked in aconite poisoning than in the other, and depends probably on the insensibility of the lips ; the saliva in contact with them is not felt, therefore no effort is made to swallow it. There is a peculiarity in the vomiting after aconite, which may help to confirm the diagnosis ; violent efforts are made to empty the stomach with very little result ; all the signs, however, connected with this symptom depend so much on the state of purity or impurity of the prepared extract, that they can only be regarded as auxiliary aids.

"The distinguishing characters of the physiological symptoms produced by these two poisons may be thus summed up and contrasted :—

DHATOORA.	ACONITE.
1. Dilatation of the pupils, which increases until the iris is a mere thread. Limited and irregular contractions do not take place while the influence of the poison continues ; when this passes away, the pupil gradually resumes its normal form.	1. Dilatation of the pupil, with a constant tendency to limited contractions, which may be increased by exposure to light. The dilatation may give place to contraction while the influence of the poison is at its height.
2. The paralysis is that of a drunken animal, and is always associated with impairment of the mental powers.	2. Paralysis generally commences in the posterior extremities, and may be extreme without any apparent impairment of intellect.
3. Insensibility to pain, when pinched, does not occur until the animal is unconscious of everything around.	3. Insensibility to pain is an early symptom, and may be extreme while the intellect and power of locomotion are still unimpaired."

In the same Monograph Dr. Palmer has made the following valuable remarks upon *the Chemical Means of detecting Aconite and Datura* in cases of poisoning. He remarks: "It is customary in medico-legal text books to describe the physical and chemical characters of the several poisonous alkaloids in a state of crystalline purity. As, however, I have never been able to obtain, in any actual case of poisoning which has come under my notice, even a microscopical quantity of the alkaloid in this pure condition, it will only be necessary to allude to those tests which can be applied when the alkaloid has been as completely as possible separated from all extraneous matter. To effect this, I would recommend the following process to be adopted in all cases of poisoning, where there is reason to believe either aconite or any plant of the atropaceous order has been employed. The stomach, after being cut into very small pieces, should be placed in a bottle with proof spirit slightly acidulated with acetic acid; the contents of the stomach, having been previously submitted to a careful physical examination, should be mixed with rectified spirit, and placed in a separate bottle with a few drops of acetic acid; both bottles should then be set aside to macerate for twenty-four hours, after which the spirit should be filtered from each into a third bottle, and a fresh supply added, as before, which should in its turn be also filtered off after a period of twenty-four hours. Three such macerations will suffice to separate any alkaloid. The several portions of filtered spirit, having been mixed together, should now be evaporated in a basin of wedgewood-ware, the first two-thirds on a sand-bath, the last third in a water-bath. The somewhat bulky residue should, when cold, be gradually and carefully mixed with rectified spirit, until a uniform pasty mass is obtained, after which a large quantity of rectified spirit should be suddenly added; this will precipitate much of the bulky matter, and retain the alkaloids in solution; this solution should be filtered, re-evaporated to dryness in a water-bath, and the residue so obtained be again treated with rectified spirit, filtered and evaporated as before. If the resulting residue appears to contain much fatty matter, it may be boiled with a little distilled water acidulated with acetic acid; this mixture should then be similarly filtered and evaporated on a water-bath. The residue may be further purified by being treated once or twice, in a similar manner, with absolute alcohol, instead of rectified spirit. Finally, the residue should be rendered neutral or faintly alkaline by the addition of a week solution of carbonate of soda in distilled water, and shaken violently for half an hour, with three or four times its bulk of ether, in a well-corked bottle; this ether should then be poured off into a small evaporating dish, and replaced by a similar quantity of fresh ether, which, after three hours, should, in its turn, be poured off into the same dish, replaced by a third supply, and allowed to remain for twenty-four hours, after which it should also be poured into the same dish, and allowed to evaporate spontaneously. The residue thus obtained should be treated with warm distilled water, slightly acidulated with acetic acid, and filtered to separate it from any remaining fatty or resinous matter; the filtrate so obtained will contain an acetate of the alkaloid sufficiently free from impurities to be tested physiologically and chemically."*

* Baboo Kanny Lall Dey has kindly given me the following modification of Stas' process which he has found very effective in separating *Daturine*. Stomach cut into small pieces, with its contents, vomited matter or food, is treated with about 8 or 10 oz. of distilled water acidulated with about a drachm of acetic acid. The substance is next treated in a capsule, till its temperature is raised to about the boiling point; it is then allowed to cool,

"In the first place, a small quantity should be applied to the eye of a kitten; if, after a period varying from half an hour to two hours, it has caused dilatation of the pupil, it may be considered highly probable that the suspected stomach contained either aconite or one of the atropaceous order of plants; practically, it may be assumed that either belladonna, *dhatoora*, or aconite was present; for hyosciamus, the only other commonly-used genus of the atropaceous order, is seldom employed as a poison. The alkaloids atropia and daturia are now generally considered to be identical; the production of dilatation of the pupil, therefore, affords tolerably good evidence of the presence of either aconitia or the alkaloid, which is supposed to be common to belladonna and *dhatoora*. A little of the solution rubbed on the delicate skin on one side of the lower lip, will, if aconite be present, produce such a diminution of its sensibility to pain, that a very decided difference will be appreciable when the point of a needle is pressed upon the part so rubbed and the corresponding part of the opposite side. This is in most cases sufficiently characteristic of the presence of aconite, as the other alkaloid would not give rise to such numbness if rubbed on in any quantity. Further evidence may, however, be obtained by injecting the solution into the stomach of a kitten or puppy, as in the cases quoted above. The further aids I have been able to obtain from chemical tests, have not been sufficiently constant or satisfactory to enable me to place confidence in them in any case; yet, as they may afford a certain amount of collateral evidence, they should be applied whenever a sufficient amount of the poisonous matter can be obtained, in addition to that required for the physiological tests.

"In the following chemical experiments, I would premise that the

---

and is transferred to a beaker containing 6 to 8 oz. of rectified spirit. After maceration for 24 hours, the fluid portion is filtered, and the filtrate is evaporated nearly to dryness on a water-bath. The extract thus obtained is digested with absolute alcohol, to dissolve the alkaloid, and to coagulate the albuminoid, gummy, and other bulky substances. The alcohol, holding the alkaloid in solution, is again filtered and evaporated to dryness on a water-bath. This process is repeated once more, if necessary. Thus the alkaloid is freed from the major portion of the impurities, and is obtained in a concentrated form. The extractive thus obtained is dissolved in water, rendered alkaline by carbonate of soda, and is removed into a small flask with a sound cork. Ether is next added (about three or four times the bulk of the solution), and the flask is smartly shaken for about half an hour, and then allowed to rest.

The ether separates from the fluid in a distinct layer. This is drawn into a capsule with a pipette.

The ethereal portion holding the alkaloid in solution is left to spontaneous evaporation which leaves an extract on the capsule.

This extract is dissolved in water which may be acidulated with a drop of dilute muriatic acid, and heated moderately on a sand-bath. The solution now holds daturine in an almost pure state.

This, when injected into the stomach of a cat, produces all the symptoms of Datura poisoning, within a short time, when the solution is strong; but dilates the pupils only (very distinctly though) when it is weak.

When this is dropt into the eye, the pupil of that eye becomes markedly dilated.

several solutions tested were made by the above-described modification of Stas' process, from aconite root, *dhatoora* seeds, and extract of belladonna ; and also that the presence of the active principle in the solutions was in every case ascertained by the above-named physiological tests before the chemical re-agents were added."

"The chemical tests which have been examined are the iodo-hydrargyrate of potassium, sulphuric acid, bichloride of platinum, chloride of gold, picric acid, and tannic acid. The first of these, *viz.*, the iodo-hydrargyrate of potassium, is made by carefully adding a solution of bichloride of mercury to a solution of iodide of potassium, until the precipitated biniodide of mercury is no longer re-dissolved. A little of the so-formed solution is generally described as capable of precipitating *any* of the alkaloids from their solution ; if, therefore, no precipitate was caused by this re-agent in a solution prepared as above, it would not appear unreasonable to conclude that no alkaloid was present. I, however, feel able to state, from repeated observations, that a solution, prepared as above described from the seeds of a *dhatoora*, may be sufficiently strong to cause dilatation of the pupil in twenty minutes, and yet produce no precipitate when treated with the iodo-hydrargyrate of potassium ; the unsatisfactory character of this test, however, arises from the fact that it does sometimes cause a distinct yellowish-white precipitate in the *dhatoora* solution. I have frequently observed that if this re-agent be applied *immediately* after the residue of the etherial solution has been dissolved in acidulated water, a precipitate will be formed ; while, if the same solution is allowed to stand a few hours, it no longer gives a precipitate with the re-agent, though it still retains the power of dilating the pupil. The same re-agent always produces a similar yellowish-white precipitate in solutions prepared from extract of belladonna; it also always produces a more abundant cream-coloured curdy precipitate in solutions prepared from aconite. It has been said that these several precipitates may be distinguished from each other under the microscope. I have been unable to confirm this statement : the test tubes containing the several precipitates, after being allowed to stand for twenty-four hours, present different appearances to the naked eye, but when a little of the precipitate is examined under a magnifying power of about 200 diameters, it appears to be resolvable, in each case, into minute, transparent, spherical granules, remarkably uniform in size, but more or less aggregated, in proportion to the amount of precipitate present. To the naked eye, the precipitate, in the case of aconite, appears as a flocculent cream-coloured curdy mass, gently floating in the lower portions of the liquid ; in the case of *dhatoora* and belladonna, the smaller quantity of precipitate not only subsides entirely, but also becomes adherent to the bottom of the tube, and has a rather bright yellow colour when looked at from below."

"If a solution of sulphate of atropia, in the proportion of one grain to an ounce of water, is treated with the same re-agent, the precipitate formed presents precisely the same appearances to the naked eye ; but, when examined microscopically, a number of bright yellow scaphoid crystals will be seen lying in the midst of the spherical granules. If similar crystals could be obtained from small quantities of *dhatoora* seeds or belladonna, treated as above described, this would be sufficiently characteristic to distinguish them from aconite in any case which would occur in practice. I have, however, only been able to obtain them when the pure alkaloid itself was used."

"The next test which had been described as capable of distinguishing atropia or daturia from aconitia, is boiling sulphuric acid. This is said to produce a brown colour and suffocating fumes with aconite, while with atropia it gives rise to a pink colour and a sweet odour. In the minute portions which have to be operated upon in actual practice, I am afraid this test would not afford much help where any doubt previously existed ; the presence of any organic matter will give rise to a 'dark brownish colour,' and fatty matters will cause 'suffocating fumes.' More stress has, however, been laid on the usefulness of bichloride of platinum to distinguish between solutions containing aconite and atropia. A chemist and toxicologist of such experience as Professor W. Herapath appears to state in a contribution to No. 3, Vol. VII. of the *Pharmaceutical Journal,* that solutions of atropia may be distinguished from those of aconite by the chloride of platinum ; this re-agent causing a precipitate when atropia is present, but none with aconite. Again, in a little book lately published as 'The Toxicologist's Guide,' I find that the non-precipitation by chloride of platinum, when added to a solution of an alkaloid, is considered to be characteristic of aconite. If these statements could be confirmed in actual practice, this re-agent would afford a very valuable aid in the cases of poisoning under consideration. I am, however, obliged to consider this test as utterly useless and unreliable, as will be presently shown. The fact is that the alkaloids are complex bodies which are liable to undergo great and rapid changes ; it appears probable from analogy, and also from experience, that their chemical properties may vary considerably within certain limits, while their physiological action remains unaltered. This is probable from analogy with the allotropic conditions of non-metallic elements, and with the homologous forms of narcotine which have been investigated ; it is further probable from the experience related above, *viz.*, that a solution prepared by Stas' process from *dhatoora* seeds will sometimes yield a precipitate with iodo-hydrargyrate of potassium, while at other times it will not, both solutions being equally capable of causing dilatation of the pupil. If this hypothesis is accepted, until approved or disproved by the advance of our knowledge of the chemistry of the alkaloids, it will explain why such observers as Herapath and Grove should have stated in the pages of the same journal, the one that aconitia *is*, and the other that it *is not*, precipitated by chloride of platinum. I have before me records of nine applications of this re-agent to solutions of aconite and atropia prepared and tested physiologically as above described ; the results in each case are tabulated below :—

Action of Solution of Bichloride of Platinum on Solutions of Atropia and Aconitia.

	Solution of Aconitia.	Solution of Atropia.
1.	Whitish precipitate.	No change.
2.	Dark purple colour, but no precipitate.	Milky precipitate.
3.	Ditto ditto.	Ditto.
4.	No alteration of colour ; flocculent precipitate.	Cloudy-whitish.
5.	No colour ; no precipitate.	No change.
6.	No colour ; precipitate after eight hours.	No change.
7.	No change.	No change.
8.	Precipitate after standing twenty hours.	Cloudy.
9.	No colour ; no precipitate.	No change.

"The chloride of gold test has appeared to me still more variable and uncertain in its actions. The tannic acid test is perhaps more useful, though still unreliable, as it precipitates both aconitia and atropia ; the precipitate in solutions of aconitia of similar strength is, however, more abundant than that produced by this re-agent in solutions of atropia."

CANNABIS SATIVA.

Indian Hemp, Bhanga, Gunjika, Bijya,—Sans., *Bhang ;* Hind., *Ganjar ;* Beng., *Ganja ;* Dec., Tam., Malay, *Tsjeroo-cansjava ;* Mal., *Gangah ;* Tel., *Mat-kansha ;* Cey., *Kinnub ;* Arab, *Bin ;* Burmah, *Guiji-lacki-lacki ;* Malay, *Kinnabis, Defroonus ;* Youanee, Birdwood. *Churrus* and *Momeea* (the concrete resinous juice) ; *Bhang, Subjee, Sidhee* (the larger leaves and capsules without the stalks) ; *Gunjah,* the dried plant which has flowered, and from which the resin has not been removed.

The practice of smoking and eating gunja is of great antiquity and exceeding prevalence in the East. We are told in the Taleef Shereef, that the author of the *Dharà Shekoi* says that, when he was digging the foundation of a house in Bengal, he found a board, on which the effects of this drug were written ; and on which it was recorded that Mahadeb used constantly to eat of this. Baboo Kanny Lall Dey says that, in the present day, the gunja-smokers of Calcutta always take the name of

Mahadeb before passing the hookah round. The *Assassins (Haschischi)*, the homicidal followers of the "Old Man of the Mountains," whose descendant Sir Charles Napier recognised in Aga Khan of Bombay, are held to have derived their name from the use of *Hashish*, or hemp-tops.* Pala d'Aquilla says that, "in India, *Bangue* is a receit much in use, especially with slaves and souldiers, making them drunke merry, and so to forget their labour." Many passages in the Seir Mutaqherin show that this vice was of great prevalence in Mussulman India a century ago. The translator says that the tops of the hemp "being pounded with water and a mixture of some spice, afford a thick liquor of a dirty green (Bhang) with which low people procure themselves a flush in the cheeks and eyes, and a momentary flow of spirits that borders on intoxication ; but it is to fall again into a greater lowness of spirits than ever. It is fifty times cheaper than gin is in England ; and, being a narcotic, it answers the purpose of a provocative, a denomination under which anything will go down with an Indian." The author says of an indigent miscreant—"He was richly deserving to keep a shop of bang, because such an establishment may be kept with a capital of no more than two shillings, or one rupee. It is only some mats stretched under some trees, where the *bangeras* of the town, that is the vilest of mankind, assemble to drink bang, which possesses such intoxicating charms that there is no parting any more with it, when a man has once used it for a couple of weeks. But, in two years' time, it always reduces a man to a skeleton, and stupefies his mind totally."

The use and medicinal and toxnological effects of *Cannabis Indica* have been so fully described by Dr. O'Shaughnessy, in his Memoir presented to the Medical and Physical Society of Calcutta in 1839, and in his Bengal Dispensatory, as well as in Dr. Taylor's treatise on Poisons, that it is unnecessary to repeat them here, although they will have to be referred to in the Chapter on INSANITY. Not long since a French poet, M. Baudelaire, left behind him a curious record of his own experiences as a *haschish*-eater.† He divides the symptoms of hemp intoxication, according to their intensity and importance, into two classes. The first of these he speaks of under the name of the *theatre* of *seraphim*. This is merely a heightened and transformed state of ordinary consciousness in which surrounding objects are continually present to the mind ; but furnish, as it were, the texture of a strange and variegated embroidery of fancy. In this stage of its influence, *haschisch* affects only the senses and the contents of the sensuous imagination. The first indication of the

---

* Royle Birdwood.

† I have not been able to meet with "*Les Paradis Terrestres*" itself. The above description is cited from a popular Journal.

activity of the drug is a child-like gaiety, an irresistible tendency to find comical resemblances, and contrasts in everything which surrounds the patient. A sense of the exquisite oddness of the most familiar words, things, and persons. A sort of courteous benevolence accompanies this state of feeling, founded on the persuasion that every one else is in the same state of sensitiveness and nervous tension as the patient himself. To this phase of humour and urbanity there succeeds, in the first place, an interval of tranquil rationality, which, however, is merely a prelude to further excitement. The extremities now become intensely cold, the limbs lax and inanimate. The eyes are enlarged, and seem drawn in all directions by "an implacable extacy." The face loses colour, and the lips are drawn inwards by a convulsive aspiration. Deep sighs escape from the chest, "as though the old body could not bear the activity and desires of the new soul." The sensation of cold reached such a pitch in one case that the patient at last believed himself completely frozen, and felt an indescribable moral satisfaction in conceiving himself a statue cut out of a block of ice, though the time was summer, and the place a crowded theatre. In this experience occurs the strange sensation—known to many persons as the result of late hours and an over-dose of tea—of seeing everything as through the big end of a telescope. The objects seen appear to be at an immeasurable distance, and yet perfectly distinct in outline and colour. The effect reminds one of Meissonnier's pictures, or of a much-reduced photograph of an engraving. The despotism of analogies, correspondencies, associations, profound meanings, a whole universe of artificial mysticism, comes in at this stage. Then the intense sympathy with all these inner-meanings of objects leads to a quasi-pantheistic identification with them. Thus, suppose you are smoking, you watch the curls of smoke, you sympathise intensely with the idea of slow, successive, eternal evaporation. In another moment, without ceasing to be the smoker, you begin to be the matter which is evaporated, and you feel yourself crouched together in the bowl of your pipe being smoked by yourself at the other end !*

In the Chapter on INSANITY it will be shown that the practice of gunja-smoking is ascertained to be the cause of a very large proportion of the cases of acute mania admitted to the native Lunatic Asyla of Bengal.

Baboo Kanny Lall Dey showed, in 1868, that there were, then, in Calcutta, twenty-three shops for the retail sale of *gunja*, and eight others in the suburbs.

---

* For much curious information regarding the practice of gunja-smoking and bhang-drinking, in Calcutta and Lahore, *see* Baboo Kanny Lall Dey's Memoir and Dr. Honigberger's book, p. 153.

According to the same authority, the Excise Revenue of the Lower Provinces in the year 1865-66, drawn from the various preparations of Hemp, was as follows :—

Churrus	Rs.	5,492
Sidhee, Subjee, and Bhang	„	6,834
Majun	„	2,650
Gunja	„	7,65,626
	Total, Rs.	7,80,612

The gunja is never smoked without tobacco. The two are kneaded together with the thumb in the palm of the hand. So that this action is at once recognised by every gunja-smoker as signifying his habit. Baboo Kanny Lall Dey notices it as a remarkable fact that, in Bengal at least, the votaries of gunja, as a rule, always smoke the drug in company, and never singly. He says that a gunja-smoker may often be distinguished by his appearance, which is always dry and ricketty, eyes sunken, and cheeks flattened. Gunja fumes are believed to possess the property of drying up the humors of the body, and giving the persons who inhale them a faded look. A gunja-smoker can never be plump, and, if the habit of excessive indulgence be long persevered in, it brings dysentery and diarrhœa. These evils are, in a great measure, counteracted by a wholesome diet of milk and ghee and confectionary having a large share of these oily ingredients. He holds that none of these effects are perceived in churrus-smokers. He does not know whether the resin has any property of mitigating the evils produced by gunja; but he believes that the indulgence in this drug seldom or never grows into a passion (p. 10). He also remarks that a peculiarity of gunja smoking is that it makes the person, with whom the indulgence has become a habit, choleric and irascible, rough in manner and in speech.

I have always found, in practice, that, if not allowed his drug when sick, the opium-eater almost certainly dies. Whereas I have never allowed hemp to any of the multitudes of avowed gunja-smokers whom I have treated, except in cases of great suffering, where every attainable means of alleviating pain is needful. I have never been able to perceive any ill effects from sudden discontinuance of the habit of gunja-smoking.

It is probable that death may not unfrequently result from over-doses of gunja, but I have only met with a single allusion to a fatal case.

Baboo Kanny Lall Dey has made particular enquiry of some of the oldest gunja-sellers in Calcutta, who are unanimous in declaring that they have never heard of an instance of fatal poisoning by this drug. It may be said that these men have an interest in maintaining this view, but, as no native would make such an assertion regarding opium, I give their statement some weight.

In the foregoing Chapter, cases are detailed (at pages 169, 181, and 199) in which *dhatoora* was given, in what appears to have been *Bhang*, the common fluid preparation of hemp used in the Upper Provinces, and it would seem that the mixture is a very deadly one. It is not evident, however, that the criminals intended to do more than administer the stronger poison in a favourite intoxicating drink, the effects of which might possibly be expected to conceal those of the *datura*.

The crime of murdering persons while intoxicated by hemp is one which might be expected to be of frequent occurrence among a people, the lowest and most depraved of whom are continually drugging themselves with this narcotic. I have, however, only met with one recorded instance, in which a man about seventy years old, living at Mynpoorie, was convicted of having murdered one Himmut Khan by strangling him while in a state of intoxication from the effects of *bhang*.*

In 1860 Dr. James Wise, the present Civil Surgeon of Dacca, wrote to me, from Muttra, that he had lately met with several cases in which *complete loss of speech, not of voice*, followed intoxication from hemp in confirmed smokers of that drug. One of these occurred in a kidmatgar, who had been addicted to this vice for years. Having been deprived of it for some time while out in the district, he recommenced smoking it on his return to the station. One morning he was found lying insensible, with a cold, clammy skin, breathing slowly. He recovered from this after emetics and purgatives had been given, but his speech was lost. He understood what was said, and made vain attempts to speak. He continued so at least up to the time at which Dr. Wise wrote to me—five weeks subsequently—well in physical health, but dumb.

Another case was that of a syce. He went to the maidan one morning; while returning he fell down. When picked up, he was dumb, and could not walk. He had a vacant stare, had no signs of paralysis, and was otherwise in good health. After strong purgatives and blisters to the nape of the neck, he recovered his speech, and was discharged to duty.

The following case † occurred to Assistant Surgeon Cockerell. A woman was sent, by the Sub-Magistrate of Itchapore, for his opinion whether she was really dumb or merely pretending; her friends said that she went out one day to the jungle in good health, but returned unable to speak. She intimated by signs that two men had caught hold of her, forced open her mouth, and put some powder upon her tongue; then, holding a knife to her throat had robbed her. She called out at first and then lost her voice. The robbers, on being found, confessed, and were sentenced. She had no power of motion over her tongue, and could only swallow by throwing the food far back into the mouth, and pushing it with her fingers.

---

* Nizamut Adawlut Reports, N. W. P., 20th July 1852, p. 689.

† Madras Quarterly Journal of Medical Science, April 9th, 1866, p. 356.

Mr. Cockerell attributed the local paralysis to excessive fright ;—possibly the case may have been one of drugging.

Several narcotic poisons, and especially datura, interfere greatly with articulation even to the production of complete aphonia ; but, considering the lamentable frequency of the vice of gunja-smoking, it is remarkable that, in my own practice, I have only met with one case similar to those described by Dr. Wise. Possibly hemp only produces this effect in persons whose brains are prone to those neurolytic conditions which lead to aphasia.

Dr. E. C. Bensley has noticed that very moderate doses of Tincture of Cannabis are liable to cause rather serious symptoms in delicate women in India ;—fainting followed by sopor and collapse, pallor, coldness of the surface, exceedingly weak pulse (see M. Baudelaire on the Cold Stage of *haschish* intoxication, *supra*, p. 221), and dilatation of the pupils.*

Majoom, Majoon, or Majun

Is a sweatmeat prepared with hemp. Various formulas are given in the Taleef Shereef (p. 51), and by Ainslie, who gives a Madras preparation, which also contains "flowers of the thora apple" and "powder of nux-vomica." Ghee and sugar are indispensable ingredients of the Indian Majoom. The Arabs use *davamesh*, a sweetmeat prepared in a similar manner by boiling the hemp flower in butter.

John Bristow states, in his Memoirs already cited, that "In the month of September 1781, about six months after my imprisonment, the Nyar, a Bramin, and the commander of our guards, entered the prison early in the morning, and selected Sergeant Dempster, with fifteen more of the prisoners, among whom were two young boys, drummers of the 73rd Regiment ; struck off their irons, and, without deigning to utter a word, carried them away, for the purpose, as I afterwards understood, of circumcising them. They resisted a long while, and bore very cruel treatment before they submitted to this operation ; nor did they submit at last until they were stupefied with *Majum* (a strong opiate) which they had been forced to swallow."

"The treatment the first victim had undergone served in some degree to apprize us of the inutility of resistance, with horror and indignation we swallowed the narcotic potion, and those whom the dose had no effect upon were forcibly seized and pinioned by stout Coffres, whilst the operation was performed."

It is remarkable that, in a manuscript copy of a deposition made by an eunuch taken at Gwalior, on the 7th March 1853, given me by my friend Dr. Hugh Macpherson, it appears that the unfortunate being stated, "At

---

* Ind. Med. Gaz., 1st July 1866, p. 175.

first Bhang, an intoxicating drug, was administered to me, and then the genitals were mutilated."

We have here evidences of the wide-spread existence in India of an anæsthetic plan which, although very rude, was quite equal to anything known in Europe previous to the employment of Ether.

This preparation of hemp is well known at Bombay. We read, at p. 87 of Bellasis' Reports, of one Luxumee, of Ahmednugger, who, in 1833, deliberately led a child of seven into the bazar, where she bought some majoom, a stupefying drug, of which she made the child partake, and then took him outside the village, and murdered him for the sake of his ornaments.

Five or six years ago, I was called at night to visit two young Calcutta Baboos, brothers, who were rather violently affected by taking an undue quantity of majoom. Previous to my arrival they had been violent and combative, but I found them in a state of not very intense sopor, which was readily dispelled by active emesis and cold affusion.

Dr. P. Cullen, of Hoshungabad, Central Provinces, has given two cases of poisoning by "Majoon or Majum."*

It will be observed that the symptoms were rather those of *Datura* than of *Hemp* poisoning; and that Ainslie gives *Datura* as one of the constituents of majoom. So also Dr. Honigberger, writing of the practice at Lahore, says, that some people adulterate the majoon with the seeds of Datura (p. 155).

Case I.—Mussamut Allarukee, aged thirty years, was brought to hospital, between 11 and 12 o'clock on the night of the 3rd of April, in a delirious state, caused, it was stated, by eating some sweetmeats about six hours previous to admission. Her friends had given her some tamarind syrup mixed with dhye, which had produced vomiting. On admission, her symptoms were :—pupils considerably dilated, but sensible to the light ; pulse 90, rather feeble; temperature of body, rather lower than natural ; could sit up, but not stand ; talked incoherently, and kept picking at the bed-clothes ; when the light was held near her face, she would put out her hands as if to lay hold of it, but appeared unable to direct her movements properly, and, after various vain attempts, would make a sudden grab at it. A sulphate of zinc emetic was administered, but it was with the greatest difficulty she was got to swallow it, and cold was applied to the head. She was made to inhale occasionally a little carbonate of ammonia. She vomited a little in about two hours' time and then fell off to sleep. At 8 o'clock the next morning she was well.

Case II.—Mussamut Buggeah, aged fourteen years, daughter of the above, was brought to hospital with her mother, and was said to have

---

* Ind. Med. Gaz., June 1st, 1868, p. 131.

partaken of some of the same sweetmeat, but had not had anything given to her, nor had she vomited. On admission, her symptoms were of the same kind as those of her mother, but much more severe; she was nearly comatose; pupils dilated, and insensible to light; pulse 120, surface cold, and breathing slightly stertorous. She was treated nearly as her mother was, but the emetic operated freely in about half an hour, and she lay insensible all night. By 8 o'clock the next morning, the somnolence had worn off, and she laughed and talked in an incoherent manner, and tried to lay hold of things, and was in a state resembling that of her mother on admission. Her pulse was now 72, and of moderate volume. A purge was administered, which operated freely, and, by the evening, she was much quieter. She slept well during the second night, and, on the morning of the 5th April, was quite well.

OPIUM.

The Plant,—*Chosa*, Sans.; *Post*, Hind.; *Pasto*, Beng.; *Casa-casa*, Tam.; *Cassa-cassa*, Tel.; *Aboonôm* (father of sleep), Arab. The pounded Herb,—*Boosa* Vulg. The Capsules,—*Post*, Vulg. The Seeds,—*Cascus*, Vulg. Opium,—*Afeem*, Hind. and Dec.; *Afiun*, Hind. and Pers.; *Abinie*, Tum.; *Afeeoon*, Arab and Malay (BIRDWOOD.)

The vice of opium-eating is a very ancient practice in India, especially among the Rajpoots. Todd frequently alludes to it in his Rajasthan. The date of the introduction of opium into India cannot be traced. The act of *eating opium together* was the form by which rival clans became reconciled, and personal friendships were declared. "*Umul lar kana,*" to eat opium together, is the most inviolable pledge, and an agreement ratified by this ceremony is stronger than any adjuration. If a Rajpoot pays a visit, the first question is *Umul kya?* Have you had your opiate? *Umul kao* "Take your opiate." On a birth-day, when all the chiefs convene to congratulate their brother on another "knot to his years," the large cup is brought forth, a lump of opium is put therein, upon which water is poured, and by the aid of a stick, a solution is made, to which each helps his neighbour, not with a glass, but with the hollow of his hand held to his mouth. A Rajpoot is fit for nothing without his *umul*, and Colonel Todd often dismissed his men of business to refresh their intellects by a dose, for, when its effects are dissipating, they become mere logs. Opium, he adds, is more necessary to the Rajpoot than food. We are told of Nahur (tiger) Khan, that when the Mogul tyrant condemned him to enter a tiger's den unarmed, he exhibited to the king of the forest a pair of eyes which anger and opium had rendered little less inflamed than his own, upon which the animal put down his head, turned round, and stalked from him. So also when an attempt was made to foil Abhye, prince of Rahtore, the first swordsman of Rajwarra, by challenging him to smite off the head of a buffalo of unusual size, he accomplished the task after swallowing a double dose of opium. Todd considered that the abuse of opium by the Rajpoots is comparatively recent, not dating back more than three centuries. In early times they merely bruised the capsules, and steeped them for a certain time in water, drinking the infusion, which they called *tejarro*, and not unfrequently *pos*, the poppy. Purchas says,* " Opium is the juice of the heads of blacke poppie beeing cut ; a dangerous drugge, vsed much in Asia and Africa, which makes them goe as if they were halfe asleepe. They suppose I know not what coniunction and efficacy both of Mars and Venus therein ; but, being once vsed, must daily be continued on paine of death, which some escaped in Acostaa's Company by the helpe of wine."

Forbes is in accordance with all old authorities when he says that " opium taken before a battle inspires temporary courage, or rather a dreadful phrenzy."

It has long been recognised as a strong poison in Rajpootana in the form of *the Kasoomba Draught.*

Baboo Kanny Lall Dey's Table of the Excise Revenue of the Lower Provinces, in 1865-66, shows that the license fees on account of abkarry, opium, and chundoo, or purified opium, in that year, amounted to Rs. 19,24,832 out of a total excise revenue of Rs. 49,39,439.

In a police enquiry upon a question of the payment of license tax which took place in Calcutta in May 1870, it appeared that one Ramnarain Daw, an opium dealer, had no less than *fifteen* shops in various parts of the town. Immediately afterwards, another dealer brought forward the keepers of *seventeen* other shops, falsely representing that they were his servants.

Prevalent as the vice of opium-eating, with all its direst consequences, is in Bengal, especially in the Eastern and Southern districts throughout Assam and in Behar,—vast numbers of infatuated wretches having accustomed themselves to consume from 6 rutties (9 grains) to a rupee's weight (180 grains) of nearly pure opium daily,—we have no grounds for believing that the drug is frequently used, in those parts of the Lower Provinces in which opium is not grown, as a means either of suicide† or

---

* Op. Cit., page 570.

† The only case of attempted suicide by opium which occurred within my observation, during the first seven years of my practice in Bengal, was that of a respectable Hindu woman who, in a paroxysm of anger, swallowed a rupee's weight (180 grains) of good opium, hastily rubbed up in oil. (Dr. Honigberger says that, in the Punjab, persons intending suicide mix opium with oil, with a view to baffling medical aid.) I saw her early, and, as the drug had been swallowed nearly in a solid state, emetics were chiefly relied upon. She fortunately consented to take these; but although vomiting was kept up during a great part of the day, she remained for many hours in considerable danger.

During the last nine years, I do not think that I have received more than, onan average, one case of opium poisoning a year in my wards in the Calcutta Medical College Hospital.

of murder. In opium-growing districts the drug is much more often used with intention to cause death. Opium poisoning is also common in the Upper Provinces. To take a single example in his Report for October 1852, March 1853, the Sub-Assistant Surgeon of Delhi mentions that, out of nineteen cases of poisoning sent by the Police to the Dispensary during that period, fourteen were instances of poisoning by opium.*

Baboo Kanny Lall Dey finds that, between 1854 and 1870 (omitting the year 1866), *fifty-four* cases of opium poisoning have come before the Calcutta Chemical Examiner.

In 1856, Dr. H. W. Jones sent me from Sandoway the following important case of accidental poisoning by *opium applied externally to a wound.*

A Burman boy, about nine or ten years of age, was struck on the forehead with a brickbat, causing a nasty gaping wound about an inch long. His parents, about three hours after, stuffed it with opium, about a quarter tola weight, with the view probably of assuaging the pain and inflammation. On the 3rd day he was brought to me in a semi-comatose state. When spoken loudly to, he opened his eyes, but soon relapsed into his drowsy lethargic state. His eyes were covered with a thin film and seemed but little sensible to light, and he appeared in the condition of one in a sound sleep. The breathing was natural but heavy, and the body cold, and partially bedewed with a clammy sweat.

By active treatment these symptoms were subdued, but irritative fever set in, from the effects of which he very narrowly escaped. He is now perfectly recovered. This is the first case I have met with or even known of the external application of the drug producing effects analogous to its internal administration. It is true that in this case all the symptoms were not fully developed, but they would, doubtless, have been so if the poison had not been timely removed. Another point of interest in this case is the length of time (about forty hours) that elapsed before the development of the symptoms.

Belladonna, when applied externally, is capable of entering the circulation in like manner. Several rather severe cases resulting from the application of atropia to the eye have occurred within my notice. Many years since I applied a belladonna dressing to an excessively painful blistered surface on the chest of a brother officer in very weak health. Moderate, but perfectly distinct, symptoms of belladonna poisoning followed.

Several testimonies concur in declaring that opium was commonly employed among those tribes who systematically destroyed the lives of their female children. Mr. Montgomery† enumerates, among the other means

* The remaining cases were three by Dhatoora, and two by Arsenic.

† Punjab Papers on Female Infanticide.

resorted to in Goojerat, the administration of a small pill of opium to the child, which destroys life in a few hours ; more recently, it has been the practice to effect the same result by rubbing the mother's nipples with opium. Again, a native authority states that, "opium is not unfrequently made the instrument through which the Rajpoots perpetrate the horrifying deed. The manner of doing it is thus related :—The mother applies it to the nipples of her breast, and it is insensibly imbibed with the milk by the infant, and has the effect of extinguishing its life. A Rajpoot, who is in my service, told me, when I asked him for some information upon this topic, that his countrymen stick a bit of the drug to the roofs of their infants' mouths, and allow them to remain in this dangerôus position for a minute or two, during which the heat of the mouth melts the drug, and it is taken into their system, and hurries them into eternity."*

The Police Commissioner's Report, L. P., for 1851, refers to a case in which a woman administered opium forcibly to a child with whose mother she had quarrelled. She became insane during the investigation. The same officer's report for 1843 also alludes to the case of a mother who administered opium to her own infant, under the impression that its death would be on the head of her brother-in-law, with whom she had had a dispute—a description of crime very frequent among natives, to which allusion has already been made (p. 71), and which will be reverted to in the *Chapter on Wounds inflicted after Death.*

The Chemical Examiners' records, antecedent to 1856, supply us with only three cases in which the presence of opium in suspected matters, or in the stomach after death, was fully and unexceptionably demonstrated. In the first of these, a packet was sent down for analysis by the Magistrate of Shahjehanpore, with a request for information as to whether the poison (should any exist) could have been poured down the deceased child's throat after death. Dr. Mouat found the packet to contain a small quantity of a dark brown powder, in which he detected a minute amount of opium. The Chemical Examiner replied that it would be difficult, if not impossible, to pour any substance down the throat after death, without the use of a tube, or some other mechanical contrivance. The entire absence of any details connected with the history of the case, however, prevented him from giving any more positive opinion on this point.†

In the second case, the Sub-Assistant Surgeon of Ramree forwarded two bottles, containing the contents of the stomach and bowels of a Burmese, whose death was said to have been caused by taking crude opium.

---

* Coverjee Rustomjee Mody, Prize Essay on Female Infanticide, Bombay, 1849, p. 11.

† This question is not unfrequently mooted in India, although I cannot point to any second instance in which it has been made a matter of public inquiry. For self-evident reasons, it is one which can rarely present any difficulties to the medical officer, if suggested previous to his examination of the body.

Nearly all the symptoms and *post-mortem* appearances were reported as those usually met with in cases of narcotic poisoning. Mr. Siddons, on submitting the contents of the bottles to analysis, detected the presence of Meconic acid and Morphia.

In February 1853, the Civil Assistant Surgeon of Gya forwarded the stomach, with its contents, of a man who was "supposed to have met with his death from poisoning by opium." Mr. Siddons's examination of the suspected matters resulted in the detection of Meconic acid and Morphia.

Two other less demonstrative cases appear in the records. In the first of these, the stomach and its contents, of a man, the *post-mortem* examination of whose body revealed every sign of poisoning (it is not said by what) were forwarded by the Civil Assistant Surgeon of Azimgurh. Dr. Mouat found that the contents of the stomach were reddish-brown in colour, and appeared to consist of half-digested food. This matter smelt strongly of opium, which he detected in it ; but, in the entire absence of any history of the case, it was impossible to say whether that drug was the cause of death.

In February 1854, the Civil Assistant Surgeon of Chittagong forwarded the contents of the stomach of a Mussulman, who was stated to have been in good health up to the day preceding his death, when, at 8 A. M., he took food. At 2 P. M. he complained of pain in the stomach and lay down. He continued to complain until 3 on the following morning, when he became insensible, and died in two hours. His mother accused his wife and mother-in-law of poisoning him ; they stated, that he died of cholera. On examination, 37 hours after death, the body was found to be stout and in good condition, with no marks of violence ; countenance composed, pupils dilated, dark bloody fluid oozing from the nostrils. On dividing the scalp, blood flowed freely. The membranes and substance of the brain were highly congested, there were slight serous effusion beneath the arachnoid, and considerable effusion of bloody serum in the ventricles. The vessels of the base were also congested. *Heart* natural in formation, the right ventricle contained a quantity of dark coagula, the left a smaller quantity. The coats of the large vessels were unusually red. *The stomach and intestines* were distended with flatus. The stomach contained a small quantity of viscid blackish substance, possessing a peculiar odour, and mixed with a few flakes of apparently half-digested food, and shreds of woody fibre. There were no traces of inflammation in either the stomach or the intestines, the mucous coat being pale. Both large and small intestines contained abundance of healthy fæces. The *bladder* was distended with urine. The tongue and nostrils were stained of the same colour as that of the matter found in the stomach. Dr. Beatson inferred, from these appearances, that death had been caused by some narcotic poison. Dr. Macnamara ascertained that the suspected fluid contained some alkaloid, soluble in dilute [muriatic ?] and Acetic acid, and precipitated from its acid solution by Ammonia. He examined the crystals under the microscope, and believed them to be those of Morphia ; but, owing to their small quantity (the fluid received not being more than two drachms), enough of the fluid could not be obtained to be treated with the liquid tests for Morphia. From similar causes, Meconic acid could not be detected. He, therefore, although firmly believing that Morphia was present in the liquid, would hesitate to affirm the fact on oath.

I have not met with any facts which would lead to a belief that opium is used, in this country, to facilitate the commission of theft. The action of the drug is less rapid and certain than that of the datura, its taste and smell are well known to all natives, and can scarcely be disguised, and persons habituated to the practice of opium-eating are not easily hocussed.*

In 1853, one Musst. Newlee confessed before the police and the joint magistrate of Shahjehanpore that, having been beaten by her husband, she mixed a pice weight of opium in *dal*, which he partook of and went to sleep : she then struck him on the neck, face, and back, and he died immediately. The civil surgeon found that the deceased's lower incisor teeth were knocked in, and a portion of the jaw broken ; and that there were other superficial wounds apparently inflicted after death. The deposition mentions that these injuries were not sufficient to account for death. The stomach was full of food, but no trace of poison could be found. At the Sessions Court, the prisoner denied her former confession, saying that it was made through fear. The judge observed that the conclusion of the medical officer, that the wounds on deceased were not sufficient to account for death, prevented the supposition that death was caused by them alone ; but his conclusion, that they were caused after death, because there was no hæmorrhage from them, was not, he considered, obvious, because the witnesses to the sooruthal mentioned that there was much blood spilt on the charpoy. He noticed that it did not appear that the food had been analysed ; therefore, the assertion that there were no traces of poison, did not, in his opinion, lessen or invalidate the conclusion afforded by the circumstances of the case, and the prisoner's confession that opium was administered. If the deceased had not been in a state of stupor, it would be difficult to understand how he should have remained lying quiet on the charpoy while a number of painful, but not disabling, wounds

* In a case of theft by administering poison tried at Allahabad in 1854, the prisoner declared that the prosecutor, while in his company at a brothel, eat one part of a small quantity of opium of which he (the prisoner) ate two parts. According to the prisoner's account, however, the prosecutor did not become insensible until the following day, and it was shown in the evidence that the state of insensibility continued three days. The drug given was, probably, Dhatoora.—*Nizamut Adawlut Reports*, N. W. P., 23rd Jan. 1854, p. 42.

were inflicted upon him. The quantity of opium, weight of one pice, would be about ten and-a-half mashas, or, in apothecary's weight, nearly three drachms ; this would furnish to even a small portion of the dish of dal more than sufficient of the drug to destroy life. The judge considered that there remained doubt as to whether the death of the deceased was caused by the poison, and whether the crime proved should be murder by poison, if death were caused by that and the wounding together ; it seemed quite possible that injuries, otherwise of trivial effect, should have proved fatal to a man in the dangerous stupor caused by opium, and which is so often succeeded by fatal insensibility. Sentence,--Death.*

Cases in which *Children are drugged with Opium by their Nurses* are, unhappily, of by no means unfrequent occurrence in India. Two cases of the kind have happened within my own knowledge, although not in my practice. I believe that, in one of these cases, death resulted. The other occurred, shortly before the appearence of my last edition, in the practice of my late friend Mr. Bedford, of the General Hospital. The infant was completely narcotised, and was restored with great difficulty.

I am told that Dr. C. Mackinnon, when at Dum-Dum, found a piece of opium as big as the end of the little finger in his infant's mouth. Dr. De-Crespigny says that, at Rutnagherry, young children "are frequently drugged with opium to keep them quiet."

Mr. James Taylor mentions that the practice of giving opium to infants is very common among hired Mussulman nurses. It is commenced when the child is a few days old, and is generally continued until it is four years of age. The drug is administered under the impression that it defends the child from cold ; but, more often, with a view of quieting it when troublesome ; and the practice is frequently carried by native nurses into European families. Deaths from an overdose are, he believes, of frequent occurrence. Within eight months, he had seen two instances of infants, under the age of ten months, who were thus accidentally killed by it, and he knew of another case, in a European family, where the parents attributed the loss of a child to it.†

A few years since, one of the medical officers at Allahabad complained of "certain savage customs" prevalent in that city, whereby, at or about the second month of its infantile life, every child is made to take opium, or some other narcotic, or wine, to lull it to sleep. "This unnatural and cruel practice," he says, "has gained so firm a footing, in

---

* Nizamut Adawlut Reports, N. W. P., 23rd June 1853, p. 787. It seems likely that the opinion of the Medical Officer, that the wounds were inflicted after death, was based upon physiological observation of their condition ; and it appears probable that wounds, especially superficial wounds, inflicted upon a person labouring under that extreme condition of cerebral and pulmonary congestion which precedes death from poisoning by a narcotic, would not present the usual appearances of wounds inflicted during life.

† Op. Citat, p. 263.

that city in particular, that even the rich mothers, who can easily afford maid-servants for their children, nay, who have them already, indulge in it frequently. If for a time they abstain, it is with no very good results. The ample opportunity, offered to the mother by this inhuman course, and the very few number of times she is required to suckle her child, induce her soon to overlook the evil and dangerous consequences, and to resume the task of destruction."*

Mussamut Bala, of the city of Bareilly, was tried, in 1854, for the wilful murder of the infant (38 days old) of a native, by administering opium. The woman had been engaged to suckle the child, and the father deposed that, four or five days previous to its death, she refused to continue in service. The Sub-Assistant Surgeon stated that he found the child dying with the symptoms of opium poisoning, and affirmed that the prisoner made confession in his presence of having given to the infant a piece of opium of the size of a pea. The judge remarked that it is a well-known fact that it is not the custom of the people of that country to administer opium (though it is frequently in use by them as a sedative medicine to children) to infants under forty days old. The father, however, appears, at first, to have confirmed the woman's statement that the infant had been in the habit of taking a daily dose of opium, and that she had unwillingly increased the dose beyond the ordinary or daily portion. He added that he regarded the result as accidental, and that he wished to lay no charge against the nurse. He afterwards, however, asserted to the contrary. The Superior Court acquitted the prisoner.†

In these cases, the opium, reduced to a paste, is usually smeared upon the child's tongue, where its characteristic brown appearance should be sought for.

Baboo Kanny Lall Dey has obliged me with the following note of a modification of Stas' process, which he is in the habit of using in the detection of opium.

Stomach, cut into small pieces, with its contents, vomited matter, or food, is heated with about 8 or 10 ounces of distilled water acidulated with a drachm of acetic acid.

The substance is next treated in a capsule till its temperature is raised to about the boiling point ; is then allowed to cool and is transferred to a beaker (wide-mouthed bottle) containing 6 or 8 ounces of rectified spirit. After maceration for 24 hours the fluid portion is filtered, and the filtrate evaporated nearly to dryness on a water-bath. The extract thus obtained is digested with absolute alcohol, to dissolve the alkaloid and to coagulate

* As cited in Chambers's Papers for the People, Vol. II., p. 16.—*The Sanitary Movement.*

† Nizamut Adawlut Reports, N. W. P., 30th March 1854, p. 331. See also a case in which a wretched woman of Muttra was believed to have endeavoured to destroy her infant by opium, and then exposed it in a dry well.
Ibid, 23rd Dec. 1852, p. 1441.

the albuminoid gummy and other bulky substances ; the alcohol, holding the alkaloid, is again filtered and evaporated nearly to dryness on a water bath. This process is repeated once more if the major portion of the impurity still remains. Thus the alkaloid is freed and is obtained in a concentrated form.

The extractive thus obtained is dissolved in water, is rendered alkaline by carbonate of soda, and is removed into a small flask with a sound cork. Ether is next added, about 3 or 4 times the bulk of the solution, and the flask is smartly shaken for about half au hour, and then allowed to rest. The ether separates from the fluid in a distinct layer, this being drawn into a capsule by a pipette. The ethereal portion, holding the alkaloid in solution, is left to spontaneous evaporation which leaves behind an extract.

The ethereal extract thus obtained is treated with water and moderately heated on a sand-bath. While hot, two or three drops of dilute hydrochloric acid is added to it. If opium is present, it will be indicated by the development of a rich purple colour, the intensity of which varies according to the amount of the poison present in the original fluid operated upon ; the absence of such colouration indicates that opium is not present.

This purple colour is altogether a different one from the blue tinge produced by the action of mineral acids upon narceine as described by Dr. Pereira. It seems that the colour, which I have observed, is owing to the action of dilute hydrochloric and upon some other constituent of opium which is soluble in ether. It disappears when the fluid is rendered alkaline, and returns if acidified again. This test will answer just as satisfactorily with dilute sulphuric acid, but dilute nitric acid does not suit the purpose. This method of detecting opium can be successfully employed in all Indian varieties, *viz.*, Bengal, Patna, Malwas, &c. It is not so, however, with Turkey opium ; no such colour is produced when the latter is treated in this manner. This is the more to be regretted, as the test is a very delicate one, enabling us to detect the presence of such a minute quantity as one-fiftieth of a grain of crude opium.

QUESTION OF THE RECIPROCALLY ANTIDOTAL ACTION OF OPIUM—DATURA, BELLADONNA.

In the Edinburgh Medical Journal, June 1860, Dr. Thomas Anderson, now Curator of the Calcutta Botanical Garden, published a Memoir on *Opium as a remedy in Poisoning by Datura*, which has subsequently led to some very interesting enquiry.

Dr. Anderson remarks that Mr. Benjamin Bell, in an article (read before the Medico-Chirurgical Society of Edinburgh) on "The Therapeutic Relations of Opium and Belladonna to each other," published in No. xxxvii. of the *Edinburgh Medical Journal*, for July 1858, directs attention to the doctrine propounded by him some years ago, that opium and belladonna exert an opposite influence on the human system, and that thus one may be used to counteract the other, even though administered in a poisonous dose. In the summary given at the commencement of his article, of the origin of this opinion, he mentions some apparently (and, to Dr. A.'s mind,) perfectly conclusive experiments made by him in 1853 (*Ranking's Half-yearly Abstract*, vol. xxii., p. 303), on the action of belladonna in poisoning by opium. He further gives very interesting details of two cases of partial poisoning by atropia, which he treated successfully by the injection of morphia. While conducting his experiments in 1853, he became convinced that the converse doctrine must be true, *viz.*, that opium would counteract the action of belladonna, and of all the solanaceæ with like properties, such as the species of datura and hyoscyamus, and perhaps tobacco.

In Britain, poisoning by belladonna, or by henbane, is so exceedingly rare an accident, that it was vain for him ever to expect to meet with a case of either. However, in 1854, he proceeded to India, where poisoning by datura is of every-day occurrence; and he determined to test his theory by administering opium to the first suitable case he should have an opportunity of treating.

He publishes the following case as illustrating his theory of the impossibility of these two classes of poisons exerting their action simultaneously on the brain, and is, moreover, the converse of his former experiments, and at the same time supplementary to Mr. Bell's.

The 43rd Bengal Native Infantry, of which he was then the medical officer, while on its passage from the Punjab to Calcutta by boats, on the River Ganges, halted for four or five days at Futtehghur, in the beginning of December 1855. The sepoys were of course allowed to go on shore, and many of them visited the large bazar in Furrackabad. One of the sepoys, a man well known to him, was found by his comrades lying by the roadside, in a state of high delirium, and was brought to the hospital boat. He had been seen partaking freely of sweetmeats (the Hindoo eats them by pounds weight at a time) in the bazar, some hours before he was found; and the men at once ascribed his condition to poison administered in the sweetmeats. The many varieties of native sweetmeats poisoned with datura and bhang, one of the preparations of Indian hemp, are well known in all large Indian towns, and are used to cause death or stupefaction, so complete, as to allow of robbery or violence being committed; and a sepoy, when in undress, usually displays valuable ornaments sufficient to tempt a thief or thug. Even without this knowledge, the symptoms were so marked, that he had no difficulty in forming his opinion of the cause of the patient's condition. He saw him immediately after he was brought to hospital, and found him in the following state: He was reclining on his back in bed, in a wakeful muttering delirium, unbroken by an interval of even transitory consciousness. His face was much flushed ; the eyes were reddened and wandering, and the pupils were brilliant, widely dilated, and quite insensible to light. The pulse was much accelerated and small. He continually twitched his extremities, but especially his hands, and every now and then pinched and tugged at the bedding. Though utterly unconscious to real external objects, the brain was evidently active, with continual visions before the eyes, as his mutterings and frequent clutchings referred to imaginary objects. He was not in the least degree violent, and required no restraint, but merely an attendant to keep him covered during his restless tossings about.

He swallowed any liquid put into his mouth, but exactly as patients in delirium tremens do, in one convulsive mouthful.

In an hour after his arrival at the hospital, Dr. Anderson began the administration of opiates, and prescribed one grain of the muriate of morphia in solution, to be given every hour, beginning the first dose at 2 P.M. He watched the effect most closely, taking the state of the pupil as his principal guide.

Eight doses were given before he could observe any result. After the eighth dose, about 11 P. M., he noticed that his attention could be fixed for a moment, and that the muttering could be arrested by loudly talking to and shaking him ; that the hands were less tremulous.

Still, no impression had been made on the widely-dilated pupils, and he was evidently as wakeful as ever. Dr. A., therefore, before retiring for the night, directed the continuance of the morphia until the morning, with orders to discontinue it so soon as sleep threatened to come on. He did not see him again until six in the morning, when he found all his delirium gone, the tremulousness much relieved, the pupils almost reduced to their natural state, and the patient surrounded by his delighted comrades, who were listening with wonder to the native doctor relating to them how "dhatoora" poisoning had been cured by "apheem" (opium).

Though he was able to talk, and was nearly well, Dr. A. considered it advisable to persevere with the treatment until sleep had been obtained. This did not supervene until three doses more had been given.

After several hours' sleep, he awoke perfectly well ; and after two days' more detention in hospital, he was dismissed "fit for duty ;" and while Dr. A. remained with the regiment, was never again in hospital. In all, 15 grains of the muriate of morphia had been administered in 18 hours ; and with reference to the largeness of the amount, he took care to inquire concerning the habits of this sepoy, and found that he used opium in no form whatever.

In this case, as well as in the experiments published in his former paper on this subject, the amount of the narcotic used as the antidote, whether belladonna or opium, to restore the normal condition of the brain, would, by itself, have been a poisonous dose. This tolerance of the one poison, produced by the presence of the other poison in the system seems to him to be a strong additional argument in favour of his theory.

It also induces him to go further, and to believe that all narcotic poisons with distinctly opposite actions, and destroying life by their effects on the nervous centres, will, when present in the body together, counteract each other, until eliminated from the system by the excretions.

For example, the distinct coma-producing narcotics, such as opium, will, he believes, in all cases be counteracted by the poisonous solanaceæ; and, as a remedy to the action of strychnine, he would hope for success from the use of conia, or preparations of hemlock itself; and of course, in all these cases the opposite would hold true.

Unfortunately, no correct conclusion can be drawn from experiments made on the lower animals, as they are variously affected by narcotics. To dogs and cats he has given morphia in enormous doses without producing almost any effect; and to them five and six grains of atropia prove quite harmless. Rabbits will feed for months on belladonna leaves, and have their pupils dilated all the time, but otherwise they are not affected. Blackbirds eat belladonna berries in large quantities and do not die.

It is, therefore, only to experiments on man that any value can be attached.

Dr. Anderson urges his brethren never to give up hope of the most desperate case of opium-poisoning; but after the failure of the usual means, such as emetics, the stomach-pump, electricity, etc., to endeavour to produce, as rapidly as possible, the first symptoms of the action of belladonna on the system, by the administration of atropia, either internally, or by injection under the skin, as indicated by Mr. Bell. His firm conviction was that, in all such desperate cases (desperate as regards the old treatment), this plan, when boldly adopted, would be invariably successful.

He had just heard that Dr Carnegie, medical missionary in China, in a letter lately received from him, mentions a case of poisoning by opium which he had just cured by giving belladonna.

Since Dr. Anderson's views were first promulgated, the question has received attention from many practical investigators in India and at home. The results obtained are very contradictory. In favour of the view we have cases by (1) Dr. Ranking of Madras, who gave Sydenham's laudanum, with apparently beneficial effects, to a lady poisoned by a decoction of dried belladonna leaves recently brought from France.* (2) Several cases of opium poisoning, in which the subcutaneous injection of atropia in quantities of from $\frac{1}{48}$th to $\frac{1}{4}$th of a grain was had recourse to with apparent benefit.† (3) In 1869, my friend Dr. Scriven, Principal of the Lahore Medical

* Mad. Quar. Jour. of Med. Science, Vol. X., 1866, p. 401.

† British Medical Journal, Jan. 8th, 1870, p. 34, from American Half-yearly Compendium of Med. Science.

College, employed a solution of atropia dropped into the mouth and eye, and by enema in a boy poisoned by laudanum, who recovered.* Again, in 1870, Mr. Scriven employed quarter grain enemata of atropia twice in the case of a man who had swallowed about eight grains of opium. This appeared to assist in restoring sensibility.† (4) A case of poisoning by belladonna, in which laudanum, in what must otherwise have been poisonous doses, was administered to two young children by Dr. Bernard Kavenagh ; the children recovered.‡ (5) Entering the Medical College Hospital, on the 20th of November 1868, I found two young native women, who had been drinking all night long with their friends, in a marked state of datura poisoning. One of them was extremely excited, but her case was not severe. In the other there were alternations of delirium and insensibility. I saw her three hours after admission. She was almost insensible, but tossed about uneasily; the abdomen was swollen, the pupils were widely dilated, the pulse had been for some time very weak, and she was upon the verge of collapse. I gave 25 minims of laudanum ; and, in less than an hour, all anxiety regarding her recovery was removed from my mind, as she rallied completely, although the pupils continued to be dilated, and moderate symptoms of datura poisoning remained. She also took a 20-minim dose at night. The other patient was similarly treated with no marked result. They were discharged well in three days.

Against these may be placed the following cases and arguments. At 10 o'clock on the night of the 13th December 1868, James Browne, a patient in the Calcutta Medical College Hospital, while convalescent from fractured ribs, poisoned himself with what appears to have been solid opium obtained from outside. Six hours afterwards, all ordinary treatment having been used in vain, I saw him at 4 A. M. He had been completely comatose for four hours. The pupils were utterly insensible to light, small, but not extremely contracted. Face much congested, pulse of fair volume, but very irregular. I injected *three* minims of a solution of atropia (gr. iv to the fluid ounce), hypodermically, at the epigastrium. 4-15.—Condition unchanged. *Three* minims more were injected. 4-40.—Pulse more irregular, patient otherwise the same, *three minims* of the solution were dropped into the mouth. 4-45.—Pulse somewhat improved, *pupils have begun sensibly to dilate*, condition otherwise the same. 4-53.—Respirations 23, unequal, somewhat stertorous, pulse 110, unequal. 5-5.—The size of the pupils is at least doubled since the atropia began to act. They are dilated beyond the medium, and are quite insensible

---

* Ind. Med. Gaz., Sept. 1, 1869, p. 182, Dr. Scriven's paper containing reference to other cases, not cited above.

† *Ibid*, March 1, 1870, p. 54.

‡ Med. Press and Circular, and Ind. Med. Gaz., Nov. 1, 1869, p. 237.

to light. 5-10.—Pupils widely dilated, condition otherwise the same. 5-20.—Pupils widely dilated. Some failure of pulse. 5-40.—Pulse sinking considerably. Enema of two measures of brandy in an equal quantity of hot water. 5-45.—Coma and collapse increasing. The dilatation of the pupils is still increasing, and is now quite equal to the dilatation recently observed in two severe cases of datura poisoning. Repeat the enema, stronger. 6-5.—Collapse advancing. Repeat the enema. 6-12.—Expired. The size of the pupils did not alter. I allowed the body to remain in the ward that my colleagues might observe the great dilatation of the pupils at their morning visit.

This case distinctly proves that, in opium-poisoning, the presence of atropia in the system may altogether change the condition of the pupil, without in any way alleviating the other symptoms of opium-poisoning.

The converse of this case occurred in the practice of Dr. S. W. Grose of Philadelphia ;* the result of which was that, the patient having been poisoned by three grains of atropia, "a grain and-a-half of morphia, used hypodermically during the space of half an hour, merely intensified the poisonous effects of the atropia, and still further jeoparded life." "A scarcely perceptible contraction of the pupil" after the injection of the second half grain of morphia ; but as the patient became worse, "the pupils regained their natural size."

I regard these two cases as being strongly confirmatory of Dr. Harley's conclusions.

1. "That" [upon collation of the cases] "the evidence of antagonism between opium and belladonna in any given case is inconclusive." [I would reserve the point of action on the iris.—N. C].†

2. "Belladonna has no influence whatever in accelerating the recovery from the poisonous effects of opium.

3. "That somnolency, stupor, narcotism, and coma, the essential effects of the action of opium, are both intensified and prolonged by the concurrent action of belladonna.

4. "That belladonna is powerless to obviate the chief danger in opium-poisoning,—*viz.*, the depression of the respiratory function."‡

---

* American Journal of Medical Science, October 1869, p. 401.

† Dr. Taylor says that, "in the later stage of opium-poisoning, and when progressing to a fatal termination, the pupils may be found dilated."

I do not think that this applies to my case, in which the action of atropia was clearly developed in forty-five minutes. In Scriven's case a little of the solution of atropia was dropped into the left eye, the right eye being reserved for watching the constitutional effect of the alkaloid, the pupils being contracted. The left pupil dilated rapidly, and fully under the influence of the atropia, the pupil of the right began to dilate in an hour. After recovery, the pupils of Mr. Scriven's patient remained dilated as those of Baker did after death. As the former recovered, the right pupil was the first to recover its normal size.

‡ The old vegetable Neurotics, p. 309.

It will be shown, in the chapter on INFANTICIDE, that TOBACCO has been systematically used in the Gwalior and Agra Districts, &c., as a means of destroying young infants. The first of the following cases is even of a darker character. The second is merely a comparatively recent instance of this ancient atrocity. Mussamut Jumna was tried at Agra for the wilful murder of her new-born male infant by administering to it pounded Tobacco. The chowkeedar of the village, in which the woman had resided for many years, stated that she was a widow. A report having arisen that she had given birth to an illegitimate child, he went and taxed her with the fact, which she denied. Upon his repeating his inquiries, she, after some demur, produced the child's body in a basket. Blood was flowing from the nose. No *dhye* (as is usual) assisted at the birth, nor was the fact of her pregnancy even reported by her or her mother, but he subsequently admitted that, some time previously, the woman went with him to the thannah, and the prisoner promised that, if a child was born, it should be properly cared for ! Two witnesses testified to her having confessed that she gave the child tobacco. She confessed this to the police, and before the magistrate, but maintained on trial that the child died from natural causes very shortly after birth. She was found guilty and sentenced to imprisonment for life in transportation.*

In the same year the suspicions of the police at Agra were excited by the fact that the pregnancy of the wife of one Ghasoonder, a Rajpoot thakoor, had not been registered, as required by rules shortly before promulgated by the magistrate with a view to check the prevalent crime of infanticide. Consequently, when the chowkeedar reported the birth and immediate death of the child (a female), an immediate investigation took place, and the grandmother of the child admitted before several witnesses, who attested her written confession, that she had killed the child by giving it tobacco. The prisoner was sentenced to imprisonment for life.†

Tobacco injurious as an emetic in a case of poisoning by opium.—*Bombay Dispensary Reports*, Vol. II., p. 4.

Dr. Burton Brown suggests that search for the leaf should be made in the mouth and throat.

STRYCHNOS NUX-VOMICA.

Veeshamoostie, Kulaka, Sans. ; *Koochila*, Hind., Beng. ; *Kajra, By. Kariram*, Mat. ; *Yettie-marum*, Tam. ; *Moostighenza, Musadi*, Tel. ; *Koodakad-doorutta*, Cey. ; *Kha-boung*, Pegu ; *Iza-rakee*, Pers. ; *Falooz mahee, Khanek-ul-Kelb*, Arab. (BIRDWOOD.)

---

* Nizamut Adawlut Reports, N. W. P., 6th Nov. 1852, p. 1311.

† *Ibid*, 9th Dec. 1852, p. 1463.

The nux-vomica (Kusta, Kupilu) is mentioned in the Shastras as prepared by being steeped for three days in congee water, and then mixed with mustard oil and other medicines.*

The general medico-legal circumstances attendant upon poisoning with Nux-Vomica are too well known to demand repetition. The *Strychnos Nux-Vomica* is "a native of Coromandel, Ceylon, and the Bengal jungles;" it was noticed in the woods of the Carnatic by Fryrer about the year 1671. According to Dr. de Crespigny Nux-Vomica seeds are abundant at Rutnagherry (Concan) and a basketful may be obtained for a few pice.

Nux-Vomica Eating.

Mr. Baker says that the natives of Hindoostan often take the Kuchila nut morning and evening, continuously for many months, beginning with the eighth of a grain, and gradually increasing the dose to an entire nut, or about 20 grains [!]. If taken immediately before or after meals, no unpleasant effect is produced; but, if this precaution be neglected, spasms are apt to ensue.†

Mr. A. Gibson mentions having heard that some of the more debauched among the Rajpoots of the province of Guzerat use the *Nux-Vomica* as a stimulus, and this to the extent of two seeds daily, but the practice is not general. *Sketch of the Province of Guzerat Transactions of the Medical and Physical Society of Bombay, No.* 1, *p.* 35.

In his report on Rutnagherry Dr. de Crespigny says that opium and bang are not in much requisition there, but there are consumers of Nux-Vomica and Thorn apple.‡

With hakeems, nux-vomica is given, in the present day, to supplant the habit of eating opium ; this practice is spoken of in the Taleef Shereef, p. 49.

Professor T. W. Wilson, late of Calcutta, mentioned to me a very remarkable and important case of one of his own native doctors who, being a great sufferer from chronic rheumatism, was in the habit of grating the *Nux-Vomica* into water in sufficient quantity to produce rigidity of the body. When his body became rigid, he remained quite sensible, and the pain of the rheumatism ceased :—a fact well deserving of attention, as showing, I believe for the first time, that nearly the full action of the drug may be produced upon the nervous system, without necessarily endangering life.

---

* Wise.

† Transactions of the Medical and Physical Society of Calcutta.

‡ Bombay Med. and Phys. Trans., No. IV for 1857-8, p. 77.

The late Mr. Piddington, Coroner of Calcutta, gave me the following paper :—

" *Strychnia an Accumulative Poison.*

" On the 3rd November 1849, a stout, young, and healthy-looking Up-country Brijbassy, a prisoner in the House of Correction, named Rutten Sing, died suddenly " of fits." He had been sent to jail only four days before his death, and he told the Superintendent, on entering, that he could not do without some sweetmeats daily made by himself; which of course could not be allowed in a jail. Due enquiry was held, and Dr. Macpherson made a careful *post-mortem* examination of the body, but could detect no assignable cause of death, and the death remained a mysterious one to us all for a length of time. I happened however to mention the case to my friend Baboo Rajendra Lall Mitter, then Librarian of the Asiatic Society, who was formerly a distinguished student of the Medical College, and he informed me that a similar case of a sudden attack of fits (resembling epilepsy) had also occurred in a stout, healthy Up-country man in the employment of their family, and that it was with great difficulty and much care that the man recovered. He added that he had learned, upon close enquiry, that this man and many of his countrymen were in the habit of taking daily a small dose of the powder of Nux-Vomica to increase their health and strength for their wrestling exercises, and that he thought it not improbable that the Strychnia of the Nux-Vomica had acted as an accumulative poison, and produced the fits. In the jail case, quoted above, the spasms may probably have been accelerated, as the morbid symptoms of opium-eaters are brought on, by the sudden privation of the drug.

" The above is a correct record of the case of our Durwan.

(Sd.) " R. MITTER."

Moulvie Tumeez Khan Bahadur tells me that it is quite common in Bengal, not only among Hindus, but also among Mahomedans, to use Nux-Vomica as an aphrodisiac. A seed is placed for two or three days in the earth under a pot of water. The bark thus becomes easily separable; then, with a pair of scissors, the seed is cut into very fine chips, not thicker than the nail. One of these is taken with *pan* once and sometimes even twice daily.

Mr. Piddington gave me the above case expressly for the purpose of showing that Strychnia is not a cumulative poison. Dr. Taylor appears not to subscribe to this view (Poisons, p. 777). Standing alone, the above case may not be fully demonstrative, but it remarkably supports the observation made by Dr. John H. Power in the case of a young woman who took Strychnia for a nervous affection of the extensor muscles of the fore-arms. The flexor muscles were in a state of contraction, the hand was clenched. She was ordered the sixteenth of a grain of Strychnia in pill every six hours. She stated that she took about 30 pills. One morning she said that she had a confused feeling in her head and indistinct vision, and that she could not walk. She then had a general jerking of the muscular system, the lumbar mass acted violently, resembling opisthotonos. There was corrugation of the forehead, with peering of the eyes, flushing of the face, and dilation of the pupils.

One of Dr. Power's inferences from this case is that "Strychnia may become cumulative in the system."*

Dr. Fleming believed that the drug was seldom, if ever, employed in medicine by the Hindus, on account of its dangerous properties. He adds, however, that it is sometimes used for a very pernicious purpose by the distillers, who add a quantity of it in the process of distilling *arrack*, to render the spirit more intoxicating.

Commonly as the Nux-Vomica finds a place among the bazar drugs of Bengal, it would appear that it is by no means very frequently employed, in this country, as a means of destroying life. The Chemical Examiners' Records, previous to 1856, only contain two cases in which there was any satisfactory reason for concluding that death had resulted from the administration of this drug.†

One of these cases is perfectly clear and convincing.‡

In 1853, the Magistrate of Goruckpore forwarded the contents of the stomach of one Mungoo, Mehter, together with a letter from Dr. Aitchison, the Civil Surgeon, to the following effect: On the 1st June, at 9 A.M., the man drank off a bottle of common bazar spirit, which he had purchased the night before in the Goruckpore bazar. Immediately after drinking the liquid, he remarked to a bystander, "Something is wrong; this shurab is intensely bitter." Soon afterwards, spasms came on, and frightful convulsions; there was perfect opisthotonos of the whole body. *Intellect was entire throughout*. On the abatement of the tetanic convulsions, coma succeeded, and he died in three-quarters of an hour. The liquor, which caused death, cost only three pice, whence Dr. Aitchison inferred that it could not have been very strong or intoxicating. Dr. Mouat found that the bottle contained about six ounces of a Brownish turbid fluid, in which, with very great difficulty, he succeeded in detecting a trace of

---

* Dublin Med. Press., Jan. 7, 1859.

† In the first of these cases "a bottle containing a small quantity of the contents of a stomach" was sent from Deyrah, for Chemical Examination in 1853, without any information regarding the particulars of the case. Dr. Mouat found that it gave evidence of the presence of a powerful vegetable bitter, which presented nearly the characters of *Strychnine*, but the quantity was so extremely minute as to prevent him from ascertaining this with such undoubted certainty as is absolutely necessary in a medico-legal case.

‡ An important case of *Poisoning by twelve grains of Nux-Vomica* taken by a native "to cure an ulcer on the back," recovered from, will be found in the Transactions of the Bombay Medical and Physical Society, for 1853-54, p. 321.

Strychnia;—if, as he writes, the test for that substance is to be relied upon. After separating the organic matter present, he evaporated half the fluid to dryness, and endeavoured to obtain, from this residue, crystal of Strychnia. In this he failed, as the amount present must have been extremely minute. He then treated a very small portion of this residue with strong Sulphuric Acid, and added to it a grain, in powder, of the Ferrocyanide of Potassium (Red Prussiate of Potash). Upon mixing these well together, in a watch glass, a scarcely perceptible change of colour to violet was produced. He then repeated the experiment with another portion, substituting the Bichromate for the Red Prussiate of Potash. The characteristic violet colour was immediately produced; and, as it is now regarded by eminent chemists in Europe as the most delicate and certain test of the presence of Strychnia, he was led to believe that the individual had been poisoned. Dr. Mouat further recommended an enquiry as to whether the practice of distilling Alcohol with the powdered bark of the Strychnos or with Nux-Vomica itself, is known to be practised by natives in the bazar of Goruckpore. He thought it difficult to suppose that it would be resorted to for other than criminal purposes, as its intense bitterness would cause its immediate detection by any one not in a state of intoxication. We have seen, however, that Dr. Fleming long ago ascribed this practice of drugging *arrack* to a design of somewhat less criminal character.*

Baboo Kanny Lall Dey tells me, of an old patient of mine with hemiplegia, that he has been using daily two half nut doses of Nux-Vomica, and is gradually improving in strength. Some time ago, his wife, by mistake, gave him two nuts at once, which produced a violent tetanic attack, without loss of consciousness. A strong infusion of tamarind pulp was administered, as a supposed antidote,† and the cold douche was employed. The patient began to recover after four hours from the commencement of the symptoms; occasional starting and slight headache continued till next morning, when they were removed by a cold bath.

STRYCHNIA.

A remarkable case in which a European poisoned himself in Calcutta with Battle's Fly Poison (one part Strychnia and two parts Starch) occurred

* More than one suspicious case of death, occurring shortly after drinking bitter spirit, will be found in the Nizamut Reports, as the following:—Certain persons invited one Ramdoolub, with whom they had a dispute, to their house, and welcomed him with wine (spirit?) of which they all partook. The wine first brought being speedily despatched, one of them remarked that he had a bottle of better wine; and sending for it, poured a small quantity of it into a vessel, and presented it to Ramdoolub who, on drinking it, observed that it was very bitter, and shortly after, exclaiming that he felt his body on fire, and that he had been poisoned, became senseless, and expired in a few hours. It was considered that the deceased died by excessive drinking.

† Infusion of tamarind is generally employed as an antidote in over-doses of gunjah or bhang.—*Baboo K. L. Dey.*

in November 1867. Stas' process (modified) did not prove the presence of Strychnia in the stomach, but one-eighth of the watery solution which was obtained was placed in the mouth of a well-developed lizard ; the reptile died, with four distinct convulsions, within ten minutes.

Baboo Kanny Lall Dey remarks that, as lizards are muscular reptiles easily obtainable everywhere in India, they are best suited for experiments in detecting, physiologically, minute quantities of Strychnia.

I have seen two cases of poisoning by the alkaloid of Nux-Vomica in natives treated in the Medical College Hospital. One of these occurred in Dr. Chuckerbutty's wards early in May 1870. The man, who had access to Europe drugs, took half a grain, believing it to be morphia. He recovered.

The other case came under my own care, and I have reported it fully in the Indian Annals of Medical Science for 1866, as *an illustration of the antidotal power of Tobacco in Strychnia poisoning*. The patient, a Mahomedan girl about 11 years of age, placed about three grains of Strychnia in her mouth. She endeavoured to spit it out, but must have swallowed a considerable quantity, as strong symptoms set in within about half an hour. Fortunately she had taken a full meal of rice shortly before.

The danger was so imminent, that I considered it my duty to administer altogether those agents which, having been recommended in strychnine poisoning, came most readily to hand. They were not incompatible with each other ; and, although it may be questioned how far each aided in or retarded the recovery, I think that the *modus operandi* of two—the Lard and the Tobacco—was distinctly apparent.

As much animal charcoal as could be mixed with melted lard without destroying the fluidity of the latter was given in tablespoonfuls. The quantity of this filthy mixture swallowed was probably not less than a pound. It appears, on Dr. Taylor's authority, that the efficacy of *Animal Charcoal* in strychnia poisoning is uncertain. In the present case, it is extremely questionable whether it had any good effect whatever. *Lard* was first recommended by Dr. W. N. Pindell, who, in the "American Journal of Medical Science" for October, 1855, reported that, in dogs, this fat, swallowed in large quantities, acts as an antidote to strychnia. I have also a reference to the successful use of *Oil* under similar circumstances, but I cannot now find the *first number of the California Medical Journal* in which the observation appeared.

In 1856, doubt was thrown upon the antidotal power of lard. Dr. William H. Hammond wrote as follows to the editor of the "American Journal of Medical Science" (No. 65, page 273) :—"I must tell you that "I have tried Dr. Pindell's antidote to strychnia—lard. I gave two "grains of the poison to one dog, without the antidote, and two to an-"other, with the addition of a pint and-a-half of melted lard. The best "of the joke is that *the latter* died in four hours, and the former, miser-"able worthless cur, who doubtless was too mean to die, is still running "about in the finest possible state of health. So much for lard. We are "of opinion here that strychnia is quite harmless, unless lard is indulged "in."

The argument here is too self-evidently weak to need criticism. Melted lard appears well calculated, when taken early, to counteract absorption. I do not believe that it was of any use in my case,—it was given late, and it and the animal charcoal, massing together in the stomach, operated as a bulky mechanical irritant to which the pylorus refused exit for a long time. Causing such embarrassment, it recalled to one's recollection Plutarch's allusion to the action of bullock's blood as a poison, and the assertion that this was the agent which destroyed Themistocles. It is very possible that distension of the stomach by a firm coagulum, to such a degree as to prevent vomiting, might cause death ; and a much larger quantity of melted lard than we gave to this girl might have acted similarly.

I feel confident that, in this case, the poison took full possession of the nervous system, the contents of the stomach never having been thoroughly evacuated as long as tetanic symptoms lasted, and that recovery was wholly due to the antidotal action of Tobacco. Nothing short of death by trachealismus in tetanic eclampsia could well have been more fearful than the spasms which this poor little creature endured. I employed this antidote upon the suggestion afforded by the case related by Dr. O'Reilly, U. S.,* which is that of a man who, having swallowed six grains of strychnia, took upwards of an ounce infusion of tobacco leaves, given in small doses at intervals, and recovered. He had previously taken an emetic which had caused copious vomiting. Much less efficacy must be attributed to the emetics in my case.

I believe that the very large quantity of infusion of tobacco swallowed by this child, *viz.*, at least 355 minims, or nearly five fluid drachms of infusion of a drachm to the pint of boiling water, could not have been safely taken within three hours, and that the repeated doses could not so long have failed to produce vomiting or any other evidence of nicotism, had the power of this agent not been met and for a long time resisted by that diametrically opposite condition of the nervous system which strychnia gives rise to. This case appears to me to confirm in the strongest possible manner the general correctness of the arguments of M. Brown-Sequard, Claude Bernard, and Dr. Haldane, to the effect that strychnia does not act as a direct excitant of the nervous system, but it exaggerates excessively the reflex functions of the spinal cord, so that the slightest irritation produces tetanic convulsion. And it appears to produce the augmentation of the vitality of the spinal cord in two ways :—1st, by

---

* *Medical Times and Gazette*, June 12th, 1858, p. 600, and Taylor on Poisons, *Second Edition*, page 783.

increasing the amount of blood in the spinal cord, by paralyzing the muscular coats of the vessels which supply it ; and, 2nd, by acting in a special manner on the tissue of the cord.*

When the foot of a frog is examined under the microscope, the circulation is seen going on in the well-known manner ; if now the animal be poisoned by nicotine, the arterial system becomes immediately emptied, in consequence of the powerful contraction of the arteries. The heart, however, continues to beat, and the stoppage of the circulation seems the result of an effect produced upon the blood-vessels themselves. The explanation of this phenemenon is to be found in the result of experiments performed upon the sympathetic nerve. When the sympathetic is cut in the neck, the parts supplied with branches from it become the seat of a more vigorous [?] circulation, in consequence of the coats of the blood-vessels which had been paralyzed by the section of the nerve becoming dilated and allowing more blood to pass through them. If, on the contrary, the cut end of the sympathetic be galvanized, an opposite effect is produced,—the circulation in this part is diminished, because the coats have contracted under the application of the stimulus, and the calibre of the vessels has, consequently, been diminished. This second effect is precisely what is produced by nicotine ; and, accordingly, it seems highly probable that the fatal effects of the poison are due to an action on the great sympathetic, and, through it, on the vascular system.†

Dr. Irving, of Allahabad (citing a case in the Indian Medical Gazette for December 1866, in which Dr. Adam Taylor observed that three doses of one-twentieth of a grain of strychnia each produced tetanic effects in a sepoy with malarious fever), mentions that, in a European lady who suffered from neuralgic symptoms which terminated in paralysis and death, one dose of one-twentieth of a grain of strychnia produced violent tetanic convulsions, with frightful twitchings of the face and mouth. In about three hours the symptoms passed off without treatment.‡

Dr. Taylor thinks it probable that, in such cases, elimination is either arrested or imperfectly performed (M. J., p. 335).

Kuchila ke Molung.

At p. 375 of the Bengal Dispensatory, and p. 108 of the Pharmacopœia of India, Sir William O'Shaughnessy Brooke and Dr. Waring have described the poisonous properties of the leaves of a viscum growing on nux-vomica trees in the neighbourhood of Cuttack. These leaves were, for

* See Brown-Sequard, Lectures on the Principal Forms of Paralysis of the Lower Extremities, p. 50.

† Claude Bernard,—Sur les Effects des Substances Toxiques, p. 399. Dr. D. Rutherford Haldane, the Modern Practice of Medicine, Ed. Medical Journal for February, 1865, p. 682.

‡ Indian Medical Gazette, April 1st 1867, p. 102.

a time, used as a substitute for nux-vomica by Dr. Duncan Stuart and others. They were found by Sir W. O'S. Brooke to contain strychnia and brucia.

The following case of poisoning by these leaves by Baboo Rajendra Lall Mittra, was handed to me many years ago by the late Mr. Piddington, Coroner of Calcutta :—

Some time in the autumn of 1840, a stout, athletic English sailor was admitted into the Medical College Hospital, and had, for four or five days successively, taken half-drachm doses of cubeb powder, three times a day. The disease for which he was admitted (gonorrhœa) was slight, and he used frequently to walk about in the hospital compound, and display his pugnacious habits by attacking the servants. One morning, by some unfortunate mistake in the dispensary attached to the College, he had given to him, instead of the usual medicine, three packets of the powdered leaf of the *kutchla molung.* (Viscum monoicum), a parasitic plant that grows on the nux-vomica tree. At 9 A.M. he sat on his bed side, took one of these packets from under his pillow, mixed its contents with a little water, and, while swallowing down the mixture, fell back and screamed out, "I am poisoned !" From that moment to the hour of his death, he never uttered another word ; every attempt at speech being frustrated by the most violent fits of convulsions. The paroxysms recurred about 2 or 3 times every minute, and each time lasted about 10 to 15 seconds ; the body being, during the exacerbations, thrown into such violent agitation that six bearers were unequal to the task of keeping it in bed. Recourse was had to the stomach pump, but it could not be used, as every touch on the body accelerated the return of the convulsions, and put the patient into the most agonizing tortures. The sitting of a fly on his body had often the same effect. Some attempt was made to administer anodynes, but that too failed, and he died at 1 P. M., after suffering the most excruciating pain for four consecutive hours. The scene was so impressive that, after sixteen years, I have now as vivid a recollection of it as if I had seen it yesterday.

This is evidently the case mentioned to Dr. Waring by Sir W. O'S. Brooke, but Sir William says that the man was "killed in less than an hour and-a-half" (p. 108).

Sudden death in the First Spasm of Tetanus.

At the time of Palmer's trial, there was great enquiry for a case of this kind. Allusion was made to the case of a negro servant at Edinburgh, who, while waiting at table, cut his hand with a broken glass, and immediately expired in tetanic spasm ; but I do not think that the instance was very clearly proved. My late friend Dr. Allan Webb, of Calcutta, gave me the following particulars of a very typical case of this description, which occurred while he held medical charge of *La Martiniere* School.

An apparently healthy boy, one of the pupils, was seated on his bed, having a small sore on his foot dressed by the Native Doctor. Having applied the dressing, the Native Doctor was leaving. He walked straight to the door ; but, as he was passing out, he heard a noise from the bed. Turning, he saw the boy supported on his occiput and heels, his body being arched up in opisthotonic spasm. He ran to the bed, the body sank, and death was immediate. The first case of tetanus which I attended in India proved fatal in less than twelve hours ; and, although cases parallel to Dr. Webb's must be very rare, it is evident that a disease which has power to kill by trachealismus or by cardiac spasm is always liable to destroy life, as it did in Dr. Webb's patient, by a single paroxysm.

ALCOHOLIC POISONING.

Apart from the cases of poisoning by drugged liquor alluded to at pp. 138, 191, 243-44, Alcoholism must have a place among the frequent causes of poisoning in India.

It is well known that, even in a cold climate, one who may be so mad as to attempt to drink off a quart of brandy at once will probably fall insensible, and expire almost in the act.

In a case like the following, death must occur rapidly—probably with effusion of alcoholic fluid into the arachnoid cavity :—

"Henry Ritmire, aged twenty-five, hawker from Bungay, has died at Hackney from 'alcoholic poisoning.' The wife of the deceased stated that, between Kingsland-gate and the Marquis of Lansdowne tavern, Hackney, he drank twenty-four quarterns of rum, and did not then seem drunk, and afterwards fourteen more half-quarterns, besides a quantity of beer at different times during the day. This took place on a Sunday, and he died the following morning."

Cases of this kind are by no means rare in India and other tropical climates. One occurred to Mr. B. S. Chimmo, in medical charge of the 20th Regiment Madras Native Infantry at Aden.*

A man of bad character, and accustomed to drink ardent spirits, broke open a cask of arrack while on the Commissariat Guard.

It was not known how much he had drunk, and, when he was seen, it was useless to use the stomach pump ; the heart's action had almost ceased, he was cold and covered with perspiration, quite insensible, features contracted, complete collapse. Gentle stimulants, cold to the head. When reaction took place, it was accompanied with determination of blood to the lungs. He was largely bled, the blood was of a highly florid red color. He died in 24 hours.

---

* Medical Reports Selected by the Medical Board, Madras, 1850, p. 232.

It is probable that many who are supposed to die from Alcoholic Poisoning are, in reality, choked by vomited food lodged in the bronchial tubes. On this question see the Chapter on Suffocation.

The following is an example of a very common case in Calcutta. On the 28th of October 1869, John Brennan, a seaman, was found by the police at 7-30 P.M. staggering towards the Scotch Church. He fell down, and was removed in a stretcher to the lock-up. He was not violent, and did not resist. A shipmate said, "I was locked up drunk. About 12 o'clock at night, I saw Brennan in the same cell ; he appeared either drunk, or dead drunk ; I called him by name, he did not answer, so I got a drink of water and went to sleep again. In the morning I went to shake him and found him stiff and cold."

The forehead, back of neck, and whole of body and limbs generally exhibited extreme hypostatic congestion ; the pupils were dilated. The brain was highly congested, both internally and over the surface ; the latter almost amounting to extravasation of blood ; the lungs, heart, and liver were highly congested ; the stomach was empty, but, on opening it, the smell of alcohol was very marked ; the internal surface of the stomach was highly congested. *Verdict*—" Apoplexy induced by excessive drinking."

In Calcutta, it is usual to send men who are found dead drunk in the streets to the hospital, and I am sure that many lives are thus saved during the eight hot months of the year in which these unfortunates' danger is doubled by a tendency to insolation. I have several times passed hours with one of these patients, extremely doubtful of his recovery, and only restoring him by artificial respiration.

It is probable that tropical heat seldom, if ever, kills any one in whom some other cause has not produced either blood poisoning or great exhaustion of nerve force. In India, the drunkard has to struggle against these states in combination, and is probably also the subject of more or less cholemia or uremia. I have noticed that while, generally speaking, *delirium tremens* is very amenable to treatment in moderately cool weather, those cases which occur in " sunstroke weather," especially between the beginning of May and the 20th of June, are mostly fatal.

PLUMBAGO ROSEA.

Vern., *Lal Chitra, Chitraca* (*Racta Chitraca,* Fleming); Sans., *Chitra molum* and *Kodivaylee ;* Tam., *Chiturmol ;* Duk., *Chita ;* Hind., *Chitra ;* Beng., *Shiturridge ;* Arab, *Tumbe codiveli ;* Hort. Malab.* This acrid plant, as well as the P. EUROPEA,—Vern., *Chitra Vani,* Sans. ; and the P. ZEYLANDICA, *Chita,* H.,—is cultivated in gardens throughout India, and a paste made with the roots is employed in native, and even in European, practice, as a very active but painful and uncertain vesicatory. It is also

* O'Shaughnessy.

employed as an internal medicine by native practitioners. Dr. Shortt says that, in Madras, "it is a universal remedy in dysmenorrhœa." For its other therapeutic uses, see Waring's Pharmacopœia, p. 169, and the Taleef Shereef, p. 76. Great light has been thrown, by the research of Sir W. O'Shaughnessy Brooke, upon the use of the Lall Chitra as a poison, especially as administered by the Natives with a view to procure abortion. It is mentioned in the Bengal Dispensatory, that an essential principle, *Plumbagin*, was discovered in these plants, by M. Dulong, in 1824. It abounds chiefly in the bark of the root, and is thus prepared :—The bark of the root is acted on by ether, the ethereal tincture mixed with water, and the ether recovered by distillation. The watery liquid is then boiled, and filtered while hot ; on cooling, crystals of *Plumbagin* are deposited ; the process is to be repeated as long as crystals are procured. Plumbagin occurs in brilliant yellow crystals of sweetish, but acrid and hot taste, easily fusible, partially volatile, scantily soluble in cold, freely in boiling water, very soluble in alcohol and ether, in the concentrated acids, and in alkaline solutions, with which it strikes a deep red color ; with hydrate of alumina or sub-acetate of lead, a crimson red-colored precipitate is formed, which constitutes a very valuable and delicate test, available in medico-legal inquiries. "The root, in its various forms," continues Sir William, "is much employed as a poison in India, and, as an irritant to occasion abortion, it is introduced into the vagina and applied directly to the neck of the uterus."* In a criminal case of the former kind, in 1837, he succeeded in detecting the poison by acting on the contents of the stomach with alcohol, concentrating the tincture, re-dissolving in a small quantity of boiling water, and adding the sub-acetate of lead, by which the very characteristic red color was immediately occasioned. It is, however, mentioned prominently by this authority, that there are other yellow coloring matters which, with alkalies, present analogous appearances ; but that, to any one who takes the trouble of comparing the effect in a series of experiments on such articles as turmeric, rhubarb, calumba root, the mishmee teeta, &c., no difficulty will arise in his decision, if plumbago be present. Rhubarb, perhaps, approaches nearer than any other ; but, with caustic magnesia, rhubarb gives a yellowish brown, while plumbago gives a crimson sediment. In illustration of the delicacy of this process, he adds that five grains of powdered plumbago were mixed with eight ounces of putrid blood and filth from the dissecting-room ; dilute sulphuric acid was added, and the mixture warmed and strained through cloth. A nearly colorless solution was obtained ; this was treated with ether, and the ethereal solution separated ; on mixing this with a weak solution of potash in water, the characteristic crimson color at once appeared.

---

* It will be seen, in the remarks on Criminal Abortion, that this root is frequently used with far more violence than is here described.

The records contain two instances in which *Men* were poisoned by the Lall Chitra. In May, 1843, a woman living in Howrah confessed that, being on ill terms with her husband, she pounded a small piece of reddish-colored root which had been given to her, and, mixing it with milk, gave it to her husband, who was taken ill in about two hours after swallowing it, and died after having vomited ten times, and being purged once. The Civil Assistant Surgeon observed a slight flush of inflammation on the surfaces of the stomach and small intestines. The stomach was preserved unopened, but the mucous membrane of the intestine continuous with it was observed to be highly injected. On opening the stomach, Dr. Mouat found a small quantity of fluid of a deep coffee-color with a few grains of half-digested rice. The surface of the organ was much corrugated, and covered with small patches of inflammatory blush. On analysing the contents of the stomach, some of the matter vomited, and the remains of the food said to have been taken by the deceased, Dr. Mouat could detect no trace of any mineral poison, but obtained distinct evidence of the characteristic appearance produced by the Lall Chitra.

In October, 1853, the Civil Assistant Surgeon of Azimghur forwarded the stomach, with its contents, of a man supposed to have died by poison, together with a substance found near the body and supposed by the police to be poison. The stomach was received by Dr. Mouat in an advanced state of decomposition, but still exhibited traces of inflammation, and was found to contain Lall Chitra. The substance sent was also found to be a portion of the root of the Plumbago Rosea.

In some ascertained cases, the Lall Chitra has been given *internally* as an abortive, *vide supra*, p. 116, and Waring's Pharmacopœia for India, p. 170. Further reference of the use of this poison will be found under the head of "*Criminal Abortion.*"

NERIUM ODORUM.—Vern., *Kurrubee;* Hind., in Bengal, *Sheth Kurrubee.* (O'SHAUGHNESSY).—Also *Kaner, Kunnar,* or *Kunere.*

Karravera, Sans.; *Hyamara,* Hind.; *Lal-kharubee,* Beng.; *Kunher,* By.; *Tsjavonna-aralee,* Mal.; *Arali,* Tam.; *Ghenneru,* Tel. (BIRDWOOD.)

Its uses in native medicine are given in the Taleef Shereef, p. 129. Baboo Kanny Lall Dey says (p. 78) that the root of the white *Oleander* is reputed in Bengal as the best antidote for snake-bite, and is also used for purposes of criminal abortion. Sub-Assistant Surgeon Koylash Chunder Chatterjee informed me that he was told by a native midwife at Bareilly that she used the root *(Koroopee Jhur)*, upon her own daughter, introducing it at the sixth or seventh month. She also gave a large cup of the decoction. The girl aborted in a few minutes, but eventually died. *See the Chapter on Criminal Abortion.*

Dr. Honigberger says that the root of the hill plant is much more violently poisonous than that of the garden kind, and that jealous women frequently have recourse to it; in fact it is proverbial among the females of the hills, when quarrelling, to bid each other go and eat the root of the *Kaneer*. Ainslie also says that it is but too often resorted to for the purpose of self-destruction by the Hindoo women when tormented by jealousy. Mr. Broughton says that it is well known and extensively resorted to in the Bombay Presidency as a poison, the expressed juice from the red variety being considered the strongest and most fatal. I heard from the late Mr. Hayes, of Medical College Hospital, and from Dr. Collis, that the root is much used as a poison in the neighbourhood of Umballa, being sometimes given in coffee. Dr. Birdwood mentions that the camel eats the sweet-scented Oleander, but it is nearly always fatal to him ; and we are told by Ainslie that it is sometimes called the Haymaraca, or hare-killer.

In 1843, a very interesting case of fatal poisoning by the root of the Nerium, which abounds in gardens all over India, was sent to the Chemical Examiner, by Dr. A. Greig, of Seetapore. On the 9th March 1840, at about 11 o'clock A.M., a man, aged about 50, was brought to Dr. Greig on a charpoy. He was apparently senseless and unable to answer questions. The pulse was preternaturally slow and soft, but regular, with an inclination to stop. On inquiry, it was found that he had eaten some of the root of the *Kaner*, Nerium Odorum, mixed with some mustard oil, about an hour and a half before, with the intention of destroying himself, on account of some domestic quarrel. He was stated to have vomited a considerable quantity of the mixture soon after taking it. He was ordered to be moved about, and draughts of warm water were given to produce vomiting, until the arrival of an emetic from the hospital. Free vomiting was induced by these means. The matter ejected was of a yellow color, and oily consistence. Under this treatment, he revived considerably. He never admitted that he felt any pain in the region of the stomach. Some hours afterwards (in the evening), he relapsed into a state of insensibility. He was immediately taken to the hospital, and treated with stimulants and frictions. A mustard poultice was applied to the epigastrium, and an enema of warm water given. He improved during the night ; and, on the morning of the 10th, Dr. Greig found him able to sit up. His pulse was natural, he expressed himself quite well, and wished to have some food. About two hours afterwards, however, he was reported to have died suddenly, after making some exertion. The body was examined five hours after death. There was no emaciation. The eyes were deeply sunk : the muscles were hard, contracted, and moved with difficulty. The heart was found of the natural size ; its cavities, the ventricles especially, were filled with black fluid blood. The lungs were natural. The stomach contained a quantity of a dark yellowish fluid, having somewhat the odour of tamarind. On its internal surface, near the cardiac and pyloric orifices posteriorly, were found small patches studded with red points, and one or two slight abrasions of the mucous membrane. The liver appeared somewhat distended, the spleen and intestines were natural. It was ascertained that he had procured the bark of the root from Dr. Greig's own garden, and had beaten it to powder before mixing it with oil. The quantity taken could not be correctly ascertained, but must have been at least two or three ounces, judging from the extent of the cut surface of the root of the tree from which he obtained it. Dr. Greig considered that the poison operated fatally by its directly depressing influence upon the nervous system.

A remarkable case of poisoning by *Oleander* was tried at Cawnpore in 1855. A woman, Deonee, was charged with the wilful murder of her husband, aided by Dhowkalla, her paramour. The prisoner confessed that she had purchased what she called opium, and that it was given to her husband in his food. The Civil Surgeon positively affirmed that the deceased died from the effects of some strong irritant poison, not of opium, its effects being not at all similar to those produced by narcotics; and that it was, most probably, a vegetable poison, which he believed, from the appearance of a small portion which adhered to the *Chukkee,* or grinding-stone, to be the bark of the plant known as *Kunere,* a variety of the *Oleander* family, which he stated are included botanically under the class "Nerium," of which there are five different species, all natives of warm latitudes, and several very common in India; the whole plant is thought to be poisonous, but especially the bark of the the roots. It was proved that the substance pounded on the stone by the male prisoner was of a black color, and in size about a finger's length and breadth. Further that the powdered drug was replaced in the rag in which it was brought from market, and was, in the victim's absence, mixed with the rice and milk which his wife had provided for his supper. When the man had eaten of this *keer,* he complained of its bitter taste, to remove which he chewed some sugar cane and a carrot, and was seized with violent purging and vomiting, and died during the night. The female prisoner threw away what remained of the poisoned food, washing the dishes in which it had been cooked. The medical officer expressed an opinion that the substance administered was not Arsenic. He had observed similar symptoms in a previous case of poisoning by *Kunere.* Both prisoners were sentenced to transportation for life.*

In 1868, Dr. James Cleghorn sent me the following notes of two fatal cases of Oleander poisoning, which occurred to him when officiating as Civil Surgeon of Berhampore.

The bodies of two men were found in the house of an old prostitute, living in the Moorshedabad District at a place called Hurryparrah, and were sent into the Civil Station for examination. The men were seen

* Nizamut Adawlut Reports, N. W. P., 13th March 1855, p. 345.

entering the house in their usual state of health, and, as their stay in it was unusually prolonged, the house was searched and their bodies were found lying on the floor, with vomited matter scattered about.

Both were about twenty-six years of age, stout, muscular, and well developed.

Post-Mortem on body of Dalgobind.

No external marks of violence.

Brain.—Engorgement of venous sinuses. Puncta sanguinea abundant, otherwise apparently normal.

Chest, Heart.—Vessels on exterior surface congested. Right ventricle distended with dark fluid blood, valves and interior surface healthy.

Abdomen.—Stomach contained two ounces of grumous fluid. Congestion of vessels on posterior surface of great curvature. A well-defined spot of congestion on posterior surface of cardiac end ; a similar patch near pyloric orifice.

Liver.—Large vessels congested, otherwise apparently normal.

Spleen.—Enlarged to four times its natural size, very much congested, soft, and pulpy (probably the result of malarial influence).

Intestines.—Small ; contained numbers of Ascaris Lumbricoides. Mucous surface throughout of a dark color, large veins very distinct. Large patch of congestion on upper part (mucous surface) of duodenum, surface velvety. Spots of congestion scattered through jejunum and ileum. Villi well marked in upper part of former. Large spots of congestion in sigmoid flexure.

Kidneys.—Intensely congested.

Æsophagus.—Covered with dark-colored mucus.

When conducting this *post-mortem*, an Assistant Surgeon, who was present, was desirous of passing a Catheter and, in trying to do so, found that the urethra was filled with purulent matter, and directed my attention to it. This is important in connection with the confession of the woman.

Post-Mortem on body of Jundoo Chung.

No external marks of violence. Dried blood in nostrils and mouth.

Brain.—Apparently healthy.

Chest.—Two ounces of serum in pericardium. Both ventricles filled with fluid blood.

Lungs.—Healthy, *p. m.* congestion at posterior part.

Abdomen.—Stomach contained a small quantity of grumous fluid. On the anterior and posterior surfaces of peritoneal coat, covering cardiac end, well marked spots of congestion. Mucous surfaces corresponding to these were covered with specks of stellate congestion.

Liver.—Enlarged, especially right lobe. Large veins filled with blood.

Spleen.—Enlarged to twice its natural size (probably malarial).

Bowels.—Normal, except that in parts of them the vessels were congested.

Kidneys.—Healthy.

Upper part of fauces covered with blood.

The Urethra was not examined.

A few days after the discovery of the bodies, the woman in whose house they were found gave herself up to the police. She said that three men came to her to be cured of gonorrhœa, from which they said they were suffering; that she gave them in milk the powdered root and bark of "*kurrubee*," a popular remedy for venereal and skin diseases; and that, soon after taking it, they became sick, vomited, complained of pain in the abdomen, writhed about the floor, and latterly became sleepy. She got frightened, and ran away before they died, and of her own free will gave herself up to the police.

I concluded from the *post-mortem* examination that the men had been poisoned, and had the stomach, its contents, &c., of each, packed up, to be sent to the Chemical Examiner, Calcutta, for examination; but, as the authorities considered that the confession of the woman was sufficient, these parts were not sent. The woman was acquitted, as she evidently had no evil intention when she gave the "*kurrubee*."

The woman showed the tree from which she had taken the poison (portion of the root and bark), and the inspector of police showed me the leaves, which, being sent to Dr. Thomas Anderson, were indentified by him as those of Nerium Odorum. The woman herself called the poison *kurrubee* and said that the tree had *red* flowers.

The following case was reported by Mr. Broughton, Civil Surgeon of Kholapore (Bombay Presidency)* :—

Kurdaree bin Dhoba, a woodcutter, aged thirty-five, of slight and delicate appearance, was brought to the civil hospital at Kholapore, on the morning of the 9th of August 1858, in a state of insensibility. It appeared from the evidence of his wife, who accompanied him, that a quarrel had arisen between them in reference to the *res angusta domi*, and that he had swallowed a cupful of *Kunere*. From subsequent investigation, it was ascertained that the cup contained a little more than an ounce of expressed juice of Oleander, and that at the time of drinking the poison he was standing five yards from his door, towards which he walked immediately, and fell senseless at the threshold. On admission, his face and eyes were flushed, head hot and perspiring, with stertorous breathing, and foaming at the mouth. This was accompanied by violent spasmodic contractions of the muscles of the entire body, but more remarkable in the superior than in the inferior extremities, and also more developed on the left than on the right side. The effect of this was remarkable, and new to me as a pos-

* Trans. Bombay Med. and Phys. Society, No. IV., N. S., for 1857-8, P. IV. of *Appendix*.

ture of disease. During the intervals of spasm, the patient lay evenly upon his back ; and, when action commenced, the superior contraction of the left side threw him over on his right, in which position he remained during the paroxysm ; after the subsidence of which he fell back into the natural posture of exhaustion. Emetics of antimony having failed, sulphate of zinc produced the ejection of large quantities of greenish matter. Insensibility remaining, with quick pulse and hot skin, leeches were applied to the temples, and sulphate of magnesia given as an aperient. The bowels were moved, although involuntarily, and the evacuations were watery, greenish in color, containing but little fæculent matter. The spasms returned at intervals of an hour, and were apparently produced by any attempts to move or rouse him. Towards evening, the spasms decreased, the face became pale, the pulse sunk to a thread, the eyes shrunk into their sockets, and the extremities rapidly became cold. Frictions, mustard poultices, with hot bottles, ammonia and camphor restored the circulation, but insensibility continued, and the bowels were moved involuntarily. In this condition he remained the whole of the next day ; the spasms were less violent and diminished in frequency. He swallowed the ammonia, camphor, and magnesia, which were continued, but the urine and the evacuations still passed involuntarily. In the evening of the 10th, reaction was established, the skin became hot, and the pulse increased ; there were no spasms, but insensibility remained as complete as before. A full dose of castor oil was given, and the bowels acted freely, after which he seemed to be in quiet sleep. He awoke on the morning of the 11th, restored to speech and reason. Weakness only remained as the natural consequence of so violent a seizure. He has since entirely recovered, and is not, I fear, particularly grateful for his recovery, as he anticipates a recurrence of domestic trouble. He assures me, however, that he recollects nothing from the moment he swallowed the draught, and could form no opinion of the time which elapsed since the suicidal attempt and his recovery.

The following case of Oleander Poisoning, treated in the Calcutta Medical College Hospital, is related by Baboo Dwarkanath Mookerjee * :—

Sreenauth Chuckerbutty, aged twenty-nine, was brought into hospital in an apparently unconscious state, on Friday, 3rd August 1866, at 1 P.M. At the time of admission his trunk and limbs were found somewhat rigid, the jaws spasmodically closed, and the pulse very feeble, and exceedingly slow, beating about thirty per minute. The previous history of the case is as follows :—At about 8 oclock that morning, the patient took more than a quarter of a *tolah* (180 grains = 1 tolah) of the fresh root bark of *Sheth Kurrubbee*, rubbed up with black pepper, and divided into three pills. This he was advised to do to get rid of a chancre and some syphilitic eruptions on the skin, which had not yielded to prolonged treatment.

* Indian Medical Gazette, September 1, 1866, p. 258*a*.

Within half an hour of taking it, he began to feel giddy and very heavy, and was obliged to lie down in bed. This was shortly followed by a general uneasy sensation, and considerable restlessness. Soon afterwards he began to get fits, in each of which his trunk and limbs became rigid and contracted, and the hands clenched, with the thumbs flexed inwards on the palms. Profuse perspiration and a sensation of constriction round the chest also accompanied each paroxysm.

A short period of partial relaxation succeeded each of them. During the third or fourth fit, the muscles of the jaws began to be affected. He had no regular paroxysm in the hospital, but came in with a severe locked-jaw, and some rigidity of voluntary muscles, which continued for a few hours. Previous to his admission, he had light fits. Constant muscular twitchings were observed all over his body, even four or five hours after he was taken in. On admission, he was ordered half a drachm of sulphate of zinc in warm water as a brisk and quick emetic. He was reported to have vomited several times at home. A fœtid enema, and counter-irritation along the spine by means of sinapism, were also had recourse to. The rigidity of all the muscles gradually gave way, and they were restored in a short time to their original state of relaxation. With a view to eliminate the poison that was evidently circulating in the blood, a constant drain was kept up from the kidneys by a course of diuretics, which were continued for three days. The next morning he declared himself to be quite easy, except that he had slight heaviness about the head, which, however, passed off in the course of another day. He remained in the hospital for more than a fortnight, for the cure of the original complaint for which he had taken the drug, and he quite recovered from the effects of it. It appeared from his statement that the sensibility of vision, hearing, and touch were all more or less heightened by the effects of the Oleander. He stated that he never lost his consciousness, but that his mind was quite clear throughout.

Baboo Kamikhya Nath Acharjee reports* the case of a boy to whom a quack had administered the powdered bark of the root of the N. Odorum, while he was suffering from intermittent fever. In three or four hours the patient "was attacked with tetanus." He was found "free from fever, and quite sensible, his jaws spasmodically closed, and the muscles of his body rigid and contracted." He recovered under blistering, purgatives, and diuretics.

I have been informed that the late Dr. John Bowhill also noticed the symptoms of Nux-Vomica poisoning in a case of Oleander poisoning.

Baboo Dwarakanath Mookerjea draws attention to the tetanic symptoms, in the case of Sreenath Chuckerbutty given above, as evidence that Oleander, in a great measure, resembles strychnia in its effects on the system.

---

* Indian Medical Gazette, Aug. 1866, p. 218.

In his case, all the urgent symptoms (as in cases of strychnia poisoning) were developed suddenly, and the muscles of the jaws were likewise the last to be affected. When the symptoms began to subside, they did so rapidly.

He adds: "The marked difference between the morbid effects of Oleander and those of Nux-Vomica consists in the condition of the pulse. In the latter case it is generally unaffected, becoming slightly quickened only during each fit; but in the former its preternatural slowness was a well-marked feature. The writer of the case in the Indian Medical Gazette does not make any mention of it, but Dr. Chevers, in his work on Medical Jurisprudence, distinctly alludes to it; and my friend Baboo Kanny Lall Dey observes the same thing in another case, which occurred in the Medical College Hospital, under the same physician, more than two years ago. Besides its action on the nervous system, therefore, the poisonous principle of Oleander seems to have a special depressing influence on the heart."

Commenting upon this similarlity in the physiological action of the two poisons, Baboo Kanny Lall Dey notices that Oleander belongs to *Apocyneæ*, a family of plants closely allied to that of Nux-Vomica—the *Loganiaceæ*. According to Dr. Fraser (Trans. of the Royal Society of Edin., Vol. XXIV.) the Nerium Oleander Antiaris, Tanghia, Digitalis, and Black Hellebore produce, first, irregularity and acceleration of the heart's action, then a diminished frequency caused by protraction of the ventricular systole, and, finally, stoppage of the contractions by cessation of the dilatation of the ventricles, which then remain contracted, white and perfectly empty.

It will be noticed that, in the three fatal cases by Drs. Greig and Cleghorn given above, the hearts were not in the state observed in Dr. Fraser's experiments. The men probably died from asthenia. In the animals experimented upon by Dr. Fraser the cause of death was evidently cardiac spasm.

THEVETIA NERIIFOLIA,

A West-Indian Shrub, domesticated in India and cultivated under the name of *the Exile* or *Yellow Oleander.*

"The kernels," says Dr. Waring, "are extremely bitter, and when chewed, produce a slight feeling of numbness and heat in the tongue; by expression, they yield a clear pale amber-colored, slightly viscid, acrid oil, which is sometimes recommended as a cathartic by the natives, but it produces violent vomiting and hypercatharsis (Dr. Shortt)." An interesting case of poisoning by one of these kernels is recorded by J. Balfour (*Madras Journal of Lit. and Science,* 1857, Vol. III, N. S., p. 140). Recovery ensued; but, from the symptoms detailed, the plant evidently belongs to the class of acro-narcotic poisons, (p. 139).

Baboo Kanny Lall Dey informs me that a case of poisoning by these seeds was brought to his notice by a medical friend who attended it. A boy, about four years old, while playing under a *Thevetia Neriifolia* tree (*Cheena korobee*), picked up and ate one of the seeds, which much resemble the almond. In a short time vomiting commenced, but there was no purging. Within half an hour, he became insensible, the body was covered with cold clammy sweat, the countenance was pale, and the eyes deeply sunken ; and, within two hours, he died convulsed. No *post-mortem* examination.

POISONOUS HONEY.

Dr. Taylor mentions (Poisons, p. 782), that it is said that the honey of bees, which feed upon the flowers of *Oleander* in certain districts, is liable to produce injurious effects. Dr. Bidie, of Madras, has recorded* his own experience of the disagreeable effects produced by eating some honey, procured from the Coorg jungle, in the joint of a bamboo. It looked clear and wholesome, and had the usual smell and taste. On three successive days he took about a teaspoonful at breakfast. On the second and third day he felt a disagreeable itching over the whole body. On the night of the third day he awoke with intense headache and a feeling of constriction about the forehead. The headache continued severe until evening, when it left, but the sense of constriction about the forehead remained. The itching had become worse, and he noticed numerous red spots all over the body. On the fifth day he felt quite well, except that the itching was very troublesome. On the sixth he again took some of the honey at breakfast. Shortly afterwards he was purged, and his whole body became covered with an exanthematous eruption of prominent, irregular red patches, most conspicuous on the face, back of the hands, and about the larger joints. The headache and constriction of the forehead returned, and he suddenly became very sick, and felt so prostrated in strength that he could hardly walk a few yards to a couch. There was no desire to vomit, but a sickness and prostration so intense that he could hardly move a limb, or even speak. This condition lasted for about three hours. He then had a short sleep, and awoke to find the headache much relieved, and the sickness quite gone. The eruption had partly disappeared. There were, however, intense thirst and a feeling of soreness in the throat, and the voice was quite hoarse. Although he was accustomed to eat English honey, it never produced such effects. The eruption continued to appear and disappear, and to be troublesome for some time.

COPPER.

Cooking vessels of this metal being universally employed by Europeans, and by most East Indian and Mussulman families throughout India, (except by a few, who use earthen pots for greater security), cases of poi-

---

* Madras Quarterly Journal, Oct. 1861, p. 398.

soning by Copper not unfrequently occur, where, by the carelessness of servants, the usual precaution of having these vessels newly tinned every month is not observed. In such cases, the salt, or acid, or oily matter contained in rich soups, stews or curries, which require long boiling, acts chemically upon the exposed copper surface, and becomes highly poisonous. It is now well understood that keeping the exposed surface of the copper perfectly bright and clean, is no safeguard against these impregnations. I was acquainted with a family among whom very severe cases of poisoning from this cause, fortunately not terminating fatally, occurred *twice*, within six years.*

VERDIGRIS, *Subacetate of Copper*.

A case, in a which a man swallowed a considerable quantity of *Subacetate* of Copper, and afterwards *about half an ounce of Essential Oil of Peppermint*, is recorded by Mr. Raleigh.† He was admitted into the General Hospital in a perfectly comatose state ; breathing stertorous ; pupils dilated to the utmost possible extent ; pulse slow, hard, laboring, but not full ; countenance bloated and purple ; foam issued from the mouth ; skin warm ; all mental and voluntary power completely suspended. The case was at first believed to be one of apoplexy, and was treated accordingly. On the following day, he became perfectly sensible, and began to suffer from marked symptoms of irritant poisoning. Under

---

* In this country, where copper vessels are used so very extensively, the following conclusions, appended by Sir Dominic Corrigan to some cases of *slow poisoning by Copper*, published in the *Dublin Hospital Gazette in* 1855, may be found valuable : 1st.—They show us that Copper, or its carbonate, will act as a slow poison by absorption, undermining the constitution, producing emaciation, catarrh, and loss of strength, and leaving the system in a state little capable of resisting the ordinary exciting causes of many diseases. 2nd.—The symptoms, although not acute, are well marked ; emaciation, cachectic appearance, loss of muscular strength, colic pains, cough without physical signs to account for it, and the peculiar characteristic sign of retraction of the gums, with a purple, not a blue edge. 3rd.—In none of the cases, although there was muscular debility, was there either acute colic with constipation, or the local paralysis that so often results from the poison of lead, and the color of the gums was quite distinct from that produced by lead. 4th.—Copper, in slow poisoning, seems to exert its deleterious influence mainly on the nutritive functions or assimilation, including absorption and secretion ; while lead acts energetically on the nervous system of both organic and animal life, exhibited in its action on the former by the obstinate constipation, and on the latter by the violent pains of lead colic, and by the production of its peculiar paralysis. 5th.—The knowledge that Copper, or its carbonate, is capable of acting as a slow poison will be useful, as it may lead us to discover the nature of some, at first sight, anomalous diseases, that might otherwise elude our diagnosis. The tint of color produced on the gums, whether by Copper or Lead, remains a very long time. It had not disappeared from any of the cases narrated, as long as they were under my observation. In the case of a policeman, who has been very lately in the Whitworth Hospital, the blue color produced by Lead was very distinct. He had been in the police force two years. Previously to his becoming a policeman, he had been a painter."

† Transactions of the Medical and Physical Society of Calcutta, Vol. V., p. 129.

treatment, the irritable state of the stomach abated on the fifth day, and considerable inflammation of the fauces and lining membrane of the trachea supervened, which continued to trouble him more or less for about a month. The earlier symptoms in this case appear to have been attributable to *poisoning with the Oil of Peppermint.*

The late Dr. Thomas Moore has described* an affection which prevailed among a batch of Indian laborers returning from British Guiana to Calcutta, which had the character of acute gastritis and enteritis with many of the characteristics of acute idiopathis dysentery. It was discovered that the coolies' food, rice and ghee, was allowed to grow stale and rancid in copper vessels, the inner rims of which presented an incrustation of verdigris, sufficient in quantity to be scraped off with a pen-knife. Two of the cases proved fatal; one of these lingered for a few weeks, and died of chronic ulceration of the intestines, the other terminated fatally soon after the introduction of the poison into the stomach.

As the reports of antopsies in poisoning by Copper are few, and as Dr Moore was a very accurate observer, I cite the *post-mortem* examination in full.

Extensive and deep-seated inflammation of the mucous membrane, and of the subjacent tissues, was found on the internal surface of the stomach. This inflammatory condition of mucous and sub-mucous tissues extended from the cardiac orifice to the pylorus, and for the distance of an inch and-a-half on the internal surface of the œsophagus, close to its termination in the stomach. The shades of red varied in different parts from a bright vermillion, or bright scarlet, to a deep red, or violet color. The patches of dark red, approaching to a brownish tinge, were small, circular, circumscribed, and situated in general beneath the mucous membrane of the posterior wall of the stomach. The mucous membrane corresponding to these patches was soft, tumid, pulpy, but not excoriated. The surface of the membrane was free from the appearance of having sloughed. At the pylorus the membrane was intensely inflamed and glistening: tumid from a quantity of serous fluid exuded beneath the sub-mucous cellular tissue. In the duodenum the appearances were those of intense redness, state of excessive injection, and congestion of the tissues by a sero-sanguineous fluid. This enfiltration did not extend beyond the transverse portion of the intestine. In the mucous membrane of the small intestines, circumscribed patches of redness were found scattered irregularly over its surface. The mucous membrane of the large intestine presented a few of these circumscribed patches of vascularity. In the rectum, the inflammatory action had commenced, but was limited in extent. Within the peritoneal sac somewhat more than eight ounces of saffron-colored fluid

* Selections from my Medical Note Book, 1852, p. 141.

were found. The peritoneal coat of the jejunum and ileum was numerously studded with minute circular dots or specks of a bright red color. On the upper surface of the arch of the colon, and on its ascending and descending divisions, these crimson-red circular spots were numerous. Between the peritoneal and muscular coats of the stomach, an irregularly-shaped patch of effused blood was noticed. On the lateral and inferior surfaces of this viscus, vascularity of the peritoneal coat, with sub-peritoneal exudations of blood and lymph was traced to a short distance. The folds of the peritoneum were not agglutinated together by lymph—lymph was not found in the peritoneal sac.

CUPRI SULPHAS.

In 1841, Dr. O'Shaughnessy mentioned that cases of poisoning by Sulphate of Copper had occurred in Calcutta. That gentleman discovered that one of three suspicious powders forwarded to him for examination by the Civil Surgeon of Hooghly was ACETATE OF COPPER (*Zangar* and *Pitrai*, H. *Pitalata*, S. Fleming.)*

Tutiya, H., *Tutt'ha* (Fleming)—Is mentioned in the Shastras as one of the mineral poisons which may be used, in a diluted form, as medicines. A case came under my notice, about eighteen years since, in which there was reason to believe that death had been accelerated by rather small doses of Sulphate of Copper injudiciously prescribed. The body of an unhealthy-looking native, who had been under treatment for bowel complaint by a kobiraj, and had died rather suddenly, was brought to me for examination. I could only discover marked signs of irritation in the mucous membrane of the stomach. This organ was nearly empty, as there had, doubtless, been some vomiting. I could not detect a trace of copper in its scanty contents, but one or two shreds of vegetable matter retained a deep green color, not usually found after the process of digestion has commenced. Two or three pills, containing very coarsely pounded Sulphate of Copper, mixed with some green succulent vegetable matter, were sent in, as specimens of the medicine which deceased had taken. It appeared probable that none of the pills had contained more than a grain and-a-half or two grains of the Sulphate ; but, although a large dose of this salt may, of course, be given as an emetic, it is probable that doses of one or two grains, *coarsely powdered*, repeated frequently, would cause death, by gastric and intestinal irritation, especially if prescribed when the mucous membrane of the intestinal canal is in a state of

* I find it mentioned in one of the Nizamut Adawlut Reports, N. W. P., that the water in which a copper pice has been boiled is considered by the natives of that part of the country as a useful emetic. It is almost needless to say that, if tolerably pure water be used, it can receive no metallic admixture in this process. See also p. 127 of this vol., on the use in Madras of Sulphate of Copper with Lime Juice as an emetic, with fatal result.

According to Dr. A. Walker, in cases of poisoning demanding immediate emesis, natives, in the Bombay Presidency, place a few copper pice in some tamarind infusion, which is stirred about for a minute or two, and then administered.

vascular excitement. The case was, I believe, viewed upon my report as one of misadventure.

A rather doubtful case of poisoning by some salt of copper occurred in February, 1854. The Civil Assistant Surgeon of Umballa forwarded two pills for examination. It was stated that one pill of the same kind had caused the death of an individual in that district, who had received it from a "Kahar" on the road. The native doctor who examined the body stated that he was unable to detect any marks of poison, and that death had occurred by other and natural causes ; his report, however, was not relied upon. Dr. Macnamara found a small quantity of copper in each of the pills.

EMPLOYMENT OF POISONS BY NATIVE PRACTITIONERS.

There is every reason to believe that the ignorant native doctors in this country by no means unfrequently administer poisonous drugs, in the treatment of disease, with so much indiscretion and recklessness as to cause death. As such cases occasionally, though rarely, are found to call for medico-legal investigation,* a brief allusion to the chief of the deadly remedies employed by these Korbirajira and Hukeems will not be out of place here.

THE BISH BOREE, OR BISH BAREE.

This preparation appears to be almost universally resorted to, by the Bengalee practitioners, in cases of fever, where the symptoms do not yield readily to milder remedies.

In an interesting paper on this subject,† Baboo C. C. Moitre, Sub-Assistant Surgeon, Nattore, mentions that, although it is a matter of great difficulty to ascertain the composition of Bish Baree, it appears, from his inquiries, that the following substances are its principal ingredients :—*White Arsenic, Sulphuret of Arsenic, Sulphur, Mercury,* and the *Seeds of the Croton Tiglium* pounded. There are, he adds, various forms of Bish Baree, some containing the mildest vegetable poisons, others the more powerful. *Snake Poison*‡ is said to be an ingredient, but the

---

* In October 1853, Dr. Mouat received for chemical examination the stomach of a native who had, by mistake, swallowed a fluid medicine prescribed by a hukeem for external use, in consequence of which he died the same evening with symptoms of irritant poisoning. The Chemical Examiner failed to discover any poison recognisable by chemical tests in the inflamed stomach, and considered that the irritant matter had probably been ejected by vomiting. He very justly added that the case was evidently accidental, and that no criminality could attach to the hukeem, as such accidents might happen and have happened, in the hands of careful, conscientious, European practitioners.

† Bengal Hurkaru Medical and Scientific Gazette, May 22nd, 1852.

‡ European Physicians residing in the East have, in several instances, allowed their scientific ardour to outrun their discretion in experiments upon Snake poison, as an internal remedy. Mead, as cited by Dr. Taylor, described the *viper poison* as having a sharp burning taste. When a drop, undiluted, was placed on the tongue, the organ became swollen, and there was a sensation of soreness which remained two or three days. Russell applied one drop of the poison of the *cobra* to his tongue, and found it tasteless. It is com-

quantity used cannot be ascertained with certainty,—*Musk* is not unfrequently used; the whole of these ingredients are not always compounded into the same mass; any two or three of these form a *boree.*

The Baboo regards the Bish Boree as a powerful excitant, determining blood to the head, and increasing the frequency and fulness of the pulse, acting on the pulmonary organs as an irritant, producing at first a dry cough and subsequently accumulation of mucus in the bronchial tubes. It also acts as a powerful irritant on the abdominal organs,—vomiting, diarrhœa, and hiccup being the usual effects of its exhibition. It exercises a similar influence on the bladder and kidneys, inducing strangury and diminishing the quantity of the urine. It can, sometimes, give rise to retention of urine. Still, singularly enough, the Baboo considers that when due caution is observed to prescribe this medicine only in cases "where there are local complications existing"—its effect being more or less that

---

monly said that it may be swallowed with impunity, but Dr. Hering found, while residing at Surinam, that, on taking even small doses of it, much diluted with water, very perceptible effects were produced; such as pains throughout the body, abundant secretion of mucus from the nose and œsophagus, and diarrhœa (Treatise on Poisons). Dr. Jetio asserts that snake poison, though tasteless, is not harmless when taken into the stomach.

In June 1870 I was, by the kindness of Dr. Fayrer, present at a series of experiments in which fresh cobra poison was introduced into the stomachs of a dog and a fowl, and into the eye of a dog. These animals died with all the symptoms of Cobra-poisoning, except that these made their appearance much more slowly than in animals which were bitten at the same time by the same snake. There exists in India an idea which is, to say the least, curious. Baboo Kanny Lall Dey saw a woman very ill after eating a mango, which they firmly believed had been bitten by a snake! My friend Dr. Francis lately raised* the question whether the milk of an animal bitten by a poisonous snake is not poisonous, and he brings forward some rather strong facts and arguments towards proving that such is the case. Dr. Honigberger says that his mehter, who ate all the fowls which he killed in a series of experiments on venomous serpents at Lahore, fattened on the diet.

Dr. Honigberger appears to be a believer in the medicinal virtue of serpent poison. He tells us that, on one occasion, he prepared it from the virus of the Aspis Naja; another time, he procured it from that of the Aspidoclonion; from whichever obtained, there appeared to him to be little difference in the effects produced. He prepares it by expressing a drop of the limpid fluid from the poison gland of a living snake, cunningly secured, upon a small lump of sugar; this is instantly deposited in a porcelain mortar and subjected to trituration with a few drops of spirit. The powder, when shaken up in a drachm of proof spirit, is fit for use. It is to be kept from the light, and to be well shaken up before it is administered. One drop constitutes a dose. Even in this homœopathic quantity, the remedy appears to have been worse than the disease—"Rumbling in the bowels,"—for which it is alone recommended.

In the list of poisons used in Bengal obtained by the late Mr. Bedford, apparently from a Kobiraj, is the following. I print it *verbatim* with the amusing English of the transcribing clerk.

"Kaytasaper Bees or Black Snake Poison—Same as Hulla-hull. This is used in Medicine, but require put it first in mustard oil, make it dry on sunshine, then put again for seven days in due [dew], then little juice of nim leaves into it, then make it dry again, also I require five boils—Roe fish, Goat, Buffalow, Bushee Hog, and Pikocks."—A quarter of a grain of this Shakesperian extract is sufficient to kill a man.

* Ind. Med. Gaz., for June 1st and August 1st, 1868.

of a stimulant irritant upon almost all the organs of the body—"it is a very useful agent ;—Ammonia is not half so efficacious !"

The late Baboo Isserchunder Gangooly also wrote a brief account of the Bish Boree, which he said is a generic term comprising a large group of medicinal preparations, the chief of which is *Aconite*, though many metallic substances enter into their composition, the principal of which are Mercury and Arsenic. This gentleman also considered that there are some of the *Rusauns* which are much more powerful stimulants than any which are to be found in our Pharmacopœia. The chief of these are Baboo Gopaul Bose's *Nas ; Kalanul ; Soochika Pills ; Jurangkoosh Pills ;* and *the Rambawn Pill.* Some of these contain Arsenic, Poison of the Black Cobra, Opium, and Sulphate of Copper ; and others Aconite, Realgar, &c.*

I have only once had an imperfect opportunity of noticing the ill-effects of this nostrum,—in the person of a Sherishtadar of high caste, whom I visited in the last stage of fever, although he obstinately refused to submit to treatment by our medicines. I found him supported by pillows, speaking very rapidly and incoherently, but in a low and broken voice ; his eyes were sunken, but inflamed and ferretty ; his skin dry and tight, but not remarkably hot ; his tongue parched, shrunken and vividly red at the edges, evidencing severe gastric or intestinal irritation. The atmosphere of the room in which he lay was intensely hot and close, and loaded with the odour of *musk.* The brahmin who sat beside him interdicted all interference with his case, except the administration of a dose of quinine, which he, however, instantly spat out. He died in a few hours. My friend Dr. Herbert Baillie, then of Hooghly, informed me that he had succeeded in saving more than one patient poisoned by the Bish Boree or *Rusaun* treatment. Previous to death, the state of excitement described above gives place to collapse. Having been called to patients in this latter stage, he has succeeded in arousing the vital powers by the prompt use of Ammonia and other diffusible stimulants.

PREPARATIONS OF MERCURY.

Cases of poisoning by those medicinal preparations of MERCURY which are in common use among the inhabitants of India,—as by the RED SULPHURET (factitious cinnabar), *Hingool* (vermillion), *Shengerf* H. (Fleming,) "*Darshikna,*" similar to our corrosive sublimate (Honigberger), and by *Rascapúr*, a mixture of calomel and corrosive sublimate,†—are

---

* Bengal Hurkaru Medical and Scientific Gazette, for 7th February and 18th December 1852.

† A case of supposed poisoning by *Rascapúr* or *Rushcapoor* was tried Up-country, a few years since. It deserves special attention, as involving a caution against reliance upon the statements of inexperienced chemists in questions of life and death. Gouree was tried for the murder of Musst. Wazeerun, a prostitute, by poison. It appeared that the prisoner, who had an illicit intimacy with the deceased, visited her on a certain day, enticed her out, and

not likely to call very frequently for the opinion of the medical witness. Dr. B. Brown alludes to one case in which *Rascapúr* was used for the

---

gave her sweetmeats. After eating these, the woman began to complain of having cramp in her limbs and tongue, and was purged. She was taken to the Cotwalee, where she deposed on oath that Gouree, that morning, gave her something in *sheereenee*, and that her feet and arms were cramped, and her stomach was griped. When he gave it to her, he coaxed her, and said that she was not to give any to her female companion. He gave her two pieces *(do danah)* and some broken pieces of *sheereenee*. She died shortly after her admission to the Dispensary. The Sub-Assistant Surgeon is reported to have given the following extraordinary chemical evidence (in the absence of the Civil Surgeon): "The deceased was, on her arrival, in a state of insensibility. Hearing that she was supposed to have taken poison, he extracted the contents of her stomach by the stomach-pump. He took a small portion of the contents, and, having mixed a small quantity of *nitric acid* and *of carbonate of potass with it* [!], boiled the whole together, then filtered; and, after filtering, boiled the liquid to the consistence of a syrup; that he then applied hydro-sulphuret of ammonia to the syrup which immediately precipitated a black substance, *which was the sulphuret of mercury*," [Not a single word is given in substantiation of this assertion];—"that, from this test, it was clear that corrosive sublimate had been administered; that he also submitted the syrup to another test, *viz.*, hydriodate of potass, which should have occasioned a red precipitate, but it did not; that this was probably owing to the substance which was administered being *Ruskapoor*, which is not pure corrosive sublimate, being mixed with calomel; that he also submitted the syrup to other tests, *viz.*, ammoniaco nitrate of silver, ammoniaco sulphate of copper, and protomuriate of tin; but that the result in all was not satisfactory, and from the same cause." That the woman came to her senses after the stomach-pump was used, and spoke a little to an old woman who was in attendance on her, and then relapsed into her former state, in which she continued up to her death, which took place about an hour after her admission into the Dispensary; that he did not ask her any questions during the interval; that he (this was at the conclusion of his deposition) did ask her some questions during the interval; and, in answer, she stated that she felt intense burning pain in her belly and cramp of all the members of her body; that these were the ordinary consequences of taking *Ruskapoor;* that he examined the body after death in company with the Civil Surgeon; that there was a slight degree of vascularity on the internal coat of the stomach; that he could not say if the other organs were in a healthy state, as he went away before the Civil Surgeon had concluded the examination of the body; that, in his opinion, deceased died from *Ruskapoor* having been given her,—this is an impure native preparation of corrosive sublimate; that purging is a common consequence of corrosive sublimate having been administered; that, if corrosive sublimate be given in a pure state, the effects would be apparent in five or six minutes; but, if given in an impure state, in a longer time; that there would have been a greater degree of redness of the stomach, if the corrosive sublimate had been pure; that he could form no opinion as to the quantity of *Ruskapoor* which must have been administered, though he can safely state that more was administered than would have been given as a medicine; that a quantity of *Ruskapoor* sufficient to cause death might be administered in a little sweetmeat; and that, amongst the contents of the stomach, some cream-like substance was observed, that might have been sweetmeat *(para)*. The jury acquitted. The sessions judge convicted. That the deceased died from having taken *Ruskapoor*, there could, he thought, be no doubt, on the evidence of the Sub-Assistant Surgeon. It was true that all the tests applied were not satisfactory in their results; but a sufficient cause for their not being so was assigned. The result, however, of one test was most satisfactory, and the usual symptoms consequent on *Ruskapoor* being administered, *viz.*, purging, cramps, a burning sensation in the stomach, and a redness of the coats of the stomach, were observed. The strength of the general evidence, as showing that the woman was destroyed by poison administered by the prisoner, was then insisted upon. The judge believed that the jury acquitted,—*as they had not confidence in chemical tests.* He recom-

purpose of poisoning in the Punjab. It was mixed with bread. In a case of criminal abortion at Tipperah, it appeared that the accused administered to the woman, with other things, some pills containing a portion of *crude mercury in a state of minute division.* An interesting case of poisoning in a native by Corrosive Sublimate, which had been used for preserving the skins of birds, is recorded by Mr. J. Murray.*

The utter rashness with which the native practitioners carry on their (in itself not ill-devised) plan of Mercurial Fumigation in cases of syphilis, is undoubtedly such as, in many cases, might call for the interference of the law, the result being death by salivation or cancrum oris, or at best, sloughing of the gums, and expoliation of the alveoli followed by excessive adhesion of the injured surfaces; still it is probably not, in reality, more criminal than the wholesale system of salivation which obtained in some of our own syphilis wards five-and-thirty years ago. Several of the Chemical Examiners' Reports mention the detection of traces of mercurial preparations in suspected fluids, but reveal nothing which could be regarded as evidence of poisoning by Corrosive Sublimate.

THE EMPLOYMENT OF MIXED POISONS.

A considerable number of facts from time to time transpire indicative of the prevalance of the employment, among the natives, of various poisons—animal and vegetable, irritant and narcotic—compounded together for purposes of murder or self-destruction. Several allusions to the use of mixed poisons by road-poisoners and others have been made in this work—especially at pp. 168, 178. A case strongly pointing to this practice occurred to Dr. Herbert Baillie, a short time previous to the publication of the last edition of this work. A man was brought to the

---

mended that the prisoner should be sentenced to death. The Judges of the Superior Court considered the crime to be proved against the prisoner by the evidence in the case, and the traces of poison found in the analysis of the contents of the stomach of deceased.

It cannot be doubted for a moment that the general facts adduced in the trial fully proved that the woman's death was caused by poison. It is equally certain, however, that the chemical evidence (as it stands in the printed report) adds not the smallest imaginable weight to those facts. It proves, in short, nothing whatever. The mere fact of a black precipitate resulting from the addition of hydro-sulphuret of ammonia to a portion of the contents of the stomach—standing alone—is *not* proof that the suspected fluid contained corrosive sublimate,—(this being the least reliable test for the poison in question †)—especially when no reason is given us for believing that the metal was subsequently obtained from this precipitate. This may, possibly, have been done, and then the experiment would have been conclusive; but, as it would appear that the whole chemical process is given in the report, and as,—judging from the fact of the operator having expected to detect corrosive sublimate in a fluid by treating it first with nitric acid and carbonate of potass and afterwards with ammonio-nitrate of silver, and ammonia-sulphate of copper,—it is evident that his chemical knowledge was, to say the least, confused, it may fairly be considered as altogether doubtful whether mercury was discovered, or was present in the stomach.

* Transactions of the Medical and Physical Society of Bombay, Vol. I., p. 322.

† Taylor on Poisons, p. 410.

Hooghly Immambarrah Hospital with several incised wounds, apparently self-inflicted, all on the left side of the neck and chest. He appeared to be under the influence of some powerful narcotic, and gradually sank, without having shown any symptoms of irritant poisoning. Upon *post-mortem* examination, however, a large quantity of *white arsenic* was discovered in the stomach. Although no other poison was discoverable, it can scarcely be doubted that the dose of arsenic had been qualified by a large addition of some narcotic, probably *Datura*.

Dr. Morehead, of Bombay, has recorded the case of a Hindu goldsmith who was found comatose in the public street. When admitted, his pupils were dilated, the breathing was natural, the pulse frequent ; there was no appearance of injury or disease. An emetic acted readily, and he became sensible. He vomited several times during the day, and passed two or three motions of gelatinous-looking mucus. Towards evening, the pulse became very feeble, the breathing hurried, the thirst and anxiety considerable, with considerable retching. He died twenty-three hours after admission. He merely stated that he had eaten some sweetmeats the night before he was brought to hospital. Arsenious acid was found upon analysis of the contents of the stomach. The traces of the irritant action of this poison were very distinctly marked in the stomach, small intestines, and cœcum. Dr. Morehead adds that, upon admission to the hospital, this case was viewed as one of narcotic poisoning, and was treated as such. Subsequently, its nature was sufficiently evident. While the narcotic symptoms were present, his attention was attracted by the circumstance that there was a fixed frown on the countenance, an expression of suffering not usual in simple narcotism, and to which probably more importance as a diagnostic sign should have been attached.* This case has been cited by Dr. Taylor,† in illustration of the opinion that narcotism may result from the introduction of arsenic into the system. It will, however, be observed, that the head-symptoms were present only at an early stage of the case ; and that, for many hours previous to death, the symptoms were those of irritant poisoning. Doubtless the arsenic was taken combined with some narcotic.

In 1842, Sir W. O'Shaughnessy Brooke remarked that "In India, compounds of acrid [poisons] and narcotics are often employed, by which the vomiting is checked while the poison is doing its work."

In 1830, Fatima, aged sixteen, was tried and found guilty in the Zillah Court of Dharwar (Bombay Presidency) for administering to her husband in his food a quantity of *Arsenic* (Safaid Soomul) and *Sugar of Lead* (Moordarsungko) which is said to have been mixed with the poisonous milk of the Seind tree (*Sehind* a species of Euphorbia—*Watson*).‡

* Trans. of the Med. and Physical Society of Bombay, for 1845-6, p. 100.

† Medical Jurisprudence, 5th Ed., p. 9.

‡ Bellasis's Bombay S. F. A. Reports, p. 37.

Cases in which the symptoms led strongly to a belief that the poison administered was a mixture of *Aconite and Datura,* will be found in the records of the Chemical Examiners; but, as this was not absolutely proved by analysis, their details need not be given here. Portions of *Aconite and Nux-Vomica* were found among several substances detected upon the person of a man who attempted to destroy himself at Allahabad with a wish to bring discredit upon his relations.

I am indebted to the kindness of the Hon'ble Elphinstone Jackson for the perusal of the record of the sessions trial of Mussamut Lagni, who was condemned at Purneah in March 1870, for poisoning her husband. The case was full of medico-legal difficulty, but *White Arsenic and Singia (Aconite)* were traced to the woman's possession, and the evidence tended in a measure to show that death was caused by a mixture of these poisons.*

Dr. H. Baillie, when at Hooghly, kindly gave me the case of a patient whom he treated in March 1854, suffering from the effects of a mixed poison, the chief constituent of which appears to have been *Hellebore.*† The patient, a young man, was found in the street, apparently in the collapse stage of cholera. The skin was cold and clammy, that of the fingers was shrivelled, and the nails were of a bluish hue. He was constantly purged and vomited incessantly. It was observed that the vomiting differed from that of cholera, inasmuch as it was far from free, and the ejected matter was a thick tenacious mucus. He seemed to champ with his mouth, which was covered with this ropy mucus. He said that it was vain to think of saving him, as he had a few hours previously taken poison—*Meeta-Bish*‡ which he had procured from a native druggist. He added that, for two hours after taking the poison, he perceived no uneasiness: he then felt a burning sensation in the throat and stomach, which was shortly followed by violent efforts to retch, which had increased in severity up to that time. The pulse was scarcely perceptible, the tongue had a white dry fur down its centre, its tip and edges appeared raw and red. He complained of a sense of constriction about the fauces and intense thirst, all attempts to satisfy which immediately brought on retching. There was some epigastric tenderness on pressure. His countenance had a remarkably odd, almost comical expression, from the first; the eyelids were nearly closed, and he seemed to be peeping through the lashes. He recovered slowly under the use of counter-irritants and moderate stimulants. A portion of some vegetable substance was found

---

* A witness stated that *Singia* is buried in fields in which rice does not grow, and is also given to cattle in sickness. The accused also said that "it is sown with dhan and given to cattle when they are ill."

† The Kalakootki of the Bazars, Birdwood, pp. 3—48.

‡ This is the common designation of Aconite, but he may have been mistaken in the name, or may have been supplied with the root of *White Hellebore* instead.

in the corner of his chudder. On being sent to Dr. Falconer, this was found to belong to a species of Veratrum. The man stated that he had mixed some of it with other poison received from the native dealer, and had taken both together.

As Dr. Baillie observes, the symptoms closely resembled those of poisoning by Hellebore.

Mr. J. Mills has reported* the case of a man in Belgaum. Having been found sleeping, a poison was poured over the upper part of his body. Examining him six days afterwards, Mr. Mills could hardly believe it possible that strong mineral escharotics had not been applied. Wherever the poison fell, the skin was entirly destroyed, and a deep black slough was formed. A small quantity of the poison had fallen on the foot, and there a similar deep slough had formed. The surfaces appeared to be doing well for a time, but he sunk in a month.

The constituents of the poison were ascertained to be *Nerium Odorum, Plumbago Zeylandica, Semecarpas Anacardium.* "In addition there were sulphate of copper beetles (genus *mylabris*) and a snake"—supposed to have been *Amphisbœna.*

RARE CASES OF POISONING.

The Records of the Chemical Examiner's Office and the Medical Journals contain various interesting details of cases in which poisons, not commonly used in India with criminal intent, were employed.

OXALIC ACID.

Two remarkable instances of death from this poison are preserved.

In June 1852, Mr. Siddons received from the Calcutta Police a bottle, said to contain the stomach and other viscera of a native woman, supposed to have been poisoned. Upon analysis of the contents, he found a very large quantity of Oxalic Acid, quite sufficient to produce death. In a note appended to the memorandum of his deposition, Mr. Siddons observed—"This is a very remarkable case. The woman was a dhoby's wife, and these people use oxalate of potash to remove iron stains: this shows the march of intellect, and with it crime."

I am indebted to Mr. Burgess, of Howrah, for having obtained for me some interesting information on this point. He finds, by inquiry of several dhobies, that they generally endeavour to remove iron moulds by a mixture of lime-juice and common salt. When the repeated use of this fails, they resort to *Oxalic Acid,* which always succeeds, and which they call the "*burrah fit duwah.*" He had just before seen a phial of this acid in the possession of one of them.

---

* Bombay Med. and Phys. Trans., No. V., N. S., for 1859.

In September 1853, a cook in the service of one of the apothecaries, attached to the artillery division, Mooltan, was found dead in the cook-room, with his face to the wall and his right hand clasped over his stomach. On inspection, no external marks of violence were discovered. The body was that of a stout able man. The fingers and mouth had both been convulsed. The stomach was contracted strongly from spasm. Its contents were only a few grains of *dal*. The mucous surface of the lower arch was greatly and recently inflamed. Both cerebrum and cerebellum were greatly congested ; there was some slight effusion of serum beneath the pia-mater. No actual effusion of blood had occurred. The body presented no other unnatural appearances. The medical officer believed that the congestion of the brain was fully sufficient to produce death, and that the sudden inflammation of the stomach was certainly due to the presence of an acrid substance, on which account, he advised that it should be sent to the Chemical Examiner. Upon analysis, Dr. Mouat detected the presence of a very minute quantity of Oxalic Acid. Dr. Mouat suggested that, as the deceased was the servant of an assistant apothecary, he may have had access to the medicines in the hospital dispensary, and have taken the Oxalic Acid in mistake for Epsom salts, should there have been any of the former drug in store.*

The Chemical Examiner added that this is a very rare form of poisoning in India, this being the second case that has come within his knowledge in the last fourteen years.

SULPHATE OF ZINC.

According to Dr. O'Shaughnessy, cases of poisoning by this salt have occurred in Calcutta, but I cannot discover the records of any.

SULPHURIC ACID, *Gundac-ca-Atr*.

In May 1853, a native at Pilibheet, near Bareilly, while in the act of eating some sweetmeats, which had been proferred to him, complained of feeling a peculiar burning sensation in the back of his throat. He went back to the house where he had received the edible, and accused the man of having poisoned him. He died in four hours, having exhibited all the signs of irritant poisoning. On examining a portion of the sweetmeat, Dr. Mouat found that it contained a considerable quantity of Sulphuric Acid. He added that this was the first instance of poisoning by Sulphuric Acid that he had ever heard of in India.

Several cases of poisoning by this acid have occurred in Calcutta.

In the case of a young native woman who swallowed a mouthful, I, having begun to use nutritive enemata, was encouraged by my friend Dr.

---

* It is, however, difficult to perceive what purpose Oxalic Acid could serve in the dispensary of a Military hospital.

Ewart to give no other nourishment for six weeks, with the exception of a teaspoonful of iced milk occasionally, in which, latterly, isinglass was boiled.

TERMINALIA BELLERICA.—(BELLERIC MYROBALON).

Vern. *Beheyra*, Hind. ; *Behira*, Sans.—O'Shaughnessy describes the tree as growing in the mountainous parts of India, and as common in Mysore. "Drupe oval, somewhat five-angled; size, when dry, of a gall nut ; color, dirty brown ; size of a nutmeg, and fleshy, when fresh, with a grey silky down, very astringent; *kernels eaten and deemed intoxicating;* bark abounds in gum. Ainslie reckons the fruit as a stringent, tonic, and attenuant. Dose one or two direms." The only cases of poisoning by the *Bahira* have been recorded by Mr. C. E. Raddock, Sub-Assistant Surgeon, in charge of Malwa Bheel Corps. Three boys, from five to nine years of age, picked up and ate some of the dry nuts near the house of a Chumar who had brought them from the jungles for the purpose of coloring leather. Two of these boys became drowsy, complained of headache and sickness at stomach, and vomited freely a thick white frothy mucus. The third, a rather weakly boy of seven, was first seen by Mr. Raddock on the following morning. He was in his father's lap, and appeared as if asleep ; the legs and arms were relaxed and bent ; eyes closed, breathing soft. There was total insensibility; shaking and calling did not make him stir in the least, or answer. The pulse was scarcely perceptible, action of the heart frequent and weak. Body of natural warmth, legs cold, eyes rather glistening, pupils fixed, neither contracted nor dilated, jaws closed, and only to be opened by much force. This child had eaten the largest quantity of kernels—between 20 and 30. At the time, or subsequently, nothing was complained of. He played all day and at night before going to bed ; went to sleep, and was not noticed until next morning, when he was found insensible, and was supposed to be dead. With difficulty he was made to vomit three or four times, the eyes opened with a heavy dull expression, and closed again ; though he relapsed, his condition was now improved, the insensibility was not so deep, and his hand was moved to his throat. Small quantities of strong black tea were administered. About 10 A.M. he became sensible, opened his eyes, and answered when spoken to ; towards the afternoon he walked about and improved greatly. At 5 in the evening he was sensible but drowsy, pulse small and rapid, complained of being giddy, had vomited twice since morning, with relief to the symptoms. His recovery was speedy. Mr. Raddock justly infers from these cases that the *Bahira* is a mild narcotic poison. In the last-mentioned case he is convinced that it would have proved fatal, had the stomach-pump not been used, or had emetics failed. He adds that, in two of the boys who ate about the same quantity, no effects were produced till about eight hours after, and the poison was got rid of by vomiting. In the third, who ate the most, no effects were produced in 12 hours; at least, no vomiting resulted, and, during sleep, insensibility came on.*

Dr. Burton Brown, in citing this case, says that the *Terminalia Bellerica* is sometimes added to spirit in bazars, in conjunction with the *Chebulic Myrobalon (hara)* and the *Emblic Myrobalon* (*anola*), so that it is possible that an accident might occur from the use of spirit so drugged (p. 106).

Royle and Birdwood merely say that the seeds of the *Terminalia Bellerica* are eaten as nuts. O'Shaughnessy, however, adds that they "are deemed intoxicating."

EUPHORBIACEÆ.

Dr. H. Cleghorn, of Madras, has obliged me with the following note :—

There are several species of EUPHORBIA, as the *E. Neriifolia, Antiquorum, Acaulis,* and others which abound in a milky caustic juice. This produces a blister, when rubbed on the integuments ; and serious inflammation if dropped into the eye. Several cases have happened within my knowledge, where the sight has been endangered from this cause. See also Article on *Administration of Mixed Poisons*, p. 269.—Case of Fatima.

CROTON TIGLIUM.

Dr. Clemenger told me that he has heard of the Croton Oil Seed being used as a poison by some of the Punjaub tribes ; but he could only speak of this as a rumour, not having heard of any distinct case.

In February 1870, it was stated in the Calcutta Papers that a native doctor of Jubbulpore, in order to mark his sense of the inadequacy of the fee paid him by a native woman, gave her child some molasses with a few Croton seeds in it. The child shared it with two of his play-mates. All three fell seriously ill, and one of them died. The native doctor had been arrested.

My late assistant, Baboo Buddinath Brummo, knew a case in which a Calcutta Kobiraj dosed two men so severely with pills made of Croton seeds as to cause death in a few hours by hypercatharsis.

Dr. Wallich used to mention in his lectures the case of a *Mallee* (gardener) who chewed the seeds and purged to death.

The Rev. Mr. Mason mentions that, when the operation of these seeds is excessive, the Burmese native doctors give the patient the juice of the sour lime which counteracts the effect of the seed.

* Indian Annals of Medical Science, April 1855, p. 709.

JATROPHA CURCAS.

Mr. Morrett, of Salem (Madras Presidency), has fully detailed [Madras Quart. Jour. of Med. Science for July 1861, p. 37] the case of a healthy young English gentleman, who ate fifteen or twenty nuts of the Jatropha Curcas. The taste did not arouse suspicion. In an hour and-a-half, burning sensations in the throat and stomach were felt, attended with great restlessness. There was profuse purging, with great pain and vomiting, by which portions of the nut were rejected. In another hour and-a-half there were severe cramps of the lower limbs. The purging now ceased. The cramps were so violent that frequently the patient sprang in agony out of bed, and stamped his feet with all his force upon the ground as if to flatten them. The cramp distorting them. The cramps affected, with less severity, the muscles of the arms, abdomen, and back. Occasionally there were convulsive twitches of the back, almost like those in tetanus. He gradually became perfectly deaf. There was also impairment of sight. The pulse was very small, thready, and weak. Skin cold, damp, and clammy; features sunken and contracted. *Treatment.*—Hot brandy and water, warm bath, anodyne frictions, and hot bottles. In about seven hours reaction set in, and he slowly improved. Throughout the following day he remained totally deaf, and had slight cramps. Next day he was awakened by the church bell, and was quite convalesent. Although during his illness, he had appeared quite conscious, he had no recollection whatever of what happened later than the profuse purging. Several other young gentlemen were in like manner affected in a less alarming degree, having taken fewer of the nuts, but in none of them was there deafness or loss of memory.

JATROPHA MULTIFIDA.

Dr. Waring once saw a case of poisoning from three of these nuts. Violent vomiting and purging, intense pain and heat in the stomach, and great prostration of the vital powers were the principal symptoms. The patient, a young man, recovered under the use of lime-juice diluted with water and stimulants. These *French physic nuts* are regarded as even more powerfully purgative than those of the purging Croton. Under the name of *coral plant* (so called from the peculiar coral-like appearance of the flowering tops), it is often cultivated in the gardens of Europeans in India.

I am also indebted to Dr. H. Cleghorn for the following notes :—

" Hura Crepitans—the *Sand-box Tree,* introduced from the West Indies, is not uncommon at the presidency towns. The seeds are violent, dangerous purgatives, and the fruit is therefore unsafe in the hands of children, who are not unfrequently seen playing about with it.

" There are several species of Arum, requiring examination, of a suspicious, if not of a poisonous, nature. On one occasion five Mysore villagers were poisoned by partaking of the acrid rhiizomes of an arum, imperfect specimens of which I sent to Dr. Wight for identification, but he could not distinguish the species. If the roots had been boiled, the fatal results would not have occurred,—(as is well known) the deleterious property is easily driven off by heat."

Baboo Kanny Lall Dey tells me that a man went to a drug-dealer for a remedy for gonorrhœa, and got, what appears to have been, the root of one of the *aroideæ.* He died with symptoms of poisoning.

I am indebted to the same gentleman for the case of a man who is said to have died after eating some raw kuchoo (*arum*). The portion of arum plant sent for examination produced no ill effects upon a cat. It, however, appeared to be made up principally of very young leaves, in which the Assistant Chemical Examiner considered the poisonous secretion of the plant would exist in only very small quantities. Older portions of the plant might, he considered, have produced deleterious effects.

HYOSCYAMUS NIGER.

Khorassanee Ajwan, Hind. ; *Khorassanie Omum,* Tam. ; *Showkran,* Arab. ; *Sapht,* Egypt., Bunj. ; *Budjir-ul-bung, Tokhem-bung-roomee,* Pers.—Birdwood.

Henbane has been fully cultivated in India for medicinal purposes.

The *seeds* (*Khorasani Ajwain,* Hind.; *Korasani Omum,* Tam.) are common in the Indian bazars. They are stated to be imported from Turkey, and are prescribed by the Hakeems " to soothe the mind, procure sleep, and keep the bowels gently open in cases of melancholia and mania." (*Ainslie* and *Waring.*)

Dr. Birdwood mentions (p. 223) that the seeds of common Henbane are frequently used criminally in Bombay.

Hyoscyamus Insanus—Is a common plant in Belochistan, where it is known by the name of *Kokibung* or *Mountain Hemp.* Waring (p. 180) says that its powerfully poisonous properties are well known, and that it is stated to be smoked in small quantities by debauched faquirs, and to be used also for criminal purposes. The chief symptoms produced by it are dryness and constriction of the throat and furious delirium (*Stocks* in Hooker's Journ of Bot., 1852, Vol. IV., p. 178). Dr. Waring suggests that it is desirable to know more of this plant and its properties.

BELLADONNA.

Royle describes the *Atropha Acuminata,* a species nearly allied to the *A. Belladonna,* as occurring in Kunawar, on the northern face of the Himalayas.

I have already noticed cases of Belladonna poisoning which have occurred in India by solution of atrophia applied to the eye, and by Belladonna ointment placed over a blistered surface (p. 228), and by a decoction of the leaves brought from France (p. 237).

In February 1870, I saw in Dr. Chuckerbutty's ward a Bengali boy of eleven, who (as the ticket which Dr. Chuckerbutty has kindly given me shows) took about a quarter of an ounce of equal parts of Anodyne and Belladonna liniments. The symptoms were great drowsiness, wide dilatation of pupils, skin of natural temperature, a pulse so small and weak that it could not be counted. In this case some antagonism between the Opium and the Belladonna might have been anticipated; but, on the contrary, the worst effects of both were developed. In eight hours and-a-half after the liniment was swallowed, the report shows that emetics had failed to act; he could not swallow; the jaws were locked; foam issued from the mouth; he was perfectly comatose; the extremities were cold, and there was no pulse at the wrist. Galvanism, Sinapisms, hot bottles. It was not until four hours subsequently that pulsation at the wrist and vital heat began to return, and he became conscious. He now gradually rallied; but, twenty-four hours after taking the dose, the pupils were still a good deal dilated, although less than on the previous day, and the pulse was very weak and small. During the next twelve hours he was feverish, did not sleep well, and complained of great soreness over the whole body. When he was discharged on the fourth day, there was still some dilatation of the pupils.

Just as these sheets were going to press, I received from a young brother-officer and friend, who is surgeon to a distant agency, a very remarkable account of the symptoms of Belladonna poisoning lately experienced in his own person. Dr. ——— suffered from rectal neuralgia in the site of a removed pile. Four grains of extract of Belladonna, rubbed up with an ounce of water, generally gave immediate relief; but, the extract which he had being old and very dry, he obtained a fresh supply from Calcutta. He used four grains of this. In about an hour and-a-half, while at luncheon, he noticed a sudden loss of the sense of taste, nothing that he took into his mouth had any taste, but still there was a peculiar unvarying taste in his mouth, which remained quite unaffected by the now flavorless wine or food. He now attributes this to arrest of salivary secretion. The next symptoms were flushing of the face to a painful degree, with violent palpitation of the heart. He imagined that he was suffering from a paroxysm of fever. Returning to his own house, he looked at his face in the glass; it was intensely red. The pupils were widely dilated, and others described that there was a peculiar glistening of the eye. Vision dim, myopia, could not read at the usual distance. Tongue dry, skin intensely hot and dry, pulse 130, irregular, giddiness, and a sinking sensation at the epigastrium. Felt rather excited than depressed, but the violent action of the heart was very trying. The great dilatation of the pupils first caused his mind to revert to the Belladonna.

He employed a cold-water enema, took twenty drops of laudanum, and, not liking to remain alone, went over to the Residency, where the appearance of his face and the peculiarity in his eyes being noticed, he was persuaded to lie down. He now and then began to feel a little easier, though his skin was as hot as fire, with intense burning heat of the palms of the hands and soles of the feet. He sent for the native doctor, and took half-drachm doses of Nitric Ether and solution of Acetate of Ammonia every quarter of an hour. The size of the pupils had now much diminished, the palpitation was not so severe, but vision was still defective. After taking the mixture for an hour, profuse diaphoresis and diuresis occurred; and, after that, he became easier, although the pupils were still much larger than natural. The attack was followed by intense headache and nervousness, with disturbed sleep at night. He felt rather shaky next day. Dr. ——— has not since been troubled by the neuralgic affection.

CHLORODYNE.

This compound, which contains opium, chloroform, and prussic acid (Taylor), has been rather frequently swallowed in poisonous doses in this country; but, when Dr. S. C. Mackenzie published the following cases in June 1868,* he could only trace one other recorded instance,—in the *Lancet*, Vol. I, 1868. The administration of this compound to their children by mothers cannot be too strongly discountenanced.

Case I.—E. G., aged thirty-three, a Eurasian female, was admitted on the 4th June 1867, at 7 A. M. During the early part of the morning, she had quarrelled with her husband, and, while in a fit of rage, she drank an ounce of chlorodyne. When admitted she was perfectly comatose, her breathing was stertorous, and pupils contracted. The stomach was emptied by the stomach-pump, and strong coffee and other stimulants were freely administered. As she could not be roused, galvanism was applied to her body, and mustard to her extremities. These remedies proved of no avail. She gradually sunk, and died at 2-30 P. M. The autopsy was made by the Police Surgeon nineteen hours after death. The vessels of the brain were found to be much congested, and both cavities of the heart were full of dark blood of the color and consistence of black currant jelly.

Case II.—L. C., aged nineteen, a Eurasian female, was brought by her friends to hospital at 9 o'clock on the morning of the 5th September 1867. Her step-mother had found fault with her; she swallowed the contents of a bottle of chlorodyne, supposed to contain one ounce. When admitted she was sensible, but drowsy and stupid, her pupils were considerably contracted,

* Indian Medical Gazette, June 1st, 1868, p. 131.

and were not affected by light. An emetic was immediately administered, by which the stomach was emptied of a large quantity of semi-digested food impregnated with the odour of ether. Strong coffee was given, and she was made to walk for about thirteen hours when the narcotic symptoms passed off, and she was allowed to rest. Two days after she left well.

Case III.—J. M., a police constable, aged fifty (but much older in appearance, and much emaciated, apparently through disease), was admitted quite insensible, at 9 P.M., on the 13th September 1867, with stertorous breathing, a cold clammy skin, and pupils contracted to the size of a pin's point. All endeavours to rouse him proved fruitless ; he gradually sunk, and died in four hours after admission. It was found that the vessels of the brain were congested, the heart full of dark blood, the whole intestinal canal much inflamed, with a few ulcers in the ileum. He had been suffering from dysentery and, feeling worse, he procured an ounce of chlorodyne. He began to take it in small doses ; but, finding it relieved the pain, he continued to take it until, by the afternoon, he had finished the ounce. He was found by his wife, late that evening, insensible.

Case IV.—H. G. W., aged sixty-three, was admitted at 11 A.M. on 8th November 1867, with all the symptoms of narcotic poisoning. He had been drinking very hard for four or five days previously, and, while in a state of *delirium tremens*, took seven drachms of chlorodyne. An emetic of sulphate of zinc on admission, and frequent doses of strong coffee during the day. Being sensible, he was made, not without much difficulty, to walk about for twelve hours. The narcotic symptoms then passed off. He was relieved of all narcotic symptoms by the 10th.

A moderate case of chlorodyne poisoning was treated in my wards in April 1870 ; and, in the following month, it was reported that a gentleman at Madras had killed himself by swallowing this poison while in a state of insanity.

CAMPHOR.

Karpura, Sans.; *Kafur*, Arab, Hind., Dec., Malaya ; *Ghansar*, Hind.; *Carpooram*, Tam.; *Payok*, *Paroak*, Burmah; *Baroos*, Malaya.—BIRDWOOD.

The following details were sent to me in February 1869, by Dr. Bateson, of Umballa,—

A man was supposed by the police to have been given opium in some native sweetmeat *(nuddoo)* and to have died two days afterwards. He, however, walked 4 coss (8 miles) home after eating the *nuddoo* and opium. He had mortgaged his land to the people who, it was suspected, gave him the opium.

At the *post-mortem* examination the eyes were much sunken in the head, as in a case of cholera. All the organs, save the stomach, were perfectly healthy ; the inner coat of this viscus was very vascular in striated patches, running from congestion centres ; small intestines healthy ; the large gut contained a little fœces. The stomach and liver were sent to the Chemical Examiner, who reported : " A large amount of solid camphor *(kapoor)* was found in the contents of the bottle containing the stomach sent. Evidence of the presence of camphor, but of no other poison, was also found in the liver sent."

I saw a case of (moderate) camphor poisoning in Dr. Chuckerbutty's ward, in September 1869. A student, *ætat* 18, took, at 9 A.M., a pice worth of camphor, which was recommended by a quack as a cure for flatulence and dyspepsia. In about half an hour he felt giddiness and a burning sensation all over the body, and especially in the eyes. He then fell into a profound sleep, and remembered nothing more ; but the man who brought him to hospital said that he could not open his mouth, and had severe spasmodic twitchings in the muscles of the arms.

On admission at 1-13 P.M., he was quite sensible, but complained of giddiness and great lassitude. Temperature normal, pulse 76, respiration tranquil, pupils slightly dilated and responding to light. Upon the action of an emetic, the vomited matter did not smell of camphor, but, during that day, his breath did. There were, subsequently, headache, drowsiness and some difficulty in micturition and pain in the loins. He was discharged well on the next day.

QUININE.

The following important case of poisoning by Quinine is given by Mr. O'Connor, Civil Surgeon of Nowgong, Assam.* Mr. B. fell insensible in his bath-room; there was no perceptible radial pulse, and there was only a slight tremulous movement at the præcordia. A mucous fluid was running from the mouth and nostrils, eyes closed, skin cold and clammy, hands clenched. He had been taking quinine two days for intermittent fever.

He was slowly roused by ammonia and brandy. He could not speak coherently for more than an hour. He explained that, his quinine mixture having been expended, he recollected to have seen a bottle of quinine in a cupboard. He took a wine-glassful of this, and immediately fell down in the state of syncope in which he was found. The bottle was found to contain a saturated solution of quinine in dilute sulphuric acid. The wine-glassful contained 240 grains of quinine. There was a label on the bottle directing that from 5 to 15 minims should be taken in a glass of water. He remained deaf until he left Nowgong, and he soon afterwards died.

POISONOUS FUNGI.

My friend, Dr. Charles Palmer, of Calcutta, has obliged me with the following interesting note, which certainly appears to point to the exist-

* Ind. Med. Gaz., July 1, 1867, p. 181.

ence in Bengal a fungus resembling the mushroom in form and flavor, and possessing the intoxicating principle *(amanitine)* which has rendered *Amanita Muscaria* so remarkable.*

The following instances of poisoning by mushrooms occurred many years since (1853). I regret I have no notes of the cases, and am consequently wholly dependent upon my memory.

In June 1853, I had been absent for a couple of days from my station, Jessore; and, on my return, was requested by the Collector to visit Mr. C. S., the Assistant Magistrate and Collector, who, the previous morning, had conducted himself in a very extraordinary manner in the Collector's Court, was apparently very drunk and was sent home by the Collector. Mr. C. S. was a young civilian, very accomplished, and of refined taste, temperate in his habits, and it appeared improbable that he could have been drinking to excess at this early hour, 11 A.M. I immediately visited Mr. C. S., and found him in a state of great depression and distress, from the recollection of the occurrences of the preceding day. He informed me he had had his breakfast as usual; had a small bottle of claret which he always took, and was not aware of having partaken of anything unusual and certainly not to excess. That he went to Cutcherry at the usual hour, and felt unable to control his actions; felt drunk; every thing and person appeared ludicrous; he laughed immoderately in open court, joked with the Omlahs, and ridiculed in an absurd way his superior officer, the Collector, by whom he was taken to his house. After some hours he recovered, considerably depressed from the effects of the stimulant, and from the feeling of shame at having made such a ridiculous spectacle of himself before his court, but more so, as he assured me, that this was the third time a similar attack had seized him, and he feared he would go mad, for he could not, with the utmost effort, control his actions, and had been seized in precisely the same manner at the same time of the year, three years in succession. Mr. S. was in such wretched spirits about this that I thought it right to remain with and watch him, and told him I would go home and dress, and return to tiffin. This I did, and this leads me to the second case, my own. During tiffin I felt myself unusually excited, and at once enquired how much beer I had taken. I found that I had had about half a bottle, and no other beverage such as sherry; but we had stewed mushrooms, and the truth at once flashed across me, that my friend had been intoxicated with mushrooms. He now told me he had had mushrooms for breakfast the previous day, and recollected that, on the former occassions, when similarly seized, he had eaten mushrooms provided by the same servant. I can-

* I have never heard of any instance but this in which Europeans in India were poisoned by mushrooms, although they are rather liable to disagree. It is strange that, anxious as the poor are to gather every edible product that the soil of India affords, very few natives will eat mushrooms—which they call *beeng ke chatta*, toads'-umbrellas.

not describe the joy my poor friend exhibited when I told him I had discovered the *fons et origo* of his madness, and that I was myself rapidly getting mad too! The Fungi had been gathered from the ground covering the roots of trees, not from open plain, and Mr. S. did not partake of them at this meal. As he had got over his three bouts of mushroom with no permanent ill-effects, I declined finishing my bottle of beer, but went on with the mushrooms: the effect was very convincing and rapid. I was, in short, soon in a state of most exhilarated and pleasant intoxication. Two friends, one the Clergyman, and the other the Magistrate of the station, who dropped in to inquire for Mr. S., could not be persuaded but that my intoxication was the result of alcohol. My symptoms were identical to those described by Mr. S.; every person appeared ridiculous, the most ordinary remark was full of fun and wit, and my immoderate laughter provoked equal merriment in others. I took a drive in the evening, and I never before or since have seen the lights and shades cast by the setting sun so brilliant, and every object looking so perfectly beautiful. These exaggerated sensations continued for some hours; indeed at the request of my friends I put an end to them by taking a full dose of ipecacuanha, and thus got rid of a considerable quantity of the Fungi still undigested. I experienced no after ill effects whatever.

The species of Fungus partaken of must, I presume, have been the *amanita*, and the almost immediate effect is a fact worthy of note.

CUCURBITACEÆ.

Dr. Burton Brown includes the Cucumis Colocynthis, Cucumis Pseudo Colocynthis, and Cucumis Hardwickii, among Indian poisons.

The whole of the Cucurbitaceæ are of questionable wholesomeness, although several of the species form staple articles of food to millions in India. Against *Lagenaria vulgaris*, the Kuddo, which almost every one eats, Dr. Birdwood notes: "Lindley states that some sailors were once poisoned by beer which had been standing in a hollowed bottle-gourd; and that there is reason to believe that some, if not all the edible sorts of Cucurbits owe their freedom from poisonous properties to cultivation, for some in a wild state are found to possess them in much activity" (p. 158).

Dr. A. Walker mentions that, although the natives of the Bombay Presidency use the edible Cucurbitaceæ very freely, they are strongly impressed with a belief in their unwholesome nature, and rarely fail to attribute any severe sickness to an abundant crop of them.

Royle says, in his work on the Himalayas (p. 219), that the wild and bitter variety of *Lagenaria vulgaris*, called *toombee*, and used for making fukeers' bottles, is considered poisonous. He was informed by an intelligent native doctor at Seharunpore that he had seen a case of poisoning from eating the bitter pulp of *toombee*, in whch the symptoms were those of cholera. Some years ago an aged officer, residing in the Hills, died in a few hours with violent symptoms of irritant poisoning after (if not in consequence of) eating *kuddo* pie.

Native Surgeon R. Moodelly mentions (p. 316), that he has heard of the death of an individual from the use of the Seeds of a *wild cucumber* as a purgative.

Trichosanthes Dioica, the *pulbull*, *potole*. Baboo Kanny Lall Dey says, that the root acts like *elaterium*, for which it may be substituted. Sub-Assistant Surgeon Koylas Chunder Chatterjee told me that the wild variety is poisonous, as is the *potole* root is in an over-dose. My assistant, Baboo Tarucknath Ganguly, informs me that cases of violent hypercatharsis, from such doses, occur frequently in Bengal villages.

GAMBOGE.

Mr. A. Jamsetjee has published the case of a delicate Parsee female, aged nineteen, who took about *three drachms** of Pipe Gamboge (value three pie) for the purpose of self-destruction. When, some five hours afterwards, she was collapsed from the violent vomiting and purging, which commenced about two hours after taking the drug, the matters passed were of a deep yellow color, and the pain and suffering were very great. Stimulants were given and frictions employed, and the collapse passed off ; but the evacuations continued frequent, with straining and griping, and were chiefly of yellow mucus for some days afterwards. She recovered slowly.

SANTONINE.

Two cases have been recorded† by Mr. Chipperfield, of Madras, in which Santonine produced distinct symptoms of constitutional poisoning. A very sickly native girl, *ætat* 13, having previously used this medicine, took three grains of Santonine in three drachms of castor oil. The results were hypercatharsis, vomiting, and extreme prostration. The evidences of poisoning were a semi-comatose condition, extreme dilatation of the pupils, urine of an intense yellow color. There was very great vertigo, everything appeared to be dancing round her, though she could see nothing distinctly ; all objects had a green hue.

A European child, a robust little boy aged five years, took three grains of Santonine in sugar, at bed-time. Soon afterwards he fell asleep, but awoke in about half an hour, got out of bed, and with the most uproarious mirth rushed into the room where his parents were taking dinner. His

---

* Bombay Med. and Phys. Trans, No. 2, for 1853-4, page 340.

† Madras Quar. Jour. of Med. Science, October 1862, p. 448.

head was very hot, and his pupils were widely dilated, he appeared a good deal excited, and asked for wine, which was refused him. He was desired to go to bed again, which he did, but he could not sleep, and said the cot kept dancing with him. He became still more excited, related humourous and fanciful anecdotes, laughed loudly, and at last retired to rest with his mother. As soon as he lay down he declared the cots and the room were going round with him, that his mother had turned into a green woman, that the sheets were green, and the walls were green. He became a little fractious, and complained of great thirst. After drinking a quantity of iced water he fell asleep. During the night he was much disturbed by dreams and awoke several times, and asked for water. In the morning he was quite well. A dose of senna was given him, but he passed no worms.

Mr. Chipperfield cites a case of Santonine poisoning, by Dr. Lohrman, in the London Medical Review, for July 1862.

GLORIOSA SUPERBA.

Kurreeare, Cariari, Hind.

According to Dr. Waring (p. 242), Hermann, Roxburgh, and others speak of the root of this handsome climbing plant as violently poisonous, but none of these authorities furnish any details of a case in which its ill-effects have been observed. A belief in its poisonous properties is, however, common amongst the natives of all parts of India. Dr. Bidie informs Dr. Waring that, in Mysore, he found *Bish (root of Aconitum Ferox)* largely adulterated with the roots of this plant. In Travancore, a remedy held in esteem in the treatment of gonorrhœa is a white farinaceous powder obtained from this root by bruising and repeated washing and maceration. Dr. Waring adds that it is very desirable to obtain further information with regard to its properties. Dr. Birdwood mentions that it is said to be a substitute for Colchicum.

Only two cases of poisoning by this root (both fatal) have come before the Calcutta Chemical Examiner, both the transmitting letters being, by a very singular coincidence, dated the 24th October 1867. The details of both are unfortunately slight.

Case I.—Dr. R. D. Logg, Civil Surgeon of Pertabgurh, sent down portions of the fresh root, stalk, and leaves of a creeping plant bearing a seed, and called by the natives *kuryaree,* together with the contents of the stomach of a woman who destroyed herself by swallowing a m—— [*masha ?*] of the same. The notes of the *post-mortem* examination are considered to show that the action of *Kurreeare* is that of a narcotico irritant poison.

Case II.—Dr. Chandra, in civil medical charge of Deoghur (Sonthal Pergunnahs), sent on from Mr. J. T. Blumhardt, Assistant Commissioner of Goddah, the roots and seed-vessels of the "Gloriosa Superba" (Urdu

Kareearee ; Bengali, *Ognishikha*). "About two tolahs weight of the root was administered with some *salt* and *red-lead* to the deceased Deba Pahariah."

QUERCUS FEROX.

It is mentioned in the Police Report, L. P., for 1843, p. 40, that "two persons, a wife and her paramour, who poisoned the husband of the first by administering to him in his food some *Hurrema meeta (Quercus ferox)*, had been sentenced to suffer death.

Piddington gives *Hurineea-batana* (for which "*Hurrema*" is probably a misprint) as the vernacular name of *Quercus ferox.* This is a large timber tree, native of the Chittagong Hills, *vide Roxburgh Flora Indica*, Vol. III, p. 639.

DAPHNADS.

India produces several poisonous members of this genus (see Royle, p. 321). Dr. Birdwood thinks that the root of the bazars may be obtained from more than one Daphne. Dr. Burton Brown mentions one species, *Gundhera,* which is the root and stem of a shrub growing in the Hills, which acts as a powerful irritant. It is recognised by the peculiar woody tissue which forms the inner bark, and which is composed of long white fibres easily separable from the wood. It has a peculiar acrid taste, and causes vomiting and death from inflammation of the stomach, but its other symptoms are not well known.

MUDAR.

Calatropis Hamiltonii.

Arka, Akund, Svaytaurkum, Sans.; *Ak, Mudar,* Hind.; *Rowee,* By.; *Yecada,* Can.; *Yercum, Vullerkoo,* Tam.; *Neela-jeeleeroo,* Tel.; *Mooduwara,* Cey.; *Maioh,* Burmah ; *Oshmar, Oschar,* Arab ; *Bejd-eloschar, Erminion ?* (Kercher), Egypt. White variety,—*Alarka,* Sans. ; *Shwet akund* and *Urka,* Ben.; *Tellajelladoo,* Tel. ; The Sugar, *Sukkur-ool-ashur,* Vulg. The Spirit,—*Bar,* By. (BIRDWOOD.)

In the Chapter on Infanticide in the last edition of this work, mention was made of the practice of murdering new-born female infants by forcing the milky juice of the *mudar* down their throats. In the Indian Medical Gazette for April and June 1867, pp. 106 and 148, Mr. McReddie, medical officer of Hurdui, again drew attention to this mode of infanticide, and suggested that an investigation should be made with a view to the detection of this poison by chemical analysis. He, at the same time, gave the results of some experiments upon puppies. Mr. McReddie infers from them that mudar juice is acrid, but that it is not, as it is supposed to be by the natives, a narcotic poison.

SEMECARPUS ANACARDIUM.

Nrooskura, Bullatakee, Sans. ; *Bhela, Belawina, Bhelaman, Bhelawan,* Hind. ; *Gheru,* Can. ; *Kampira,* Mal. ; *Shayngcottay, Shayrangcottay,* Tam. ; *Nellajidi, Jeedighendzadoo, Bhallataki, Bhallatamu,* Tel. ; *Kiribadulla,* Cey. ; *Chai-bin,* Pegu. (BIRDWOOD.)

A case in which a singular vesicular eruption was produced by the external application of the juice of the *Marking Nut,* will be found recorded by Mr. A. Gibson, in the Transactions of Medical and Physical Society of Bombay, Vol. I, p. 332. See also p. 271 of this volume, in which the juice, mixed with other vesicants, caused fatal blistering.

Dr. Balfour says, *(Timber Trees of India)* that the juice of the tree is so acrid that wood-cutters are unwilling to cut the tree until after it has been killed by ringing the bark ; this acridity also renders the wood dangerous to work.

Sir W. O'Shaughnessy Brooke found that a minute drop of the juice, placed on the back of his hand, occasioned the eruption of an herpetic blotch, intensely itchy, and scaling from the centre towards the circumference, which did not disappear for eight months, and left a scar like that of a boil (p. 280).

Dr. Honigberger notes (p. 228) that, at Lahore, he discovered that some of the prisoners rubbed the juice of this nut on their eyes ; others had rubbed it on their bodies. The former were, apparently, suffering from incurable ophthalmia, the latter from a kind of ring-worm. By this means they contrived to remain on the sick list, eating and drinking without being necessitated to work.

According to Dr. Percival Lord* the Marking Nut, brought from Goa, is applied externally, as a rubefaciant, for chronic rheumatism, indolent swellings, &c. The natives also use it in some of their aphrodisiac mixtures, and it is said to be safely taken internally if mixed with cocoanut-oil. Dr. A. Walker† says that this juice is very generally employed by the natives as an epispastic, and is also taken internally in venereal complaints, the belief in its efficacy in these being, most probably, derived from the old doctrine of signature which prevails in India as a popular notion. He adds that every one who has had any practice among natives (Bombay Presidency) must have seen the troublesome and sometimes fatal consequences produced by its abuse. Its effects on different individuals are strangely dissimilar ; on some it acts simply as a blister, while on others deep ulcerations with sloughing and even death itself (if the scrotum be the part on which it is put) are the results of its application ; even sleeping under the tree is said to be attended with very troublesome conse-

* Bombay Medical and Physical Transactions, for 1841, p. 117.

† *Ibid* for 1840, p. 68.

quences. By subjecting the juice to a species of distillation, it is said to be rendered more manageable as an epispastic. The whole nut is given to horses in farcy. The native farriers commence by giving one a day, and gradually increase the dose by one, till they reach fifteen, which is the maximum given. They then decrease the quantity by one; they think it a good remedy.

Dr. J. Newton (cited by Waring) mentions that the bruised nut, applied locally to the os uteri, is one of the means in use amongst native women for procuring abortion.

POUNDED GLASS.

Baboo Kanny Lall Dey informs that, about ten years ago, some cooked *sag* (spinach) was sent to Dr. Macnamara for inspection. He detected a large quantity of powdered glass in the mess. It was proved that the kidmutgar who served the dish introduced the glass with the intention of poisoning his master. On the 28th of November 1869, an Italian woman, *ætat* 20, was brought to the Medical College Hospital, said to have swallowed about three drachms of powdered glass with suicidal intent. The bowels were constipated. As there were no symptoms, she took an ounce of castor oil and left. Dr. R. Haines has published an interesting case in which a Mahratta artist of Bombay, having been seized in the act of committing a robbery, managed to break up and swallow a quantity of bottle glass. The remainder of the bottle was produced—a reddish brown quart bottle, such as Rhenish wine is imported in. He merely complained of a little pricking sensation in the throat and stomach. He was made to vomit, but no glass was ejected. He took castor oil; the stools were yellow and loose, not bloody. At the bottom of the vessel were found a number of pieces of thin bottle-glass, precisely corresponding with the remains of the bottle shown by the policeman. There were about twenty fragments of various sizes, the largest an inch long by a quarter of an inch broad, the smallest as large as a grain of rice. There was considerable tenderness at the epigastrium which continued more or less until his discharge on the 8th day.

Mr. Haines remarks that cases of this kind are by no means unfrequent in that part of India, the idea of the poisonous nature of pounded glass being even more generally received among the natives than in Europe. It is generally taken for the purpose of committing suicide. One or two other such cases have come under his observation since the one above mentioned. Where such large fragments, slender and sharp-pointed, have been swallowed, some degree of danger, he thinks, must always exist of the pieces sticking cross-wise in some portion of the intestinal tube, and producing ulceration, which might lead to the laying open either of a large vessel or of the cavity of the peritoneum. Hence, he insists, it will always be advisable to keep the patient under observation for ten or twelve days, by which time symptoms of such ulceration, if it existed, would manifest themselves.

In Mrs. Florence Marryat's recently published book "Gup," allusion is made to a woman at Bangalore who poisoned some intruding dogs with ground glass, and they died in great pain. In his report on Cattle Poisoning, Dr. Walker, Chemical Examiner, Allahabad, mentions what he appears to have considered a trumped-up case, in which pounded glass was submitted as the poisoning agent.

It is very singular, however, with how much impunity fragments of glass have frequently been swallowed. It seems to have been a rather common practice among mountebanks and drunkards, in the last century, to eat the glass after drinking its contents. Sound teeth and strong jaws appear generally to have afforded these idiots an impunity which they scarcely deserved.*

In March 1856, a street mountebank placed himself before my window in Calcutta and, to my full belief, eat part of a common black bottle.

There cannot be a doubt that powdered glass is a powerful mechanical irritant, although Taylor shows (Poisons, p. 15) that its effects vary much in different cases. I suspect that this depends almost wholly upon the degree of levigation. A woman swallowed a quantity of coarsely-powdered glass, in order to "scour out" her stomach. Intense pain in the stomach came on with tenderness ; the pulse became small, 100 in the minute, and there were thirst and pallor of countenance. An emetic was given, a part of the glass was rejected. Afterwards stimulants and Aqua Lauro-Cerasi were employed ; the next day the urgency of the symptoms had passed of, and she completely recovered.†

A writer in *Notes and Queries*‡ mentions that he has heard of several persons whose death was attributed to mechanical poisoning with pounded glass. He knows that this material has been too commonly employed (chiefly by jealous negresses) on the west coast of Africa, to ensure the death of a rival or a faithless lover,—the finely-powdered glass being introduced into some favorite food, the native "foo foo" for example.

---

* The well-known expressions "crush a cup of wine," "crush a pot," "crack a bottle," are probably founded upon this practice. Linschoten, the naval historian, says of Sir Richard Greenville, the brave admiral : "He was of so hard a complexion that, often, when he had other captains for his guests, he would carouse three or four glasses of wine ; and then in a bravery take the glasses between his teeth, crush them in pieces and swallow them, that the blood sometimes ran out of his mouth. This was told me (adds Linschoten) by divers credible persons who had many times seen him do it." Some Arab jugglers, calling themselves of the tribe of Aissahouha, lately in London professed to masticate tumblers. The editor of a leading medical journal considered that this was a mere trick, as one would not be likely very long to survive the real performance.

† N. Sydenham Society's Year Book for 1863, p. 401.

‡ Third Series, Vol. II., p. 159.

DIAMOND DUST.

Although this material has no place, in Dr. Taylor's treatise, among the mechanical irritant poisons, it is certain that a belief in its deadly potency existed long ago in Europe, and that the same idea is, at present, of considerable prevalence in India.

It is considered that the *Powder of Succession* of the Italian poisoners was diamond dust. Benvenuto Cellini relates that an attempt was made to poison him, when in prison at Rome, by the administration of pounded diamond in his food, and that he escaped in consequence of the accomplice reserving the valuable diamond for himself, and substituting powdered glass. He says that the diamond is not poisonous in itself, but that it acts mechanically by perforating the intestines, which no other sort of stone or glass can do.* He adds that it was not to produce its effect for four or five months. One of the Duke of Orleans's old servants told Voltaire, of Henrietta, Duchess of Orleans, who died in 1680, with symptoms of acute irritant poisoning, that "the poison was a diamond reduced to powder, and strewed with pounded sugar over some strawberries." †

Captain Burton has noted that the Hindus of the present day consider that the diamond is poisonous. Baboo Kanny Lall Dey confirms this. He says that Sir William O'Shaughnessy Brooke mentioned, in his lectures at the Medical College of Calcutta, that he was once called to an Armenian gentleman of this city, who had swallowed a whole diamond, with the intention of destroying himself. A purgative removed the stone which was, very properly, presented to the Physician. Baboo Kanny Lall Dey also tells me that, a native of wealth going to prison with a diamond ring on his finger, it was considered that the reason for taking it away was lest he should use the stone as a poison. Sub-Assistant Surgeon Meer Ashruff Ali, Teacher of Midwifery in the Calcutta Medical College, informs me that he attended a Greek lady at Agra who, in a fit of passion, attempted to kill herself by swallowing a diamond of about the value of a hundred rupees, which she had taken for that purpose from a ring. He adds that the idea of the poisonous quality of this gem is now prevalent even among women in Bengal, and that it was reported in native society that an European gentleman, in Lord Dalhousie's time, who had got into trouble in the Central Provinces, destroyed himself by swallowing a diamond. He believes this idea to be principally due to a confusion of the words "*Zewar, Jauhar,*" Jewel, and *Zahr*, Poison, and also to the fact that, in several dramas by Kali Das and others, the diamond is represented as a poison. My House Physician, Baboo Taruknath Ganguly, has obtained for me the following passage from one of these plays.‡ A wronged woman

* Autobiography, Chap. XIII.

† Life of Louis XIV, p. 101, Vol. I.

‡ "Biddabha Bibaho Nattuck," by Baboo Womesh Chunder Mitter.

exclaims: "It is said that diamond destroys life." *(Addressing the diamond ring presented by her lover)* "Ah most beautiful ornament! A moment more and thou wilt destroy the life of her whose finger thou adornest, thou wilt kill the love which it was thy commission to preserve!"

Upon this point that eminent Sanskrit Scholar, the Raja Kalikrishna Bahadur, informs me that he, and also a learned and experienced Kaviraj (physician) of Calcutta, consider that diamond dust can only injure as a mechanical irritant. The Raja heard long ago of instances, in Calcutta, of death caused by swallowing diamond, "and he believes that they are authentic." He adds—"In ancient writings we meet with similar occurrences, which are consistent with reason."

The Raja cites a work, "*Bhavaprakasha,*" to the effect that the diamond, when properly calcined, increases life, energy, health, beauty and happiness, and undoubtedly destroys all sorts of maladies. It also increases the sight of the eyes. Another work, the *Raj-bullabha,* mentions that the diamond has the properties of causing purging, vomiting, dulness and astringency, and of being agreeable to taste.

We are told* that, when Ajmir was invested by De Boigne, the faithful Governor, Dumraj, a Rajpoot, placed in the dilemma of a disgraceful surrender or disobedience to his prince's summons, swallowed diamond-powder. "Tell the Raja," said this faithful servant, "thus only could I testify my obedience: and over my dead body alone could a Southron enter Ajmir."

These facts gain considerable importance when placed in co-relation with the following case which occurred at Sylhet in 1855. Mussamut Fool Bebee was tried for having murdered Sullimoollah (with whom she had formerly cohabited, but who had offended her by marrying another woman) by giving him something in a cup of milk which brought on fatal vomiting and purging. The body was in too decomposed a state to admit of examination.

The prisoner confessed that she administered a powder of ground diamond to the deceased in milk, soon after which he became ill and died the next day. She declared throughout, that the poison had been given to her by another to administer, but that she gave it to her master as medicine, he being ill of fever. She never admitted that she had given poison to kill from anger at her master having married another, when he had promised to marry her. It was, however, in evidence that she used to declare that deceased had brought her to his house with promise of marriage, and that she administered a poison in milk which killed him a few days after his marriage, and she stated that the person who gave her the powder to administer told her to mix it *secretly.* She was convicted of murder by poison on violent presumption, and sentenced to imprisonment for life.†

* Todd, Vol. II., p. 134.

† Nizamut Adawlut Reports, May 4, 1855, p. 503.

Doubtless, this woman believed that what she gave was diamond dust. It may, however, be doubted whether it was not some ordinary poison such as arsenic, especially as it was given in milk. Still this case and the following one are of sufficient significance to prove that the tendency to employ diamond dust as a poison still exists in India. About eighteen months ago, an Up-Country dealer in jewels, residing in the Burra Bazar, was brought to the Medical College Hospital having, it was stated, swallowed *diamond dust;* as there were not any symptoms he left, after having taken an aperient.

HAIR, &c.

The late Dr. Cantor informed me that the administration, in curry or other soft food, of very finely-chopped human hair is a recognised mode of slow poisoning in Singapore, especially by women intent upon destroying their husbands. Paris mentions (Vol. II, p. 145) that it has been asserted that human hair, chopped fine, constitutes the active ingredient of a slow poison frequently employed in Turkey, and that it induces, by irritation, a chronic disease resembling cancer.

Dr. Honigberger mentions that there exists an idea, Up-Country, that tigers' smellers are poisonous, and General Ramsay informed me that such a notion is prevalent. There cannot be a doubt that, chopped up rather finely, these coarse bristles would act as a mechanical irritant.

Baboo Kanny Lall Dey tells me that hair is sometimes used by cattle-poisoners. It is well known that cattle and camels are not unfrequently killed by the formation of large hairy concretions in their stomachs. And, of late, more than one case has been reported in the English journals of women whose death has been caused by the habit of swallowing their own hair.

Dr. Francis Macnamara informed me, in 1856, that he had lately received for examination certain pills, supposed to contain poison, which appeared to be chiefly made up of prickly particles of grass. The mass was regarded as a mechanical irritant without trace of any chemical poison.

Dr. John Murray, Superintendent of the Madras Lunatic Asylum, has recently communicated* a case of fatal peritonitis and bowel-obstruction caused in a native insane woman by eating the husks and seeds (with which the colon was completely filled throughout its whole course) of the *Guazama tormentosa*, a tree devoid of poisonous property.

It frequently happened, in India, when it was customary to make teats of wash-leather, that infants swallowed the piece of SPONGE which was tied at the mouth of their nursing bottles. The accident generally caused much alarm; but, in two cases which I saw, the foreign body was passed in a few hours without causing any inconvenience. The general use of gutta-percha teats has, perhaps, put an end to these accidents.

---

* Madras Monthly Journal of Med. Science, May 1870.

CARBONIC ACID.

It appears probable that the incautious manner in which the natives burn charcoal in close ill-ventilated rooms must, not unfrequently, lead to fatal results, at least where the practice is followed in brick houses—the smaller huts are rarely sufficiently air-tight to prevent the escape of the gas. Dr. Baillie, when stationed at Hooghly, mentioned to me a case of this kind which occurred in his practice. He was in attendance upon the infant of a wealthy Hindu suffering from an ordinary attack of fever. After the usual symptoms had been abated, he was surprised to find that the child always appeared to be drowsy. On one or two occasions, he found that the atmosphere of the small brick room in which the child lay was unusually close—and that the child appeared to revive when the windows were opened. On about the third day, he found the child lying upon the lap of a nurse, who was seated on the ground close to a pan of charcoal, with the fumes of which the room was almost unsupportably redolent. The infant lay torpid, as usual—but soon revived and did well in a clear atmosphere. It subsequently appeared that the child had been thus exposed to the influence of the poison for several days.

Baboo Kanny Lall Dey tells me of the case of a woman who took a young infant to nurse. She lay down with the child at night in a small close upper room in a brick house—a pan of ignited charcoal stood by. In the morning the child was found to be dead, and the nurse insensible.

During the rains, charcoal pans are much used in European houses for drying towels, &c., which are spread on a bamboo frame over the pan. I have found my own children sitting round a carbonic acid manufactory of this kind, when the air of a lofty room had become very perceptibly vitiated by carbonic acid.

It was reported in the Calcutta Papers in May 1856 that, several deaths having recently occurred by persons descending into wells for lotas which had been dropped, the Chief Magistrate, at the recommendation of the Coroner, had ordered a notice to be given by beat of tomtom throughout the native part of the town, warning the people of the danger of going down into wells, without taking the precaution of ascertaining whether a light will burn near the surface of the water. It would seem that this mode of warning is an old custom which had fallen into disuse.

As this copy lies before me, the same evil is complained of in the morning Papers.* It is stated that, during the past few months, there have been reported, in both the town and suburbs of Calcutta, several deaths from this cause. A native went down a well in Bortollah, to pick up a brass spoon, and lost his life. Another case, in Toltollah, would also have been

---

* *Indian Daily News*, 31st May 1870.

fatal had not some lascars promptly let down a rope and pulled the man up in a state of insensibility. These accidents are most frequent in the hot weather before much rain has fallen, when the wells are nearly dry.

TARTARIZED ANTIMONY.

I mentioned in my last edition an instance in which a family, residing near Calcutta, had suffered greatly from the stupidity of a native servant, who added a quantity of this preparation, which he found lying about, to a curry, mistaking it for salt !

Native Surgeon Moodelly gives, in the paper already cited, the case of an enfeebled native woman in whom a dose, little exceeding a quarter of a grain, of tartar emetic produced serious symptoms of poisoning. In March 1868, four Mahomedans who had been eating a mess of rice, dal, and curry together, were attacked in half an hour with rather violent symptoms of tartar emetic poisoning, and were brought to my ward. The symptoms were severe vomiting, purging, burning sensation at the epigastrium, cramps in the arms, great prostration, thirst. They recovered quickly.

HYDRATED OXIDE OF LEAD.

The practice of keeping drinking-water in long-necked leaden bottles, which do not admit of being properly cleaned out, most undoubtedly has led to much severe illness in this country. Filtered rain water of great purity, almost perfectly free from saline matter, being commonly in use, the chemical action of this fluid upon the containing leaden vessels must be incessant. About eighteen years since, having to prepare some medicine at a patient's house, I called for water, which was brought in a leaden surai. Upon pouring it out, I was startled to find it perfectly milky from admixture, as was afterwards proved, with a very large quantity of Oxide of Lead. It was found that the water (about half a pint) had been standing in the vessel for nearly a week. Had the invalid called for this draught in the night, it would, in all probability, have destroyed life.

When in medical charge at Howrah, I was consulted by a gentleman for a weakness in one of his feet. On endeavouring to plant the foot firmly on the ground, one of the muscles of the sole, probably the adductor pollicis, appeared to fail suddenly ; he was therefore compelled to rest in walking on the heel and outer side of the foot. This had come on gradually without any hurt, that he was aware of, or other apparent cause. Being almost at a loss to account for this, I inquired whether his servants kept his drinking-water in leaden vessels. He at once replied that he had purchased one at Moulmein, and had used it constantly until a short time previously, *when the neck had come off.* There was no appearance of a lead line upon the gums, and, as he appeared in robust health, I merely recommended frictions and the salt-and-water douche, and advised him to wear an inflexible sole. The weakness gradually wore off, and he has since walked firmly.

In June 1870, Dr. W. Palmer, Officiating Chemical Examiner to Government, having heard that a child living in a Calcutta house, wherein the new water supply was conducted by means of leaden pipes, had suffered in a way not unfrequently induced by lead-poisoning, instituted a series of experiments, and reported to the Justices that the water contained metallic lead equalling 57 of a part to one million parts. An individual might thus swallow in a month, a quantity equalling six-tenths of a grain of sugar of lead. He considers that, as lead is a cumulative poison, the child suffered from the effects of the poison, as the proportion of lead contained in the water varies with varying circumstances. He, therefore, maintained the necessity of forbidding the use of lead pipes, except those lined with tin, which, if properly made, effectually prevent contamination.

The following case of lead poisoning was sent me by Dr. Wise of Dacca in 1865.

Colica Pictonum. Gondial Singh, a native of Hindoostan, but for several years a Chowkidar at an Indigo factory in this district, suffered from Syphilitic disease and from an eruption attended with much itching. One of the head servants at the factory gave him an infallible (?) cure in the following :

Moorda Sung (Litharge)	1 tolah
White Sugar	1 pan

These, after being mixed, were divided into seven powders, and one was ordered to be taken every day. Each powder contained a little over 25 grains of Litharge. The first dose was taken on the 6th February, and for five days he daily swallowed one. He then became seriously ill, with violent pain at the navel, constipation, vomiting, trembling of the extremities, and *retention of urine*. For three days, he says, he passed no urine, and for eight he had no stool. Warm poultices of neem leaves caused a free discharge of urine. On the 13th March I first saw him. He was then unable to stand or to raise his arms. He complained of a twisting pain around the navel, his bowels were obstinately costive, but there was no distension of the abdomen, nor retraction of the muscles. A distinct blue line was found running parallel to, but at the distance of a few lines from, the edge of the gums. No bad taste in the mouth was complained of. There were great emaciation and debility. From the above date until his death on the 27th March, emaciation proceeded rapidly. Paralysis of the muscles of the arms, causing the characteristic *drop-wrist*, was well marked. His bowels remained obstinately costive, except when purgatives were given.

The treatment adopted was Castor-oil with Croton-oil, Iodide of Potassium with Citrate of Quinine and Iron. Latterly galvanism was tried.

Moorda Sung, mixed with ghee or wax, is a favorite application of the Kobiraj in diseases of the skin. It is rarely used internally.

Two cases of Colica Pictonum in natives have been reported by Dr. W. S. Charters.* The patients were two suwars, who had been some time previously under Dr. Charters' treatment for syphilis, but who had recently (each) taken three white powders, one on three successive days, prescribed for them by a Fukeer. This man made no secret of his prescription, and said that he had been constantly in the habit of giving such medicine with impunity, prescribing, at the same time, certain rules and restrictions regarding diet, which, he said, they had neglected to follow and had suffered in consequence. His receipt was as follows :

1 tola (about 3 drachms) of "Bans Lochan" "Bamboo eyes," small nodules found in the pith of some species of bamboo.

2 tolas of "Moorda Sung," (Litharge) rubbed up together, and made into three powders. One powder given daily, in a portion of rice and ghee, for three successive days.

Dr. A. Smith has published an account of *an epidemic of Colic apparently caused by the presence of Lead in the sugar and arrack* served out to the men of H. M. 37th Regiment, at Newera Elha, Ceylon, in 1862.—Monthly Medical Journal, March 1853, p. 202.

A fatal case of *colica pictonum* is given by Dr. Morehead in the first volume of his treatise.

HYDROCYANIC ACID.

Up to the time of the publication of the last edition of this work in 1856, no case of poisoning by Prussic Acid in India had been reported. Subsequently there have been several—the first having been that of an assistant in the Calcutta Medical Stores Department. Baboo Kanny Lall Dey has noticed that those who have selected this poison have generally been persons of some education.† He has had four cases brought under his notice within the last two years.

For the detection of this poison in the viscera he recommends that they should be preserved in strong spirit which tends to retain the Prussic Acid in the tissues. Subsequently the distillation process can be adopted, the acid distilling off with the spirit, in which it is detectable by the usual liquid tests. The spirit can be easily driven off from the distillate, while

---

* Trans. Medical and Physical Society of Bombay, 1853-54, p. 340.

† Dr. Honigberger hazards the statement that "Maharajah Sheer Sing, having heard of this poison, procured a phial from Agra, probably for the purpose of poisoning his minister the Rajah Dhyan Sing; but, on his majesty's having been informed that I was aware of his having received the poison, he pretended that he had sent for it to try some experiments on dogs; and handed to me the phial unopened. Very soon after, the enigma was solved by their mutual destruction." (Vol. II., p. 288.)

the escape of the acid may be prevented by fixing it with re-agents forming stable compounds, *viz.*, Nitrate of Silver and Sulphide of Ammonium.

CYANIDE OF POTASSIUM.

The introduction of this salt for photographic and electro-plating purposes has been followed by several cases of poisoning by its means. One of the earliest was that of a European, at Kurrachee, noticed by Dr. B. Brown. The symptoms were complete insensibility, pulse almost imperceptible, breathing slow, pupils dilated, and rapid death.

Dr. Brown mentions that this salt had (in 1863) been actually made in Lahore by natives, so that an accident might easily occur.

Five years later, in 1868, the wife of a Mahomedan electro-plater, living in Mirzapore, a Suburb of Calcutta, destroyed herself, by swallowing this salt of native manufacture, as Baboo Kanny Lall Dey found on analysis that it was very impure, and contained much of the undecomposed Ferrocyanide. A portion of the stuff was found and was produced in Court. Baboo Kanny Lall Dey tells me, that it is an impure mixture of Cyanide and Ferrocyanide of Potassium. The native gilders prepare it by imperfectly roasting a mixture of Ferrocyanide of Potassium and impure Carbonate of Potash.

The Madras Medical Journal, for May 1870, p. 395, notices two cases of suicide by this salt which had recently occurred in Madras. In one of these a respectable womam, irritated by some family squabble, sent out to the bazar for "*rat-poison;*" her messenger received, without question, a lump of Cyanide of Potassium; she swallowed about ten grains of it, and died.

NITRATE OF SILVER.

The following rare case of poisoning by this salt is recorded* by G. C. Chatterjea, M.A. and M.B., of Azimgunj :— He prescribed, with due precaution, a solution of the nitrate (a drachm to the ounce) for a sloughing sore on the scrotum. The patient, a very ignorant old man, divided it into four parts and took one, containing 15 grains, and two doses more within the next two hours. He was then seen,—45 grains had been swallowed. He complained of an indescribable burning sensation in the stomach, eyes red, forehead covered with perspiration. Pulse quick, and respiration hurried. Tongue devoid of epithelium. Mind clear, but he was unable to speak. He was made to swallow a large cup-full of milk, and a strong solution of common salt. Milk and eggs caused vomiting. At first thick tenacious mucus, subsequently mucous casts of different forms streaked with blood. This continued for about an hour when the burning sensation somewhat abated. Vomiting was maintained by large draughts of milk with relief. In about three hours he felt comfortable, and fell

---

* Ind. Med. Gaz., March 2nd, 1868, p. 61.

asleep. Next morning the bowels were cleared by a saline purge. On the third day he had rather a sharp attack of dysentery, but made a good recovery.

CHLORIDE OF ZINC.

Two cases of poisoning by Burnett's solution have occurred in the Medical College Hospital. In one of these, which came partly under my own care, a student drank about two ounces, mistaking it for syrup. He was immediately treated, but death occurred in about a week from sphacelus of the coats of the stomach. In two other cases which have occurred in Calcutta, the patients' escape (after severe vomiting) appears to have been due to the fact that the solution was accidentally swallowed immediately after dinner.

CHLORIDE OF CADMIUM.

The following case of poisoning by the above-named salt has been published by Mr. Hinder of the Calcutta Native Hospital.* It is, I believe, happily unique :—

Sheik Laljaun, a slender lad, about 14 years of age, was brought to hospital on the 2nd March 1866. On admission, he was in a state of perfect collapse, with a cold clammy skin ; radial pulse scarcely perceptible ; respiration feeble, slow, and sighing : no stertor ; face considerably disfigured, owing to considerable chemosis of both eyes, to such an extent as to prevent closure of the lids, completely hiding the pupil ; lips everted, the mucous membrane of the mouth being pale and sodden ; tongue swollen, greatly resembling the distended belly of a frog ; lay apparently unconscious, though, when shaken and roused by dashing cold water on the face, he replies rationally, in a hoarse whisper, to any questions put to him ; there was extreme restlessness and throwing about of the limbs; deglutition impeded ; with considerable difficulty he could be got to swallow a little milk and water—this was due in all probability to a similar condition of parts existing in the pharynx, as was seen in the mouth.

His mother stated that her son had been rigidly observing the Mahomedan lent and, on its completion, finding his appetite fail, he proposed to take a purgative, and, for this purpose, he purchased from a native vendor of drugs a pice worth of senna leaves, and a pice of Epsom salts (sulphate of magnesia), the latter being equal in quantity to four drachms and twenty grains, half of which he took in a decoction prepared from the senna leaves. "Immediately on swallowing it he began to spit and vomit, throwing himself on the bed, rolling about, and complaining much." He died about one hour and-a-half after taking the dose.

---

* Ind. Med. Gazette for June 1866, p. 156.

On tasting some of the supposed Epsom salts, Mr. Hinder experienced, almost instantaneously, a sharp raw sensation throughout the tongue, as though it were bared of its epithelial covering, with constriction and dryness of the fauces, followed by a spasmodic pain at the epigastrium, attended with nausea and spitting.

Dr. W. Palmer, Officiating Chemical Examiner to Government, said that one of the two packets was found to contain Chloride of Cadmium, the other contained a mixture of about equal parts of Chloride of Cadmium and Sulphate of Magnesia. Examination of the contents of the stomach did not reveal evidence of poison or any indication of the cause of death. Chloride of Cadmium is such a rare salt that little or nothing is known of its action; to test this, he gave to a cat about 30 grains of the mixture. The cat died in less than five minutes. The salt is very rare indeed, and he doubted if it could be bought in all India under its proper name. He had a small quantity in the laboratory of the Chemical Examiner's department. Iodide of Cadmium is used in photography, and may be purchased, but he could not find that the Chloride had ever been used. It is an expensive salt. It appears to kill through the nervous system; the cat struggled, apparently unconsciously, for a few minutes, and then became motionless. The action was almost immediate. He would expect to find all the blood-vessels of the nervous system highly congested, and that would be the immediate and apparent cause of death.

Dr. Woodford found the vessels of the brain excessively engorged with blood. The left lung was congested, and the stomach contained a few ounces of mucilaginous-looking fluid. In his opinion the deceased died from congestion of the vessels of the brain.

TELINI.

(*Mylabris Cichorii.*)

Dr. Burton Brown says that this very efficient Indian substitute for *Cantharides* is rarely employed in this country as a poison, but that it is occasionally given to produce abortion, or to relieve impotency; and, when so employed, it may produce dangerous symptoms. In one case these flies were applied externally for the purpose of injury, and in another several were found in spirit, probably added to produce greater stimulating effect (p. 90). Colonel Todd's work contains ample evidence of the existence in Rajputana of the idea that the deaths of several historic personages have been caused by wearing *Poisoned Robes*. It is believed that the son of Jeswunt, the formidable Rahtore prince, was thus done to death by a robe of honor presented to him by Arungzeb. So also Raja Bukht met his death, a learned *vedya* declaring, from the first, that he was beyond the reach of medicine. The Queen of Ganore, having been taken prisoner in her last stronghold on the Nerbudda, complimented the victor on his gallant conduct and determination in pursuit, adding that he merited her hand for his bravery, and might prepare for the nuptials. Robed in the marriage garb presented by the Queen, he hastened to obey the mandate. He was desired to be seated, and in conversation hours were as minutes while he gazed on the beauty of the queen. But presently his countenance fell, he complained of heat ; punkas and water were brought, but they availed him not, and he began to tear the bridal garments from his body, when the queen thus addressed him. "Know, Khan, that your last hour is come ; our wedding and our death shall be sealed together. The vestments which cover you are poisoned ; you left me no other expedient to escape pollution." While all were horror-struck by this declaration, she sprang from the battlements into the flood beneath. The Khan died in extreme torture (Vol. I., p. 626).

Any one who has noticed how freely a robust person in India perspires through a thin garment can understand that, if the cloth were thoroughly impregnated with the *cantharidine* of that very powerful vesicant, the *Telini*, the result would be as dangerous as that of an extensive burn.

FISH POISON.

Dr. Collas, of Pondichery, kindly sent me, in 1861, a printed account of the dangerous properties of the *Gobus Criniger* (Cantor's Malayan Fishes, p. 1166), sold in the Bazars of Pondichery. A Mussulman police peon, his wife, and little daughter, were attacked with vertigo and very great feebleness in the limbs, after having eaten a curry made of these little fish by the child. It was also stated that three fowls which had eaten the fish died in a short time. The family were well by the next morning. Entertaining doubts of their having been poisoned, as these fish are eaten in great quantities by the natives, Dr. Collas instituted a series of experiments with fowls. All the fowls which ate the entire fish, the head, livers, or intestines, died. Two fowls only escaped with life, having eaten only the caudal portions of the fish, and they for a short time displayed stiffness in walking. The fowls which died gradually lost the use of their lower limbs, fell on their sides, and died without convulsions. All the several dogs to which the fish were given threw them up with severe and repeated vomiting.

Dr. Collas remarks that, in preparing these fish for the pot, the native females take extreme care completely to remove the head and intestines, and to wash the fish thoroughly. This supports Dr. Taylor's remark (Poisons, p. 551), that the cause of the poisonous property of several fish in the tropical seas, such as the Conger-eel and the Yellow-billed Sprat, has been assigned to the food taken by the fish (acrid mollusca). This he, however, adds is a mere hypothesis.

Dr. Fayrer informs me that, recently, eleven girls at the European Female Orphan Asylum in Calcutta were poisoned by eating a *Rohee fish* caught in their own tank. This fish is a common article of food in Bengal, and I have not heard of any other instance in which it has proved noxious. Nine of the girls vomited repeatedly, one fell insensible and remained for an hour in a fainting state. She did not vomit. In twelve hours after the first faint she had a similar attack. The other child was not taken ill until twenty-eight hours after eating the fish. She remained in a partially fainting state; she vomited slightly. The matron, who ate of the fish, suffered from diarrhœa, but did not vomit.

Dr. Fayrer has also mentioned to me that a Greek family, in Calcutta, were severely poisoned by eating *Caviaire* preserved in tin; their symptoms were nearly those of cholera. The Caviaire was much decomposed and fall of *acari*. This case appears to be nearly allied to those of poisoning by German Sausages.

While this sheet was going through the press, a delicate European woman, who had been confined only a month previously, was brought to my ward with symptoms of Fish Poisoning (vomiting, diarrhœa, cramps in the limbs, and prolonged faintness, in which she appeared to be deprived of speech). She was well the next day. The symptoms commenced in about three hours after having eaten a small *crab*.

ANAMIRTA COCCULUS.

Kakmari, Sans.; *Kakmari*, Hind. Dec., *Bacaen-ka-phal*, Calcutta; *Jermœ*, Hind. Guz.; *Kaka-collei-verei*, Tam.; *Kakichimpoo-vitteloo*, Tel.; *Pola Kaandaka-conuveh*, *Garalaphala*, Mal.; *Tuba-bidji*, Malaya. (Birdwood.)

Dr. Birdwood mentions that the berry of *Cocculus Indicus is said to be largely employed by the liquor retailers of Bombay*, and that, in the Ghurwal mountaius, an ardent spirit is distilled from the root of *Cissampelos Obtecta* (page 205). Royle mentions (page 61) that the berries of both *C. Flavescens* and *C. Lacunosus* are used in the Eastern Islands for poisoning fish.

In the "Notes of North Cachar," already cited, we are told that the Kookies use a poison called *Deo-bi* to kill fish. It has an intoxicating effect upon them, floating them upon the surface, when it is thrown into the water. This is probably *Cocculus Indicus*, as its *habitat* extends to their Hills.

A writer in the *Indian Daily News*, for June 20th, 1870, says: "During May last, a Civil Officer of the Central Provinces informed me that a cart-load of large and small fishes had been taken by being stupefied with the root of a native herb. This practice is being extensively carried on all over the country, and no law exists by which the perpetrators can be punished. The greatest loss is not caused by those larger fish that can be counted by thousands, and used as food; but the tens of thousands of young fry that are killed at the same time and thus wasted, when otherwise they would have, for the most part, grown to some size."

Sir W. O'Shaughnessy Brooke insists that "it is well known that fish thus caught" [by *C. Indicus*] "are exceedingly dangerous."

POISONOUS GRAIN AND LEGUMES.

Rice.

In 1820, Dr. Robert Tytler published a work, entitled "***Remarks upon Morbus Oryzeus or Disease occasioned by the employment of noxious Rice as food; comprehending a narrative of facts connected with the disease which occurred in the district of Jessore;***" in which he argued, with great ability, that the outbreak of the epidemic Cholera in 1817 was "entirely owing to the general employment of an *unwholesome crop*," the natives being driven, in consequence of an unusually rainy season, to cut the rice before it was ripe, and to eat it before it had been kept sufficiently long. His arguments certainly appear to go far towards proving that, in the presence of a cholera epidemic, this unwholesome grain acted as an immediately *exciting* cause of the disease. Dr. Tytler also published* a supplementary paper, in which he maintained that what is called in the Upper Provinces the *Kun*, and in the Lower the *Koora*, or inner pericarp of rice, "*is a rank poison.*" All practical men recognise the fact that imperfectly husked rice is very unwholesome, but I do not find in our medical literature any observations in continuation of Dr. Tytler's upon the evil effects of atah and other flours adulterated with *Koora.*

It is a fact practically understood by every native of Bengal that *new* rice cannot be eaten with impunity, as it generally proves indigestible, and is liable to give rise to diarrhœa, dysentery, and other evidences of intestinal irritation. The use of very new rice has generally been forbidden in the Jails of Bengal, but it is considered that the grain is not perfectly wholesome until it has been carefully stored for two years. The late Mr. F. P. Strong, Surgeon to the 24-Pergunnahs, whose attention for many years was directed to the important subject of dieting prisoners, has shown,† by tabular statements, that an inferior kind of grain, known in the neighbourhood of Calcutta as "*deesee*" rice, is so unwholesome as to be positively destructive to the lives of those who eat it constantly. It cannot be doubted that inferior rice, apart, it would seem, from any positive disease in the grain, is a very dangerous article of food, especially to those unaccustomed to its use. Dr. McNab published, in 1838,‡ some valuable remarks

---

* The Ghost of the Asiatic Mirror, Oct. 21, 1820, p. 344.

† Indian Annals of Medical Science, No. V., for October 1855, p. 168.

‡ Quarterly Journal of the Calcutta Medical and Physical Society, July. Dr. Finch considered that the injurious effect of a mixed rice and atah diet had been overrated.—*Trans. Medical and Physical Society*, Vol. IX., Part 1, p. 20.

on "*Bad Rice when used as food productive of Dysentery and other Alvine Affections.*" His observations were chiefly made among sepoys who, on their arrival in Bengal from the Upper Provinces, had their wheat flour *(Ata)* adulterated with ground rice of a cheap and inferior kind. Dr. McNab states that,—"When the disease was at its worst in the regiment, the symptoms became exceedingly distressing, very many had excessive torminæ and tenesmus with stools consisting entirely of blood and mucus in white flakes, destitute of a single trace of feculent matter. From 16 to 20, or even 24, were not uncommon occurrences in the course of the night, leaving hardly half an hour's interval between each evacuation. The calls were urgent, and required instant obedience. On pressure, few had pain above the pubes, or indeed in any other part of the abdomen ; the sensation in the former place was characterized as an impatient sort of uneasiness, so to speak, which did not amount even to tenderness : none felt sick at the stomach, some complained of dry tongue with thirst, and slight increase of surface heat ; whilst others, though the local symptoms were, perhaps, equally intense, suffered but little general disturbance of the system. The pulse, in most instances, had an accelerated beat.". . . "The tongue, excepting where pyrexia existed, was usually moist, though coated to a greater or less degree ; the fur being sometimes of considerable thickness and of a pale yellowish color. When dry, the color of the tongue inclined to redness."—In short, the disease was simple uncomplicated Dysentery, arising entirely from irritation of the intestinal mucous membrane. *See also p.* 307.

Paspalum Scrobiculatum.

Dr. R. Tytler reported* upon a grain called *Kodoo*, commonly grown in the Tirhoot district and in the Upper Provinces, but which he had not observed in the Dooab, and which the natives regarded as a species of rice. He was informed, at Mozufferpore and Bilsund, that the use of this grain is frequently attended with violent cramps, intoxication, and madness, as if the person had been taking *bhang*.

Dr. Kenneth Mackinnon, in speaking of the diseases most prevalent among the native inhabitants of Tirhoot, says : "I have met with one case of genuine dry gangrene ; and I am inclined to think further observation will show that the diseased grains in this country will sometimes show a kind of ergot, and that will, I suppose, produce the dry gangrene. Other writers have stated that a permanent contraction of the knee-joints is a frequent consequence of eating some kinds of Kodoo,—the *Paspalum Frumentaceum*." [*P. Scrobiculatum.*] "Numbers of people so affected are to be seen here."†

* The Ghost of the Asiatic Mirror for October 21, 1820, p. 349.

† On the Public Health, Climate, Hygiene and Prevailing Diseases of Bengal and the North-West Provinces, p. 36.

This question of the poisonous effects of the Kodoo has been revived by Dr. Bonavia, of Lucknow.*

Dilawal Khan, beeshtee, says that, on the 16th January 1866, he bought some "bajra" flour *(pencillaria spicata)*, made it into cakes, and ate about one cake and-a-half, which are equal to about a quarter of a seer of the flour. They were eaten at 7 P.M., and at 9 o'clock he vomited, and again about midnight. He also was purged twice. He had vertigo, and was uncomfortable all night, with pains all over his body. On the 17th he could not stand, from vertigo. On the 18th he was still uncomfortable, and drank some "mattha" (butter-milk). On the 19th he was all right, but did not quite feel as usual. Debee ate some of the same flour on the 17th, two *roties* mixed with potatoes, equal to about three-eighths of a seer of the flour. They were eaten at noon, and at 2 P.M. he began to feel heat and puffiness in his stomach. At 4 P.M. his bowels were moved, and at 6 P.M. he vomited nearly all he had eaten. All night he was lying down with vertigo, and pains all over his body. On the 18th he had still vertigo and stiffness of limbs. He drank half a seer of butter-milk. On the 19th he was all right. Nabboo, beeshtee, on the 16th, ate a quarter "rotee" made of the same flour; soon afterwards he vomited, and was purged once. He had also vertigo and pains in his body, and remained uncomfortable till the 18th. On the 16th, beeshtee No. 1 gave a bit of cake to a dog which was near. In half an hour the dog vomited, and could not keep his legs. On the 17th, Debee gave a bit of cake to a monkey. It purged the animal, and from signs about the monkey's mouth, Debee thinks he must have vomited also. The old woman who sold the "bajra" flour said there was "Kodoo" flour *(Paspalum Scrobiculatum)* mixed with it. All the men, together with the old woman, were sent to the magistrate. In the Court many persons said the flour had "Kodoo" in it, and that was the reason it produced poisonous effects. The magistrate stated, "*New* Kodoo, I have always understood, produces the symptoms complained of by your servants. Ask any native. I never heard the fact disputed. The flour was examined here, and said to be mixed with 'Kodoo.' Chundee, garariah, lives at Bantra. He says, 'near his village "Kodoo" is extensively cultivated.' There is no difference in effect between new and old Kodoo, but when the ears of Kodoo are ripening about September, and rain falls, it is called *Matawna Kodoo*. It is always deleterious, and produces the effects above described, and some people die of it. *Matawna Kodoo* is never eaten ground into flour, but as rice, and is well *washed* before being cooked. Then it produces no bad effects."

Dr. Bonavia suggests that the newness or oldness of "Kodoo" has little to do with its poisonous qualities; but that, after rainfalls, when the

* Indian Medical Gazette for July 1867, p. 179, "A case worthy of further and more accurate investigation."

ear is ripening, some fungus is formed, the spores of which, if the Kodoo is ground, are mixed up with the flour. But if the *Matawna Kodoo* be well washed in the state of rice, the spores of the fungus are washed away, and it becomes harmless. *See also p.* 307.

Lathyrus Sativus.

Dr. Buchanan Hamilton noticed* that there is a species of lameness, called *kungi* in the Sanscrit language and *maghniga langra* in the vulgar dialect, as it is supposed to be peculiarly prevalent in Magadha; and in fact it is very common in Patna and its immediate vicinity; but he observed it nowhere else, although he was told that it prevails in every part of both districts. It attacks all ages and both sexes, and, after continuing a year or two, is considered incurable; but some have recovered after having been affected for several months. It seems to consist in a weakness and irregular motion of the muscles moving the knees, which are bent and moved with a tremulous irregular motion, somewhat as in the chorea, but not so violent. When the disease has lasted some time, and has become confirmed, the legs suffer emaciation. It is not accompanied by fever, but in the commencement is often, though not always, attended with pain. It is attributed by some to eating *khesârree* (*Lathyrus Sativus*), but this, he says, seems fanciful, for although in Magadha this pulse no doubt enters largely into the diet of the poor, it does no less so in that of those in Mutsya (Dinajpur), where the disease is as rare as in any other part of the world. By others it is attributed to sleeping on *Kodoo* straw, an opinion which deserves more attention, for the grain of some fields of Kodoo possesses narcotic qualities, probably owing to some weed intermixed with the real grain, and the stems of this weed may emit narcotic exhalations very capable of affecting the health.

General Sleeman appears to have been among the first who directed attention to the injurious consequences resulting from the use of *Lathyrus Sativus* amongst the people of Central and Northern India. He states that, in 1829, the wheat and other spring crops in the villages about Saugor, were destroyed by a severe hailstorm; in 1830, they were deficient from the want of seasonable rains; and, in 1831, they were destroyed by blight. During those three years, this *teoree*, or what, in other parts of India, is called *khesârree* (a kind of wild vetch which, though not sown itself, is left carelessly to grow among the wheat and other grain, and is given in the green and dry state to cattle), remained uninjured, and thrived with great luxuriance. In 1831, they reaped a rich crop of it from the blighted wheat fields; and subsisted upon it during that and the following years, giving the stalks and leaves only to their cattle. In 1833,

---

* Montgomery Martin's Eastern India, Vol. I., p. 115.

the sad effects of this food began to manifest themselves. The younger part of the population of this and the surrounding villages, from the age of 30 downwards, began to be deprived of the use of their limbs below the waist, by paralytic strokes, in all cases sudden, but in some more severe than in others. About half the youth of this village, of both sexes, became affected during the years 1833-34; and many of them lost the use of their lower limbs entirely, and were unable to move. The youth of the surrounding villages, in which the *teoree*, from the same causes, formed the chief article of food during the years 1831-32, suffered in an equal degree. Since the year 1834, no new case had occurred; but no person, once attacked, had been found to recover the use of the limbs affected; and Col. Sleeman's tent was surrounded by great numbers of the youth in different stages of the disease. Some of them were very fine-looking young men, of good caste and respectable families; and all stated that their pains and infirmities were confined entirely to the parts below the waist. They described the attacks as coming on suddenly, often while the person was asleep, and without any warning symptoms whatever; and stated that a greater portion of the young men were attacked than of the young women. It was the prevailing opinion of the natives, throughout the country, that both horses and bullocks, which have been fed much upon *teoree*, are liable to lose the use of the limbs.*

Subsequently, Dr. Kinloch W. Kirk published some interesting remarks upon the injurious effects of this *khesârree* dâl upon the poorer inhabitants of Upper Sindh. His attention was first directed to the subject by a villager bringing his wife, about thirty years of age, to him with paralysis of her lower extremities; she had been so afflicted for the last four years. The man said,—"It is from *khesârree;* we are very poor, and she was obliged to eat it for five months on end." Dr. Kirk had never heard of such effects before from any grain, and asked whether it was good of its kind. Finding it was so, he sent the man into the bazar to bring him a handful, which he subsequently showed to some respectable natives, and was told that disease from its use was very common all over the country. The villagers said that, if they sowed a better kind of grain, it would be plundered by the Beloochees from the hills, but that they would not take this. He did not enter a village in Sindh where this vetch was not to be found in the bazar, and daily used by great numbers of poor people, nor where several were not rendered most helpless objects by the use of it. Their general health seemed good, their only complaint being that they had no power in their legs, but they moved about lifting themselves on their arms. *Khesârree* they described as causing "*Badee,*" or severe pains in the joints like those of acute rheumatism in the first instance, but gradually changing into the permanent affection described, the seat of

---

* Op. Citat, Vol. I., p. 135.

which is probably in the lumbar portion of the spinal cord. Under the use of a poisonous food of this kind, the injury which meets the eye is nothing to the unseen evil, which does not terminate with the individual, but extends itself to the children of the third and fourth generation. All natives know that this dâl is a poison, and eat it only *because it is cheap*, thinking that they can stop in time to save themselves from its consequences. Dr. Kirk adds an expression of confidence that, could the amount of the evil be known, it would awaken the sympathy of Government in behalf of the people who are compelled by want to endure it; indeed he considers that it would be a boon were its cultivation suppressed entirely.*

In 1857, I requested Dr. Kirk to favor me with any information which he might have collected, in addition to that on Khesarree Dâl which he gave in his Medical Topography of Upper Scindh.

He, accordingly, most obligingly drew up the subjoined paper, and sent it to me, desiring that I would "make use of it in any shape I pleased." A brief abstract of its contents was published, some years since, by Dr. Mouat; but the entire paper well deserves a place in our literature.†

In his letter, Dr. Kirk sent me the subjoined additional information regarding poisonous legumes and unwholesome rice :

"It is not admitted, much less established, that Urhur is a cause of leprosy,—I firmly believe in the accuracy of my opinion, and only offer it as a suggestion, however. This very morning, I found two lepers begging near my gate; they came from Dutteah. Their fingers had nearly disappeared. I talked a little to them, and both admitted that the Dâl used before getting ill, was Toar (or Urhur) *with* the skins. I cannot help thinking that the Delhi Emperors brought this Dâl from the West. The Rajpoots hate the Mussulmans and always have—and this pulse is not to be found in Rajpootana till you reach its northern districts, and its not being found wild in India appears to show that it does not belong thereto.

---

* Medical Topography of Upper Sindh, p. 60. For ample particulars of similar effects resulting from the use of the *Lathyrus Cicera* and the *Ervum Ervilia*, or Bitter Vetch, in several of the continental states of Europe, *see* Taylor on Poisons, p. 535.

† This Memoir derives a strong additional interest from the fact that its able and estimable author composed it, at the request of a stranger, not many days before the Mutiny of 1857 involved him in its destruction ;—at a time when, warned and resolute, he stood calmly prepared for either fate. He concludes the letter, in which he transmitted the article to me, with these words,—penned on the 18th of May.—"The worst we can do is to despond. I pity the poor European Soldiers who must be exposed, and who cannot escape much suffering and loss of life, even with the greatest exercise of strictness and foresight."

Twenty-eight days later, on the 15th of June, the treacherous villains, to whom he had so often ministered in suffering, had despatched this wise, humane, and valiant spirit to his high reward.

"I asked Dr. O'Brien, who has been in India since he was a child, as well as some natives, about Kodoö. It appears that persons after a meal of it, feel *soost* and sleepy, and Dr. O'Brien tells me that, when liable to diarrhœa, even people of the better classes eat it, on account of its binding effect. I have no experience of it, however, and I do *not* believe in the suspicion that sleeping on its straw is hurtful, except under conditions that would make straw of *any* kind hurtful. I have, moreover, talked to hundreds of people with the affection of the lower limbs arising from Khesarree, and feel sure, that Khesarree is the *only* cause. I have, as you will see, suggested reasons for differences of result from eating this food.

"In respect to new rice, I find I mentioned its effects in my Sindh paper. There is a good deal of harm done by the use of it over India, among Europeans who do not know the importance of attending to it.

"Good rice should be kept three years before use; of second quality it should be kept two years, at the least. During the time of keeping, the grains appear to lose something in the shape of a white powder that forms upon their surface. This is carefully removed by beating and rubbing with coarse flour every year.

"Rice under-kept boils *thick* in the grain, and so gummy that the grains stick together; but when of good quality and condition, the grains elongate remarkably by boiling; they do not stick together, and they have a pleasant mealiness in the mouth.

"The effects of new rice are, heart-burn, dyspepsia, flatulence, colic, and sometimes diarrhœa, together with local affections of the colon and hœmorrhoidal diseases."

[It is a fact that the poorer the rice as a food, the less does it need keeping; all the better sorts need long keeping.—N. C.]

"The principal leguminous seeds, bearing the general name of Dâl, which are in use throughout India as articles of diet, are named in the following list :—

Urhur or Toar	...	*Cytisus Cajan.*
Oordh or Marsh	...	*Dolichos Pilosus.*
Moong	...	*Phaseolus Mungo.*
Motth	...	*Phaseolus Aconitifolius.*
Chunna or Gram	...	*Cicer (or Ervum) Arietinum.*
Khesarree, Kussah Muttur, or Keraow	}	*Lathyrus Sativus..*
Mussoor	... ...	*Ervum Lens*

"Of these, the Urhur is in highest estimation; though, on account of its expense, not the most generally used. The wealthy natives, throughout Central India, seldom use any other Dâl, and such Europeans as occasionally partake of it, admit that it is the most relishable of all the pulses. I have always heard it mentioned as *remarkably nice*.

"Among the poorer classes, many eat this Dâl occasionally—and in the cold weather especially, under an impression that its use enables them to resist cold, a long-continued reaction or glow succeeding a meal of it. But this reaction is often so severe in degree, as to constitute considerable general disturbance which, after a time, is accompanied by impaired health, and rheumatic affections.

"Many who use this food occasionally, and chiefly among the lower classes whose usual diet is poor, entertain for it a morbid relish which grows so upon them, that, in time, they feel convinced they cannot do without it, and, accordingly, make a meal of it several times a week.

"Such people often bear on their persons marked evidence of its bad effects. But the increasing relish entertained for the food makes them unwilling to discontinue its use.

"Such people invariably have the Dâl cooked without separation of the skins ; while others, rich or well-to-do in the world, as invariably have the skins removed before cooking by careful soaking and washing.

"The simple circumstance of eating the skins or otherwise with the Dâl makes the most marked difference in the effects of this food on the system. Under the best of circumstances, it cannot be considered really wholesome for every-day use, but the skins being physiologically and mechanically unwholesome, when they are not separated, this food becomes a slow but certain poison.

"It appears from all I have observed and heard of its effects, that such persons as commence using it, who have not hitherto been accustomed to it, are more apt to suffer from it severely than others to whom it has been long a staple article of diet. A recruit, for instance, who has never tasted it at his home, soon breaks down in his corps from its frequent use.

"The following symptoms which arise in the course of using Urhur Dâl are given in the order in which they show themselves. Urticaria, sense of heat in the stomach, redness of the lining membrane of the mouth, apparent elongation of the teeth, discoloration or bronzing of the skin, sponginess of the nails, burning of the hands and feet, a dry harsh and cracked condition of the cuticle of the hands and feet. Deep cracks (longitudinal) in the heels, rheumatic pains, thickening of the periosteum, especially of the shins, with rheumatic changes in the joints, white spots indicating a leprous taint appearing about the body, but chiefly on the palms of the hands, and on the lips, and lastly, all the characters of confirmed leprosy.

"I was once led to question many lepers as to their diet, under a suspicion that the supposed scarcity of salt had something to say to their complaint, and learned that they ate as much salt as other people, and as much as they pleased ; that their disease was, most commonly, preceded and accompanied by the use of Urhur Dâl, though inherited taint and syphilitic affections were also evident precursors. Many years of continued attention to this subject only confirm the opinion I then formed of the effects of this substance as an article of diet. The following instance occurred to me about a month ago, as I was marching through Sirsa, a village in Rajpootana. A man *ætat* forty, hearing I was a medical man, came to consult me about some leprous spots on his person, which had been present four years. Urhur, he said, was not grown in his district, and is not to be had in the bazars. He had spent a year in Malwa, where it is common, and where he ate it almost daily. It was while he was in Malwa that the spots showed themselves; there also he had suffered from rheumatism. On his return to Rajpootana, he had never again seen the Urhur; his spots remained, but were not getting worse, and his health was very good.

"Many similar instances have occurred to me, which, though valueless when taken singly, all point in one direction, and tend to support the opinion I have here offered.

"The rich people who use this kind of Dâl suffer comparatively little, on account of the skins being completely removed before cooking. But even they appear to be injured by it. They are all morally and physically deteriorate. Heirs are constantly failing in families, and even leprosy is not uncommon among them.

"There are several varieties of this plant; but as it has not been found except as the result of cultivation, it is evident that it is not indigenous, but must have been introduced into India—and it would be interesting to know when!—and to observe its effects since that time on the high families of the country.

"The Oordh Dâl is in more common use than any other throughout the country. It may be had in every bazar. It is the staple article of the kind among all classes, except the highest and the lowest.

"It is eaten both with and without the skins; those who are very poor, or very saving, invariably eat skins and all, and it is supplied for use in our jails with the skins. This is a great mistake, for there is no nourishment contained in them; anything they give out, in cooking or while digestion is going on, is of a poisonous nature, and their mechanical properties render them highly injurious to men who are liable to chronic purging, and dysenteric affections.

"The skins have an effect in causing colic and indigestion, and as secondary results, rheumatic affections, harshness and dryness of the cuticle of the hands and feet, often accompanied by deep cracks. The nails, too, become spongy.

"By the removal of the skins, however, this Dâl becomes wholesome to all but invalids, and is a most excellent and pleasant food.

"Moong, after removal of the skins, is the most wholesome of any pulse in use in India. Boiled to a thin pulp, it becomes an excellent food for invalids and children. It is light and easy of digestion, and often infinitely more grateful than the slops frequently forced upon the former.

"It is the only kind of Dâl that should be permitted to be brought to the tables of Europeans in India. The natives consider it a poor food; and, though they often eat it and admit its wholesomeness, they like to recur, at short intervals, to the richer varieties of Dâl. The fine powder of Moong, added to that of Barley, is often used instead of the very expensive ***Revelenta Arabica,*** and certainly leaves nothing to be desired, in respect to cheapness, lightness, and wholesomeness.

"Motth is eaten by the poorest ryots, and one reason for the estimation it receives is that its straw is an excellent food for cattle ; there is, therefore, a double purpose in growing it. It is a poor food, very heavy of digestion, less wholesome than Oordh, and causing what the natives call *dădee* with all the evils that attend the use of Oordh.

"Chunna is not in general use as a Dâl. It is very heavy of digestion. The same may be said of the Mussoor, though I understand there are varieties of the latter which are esteemed light and wholesome. I have heard of a Hill variety reputed very digestable.

"The least wholesome Dâl is the Khesârree, which is only found in the poorest villages, where its use is confined to the lowest and most miserable of the population. The depth and extent of misery in a village may be estimated, readily, by the quantity of this pulse found in the bazar. If the people are in anything like comfort, this grain may be sought for in vain ; whereas its abundance indicates wretchedness.

"Its use, for even a short period, often causes serious injury to the general health. Rheumatism often comes on after a few months' use of the food, which, latterly, appears to settle in the loins, the posterior muscles of the thigh and leg lose their power, and the injured man walks dragging his toes along the ground. In this state he may remain for the rest of his life ; the continued use of the food, however, leads to complete paralysis of the lower limbs, the injured person then lifting himself about on his hands.

"The bad effects resulting from this Dâl come on insidiously, but not suddenly, and the poor people who are obliged to eat it, think they can discontinue its use in time to save themselves from its evil consequences. In this they are sometimes mistaken, and victims to its use are to be found in every commnnity who have to appeal for support to this wretched food.

"The first case that fell under my notice of injury caused by the use of Khesârree, was in a woman, who was brought to me at Shikarpore in 1845, who could, with the greatest difficulty, move with the aid of crutches. She was unable to lift her toes from the ground, and could scarcely get one leg past the other. She had been helpless, in this way, for four years. The husband explained the cause, as consisting in neither blow nor fall, or other injury, but in the destructive effects of this food—a specimen of which he brought me from the bazar. I showed this to well-informed natives, and learnt from them the undisputed truth of its poisonous properties, which was most amply confirmed by what afterwards fell under my notice in every village I had an opportunity of visiting in Upper Sindh, where the resulting injury was in every degree, from a slight dragging motion of the lower limbs to complete paralysis; in which latter case, the unfortunate objects lifted themselves about on their hands, in which they held small wooden clogs.

"Since returning to the Provinces, I have often seen men in the same condition, and have made a point of questioning the sufferer in each case; and without exception, where we fairly understood each other, Khesârree was the admitted agent. I visited once the Undha Khana at Benares with the magistrate of that place, to whom I had spoken of the effects of this food, and there were two men whom I pointed out as injured in this way before I had spoken to them, and their own report confirmed at once the opinion I had formed.

"The gait of such persons is so characteristic that, when once observed, it will hardly be forgotten; the toes are turned slightly in, and dragged on with difficulty lifted from the ground; the limbs and joints appear loose, weak and agitated, and *give* so much at every step that, while the person is walking, the figure has a continued up-and-down motion. The appearance of a person so affected, while walking, reminds us of Chorea—but the two complaints essentially differ.

"This affection of the limbs has, by some, been attributed to other causes—one of which is supposed to be sleeping on Kodoo straw. I may say, however, after talking with hundreds of such patients, my conviction is that the use of Khesârree, if not the only, is almost the only, cause.

"Two very important questions naturally arise, which are—finding large communities consuming this food,—'Why do only a comparatively few people suffer in the manner described?' 2ndly,—'Why does one district suffer more than another where this food is extensively eaten?'

"We must remember that the parties who eat Khesârree are the very poorest, that they do not eat it exclusively, but appear only to bring up with it the balance they are short of other food; that this other food may be poor in kind and deficient in quantity or otherwise; and that susceptibility to injury must have a relation to the state of health of individuals.

"The person least likely to suffer is he whose health is good, who takes the least quantity of Khesârree and for the shortest time, and who has, besides it, other food of wholesome quality; whereas, the most susceptible is, naturally, he whose health is already weakened by want and other causes, such as those productive of low fever, who, while he eats Khesârree, has little else to eat, and that little of poor quality, and especially where the person is driven to eat the skins with the seeds: for we may expect naturally that, as in other pulses, the ill-effects of this food are most marked where the skins are eaten. This, however, is only an inference.

*

"The circumstances and susceptibility, therefore, of no two families can be precisely alike.

"There is, moreover, another matter to be considered which may help us to understand the second question. There appear to me—after consultation with natives and botanical reference to the herbs so called—to be several distinct varieties, and most likely distinct species bearing the name. We have the grain of white, green, variegated, spotted and black colors. Now the white is, certainly, not a *Lathyrus*, and the other varieties, except the black, are probably crosses, where the pollen of the white has impregnated the flower of the black-seeded varieties.

"Even in respect to the *Lathyrus Sativus* (the black-seeded sort and the only true Khesârree) I find, on referring to Roxburgh, that there are two varieties, between which there is a marked botanical difference.

"It is, therefore, evident that there is much to account for a very marked difference in the effects of the grain that goes by the name of Khesârree, independent of the varied susceptibility and circumstances of those who consume it.

"Under the head 'Lathyrus' some very interesting information is given in Loudon's Encyclopædia of Plants, from which it appears that, eaten in the proportion of a quarter or even a half mixed with wheaten flour, it is reported harmless; that the effects of the food, as witnessed in man, are also observable in the lower animals; and a mule plant is mentioned between the *L. Sativus* and a *Cicer*. It would appear, moreover, that, in certain countries of Europe, the effects are as varied as they seem to be in India. In some, however, they have proved so destructive that Governments, in their alarm, have, at times, forbidden the use and culture of the food.

"I think, then, considering all that has been stated in respect to Khesârree, its hurtful effects depend as much on the concomitant circumstances of its consumers, in respect to all that can possibly influence health, as on the direct influence of this food itself on the system."

Dr. James Irving, of Allahabad, has published* some important additional facts, illustrative of the dependence of palsy of the lower limbs upon the use of Khesârree Dâl, especially in Pergunnah Khyraghur, in Zillah Allahabad, where, out of a population of 70,800, there were no less than 889, or 1·25 per cent., affected with paralysis. In this locality the Khesârree grows in all seasons, varying in luxuriousness of growth only according to the season, and *affording the only certain provision of life.* A remarkable peculiarity in this form of paralysis is that the great majority of sufferers are *males.* Thus it appears that, in Barra, of a population

* Indian Annals of Medical Science, No. XIII., p. 127.

of 33,951 males, 2,087 were paralysed, or 6·11 per cent. ; while, of 22,658 females, only 134, or 0·59 per cent., were paralysed. Dr. Irving traces the existence in other districts, Banda, Mirzapore, Gyah. He brings forward the suggestion that the disease, so well known as *Kumree*, which spoils so many horses—"gone in the loins,"—in Bengal and in other parts of India, is probably due to feeding upon grain largely adulterated with Khesârree Dâl.

Leera in Barley.

Dr. R. Tytler has given* some account of a disease termed Leera, which affects Barley during its growth in the Upper Provinces, and which is said to destroy an immense quantity of grain annually. The vitiated substance is supposed to be an organic body which makes its appearance in the earliest stage of the grain's growth, and gradually increases until the ear is fully formed, and filled with a black matter. The disease does not resemble that called the "black rust" in Scotland ; but is more like the ergot of rye, when the spur is short, and affects nearly all the pickles of the ear. The diseased grain is represented as being extremely poisonous. Several chickens having eaten of it, all died in about twenty-four hours. It does not appear in the wheat of India, but an analogous disease is observed in *oats*, and occasionally, in the cones of *Bajrah* (*Penicellaria Spicata*), in which latter case it is named *Kindol.*

EXAMINATION OF THE MEDICINAL STOCKS OF BUNNEEAS, &c.

It will not unfrequently happen that the civil surgeon will be required to examine and report upon the medicinal stock of a native trader seized under suspicious circumstances. This will generally comprise a variety of charms, the teeth of alligators, the dried teats of the jackal, or of some animal of like size, scales of the manis, tigers' claws, &c., &c., together with a few inert substances, such as chunam (lime), iron-rust, tabashir, &c., and several poisons,—white arsenic (perhaps bearing marks of scraping on the edge), orpiment, realgar, crude antimony, dhatoora seeds, gunjah leaves, churrus, and the roots of aconite and hellebore. The following is a list of this kind from the records : "1.—Ordinary bazar spirit. 2.—The liquid had disappeared, the lumps are vegetable matter, nature cannot be positively stated. 3.—Sugar slime. 4.—Oil of Cinnamon, ditto of Peppermint. 5.—Dhatoora Seeds. 6.—Pills, which, on analysis, yield oxide of lead. 7.—Dhatoora fruits entire, with seed. 8.—Vegetable powder, nature cannot be positively stated. 9.—Yellow Sulphuret of Arsenic (Hurtal) and Sulphuret of Copper. 10.—A quantity of the roots

* Calcutta Medical and Physical Transactions, Vol. V., p. 441.

of the Sungya Bikh (*Aconitum Ferox* of Nipal), a deadly poison. 11.—Vegetable powder, nature cannot be positively affirmed."

The following articles are reported to have been found in the possession of an unfortunate, who was apprehended under suspicion that he was the Nana : White Arsenic, Yellow Arsenic, Opium, Tin and Mercury prepared, Red Oxide of Mercury, Dhatoora, Bhang, Ajwain and Black Pepper, Poppy Seeds, Indigo, Frankincense, Sulphur, Aloes, Camphor, Catechu. Poppy Heads, Bruised Cardamoms, Alum, Lead, Earth used by Goldsmiths, Pill, composition unknown, Black Pepper, Massallah, Rosin, Snuff, Beads, String worn by Brahmins, Salt, Sugar, Tobacco, Bhillaray (*bilhara—juniper ?*), White Sandal-wood, Attah.

In the article already cited, Native Surgeon Moodelly, of Nellore, justly animadverts upon the careless manner in which the Hakeems of Madras keep their medicines. They are unlabelled, and harmless drugs are often kept in contact with the most subtle poisons in the same sack. The men go by their physical appearance (many cases of poisoning have thus occurred in Calcutta), and in apportioning the dose they guess, but do not actually weigh.

The recklessness with which chemicals are sold in the Indian bazars, by dealers quite ignorant of their properties, has been more than once illustrated in preceding Chapters (*vide supra*, pp. 110, 296, 297). We find it reported in Allen's Asiatic Journal for August 1838, that "Dr. O'Shaughnessy has discovered, *on sale in the bazar*, a large quantity of *white vitriol* marked 'Epsom Salts,' with forged labels, and seal of 'Bristow and Edmonds, London,' on the bottles. The dealer, on being questioned, stated that he purchased a cask of the salt about two years ago, at one of the auctions, and last month he bought 1,000 lbs. of another sample, from an American captain ; that the contents of the cask and a part of the last purchase were *mixed and sent to the Upper Provinces for sale !* and that small parcels had been disposed of in Calcutta."

The same kind of thing has gone on in Calcutta ever since, and I have met with more than one instance only less flagrant than the above. A druggist or photographer dies, or becomes bankrupt, the stock is sold off, and then every white non-delinquescent salt becomes either Epsom or Glauber's salts !

But few general rules can be laid down with regard to *The manner in which poisons are generally administered in India*—Our criminal records affording instances in which they have been given in nearly every kind of food and drink common among the natives ;—in water, wine, spirits, sherbet, suttoo, or parched grain, dâl (lentils), rice, kuddoo and other turkarees (vegetables), in goor (treacle or coarse sugar), in sweetmeats, &c., &c. The last is, however, a favorite mode of concealing poison among the natives.

We have seen that Dhatoora Seeds are frequently concealed by being given with capsicum and the pulp of the *baigun*, and that dall has been selected, on account of its color, as a vehicle for Yellow Arsenic.

In Todd's work there are several references to the administration of poison in *Pan*. Pirthi Raj, visiting, after a desperate battle, his uncle Soorajmul, who had rebelled against him, did not hesitate to eat the *pan* on taking leave (1—297). The chief of Saloombea having incurred the suspicions of Ursi Rana of Boondi, the Rana commanded him to eat the *pan* leaf presented on taking leave. He remonstrated, but in vain ; and with the conviction that it contained his death-warrant, he obeyed, saying "My compliance will cost you and your family dear !" To this and other acts is ascribed the murder of Ursi (p. 435).—Several cases of poisoning and drugging in *pan* have been given in the preceding pages.*

Herklotts says that philtres (which, as we have seen, are not unfrequently poisoned) are so often given in *pan* that, when a man is submissive to a woman and overlooks her bad conduct, the common saying among the valgar is "she has fed him with betel-nuts."

The *Majoon*, a compound of sugar, butter, flour, milk, and sidhee or bang,† a preparation of the *Cannabis Indica*, can probably be purchased in nearly every bazar in India, and is known to every native ; and it is to be feared that other confectionary, containing Opium, Dhatoora,‡ &c., may also be prepared by nefarious dealers,—although acquaintance with such deadly sweets is entirely ignored by nearly all who are questioned upon the subject. Numerous cases might be cited in which Arsenic, Dhatoora, and Aconite have been mixed in sweetmeats for criminal purposes.

OUTWARD ASPECT OF THE BODY AND COUNTENANCE IN DEATH FROM POISONING.

The reports sent into the Nizamut, about thirty years ago, are replete with evidence of the existence of a general belief, not only in the minds of natives, § the police, and of the judicial officers, but also among the

* Dr. S. Coull Mackenzie tells me that he has received several patients at the Medical College Hospital, who declared that they had been poisoned in *pán sooparee*. None, however, exhibited symptoms. I, therefore, merely allude to this as an illustration of criminal practice.

† O'Shaughnessy.

‡ Dr. O'Shaughnessy's informant on the manner in which Majoon is preparèd said that, sometimes, by special order of customers, he introduced Dhatoora seeds, but never Nux Vomica.

§ In a trial for poisoning (probably by Aconite), in Assam, a native witness said: "The deceased had not previously been ill, but, on examining the body, from the throat to the chest and tongue was black." A native doctor deposed: "saw no wound, but found from the face to the waist as well as the back, black; questioned the neighbours, from whom he heard that the deceased had had a burning sensation, and that his feet and hands were

medical witnesses, that ***certain outward appearances are to be received as indications that death has resulted from poison.*** Thus we find it inquired: "Are you of opinion that any poisonous substance taken internally would have caused the rapid decomposition of the body; and what appearances does the body of a person, being a native of this country, generally exhibit on being poisoned?" The reply is—"I do not think that poison would much accelerate decomposition, but different poisons would have different effects upon the body. The face and features of a person who had died from taking poison would be distorted, and show an expression of pain," &c. Again it is questioned—"It is stated in the evidence that the body turned black, and blood flowed from the eyes and nose;—are these symptoms usual in cases of death from poison, or indications of the same?" The reply is—"The body would turn black in cases in which mineral poison had been administered, but I think not in cases in which vegetable poison had been employed. The bleeding from the eyes and nose is not uncommon after death in other cases." The medical witness in another case says—"The nails were blueish, which is another mark of poison." This gentleman elsewere says—"The general appearance of the body was as though poison had been administered. The nails were black, and the skin unusually pallid." It was believed, for many centuries,* that the bodies of individuals who had

---

drawn up; is of opinion that the deceased died from the effects of poison."—*Nizamut Adawlut Reports*, October 16th, 1856.

Four years ago a medical friend enquired of me, "Do you know of any indigenous product—a poison, mineral or vegetable—that could, by being taken internally, render the body blue in color? I ask this in connection with a legal case in which criminal abortion was produced, and where the bodies of the mother and the fœtus were reported to be blue *throughout*." This was doubtless mere hypostatic congestion.

* According to Tacitus, Britannicus was destroyed by a poison, concocted by Locusta, by command of Nero, which acted instantaneously, the unfortunate youth appearing to be stricken down by epilepsy. Dio Cassius mentions that an extraordinary lividity overspread the face of the corpse, which it was attempted to conceal by the application of a pigment. William Mentieth, Archbishop of York, dying rather suddenly in June 1154, it was reported that he had been poisoned in the chalice at mass, or in the water in which he washed his hands before consecration. As Bishop Goodwin gives it,—

Et ut ipsum privent vita,
Celebrantes aconita,
Propinant in calice.
Toxicatur a profanis
Ille potus, ille panis,
Per quem perit toxicatum.

His teeth and nails turned black before he died.

We are told by Guicciardini that, when Pope Alexander VI died, about a week after swallowing a poison which he had prepared for some of his Cardinals, his body became a most frightful spectacle; it was so very black, swelled and deformed, that it could scarcely be known; the nose appeared full of putrefied pus flowing from it, the mouth hove up in a frightful manner, and the tongue became monstrously swelled, so that it filled the whole mouth. It was a sight so very shocking and horrible, that people were not able to look on

died under the effects of poison exhibited, outwardly, certain tokens of its operation. In their entire innocence of either chemical or pathological knowledge, the ancients clung with absolute reliance to this error, which affords a very singular example of false induction, inasmuch as, while the inference was erroneous, the observation whence it was deduced was perfectly correct: the rapid progress of decomposition noticed in the bodies of strong and full-blooded persons suddenly cut off by poison being contrasted with the comparatively slow and dry decay of those dying from exhausting chronic diseases, or from wounds attended with profuse hæmorrhage. The appearances which were, of old, regarded as so characteristic of death by poisoning are the natural evidences of rapid decomposition in a body of full habit. It is certainly true that some *animal* poisons, which act fatally by disintegrating the blood, appear to favor the rapid advance of *post-mortem* decomposition. This may be the case with the poison of some snakes, it is certainly so with urea. It was remarked

---

it, nor to endure the pestilential stench that came therefrom, so were obliged to turn their heads aside and retire. Apart from the effects of poison, this was simply the natural progress of decomposition in the remains of a gross-bodied sensualist, exposed to public view in the middle of a Roman August. So, in the case of one of Alexander's victims [?], the Cardinal of Sienna, we are told that, after his death in confinement, his body was allowed to be buried publicly; but care was taken to have it well wrapped up and covered; but, upon his mother's suspecting foul play, and boldly uncovering it, there were plainly discovered to the spectators the visible marks of his having been poisoned. So when the Duke of Burgundy desired to raise a report that John Dauphin of France (1417) was poisoned, he wrote:—"One evening, our most redoubtable lord and nephew fell so grievously sick that he died forthwith. His lips, tongue, and face were swollen; his eyes started out of his head; it was a horrible sight to see, for so look people that are poisoned." Similar appearances are said to have led to a close investigation of the deaths, in 1536, of the Dauphin Francis, son of Francis I.; and, in 1522, of the Cardinal de Medici, both of whom appear to have died from the effects of poison. So again the libellous Eaglisham asserted, as a proof that poison had been administered to James the First, that the king's body and head swelled above measure; his hair, with the skin of his head, stuck to his pillow, and his nails became loose upon his fingers and toes. The same person, in attempting to show that the death of the Marquis of Hamilton had been brought about in like manner, says:—"No sooner was he dead, when the force of the poison began to overcome the force of his body, it began to swell in such sort, that his thighs were swollen six times as big as their natural proportion, his belly became as big as the belly of an ox, his arms as the natural quantity of his thighs, his neck as broad as his shoulders, his cheeks over the top of his nose, that his nose could not be seen or distinguished, the skin of his forehead two fingers high. He was all over of divers colors, full of waters, some white, some black, some red, some yellow, some green, some blue, and that as well within his body as without. His mouth and nose foaming blood, mixed with froth, of divers colors, a yard high." Here we have merely an account of the appearances resulting from rapid decomposition intentionally exaggerated *ad captandum*. Still again, Sir Henry Halford, in commenting upon the death of Britannicus, says:—"I remember to have seen [1780] the face of Sir Theodosius Boughton, when the corpse had been disinterred, in order to be examined for the satisfaction of the Coroner's Jury, and its color resembled that of a pickled walnut."

Appearances of this kind are seen by Civil Surgeons in India every week, in bodies brought in for examination during the hot weather, in cases where there exists not the slightest reason to suppose that death has resulted from poison.

by myself and others, many years since, that the bodies of persons dying of renal disease often become excessively offensive, even before the vital heat has entirely left them. It is also stated that animals bitten by certain venomous snakes become enormously swollen in a few minutes, and remain so after death. This has not been observed to be the case in India ; but I am informed by a friend who spent some years in Australia that he has twice observed this result in a dog and a horse which died from snake-bite in that country ; still this point remains open for investigation.

Dr. Fayrer's experiments show that the blood of animals killed by the poison of the cobra, a *colubrine* snake, coagulates after death ; whereas, in death from the bite of Russell's viper, a *viperine* serpent, there is no coagulation. This may, perhaps, influence decomposition. At my request Dr. Fayrer had the body of a young dog which I had seen killed by a strong cobra on the afternoon of the 4th June (the hottest time in Calcutta) kept for fifteen hours. Mr. Sceva, of the Asiatic Societies' Museum, wrote :—"No part of the body was swollen ; on the contrary, it appeared to have shrunk, and was very stiff." One or two similar experiments with viperine snakes (of which none were then available) would be useful as evidence on this point. There is not the slightest ground for believing that mineral or vegetable poisons have any tendency to hasten decomposition. Dr. Taylor says :—"The bodies of persons poisoned are not more rapidly decomposed, *cæteris paribus*, than those of others who have died a sudden and violent death from any other cause whatever." With regard to *Distortion of the Countenance after death*, nothing of the kind can possibly occur—except from merely mechanical causes. Whatever amount of agony may precede death, all nervous action, and, with it, all suffering, and all expression of pain by muscular contraction, must cease with the cessation of life. Where the eyes remain open, and the jaw is not secured, the face will assume a ghastly appearance, when rigidity sets in ; but no practised medical man would mistake this for an expression of pain, or for distortion produced during life.

In ancient times, these erroneous opinions did infinite mischief. And, in the present day, they cannot be too strongly discountenanced, when occurring among non-professional persons.

MODE OF TRANSMITTING SUSPECTED MATTERS FOR CHEMICAL EXAMINATION.

Writing in 1856, I remarked—"In India, unfortunately, but little systematic arrangement has hitherto been observed in sending in cases of supposed poisoning for investigation, whether to the civil stations, or to the office of the Chemical Examiner. Suspicious portions of food and matters stated to have been vomited are, commonly, sent in by darogahs, in open vessels, with which nearly any person might tamper with scarcely a chance of detection, and in unsealed coverings of leaves or paper. Again, no systematic plan whatever is adhered to in the manner of transmitting packets from civil stations to the office of the Chemical Examiner. The Government Regulation is that such packets of suspected matters, together with full reports of the details of the cases, should he transmitted to the Chemical Examiner *direct* through the magistrate.* This rule is generally attended to ; but, not unfrequently, the medical officers send the packages with their reports direct to the Chemical Examiner. The pages of this officer's records are filled with remonstrances upon the hasty and insecure manner in which suspected matters have been packed and transmitted,— the vessels have not been air-tight, their mouths have not been properly tied as well as sealed, the corks have started out ; or the putrid matters, not having had strong spirit poured upon them, have burst the bottles,— or jars enclosed in boxes, without proper care in packing the interstices closely with tow, cotton, or hay, have broken, and the horribly putrid contents have exuded in every direction. It is evident that, although the transport of glass or earthen vessels many hundred miles by hand is, of course, attended with considerable risk of breakage, many of these accidents might be avoided, if certain rules and precautions were adhered to." I retain these remarks because, although matters are generally far better arranged in the present day, the errors here referred to are still, now and then, committed.

The Medical Authorities have, on several occasions, during the last thirty years, issued circulars calling the attention of medical officers to the proper mode of packing morbid preparations and suspected matters. In their circular letter No. 131, dated 31st May 1852, the Medical Board, under instructions from Government, acquaint Medical Officers :—

"That they are to consider it to be their duty on all occasions of *post-mortem* examination in which the signs are such as, in their opinion, to require that the contents of the stomach, or portions of the stomach itself, or of any other part of the body, should be transmitted to the Presidency to be tested by the Government Chemical Examiner, either to put up with their own hands these suspected substances in a suitable vessel, or see them put up at once by an assistant or subordinate, and after affixing as many impressions of their own seal as they may think necessary to guard, as far as possible, against the vessel being opened or tampered with, without detection, to dispatch them," &c.

Shortly before my last edition appeared, I made the following suggestions to the magistrate of the Howrah district, for the guidance of darogahs, in transmitting matters for chemical examination :—

In cases of poisoning, darogahs are in the habit of sending in cooking vessels containing suspicious food, either open or slightly covered with leaves. I would

---

* See Government Orders, Circular 129, April 4th, 1843 ; Circular 110, June 24th, 1842.

recommend that a few wide-mouthed stoppered bottles should be supplied to each thannah for the conveyance of such matters. The darogah should be ordered to see that a portion of the contents of the cooking or eating vessel is carefully placed in a bottle, especial care being taken to drain in all sedimentary matters. (Portions of the earth upon which persons supposed to have been poisoned have vomited, or upon which suspicious food has been thrown, should also be carefully collected and sent in.)

The bottle, being then stoppered, should have its mouth securely tied over with thick waxed cloth, and strong twine passing across the stopper. The cloth and string should then be completely covered with sealing-wax, upon which the office seal of the thannah should be impressed. The bottle, enveloped in waxed cloth, should be sent in by hand.

It is highly advisable that every Civil Surgeon should be supplied with a few glass or porcelain jars, manufactured for the express purpose, out of materials in which the absence of arsenic, barytes, lead, &c., had been clearly ascertained by chemical examination. These would be best secured by the earthen stoppers set in iron which are generally used for English preserve pots, intended for exportation to hot climates. These, together with strong spirit, leather, twine, and hard sealing-wax, should always be ready in the inspection-room, and all suspected matters should be placed in these vessels, and secured and sealed therein by the Civil Surgeon himself, before he quits the room in which the body has been examined. Every bottle should not only be sealed with distinct impressions of the Surgeon's and Magistrate's seals, impressions of which should accompany the letters to the Chemical Examiner, but should also be labelled or be accompanied with a memorandum of the matters sent, the station, the names of the Magistrate and Civil Surgeon, and the dates of their letters, with reference to the case despatched to the Chemical Examiner. The practice of enclosing the letters in the parcel containing the suspected matters is highly objectionable. In many such cases, the contents of the bottles escaping, have completely saturated the letters which, in one or two instances, have required to be subjected to a tedious chemical process before their contents could be rendered legible.

The following judicious directions for securing packages to be transmitted to the Chemical Examiner, were published by Dr. O'Shaughnessy in 1842 :—

" *Preservation and Despatch of Suspected Matters.*—Three objects should be carefully attended to in the despatch of all suspected matters : the proof of identity ; the impossibility of any interference during transit ; and, thirdly, preservation from decomposition.

" I have frequently received articles for analysis in bottles merely corked in wooden boxes, secured by a few nails, &c. In more than one case, the contents of the bottles had partially escaped, or those of various parcels were mixed together.

" It is obvious that it would be exceedingly difficult to convict any accused party on evidence given on the analysis of such articles.

" Articles for analysis should be, whenever practicable, enclosed in glass bottles accurately corked, tied and sealed with hard wax, and by the private seal of the Surgeon or Magistrate. Bottles should be enclosed in a thick layer of raw cotton, and all placed in tin, and soldered up. When wooden boxes must be used, these should be sealed and taped at every opening, below as well as above. All liquid and animal matters liable to decomposition should be put up in, or mixed with, the strongest spirit available. This effectually prevents decomposition, and, without interfering with the subsequent analysis, thereby obviates many serious accidents. I have known two instances of bottles bursting, and the contents being totally lost in transit by the fermentation of their contents. In Major P.'s case, one of the bottles exploded in the Laboratory with a loud report, and the contents were lost, except a small portion."

The following instructions were issued by the Government, at Dr. Macnamara's suggestion, in 1862. Dr. Macnamara complained of the following irregularities :—

" Substances have been sent to me without any accompanying letter, but merely a label on the bottle stating that its contents are so and so, sent for analysis.

" The same box may include the stomachs of two or more individuals, in separate bottles, but with no labels or marks affixed to indicate which is which.

" There may be no label on the bottle, and no means of identifying the parcel but by the franking signature on the outer cover, and if this be illegible, as it often is, by reference to the Dak Peon's Book, which only shows the place whence the parcel comes.

" The label on the bottle may be signed by one official, the parcel franked by another, while the letter which has reported the despatch of the substances is signed by a third.

" The letter regarding the parcel is not unfrequently enclosed in it.

" Then, as regards the sealing and packing of the suspected substances, this is often very defective.

" The substances are only loosely corked, or put up so badly, that the bottle could not fail to break during transit ; it is very seldom that the substances are carefully sealed.

" I have also to complain of the meagre reports of cases which are sent to me, and indeed I have often to write for them before receiving any of the details of symptoms or *post-mortem* appearances which are frequently such useful guides to the direction which analysis should take.

" The following are the points which I think should be attended to in transmitting substances to the Chemical Examiner for analysis :—

" The suspected substance should be, when practicable, inclosed in a glass bottle fitted with a sound cork, or in a well-stoppered jar, and the medical officer who makes the *post-mortem* examination should see the cork tied down, and should seal it with his own seal. An impression of the seal should be sent to me in the letter reporting the despatch of the parcel. It would be well, at any rate, in the hot season, that matters liable to decomposition should be put up in spirit. The bottle should be enclosed in a thick layer of raw cotton, and tightly packed into a tin case or box. The box itself should be carefully taped and sealed. Every bottle or packet containing substances sent for analysis should be carefully labelled, and the official who despatches it should write across the label (adding his signature) the nature of the contents, and a reference to the number and date of the letter in which it has been referred to.

"The letter regarding the case, signed by the official who has signed the label, and containing the impression of seals, should be always sent separate from the parcel containing the suspected matters, and it should contain, for the guidance and information of the Chemical Examiner, the fullest possible details regarding symptoms and *post-mortem* appearances."

The following instructions, suggested by Dr. Hutchinson, Civil Surgeon of Patna, in 1865, are in continuation of those given above at p. 32 :—

In cases of Suspected Poisoning.

1. Bring away under seal any food (especially atah or sweetmeats), drink, tobacco, or drugs which may be in the house or near the body.
2. If vomiting has occurred, sweep up with a clean rag any vomited matter which may be on the person or bed, and seal up the rag in a packet.
3. Bring away under seal, any clothing, matting, wood or mud flooring into which any vomited matter soaked.
4. As carefully bottle and seal the contents of any vessel containing vomited matter.
5. Ascertain the exact time between the receipt of food, drink, or medicine, the appearance of symptoms, and occurrence of death.

IDENTIFICATION OF MATTERS SUPPOSED TO CONTAIN POISON.

The following extract from a letter addressed by Dr. Mouat to the Magistrate of Agra in July 1853, involves an important question with regard to the non-validity of evidence deduced from the chemical examination of suspected matters insecurely preserved and transmitted, without sufficient proof of their identity :—

"I have long been of opinion that evidence derived from suspected substances sent to Calcutta for examination is of no value, and would not be admitted in any Court of Justice on the Continent of Europe, where a greater degree of care and guardedness is required in all medico-legal cases than in England or in India. No precaution whatever is taken to prove the real identity of the substance, and most cases are unaccompanied with any history or other detail. Strictly speaking, the identity of the substance should be deposed to, and it should be examined in Court, that the examiner may be subjected to cross-examination, regarding the process upon which he bases his judgment. As this is impracticable in this country, the Civil Surgeon should, I am of opinion, swear to the substance when properly packed in open Court, and it should then be again covered and sealed by the Magistrate. The Chemical Examiner, upon receipt of the package, should prove the receipt of the substance so identified with unbroken seals, and should attest his own examination before a Magistrate: even this, I fear, will not render his testimony of primary value; as he cannot be subjected to cross-examination for the benefit of the accused party. I am unacquainted with the laws in India regulating this matter, and cannot, therefore, say how far the proceeding, above suggested, may be deemed practicable or advisable. Nothing can, however, be more unsatisfactory than the present manner in which such cases are sent to the Chemical Examiner for report."

Evidence of the identity of poisoned matters is strictly required in the Sessions Courts. In a case of road poisoning tried at Moradabad in 1852 [already quoted at p. 168], the superior Court decided that "the sugar sent to the Civil Surgeon for examination and report, with which *Dhatura* and *Nux Vomica* were stated" [by that officer] "to have been mixed, should have been produced upon the trial and sworn to, and evidence should have been given to show that it was the same which was found in the house of the prisoner Kishnoo; also in whose custody it had since remained, and that there had been no opportunity of its being tampered with or changed. In these respects, the record of the trial was defective; and there was also no proof of the sugar in question having ever been in the possession of the" [other] "prisoner Jhana."* In a case of poisoning by arsenic, tried at Bareilly in the same year, the Judges of the higher Court requested that the Sessions Judge would ascertain what means had been adopted by the Magistrate for the prevention of any tampering with the contents of the stomach,—the sealing up of which, it would seem, he had left to his Nazir,—instead of having this important duty performed in his own presence. It was explained that the body was sent for examination to the Sub-Assistant Surgeon, who, being shortly afterwards removed to Calcutta, was unable to analyse the contents of the stomach. The Sub-Assistant Surgeon was, therefore, ordered to send the bottle containing the stomach to the Joint Magistrate; this he did, and it was received and re-sealed in the presence of the Joint Magistrate and also before four witnesses; the bottle was then made over to the Nazir of the Court to keep in his custody until it could be sent to Dr. Kirk, at Bareilly, to analyse. There was no possibility of the contents being tampered with, as a special peon took the bottle to Bareilly with a letter to Dr. Kirk.† Again, late in 1854, the Sessions Judge of Moradabad remarked, in a case of poisoning by Aconite, that—"in the Magistrate's record was a letter to his address from the Civil Assistant Surgeon of Moradabad, reporting that the *dâl* which he had examined contained particles of the poison above named. There was no proof in his record, or any evidence in his [the Judge's] Court to prove that the *dâl* referred to in the letter was a portion of that which had been cooked by Raheeman, of which she and the principal witnesses in this case had partaken; and he was, therefore, under the necessity of suspending the trial. He directed the Magistrate to furnish the required proof, his order being contained in a proceeding which was very explicit. The Magis-

---

* Nizamut Adawlut Reports, N. W. P., 21st August 1852, p. 853.

† *Ibid*, 2nd September 1852, p. 960.

trate replied that he was unable to comprehend what proof was required; and that it would be as reasonable to send up witnesses to prove that swords or lattees, sent to Court with any Sessions case, belonged to the prisoners, as to furnish proof that the *dâl* sent to the Civil Assistant Surgeon was part of that which had been found by the police on the premises of the persons who had been intoxicated or poisoned. He, however, ordered the Kotwal to send any witnesses that might be procurable, and directed the Civil Assistant Surgeon to attend at the Judge's Court." The proof of identity failed.*

MEDICAL EVIDENCE IN CASES OF POISONING.

About eighteen years ago, the validity of the written evidence of the Chemical Examiner, in cases of poisoning tried in the courts of the mofussil, began to be questioned. In October 1852, and again in the following September, the Sessions Judge, Saugor and Nerbudda Territories, brought, before the Sudder Court of the North-West Provinces, a difficulty in respect to references authorized to be made to the Chemical Examiner to Government at the Presidency for information "*which, when acquired, there is no available mode of embodging into legal evidence, recordable by the Court trying a criminal case, or of any effect on the result of the trial.*" The local means of analytic examination are, he observed, in most instances, notoriously inadequate to the discovery of the nature of substances (even mineral) supposed to be poisonous, with any such degree of certainty as would amount to legal evidence of the fact. In cases of supposed poisoning (unhappily far from uncommon) the prosperous or adverse issue of the inquiry may often entirely turn on the availableness of such professional testimony.

The Court replied that the difficulty commented upon by the Sessions Judge is common to all the Courts of those Provinces, in all of which the want of the evidence of a Chemical Examiner is not unfrequently felt. As, however, the opinion of such an officer is of no value, unless it can be made available evidence, and as no apparent means existed by which this end could be obtained, as regards analysis made by the Government Examiner in Calcutta, the Court would suggest that, in all cases where such evidence might be required, the reference should be made to the Civil Surgeons, whose analysis, though, perhaps, not so scientific as one by the Chemical Examiner, would at all events, *quantum valeat*, be susceptible of proof on trial.

At that time, however, medical officers in civil employ were furnished with no other chemical re-agents and apparatus than those which might happen to be included among the medical stores of their hospitals.

---

* Nizamut Adawlut Reports, N. W. P., 27th November 1854, p. 766.

A decision of great importance, as bearing upon this point, was delivered by the Judge of Allahabad in May 1854.* A road poisoner, having halted for the night with two travellers whom he had met with on the way, his companions were attacked with vomiting and purging, and died in the morning. The prisoner attempted to escape, but was brought back and searched, when a packet of powder was found in his kummerbund, together with some strings of pearls, which latter he admitted to have belonged to one of the deceased travellers. The Civil Surgeon examined the bodies, and deposed that the men had died from poison. He abstained from giving an opinion as to the description of poison used, and from analysing the powder and a portion of the flour of which the deceased persons had partaken, on account of his not being provided with proper tests for such purposes ; and he forwarded the stomachs, the powder, and the flour to the Chemical Examiner in Calcutta, with the view of having the question determined. The Chemical Examiner reported that the powder and flour both contained arsenic, and that the stomachs also contained arsenic, and in very considerable quantities. On the application of the Deputy Magistrate, the Judge proposed to the Sudder Court to convert this report into legal evidence by calling upon the Chemical Examiner to swear to the truth of the report, before a Magistrate in Calcutta, in the presence of two witnesses, to be sent to Allahabad, to give evidence on the trial to the genuineness of the affidavit. The Court rejected this proposal, on the ground that this course was met by the insuperable objection that there would be no opportunity of cross-examining the Chemical Examiner, the real witness as to facts ;† and directed the Deputy Magistrate to send for the stomachs, powder, and flour from Calcutta. This was done, but the Chemical Examiner reported that everything had been thrown away as soon as the analysis was finished. As the report of the Chemical Examiner was not considered evidence in the eye of the law, and the nature of the powder was not tested by any witness at the trial, the case had to be treated as if no powder had been found on the person of the prisoner. The Civil Assistant Surgeon

---

* This case has already been referred to at page 116.

† I find, in the records of the Chemical Examiner, that the same objection to receiving that officer's deposition on affidavit was made on several occasions previous to this. The law on this subject was laid down in C. O., Nos. 110 and 146, of Vol. III.,—"Magistrates are not to call upon the Chemical Examiner to make affidavits before the Chief Magistrate of Calcutta, regarding any matter referred for examination, as such affidavits are not legal evidence." It would appear, however, that such an affidavit had some weight as corroborative evidence. In a case of poisoning by arsenic tried in 1852 before the Sessions Judge of the Saugor and Nerbudda Territories, the Judge reported that the testimony of the Officer in civil medical charge, as to the appearances presented on dissection of the stomach, corroborated by the clear evidence, on affidavit, of the Government Chemical Examiner, to the detection of a quantity of arsenic in the contents of the stomach, left no doubt at all, in connection with the proved facts of the case, that the death of the deceased resulted from poison.—*Nizamut Adwalut Reports, N. W. P.*, 8th March 1852, p. 160.

deposed, upon the evidence afforded by his dissections, that the men died of poison of an irritant nature, such as arsenic. Upon this and the other very clear evidences of criminality brought forward in the trial, the prisoner was sentenced to death.*

Consequently upon the delivery of the opinion of the Sudder Court of the North-West Provinces cited at the commencement of this Chapter, Mr. C. G. E. Ford, Civil Assistant Surgeon of Nursingpore, suggested that, in accordance with the custom of the Madras Presidency, small analytical chests should be supplied for the use of Civil Stations in this Presidency. Upon this, the Medical Board recommended to Government that a supply of small cases containing the most useful tests for poisons should be procured from Europe. Forty boxes of this kind were supplied in February 1855, and were distributed to the principal Civil Stations in Bengal and the North-Western Provinces.

Very little was done in this way; and, subsequently, Chemical Examiners were posted at Lahore and Allahabad.

The law now provides that:—

"Any document purporting to be a report from the Chemical Examiner to Government upon any matter or thing duly submitted to him for examination or analysis and report in the course of any criminal trial, or in any preliminary enquiry relating thereto, shall be received in evidence at a trial by the Court of Session, if it bear the signature of such Examiner, and no proof of such signature, or that the person signing holds such office, shall be requisite, unless the Court shall see reason to doubt the genuineness of the document."—*Code of Criminal Procedure.*

"Government have appointed an Additional Chemical Examiner in Bengal, and have directed that his certificates shall be received in all cases where those of the Chemical Examiners have been received heretofore." —*B. G. Cir., No.* 2018, 1865.

Another frequent and very just cause for complaint, by the Chemical Examiners, for many years arose from the scantiness of the information furnished to them regarding the history of the suspected cases or matters under investigation. The rule, however, upon this point is sufficiently strict and definite, as laid down in a Government Minute of the 18th January 1854:—

"Read letter No. 45, from the Chemical Examiner to Government, dated the 9th instant, requesting, for reasons stated, *that all cases forwarded to the Chemical Examiner for analysis and report may be accompanied by the fullest details that can be procured for his information and guidance.*"

An order was passed to this effect.

---

* Nizamut Adawlut Reports, N. W. P., for May 1854, p. 570.

A repetition of this order will be found in Skipwith's Magistrate's Guide ; 902, and C. O., Sup. Pol., L. P., No. 6 of 1843.

In accordance with this rule, a few Officers furnished not only very full details of the histories of the cases, and of the appearances discovered on dissection, but also extracts from the depositions of witnesses and other data, whereby the Chemical Examiner was enabled to perceive in what direction his investigations should be specially directed. More frequently, however, the details sent were extremely meagre and unsatisfactory ; and, in a very great number of instances, all information was evidently intentionally withheld, the transmission of suspected matters for chemical examination being simply notified in the letters of the Magistrate and Civil Surgeon. For some time after I had begun to peruse the Chemical Examiner's records, I felt quite unable to account for the very general prevalence of this latter practice. This, however, was explained by a very able and experienced brother officer who, in reply to my question upon this subject, assured me that the transmission of details was considered as an unnecessary interference, which might be viewed as intended to bias the opinion of the Chemical Examiner. If it be possible that so mistaken an idea can still linger in the mind of any officer, it is but necessary to repeat that it can only be acted upon in violation of the first laws of Medical Jurisprudence, and in transgression of an express Government order.

No such cause for complaint now exists : the Police Reports and all other available information are now sent to the Chemical Examiner ; but, in the interests of Medical Jurisprudence, it is greatly to be regretted that these documents are not filed in the offices of the Chemical Examiners.

LAW IN FORCE FOR THE PUNISHMENT OF THE CRIME OF POISONING IN INDIA.*

It is laid down in Section 328 of the Indian Penal Code that—

" Whoever administers to or causes to be taken by any person, any poison or any stupefying, intoxicating, or unwholesome drug, or other thing, with

* *Laws in force previous to* 1860.

Any person against whom the crime of wilful murder, by drowning or poisoning, may be established—" Penalty"—to suffer death by *Seasut.—Regulation VIII. of* 1799, *Section* 5.

The simple offence of administering poison, with intent to commit murder, if unattended with any aggravated circumstances, may be disposed of by the Sessions Judge—" Penalty "—imprisonment not exceeding seven years—*Regulation LIII. of* 1803, *Section* 2, *Construction No.* 755, *February 7th*, 1833.

A person administering an innoxious drug, under the impression that it is poison, incurs punishment by *Tazeer*, under the Mahomedan Law.—*Macnaghten's Reports, Vol. I., p.* 307.

According to Moulvee Siraj-ool-Huk's exposition of the Mahomedan Law, " the killing by poison, in whatever manner it be given, is not deemed wilful homicide ; that the fine of blood is payable, as for manslaughter, if the poison be compulsively put by another into the mouth of the deceased ; but that, if the deceased took the poison into his own hand, and eat or drank it, without compulsion, though he did not know it to be poison, the giver

intent to cause hurt to such person, or with intent to commit or facilitate the commission of an offence *(see Act IV of* 1867, *s.* 1*)*, or knowing it to be likely that he will thereby cause hurt, shall be punished with imprisonment of either description for a term which may extend to ten years, and shall also be liable to fine."

The words "other thing" must be read "other unwholesome thing." Hence administering a substance, as to whose nature no evidence was given, which was intended to act as a charm, was held to be no offence (1 W. R., C. C., 7)—Mayne's Penal Code, 5 ed., p. 221. See also this authority for the ruling in a case where the prisoner had administered a drug to a female, with intent to excite her sexual passions, in order that he might have connexion with her, and in which the conviction was confirmed.

---

is liable to discretionary punishment only." He adds, however, that the opinion of Tukavee, *viz.*, "that, if a person mix poison with food, and give it to another, who eats it, without knowing it to be poisonous, and dies, the giver of the poison ought to suffer death by *Seasut*," should prevail, "as the mixing poison with food is a heinous offence, such as is declared punishable with death for the security of mankind."—*Macnaghten's Reports, Vol. I., p.* 60.

Administration of Poisonous Drugs with a view to Robbery.

All cases in which the prisoners may be convicted of administering poisonous drugs to persons, with a view to robbing them while in a state of insensibility, whether death shall have ensued or not, come within the provisions of Clause 4, Section 8, Regulation XVIII. of 1817; and the Sessions Judge must pass sentence of imprisonment in transportation for life, and refer the case, if the prisoners are convicted, for the final sentence of the Nizamut Adawlut.—*C. O. No.* 291 *of Vol. I., Construction No.* 365, *N. A. R., Vol. III.*, page 333.

As thuggee officers are vested with magisterial powers, with respect to the specific crimes of thuggee and poisoning, so persons committed on a charge of poisoning may be tried by the Sessions Judge specially appointed for the trial of thugs.—*Construction No.* 1107.

Persons accused of robbery and murder, or of either of those crimes, under circumstances justifying a suspicion that the crimes have been perpetrated by persons engaged in a systematic combination for such purposes, are to be made over to the Assistant to the General Superintendent for the Suppression of Thuggee, who will commit the persons so transferred to be tried before the Special Sessions Judge for the trial of thugs, and will make investigations as to the existence of combinations of the kind described, with a view to the suppression of the offences to which they give rise. [This order was circulated in the Behar district only, but appears applicable to all the Provinces].—*C. O. No.* 92 *of Vol. III.*

The above rule is applicable only to the crime of administering *poisonous* drugs to persons, with a view to robbing them when in a state of insensibility; and does not include the offence of administering drugs and substances of a merely *intoxicating* character, and not of a nature to endanger life, for the purpose recited; consequently those cases only are referrable to the Nizamut Adawlut in which the prisoners are accused and convicted of having administered *poisonous* drugs.—*C. O. No.* 64 *of Vol. III. N. A. R., Vol. V.*, page 121.

In such cases an indictment is defective, if the name only of the drug used be given, and its designation of poison be not specifically adduced. Such indictments, therefore, are to be worded simply "administering poison or poisonous drugs with intent," &c. (according as either of the above rules applies to the case), the article given, whether Dhatoora or other substance, being adduced in the evidence in support of the charge.—*C. O. No.* 83 *of Vol. III.*

The provisions of Clause 5, Section 8, Regulation XVII. of 1857, are not applicable to cases of "administering *intoxicating* drugs, and theft."—*Construction No.* 1324.

Held, by the majority of the Court (*dissentiente* Seton-Karr, J.), that the offence of administering deleterious drugs, without endangering life, is punishable under Section 328 of the Penal Code, and not under section 326 as grievous hurt.—*Queen* v. *Joygopal*, 4 W. R., Cr., 4, Cowell and Woodman, p. 589.

When a poisonous drug was administered to a woman to procure miscarriage, and death resulted, and it was not proved that the accused knew that the drug would be likely to cause death, &c., they were acquitted by the High Court of murder, and convicted of an offence under section 314 of the Penal Code.—*The Queen* v. *Kalla Chand Gope and another*, 10 W. R., Cr., 59, Cowell and Woodman, p. 537.

A man and dog die a few hours after eating the same food, but no traces of poison are found in their bodies, or in the possession of the accused. The mode of investigation by the Police and by the Magistrate in such cases fully laid down.—*Chutto Chumar, appellant*, 1 W. R., Cr., 3, Cowell and Woodman, p. 538.

There is no Law in India prohibitory of the Sale of Poisons.

The necessity for such an enactment was largely canvassed by the Governments of the three Presidencies of India in 1865. For a history of the measures taken towards this end in Madras, see Madras Monthly Journal for May and June, 1870, pp. 395, 478.

According to Dr. Wallich, the sale of Aconite Root appears to have been prohibited under the native Governments, on pain of heavy penalties, except to persons well known, or by authority.

Note on Cattle Poisoning.

The following is an abstract* of a recently published report on this subject, by Dr. Walker, Chemical Examiner to the Government of the North-Western Provinces :

Dr. Walker says that, during 1867, only one case was sent to him for analysis, five in 1868, but one hundred and seventeen in 1869. Eight districts—seven in the North-Western Provinces, and one in Oudh—contributed to the latest aggregate. The largest numbers were from Ghazeepore, Azimgurh, Allahabad, and Jounpore. The exact figures are as follow:—

District	
Ghazeepore	43
Azimgurh	26
Allahabad	19
Jounpore	18
Mirzapore	5
Benares	3
Fyzabad	2
Meerut	1
Total	117

* As given in the *Indian Daily News*.

The circumstances were invariably the same. A chumar charged with having placed some stuff before a bullock or cow in a surreptitious manner, or a chumar suspected of being concerned in cattle-poisoning, having his person and his house searched, and certain suspicious substances discovered in his possession. "In only two cases," says Dr. Walker, "had I information that the death of any animal had resulted from poisoning, and in only one of these two was a portion of the viscera of the poisoned animal sent to me for examination." In 28 of the 117 cases, there is no evidence of any poison being present; indeed, many appeared to have been clumsily trumped up. In one instance, from Allahabad, a bunch of castor-oil leaves had been rolled up; in another, from Azimgurh, a piece of arsenic as big as a walnut had been enclosed in leaves, it being almost as probable that a bullock would chew it as that he would masticate a piece of quartz of the same size; in another, from Ghazeepore, pounded glass was submitted as the poisoning agent; in a fourth, from Jounpore, alum; and in a fifth, from Azimgurh, some common salt. Even in the cases where arsenic had been detected, it was found in so small a quantity that it could not possibly have been administered by an expert with the intention of causing the death of a bullock or cow. In the majority of the cases, however, arsenic was found made up in such a quantity and in such a form as might have caused the death of, and be readily eaten by, a bullock or a cow. The poison was usually pulverized and kneaded into a ball with some coarse atta; this was rolled up in grass, or leaves of bajra, or mowha, or castor-oil. It is natural to doubt—only two cases of death having been reported against so many suspected cases—that the large number referred to should be regarded as evidence of systematic poisoning. The sudden increase may be explained by extra zeal and vigilance on the part of the police in consequence of the special orders of Government in those districts which are supposed to be peculiarly infested by cattle-poisoners. And it only requires a suggestion to induce an ignorant ryotry to entertain the idea that the cattle are being poisoned, or done to death by witchcraft or any other means than the hand of Providence. The "mysterious dispensations of Providence" do not, nevertheless, account for the presence of arsenic in the majority of cases submitted to the Chemical Examiner. Amongst them were several which indicated plainly the extent to which the ignorant suspicions of the peasantry might exaggerate the matter. In three, a piece of cloth was asserted to have been used by chumars to cause the death of cattle; and, in a fourth, a piece of split bamboo, *eighteen inches long*, was declared to have been given to a bullock, to have caused purging, and to have, finally, passed through the intestines of the animal. The stick was sent to be reported upon—that is, as to what poison could be on it! Dr. Walker suggests, as an experiment to determine the existence of extensive cattle-poisoning, that as, with very few exceptions, the poison used, or said to be used, is arsenic, it would be no difficult matter to ascertain whether an animal has died from the effects of arsenic or not; and that, when the Civil authorities of a district are apprised of a sudden increase in the mortality of the cattle of a particular locality, an intelligent native doctor might be deputed from the nearest station to make a *post-mortem* examination, and be instructed to secure in a bottle a piece of the third stomach, of the liver, and of one kidney, of two or three of the animals, making the bottle over to the magistrate. Large pieces would not be required. The pieces taken from each animal might be bottled in strong country spirit. "Until this is done," Dr. Walker observes, "it will always be open to doubt whether increased mortality arises from disease or from poisoning, as it is always open to designing men, or ignorant sufferers from a prevalent epidemic, to accuse some social pariah of the crime of poisoning the village-cattle. This, at least, is as likely to result in the India of to-day as the burning of decrepit old women, under similar circumstances, in our own country two hundred years ago."

WOUNDS, HURTS, AND PERSONAL INJURIES.

Legal Definitions.

The legal definitions of "*Grievous Hurt*" and of "*Assault and Criminal Force*" are laid down, respectively, in *Sections* 319 *et seq.*, and 349 *et seq.*, of the Indian Penal Code (Act XLV of 1860).

LETHAL WEAPONS COMMONLY EMPLOYED IN INDIA.

Regulation XX of 1817, Section 14, required that the weapons with which injuries have been inflicted shall be produced. As any *probable* weapon may be sent in, when the real one is not forthcoming, caution is needful in giving an opinion as to whether the wound in question was probably caused by the weapon produced. On this point consult Nizamut Adawlut Report, September 16, 1857, pp. 471-73.

I am indebted to Dr. Robert Faure Hutchinson, Civil Surgeon of Patna, for the following notes on Lethal Weapons, especially those employed in Behar. (Also *vide supra*, pp. 9 and 10.)

ON LETHAL WEAPONS.

The lethal weapons in use in these Provinces, and I fancy throughout this Presidency, may be classed under three heads:

I.—Those capable of inflicting contused or lacerated wounds, such as the bludgeon and club.

II.—Those capable of inflicting incised wounds, such as the sword, the halberd or battle-axe, the axe, the bill, the chopper, the sickle, the knife, and the razor.

III.—Those capable of inflicting punctured wounds, such as the spear, the arrow, and dagger.

I. 1.—The *Bludgeon ;* synonyms O. H. and B. *Lathi.* This formidable weapon, carried by every traveller and by every rascal bent on mischief, is a stout bamboo staff, of good weight, and generally measuring from four to five feet long ; it tapers, the thick end measuring about two and-a-half and the thin end about one and-a-half inches in diameter. It is used as a walking-stick, or is carried on the shoulder ; in either case, the thin end is always held ; when used offensively, the weapon is grasped towards the thin end with both hands, and is then wielded with tremendous force, and can inflict injuries of every gravity. The head is most frequently assailed; but, owing to the contour of the skull, the contused wound inflicted rarely measures more than two and-a-half or three inches in length, the skin being generally divided to the bone. As the blow is generally received in the erect posture, the vertex *parietes* are generally involved, the forehead and *occiput* generally escaping ; hence lathi-wounds of the head are generally accompanied by considerable hœmorrhage from the divided twigs of the temporal arteries. The edges of the wound are almost always ragged and irregular, but I have known a lathi to cut the skin as clean as a knife. As the lathi is in every one's hand, so the majority of cases sent to the Civil Surgeons are lathi cases, varying in intensity from the broken scalp to the crushed-in skull, from the simple to the compound and comminuted fracture. As the valorous native does not hesitate to smite a prostrate foe, the butt-end (*kunda*) of the lathi is often resorted to, and a very ugly pounding results. Among the grave injuries inflicted by a lathi-blow, I may note ruptures of the heart, liver, and spleen; the latter not at all uncommon. When the thick end of a lathi is bound with iron, it becomes a tremendous weapon of offence called the *lohbanda*, and can inflict frightful injuries, which, confined to the head, are invariably fatal, the blow being almost always accompanied by depression or fracture of both tables. A split bamboo (*bánree*) is an awkward weapon, and is used in *dom* fights. On one occasion I examined a body, in which the 7th and 8th ribs on each side were fractured, and the liver and spleen ruptured ; the skin over the right fractures was marked with parallel and close-lying *striæ* impressed by the similar fibres of the split side, and by them I recognised the nature of the weapon used, and my supposition proved correct.

2. The *Club, Sonta,* is a stout cudgel made of bamboo or some hard wood, nearly three feet long, and like an exaggerated rolling-pin. It is not often carried ; and, therefore, not frequently used ; nor are the injuries serious, broken skin being the utmost.

I have met with one case of murder, in which the head of a boy was pounded in by the stone pestle (*lorha*) used with the grindstone (*sill*).

[Messrs. Cowell and Woodman notice (p. 539) a case in which a man, being struck a violent blow on the temple by a heavy pestle, instantly died.—N. C.]

II. 1.—The *Curved Sword or talwár*, as opposed to the straight sword, or *kirich*. Though, under the Arms Act, the carrying of a talwár is illegal, yet this weapon is very commonly met with, and is capable of inflicting tremendous injuries. The cuts are always clean, and easily amenable to treatment. Sword-cuts, owing to the curve of the weapon, can always be recognised by being, as it were, saucer-shaped in profile; the depth of the saucer varying with the force used, and the locality receiving the wound.

The talwár is frequently used for inflicting made-up wounds; but a practised eye will always at once detect such impositions, for these wounds are always inflicted in localities where a sword, drawn in anger, could not possibly reach. Thus I recollect a case of a cut at right angles across the left calf high up, which the fellow said had been inflicted during pursuit. Now, had the sword reached, under the circumstances, an oblique cut might have been inflicted, but the man said he was wounded while running, therefore the left heel must have been in the way, and would probably have received the cut. A made-up sword-wound has always a little tail at one end, showing that it has been a deliberate draw, and this remark applies equally to wounds self-inflicted by the knife or razor, especially to the latter. A case in point had this tell-tale. The man declared that he had been wounded by a sword, and, true enough, there was a cut across the front of the thigh six inches long, but only penetrating, *all along*, into the subcutaneous fat. I at once declared that this was a made-up injury, for no hostile sword could have inflicted a wound of such magnitude without the muscles having been cut into in the centre of the wound. With a little care and thought the sequence of sword-wounds can be clearly laid down as in the following case, which also illustrates the tremendous injuries which a sword can inflict. It is abstracted from my *Post-Mortem* book: "Body of an old woman. An enormous gash has cloven the right breast and right side of chest; right hand cut in two obliquely; cut extending downwards and outwards; enormous gash down right side of neck penetrating chest. A gash down right cheek in front of right ear, dividing right ramus of lower jaw. As the gash in the neck is deeper behind than in front, I believe the wounds were inflicted in the following sequence. First the poor old woman was felled from behind by the blow on the neck; when down, she would raise her right arm in helpless defence, and then came the tremendous blow severing the hand, and cutting into the right breast. The blow on the face was given last, as a *coup de grace*, and from behind."

Subsequent investigation determined the exact truth of my supposition, for the poor woman was literally cut up as I described.

[Although the talwár has a sharp point, this is seldom used. An exceptional case is found in the Bengal Police Report for 1866, p. 302, where it is stated that "the medical officer's certificate, after examination of the body, corroborated the statement of the eye-witnesses, who stated that, because the *joopree*, or shed, in which Ramdoyal was lying, was so *low*, the murderers could not cut him with their swords, but had *stabbed* him with the points.—N. C.]

2.—The *Halberd*, or battle-axe, is the only English term I can find for this well-known weapon, the progenitor of the harmless, but imposing halberds of our "beef-eaters." I allude to the *garássa* or *gandása*, of which there are three varieties; two consisting of a crescentic or double cresentic blade attached to the thick end of an ordinary lathi, and the third, a truncated form of the first, with a heavy oblong blade, the ordinary chaff-chopper of the country; the blade is generally let into a heavy wooden handle.

The first of the three is the form most frequently seen, and ugly wounds are inflicted with it. It is, *par excellence*, the weapon of watchmen or Chokidars, so that whenever these valorous guardians have been engaged in a scrimmage, you may always look out for *garássa* wounds.

The chopper may become a tremendous weapon of offence. In a recent case, a man was assailed, while asleep on his right side with his left hand resting on his head, the first blow crushed through left index and middle fingers, and through the outer table of the occipital and left parietal bones. The second blow inflicted a hideous gash six inches long, cutting through the left eye and across the root of the nose, and into the right antrum, and revealing depths I feared to gauge with the probe. Wonderful to say, the man recovered without a single bad symptom, the only traces of the tremendous blow was a sightless, but not disfigured eye, and a cicatrix half an inch long on the root of the nose. No human being, not in the secret, could have sworn that the man brought to me and the man in Court were one and the same individual.

I have had no experience of the axe (*koolhári*) or bill (*dao*); but have met with one or too ugly tears inflicted by the serrated sickle, or *hussooa*. The sharp sickle, or paring knife, used by pasees in trimming and tapping the tar palm, is the common weapon in their fights, and inflicts ugly cuts, which, however, are not extensive, owing to the curve, and the sharp edge being inside. The domes use a truncated sickle for cutting up bamboos, the sharp edge being at the end, and it can inflict severe wounds. The knife (*chooree*) and the razor (*astoora*) are ready to the hands of butchers and barbers, and are most frequently used in inflicting designed injuries. Like designed sword-cuts they can always be recognized by being inflicted with a wavering, faltering hand, in most inaccessible positions, and the tell-tale fag-end is almost always present. But both are frequently used as murderous weapons, and with deadly effect.

In a murder case, the fatal and only wound was a deep cut, two and-a-half inches long, and one inch deep, extending from below the right angle of the lower jaw obliquely across towards the larynx, dividing the carotid artery. An attempt was made to prove that a sword had inflicted the injury, and the sub-divisional native doctor swore to this: When called upon, I maintained that no talwár, however skilfully wielded, could inflict, in that locality, a wound of such limited dimensions, for the angle of the jaw and the right shoulder (the man was lying on his left side) would effectually protect the part; that no native knife could, at a blow, inflict a wound so short and yet so deep, but that a razor could; and so it was proved, for the man's own barber was his murderer.

III. I have no experience of wounds inflicted by the spear (*ballam* or *barchi*), arrow (*teer*), or dagger (*krees*). A murder was recently committed at Barh, with a *soolfie* a (single) barbed spear used as a harpoon in striking the larger fishes or turtle. I am told that it is very common in Bengal Proper.

Regarding weapons commonly used in Lower Bengal, I may add to Dr. Hutchinson's the notes that, in an affray at Jessore, the weapon used was an *aro*, a sharp three-pronged instrument, similar to that used in harpooning fish.

In a trespass case at Mymensingh, a man was killed by a *koanch*, an instrument with iron at the end, used by the natives for spearing fish.

Fatal wounds are frequently inflicted with *pointed bamboos*, as in the case of a Backergunge man who, being struck on the right side under the nipple, by a long sharp-pointed bamboo, used to scare away wild hogs from the crops, died after a short interval.*

Bamboos split in the ordinary manner are capable of inflicting very ugly wounds, as will be experienced, in hands and clothes, by any one who personally undertakes that very effectual mode of checking fires in native villages—the breaking up of huts and fences in front of the advancing flames.

In a trial at Shahabad, one accused of participating in a murderous affray attempted to establish an *alibi*, and accounted for a wound over the shoulder-blade by saying that it had been caused by his accidentally striking himself against a bamboo in the roof of a house. "The darogah described it in his report as being of about a hand's breadth. The judges remarked that, unfortunately, he does not appear to have been subjected by the magistrate to an examination by the surgeon, who might have been able to show how the wound was caused; there is only a slight mark."

---

* Nizamut Adawlut Reports, Sept. 9, 1856, p. 58.

[This was the appearance more than five months subsequently to the date of the darogah's report.] "And, judging from its appearance, it could not have been a wound of any great depth or extent, and it is not impossible that it may have been caused in the way he describes ; if so, it is a most singular circumstance that it should have happened at the very time when he is accused of being concerned in the affray." The judges of the Court of Appeal observe that "the account which he gives of the mode of receiving his wound, which was inflicted on the same date, is wholly incredible." * It is not said why.

Blows on the head with split bamboos inflict very clean cuts; indeed, as Dr. Hutchinson remarks, some lathee wounds of the scalp can scarcely be distinguished from incisions. In a case where Dr. Duka was of opinion that death had been caused by extensive bruises and cuts on the head, and fracture of skull causing effusion of blood in the brain from a large artery which was ruptured, the *sooruthal*, held by the police, showed that there were fourteen injuries said to have been inflicted by a *gurassa*. On being questioned by the judge, Dr. Duka said, "The soft parts of the head are scarcely a few lines deep, and it is very possible that a hard stroke with a piece of wood may cause a cut very much resembling that inflicted with a knife or sword, and I am not prepared to say, in this instance, whether a knife or sword or any sharp instrument was used or not." † So also, at Rajshahye, the civil surgeon stated, at the trial, that two wounds "fracturing the skull and rupturing or bursting open the sutures which connect the right parietal with the occipital bone" were probably inflicted by blows of a *lathee*. He had previously informed the magistrate that they might have been inflicted with a *dao*, which discrepancy he explained by stating that he was, in the first instance, given to understand that a *dao* had been the fatal weapon ; and by the observation that, in many cases, within his knowledge, of blows from a *lathee*, the fracture and cut were (as they were here) so clean as not to be distinguishable from a wound with a *dao*.‡

In all such cases, examination of quite recent wounds with a lens would at once decide whether they were, in reality, incised or contused.

Allusion has already been made, in foot-note to p. 138, to the *panjies* or *kumanchees*, as the Nagas sometimes call them, used by the Eastern hill tribes of Bengal. We are told that, when the Nagas are obliged to retreat before an enemy, they obstruct the narrow path through the jungle by these slender bamboo spikes. They always go armed with these, having a case of them attached to their waists. They are very expert and extremely quick in placing these in the ground to the

* Nizamut Adawlut Reports, August 25, 1856, p. 275.
† *Ibid*, July 18, 1865, p. 76.
‡ *Ibid*, February 2, 1857, 84.

best advantage. In time of war, they guard the paths to their villages by these. It is quite impossible to pass or go over them with naked feet; they will even penetrate a good shoe : the enemy must sit down quietly and lift them before he can advance. They also protect themselves from wild beasts with these *panjies.* A large fire is made, round which they arrange themselves, and then they form a circle of such spikes towards the country so that no animal can come near ; an elephant or tiger is stopped immediately. If the latter makes a spring, he falls in the midst of the spikes.

In describing Cooch Behar, early in the 17th Century, R. Fitch says, "All the countrey is set with canes made sharpe at both ends, and driven into the earth ; and they can let in the water, and drowne the countrey knee-deepe." *

The *gooleil-bans,* or pellet-bow, generally used as a weapon against crows, is capable of inflicting rather severe injuries. In a riot at Sylhet, in 1856, some men appear to have been wounded by the balls fired from these weapons.

Gobind Misser, of Cuttack, was sentenced to transportation for life for having taken a boy of twelve into the jungle, inflicting five wounds in his throat, and others on his chest, his temple, and ears, and robbing him of his ornaments. The boy said that prisoner had wounded him with his own *iron pen,* seven or eight inches long, and pointed for writing on tal leaves. The weapon was capable of producing death.†

WOUNDS INFLICTED BY WEAPONS COMMONLY IN USE IN LOWER BENGAL AND THE N. W. PROVINCES.

Notwithstanding the character for mildness of temper which they have gained, from superficial observers, deceived by their manners, and unacquainted with their customs and habits of thought and action, the common people of India are scarcely less apt to conclude their quarrels by severe wounding than are the more impetuous denizens of European countries. This, probably, arises from the circumstance which has been more or less operative in determining nearly every homicide since the first,—the readiness with which an offensive weapon always comes to hand ; few Bengalees are without a *lathee* (bamboo stick), *dao* (bill-hook), and perhaps a *codalee* (adze or large hoe), a *hussolee* (sickle), a *kolharee* (axe or hatchet),‡ and a *bullum* or *sain* (spear) ; and nearly every Hindustanee has his sword, and his iron-bound cudgel. The *gurassa* or *gundrasa*—a

---

* Purchas, Part V, p. 509.

† Nizamut Adawlut Reports, August 18, 1856, 237.

‡ Mahommed Jan, one of Moorshed Cooly Khan's police guards, was in the habit of having the bodies of all the thieves whom he caught split in two, and hung upon trees by the highway. Hence, we are told by Stewart, he was nicknamed the *Kolhareh.*

kind of bill or battle-axe,—and the *koorpee,* or hoe, are common both in the North-West and in Bengal.

It is of considerable importance that medical men and judicial officers should make themselves acquainted with the appearance and modes of use of the various weapons, tools, &c., employed by the natives, as questions of considerable moment not unfrequently arise with regard to the weapon with which wounds have been inflicted. Thus a dead body may present numerous gashes, in the neighbourhood of which are observed several deep stabs. An inexperienced surgeon would, perhaps, assert that two weapons had been used, or that the wounds were inflicted with the edge and point of a sword. It would probably be found that a short sickle had been employed, or a *dao* with a curved and pointed beak. In a trial at Futtehpore, the civil surgeon deposed that the wounds found upon the bodies of two persons must have been inflicted with three kinds of weapons, one of which must have been pointed like a spear. The prisoner confessed freely that, having heard that his wife and her paramour were together, he proceeded to his house with a hatchet (or *koolharee,* misnamed an axe by the surgeon, as the judge considered) which he had in his hand when he heard the news. He slew the adulterer with this hatchet, and afterwards killed his wife with the same weapon. A blood-stained dhotee was found on the person of the prisoner, and he pointed out the *koolharee* in a gutter. The sessions judge considered that the efforts made to prove the act one of culpable homicide, and not murder, failed from the improbabilities of the story, and before the evidence of the surgeon. There was violent probability, he held, that other persons, well armed, were engaged in the murder, and that the assault was premeditated, and not effected suddenly by one man armed only with a small hatchet for cutting wood. He recommended that capital punishment should be awarded. One of the judges of the superior Court was not able to discover anything which could support the opinion of the sessions judge that the prisoner must have had accomplices, or that of the civil surgeon that the wounds observed by him on the bodies of the deceased could not possibly have been inflicted with the same weapon. All the circumstances of the case tended directly to show that the prisoner alone perpetrated the acts charged, and that the only weapon he used was that produced in Court. The only conclusion, therefore, to which he could arrive, was "that the civil surgeon must have been mistaken, which might very easily have happened." The other judge saw no reason to believe that the prisoner had any accomplices in his crime. He accepted the confessions as they stood.—Sentence, imprisonment for life in transportation.*

The description of wound most frequently inflicted in Bengal is the

* Nizamut Adawlut Reports, N. W. P., April 29, 1852, p. 370.

contused scalp wound, produced by a blow with a stout bamboo. When not loaded with metal, or used with a full intention to kill, this instrument is peculiarly well adapted to inflict a broken head, without the accompaniment of a fractured skull. By far the largest number of letters, which pass between the magistrates and the civil surgeons, are relative to injuries of his kind. Scarcely a week elapses, in any large civil station in Bengal, in which one or two cases of this kind do not come under the surgeon's treatment. Although the bamboo, used with moderate force, seldom proves a deadly weapon, blows from it not unfrequently fracture the arm and collar-bones of aged natives. I have seen some hundreds of these simple scalp wounds, but do not recollect to have met with erysipelas, or any other serious result in a single case.

Blows on the head, inflicted even with a light bamboo, may, however, cause death. In 1852, a zumeendaree quarrel occurred at Banda, in which a man was killed by persons armed with bamboos, the heaviest of which weighed a pound and-a-half and was six feet long: he received a blow on either temple, fell down insensible, and died without being able to give his deposition.*

In 1854, a man of Mymensingh being at his evening meal, observed that there was too much salt in one of the dishes. As his wife was stooping down to help him, he gave her a severe blow, *with his open hand*, on the right temple; she fell, became senseless, and died shortly after. She was only eleven years old, and had been some time before unwell with fever; and, though she had recovered, she was still weak. No examination of the body could be made. The medical officer stated (as far as can be gathered from the printed report, which is scarcely intelligible), that fever might have occasioned such a condition of the brain as to render it liable to become easily disorganized by a slight concussion;—in such a case, a severe blow with the open hand might produce a fatal effect.†

A similar case was tried at Chota Nagpore in 1856.‡ A man, who was proved to have had grave suspicions of his wife's fidelity, confessed that he gave her three slaps on the head. She lay down, and he, after a while, taking a light, found that she was dead. The body was not exhumed until twelve days after death. The judge remarked that the absence of any marks of violence on such cursory examination as would in such case be made by untaught persons, does not prove that violence was not used. Deceased had been weakly since her last confinement, of twins, two or three months previously. The opinions of the judges of the Court of appeal were divided upon the measure of guilt; but, as there was nothing

* Nizamut Adawlut Reports, N. W. P., 2nd November 1852, p. 1295.

† Nizamut Adawlut Reports, 27th October 1854, p. 520.

‡ *Ibid*, May 3rd, 1856, p. 771.

on record which falsified his confession, he was convicted of culpable homicide.

The reports to the superior Courts, however, contain a very large proportion of cases in which the skull had been horribly fractured by repeated blows with a heavy weapon. In these cases, either the bamboo is employed with decided intention to destroy life, or an iron-bound lathee, or some weighty instrument used in agriculture or building, is brought, or caught up to effect the crime. It is probable that the generality of fractures of the skull, inflicted with blunt instruments by natives, are fatal. Usually, the destruction of parts (although the fractures are not always compound) is so extensive that recovery is impossible. I have only seen two cases of this kind of fracture in which life was prolonged even for many hours.*

Violent attempts to tear off the neck rings (*hassoolee*), worn by native women, frequently produce rather severe wounds, which, however, can rarely occasion any doubt in the mind of the medical man with regard to the cause of injury.

Spear Wounds are of not uncommon occurrence in Bengal, and it is remarkable, although perhaps only as a coincidence, in how many of the recorded cases the *Heart* has been transfixed with these weapons, sharp ended bamboos, &c. It is important, in cases of this kind, to be able to deliver a clear opinion with regard to the amount of *force* used in the infliction of the fatal blow. In an instance which came under my notice, I very strongly insisted upon the fact that, although a blow with a *korrah* had, unfortunately, pierced the heart, this instrument could not have been wielded by the prisoner with extreme force, otherwise it would have been driven through the chest, whereas the wound was scarcely more than two inches in depth.

In 1854, Mokim Sheikh, of Nuddea, was sentenced to 14 years' imprisonment for having killed his sister's husband, Bedoor Sheikh, with a spear called a *surkee*. Bedoor beat and abused his wife. Her brother resenting this, the two men had a scuffle, when Mokim got a spear from his

---

* One was that of a woman, who was struck on the forehead with some small blunt instrument. She survived the injury for about a month. On examination, I found that a nearly circular portion of bone, as large as a shilling, had been completely depressed upon the dura mater, the membrane had become thickened around the edge of the encroaching bone, and the frontal bone presented evident traces of active absorption upon every part of the broken circle;—it was quite evident that, but for an abscess in the substance of the brain, which had destroyed life, the depressed bone would have gradually become detached and been thrown off. In the other instance, a man had been struck on the head by his daughter with a ponderous wooden hammer, used for smoothing turfs. The injury was frighfully extensive, and I found it necessary to remove twelve or fourteen pieces of bone by aid of the trephine and Hey's saw. The man survived this operation about 48 hours. The brain was discovered to be extensively lacerated.

house and flung it at Bedoor. It pierced the right side of his chest, and he died almost immediately.*

It appeared, from the statements of the witnesses for the prosecution in a trial at Azimgurh, that a man had been seized by the arms from behind by a person named, while another thrust a *spear* into his right breast. The accused protested that the man was killed by an *arrow*, shot by one of his own party. The Native Doctor who examined the body deposed that he found a deep wound in the right breast, which was the cause of death. It was a Spear wound, not an Arrow wound.†

In a land dispute at Backergunge, Junnoo Beaparee thrust his *soolfee*, or spear, into his opponent's thigh, dividing the popliteal artery and causing immediate death.‡

A case will be found in the Chapter on *Torture*, in which a man killed his wife, by thrusting a spear through her neck, while another held her head.

In 1852, one Dyaram, of Bareilly, confessed that he had gone to the apartment of a woman, while she was asleep, had taken off her ornaments, and then murdered her by stabbing her in the neck three times with the coulter of a plough (*phalah*). This was a piece of iron rather thicker than a man's finger, about a foot in length, tapering to a point which seemed to have been broken off just at the end.§

Some years since, the body of a man was sent to me for inspection, in which I found an incised wound completely traversing the popliteal space, from side to side, under the tendons of the ham-string muscles, and dividing the artery. It was stated, with great probability, that he had been found dead near a large bow, which had been set in the jungle for tigers ; he had stepped unknowingly upon the string, and the arrow had transfixed his limb.

The people of India, both Mussulmauns and Hindus, were long remarkable for their skill in the use of the bow.‖ At present, *Arrows* are only used by the Hill Tribes. The arrows used by these people in the chase are usually understood to be poisoned with a preparation of the *aconilum ferox*, but it would appear, from our accounts of the Santhals, that the

---

* Nizamut Adawlut Reports, 28th August 1854, p. 307.

† Nizamut Adawlut Reports, N. W. P., 10th December 1852, p. 1471.

‡ Nizamut Adawlut Reports, 20th October 1856, p. 838.

§ Nizamut Adawlut Reports, N. W. P., 19th September 1852, p. 1011.

‖ We read of Buckhtyar's invading army (A. D. 1202-3) being much annoyed by the skill of the Thibetan and Hindu archers. Subsequently to the conquest of Bengal, we find Hindus and Mussulmans, especially the Mahomedan princes and the Rajas, employing the bow almost up to the time of the commencement of the British rule, although matchlocks were in use at the commencement of the seventeenth century. Long previous to this, the Mussulmans had plenty of cannon, but found them of little use, except when they got Portuguese gunners to serve them. In 1567, M. Cæsar Frederick found that the King of Pegu had "great ordanance, made of very good metal."

arrows which they use in war are not always poisoned. This is supposed to be owing to the circumstance of the process of preparing and applying the poison being somewhat long and tedious.

In 1853, Soneeah, a Hill man, was tried at Moorshedabad for the murder of a man with whose wife, it was probable, he had intrigued. He confessed that they had been drinking together. That deceased abused him on account of his intimacy with tbe woman, and tried to strangle him. He fled, and the deceased chased him for above a mile ; he then turned and shot the deceased with a poisoned arrow at a distance of *eighty paces*. Two witnesses declared that he was a good shot, and could hit an object at that distance. This part of the prisoner's statement was not altogether credited. The deceased was found with an arrow wound on his breast, fresh and bleeding. He never spoke, and died during the night. The Judge remarked that the Hill people (of that neighbourhood) always carry poisoned arrows. The medical officer's evidence showed that the wound was sufficient to cause death, even if the point of the arrow had not been poisoned.*

In the same year, a Hindu, of Manbhoom, being awaked in the night by robbers, went out of his house and was immediately struck in the breast with an arrow, and died shortly afterwards.†

In 1845, some dacoits, probably from the Hills, killed the chowkeedar of a village in Bheerboom, with an arrow. In the same year, a body of Kunjurs, armed with spears and arrows, committed a most daring dacoitee in the bazar of the city of Patna, striking down with their spears all whom they met.‡

In 1843, a Bhaugulpore Hill man, suspecting his wife of witchcraft, took her out and shot her with his bow and arrow.§

Another of these men, suspecting his brother-in-law of an incestuous intercourse with his wife, and knowing that her sister had cognizance of it, went out, met the sister-in-law, and shot an arrow at her, which went through the upper part of her arm. She escaped. Falling in with his brother-in-law, he shot him through the heart. He then shot at the man's wife, but she escaped.

Cases of this kind, from time to time, occur in the Upper Provinces.

One Duljeet, of Bussye, in the Dholepore territory, but for some time a refugee in the Agra district, was tried at Agra, for having attacked, at the head of an armed body, two men, one of whom they wounded fatally with an arrow.||

---

* Nizamut Adawlut Reports (N. W. P.), 9th August 1853, p. 187.

† *Ibid*, 18th October 1853, p. 654.

‡ Police Report, L. P., 1845., pp. 10, 62 and 89.

§ *Ibid*, for 1843, p. 19.

|| Nizamut Adawlut Reports (N. W. P.), 4th February 1853, p. 1488.

In 1847, a man, of Shahjehanpore, was shot by an arrow which "entered between the sixth and seventh ribs of the left side, and penetrated the lung and apex of the heart."*

It will be observed, from several of the above cases, that the accuracy with which these people aim at the Heart, is very remarkable.

HACKING WITH SWORD OR BILL-HOOK.

Hacking to pieces is a mode of death which appears from the Seir Mutaqherin to have been rather frequently inflicted at the Court of the Nuwab of Bengal in the first half of last century. Thus fell Meer Cossim Khan, and, perhaps, also Juggut Sett and his brother, Rajah Soroopchand So also the body of Suraj-ed-dowlah "was hacked to pieces by strokes without number" by the sword of Mahmedy-beg.

The most frightful injuries are frequently inflicted by the natives of Bengal and Hindustan with the *dao* and the *tulwar*. An unfortunate will be caught in the act of burglary or theft by the people of the village or by a chowkeedar, and will be hacked until the assailant's arm grows weary.† Or several persons will set upon one and cut him almost into shreds. Similar cases occur in the Bombay Presidency. See that of Willoo, who hacked his wife with a sword for adultery.‡

In June 1838, Mirza Hyder Shekoh, cousin to the king of Delhi, murdered his wife, the Kandera Sultan Begum, the king's niece, by cutting her in pieces with a sword,—she being at the time eight months advanced in pregnancy. The body presented a most appalling sight, being a complete mass of bloody flesh. After which he quietly left the house, and threw himself down a well near at hand. The unfortunate princess was universally esteemed. The motives for this murder were variously stated, as the criminal refused offering any defence. It was said that she declined to associate with the prince's mistresses, or refused to give half of her jewels to one of them.

---

* Nizamut Adawlut Reports (N. W. P.), 18th November 1852, p. 1335.

† I, when at Howrah, sixteen years ago, examined the body of a thief who had been treated in this manner. There was an enormous wound across the back of the skull, not quite penetrating the brain, one humerus was cut through [or rather broken through,—the manner in which a common *tulwar* divides one of the long bones very much resembles that in which a table-knife can be made to divide a marrow-bone by a slight cut and a fracture] and the elbow joint laid open and splintered. Nearly the whole of the intestines protruded through a wide gash in the abdomen; there were also other wounds. Still the unfortunate man survived these injuries for a short time. See also cases,—Nizamut Adawlut Reports, N. W. P., 2nd June 1852, p. 512. (An unarmed intruder hacked until he died, the head nearly severed from the body). *Ibid*, 30th June 1853, p. 804, twelve wounds inflicted by a youth upon a stealer of *sursoon* (mustard), of which he died in the jail hospital.

‡ Bellasis' Reports, p. 141.

The prince was tried by Mr. (afterwards Lord) Metcalfe, and hanged in the palace.*

It appeared, in a trial at Mirzapore, that one Beney Persaud, whilst lying on his charpoy, was attacked by a party of armed men, who inflicted forty-one wounds, twenty-one of which were very severe, from the effects of which he died the same evening.† A few months later, three men of Bareilly were attacked by a number of persons armed with swords, who hacked them almost to pieces. The dead bodies of two were found each to have twenty wounds, and that of the third, thirteen, one of which completely severed the head from the body.‡

A rude and savage sense of honor leads the Rajpoot to conceive that,—when he has been grossly insulted, or an injury has been done him,—"*life is no longer of any value*;"§ his opponent must be destroyed as a matter of course, and then he will be prepared to meet death himself. Numerous instances could be cited in which whole families have, in this way, fallen victims to the vengeance of Up-country natives. The subject will be recurred to in the Chapter on INSANITY. The following instance will suffice in this place. Here the extreme point of honor was carried out: the offended party, having wreaked his vengeance upon his enemy, devoted himself and his disgraced family to a common destruction.‖

In 1853, one Hoolassee was tried at Hoshungabad. It appeared that Hureeram, *malgoozar* of the village, took with him a man and four women labourers to the wheat field of Sawunt Chowdhree, the prisoner's father, a cultivator said to be in balance to the malgoozar. He went unarmed, but with the avowed object of cutting the crop. He was opposed by the old man, his two sons, and his wife. An affray ensued, in which the prisoner and the two other men killed the malgoozar by blows on the head with an axe, club, and stick. On returning to their own house, Anuntram, the prisoner's brother, stunned his own wife by striking her several severe blows on the head with a club. She, however, recovered. He then attacked his own daughter (three or four years old) and killed her by fracturing her skull, the prisoner suggesting, or at least, aiding the crime,—seizing the unfortunate infant by the leg and throwing her down

---

* *Delhi Gazette*, July 4th, 1838.

† *Ibid*, 27th April 1853, p. 590.

‡ *Ibid*, 20th July 1853, p. 896. See also *Ibid*, 14th August 1852.—(A man "hacked to pieces," while lying on his charpoy, by two persons). *Ibid*, 25th August of same year, p. 870.—(A man enticed away to a place where several persons were waiting for him, who despatched him with twenty sword-wounds.)

§ See Nizamut Adawlut Reports, N. W. P., 22nd July 1853, p. 900.

‖ Stewart mentions that Chukl Kirshom, vakeel of the Nawab of Bengal, (Cir. 1730) being ill-treated, murdered his whole family, and then put an end to his own existence.

before her insensate father, and following up the fatal blow. The party then made for the malgoozar's house, and, on the road, met an unarmed man, a servant of their first victim, whom they despatched with axe and club blows. Arrived at their opponent's house, they killed a man with sword or axe wounds, wounded a young child in the face, and despatched the malgoozar's mother by wounds which were described as "very dreadful and extensive." The father then said—"Having done for all, we must now, as Rajpoots, die ourselves"—and despatched his son Anuntram by two sword wounds on the neck, nearly decapitating him. He next called on his son Hoolassee, the prisoner, to come forward. He (craven according to the dreadful standard of courage here exhibited) swore a solemn oath that he would die after killing his father, who then, failing in an attempt to stab himself, was put to death by the prisoner, who used the sword with both hands, and almost severed the head from the body. The prisoner was soon after seized, fleeing away, with his axe in his hand.*

In many cases, both Up-country and in Bengal, the *tulwar* or *dao* is snatched up, and used with horrible ferocity upon what would appear to be very trivial grounds of provocation.

One Chittar Singh, of Furruckabad, was sentenced to death, for the murder of a female servant *pregnant by his lately deceased brother.* He was engaged cooking his dinner when the unfortunate woman put a lota of water within the circle (*chouka*) where he was sitting, by which his food was defiled. He sprang up, seized his sword, which was lying close by, and inflicted upon her "two deep wounds on the left side of the head, one on the left shoulder, and one on the upper part of the back, which had divided the spine and entered the cavity of the chest."†

Nundram Dhobee, of Sylhet, desired his sister-in-law, who was cooking, to grind down some herbs for him. She objected to doing so, at the moment, lest her vegetables should be spoiled, but asked him to wait awhile. Upon this the prisoner seized a very sharp *dao*, weighing two pounds, which lay near, and cut the woman down, inflicting ten wounds about her head, neck, and shoulders. She subsequently died of lock-jaw. He then attempted suicide, by cutting his own throat very severely. After he heard of the woman's death, he appeared to be seized with remorse, and then repeatedly attempted to hang himself.‡

Two men of Allahabad had been eating together; one told the other to take away the cooking pots. Upon his replying that he would do so

---

* Nizamut Adawlut Reports, N. W. P., 5th December, 1853, p. 1431.

† *Ibid*, 10th February 1853, p. 192.

‡ Nizamut Adawlut Reports, 3rd August 1854, p. 193.

presently, his companion seized a sword and slaughtered him with nineteen wounds.*

Somaree was sentenced to death at Tirhoot in 1855, for having, on returning from work in the fields with his *koodalee* in his hands, killed his wife with the hoe. He confessed, first, that he had killed his wife because "she had kicked the dish containing his food;" but, both in the Foujdary and Sessions Court, he said that he had killed her, because she had been unfaithful to him, would not sleep with him, and had also kicked the vessel which held his food.

Dr. Durant, who examined the body, deposed to finding seven cuts on the back of the neck, head, and shoulders. Each was a deep gash, some inches in depth, and the cut on the neck had severed the bones of the spine. The skull was not fractured, but a piece, the size of a rupee, was cut clean out of the back part of the head, severely injuring the brain, which, no doubt, was the cause of death.† There was no proof of his wife's alleged unfaithfulness adduced at the trial.

Shudu Sheik, of Jessore, was sentenced to hard labor in irons for fourteen years, for miserably cutting with a *dao* his child-wife, whom he had first gagged. There were thirteen wounds on the back of the head, neck, arms, and hands, and some fingers were cut off. At first Dr. Palmer feared that her recovery was hopeless, but she ultimately recovered. He said that, "he began talking to her, and she refused to answer." The poor little creature, a child of eleven, stated, after much hesitation, that her husband had, at midnight, asked her to let him have connexion with her, which she refused, partly from resentment at his having before causelessly abused her, and more because sexual intercourse caused her much pain. The Court was induced to put the question, as a witness, the prisoner's brother-in-law, stated it was his belief that the prisoner was incensed, because his wife was yet too young to allow him to have intercourse with her.‡

Shibram Chuny, of Sylhet, was capitally sentenced, for hacking his wife and her mother with a heavy *dao*. The elder woman died in consequence. All that came out in explanation was that the prisoner, finding a straw in his rice, abused his wife and her parents; upon her remonstrating, the violent act was committed.

This subject of acts of furious homicidal violence, committed without any apparent adequate motive or provocation, will be again taken up in the Chapter on *Cut Throat*.

A man, excited to madness by jealously or by *galee* (foul abuse), seizes

---

* Nizamut Adawlut Reports, N. W. P., 17th February 1853, p. 249.

† *Ibid*, Nov. 23, 1855, p. 814.

‡ *Ibid*, Feb. 25, 1857 p. 209.

a heavy weapon, and, with from five to twenty strokes, literally hews his victim to pieces, proving that the power—

> "His foeman's limbs to lop away,
> As wood-knife shreds the sapling spray"—

does not require the thews of a Douglas for its exercise.*

In these cases, the wounds are actually to be measured rather by the foot than by the inch. The skull is generally penetrated in more than one place to the brain; the neck is cut to the spine; a shoulder-blade is completely divided; a humerus is cut through; a hand is lopped off; the abdomen is gashed and the bowels are protruding. It is very remarkable that many of the unfortunates thus treated recover with scarcely a bad symptom. I have known patients recover from each of the above-mentioned injuries, with the exception of the second. In many of these cases the sword is only cast from the hand of the murderer after it has been snapped in two,† or when it has been "bent out of all shape" by striking against the victim's bones.‡

Judging by the cases of this kind which I have myself seen, but especially drawing inference from the very numerous accounts of similar instances which I find among the Surgeons' Reports sent into the Calcutta Nizamut Adawlut, I have, not without considerable astonishment, arrived at the conclusion, that these frightful outrages,—which have hitherto been regarded merely as acts committed in a paroxysm of uncontrollable rage, in which the murderer strikes wildly at his victim, with no other purpose than to hack him to pieces in any manner whatever,—are, especially when committed with the *dao*, done after a certain definite mode, which can scarcely be supposed to be otherwise than the result of

---

* The following is the civil surgeon's description of the wounds found upon the bodies of two men at Furruckabad, who were set upon and cut to pieces by several persons armed with swords:—"Maharaj Singh had the third, fourth and fifth fingers, and part of the *left hand, cut off*; the *right hand cut off at the wrist*, also a deep cut on the right arm below the shoulder-joint; *the left leg cut off at the knee-joint*, a deep cut on the same leg below the knee, dividing the bone; also a deep cut on the ankle, a superficial wound on the abdomen, and one on the forehead. Heera Lall had a deep cut extending across the chest, laying it open, and wounding the lungs; another on the left side of the face, extending from the lobe of the ear to the corner of the mouth; *the left arm cut off near the shoulder-joint*, also a deep cut across the palm of the left hand, another about nine inches long (?) on the back of the left hand, and one about nine inches long on the back of the right shoulder, and another on the top of the same shoulder. He was of opinion that these injuries occasioned immediate death."—*Nizamut Adawlut Reports, N. W. P.*, 5th April 1854, p. 374.

† Nizamut Adawlut Reports, N. W. P., 12th June 1852, pp. 534, 946, and 1005 (two swords broken), also 24th May 1853, p. 700, sword broken into three pieces.

‡ *Ibid*, 27th October 1852, p. 1246. A case in which a wretch inflicted twenty wounds upon a prostitute which she survived eight days.

design. In different cases, the direction and number of the wounds given will, of course, vary somewhat, but the gashes inflicted are generally many; and, considering that the victim cannot always be deprived of motion by the first blow, and that the assailant is not a practised executioner, it is very extraordinary how similar are the injuries inflicted in very many of the cases. Thus, when the victim is struck while in the erect position, blows inflicted upon the upper part of the head are usually ***vertical;*** most of the victims receive one or two ***horizontal*** strokes across the temple and side (generally the right) of the face; strokes on the back of the head and neck and on the sides of the neck appear to be ***invariably nearly horizontal;*** wounds on the shoulders, back, and upper part of the chest, are nearly as invariably ***vertical*** or ***oblique*** in their direction; the hands and arms are often cut transversely, but this evidently occurs in the efforts of the assailed to protect his head. It is within the verge of possibility that these marked coincidences are accidental;—it may be that a person, wielding a heavy weapon with all his force, naturally changes the direction of the strokes; —still it is difficult to believe that they could occur so frequently, where a weapon like a bill-hook (which is not known to be wielded after any fashion of sword exercise) is grasped by a series of individuals suddenly enraged to madness, and only impelled by an undiscriminating impulse to kill.

The murderous desire—or shall we call it ***instinct?***—evidently is to split the skull, to cut off the head, and to lay open the heart and lungs.

It has been humanely ruled that—

"Verbal abuse, which is often of the grossest nature amongst the natives of India, and is extremely offensive, amounts to a high provocation in this country; and it is consonant to the spirit of the English law, as well as to the general principles of justice, to make a distinction of punishment between cases of deliberate murder, and a sudden homicide committed in heat of blood."*

Whether the infliction, in the sudden heat of passion, of a particular kind of wound usually given under similar circumstances, will or will not be regarded by the law as, in a certain degree, an evidence of premeditation, it is not for the medical witness to decide; it is merely his duty to state that the wound evidences sufficient thought on the part of the prisoner to have led him to select a well-known mode of destroying life, and to prove that the multitude of wounds under which the deceased sank were not inflicted in mere blind and purposeless rage.

Two Garrows murdered and robbed a man. The crown of the head was shred off, and hung by the skin of the scalp; two wounds on the back, the back-bone being cut through; four fingers cut off the left hand;

* Macnaghten's Reports, Vol. I., p. 53.

both ankles cut into, but not through, the bone. The wounds indicated the use of the Garrow *lungbari*, or sword. The accused said at the foujdary that life was extinct from a blow inflicted by his uncle Bengra, before he, prisoner, struck ; and that *it was in play that he cut the body.* In his defence before the judge he said that Bengra having killed the deceased, he went forward to see if he was really dead, when he inflicted the wounds on the back and loins. He was, notwithstanding these gentle pleas, sentenced to death.* These blows were evidently inflicted when the victim was lying on the ground.

My *Commentator* directs attention to the great frequency, in Up-Country fights, of the *cut beneath the knee.* This, which is according to English feeling a foul blow, is a common sleight of Hindustanee swordsmen. By severing the artery it generally proves instantaneously fatal ; and, when not fatal, it at once brings the man to the ground, and leaves him at the mercy of his assailant.

RECOGNITION OF WOUNDS INFLICTED AFTER DEATH.

Bodies sent in to the civil surgeon for examination very frequently present marks of gnawing by Insects, Fish, and Vermin, or have been partially devoured by Dogs, Jackals, Crows, and Vultures ;—some of the appearances thus caused may interfere considerably with our means of forming an accurate opinion upon the case.

The generality of bodies are found to have heen attacked by *Ants ;* the most destructive of these are the small red kind. Where the body has been left long upon the ground, a gigantic species of black ant also attacks it. It is particularly noticeable that the insects generally commence upon any abraded or raw surface which the body may present ; and,—where there have been a number of superficial scratches, perhaps inflicted in the fatal struggle, or where the dried line left by the cord in hanging has remained uncovered,—the gnawings of these creatures into the true skin, completely along the injured tracts, greatly obscure the aspect of the parts, by removing any minute superficial ecchymoses or effusions of blood which may have existed as the only evidence that the injuries were inflicted during life. In a not extremely decomposed body, sent to me when I was in medical charge of Howrah, I found that the ants had attacked an oval ulcer on the leg, and had completely eaten away all the tissues within its circumference to the bone.

Recabi Ghazi was sentenced at Jessore in 1859, to transportation for life, for causing the death of his wife, who was found hanging, and whose body bore marks of beating and of strangulation. The prisoner admitted, before the sessions judge, that he struck his wife once, but said that she had

* Nizamut Adawlut Reports, July 11th, 1855, p. 53.

afterwards hung herself, and that ***ants had produced the appearances seen in the corpse.*** This the judge held to be impossible. The evidence of the civil surgeon showed that the beating must have been severe, bruises and extravasated blood being found on the scalp, back, neck, loins, and even on the abdomen and knees. Considerable force must have been employed, probably with a stick or blunt weapon.*

Fish, Turtle, Rats, and Water Insects are very destructive to bodies submerged in tanks and rivers. In the first case brought to me for examination in this country, I found that blood appeared to have escaped freely from what seemed to be extensive lacerated contusions of the eyelids and nose. A little further investigation, however, showed that the parts had been gnawed, probably very soon after submersion, by the fish of a small river into which the woman had fallen.

Bodies which have been left exposed in the fields for a few days are often brought in nearly devoured by ***Wild Animals.*** It appears that these creatures generally attack the limbs and abdomen first. They occasionally leave extensive wounds, inflicted previously to death, entirely untouched—even after having torn away some of the large joints. This I have noticed with great surprise, as it would be supposed that an extensive bleeding surface would first attract their attention.

The question of, whether a Wound has been inflicted Before or After Death, always one of great moment, is often of peculiar importance and difficulty in this country. It is a well-known practice in India, where a death occurs suddenly, from natural causes, to a member of one of two rival houses, for his relations to inflict various wounds upon the corpse and to place it in a spot, where it may be readily discovered, near their enemies' dwelling.† In such cases, it is known by the culprits that the body, being in a greatly advanced state of decomposition when brought in for inspection, will be viewed with considerable doubt by the medical officer ; his uncertainty, of course, telling more or less in favor of their plot.

It will generally happen, however, that wounds thus inflicted are so extensive as to render it almost a matter of certainty that, providing

---

* Nizamut Adawlut Reports, 31st Jany. 1859, p. 17.

† Indeed, it would appear that the criminals of the present day prefer the expedient of leaving the body of a person who has, in reality, been murdered. In 1843, three persons of Nowakolly murdered the daughter of one of them for the purpose of getting up a false complaint against certain parties. In the same year two brothers, of Beerbhoom, were made over for trial on circumstantial evidence, charged with the murder of their infant brother for the purpose of bringing another person into trouble.—*Police Report, L. P.*, 1843, pp. 43, 59. Again, in 1849, a man of Backergunge intrigued with the wife of another, who, to harass him, preferred a false charge of theft against him. The prisoner, in revenge, to involve the other in a graver charge, slew his [own ?] idiot cousin, and left the corpse close to the house of his enemy.—*Ibid*, 1849, p. 46. *Vide supra*, p. 71.

that they caused death, they must have done so by hæmorrhage. Here the discriminative rules which I have found of most practical use are the following: That, *cæteris paribus*, the body of a person bled to death decomposes more slowly, and with a greater tendency to desiccation, than is usual in any cases but those in which death has been attended with exhausting discharges, as in cholera, dysentery, diarrhœa or phthisis.* In cases of the latter kind, however, the emaciated appearance of the body would probably guide the surgeon, even after the recognition of internal lesions had become difficult. The Hon'ble Elphinstone Jackson has mentioned to me a recent case in which, the head of a man having been struck off, by way of human sacrifice, the whole of the blood drained away, and the deserted body became so thoroughly desiccated as completely to preserve the appearance of the wound. That the muscles of one who has bled to death have a peculiar whiteness easily distinguished from the anemiated appearance of the same parts in persons long exposed to miasmatic influences. In the former case, the muscles retain their usual consistence, and are nearly *white*; in the latter, they are flabby and of a *greyish hue*.

The conjunctivæ of the eyelids, parts which long remain moist and free from decomposition, are found unusually white when death has resulted from hæmorrhage.

In all cases, however, where recent wounds are observed in a putrid body, and no distinct marks of external or internal acchymosis, and no appearance of effusion of blood into the serous cavities or substance of the brain can be discovered, the medical officer's opinion will, of course, be given in the most guarded manner.

A very moderate insight into the criminal habits of the natives will sufficiently convince the surgeon of the vast importance of tact and caution in determining whether a wound has been inflicted before or after death, all collateral evidence being, at the same time, fully weighed. A single set of cases may be cited in illustration.

1. A thief may be beheaded while in the act of committing a robbery.
2. He may be captured, and then beheaded by the people of the house or village.
3. He may die from wounds received in the act of committing a robbery; and his accomplices, unable to remove his body, may cut off the head to disguise it.
4. Or, his accomplices may decapitate him while living.

---

* Whether desiccation of the body occurs early or late, or not at all, will, of course, depend much upon the climate, season, and hygrometric condition of the atmosphere, the amount of adipose tissue, &c. In dry climates and seasons the body generally desiccates quickly. In Seville, we are told by Mr. C. Hervey, the heat creates putrefaction easily, but it soon draws up the noxious effluvia of it, and the bodies of dead dogs and cats, which are thrown plentifully into the streets, are not offensive the day after their being exposed.—*Letters from Portugal, Spain, &c.*, 1785.

5. An innocent person may be murdered by poison, strangling, &c., and the assassins may cut off the head with a view to concealment, or with a desire to wreak their vengeance upon the insensible body.*

---

* 1. A person caught a burglar making his way through a hole which he had burrowed in a mud wall. Seizing a sword, he nearly struck off the unfortunate wretch's head, while he lay struggling in the narrow aperture.—*Nizamut Adawlut Reports*, 5th Feb. 1852, p. 158. In 1846, a Behar man, being awakened by persons who were robbing his house, took his sword and went quietly outside, and, on the burglar coming out, cut off his head with a single blow. Being then attacked by the comrade of the man killed, he laid him dead also.—*Police Report*, *L. P.*, for 1846, p. 14.

2. It will be shown, in another Chapter, that the practice of decapitating persons captured in the act of burglary is of frequent occurrence in this Presidency.

3. 4. The Report of the Police Committee (1836, p. 122,) contains a remarkable case illustrative of this point. A native of Hidgellee was called away in the night by certain persons, and never returned. On the following day, his wife inquired, of one of those who had called her husband, what had become of him. He replied that he had not called her husband. Search was then made, and the body was found in a river some distance off. There were two spear wounds in the chest. The body had been decapitated, but the head was discovered at a distance. The suspicion was that the deceased, a bad character, had been concerned in a burglary, and, getting wounded, was killed by his accomplices to prevent detection through him ; and this was corroborated by some articles of suspicious property being found near the house of deceased, having been removed from the house by direction of his widow. A long and very singular inquiry by the police ensued ; but it appears that no further light was ever thrown upon the manner in which the man had met his death. There is a very current, and probably authentic story of a traveller in India who, being awakened in the night by a robber moving about his tent, seized the intruder by his feet, as he was crawling out. The traveller pulled against the thief's accomplices, until, the opposition giving way, he dragged in a decapitated body.

5. The reports contain several cases of this description. In 1853, one Ruttee, having persuaded another man's mistress to elope with him, cut off her head and the left lower limb in a jungle, hid them, and stole her ornaments.—*Nizamut Adawlut Reports*, N. W. P., 29th Novr. of that year, p. 1430.

In 1855, Gopee Singh, of Bhaugulpore, finding an intriguer with his sister in an *urher khet*, caught him, brought him back, and strangled him. The body was found sunk with stones in a tank. The head was cut off, and one of the hands was missing. The prisoner said that he cut off the head, but that the jackals or dogs had eaten one hand.—*Nizamut Adawlut Reports*, *May* 14, 1855, p. 552.

In 1854, a widow of Bareilly left her house, and never returned. It appears that she was strangled by several persons in the jungle, that her body was concealed for three days, and was then decapitated, to prevent detection, and thrown into a blind well, which was filled in with earth.—*Nizamut Adawlut Reports*, 13th Novr. 1854, p. 71.

Two men were tried at Bareilly, in 1852, for the murder of a servant. The decapitated body was found in the nuddee, the hands and feet were bound with ropes. The sub-assistant surgeon stated that the body was much decomposed, but that there appeared marks which induced the conclusion that the head was separated from the body by cutting with a *saw*. The prisoners said that deceased had hanged himself ; and that, fearing inquiry, they had first buried the corpse and had afterwards beheaded it and sunk it in the nuddee with four ghurras.—*Nizamut Adawlut Reports*, N. W. P., 23rd July 1852, p. 727.

The corpse of a female was found in a village near Burdwan, with the head, feet, and hands cut off. A person came forward and deposed on oath that the body was that of his sister, who had been murdered by certain persons, and named his witnesses. On the arrival of the mohurer, he stated, on oath, that his previous evidence was false, and that his sister died a natural death. No further facts could be elicited.—*Police Report*, L. P., 1846, p. 67.

Under these various circumstances, the following particulars should be noticed :—

1. The body of a person decapitated in the very act of committing a robbery, or in fair fight, will, in all probability, present merely *clean* cuts (indeed the body may be found hacked all over, if the first wound was not mortal), and perhaps some contusions. The head and body will be exsanguine and the pupils dilated ; and, for some hours, the muscles of the neck will be retracted.

2. On the body of a captured thief, beheaded or cut on the neck in cold blood, there will, probably, be, judging by the reports of three recorded cases in which the punishment was committed with *koodalees,* (adzes),* the traces of repeated hacking blows or cuts. A sharp sword, inflicting a clean wound, is not likely to be used, while the struggling victim is held down upon the ground. There is a case, however, on record, in which it is stated that, while three persons held the deceased down, a fourth, " with a large knife used in sacrifices, cut off his head with one blow, and with a second divided the body at the waist." It will be shown, hereafter, that the infliction of such mutilations as these, by single strokes of a heavy weapon, is possible. Still, in the absence of medical evidence, it may be questioned whether, in the above case, the murderer only struck twice.†

3. 4. Where a man has been mortally wounded in the act of robbery, and his body has been carried away by his accomplices, who, not having, had time to bury it, have beheaded it to prevent recognition, the presence of other mortal wounds, taken with the general evidence, will go very far

---

A young man of property and good family, but of dissipated habits, of Ghazeepore, went with his brother-in-law and another to the former's house, where, while he was either asleep or drunk, he was stabbed to death. They kept the body two days, when, having decapitated it, they had it carried in a basket to a well, into which they threw it, and buried the head in an adjacent field.—*Nizamut Adawlut Reports*, N. W. P., 9th March 1855, p. 328.

One Dhurm Singh, of Bareilly, was beaten to death in his own house by, or certainly with the knowledge of Lalljeeta, his own nephew, who was supposed to be criminally intimate with his (Dhurm's) wife, and Badam Singh, with whose cousin's daughter, the unfortunate man had himself intrigued. The murderers conveyed the body away on a cart, and threw it down at about a mile's distance, where Badam nearly severed the head from the body with a sword. When found, the corpse was tied hand and foot. It was considered that the wound was inflicted to make it appear that he had been attacked and killed by robbers. It appears very probable, however (especially when the case is compared with others, which will be cited hereafter), that the wounding after death was rather intended as an expression of vengeance for an unpardonable injury.

For instances in which the bodies of murdered persons were *dismembered*,—see Nizamut Adawlut Reports, Vol. III, Part 1, of 1853, pp. 54 and 680, and Part 2 of Vol. IV., 26th September 1854, p. 427.

* Nizamut Adawlut Reports, 14th June 1853, p. 796, and 17th June, p. 810; and one in which a knife was used, *Ibid*, 1st Jan. 1852, p. 1.—Nizamut Adawlut Reports, N. W. P., January 3rd, 1852, p. 4.

† Police Report, L. P., for 1854, p. 71.

to explain the nature of the occurrence—as in the cases given at pp. 72 and 73 of this Manual. If, as would be probable, death was caused by external hæmorrhage, the head would be exsanguine, but the muscles of the neck would not be contracted, if the head were not removed very soon after death. In the fear and hurry of a pursuit, however, the fugitives might only pause for a minute or two, while their wounded companion fell and breathed his last, before they removed the head. The only manner in which the surgeon could distinguish between this last case and one in which the head of a fainting person had been cut off, or in which a person merely disabled and unable to keep up with his companions in flight had been decapitated, would be by forming an accurate estimate of the severity of the original wounds,—all collateral evidence also being called in aid.

5. Where the head is cut off several hours after death, it will probably not be altogether exsanguine, the muscles of the neck will not be contracted, the pupils will, generally, be in the condition usual after death,—neither dilated nor contracted ; it may present traces of contusions, &c. After decomposition has fully set in, the appearances will, of course, be obscured ; but, other conditions being equal, the head of a person cut off during life will swell less, as decomposition advances, and dry much sooner than one removed after death.

For remarks upon the practice of beheading those who have come to violent deaths, for the purpose of concealing their identity, vide supra, pp. 72-73.

SELF-INFLICTED INJURIES.

In accusations of crimes against the person, false evidence and simulation are so frequent throughout India that, in the case of nearly every wounded person brought before him for an opinion, the surgeon's first inquiries should be,—*Was this injury self-inflicted?* and,—*Was it inflicted in the manner alleged?*

In my last edition I remarked as follows :

" Considerable aid would be given to the investigation of police cases, involving charges of wounding, if the form of the lithographed letter which is forwarded by magistrates to civil surgeons, in cases of assault, &c., were modified as follows :

" *Sir,—I request you will be good enough to examine the wounds of ————— sent herewith, and favor me with a full report of the nature and extent of the injuries, which are stated in the* [thana or foujdaree] *depositions to have been inflicted in the following manner.*

" At present, the medical officer's reply to the magistrate's requisition generally conveys merely his own opinion of the nature of the case, probably without reference to the credibility of the wounded person's statement, and almost invariably without any knowledge whatever of the counter-statement of the accused. A precaution of this kind would certainly lead to the immediate detection of many serious attempts at fraud, which, under the present system, either succeed or are only quashed at the end of a tedious and expensive inquiry."

Reference to the form of letter now in use, *vide supra*, p. 33, will show that by the insertion of the words "*all that is at present known of the case is as follows*" has obviated this objection.

As a general rule, the natives of India, in common with most other persons, are unwilling to inflict severe injuries upon themselves for purposes of false accusation ;—there are more Neros than Scævolas or Feltons.*

* John Felton is said to have enclosed a joint of his little finger, which he had hacked off, as a proof that he was in earnest, in a cartel sent to a brother officer who had offended him. It is well that the surgeon should be aware of the degree of resolution which a person, not insane or prompted by suicidal determination, may display in inflicting pain upon himself for a definite purpose. It is well known to Army Surgeons that men, stationed for long terms in the West Indies, frequently placed their thumbs, and even their hands over the muzzles of their pieces and blew them away, with the hope of being invalided and sent home. I know an instance of a medical man who had sufficient nerve to extract one of his own firmly-set grinders with a tooth-key. Cranmer's constancy, in stretching forth his hand into the flames, need not have been cited, had it not recently been discussed as a physical impossibility. The act appears, however, to have been possible enough, seeing that the fire had already taken the victim's feet;—beyond this, the amount of pain endured could scarcely be increased. Much more resolution was shown by the woman who allowed Bonner to hold her hand over a candle until the sinews cracked. When Mandrin, the noted French robber, was broken on the wheel, he screamed violently, as the first blow fell on his collar bone :—at the second stroke, he laughed. The executioner paused, and inquired why he did this? He replied—"to think that I should fear the second blow, when the first had deprived me of all feeling."

The Seir Mutaqherin contains (Vol. I. Part 1, p. 103) the apochryphal story of a Rajpoot wife of Daoud-Khan, in the reign of Ferohsyur, who, on receiving the news of his death in the moment of victory, took his poignard which he had given her as a token of his love, and "opening her belly with a precaution and dexterity which amazed every one, she carefully drew out the child and tenderly recommended it to the bystanders ; after which few words, she expired." Pregnant widows were not allowed to burn themselves.

In visiting a country, with the customs of whose inhabitants he is not well acquainted, the surgeon, when called upon to decide whether certain injuries upon the person of a native have or have not been self-inflicted, will gain but little aid from his text book on Medical Jurisprudence. Nearly every nation has its own peculiar modes of self-destruction and self-torture.

The Japanese nobleman goes through his public career in a state of constant expectafion of cloudy times in which the self-inflicted execution by *Hara Kiri*, or happy dispatch, will bring life's fever to a sudden end. In an account of this mode of self-immolation, which he has lately given, Mr. Mitford tells us that extraordinary heroism is displayed in the *Hara Kiri*. A young fellow of the Choshin class, not content with giving himself the one necessary cut, slashed himself thrice horizontally, and twice vertically. Then he stabbed himself in the throat until the dirk protruded on the other side with its sharp edge to the front. Setting his teeth in one supreme effort, he drove the knife forward with both hands through his throat and fell dead.

The civil and quiet-mannered Malay, when insulted, at once seeks the death of a mad dog in running *Amok*. Stringent laws have been required to prevent the timid Brahmins of Hindustan from burning themselves in their enemies' territories, and from throwing themselves into wells when offended or intefered with. According to Ward, the Hindus relate that there existed, formerly, at Kasheera, a village near Nudeeya, an instrument called Kuravut, which *was used by devotees to cut off their own heads*. It was made in the shape of a half-moon, with a sharp edge, and was placed at the back of the neck, having chains fastened at the two extremities. The infatuated devotee, placing his feet on the stirrups, gave a violent jerk, and severed his head from his body!

Still, among these people, a good deal of caution and reflection is required on the part of the medical officer in many cases.

The instances which have occurred to myself did not require much discrimination.

When I was in medical charge at Chittagong, a man was brought to me with several recent wounds on the head, which he said were inflicted by a person who attacked him with a *dao* (heavy bill-hook). Some of them were about two inches long, but they did not penetrate much below the true skin, and the edges of each incision were so perfectly smooth that it was certain that they could not possibly have been inflicted with the coarse-edged weapon alleged, or, indeed, with any other instrument likely to be procurable by a native—except a razor.

At about the same time, I was called by the police to the house of a native woman who they stated was dying. I found a very trivial ragged wound on the throat, apparently inflicted with a pair of scissors. It afterwards appeared that the woman, a prostitute, had been disappointed by the marriage of a person with whom she had lived, and had wounded herself with an intention of bringing him into trouble.

In 1852, one Luchmun Doss, *alias* Khunjuna, was tried at Bareilly for a murder committed eight years previously. Several witnesses deposed that they were well able to recognize the prisoner as the murderer; one of them stated further, in identification of the prisoner, that, some time before the murder, the prisoner had a quarrel with a person named, and that, for the purpose of getting up a false charge, he cut himself with a *hussoolah* (adze) in the middle of the calf of the leg, the mark of which injury still remained on his person. The civil surgeon examined the prisoner at the judge's request, and certified that he still bore marks of such an injury. The jury found the prisoner guilty, and the sessions judge recommended a capital sentence. The Judge of the superior Court, however, proved demonstratively that the prisoner differed entirely from the real murderer in age and in appearance. He further noticed that, on referring to the civil surgeon's evidence, he found that the prisoner's scar was on the *calf* of the *left* leg ; but that, on looking at the descriptive roll [of the murderer] of 1845, his scar was on the *shin* of the *right* leg. The prisoner's immediate release was ordered.*

Certain prisoners, of Bareilly, who had cruelly butchered three unarmed men, stated that they had been struck and wounded by their victims. The judge examined the marks ;—"they were not of sword cuts, but small scratches, evidently self-inflicted, or with their connivance, to which some substance had been applied to prevent their healing."†

---

* Nizamut Adawlut Reports, N. W. P., 19th October 1852, p. 1209.

† *Ibid*, July 22nd, 1853, p. 899.

In 1854, six men were tried at Mirzapore, for having murdered four persons by sword and spear wounds. One of the prisoners had a wound on his shoulder, which the civil surgeon considered was the result of a blow partly warded off. This, however, the judge held, must be pure conjecture, and the fact that the cut was but a quarter of an inch in depth was, in his opinion, conclusive that it had not been inflicted with force; its position, just below the left shoulder, he thought, made it unlikely that he inflicted it himself; but the judge was inclined to believe that he got it done by one of the other prisoners, with a view of giving the affair the colour of an affray. All the prisoners were sentenced to fourteen years' transportation.*

In 1853, three native women and two children were found lying daed in a heap, with their throats cut, in their bungalow, at the station of Baitool. The husband of one of the females gave the alarm, stating that the crime had been committed by dacoits, who had also wounded and bound him. It, however, soon became evident that this man was the murderer. The medical officer found that his wounds were very slight. The chief was on the thigh, three inches long, in no part penetrating completely through the true skin. The officiating commissioner, who reported the case, stated that it was evident, from Dr. Chisholm's deposition, that all the blood upon the man's body and clothes and on the gravel walk could not have flowed from those very trifling wounds. His account of the way in which he received his wounds was also not to be credited; for, had he been cut at with swords, under no circumstances could the wounds have been so slight, if the weapons with which they were inflicted had not previously come in contact with something other than his body, by which the force of the blow could be lessened; but this, it was considered to be proved, was not the case, the spot where he stated that he received his wounds bearing no traces of any blows of a sword or cutting instrument having been intercepted by any surrounding object. But, whether the blows were intercepted or not, it appeared impossible that the wound and scratch on the left thigh could have been inflicted in the manner described. Their direction was such that a pursuing enemy could not have given them with a sword or other weapon; and, from the roundness of a man's thigh, a wound of the length of either the cut or scratch must have been considerably deeper in the middle than at either end; but this was not the case. Their being *exactly* parallel was also strongly against the man's story; and, from their direction, parallelism, and uniform want of depth, they were just the sort of wounds that a faint-hearted man would inflict on himself—first timidly drawing the sword over his thigh, and inflicting a mere scratch; and then, knowing that the safety of his neck

* Nizamut Adawlut Reports, N. W. P., 3rd February 1854, p. 121.

depended on his having some wound to show, half plucking up his courage and giving himself a wound, it is true, but a very slight one.*

See Dr. Hutchinson's remarks on self-inflicted wounds, *supra*, p. 333.

The most difficult cases are those in which the injuries shown in support of a false charge have been inflicted, not by the prosecutor himself, but by his accomplices or instigators.

Dr. Kenneth Mackinnon gave me notes of two very important cases bearing upon this point. A case occurred at Dinapore, in 1844, in which the servants of a medical officer were said to have been attacked and wounded by certain parties at night. The wounds were so slight and numerous, and other circumstances were so suspicious, that Dr. Mackinnon believed the injuries to be self-inflicted. The magistrate concurred in this opinion, and sentenced the servants for false complaint. The magistrate's decision, however, was subsequently reversed by higher authority, and the original defendants were punished. Dr. Mackinnon heard, years afterwards, that a native doctor confessed, at Umballah, that he had himself inflicted the wounds.

In 1839, a young lad was sent to Dr. Mackinnon by the magistrate of Tirhoot. The index finger of the right hand was severed at the joint between the first phalanx and the metacarpal bone, and the thumb also at the same articulation. Dr. Mackinnon then gave his opinion merely to the effect that a sharp cutting instrument must have been used to effect the amputation. The case before the magistrate was, that one zumeendar accused another of having met his slave-boy in a wood, attacked him, and, with *one blow of a sword*, inflicted the injury above described. It was only in his examination before the sessions judge that Dr. Mackinnon was informed how the injury was stated to have been inflicted. He gave it as his opinion that the blow of a sword could not have neatly disarticulated the thumb and fore-finger without injuring the rest of the hand (the reader will perceive this on looking at his own hand). The view of the matter led to a keen cross-questioning, when the slave-boy made a full confession that his master had cut off his fingers with a knife. The magistrate's decision, which had sentenced the party first accused to fine and imprisonment, was quashed, and the original plaintiff was punished for subornation of perjury.

In 1862, Mr. Perceval, who had been a police superintendent, stated that, when he was connected with the police in Bombay, there were two or three gangs in that city who cut and wounded each other for purposes of false accusation and extortion. They used to cut one another's necks and arms by turns, as the lot fell, and accuse some rich passer-by of having done it. The wounded rascal would cry out "Murder!" and his com-

* Nizamut Adawlut Reports, N. W. P., 25th February 1853, p. 283. A most important case, weighed and investigated with great care and ability.

panions would follow and point out to the police the abode of the alleged culprit, and confirm the charge by declaring that they were present when the crime was committed. Several respectable men were disgraced and ruined by these villains. If those accused and arrested paid handsomely on the day of trial, the prosecutors would invent some plea to enable them to escape. It fell to the lot of a youthful member of one of these gangs to have his neck cut. The person appointed to cut him was a drunken barber, who, instead of making a slight cut, inflicted a mortal wound. The gang fled, abandoning the youth, whose dying confession led to their arrest.

INJURIES INFLICTED BY WILD ANIMALS.

The destruction of life by Wild Beasts among the rural population of India is enormous.

The Mortuary Return for the N. W. P., for 1867, shows that 436 persons were killed by animals. The details are given as follows :—

	Males.	*Females.*	*Total.*
Killed by Wolves	104	117	221
,, ,, Tigers	26	10	36
,, ,, Bullocks	40	17	57
,, ,, Dogs	9	14	23
,, ,, Bears	4	4	8
,, ,, Leopards	3	...	3
,, ,, Alligators	5	...	5
,, ,, Elephant	1	...	1
,, ,, Horses	2	...	2
,, ,, Boars	1	1	2
,, ,, Jackals	1	...	1
,, ,, Reptiles	20	8	28
,, ,, other animals ...	43	5	48
Stung by Bees	1	...	1
Total ...	260	176	436

Besides the above, 1,678 deaths from snake-bite were registered.

The Reports of the Central Provinces show that, there, the number of persons killed by wild beasts in three years was as follows :—

1865	546
1866	699
1867	506

And 832 killed and 195 wounded by scorpions and snakes.

In 1867, there were killed, in the Central Provinces, 518 tigers, 895 panthers and leopards, 534 bears, 467 wolves, 475 hyænas, and 13,644 snakes. The chief mortality is among children, who are often employed to scare away birds, or to tend cattle.

The following statistics were lately collected, from various recent blue books, in the Calcutta *Englishman*.

In Oudh, wolves seem to be more formidable than any other kind of wild beast. In 1867, according to the Police Report, 5 men, 2 women, 75 boys, and 80 girls were killed by them. In the Punjab, during the same year, 30 persons were killed and 28 injured by wild animals, of which there were destroyed 15 tigers, 307 leopards, 215 bears, 3,681 wolves, and 3 hyænas. In the Central Provinces, again, 506 human lives were lost, while 518 tigers, 895 panthers and leopards, 534 bears, 467 wolves, 475 hyænas, and 13,644 snakes were put to death. In Bengal itseltf he ravages of wild animals, during the last six years, have been almost as bloody as a campaign. A tabular statement shows that, in that space of time, 4,218 persons have fallen victims to tigers, 1,407 to leopards, 105 to bears, 4,287 to wolves, 174 to hyænas, and 3,210 to other beasts, such as boars, jackals, mad dogs, buffaloes, elephants, and even deer. On the other hand the *feræ naturæ* suffered to the extent of 7,278 tigers, 5,663 leopards, 1,671 bears, 1,338 wolves, 296 hyænas, and 1,950 other animals. The grand total is, therefore, 13,401 men, women, and children, as against 18,196 more or less savage quadrupeds—a result that is by no means flattering to those who profess to have dominion over the beasts of the field and forest, the worms of the earth, and the birds of the air. This victory, besides, such as it is, was only achieved by the expenditure of £6,500 in rewards.

We are told that the most ancient and universal punishment for unchastity, among the Hindoos, was to anoint the victim's body with rancid oil and to cast her, bound hand and foot, out of the city, to be devoured by the herds of pariah dogs which surround the walls of all inhabited places in India.

The Rev. Edward Terry, who accompanied Sir Thomas Row to the Court of the Great Mogul in 1615, says that it was then customary to have malefactors torn in pieces by wild beasts (p. 372).

Dogs and jackals are able to inflict but very little injury upon the larger bones of the skeleton. It is considered that tigers and leopards usually break the bones. In a case tried in 1845, the medical officer decided that the woman could not have been killed by one of these animals, as her skeleton was discovered entire. I have great doubts, however, upon this point. In the body of a buffaloe killed and partially devoured by a tiger, the abdominal purietes only had been eaten; the animal may, however, have been scared from its prey. It is considered that the tiger, after having seized any animal, does not proceed to devour it on the spot, but at once carries it to a close covert. There are certainly exceptions to this rule. It is probable that entire human adult bodies are never dragged very far by dogs and jackals, which do not tug in concert, each animal tearing for himself; as, however, the dismemberment proceeds, separate fragments are often carried to a considerable distance. In the outskirts of Calcutta, there is scarcely any ditch, a mile inland, which does not contain human remains, skulls especially,—brought from the river to be mumbled at leisure. I remarked, at page 23 of this work, that pilgrims, fakeers, and others may die unnoticed in jungles and other remote spots, and that lunatics or sick or intoxicated persons may be thus lost in the wilds, and there be attacked and devoured by the smaller wild animals.

Mr. Ward, the missionary, in speaking of the jackal, says—"So ravenous are these animals, that they frequently steal infants as they lie by the breast of the mother; and sick persons who lie friendless in the street or by the side of the Ganges are sometimes devoured alive by these animals in the night. I have heard of persons, in a state of intoxication, being thus devoured, as they say, in the street in Calcutta.*

It is generally considered that tigers, leopards, and bears do not prey upon dead bodies. It cannot, however, be doubted that jackals, pariah dogs, &c., do attack dying or intoxicated persons.

Soon after the publication of my last edition, Dr. Baillie, then of Hooghly, sent me the following cases:

The body was that of a young man, a Hindoo of low caste. The abdomen and its contents entirely removed, together with diaphragm and heart; the lungs remained, but not blanched, as one would expect from hæmorrhage; penis and scrotum gone and upper part of thighs mangled; the muscular tissue, however, red and fresh; the cartilage of the nose seemed eaten away. The poor fellow is said to have been devoured by birds and jackals, when in a state of intoxication, but I could not determine whether death had occurred previous to or after the attack by the said scavengers. I know that they do attack persons whilst alive and in a state of drunkenness, as, on the 9th March last, an old Brahmin of respectable family at Panduah was sent in by the police to the Emambara Hospital,—on account of the whole buccal and labial region, cartilage and septum nasi, together with the tongue, uvula, and left tonsil, being destroyed by vultures, whilst the said holy man was lying insensible from drunkenness. The exposed maxillary bones had been nearly picked clean. He was fed by means of the æsophagous tube and funnel, and did not appear to suffer except from the annoyance of flies, for which account he was covered with musquito curtains. He was apparently doing well, when, on the morning of the 14th idem, he was found dead.

A very remarkable trial look place in Madras, in May 1868, in which the main point at issue was—Had the deceased died from the effects of poison, from wounds inflicted by a cutting instrument, or by tearing by wild

* View of the History, Literature, and Religion of the Hindus. Third edition. Vol. II., p. 326.

animals? I regret that the report of the case, which lies before me, is imperfect.

A Christain school girl, at Wellington, left her home after having got from her mother a knife to cut flowers. An officer and his *bandy*-man both said they had seen a soldier and a little girl making for the *Sholah* in which the body was subsequently found, nine days afterwards. The soldier, having been fully identified, was tried for the child's murder. The case was dismissed on the ground of insufficient evidence on the side of the prosecution. The following is an abstract of the [incomplete] medical evidence:

Thomas Kirkwood deposed: He is an assistant surgeon attached to 102nd Regiment, was doing duty at Depôt at Wellington, on 30th of January; made a *post-mortem* examination on body of a child in the dead-house on that day; the members of the Court of Inquest told witness that the body was that of Catherine Izzard. Dr. James was one of the members of the Court of Inquest, and he saw the body, and was present for a little while when examination was made. Witness made a note of observations,—the scalp was entirely removed, the soft parts of face were entirely removed, decomposition would not account for appearance of face, too much was removed about the neck to be accounted for by decomposition.

This must either have been caused by animals or by cutting. The body had been exposed for eight or nine days; very probably wild animals had removed the soft parts of the face. All the muscles of the neck were wanting. Upper extremities were removed, witness means fore-arms and arms; only one arm, the left arm, was present; the other was removed altogether. When witness saw the body, both arms were separated from trunk, but only one arm was produced. From the appearance of the edge of the wound, witness fancied it was removed by a cutting instrument. Cannot state positively that the arm was removed by a cutting instrument. It is possible that the arm might have been removed by some other means. Cannot suggest any other means. Nearly all the muscles and soft parts covering the thorax were absent on the right side,—portions might have been removed by wild animals, and portions might have been accounted for by decomposition. The middle of the body was covered with skin, and the extremities of the skin were well defined, being in a straight line, from which it could be inferred that it was removed by a cutting instrument. It is impossible that decomposition would have produced such an appearance. It is not impossible that wild animals might have produced the appearance, but it was not probable; portions of the body presented an appearance as if a wild animal had been at the body. There were marks of teeth. The witness then proceeded to describe that muscles and skin were absent from other portions of the body. The contents of the pelvis and organs of generation and the buttock were entirely removed, but he could not say how this was taken away. The bones of the thighs were bare up to the knee-joints [?] and both the knee-caps presented the same appearance. The witness judged from this that the flesh must have been removed carefully with a cutting instrument, as wild animals could not have produced similar appearances in both legs.

The flesh of the legs, from the knee downwards, was present. The left arm, bent at right angles, presented a dry and shrivelled appearance, which was produced by exposure to sun. Other portions of the body were in a decomposed state. The stomach was also examined, and was found to contain guavas and gooseberries, and there was no appearance of poison. The witness was of opinion that the child might have eaten poisonous berries and died, the poison might not have appeared ten days after death, and that the wounds which appeared on the body must have been inflicted after death. The witness thought that, from the state of the prisoner's arm, he could not have inflicted the wounds without some difficulty, and that the knife produced in the Court might have produced the wounds. Does not know when the prisoner left Wellington. The prisoner left Wellington, because he was ordered away.

Cross-examined.—The contents of the pelvis and organs of generation were entirely removed, is able to say the spleen was not ruptured, it is a difficult operation to remove the arm, the right arm was not present, has not seen a body that has been exposed to the attacks of wild animals, and has seen a body mutilated by a sharp cutting knife.

By the Court.—Does not think that such a smooth edge might be produced if the skin is torn after decomposition has set in.

Henry James deposed: He is an assistant surgeon doing duty at Wellington; remembers 30th of January, was present when the body was found at the Sholah about half-past five on the 29th. The body was lying on a footpath with clothes drawn backwards over the head; one leg was extended, the other leg was drawn backwards; looked at the face and hand, the soft parts were all removed, and the place where the face ought to be was in a very advanced state of decomposition; found the hat and shoes that evening about six or eight yards from the body, saw the muslin dress, stockings, and serge petticoat on the girl; remembers the Court of Inquest, the body was identified at the dead-house by Mrs. Izzard; could not form any opinion of cause of death; when witness examined the body in the hospital, there appeared marks of cutting. The way in which the flesh had been removed at the back of the knee-joint led the witness to suppose that a cutting instrument had been used. The line which was regularly cut extended all round the knee, and there was a mark on the left thigh bone as if a knife had been used. There was a scrape along the bone; witness saw marks of teeth on the body, and came to the conclusion that jackals had got at the body. The clothes appeared dirty and muddy, which made the witness suspect that the body had been dragged.

Cross-examined.—The body was at the bottom of the Sholah. The body was partly on the back and partly on the left side, as far as witness could remember.

By the Court.—Could not form any opinion from the appearance of the wounds as to whether the mutilation had been caused before or after death. If a part were decomposed, it could be torn more smoothly than if it were in its natural state.

The proneness of the *Jackal* to carry away and devour young children has already been alluded to, and is known to every old resident in Calcutta.

The following are extracts from Calcutta Newspapers of January and February 1838 (the country south of Calcutta had, not long previously, been devastated by one of those storm waves to which that district is liable). "During one week, two children were attacked by jackals in the suburbs of Calcutta,—one was killed, and the other narrowly escaped, having been snatched away from their jaws."

"A native male child, aged eighteen months, named Chunder Mitter, was killed by a jackal, in Saumpooker. The mother left him near the door, while she went to wash some clothes in an adjoining tank; on her return she missed the child, and commenced a search with the neighbours in the jungle about the house. What was her horror to perceive a jackal eating the neck! The jackal ran away on her approach. The child was quite dead."

The next paragraph is from the Calcutta *Englishman* of the 31st March 1860:

"On Friday evening last, at about 7 o'clock, a native child of five months old was left by its mother on a mat just outside her house in Manicktollah. Whilst she went within for a few minutes to do some family work, she had no sooner turned her back, than a large jackal sprang upon the child and carried it away. Some other children playing near the place at once gave the alarm, the animal being pursued was at last forced to drop its prey, but not before it had mangled the poor little creature in such a manner that he died shortly after."

Only a few weeks ago, Dr. Fayrer informed me that he had just seen a child about six weeks old belonging to well-to-do parents, which had been carried off by a jackal, but saved in time. The chief injury had been caused by the animal's efforts to drag the child between the bars of a fence in which its body became jammed. A canine tooth had broken one of the thigh-bones. The child has perfectly recovered. Wolves not unfrequently do the like in Upper India.

In out-stations, it, from time to time, becomes necessary to distinguish injuries inflicted by Elephants, Tigers, Crocodiles, and other wild animals.

The *Elephant* generally seizes his victim, raises him in the air, dashes him violently upon the ground, and tramples upon him. The results, for the most part, are that the chest is driven in, some of the larger viscera are commonly ruptured, and more than one limb usually receives a compound fracture. In other cases, the animal kicks his victim to and fro between his fore and hind legs.

The elephant has been frequently made the executioner of criminals, by the native princes of this country and of Burmah.* It was regarded as an especially degrading mode of execution. We are told, in *Peyton's Voyage*, 1614, that the king of Achen "is very cruel to his subordinates, causing them to bie throwne before elephants, himselfe commanding the Understanding Elephant to tosse the partie so oft and so high, either to bruise or kill him, as he fancieth. He hath prohibited any which arrive at his Port, without his chop, to come on shore, which a Dutch merchant neglecting, the king sent for him and laid him before the elephant (which tossed him three times, without much bruising) to teach him how to neglect the commands of kings another time."

With the Mahomedans, destruction by *Elephants* was one of the modes in which unchaste women were put to death. We are told by the Rev. Edward Terry, that "those which are brought to suffer death by elephants (some of which vast creatures are train'd up to do execution on malefactors) are thus dealt withal. First, if that overgrown beast be commanded by his rider to dispatch that poor trembling offender presently, who is *prostrate* before him, he will, with his broad round foot, immediately press him to death; but if that wretched creature be condemned *ita mori ut se mori sentiat*, die so as that he may feel tortures, and torments in dying (which are as so many several deaths), the elephant will break his bones by degrees (as men are broken upon the wheel), as first his legs, then his thighs, after that, the bones in both his arms ; this done, his wretched spirit is left to breathe its last out of the midst of those broken bones."

A parricide was sentenced by the Mogul to be "bound alive by his heels, fastened to a small iron chain, which was tied to the hinde leg of a great elephant, and then that this elephant should drag him after him one whole remove of that king from one place to another, which was about ten miles distant ; that so all his flesh might be worn off his bones ; so it was, when we saw him in the way following that king in his progress, for he appeared then to us a *skeleton*, rather than a body."

* The following account of the execution of a criminal at Baroda is given in the Bombay journals for 1814 :—"The man was a slave, and two days before had murdered his master, brother to a native chieftain, named Ameer Sahib. About eleven o'clock, the elephant was brought out, with only the driver on his back, surrounded with natives with bamboos in their hands. The criminal was placed three yards behind on the ground, his legs tied with three ropes, which were fastened to a ring on the right hind leg of the animal. At every step the elephant took, it jerked him forward, and eight or ten steps must have dislocated every limb, for they were loose and broken when the elephant had proceeded five hundred yards. The man, though covered with mud, showed every sign of life, and seemed to be in most excruciating torments. After having been tortured in this manner about an hour, he was taken to the outside of the town, when the elephant, which was instructed for such purposes, was backed, and placed his foot on the head of the criminal."

In Captain Meadowes Taylor's Confessions of a Thug, we read: "They bound him by a chain round his loins to the fore-foot of the elephant, and they tied his hands behind him, so that he could not save himself by clinging to it." . . . "The mahout drove his ankoos into the head of the noble beast, which, uttering a loud scream, dashed forward. A few steps, and my father's soul must have been in paradise."

In an execution, which took place at Baroda, a few years ago, we are told that the unfortunate man "was tied with a chain or stout rope round his body and arms to an elephant's leg, and then dragged along through the streets, until life became extinct. To make all sure, however, another elephant was brought to crush him with his feet, but this, it appears, the animal, from some feeling, would not do till the brute was goaded on by spears and fire-works and made to do it."

I believe that the animal's habit of kicking his victim to and fro between a hind and fore-leg, until the body is reduced to a bloody mass, has sometimes been resorted to.

A remarkable crime was committed in Tirhoot, in 1849. A mahout, in the service of a rich zumeendar, began to cut, as fodder for his elephant, the branches of a butt tree, the property of a man who resisted and abused the mahout—the latter drove his elephant over the unfortunate man, who was "torn to pieces" by the animal.* These cases are of importance, as, where a person is attacked by a crowd of Bengalees, unarmed with cutting weapons, the injuries inflicted are often very similar to those above described. However, a question of this kind could only occur when a body, thus mutilated, was discovered in a very remote part of the country ranged over by wild elephants.

In the *Tiger* wounds which I have seen, either a flap of integument or muscle has been torn down by the blow of the animal's claws, or a mouthful of integument, muscle, and bone, altogether as large as two fists, has been completely bitten away.

In Demmin's Weapons of War (p. 413), we have figured the *Bag-nuk*, or tiger's claw, preserved in the Meyrick collection. It is said to have been invented, about 1659, by Sivajee, and to have been used by a secret society for purposes of murder, as, counterfeiting the wounds inflicted by a tiger's claws, it diverted suspicion from the offender. If this was the case, the weapon was not used exclusively in this manner. Sivajee is said to have employed it in the most critical moment of his eventful career; and Todd says that, in last century, Zalim, regent of Kotah, not satisfied with the use of more natural weapons, occasionally made his corps of gladiators fight with the *bag-nuk*,† when they tore off each other's flesh.

In two cases where I have been compelled to amputate the limbs of persons

---

* Police Report, L. P., 1848, p. 7.

† Colonel Briggs has described this weapon, Trans. R. Asiatic Soc., Vol. II.

seized by *Crocodiles* (*Mugger*), the victim has been caught by the leg while bathing ; the limb has been marked, at regular intervals on either side, with the punctures of the huge peg-like teeth, giving it much the appearance of one that has been drawn in between wheels with wide cogs ; towards the knee, however, there have been evidences of a struggle between the man and his assailant,—the integuments and muscles are torn, but not at all in proportion to the internal injury, the bone being literally crushed into splinters, apparently by a lateral movement of the enormous jaw.

The *Alligator* (*gharial*) sometimes devours children, and occasionally seizes the legs of men who venture into the shallow waters in which these creatures abound. About two years ago, Mr. Carlleyle, Curator of the Riddell Museum, Agra, wrote to the *Delhi Gazette* that the following had been found in the stomach of a large *gharial* taken near that city :—

" About a dozen large bunches, pellets of *hair* (probably *human*).

" Sixty-eight (68) stones (rounded pebbles), averaging in size from nearly three inches to one inch in diameter.

" One large ankle bangle ring of mixed metal.

" Twenty-four (24) fragments, of various sizes, of vitreous armlet rings called '*churis*.'

" Five (5) bronze finger rings.

" One small silver neck-charm (a small defaced silver coin, with a metal loop, for suspension, attached to it).

" One *gold* bead, about one-third of an inch square.

" One largish bead, of black stone, veined with white, called " *Suleimani, manka*" (Quære, *Onyx* ?)

" Thirty (30) small red necklace beads."

All these things (barring the stones), says the reporter, must have been on the body of some young woman, or girl (if not more than one), who had been devoured by this monster ; which shows that the brute must have had an unfortunate predilection for the weaker sex. And these facts prove the fallacy and incorrectness of the generally received idea that the " *Gharial*" *never* preys upon living *human* beings.

Five severe cases of *Shark-bite* which I examined in the Medical College Hospital, in April and May (the time at which the fish come up with the freshes), presented the following appearances : two principal lacerated wounds, or lines of wound, forming segments of large circles, each forming an arc of about a foot. The upper by far the most severe, separating tissues deeply ; this is evidently caused by the fish's effort to drag its victim under water. In one case, the lower wound had a serrated upper edge, and a fine line of incisions parallel to it below caused by the drawing action of the complex rows of teeth. The presence, more or less, of these short, straight, linear cuts through the integument near the edge of a mangled chasm from which a mass of flesh has been torn away, is very characteristic of shark-bite.

I have seen one *nates* nearly removed, and a hand bitten off in a woman, the whole gluteal mass and back of the thigh entirely removed in a man. Here one stroke of a strong tooth had half cut through the neck of the thigh-bone. I doubt if any single blow, with a strong chisel on the side of the bare bone, would leave so clear and deep a groove.

A full and very interesting narrative of this latter case, with a wood-cut representing the injury done to the head and neck of the femur by the animal's teeth, has been published by Dr. Fayrer.* Dr. Fayrer considers that the shark was, in all probability, the *Carcharias Gangeticus.*

The shark either begins to devour his victim at once, or, when the sufferer is dragged out of his jaws, tears off as much flesh as his teeth will hold. The object of the crocodile appears to be to drag his victim into deep water, and first drown, and then devour him. Two large *muggers*, kept in a tank by the Raja of Burdwan, always used to drown pigs in this way. When putrefaction caused the bodies to rise, the crocodiles devoured them.

Dr. Day, of Madras, has told me of a man who had his upper arm cut all round to the bone by a coil of the tail of a *Whip-ray* (*Myliobatis*).

Captain Bacon mentions that, in 1821, a private soldier running hastily round an angle of one of the barracks in Fort William, came suddenly into collision with an *Adjutant bird*, and was spitted clean through the body by its beak : both were victims to this meeting, for the violence of the concussion broke the bird's neck, and both fell dead upon the pavement.

I have read somewhere of a like accident which occurred to a man who suddenly came in contact with a *Stork* in one of the old Netherlands towns.

BITES OF VENOMOUS SERPENTS.

Cases of *alleged* death by snake-bite are of such frequent occurrence in this country, that it is singular they should not become more frequently the subjects of medico-legal investigation. Some years since, it was stated, by the magistrate of Midnapore, that the deaths from this cause, in that zillah alone, amounted to 402 in twenty-one months ; and it was asserted, in the public prints, that 50 had thus perished, in Delhi, during the rainy season of 1853.†

The above scanty statistics prefaced this Chapter in my last edition. Since then the Government have been at considerable pains to ascertain, as precisely as possible, the mortality from snake-bite in every district; and this measure has been greatly strengthened by a letter of instructions which, at Dr. Fayrer's suggestion, the Head of the Medical Department issued, last year, to the medical officers of this Presidency.‡

* Medical Times and Gazette, June 20, 1868, p. 657.

† *Ibid* for January 1854, from the *Delhi Gazette*.

‡ Circular Memo. No. 127. of the 22nd November 1869.

The enquiry, thus organized, has already led to the collection of much valuable statistical and scientific information. Dr. Fayrer has recently published the subjoined statistics :—

"An idea of the loss of life caused throughout India yearly by the bite of the cobra and other venomous snakes, but especially the cobra, as it is by far the most common, may be formed from the following information extracted from a recent report of the Commissioner of Burdwan to the Bengal Government :—

"He says, 'The number of deaths from snake-bite, during the last nine years, is shown in the annual printed police returns to have been as follows:—

1860	... 878	1863	... 1,048	1866	... 929
1861	... 989	1864	... 1,035	1867	... 984
1862	... 1,041	1865	... 1,184	1868	... 1,144

Total, 9,232 persons killed in nine years, out of a population of 5,701,072.

"'There may be a little inaccuracy in the above figures, but they have been compiled over a series of nine (9) years, and it cannot be questioned that they show that there is a mortality of above 1,000 persons every year, in a population of nearly 6,000,000 people.'

"In the district of Midnapore—which the commissioner considers the worst—in the year 1865, there were 530 deaths from snake-bite recorded, out of a population of 1,200,000 persons.

"In the district of Beerbhoom, on the other hand, there were in one year 60 cases of death from snake-poisoning, out of a population of 743,685 persons. It appears from the report that women suffer more than men.

"In 1858, a reward of four annas was given by Government for each venomous snake destroyed in the division, and the magistrate reported in December that Rs. 1,961-8 had been paid for 1,845 snakes destroyed during the year. The reward was reduced to two annas for every poisonous snake brought in, but this was not sufficient inducement, and the numbers rapidly diminished.

		Snakes.	Rs.	As.
In 1859	...	957	124	4
„ 1860	...	217	27	0
„ 1861	...	8	1	0

"The magistrate remarked 'that there are few persons who would risk their lives to bring in a live snake for two annas.'

"In Bancoorah, another district of the Burdwan division, the magistrate proposed that the reward of two annas shall be given for all poisonous snakes brought in dead or alive. This was sanctioned with a proviso that the magistrate himself should see the snake's head cut off. The reward was raised to four annas for each snake, in 1862. On the 14th

July following, the magistrate reported that the increased reward had produced its effect—47 snakes had been brought in on one day, and 70 on another day ; Rs. 89 had been spent in less than a month.

"On the 21st July of the same year, the magistrate proposed to reduce the reward to two annas ; he says, '97 snakes were brought in on Saturday, and 118 to-day.' The duty of personally supervising the decapitation of the snakes became so irksome, that the magistrate applied to higher authority for permission to depute some one to see this done ; but the request was refused.

"On the 20th October, the commissioner reported that, from the 29th May to 14th October 1862, 18,423 snakes had been killed, giving an average of 110 snakes a day ; and he applied for a grant of Rs. 10,000 to provide for the rewards, at the same time proposing to reduce the reward to two annas.

"On the 6th January 1863, the Government of Bengal remarked that, whereas from 29th May to 14th October, 18,423 snakes had been killed ; and from 15th October to 7th December, the number had increased to 26,029, giving an average of 463½ per diem, the Lieutenant-Governor expressed his surprise that the average number of snakes killed daily should have increased during the cold weather, and the magistrate was requested to submit an explanation on this point. The magistrate explained it by ascribing it to the increased expertness of the snake-catchers, and the large number of persons who had abandoned their occupation, and taken to this comparatively lucrative mode of obtaining a livelihood. It was considered probable that many of these snakes might not have been poisonous, but the magistrate rejoined that he had exercised great care in discriminating, and that 40,000 rupees would not have paid the rewards had they been given for all kinds of snakes. From this one would conclude that the advantages of Bancoorah as a residence must be doubtful. It gives a sad proof of the fatal character of the bites of the Indian Thanatophidia, and there is reason to believe that the greater share of the mortality is due to the cobra."

The following statistics are from other authentic sources :—

	Deaths from Snake-bite.
North-Western Provinces, in 1867	1,678
Oudh, in 1867	1,127
Oudh, in 1868	1,427
Central Provinces, three years' Returns ...	1,874

In the above-named circular, Dr. Fayrer has given the subjoined list of the best known of the *poisonous* Land and Sea Snakes of Hindustan.

"*Snakes most commonly met with have ** prefixed; those less so *; the remainder are comparatively rare.*

SUB-ORDER, POISONOUS COLUBRINE SNAKES.

Family ———————— *Elapidæ.*

GENUS ** 1. NAJA: *N. Tripudians*, or Cobra: several varieties. Native names Keautiah, Gokurrah, &c., &c., &c., &c.

" * 2. OPHIOPHAGUS: *O. Elaps. Hamadryas*, one species. From Assam to west bank of Hooghly. Native name, Sunkerchoar.

" ** 3. BUNGARUS: *B. Cæruleus*, or *Krait.* From Calcutta to Delhi.

** *B. Fasciatus*, or *Sankni* (marked with black and yellow bands—Bengal generally).

" 4. XENURELAPS: *X. Bungaroides*, found about Cherrapoonjee.

" 5. CALLOPHIS: *C. Intestinalis.*

C. Maclellandii, found in Central India.

C. Nigrescens, found in the Neilgherries.

C. Annularis, India generally.

Family of Hydrophidæ or Sea Snakes.

1. PLATURUS: *P. Scutatus*, found on the Coast from Chittagong to Madras.

P. Fischeri, Ditto, ditto.

* 2. HYDROPHIS: several varieties found on the Coast. *H. Cyanocincta, Hidgelli.*

* 3. ENHYDRINA: *E. Bengalensis, Hidgelli*, Botanic Garden, Dhappa Canal. } *H. Robusta*, Ditto.

4. PELAMIS: *P. Bicolor.*

H. Coronata, Ditto.

H. Stricticollis, Ditto.

H. Chloris, Sandheads.

H. Gracilis, found at Dhappa, Calcutta.

SUB-ORDER, VIPERINE SNAKES.

Family of Pit Vipers or Crotalidæ.

1. TRIMERESURUS :* *T. Gramineus*, found in Bengal, has been found at Dhappa Canal.
   * *T. Erythrurus*,
   T. Carinatus,
   T. Anamallensis,
   T. Monticola,
   T. Strigatus,
   T. Mucrosquamatus, found in Bengal, has been found at Assam.
2. PELTOPELOR : *P. Macrolepis*, found in the Annamallay Mountains.
3. HALYS : *H. Himalayanus*.
4. HYPNALE : *H. Nipa*, or *Carawala*, found in Southern India.

Family of Vipers or Viperidæ.

1. DABOIA : ** *D. Russellü ;* Native name, *Bora*, found all over Bengal, from Southern India to the Himalayas, as high as 3,500 feet above the sea.
2. ECHIS : *E. Carinata*, found in the Annamallay Mountains, Carnatic, and other parts of India."

The late Dr. Cantor gave me a note of six species of the Genus Hydrophis, which inhabit the Bay of Bengal, *viz.*, *H. schistosa*, *striata*, *nigrocincta*, *gracilis*, *pelamis*, and *pelamoides*. Out of this number, he has observed the H. *schistosa* and *striata* to be most common, and the *H. gracilis* comparatively rare in the northern part of the Bay and the estuaries of the Ganges. *All the Pelagic Serpents are Venomous.* Dr. Cantor has disproved the accuracy of M. Schlegel's opinion that the pelagic serpents are of a more peaceable disposition than the greater number of terrestrial venomous snakes,—showing, from his own experience, that those species which inhabit the Bay of Bengal and the estuaries of the Ganges are of very ferocious habits, as well in as out of water. He refers to the record, in the Asiatic Researches, of a number of accidents, at Madras, caused by the venom of these serpents ; and also to an instance, which took place in 1837 on board H. M. Brig *Algerine*, while in Madras Roads, where the person bitten expired within four hours of the infliction of the wound.*

The subjoined detail of this case is given in Statistical Reports of the Health of the Navy, 1837—43, Part 2, East India Station, page 9.

On the 9th October, while the ship lay at anchor in Madras Roads, a water-snake was caught, measuring seven feet six inches long, and six inches and-a-half in girth at the thickest part. After the patient had handled the reptile for some time, it suddenly bit him on the inside

* Transactions of the Zoological Society of London, Vol. II., p. 303.

of the index finger of the right hand, inflicting a wound resembling that caused by the point of a pin. He declined having the wound fomented, having been bitten by reptiles of the same kind, as he supposed, in the Straits of Malacca, without any bad consequences. At 8 A.M., half an hour after the inflicting of the wound, he made a good breakfast, dressed; and about 10 o'clock went on deck. After taking a few turns, he was suddenly seized with vomiting, the matter ejected being of a dark brown color, resembling coffee-ground, and of a very offensive odour. After a short time, his pulse became small, variable, and intermitting; and the pupils were dilated, but contracted readily by the stimulus of light. The left side of the face was slightly paralysed; there was subsultus tendinum, and the skin was covered with a cold clammy perspiration; the countenance was anxious, and indicative of much distress. In consequence of the spasmodic action of the muscles of the glottis, he breathed with great difficulty. The integuments from the wound to the wrist were slightly swollen, and, on the right side of the neck and face, they presented a mottled appearance of dark purple and livid colors. A ligature having been placed above the wrist, and fomentations applied to the hand, a liniment, composed of turpentine, liquor ammonia, and olive oil, was rubbed on the throat and neck. He made frequent attempts to swallow a mixture containing liquor ammoniœ and tincture of opium, but failed. At 10-20, in consequence of the spasmodic action of the muscles of the glottis, he was put into a warm bath, which apparently relieved the symptoms, and enabled him to take a dose of the mixture, which caused him to vomit a dark ropy fluid. About twenty minutes after coming out of the bath (in which he remained ten minutes) the spasmodic action of the muscles of the neck and throat became more severe, and the whole body assumed a purple color; the breathing became very difficult, from the obstruction caused by a dark brown substance which came away in a stringy form from the air passages. By 11 o'clock he was in a state of coma; the pupils were contracted, and the pulse imperceptible at the wrist. At 11-20, not quite four hours from the time he was bitten, he died. It does not appear that any *post-mortem* examination of the body took place.

It will be remarked (adds the reporter) that the symptoms in this case very much resembled those produced by the bite of a rabid animal, although they were much more violent, and more speedily fatal.

The anatomical peculiarities by which the venomous snakes of India may be distinguished from the harmless species, as well as the characteristics of the various poisonous kinds, will be found clearly laid down in Dr. Fayrer's work on the Thanatophidia of India, commenced in No. 1, Vol. V. for 1870, of the Indian Medical Gazette.

Mr. Sylvester has pointed out briefly that the poisonous kinds are deficient in an outer or marginal row of teeth in the upper jaw, which are present in the harmless varieties, and are fixed to the maxillary and pre-mandibular bones; but their place is supplied by the grooved poison fangs. Both varieties have two palatal rows of teeth, which run from before backwards, a little outside the median line of the roof of the mouth, and are embedded in the palatal and pterygoid bones. A few exceptions, however, occur,—as in the genera "Dryophis," "Dipsus," and "Bucephalus," where the marginal teeth increase in size backwards, and several of them are traversed by a groove through which an acrid saliva is injected; but no true poison gland exists.

It is strongly believed by several experienced officers, missionaries, and others, well acquainted with the country and its people, that a vast amount of undiscovered crime is concealed (at least in Bengal) under the always plausible, and not generally controvertible, report of "*Died by Snake-bite.*" At present, the violent suspicion rests only upon the evidence of occasional cases.* Nevertheless, it appears to call for close and frequent investigation by magistrates and civil surgeons. It would be very desirable that, from time to time, magistrates should direct that, during a stated period, all bodies of persons reported to the police as having died from snake-bite, within a moderate distance of the zillah station, should be at once sent in for inquest and for examination by the civil surgeon. Whether instances of discovery occurred or not, the frequent repetition of such an order would evidently have a direct tendency to place a check upon the perpetration of secret crime under this disguise.

In cases where men are bitten by the cobra in full venom, and where a proper ligature is not instantly applied above the punctures, and the stimulating treatment, by ammonia, brandy, &c., is not had recourse to, the symptoms usually set in within an hour, and destroy life with great rapidity.

The following case, by Dr. Burder, affords one of the fullest descriptions on record of the action of cobra poison, when altogether unchecked by treatment.

A keeper at the Regent's Park, Zoological Gardens, aged thirty-one, of rather intemperate habits, was bitten, while partially intoxicated, on the upper part of his nose, by an Indian cobra. For a short time after the receipt of the wound, there appear to have been no striking symptoms, apart from his agitation and alarm at the occurrence; and he was able to walk and talk without difficulty. After *twenty minutes*, however, he began to stagger in walking, and ceased to speak intelligibly. At the same time movements, apparently convulsive, of the mouth and of the limbs were observed. He made no special complaint. He was brought to the hospital about thirty-five minutes after the accident. He was then unable to speak, and consciousness was nearly or quite abolished. He moaned, grasped his

* *Murdered and reported to have died by Snake-bite.*—The following examples have been taken without special search. *Hanged while living.*—N. A. R., Oct. 2, 1855, p. 531. *Death by Abortion.*—*Ib.*, Feb. 14, 1857, p. 162. *Neck broken.*—*Ib.*, Jan. 19, 1858, p. 41. *Strangled.*—Beng. Pol. Rep., 1868, p. 275. *Seven* cases were discovered in the Bogra District in 1868.—*Ibid*, pp. 300 *et seq.*

throat with some eagerness of action, tossed his head from side to side, and moved his arms and legs in an uneasy restless manner, not apparently convulsive. When asked, in a loud voice, if he felt pain, he made no reply, nor gave any indication of intelligence, beyond the action of placing his fingers on his throat. He was unable to support himself in a sitting posture. His face generally was slightly livid, his eyes fixed, the pupils rather large, acting sluggishly to light ; the skin was of natural temperature and moisture ; pulse 120, regular in rythm, but unequal in force, most of the beats, however, being tolerably full and strong. On the upper part of the nose were a number of small punctured wounds, from one or more of which a small quantity of blood had flowed. The eyelids of the right eye, especially the upper, were swollen and livid, the lividity extending to the right side of the nose. The eyelids of the left eye were not thus affected. There appeared to be no swelling of the tongue. Within five minutes, movements of the extremities had entirely ceased ; the respiration was 20 per minute, very shallow, without stertor, and free from any sound indicating laryngeal or tracheal obstruction. The lividity of the face had very markedly increased, a free perspiration had occurred over the body generally. The pulse continued tolerably good. In two minutes more (about forty minutes after the infliction of the bite) natural respiration had ceased, and, but for the continuance of the pulse, the man might have been pronounced dead. The pulse at this time was 32 per minute, remarkably regular both in rythm and in force, some of the beats being strikingly full and bounding. Artificial respiration and the application of galvanism were now employed and continued for fifty minutes, at the end of which time all muscular action ceased.

On examination, there was found, immediately above the middle of the nose, on either side of its centre, a horizontal row of small punctures ; on the left side four (the three next the centre being, however, mere scratches), on the right side two, larger than those on the left. Half an inch above these, was another row of punctures, of somewhat greater size,—on the left side two, on the right side one, that on the right side being again the largest. A quarter of an inch higher still, on the right side of the nose, was the largest wound of all, transverse in its direction (as were also such of the others as had any appreciable dimensions) measuring in diameter about a sixth of an inch, and in depth extending apparently through the substance of the skin. From this wound, a little blood was oozing ; the others were closed by coagula. Two hours and-a-half after the man's death, a mouse was inoculated with the blood that flowed from the wound. No effect was produced upon the animal.

The *post-mortem examination* was made thirty hours after death. A considerable quantity of frothy blood had issued from the mouth and nostrils. There was livid discoloration of the neck, face, and upper part of the chest, also of the dependent parts generally, except at the points where the pressure of the body had fallen ; here the skin was pale. There was no swelling of any part, except the right eyelids, and these were less swollen than during life. Rigor mortis was strongly marked in the lower extremities ; less so in the upper.

Bloody fluid had continued to exude from the highest wound on the nose. On dissecting back the skin, it was found that the three highest punctures on the right side had penetrated into the cellular tissue, which was infiltrated with dark blood.

In the *Brain and Spinal Cord* scarcely anything abnormal was discovered. There was little, if any, unnatural congestion, either of the nervous centres themselves or of the meninges. The lateral ventricles of the brain were filled with transparent fluid. The spinal cord, at its lower part, was softer than usual. The lungs appeared less collapsed than usual ; their posterior parts were excessively gorged with blood, being almost black on section, and exuding copiously a blackish fluid mixed with some air. The air-tubes, large and small, throughout both lungs, were filled with a black frothy fluid, and the lining membrane was generally stained of a very dark blackish color.

The *Heart* was healthy in structure. The left cavities were contracted and empty ; the right were filled with dark fluid blood, amongst which was a small quantity of very loose coagulum. There were no clots in the great vessels.*

There was no swelling about the tongue or fauces ; the œsophagus was healthy ; the *Stomach* presented patches of pale color, alternating with patches of red, the latter formed by the aggregation of pale red spots. The *Intestines* were natural.

The *Liver* was of dark color externally, and darker than natural on section ; otherwise the organ was healthy.

The *Spleen* was enormously congested, of very dark color externally, and, on section, almost black ; the substance was very soft, and from it exuded abundantly very dark blood.

The *Kidneys* were of very dark color, both externally and internally, and the cut surfaces yielded, on pressure, dark-coloured blood ; otherwise the organs were healthy.†

This case appears to establish the facts, that,—the bite of a full-venomed cobra will, if not interfered with, produce severe symptoms in about twenty minutes, and death in about fifty ; but, as the state of intoxication appears

* The reporter in the "*Lancet*" says, "The blood was altogether dark, alkaline, fluid" (this was thirty hours after death in the month of October), "and it emitted a peculiar sour and sickly smell, quite different from the odour commonly known to pervade the dead-house."

This is quite contrary to Indian experience. The blood drawn from an animal which has just died from cobra poison always coagulates firmly. The blood of animals killed by Russell's viper does not coagulate.

† Medical Times and Gazette and Ranking's Retrospect, Vol. XVI., p. 134.

to be, in some measure, antagonistic to the operation of snake poison,* it is probable that the fatal symptoms will generally set in and close more speedily; that the cobra poison acts more rapidly than any other poison known to be in use among the natives of India, with the exception of the nux vomica; but that the operation of this snake poison is not attended with any convulsive motions which could be mistaken for the opisthotonic spasms under which life fails in poisoning by nux vomica; that decomposition is not unusually rapid; and that the rigor mortis is not absent after death by this kind of snake-bite.

The Profession are well acquainted with Dr. Fayrer's invaluable series of Experiments upon Snake-Bite which have appeared in the Indian Medical Gazette, from the 2nd of December 1867, and which afford an almost inexhaustible treasury of most interesting practical facts and observations to those who may, hereafter, investigate the history of the poisonous serpents, or, as Dr. Fayrer appropriately terms them, the Thanatophidia of India. One of the many important deductions drawn from these experiments is the fact that a fair bite from our Indian Cobra or Russellian Viper, in full venom, has been incurably mortal to every animal on which the experiments have been tried, despite of all treatment, except only where the bitten part *has been instantaneously and completely excised.*

Consequently, it is only when persons are bitten by these snakes when their supply of poison is exhausted, or by less venomous

---

* That is to say, Lieut. Woodruff and Dr. Blackburn have found the administration of strong whisky, in almost unlimited quantities (a practice known as the *Western Remedy*) of very great efficacy in cases of rattle-snake bite. Dr. Gilman considers that alcohol, if brought in contact with the venom, is, to a certain extent, an antidote.—American Journal of Medical Sciences, January 1853, and Ranking's Retrospect, Vol. XVII., p. 295; American Lancet and Ranking, Vol. XIX., p. 114; St. Louis Medical and Surgical Journal, quoted in the Lancet, February 8th, 1854. Dr. Jeter, of Quincy, has administered to a girl between three and four years of age, who had been bitten, a pint and-a-half of fourth-proof brandy without any signs of intoxication ensuing. He considers the application of sinapisms over the whole body to be the next most reliable means of averting collapse.

Dr. Gilman arrived at the conclusion "that the venom of serpents destroys all kinds of organised life, vegetable as well as animal," and "that the blood of small animals destroyed by the venom of serpents bears a close resemblance to that of animals destroyed by lightning or hydrocyanic acid; it loses its power of coagulation, and cannot be kept long from putrefaction." It must be observed, however, that in poisoning by the less deadly snakes such as the English adder and even by the Australian snakes reported upon by Dr. Halford of Melbourne, powerful stimulants of nearly all kinds not only keep off the symptoms of poisoning, when had recourse to early, but appear to have, in some instances, the power of restoring vital action after the pulse has become imperceptible,—when, according to the above theory, the blood should have become disintegrated and unfit to serve the purposes of circulation and nutrition. See the very remarkable cases by Dr. Chamlers, late of the H. E. I. C., Glasgow Medical Journal, April 1853, and Ranking, Vol. XVII.; and Dr. Macrae's (of Chittagong) narrative of his own case, Ranking, Vol. XVI., p. 138. The *final* effect of the poison of some of the viperine snakes is, doubtless, to destroy the vitality of the blood; but I think that, in our attempts to restore those bitten, we should be encouraged by the belief that, although a strong poison is circulating in the blood, that fluid retains its essential chemical and vital conditions up to, and *even after*, the moment of apparent death.

For remarks on the tendency to Hæmorrhage after snake-bite, see Bombay Med. Trans. and Bombay Dispy. Rep., No. 2, p. 64.

serpents, like those of Australia, the *Trigonocephalus Gramineus* of the Nepaul Hills, and the English viper, that the reputed antidotes, liquor ammoniæ—administered by the mouth and by injection into the circulation—eau de luce, liquor potassæ, spirit, &c., can have valid curative effect.

The following facts, relative to the chemical properties of the venom of Indian snakes, have been adduced by Dr. Cantor and Mr. Laidlay. The latter has given the following memorandum relative to the venom of *Naja lutescens* (Laurenti):—"The venom was carefully obtained, so as to avoid any admixture of saliva, by compressing the venomous glands. It issued from the lower aperture of the fangs in viscid drops of a syrupy consistency, and was received as it fell from the fangs in platina capsules. The serpents operated upon were an adult *Cobra de Capello*, and one of its varieties *Naja Kaouthia* (apud Belanger). In every instance, the venom readily changed the blue of litmus to red, and restored the bright yellow of turmeric paper that had been reddened by the application of caustic alkali, an unequivocal proof of acidity. When left to spontaneous evaporation, it dried into a varnish resembling mucilage or the glare of an egg, cracking in all directions; and, on being heated, it deposited an abundant coagulum, apparently albuminous. In either instance, when re-dissolved, it retained its acid property. What the nature of this acid may be, it is impossible to determine from the small quantity operated upon; nor am I prepared to say that the poison *itelf* is an acid, although, if it be not so, it is certainly associated with one. Most probably, from the rapid disappearance of its properties by keeping, the poison itself consists of some exceedingly unstable compound, which would be totally disorganized under any attempt at isolation by chemical means."*

Long previous to this, Dr. Cantor described the fresh poison of the *Hamadryas* as a pellucid tasteless fluid, in consistence like a thin solution of gum arabic in water; and as slightly reddening litmus paper, which is also the case with the fresh poison of the *Cophias viridis*, *Vipera elegans*, *Naja tripudians*, *Bungarus annularis*, and *Bungarus cæruleus*. The same is the case with the poison of *Elaps bivirgatus*. In these observations, the assertion of M. Schlegel† that the venom is neither acid nor alkaline is refuted. Dr. Cantor accounts for the mistake by supposing, that M. Schlegel himself never had an opportunity of testing the poison of a living serpent; for, besides the five above-mentioned genera of Indian venomous serpents, he found the fresh poison of different species of marine serpents *(Hydrus)*, to possess the property of turning

---

* Catalogue of Reptiles inhabiting the Malayan Peninsula and Islands, by Theodore Cantor, M.D., Journal of Asiatic Society, Vol. XVI., p. 1040.

† Schlegel's erroneous observation is generally cited; it will be found quoted in Taylor on Poisons, p. 574.

litmus paper red. The same fact with the *Crotalus* is noticed by Dr. Harlan, who says—"The poison of the living *Crotalus*, tested in numerous instances with litmus paper, &c., invariably displayed acid properties."*

A good deal of controversy having arisen upon the microscopical condition of the blood of animals killed by the bites of venomous serpents (which blood Dr. Fayrer has proved to be so poisonous as to be capable of transmission through a series of three animals with fatal effects), I subjoin the most recent observations upon this question.

In his pamphlet on the Injection of Ammonia into the circulation, p. 13, Professor Halford observes: "Let us suppose a dog to have been bitten (by a cobra, rattlesnake, or tiger-snake) at 11 A.M., and to have died at noon. It is probable nothing strange will be seen in the blood but granular matter, for two or three hours, but then, in the midst of the germinal matter, which by this time has greatly increased in quantity, will be seen here and there nuclei with very sharp outlines, some single, others double, triple, and quadruple, many of them hour-glass shaped, as if dividing, and others again kidney shaped. At this time only the most practised observer could see the cell-wall of a few, and to do this requires a power of 1000 diameters, and good management of the light. Numerous unaltered white corpuscles, pearly and opaque, may be seen here and there. By 5 P.M. the cells will be fully formed, their numbers literally innumerable, the nucleus usually single, division and multiplication having ceased; the macula may occasionally be seen, and the cell-wall, which is of the most exceeding delicacy, fully formed. *As the cells increase, the nebulous germinal matter disappears.* Occasionally, particles of germinal matter may be seen running between the nucleus and cell-wall. It is to be understood that I am describing the condition of the blood before any re-agent whatsoever is applied; but now suppose we add a drop of magenta dye in the proportion of one part of dye to twenty or fifteen of water, then immediately the cell-wall becomes colored and distinctly visible, the nucleus more so; and, lastly, the brilliant little macula is seen at some part of the circumference of the cell, being $\frac{1}{1700}$th of an inch, that of the nucleus $\frac{1}{2800}$th inch. The cells are of this size before the diluted dye is added. From this time every further observation for several days will show the cells in great abundance, until, finally, they become destroyed; the blood at the same time getting thinner and thinner."

In a paper on poisoning by rattlesnake poison, by Dr. S. W. Mitchell, with microscopical notes by Dr. Joseph G. Richardson,† it is stated that, "In the example of a rabbit, dog, and goat, so poisoned by rattlesnake venom, as to survive its insertion from one to six hours only, whose hearts

* Cantor, as quoted in the Penny Cyclopædia, article NAJA.

† American Journal of the Medical Sciences, for April 1870, p. 317.

were allowed to remain unopened from twelve to twenty-four hours after death, the temperature varying from 75° to 90° Fahr., the blood, when removed from the cardiac cavities in such a way as to avoid all contamination, and carefully examined with a high power, exhibited cells corresponding perfectly to those described by Prof. Halford; yet that these so-called 'peculiar cells' were always mingled not only with white blood corpuscles in their ordinary 'pearly and opaque' condition, but also with those in various stages of enlargement and alteration, such as may be at any time produced in the white globules of normal blood simply by diluting the liquor sanguinis with water; and further that, in the case of the goat, when a majority of the 'peculiar cells' presented the unusual character of being multinucleated, the white blood globules, if distended by water, exhibited the same peculiarity. We may, therefore, fairly conclude that the abnormal corpuscles in these particular instances were, in relaity, only white blood globules which had undergone an alteration similar to that caused by reducing the specific gravity of the blood, and so establish a strong presumption (whose correctness Prof. Halford can alone decide) that the "peculiar cells" described by him as resulting from the poison of snake-bites are precisely analogous in their character."

I was informed, by my friend the Rev. Dr. Thomas Smith, of a fact, which is, at least, curious,—*viz.*, that the snake-catchers of Bengal appear to be all opium-eaters; and that it is a popular belief among the natives that an habitual opium-eater may handle venomous snakes with impunity.

It is said that the snake-charmers in Madras are in the habit of drugging themselves with daily doses of nux vomica. Dr. Honigberger has a curious story of a half-mad Brahmin, who professed that he had, by arsenic eating, rendered himself capable of resisting the poison of *vipers*. This religious mendicant was also habituated to smoking churrus and eating opium.

I believe that these observations resolve themselves into the facts, that those who have to do with snakes make their occupation an excuse for their vices, and that they escape being bitten because, to those who are well accustomed to them, venomous snakes are handled with the greatest possible ease and safety.

HOMICIDE BY SNAKE-BITE.

Strange as it may appear at first sight, this crime has a rather full history from very ancient times.

The *employment of Snakes in war* is a practice which extended through many centuries.

Hannibal and Antiochus defeated the Romans in a naval action by throwing earthen pots filled with serpents into their ships.

In Paradin's Chronique de Savoye, there is notice of the taking of a Saracen ship with snakes in cages, which were to be thrown among the Christians in their camp. In Martene and Durand, quoted by Southey, is an allusion to the circumstance of there being kept two serpents on board a ship of Saladin's, which were to be thrown among the Christians.

We are told, in Capgrave's Chronicle, that, among other preparations for the seige of Calais, "was *a horrible ordinauns.* Small barrelis filt full of serpents and venomous bestes, which he thoute to throw into Caleys be engynes, that when the barrelis broke, the corupt venom schuld infeste hem of the town."

Distinct mention of the crime of using snakes as homicidal instruments is made in both the Hindu and the Mahomedan Law.

"If a man, by violence, throws into another person's house a snake or any other animal of that kind, whose bite or sting is mortal, this is *Shahesh, i. e.,* Violence. The magistrate shall fine him five hundred puns of cowries, and make him throw away the snake with his own hand."—*Halhed's Code of Gentoo Laws,* pp. 262, 263.

It was enacted, in the ancient Mussulman Law, that "If a person bring another into his house, and put a wild beast into the room with him, and shut the door upon them, and the beast kill the man, neither *kisas nor diyat* is incurred ; *and it is the same if a Snake or Scorpion* be put into the house with a man, or if they were there before, and sting him to death. But, if the sufferer be a child, the price of blood is payable."

Captain Alexander Hamilton* states that, in 1709, the Nawab of Chicacul set a Gentoo, named Agapa, in the hot scorching sun, for three days, with his hands fastened to a stake over his head, and one of his legs tied up until his heel touched his buttock ; and, "*in the night he was put into a dungeon with some venomous snakes to keep him company,*" and this was repeated till, the third night, he ended his miserable life.

A well-informed writer on Witch Murders in India† says that, "In former days, under the beneficial rule of the Rajahs," witches were "sometimes, by way of a little gentle torture, crammed into a small chamber full of cobras, where they first half died of fright, and then quite died of snake-bites."

Terry states that some of Sir Thomas Roe's suite were present at an Execution by Snake-bite, which he describes as follows :

"There was another condemned to dye by the Mogul himself (while we were at Amadavar" [Amedabad?] "for killing his own mother, and at this the king was much troubled to think of a death suitable for so horrid a crime ; but, upon a little pause, he adjudged him to be stung to death by snakes, which was accordingly done. There were some mountebanks

---

* New Account of the East Indies, Vol. I., p. 375.

† Cornhill Magazine for October 1867, p. 414.

there which keep great snakes to show tricks with them ; one of these fellows was presently called to bring his snakes to do that execution, who came to the place where that wretched creature was appointed to dye, and found him there all naked (except a little covering before) and trembling. Then, suddenly, the mountebank (having first angered and provoked the venomous creatures) put one of them to his thigh, which presently twined itself about that part, till it came to his groin, and there bit him till bloud followed ; the other was fastened to the outside of his other thigh, twining about it (for those snakes thus kept are long and slender) and there bit him likewise. Notwithstanding, the wretch kept upon his feet near a quarter of an hour, before which time the snakes were taken from him ; but he complained exceedingly of a fire that with much torment had possessed all his limbs, and his whole body began to swell exceedingly." . . . "About half an hour after they were taken from him, the soul of that unnatural monster left his growing carkasse, and so went to its place."

Referring to the great mortality from snake-bite at Delhi, in 1853 (*vide* p. 365), and to the ancient laws against the employment of snakes for homicidal purposes, I remarked, in my last edition, "Had there not formerly existed frequent practices of this kind, it is almost needless to say that a special law would not have been enacted to curb them. Where we see such enormous loss of life by *snake-bite* in a stronghold of Mussulman tradition like Delhi, we may be justified in enquiring,—*are such crimes still practised?*"

The following extraordinary particulars, condensed by Dr. Fayrer from the Sessions Report, contribute one answer to the above question :

"Poonai Fatmah and Joomun Fatmah are brought to trial for having, 'on or about the 11th day of October 1868, at Hurdah, Zillah Purneah, committed culpable homicide not amounting to murder, by causing the deaths of Titroo, Menghon, and Jikree.'

"1. Etwarree Moossahar, son of Dhunpat, aged twenty years, Moossahar of Bacha, Pergunnah Soorujgurrah, Zillah Monghyr, laborer.—I cannot recollect day or month. I came to Chitrapore, Zillah Purneah, being engaged to make bricks for the Darjeeling and Caragola road, and was learning how to charm snakes from the two prisoners, Poonai and Joomun. At length, on a Sunday, the prisoners wanted to make the snake bite me. I did not wish the snake to bite me on any part of the body. They then pulled my ears in a tyrannical manner, and said, Why are you afraid? If the snake does bite, we will charm you, and recover you. Then they brought three snakes, two keraits and one keautiah ; the latter a young snake, but all were poisonous. The two smaller snakes they put aside, and one large kerait, two *haths* long, they placed in front of us, and made Titroo place his right hand on the ground, and made the snake crawl on to his hand ; but at first the snake did not bite him, then Poonai struck the snake with a cane, and the snake immediately bit Titroo on his right fore-finger. After this, in the same manner, the snake was made to bite Menghon on the right hand, and then in the same manner the right hand of Jikree. After this, in the same manner the snake was made to bite me on the right wrist; the snake then appeared to be dead. After this, the prisoners having made incantations over the snake brought it to life again, and having placed some vermilion on his head, let it go free in a paddy field. After the snake had bitten Titroo, he was attacked with great thirst, and began to foam at the mouth: he became senseless. At one *pahur* of the night remaining, Titroo was bitten, and he died half an hour before daybreak. Menghon and Jikree appeared well after Titroo's death; the poison did not seem to have affected them. The prisoners then ran away; Menghon and Jikree returned to their houses, and I heard they died there at mid-day. I was then senseless after I was bitten, my body and head began to turn round, and great perspiration commenced, with severe pain in the stomach, and my eyesight became dim; then I became senseless. I was brought from Bahadurpore to the hospital, and remained there five or six days, when I became sensible again. All this took place at Bahadurpore in the court-yard of Moosum; he is not related to the prisoners, neither did he assist them. Some five or six other men besides we four were made to sit down by the prisoners in order that the snake might be made to bite to them; but owing to the snake becoming weak, they were not bitten. Seeing all the above, they ran away.

"2. Beehoo Sirdar, son of Dookhun, aged twenty-two years, Moossahar of Manikpore, Pergunnah Secundra, Zillah Monghyr, laborer.—The prisoners, Poonai and Joomun, were, in Assin, teaching Titroŏ, Menghon, Jikree, Etbari, Laloo, &c., some ten men, snake incantations, and I was also being taught by them. At length, on a Sunday night, the prisoners produced from an earthen pot two keraits and a keautiah snake, and began to teach us the incantations, and began to make the snakes move about in front of us all. We became afraid, whereupon the prisoners said, Why do you fear? If the snakes bite you, we are *gooroos*, and will soon restore you. After this they made us place our right hands on the ground, and began to make the big kerait snakes move towards our hands. We immediately, from fear, raised our hands. Upon this the prisoners struck us with rattans, and when the snake moved to a distance we again placed our hands on the ground. Then the prisoners took the snakes near to Titroo, Menghon, Jikree, and Etwarree, and made the snake, by striking it with a rattan, bite Titroo on the fore-finger of the right hand; the throat of Titroo immediately became dry, and he became senseless; then the snake was made to bite Menghon on the fore-finger of the right hand, but Menghon did not suffer or become senseless. After this the snake was made to bite Jikree on the right hand; he did not either become senseless, but remained talking. Then the snake was made to bite Etwaree on the right wrist; he did not appear to suffer. Then Titroo died two hours before dawn, and the prisoners then ran away. We went in search of them, and at 10 A.M. we found them, and seized them in a rice-field at Gurnabaree, west of the road, and took them to Bahadurpore. We told them to restore Titroo to life again, but they could not do it, but went and sat down at a distance. Then the police came, and we made the prisoners over to them.

"I heard Menghon and Jikree died on the day following. Etwaree was placed on a cart and brought to hospital. When Titroo became senseless, the prisoners tried to recover the snake, which became torpid after biting Etwaree. The prisoners took the snakes with them when they went off. I did not see them let go by the prisoners. We were to pay one or two rupees for being taught. We were told that, if we were bitten by a snake, in repeating the incantations, and fanning the snake, we should recover.

"Two other witnesses are examined, but they give similar evidence to the preceding.

"The information and deposition of Dr. David Picachy, civil surgeon of Purneah, taken before me, J. R. Muspratt, sessions judge of Purneah, at Purneah, on this twelfth day of January 1869, who being put on his oath, saith as follows :—

"*Ques.*—Did you examine the bodies of Titroo, Menghon, and Jikree?

"*Ans.*—Yes, I did, and found that they had died from the effects of snake-poison. There was nothing abnormal about their internal organs, which could be said to be the result of disease.

"*Ques.*—In what way did the three bodies exhibit the effects of snake-poison?

"*Ans.*—Externally, there were the marks of snake-bites on their hands and arms, and internally the blood was in a fluid state, and the brain vessels deeply congested; the former state, *viz.*, the fluid state of the blood, being particularly indicative of snake-poison.

"*Ques.*—Did you examine the wound of Etwaree?

"*Ans.*—Yes, and found a scratch on the fore-arm; he was partially senseless when received into hospital, but could reply to questions I put to him. His wound and scratch looked like that which would be inflicted by a snake. I treated him with ammonia for three days, when he recovered.

"*Ques.*—How do you account for the escape of Etwaree, the other three having died?

"*Ans.*—He was the last person bitten, and must have received less poison than the others.

"*Ques.*—Was he in your opinion suffering from the bite of a poisonous snake?

"*Ans.*—Yes, he was lethargic and depressed; there was very slight swelling about the scratch. The wounds on the three dead bodies presented a livid appearance, and the corpses were swollen and in a semi-decomposed state, resulting from rapid chemical change after death by animal poison.

" *Ques. by the prisoners.*—None.

" These men were sentenced to five years' imprisonment by the sessions judge of Purneah, which sentence was confirmed on appeal by the High Court of Calcutta.

" The snakes, as described by the witnesses, are two keraits *(Bungarus Cœrulus)* and one keautiah *(Cobra de Capello)*, the variety with one occellus on the hood. The larger snake, said to be a Bungarus, bit four men ; three died, one appears to have narrowly escaped."

I believe that this crime remains unexplained.

We are told that the prison of the Châtelet, in Paris, contained, among other dreadful chambers of punishment, one of extreme horror called *la Fin d'aise* (end of ease), which was full of dirt and *Reptiles.* This might pass for exaggeration if we did not recollect that it is quite contrary to our knowledge of the habits of such creatures to expect that " Reptiles " would, voluntarily, select any roofed building, in a city, as a habitation ; and did we not read in the *Saxon Chronicle* that " The " [Norman] " Barons and Knights oppressed England with their castle works. When the (new) castles were made, they filled them with evil men, or rather devils ; and then they seized every one supposed to have any property, man or woman, and put them into these dungeons—dark, foul, and slimy places, *full of toads and adders*."

There also appears to survive in Brittany the legend of a Count who stocked the dungeon of his castle at Pencoel with vipers, and there immured those of his peasants who were so unfortunate as to offend him.*

---

* This gives significance to the curious fact, mentioned by Forbes (Vol. II., p. 19), that, in India, snakes have sometimes been made the custodians of concealed treasure. He gives a most vivid narrative of the manner in which he personally investigated the mysteries of a chamber supposed to contain treasure. Viewed from above, it was a gloomy dungeon of great depth. He desired his men to enter it. They positively refused " alleging that, throughout Hindustan, wherever money was concealed, there existed one of the genii, in the mortal form of a snake, to guard it. He at last prevailed upon them to descend with ropes. They had not been at the bottom many seconds, when they called out vehemently that they were enclosed by a large snake; their screams were dreadful, and his resolution inflexible, until at length, by keeping the upper light steady, he perceived something like billets of wood, or rather more resembling a ship's cable coiled up in a dark hole. No language can express his sensations of astonishment and terror when he beheld a horrid monster rear his head over an immense length of body coiled in volumes on the ground. The panting terrified wretches were drawn up speechless, but uninjured. Some hay being thrown down upon the lighted torches left in the cavern, consumed the mortal part of the guardian genius, as they afterwards took up the scorched and lifeless body of a large snake; but, notwithstanding a minute search, no money could be found. The proprietor had, doubtless, carried off his treasure when he fled to a foreign country. As the cells in the tower were all very small and deep, and the walls of strong masonry, it appeared wonderful to Mr. Forbes how this snake had subsisted confined in this manner.

Indian snakes are the best possible custodians of concealed treasure, being very terrible and very abstinent. Dr. Fayrer mentions that a Russellian viper lived in a cage of fine

The coincidence of the existence, first, of this practice in Hindu India; and, again, of its spread, as a Saracen custom, to Northern Europe, doubtless by the early crusaders, and to India by the Mahomedan conquerors, is very interesting.

With the above detail before us, the following, which appeared in the Calcutta Papers in October 1868, is at least curious :—

"The *Indu Prokash* relates a somewhat extraordinary incident that has come to his knowledge. It seems that a few days ago a master, with a view to punishing his boy, put him into a basket of rice, shutting the cover upon him, and kept him there for some time. The boy cried out loudly, but no attention was paid to him; and when he was taken out it was found that he had been bitten by a snake which was in the basket. The unfortunate lad died soon afterwards."

WASPS AND HORNETS.

These insects are large and numerous in this country, but are not, under ordinary circumstances, very fierce.

About two years ago there died in my ward, from chronic bowel disease, a young native woman, one of whose arms had been amputated at the shoulder joint on account of disease set up by a wasp-sting. The following report appeared in the *Home News* at about the same time :—

As Major-General Dalton, of the Royal Artillery, was driving with his family in an open carriage, on the afternoon of the 31st ultimo, a large swarm of wasps, darkening the air by their numbers, attacked his horse, stinging it in every part of the body. They pitched in hundreds about the horse, pursuing the carriage for nearly a mile, and endangering the lives of all who were in it, who, however, fortunately escaped with only a few stings. Although every necessary remedy was resorted to, the shock given to the nervous system of the horse, and the high state of inflammation produced, caused its death in forty-eight hours.

In the Chapter on *Drowning* will be found a remarkable case, in which wasps, swarming upon an unfortunate in a river, compelled him to dive until life was extinct.

SCORPIONS.

The following note appears in the Transactions of the Medical and Physical Society of Bombay, No. VII., N. S., for 1861, p. 43 of Appendix :—

"*Deaths reported to have occurred from the bites* [?] *of Scorpions.*—

---

wire gauze for twelve months, without appearing to obtain any fluid or solid food whatever. For some time, he was duly supplied, but, as snakes in captivity very frequently do, he appeared to eat nothing, all supplies remaining and going into putrefaction in the cage. When all supplies were discontinued, he remained perfectly active and very venomous, but became rather thin. At the end of the year, he was taken out and had his portrait painted. When the picture was nearly finished, he died suddenly.

In the diaries of the Superintendent of Police, Rutnagherry, three deaths were reported to have taken place from the effect of scorpion bites. 1.—20th May 1861. In Kelondey, Talooka Jhijunwell, it was reported that a Maratha male, age about thirty years, was stung on the foot by a scorpion, became insensible, and died within an hour of infliction of the bite. 2.—15th June 1861. In Boregaum, Talooka Jhijunwell, Gunna, a Coonbee boy, fifteen years old, was bitten on the right foot by a scorpion whilst ploughing; he was affected with great difficulty of breathing, and died within two hours. 3.—13th July 1861. In Doughur, Talooka Swindroog, a Maratha man, twenty-five years old, after becoming insensible, died in an hour and-a-half. No treatment was adopted in either case, but, in each instance, the scorpion was killed.

It is to be regretted that these cases are not more fully reported, as Dr. Taylor says that scorpion poison is not fatal to large animals (On Poisons, p. 575).

I find the following note: "In Scorpion-Stings, chloroform, applied on lint to the part, has proved a specific in sixteen cases—H. G."

HACKING THE NECK.

There is one mode of killing with the *dao* or *tulwar*, which is clearly a matter of customary design. Sir Thomas Roe, who visited the Court of the Great Mogul, in 1614, mentions that, on one occasion, nearly a hundred thieves, by order of the Emperor, "having their hands tied down to their feet, had their necks cut with a sword, but not quite off." Now I find that the nine years' reports to the Calcutta Nizamut contain the details of twenty-seven cases of wounding, in which the *principal* injuries were as follow: Cuts on the outer side of the neck, generally extending to the vertebræ, 8; wounds across the nape of the neck, usually also reaching to or dividing the spine, 12; wounds on the back of the skull, 4; instances of decapitation, 3.

The details of these twenty-seven cases go far to prove that the wounds were, in nearly every instance, inflicted in a deliberate and more or less successful attempt to divide the spine by blows across the back of the neck.

These wounds are nearly always of frightful severity; and, in most of the cases, other parts of the body are hacked.

In only two of the eleven cases where the wound had been inflicted quite across the back of the neck, did the victims escape the hands of their assailants. In one of these, reported by Dr. Ross, of Jessore, the unfortunate man lived several days with (in addition to eight other wounds, two of which were on the back of the head, and two completely through the shoulder-blades) a wound across the back of the neck so large that "a child's head might have been put into it." It was discovered, after death, that the bones of the neck had been injured, and that the spinal cord was surrounded with blood. Dr. Ross mentioned that the wound was such that a sudden turn of the head might have caused instantaneous death. The other individual recovered under the treatment of Mr. Scanlan, of Burrisaul, after receiving a severe wound on the upper and back part of the neck, one on the back of the head, and three others.

In another case, subsequently reported, which also occurred under the care of Mr. Scanlan, the wound penetrated to the vertebræ, injuring one of them, so that the spinal marrow only escaped by a very little. The woman had sustained other severe wounds, but, at the trial, was pronounced out of danger.*

In a more recent case, a woman prosecuted her son-in-law who had struck her a very severe blow with a heavy *dao* across the back of her neck—a large scar remained.†

In another case, a woman's life was barely saved from a blow of this kind, by the interposition of her long tresses of hair and her clothes.‡

So common is this practice of striking deadly blows on the back or side of the neck, in the North-Western Provinces, that, in the printed Records of the Agra Nizamut Adawlut, I find no less than *thirty-three cases* reported in the two years, 1852-53 ; instances of complete decapitation being excluded.§

I was, for a time, disposed to believe that, in most of the cases where this mode of killing was adopted, it was selected by the murderers as a kind of judicial punishment—the thief, the adultress, or the trespasser being regarded as a criminal upon whom condign punishment, according to ancient law, ought to be inflicted.‖

The prevalence of such an opinion, at least among the Up-Country natives, is negatived by the fact that men of very strong feelings have, in at least two instances before me, voluntarily submitted to be put to death in this manner by their relations, in preference to incurring disgrace.¶

---

* Nizamut Adawlut Reports, 20th February 1855, p. 240.

† *Ibid*, 24th August 1854, p. 301.

‡ Nizamut Adawlut Reports, N. W. P., 2nd September 1853, p. 1093.

§ In *eighteen* of these cases, the provocation was shown to be in some way or other connected with the misconduct of women (in one of these, a blind man killed his wife when asleep)—nine instances were the result of disputes, zumeendaree feuds, or abuse; one was a case of insanity. In one, a thief or intriguer (for in a large proportion of cases it is found difficult to distinguish the cases) was put to death by the people of the house in which he was caught. And, in one, a brahmin killed his pregnant wife, that her blood might be upon certain persons who had offended him. My notes of the other three cases were mislaid.

‖ This mode of self-justification is not overlooked by the criminals of India—neither is it ignored by the dispensers of the law. Thus, a man's wife having eloped with another, the husband pursued the guilty pair, and at last discovered the village in which they had taken up their abode. He concealed himself in the jungle, determined, as he avowed, to rush on them at night and kill them both. He failed in doing so, but severely wounded them. The sessions judge concurred in the futwa of the law officer, who *declared the crime justifiable by the Mahomedan Law*, and acquitted the prisoner.—*Police Reports, L. P.*, 1845, p. 69. *Vide supra*, p. 12.

¶ These cases are referred to at p. 345, and in the Chapter on *Torture*.

Still there are many cases on record in which the infliction of this punishment had rather the character of an execution than of a murder. Thus it appears to be a generally received popular opinion throughout the country, that those who succeed in apprehending a dacoit or thief in the act, have a right to put him to death while he remains defenceless in their hands. The Government have, for years, endeavoured to put down this barbarous practice, but cases still frequently occur.

One Baronee, of Sarun, stated on trial that, having heard a thief making his way into his house at night, he caught him as he was getting out of the hole in the wall. While the wretch lay half in the hole and half out of it, he tied his arms with a piece of rope, and then struck him several blows over the back of the neck with a *kodaul*, nearly severing his head from his body.* At about the same time, and in the same district (Sarun), three persons captured a thief, who had robbed the house of one of them, and knocked him down; while two of them held him down, the third brought a *kodaul* from the house and nearly hacked his head off.†

At Goruckpore, in 1852, three persons seized a man, who had made his way into their house, whether for purposes of robbery or of intrigue it appeared doubtful, overpowered him, held him down, and killed him by repeated blows with a *kodaul* on the back of the neck.‡

---

* Nizamut Adawlut Reports, 14th June 1853, p. 796. See a similar case, Police Report, L. P., for 1846, p. 14.

† *Ibid*, 17th June 1853, p. 800. The operations of the "Wall Piercers" extend to every part of India in which earthen walls and foundations are common. This mode of burglary was formerly so prevalent in the neighbourhood of Bhaugulpore that *Bhaugulpore ki Buguleea* became as well known a designation as "*Gamin de Paris.*" They are generally a miserable class of petty depredators who, urged by want, find out the room in a well-to-do homestead in which grain is kept, and, making a hole in the wall, take as much *dhan* as they can get. Others mine under the foundation so as to come out through the earthen floor of the room which they wish to enter. Knowing that, if the master of the house should have become aware of their approach, he will be standing ready with a tulwar or kodalee to give them a fitting reception, they either emerge feet foremost or push before them a *gurrah* (earthen vessel) which, in its globular form, very much resembles, under the circumstances, the top of a native's head. When this receives the first blow, there may possibly be time for retreat. Consideration of the facts that this crime is a theft rather than a burglary, and that intriguers are frequently called burglars and maltreated as such, appears to have determined our Judges strongly to discountenance the slaying of wall-piercers, thus: "Prisoner found deceased in act of house-breaking by night in his house, and killed him with a *kodali*, which he had called for, as he admitted, for the purpose. He was convicted of murder and sentenced to death by the sessions judge. The sentence being referred to the High Court for confirmation, it was held that the prisoner had been legally convicted of murder, that he had intentionally done to the deceased more harm than was necessary for any purpose of defence, and that not whilst deprived of power of self-control. But the sentence was mitigated to transportation for life, than which, it was held, no less sentence could be legally passed. The Judge, however, in a letter to Government, suggested the mitigation of the punishment, which was accordingly reduced to imprisonment for six months.—*Regina* v. *Dawan Geer*, 1 Ind. Jur., N. S., 253."—*Cowell* and *Woodman*, p. 537.

‡ Nizamut Adawlut Reports, N. W. P., 3rd January 1852, p. 4.

The converse of the above cases appeared in a trial at Bareilly. It was shown from the confession of one Khyala Sing, that he entered the house of one Hussao Sah with intent to steal, and armed with a sword. The master of the house was aroused, and endeavoured to capture the thief; a struggle ensued, in which the robber cut his opponent on the neck so severely as to cause instant death.*

A case of the kind was tried before the Commissioner of the Tenasserim and Martaban Provinces, in 1854. Its details are very remarkable, as showing the extension of this mode of punishment into Burmah. A number of Burmese wood-cutters, on the frontier, seized four Shans, on suspicion that they were elephant-stealers, tied their hands, and killed them with blows of a *dao* on the back of the neck, without completely decapitating them. They all pleaded guilty; and, in consideration of their ignorance and half-civilized state, were sentenced only to a long term of imprisonment.†

We have already seen that, in a very large proportion of the recorded cases, this mode of death has been inflicted as the punishment of sexual crime, suspected or discovered. The following is a singular case in point. A Dacca man, suspecting his wife of having an intrigue with another person, had often warned her to break off the intimacy, but to no effect. One day, returning home, he caught them in the act of adultery. They ran off, and the husband went on to the house. Shortly after, the woman came in, when he asked her where she had been. She replied, looking after the cattle in the field. He inquired—were the cattle in the jungle? "If you want to eat,—eat; I will not suffer you to live. I have often told you to break off intercourse with that man, but you have not listened to me." He then tied her right hand, and, seizing her by the left, nearly severed her head from her body with a *dao*, with which he also inflicted several other blows on her person. He then, with the weapon in his hand, gave himself up, freely confessing the deed.‡

Mention was made, in Note to page 350, of a case in which a man having been murdered in his house, evidently on account of an intrigue, the body was bound head and feet, carried to some distance, and there left, after having been chopped on the back of the neck. The above instances may throw a light upon the motive which suggested the apparently unnecessary hacking in that and in the following case. The body of a man was discovered, in the Almorah district, with the back of the neck and head cut, the throat gashed, and the nose and ears cut off. It came out, in the inquiry, that the deceased had intrigued with the wife of one Harkoa, who, it appeared, lay in wait with three others, for the deceased; seized him, struck him on the back of the neck with an axe, and despatched him. They

---

* Nizamut Adawlut Reports, N. W. P., 27th February 1854, p. 234.

† Nizamut Adawlut Reports, 27th July 1854, p. 126.

‡ Police Report, L. P., 1849, pp. 42, 43.

then bound the body to a pole and took it away to a ravine, where they hid it,—but not until the injured husband had cut the throat with a razor, and another had cut off the ears, for the ear-rings. The husband also cut off the nose (the penalty of adultery) and threw it away.*

In the following case, which came under my own notice, this crime was committed upon a defenceless person with most cruel deliberation. In August 1853, the body of an aged man was brought to me, at Howrah, with an enormous wound traversing the back of the neck transversely just above the line of the shoulders, completely dividing the spine, and nearly effecting decapitation. The lower limbs had been in great part devoured by dogs or jackals. I gave it as my opinion that the wound must have been inflicted during life, and at a moment when the deceased was either on his knees, or lying with his face to the ground ; and that it caused instantaneous death. I added that the instrument employed was probably a *dao* or heavy sword. One Petumber Dass Sewlee, upon being arrested on suspicion, admitted the murder, and named his associates. He produced two *daos* as the instruments used by himself and one of his accomplices in effecting the murder. I found that the longer of the two weapons was singularly calculated to cause such a wound as that observed on the deceased's person.†

In the majority of cases, it would appear that the wounds on the neck are inflicted in the heat of passion, in a struggle or in a chase, where the victim's limbs are perfectly free. In many instances, the wounds on the neck are the only injuries inflicted. The natives' dexterity in striking the neck may result, among the Bengalees, from their practice of decapitating goats, &c., for food and sacrifice with a single blow ; among the Up-Country men it may be attributed to more or less acquaintance with the use of the sword.‡ Still, wherever the hands and arms are uninjured, it must be a matter of probability that the victim has been tied or held.

* Nizamut Adawlut Reports, N. W. P., 30th August 1853, p. 1048.

† Nizamut Adawlut Reports, Vol. II., Part I of 1853, p. 87.

‡ Most of the heroes of India history have been remarkable for the force and dexterity with which they could strike with the sword. Thus we read of Bukhtyar's contest with a fighting elephant, in which he put the enraged animal to flight by a blow on the trunk. Of Shere Khan's killing an enormous tiger with one blow of his sabre, and of Shere Afgan's cutting off the trunk of the Emperor's elephant with a single stroke, and finishing his career by cleaving the Subadar of Bengal in two. Beheading a buffalo with a single blow is a common exploit among the Nepaulese. It appears to be a feat which requires more dexterity than muscular power. *Vide supra*, p. 226.

A friend told me that, some years ago, a party of English gentlemen (who were not swordsmen) were standing with a Mahomedan Prince on the bank of a river, out of which a rohee fish as thick as a man's thigh had just been brought. The Englishmen, taking a tulwar from an attendant, tried, successively, to cut the fish through as it lay on the ground, but, to their surprise, their heavy downward blows almost entirely failed. The Nawab, the least muscular of the party, took the sword, and before a moderate drawing-cut the fish appeared to fall in two.

It is remarkable that there are very few Mahometans, in fair circumstances, who are not swordsmen.

Among the cases of hacking the neck published in the Nizamut Reports, are several of considerable importance in a medico-legal point of view. As that of a man in Assam, who struck the child of his sister-in-law, three years old, while she was sleeping. He gave merely one stroke with a *dao*, which, however, half cut through the infant's neck, and must have caused instantaneous death. He appears to have been a weak-minded man, but not a lunatic—no cause of ill-feeling could be discovered. He had formerly smoked gunjah, but had entirely left it off. During the preceding six months he had suffered extremely from a disease, apparently of neuralgic character. It became a question whether the murder was committed to effect his own recovery,—to appease the goddess Kalee; or whether the deed was done under the influence of gunjah. There was no proof of insanity. He was sentenced to death. *

Gopal, a Brahmin, acknowledged, on trial, that he had killed his wife in the night, by striking her on the neck with his sword. She woke him up suddenly, he said, and taking her for a thief, he snatched up his sword and cut her down with two blows. The woman had *kansa* ornaments on her toes, the sound of which, it was held, he must have heard on the slightest movement. He had left his house stealthily after the deed, throwing his sword down a well, and it was only in the fouzdaree depositions that the above defence was made. At the thannah, it was merely said that he had killed his wife. The crime was regarded as murder, but he was sentenced to transportation for life.†

In the same year, Nunha, of Bareilly, asked bread of *his mother:* she refused it, with an indelicate retort. Enraged at the reply, he took up an axe and killed her with four wounds—"one on the temple cutting through the flesh; another on the face dividing the lips, and breaking two of the front teeth; another just under the neck, cutting through the bone; and a fourth, on the throat, severing the windpipe."‡

DECAPITATION.

The practice of beheading appears to have been, from very early times, equally common among the Hindus and Mussulmans, but we do not find that it was employed by any of their Governments as the national mode of executing criminals after the manner of the Turks and the Chinese.§ The Southern hill tribes of this Presidency, who are generally

* Nizamut Adawlut Reports, 16th October 1855, p. 453.

† Nizmut Adawlut Reports, N. W. P., 3rd November 1854, p. 647.

‡ *Ibid*, 17th January 1854, p. 44.

§ It is related of the tyrant Muzuffer Shah that, whenever he made prisoners of any rebels, he took pleasure in beheading them himself, and that the number of persons he is said to have put to death in this manner is incredible. Most of the other Mussulmaun

regarded as the aborigines of the country,—driven up into their narrow territories by the first influx of the Hindus, at a time which is pre-historic, but still retaining many of their original religious usages and distinctive traits of custom,—all these scattered races, the Soorys, Khonds, Koles, Santhals, Garrows, and the various tribes of Nagas, Kookies, Chuckmas, Reaugs, Mughs, &c., who inhabit the hills of Assam and those extending from Muneepore to Arracan and Burmah, behead their enemies. This fact, of course, has an important bearing upon many cases of homicide occurring in the border districts of the Bengal Presidency.

Mr. Charles Bedford tells me of a Kole who, thinking that six old women had bewitched him, placed them in a line, and cut all their heads off, except the last, who, objecting to this severe ordeal, ran away.

It appeared, in a trial at Maubhoom (bordering upon the Kole and Soory countries), that two hill men having missed their wives, and suspecting that they had gone off with a certain man, made search for them; and, after eight days, found the three sitting together under a tree eating some jungle fruits. Whereupon, they, without parley, both struck the man with their weapons, an axe and hatchet, severing his head from his body. They then attacked their wives severally, and cut off their heads by repeated blows. They then took the heads into the village and freely surrendered themselves. At trial, they confessed all with the utmost candour, evidently thinking that they acted justifiably.*

In 1849, an inhabitant of the neighbouring district of Bancoorah, becoming acquainted with his wife's criminality, warned her. His wishes were disregarded. Hearing that the meetings took place at a tank whence the woman fetched water—he, early one morning, ascended a tree on the banks of the tank, armed with a *tanghy*. The woman came, and was met by her paramour; but, other persons coming up, they went away, each returning home. He remained on the tree *that day and night, and part of the next day*, when the woman came again, and her paramour met her. He descended the tree, cut off the man's head, while in the act, then pursued the woman, cut off her head, and, tying the two heads together, was proceeding to Bancoorah to bring them to the magistrate, when he was met by some ghatwals, to

---

rulers of Bengal also had some of their criminals decapitated. The late native government of Nagpore numbered beheading among their punishments. The Mussulmauns generally took the heads of their enemies slain in battle. Khan Alum, having taken the fortress of Hajypore, and put the governor and most of the garrison to the sword, despatched all the heads to the Emperor, who immediately sent them to Dad Khan as a hint of his own probable fate. Moorshud Cooly Khan having defeated Rasheed Khan, near Moorshedabad, in 1712, ordered that a pyramid should be erected on the Delhi road, with niches to contain the heads of the enemy, as a monument of his victory.

According to the Mahomedan law, Decapitation by a sword, or similar weapon, was the prescribed punishment in sentences to *Kisas*, or Retaliation of Death, in cases of murder.

* Nizamut Adawlut Reports, 9th June 1852, p. 941.

whom he delivered himself up. He was acquitted, on the plea of justification.*

This may almost be considered as a local custom. Nineteen years later, in 1868, Shaik Buxee, of Chyebassa, murdered his wife and her paramour, and brought their heads to the deputy commissioner in triumph. The confession was at once recorded by the deputy commissioner, who committed him to the sessions. He was sentenced to death.†

In 1850, another Bancoorah man, having had an intrigue with a neighbour's wife, who had quitted him for a Brahmin, and refused to speak to him, went to her house, and asked her if she persisted in not speaking to him. She replied, "Yes," and abused him, when he caught up a *kurari*, and cut off her head by repeated blows ; he then took up the head and the *kurari* to go to the magistrate, but was seized by some ghatwals, after proceeding openly with them for a short distance. He was sentenced to death.‡

In 1844, a party of hill men made an inroad and killed and decapitated twenty Munneepoorees residing in the Company's territory.

In 1854, two Garrows were sentenced to death for having been parties in an expedition into Assam for the sake of plunder and of procuring heads, in which they took eight lives. [See p. 408.]§

The most ordinary cases of murder by decapitation in the plains are generally the results of some act of sexual immorality.

In 1852, one Sobha, of Bareilly, took a sword with which he beheaded his wife, and wounded the infant in her arms, and then struck his brother. The child appears to have died of starvation, and the brother of fever. Sobah said that his brother had intrigued with his wife.‖

In a case tried in the Saugor and Nerbudda territory in 1852, a man confessed that a married girl of eighteen or nineteen, who hadbecome pregnant by him, having urged with great pertinacity that he should take her into his house, which he was unwilling to do, lest his reputation should suffer by his connexion with a woman of inferior caste, took her to the river, where he killed her with repeated strokes of an axe, finishing by decapitating her and abandoning her body in the water.¶

In the following year, a man of the same district confessed that a married woman with whom he had intrigued for three years, becoming importunate in urging him to elope with her, which he resisted on account of his family, and being then married, he cut off her head in the jungle, after a vain attempt to throttle her with his hands.**

---

* Police Report, L. P., 1849, p. 57.

† Bengal Police Report for 1868, p. 273.

‡ *Ibid*, 1850, p. 50.

§ Nizamut Adawlut Reports, 19th June 1854, p. 743.

‖ Nizamut Adawlut Reports, N. W. P., 25th March 1852, p. 214.

¶ *Ibid*, 3rd March 1852, p. 146.

** *Ibid*, 29th Nov. 1853, p. 1420.

In 1852, a Mussulmaun, of Delhi, beheaded and almost hacked to pieces a common prostitute, who threatened to discontinue her connexion with him ;—a very common incentive to murder in India.*

In 1853, Gandiah Kahalin, of Manbhoom, confessed that,—her husband having been in the habit of beating, starving, and abusing her, and of associating with another woman,—she, on a certain night, freed herself from a post in the yard to which he had bound her and, finding her husband asleep in the house, struck him two blows on the neck with a *koralee*, and severed his head. She then dragged the body first to a shed, and afterwards to the bed of a rivulet, and threw the head into a pool. The head was not found ; traces of dragging a body were found up to the cow-house, where some spots of blood were seen, smeared over with sand. The place where the body was found was about 160 yards from the house. Sentence—imprisonment for life.†

Two men, of Nuddea, having long cohabited with the same woman, one, assisted by an accomplice, cut off the other's head with a *dao* and a knife, and threw the body into a tank. The head was not found.‡

In several recorded cases, this crime has been committed under very extraordinary circumstances. One Bheekaree, of Cawnpore, being in his house with his two children—a girl aged nine or ten years, and an infant eighteen months old, desired the girl to pacify the child. She not complying at once, he was seized with ungovernable rage, seized a hatchet, and severed the neck of his daughter, fairly decapitating her at the second blow. He then threw himself into a well. Sentence—death.§

Reference has already been made to the crime of a Hooghly man who, in 1845, had his enemy (who had intrigued with one of his female relations) held down by three persons, and with a large sacrificial knife, cut off his head with one blow ; and, with a second, divided the body at the waist.

In 1852, one Bissonath, also of Hooghly, confessed the murder of his wife's paramour, having concerted his destruction with others. After he had knocked down the man senseless with a heavy pukkah bamboo, he and his four accomplices took turns with a sharp-cutting vegetable knife, in hacking the neck, until they severed the head from the body. Dr. Ross found several wounds on the shoulder, made with some cutting instrument, and the head had evidently been severed from the trunk by blows.‖

---

* Nizamut Adawlut Reports, N. W. P., 10th March 1852, p. 184.

† Nizamut Adawlut Reports, 10th June 1853, p. 769.

‡ *Ibid*, 25th June 1853, p. 85. See also cases of decapitation apparently by *a single blow*. N. A. R., May 28, 1856 ; p. 8541 ; and *ibid*, Sept. 26 of same year, p. 649.

§ *Ibid*, 3rd August 1853, p. 943.

‖ Nizamut Adawlut Reports, 1st January 1852, p. 1.

In 1848, a Chittagong girl of about sixteen murdered her husband, an old Brahmin of sixty, by cutting off his head, whilst he was asleep, with the large two-handed knife used in sacrifices.*

In 1850, a Dome, of Baraset, in a state of frenzy, without apparent reason, came up to where his brother's wife was standing with other women, and struck off her head with a *dao*. The bystanders were too much alarmed to apprehend him; he escaped and was not again heard of.†

In May 1854, a case was tried, at Agra, which illustrated the deadly certainty with which natives accustomed to the use of the *tulwar* slay by decapitation. One Rambuksh, a sepoy, having gone with three of his comrades to witness the religious ceremonies at Gobardhun, suddenly and, as far as could be ascertained, without any provocation, drew his sword and, attacking one of his comrades, severed his head from his body, and immediately went onwards and decapitated three harmless women before he was arrested, which, however, was not effected until his left forearm was severed from his body. His companions declared that they had known him five or six years ; that he was a quiet, inoffensive man, and was not intoxicated at the time of committing this act, nor was he even suspected of being insane.‡

Dr. Kenneth McLeod tells me that there appears to be an increasing tendency, among criminals in this country, to expose the bodies of their victims on railroads, that it may appear that death has been accidental. He alluded to a case of decapitation. Medical Officers cannot be too careful in their examination of such cases. As in the instance of a gentleman who was decapitated by a train at Ashford in Kent in June last, there can be no doubt whatever with regard to the nature of the injuries inflicted by the wheels, &c.; but it will have to be decided whether these were sustained before or after death, and also whether other cause of death, as by wounds, poison, strangulation, &c., &c., is discoverable.

For Decapitation, see pp. 72, 73, 348-49-50-52.

HUMAN SACRIFICE.

The practice of human sacrifice (altogether apart from sati and female infanticide) constituted, previous to the times of Mahomedan ascendancy in India, a leading feature in the religion of the Hindus. The life of a man was the most acceptable sacrifice that could be offered to their sanguinary deities. Hence the immolations and sacrifices at Hurdwar, at the Mahadeo Hills, at Saugor Island, and at Jugganauth, and the Satis, once universally practised throughout India, and still prevalent in many of the native states. According to Col. Sleeman,

* Police Report, L. P., 1848, p. 41.
† *Ibid*, 1850, p. 63.
‡ Nizamut Adawlut Reports, N. W. P., for May 1854, p. 575.

human sacrifices were offered in the City of Saugor during the whole of the Mahratta Government, up to the year 1800. The Rev. Mr. Ward collected much important and striking information relative to this practice as prevailing in Bengal, so late as the year 1817. He was informed that, at Chitpore and at Kalighat, near Calcutta, human sacrifices had been occasionally offered up to the year 1788, and that the practice was still known to exist at other places,—as at Ksheera, a town near Burdwan, and at Brumha Neetula, near Nuddea, where headless human bodies continued, from time to time, to be found near the temples.

Baboo Bholanath Chunder, of Calcutta, speaks thus of the human sacrifices at Chitpore and Nuddea :—

"Chitpore, so called from the Kali Chitraswari of that village. She is one of those old images to whom many a human sacrifice has been offered under the regime of the Brahmins" (p. 2).

At Santipore, near Nuddea, the *Baroary* Poojah used to be celebrated with great ceremony. "In one of these Poojahs, a party of Brahmins had assembled to drink and converse under the effects of liquor ; one of them proposed to offer a sacrifice to Kali, to which the others assented ; but, having nothing to sacrifice, one cried out 'Where is the goat?' On which another, more drunk than the rest, exclaimed, 'I will be the goat ;' and at once placed himself on his knees, when one of the company cut off his head with the sacrificial knife." Next morning they took the body to the river, and had it burnt, reporting that the man had died of cholera (page 21).

Among the temples near the seat of the old native kings of Assam, in the Seebsaugor District, is the Copper Temple or Jama Serai, "a small room or cell built of stone masonry, about 10 or 12 feet wide, and surrounded at about 30 feet by a stone wall on all four sides." This was, at one time, "a very notorious place, for here numerous human victims used to be sacrificed in honor of Durga."

At Jainteapore, east of Sylhet, there is also a temple where similar bloody rites were frequently perpetrated.

In 1821, certain persons were caught in the act of carrying off a human victim to be sacrificed at Jainteapore. It appears that these men were directed by Oochung Bunggaunt Kooam (brother-in-law of the Rajah of Jainteapore) to procure a man for this purpose, and that they actually seized a person named Mon ; but, an alarm being given, they were taken prisoners. They affirmed that Koosa had, for several years past, immolated human victims. That, after ablution of the intended victim, a garland of flowers was placed round his neck, and then his head was cut off with a sword. It was added that it appears that these sacrifices were made to the goddess Kali, in hopes of procuring progeny.*

* Macnaghten's Reports, Vol. II., p. 108.

Captain Gavin R. Crawford has described a similar place in the Central Provinces.* He writes: "Whilst Superintendent of the Chunda district, in the Nagpore dominions, I heard that such sacrifices took place every third year in the neighbouring principality of Bustar, which is tributary to the Rajah of Nagpore. Being anxious to ascertain the truth of these reports, I sent a man in the disguise of a cloth merchant, in the year 1822, to procure necessary information; and he brought me a detailed account of the sacrifice, of which he was an eye-witness. I sent the statement to Mr. Jenkins, late Resident at Nagpore; he remonstrated on the subject with the Rajah of Bustar, who did not deny the fact, but promised that it should never happen again. Whether he kept his promise or not, I do not know. I give the account brought to me by Enkya Pudlwar as nearly as possible in his own words. 'I arrived at Dhuntewarra on the 19th September. The Fort is of mud, and has two gateways; within it are the temple and five huts belonging to the officiating priests. The temple is dedicated to Devi or Dhunteswurree, some name or incarnation of the goddess Kali; it is built of cut stone; it is square of 15 feet, and is 18 feet in height. In front is a portico. About six weeks before my arrival, Mypal Deo, Rajah of Bustar, had marched from Jugdulpore, taking with him one large Car (*ruth*) ornamented with pewter, and four other cars covered with nettings and garlands of flowers. His train consisted of 100 matchlockmen, 20 horsemen, and one elephant. On the 23rd of September, at 8 o'clock P.M., the following sacrifice was offered in the portico in front of the temple, the Rajah being present:

5 *Gossyns*,
10 People, *of different castes*,
600 *He-goats*, and
10 *Male Buffaloes*.'

"The victims were killed by having their heads cut off with a large sword. As a conclusion to this sacrifice, on the Dusehra, 25th September, the image of Vigra Devi (another name for Kali) was placed in the upper platform of the large car, and the Rajah and his wife sat on the lower one. They were, in this manner, dragged by 300 men to a spot near the village, where the Rajah performed the Sumya Poojah. The sacrifice takes place every third year, and the number of human victims ought to be fifteen. Should it be impossible to procure *any* victims by the seizure of travellers, or others, not inhabitants of the Bustar country, the Rajah, in that case, caused *one* of his own subjects to be seized for the sacrifice. Human sacrifices also occur in the Nizam's country. Mr. Fenwick, a gentleman who was an agent for Messrs. Palmer & Co. of Hydrabad, and who lived for many years at Madeepoor, informed me that,

* Bengal Annual for 1830, p. 321.

in the neighbourhood of that place, there is a small tract of particularly fine land, to keep up the fertility of which, the natives conceive it necessary to offer a human victim yearly. The statement of Enkya Pudlwar would, of itself, appear sufficient to prove that human sacrifices do take place; but not a shadow of doubt, as to the fact, can exist in any one's mind, after knowing that Mr. Jenkins wrote to me and stated that the Rajah, in an interview with him, did not deny it."

We have already seen that the Dacoits-proper of Bengal are votaries of Kali, and perform *poojah* to that divinity before undertaking any perilous attack. Old writers state that they, on some occasions, even vow that they will offer up human sacrifices, in the persons of those whom they murder in their depredations,* and that, if we may credit very respectable testimonies, they were frequently guilty of sacrificing human victims to Kali under circumstances of horror and atrocity scarcely credible.†

It was held, in the Rudhiradhyáya, or Sanguinary Chapter of the Calica Puran, that, through sacrifices, Princes obtain bliss, heaven, and victory over their enemies. By a human sacrifice, attended by the forms laid down, Devi is pleased one thousand years, and by the sacrifice of three men one hundred thousand years. [It is of great importance, in a judicial point of view, that it should be borne in mind that nearly all the scriptures and traditions of the Hindus concur in promising the highest blessings,—such as success in war, numerous offspring, wealth, the realization of all desires,—to him who offers a man in sacrifice.] The victim must be a person of good appearance, and be prepared by ablutions and requisite ceremonies. The performance of the sacrifice with a Chandrahassa, or Cattri (two weapons of the axe kind) is reckoned the best mode. The sacrificer must previously make use of certain prescribed texts and invocations ; an unclean or deformed person, one unwilling, one under twelve years of age, or a female, must never be sacrificed. If a human sacrifice is performed, without the consent of the Prince, the performer incurs sin. In cases of imminent danger, or war, sacrifices may be performed at pleasure, by Princes themselves and their ministers, but by none else. The victim's head is to be struck off, and offered with the blood. Previously to striking the blow, the sacrificer is to invoke the deity and to worship the victim. Having immolated a human victim, with all the requisite ceremonies, at a cemetery or holy place, the sacrificer must be cautious not to cast eyes upon the body,—the head must be presented with averted eyes.‡

---

* Tytler's Considerations on the Present Political State of India, Vol. I., p. 224.

† Asiatic Researches, Vol. VII., p. 465.

‡ See Mr. Blacquiere's translation of this Chapter, Asiatic Researches, Vol. V., p. 369.

In one of the Mackenzie Manuscripts we have an account of a people who, entering Kasi (*i.e.*, fictitious Benares), found that it was a wilderness of banyan trees. They cleared the forest, but were opposed by a local Durga, who threatened to destroy them for trespassing on her

These details will be found to illustrate, in a very remarkable manner, the proceedings of the criminals in the following case. In September 1851, an informer waited upon the magistrate of Chittagong, offering to cause the apprehension of one Joodhomonee, a Reaug, an old offender, occupying the Jaoni village of Punooa, in the hills to the North-east of Chittagong. Joodhomonee appears to have been a man of considerable influence in his tribe; and, upon an attempt being made by a large body of Hill-men under the orders of the darogah to arrest him, his people rushed out, fired at them with muskets, and drove them off. Thirteen days after this affray, Joodhomonee, with a body of armed men, entered a place called Sukhun, where some Kookies had taken up their residence a short time previously. These unfortunate persons, eleven in number, were seized; six were caused to bathe in the river, and were taken through the jungle to a place of sacrifice,—a cleared spot, staked round with bamboos about six feet high, with strips scraped up and left adhering to the stems as a kind of ornament. Five sacrificial altars were afterwards found on that spot, and one elsewhere. The sacrifice was performed by torch-light in the presence of many persons. The victims, having been bound, six of Joodhomonee's people, armed with bill-hooks, selected each his sacrifice, and, having performed a religious ceremony (*poojah,*) struck off the Kookies' heads, Joodhomonee and another salaaming at each successive sacrifice. On the following night, three more Kookies, two men and a woman, were taken to another spot, and there sacrificed in like manner. After the sacrifice, one of these murderers carried a body to the police and charged one Bhuggoe Roy, an enemy of Joodhomonee, with his death. The other bodies appear to have been thrown into the water. The sacrifice was said to be intended to propitiate the gods in favor of Joodhomonee, and to get his enemy, Bhuggoe Roy, into trouble.

Mr. Bowring, who tried this case, mentions in his report that the tribes inhabiting the Jaoni Mehals, worship fourteen *deotas,* or gods, some of which correspond to the Hindu deities, while others are local divinities. He adds—" It has long been notorious that human sacrifices to these gods are not of uncommon occurrence."* It will be at once remarked that, considering the absence of all but oral tradition upon religious ceremonies among these savages, the sacrifice detailed above was performed in remarkably strict conformity with the rules of the Sanguinary Chapter. Indeed, except in the particulars of the victims being prisoners, and one of their number being a female, every item of the ceremonial appears to have been rightly carried out.

---

domains. They promised her one thousand and eight human sacrifices from among the people of the tribe, and the title of War Goddess, so that, when the tribe should rule and fight with other Kings, her appetite for human blood should be abundantly satiated. With these terms the Durga was satisfied.

* Nizamut Adawlut Reports, Vol. II., Part 1, of 1853, p. 899.

Although I was then the Medical Officer of Chittagong, the bodies of the victims were not brought in to me fer examination ; but, according to the evidence of eye-witnesses, each head was cut off—" as if it were that of a kid."

In 1837, four Bengalees went to Kootoob Parah, in the Joom Bungoo Hills (Chittagong District), to trade, and never returned. It was declared in evidence that they fell into the hands of Joymonee Dewan, Tonooram and Allychurn, and that they were taken with their hands bound behind them by a large body of hill men with torches, armed with *daos*. As they passed, the women were heard saying that Tonooram had dreamt that, if *Indra poojah* could be performed on a rock on the top of Nooncheeree Hill, and some people sacrificed there, the treasures of seven Rajahs would be found concealed under the rock,* and that they supposed the Bengalees had been taken away to be sacrificed. Other witnesses deposed that, going to the top of the Nooncheeree Hill, they saw there a large rock, which appeared to have been partially broken, and the jungle cleared away from it. Hearing a great noise of men approaching, they hid themselves in the jungle, and saw Tonooram and Allychurn, accompanied by about fifteen Kookies, bringing with them four Bengalees with their hands bound to their waists. They ascended the hill towards the rock. Early next morning they heard the sound of a gong from the rock. Going towards it, they concealed themselves at a short distance and observed that a large quantity of red flowers were collected on it for making *poojah*. Joymonee Dewan was sitting on the rock, near the flowers, and saying, " It is time to commence the *poojah*. Let the men be sacrificed." The other two prisoners approached the four captives who were bound separately to trees and surrounded by forty or fifty Chackmas and Kookies. The second prisoner took one of the captives, and bound him by his feet to a post ; the third prisoner threw a rope about the prisoner's neck, and knocked him down with his head towards the east ; the prisoner exclaimed "*Ma! Ma!*" The third prisoner took a hill *dao*, one and-a-quarter cubit long, and struck the victim one blow on the back of the neck ; this blow, not having separated the head from the body, he cut the residue by drawing the *dao* backwards and forwards. The second prisoner took the severed head, ascended the rock, and placed the head down on the flowers ; then the first and second prisoners made their obeisance to the *poojah*. In this way, they despatched the other three captives, one after the other, the second prisoner holding each of them down, whilst

* The following appeared, not long since, in the papers. A Greek, some time ago, at Stamboul, dreamt a dream, in which the guardian demon of a certain hill appeared to him, saying that if he would sacrifice his child to him he would disclose the whereabouts of a vast treasure. The Greek took his little daughter to the hill next day, and having beat out her brains, dug for the gold in high spirits until he was arrested.

the third cut off their heads. After the ceremony, the prisoner ordered that the bodies should be bound up with pieces of rock and carried off towards the north and thrown into a large tank situated there. The special sessions judge appointed to try the case was of opinion that the whole of the prisoners were guilty of the crime of having murdered and immolated four human beings in cold blood.* The Nizamut Adawlut, not being satisfied with the evidence, acquitted the prisoners.

When Joodhomonee's case, related above, occurred, the recollection of this affair was still fresh at Chittagong. On comparing the accounts of the two *poojahs,* it is certain that, if the description of what occurred on Noončheeree Hill was fictitious, those who gave it were, at least, well acquainted with the manner in which human sacrifices are performed in that part of the country.

The *Madras Herald,* December 12, 1840, published the following account of a supposed human sacrifice, communicated by a correspondent at Ramnad, and authenticated by a respectable signature :—

" About the end of last month, a pandarum, on his return from Rammisseram, located himself in a village about five miles east of Ramnad. He gave himself out to be a great swamy; that he could work miracles ; the first of which was opening a spring of water near a tank, which he named *Gunga Theertum,* or the holy water of the Ganges. Hundreds of the deluded population, in and about this place, left their houses, in order to have their sins forgiven and their diseases cured. I rode out to see the man, as he was much talked of by the people, and was astonished to witness about two hundred people, men and women, anxiously awaiting an opportunity to have access to the 'swamy.' I spoke to him on the absurdity of his pretensions, and entreated him not to deceive the people. I also advised the people not to be so foolish as to believe that the pandarum could do them any good, for he and all mankind are sinners, and that forgiveness of sins and miracles proceed alone from God, who is the author of all good. On the evening of the 19th instant, the chucklers of the village where the pandarum resided, observing crows and vultures hovering near a group of trees, and suspecting there was carrion for them to feast upon, were tempted to visit the spot ; when, lo ! they found a corpse, mangled most dreadfully, having the left hand and right leg cut off. On the head were many iron nails driven; on the neck they found a garland of flowers, and the forehead besmeared with sandal-paste. It was a matter of difficulty to find out who the unfortunate individual was, but his handkerchief and short trousers identified him to be a peon, in the service of the zemindar, named Moothacoree. It is commonly rumoured that a certain person, named Moothacoree, was ailing, and that his relations went to the pandarum to inquire if he would recover. The panda-

* Asiatic Jour., N. S., Vol. XXXI., p. 1.

rum replied that Moothacoree would die of the disease; that nothing short of a human sacrifice could propitiate for him, and that the victim should bear the name of the sick individual. On the day after the discovery of this horrid deed, the pandarum was found absent. He had taken the alarm and started; but, through the active vigilance of the rajah's peons, he was brought yesterday, and is confined in the palace guard-room."

Government have long been actively engaged in endeavoring to put down the system of human sacrifice extensively prevailing among the Khonds inhabiting the hill tracts of Orissa. Valuable reports have, from time to time, been published, showing the character and extent of this frightful evil and the success which has attended our efforts to suppress it. I think it right to quote, from these reports,* the descriptions which have been given of the various modes in which these sacrifices are perpetrated, as it will be found that they illustrate, in several striking particulars, the modes of sacrifice, wounding, and torture adopted in other parts of India.

It must be premised that the victims of these sacrifices, or "Meriahs," must, in every case, be *bought;* otherwise they would not be regarded as acceptable offerings to the deities whom their deaths are intended to propitiate or appease. They are generally well fed and kindly treated, up to time of sacrifice.† The modes of sacrifice differ much in the several districts of Khondistan.

Mr. Russell states that, in the *Maliahs of Goomsur*, the victim, having first been stupefied with toddy, is seized and thrown into a pit, into which the blood of a hog has been previously allowed to flow. His face is pressed down until he is suffocated in the bloody mire. A piece of flesh is then cut from the body by the priest, all present follow his example. The head and face alone remain untouched, and the bones, when bare, are buried with them in the pit.

Mr. Arbuthnot reports that, among the *Codooloos*, the victim is kept in a continued state of stupefaction or intoxication from the moment of his seizure until he is sacrificed. The priest cuts a small hole in the

---

* As collected in Selections from the Records of the Government of India (Home Department), 1854.

† Camerarius tells us that, in a place hard by the city of Arles, in Provance called LaRochette, there stood two pillars, and upon them an altar of stone, upon which the people (meeting there every year, the first day of May) offered human sacrifices for the prosperity of the city. Their custom was to buy three young men, upon whom they bestowed good store of dainty victuals, and fattened them a whole year, and after, at a day appointed, they cut their throats upon this altar, and with the blood sprinkled all the people standing devoutly round about the pillars. This bloody ceremony, he adds, was abolished by Saint Trophimas, one of the seventy-two disciples of our Saviour Christ.—*The Living Librarie*, p. 214.

The coincidence between certain of the leading features in these two practices, separated by eighteen hundred years, are very remarkable, especially in the *buying* and *fattening* of the victims.

stomach of the victim, and the idol is besmeared with the blood which flows from the wound. The people then rush forward, and he is literally cut to pieces. Each person, who is so fortunate as to procure it, carries away a morsel of flesh, and presents it to the idol of his own village.

Mr. Ricketts wrote that very contradictory stories were told of the manner in which the ceremony was conducted. One of the most common modes appeared to be to bind the victim between two strong planks or bamboos, one being placed across the chest, the other across the shoulders. These are, first of all, strongly fastened at one end ; the victim is then placed between them ; a rope is passed round the other ends, which are long enough to give a good purchase ; they are bound together, and the unfortunate sufferer is squeezed to death. Life still ebbing, the body is thrown on the ground, and chopped in two pieces, below the bamboos, with hatchets. Some accounts say that, after the performance of several strange ceremonies, the divided corpse is buried unmutilated. Others say that, as soon as it is divided, those in attendance fall on and cut each a piece.

Mr. Mills learned that the victim's head and neck were introduced between the reft of a strong bamboo split into two parts, the ends of which are then secured together and held by the sacrificers. As soon as he is firmly fixed, the presiding priest advances and, with a sharp and curiously curved axe, breaks the joints of the legs and arms, at the ankle, knee, elbow, and wrist ; the surrounding mob then fall to and strip the flesh off the bones with knives. The bones of the deceased are buried where the sacrifice has been performed, and their situation is generally marked by a long pole struck into the earth just above them. Colonel Campbell says that, in *Chinna Kimedy*, the remains are burnt, and the ashes mixed with the new grain to preserve it from insects. According to Capt. MacVicar, in *Maji Deso*, the Meriah is first surrounded and beaten on the head with heavy metal bangles ; and, if this inhuman smashing does not immediately destroy life, strangulation is effected by means of a split bamboo. Colonel Campbell states that the sacrifice called "Junna" is peculiar to the Khonds of *Jeypore*. It is always succeeded by the sacrifice of *three* human beings, two to the sun, to the east and west * of the village, and one in the centre. A stout wooden post is firmly fixed in the ground, at the foot of it a narrow grave is dug, and to the top of the post the victim is firmly fastened by the long hair of his head ; four assistants hold his outstretched arms and legs, the body being suspended horizontally over the grave, with the face towards the earth. The priest then repeats an invocation, hacking, at intervals, the back part of the shrieking victim's neck. The victim is then decapi-

* The Sanguinary Chapter ordains that the human victim is to be immolated to the *East*, and his blood to be presented in the *West*.

tated, the body thrown into the grave, and the head left suspended from the post till devoured by wild beasts.

Several details in the above frightful proceedings should be kept in mind, as associating the practice of Meriah Sacrifice (although it may be only accidentally) with other descriptions of murder and sacrifice—these are, especially, the sacrifice of *three ; the compression of the chest or neck with bamboos* (bansdollah) ; and the *infliction of a wound on the back of the neck*—also a practice in Bengal, which is made the subject of a separate Chapter, *vide supra*, p. 387.*

All subsequent reports tend to show that, although this practice has probably been wholly repressed by our Government with the co-operation of the Rajahs, the popular mind in Khoondistan still looks back with regret to its *Meriah* sacrifices, and can only be prevented from recommencing them by the most vigilant supervision.

In 1863, Mr. D. F. Carmichael, acting agent to the Governor of Vizigapatam, made a tour through the hill zemindaries and Jeypore. Speaking to the Rajah of Jeypore, he alluded to the alleged existence of the *Meriah* Rite in the more civilized portions of his zemindary. It had been repeatedly stated, by the officers of the late *Meriah* agency, that influential Hindus of Jeypore secretly practised this rite, and that there was even reason to believe that the Rajah, when he installed himself at his father's decease in 1860-61, sacrificed a young girl, thirteen years of age, at the shrine of the *Goddess Durga,* in the town of Jeypore. These charges have always been stoutly denied, and Mr. Carmichael was inclined to believe that the officers of the agency had been misinformed. Colonel Campbell declared the practice to have ceased amongst the Jeypore Khoonds in his report for the season of 1853. He, however, at the same time, strongly advocated the system of yearly visitations by the European officers of Government, adding—" After ten consecutive years of intercourse with all these tribes, it is my confirmed opinion that, if the same degree of surveillance be not kept up, they will, without fail, resort to human sacrifices, and that no unaided efforts on the part of my subordinates, or even of the Rajah, will be able to prevent it. Personal influence and local knowledge, not only of the tribes, but of their language, will alone have any effect upon the Khoonds." Mr. Carmichael wholly coincided in these views.†

---

* See the case of Noboo Kor, who was capitally sentenced at Bancoorah in 1856, for killing a man with whom he had a land dispute by striking him on the neck with a koolharee (axe), shouting, as he struck, *Jye Maha Kali !* (Victory, mighty Kali !), or *Jye Ma Kalee !* (Victory, O Mother Kali), a cry which may be heard wherever sacrifices are offered to the goddess Kali. This was held to add to the evidence of his murderous intent, but the sessions judge considered that he probably used the cry much as a Mussulman would have shouted *Bismallah !—Nizamut Adawlut Reports*, Oct. 6, 1856, p. 772.

† Report to the Chief Secretary to the Government, Fort St. George, dated the 31st March 1863.

It was announced, in May 1868, that the Paik and Seit Rajahs of the hill tracts of Orissa had recently been presented with Khillats as a mark of the appreciation by the Government of their services in the suppression of *Meriah* sacrifices amongst the hill tribes; it was added that this practice had not yet wholly died out. Only recently, there were two attempts to offer the sacrifice, but the parties concerned were arrested and punished.*

In the following July, it was announced that the Khoonds appeared to have abandoned all thoughts of being able to sacrifice human beings, though they reluctantly acknowledged that all the rites formerly used at the *Meriah* were, last season, celebrated during the immolation of buffaloes.

Most positive instructions have been issued by the local authorities prohibiting the future use of any of these rites, and the Hindoo chiefs have been informed that they would be held personally responsible, should any of these ceremonies be again revived, and the circumstance not be brought to the notice of Government.

In October of the same year, it was reported that the Khoonds were engaged in disputes which might, unless carefully watched, give trouble. It would seem that such chiefs, as the Rajahs of Jeypore, Trimmopoly, and Parkakemmedy are opposed to the practice of *Meriah* sacrifices, but that their people are of a different opinion, and in favor of the old custom. It was added that the issue of such a difference as this cannot be doubtful. The influence of the chiefs, supported by the Government, must ultimately prevail.

The following report of an act, which greatly resembles the "Junna" Sacrifice by the Khoonds of Jeypore, is conveyed in a letter dated Benares, the 7th April 1865, from Mr. Goad, District Superintendent of Police, N. W. P., to the Inspector-General of Police† :—

"On the 13th instant, at 3 P.M., Fokoo Gorail, of Surrowlee village, reported at the Bulloowah Police station that, for the last five days, the 'Seers' or Mullahs of Tanda, Hussunpore, Bholowla, and several other villages, had assembled in Surrowlee village to perform a certain religious ceremony ; and that, to-day at 10 A.M., they had tied two of their own brethren to a tree, and were hacking away at their necks with axes ; and when any one tried to prevent them, they rushed at them with clubs, and cried out, 'You have nothing to do with us ; we will kill and bring to life again.' On receipt of this information, the sub-inspector, with four constables, at once proceeded to the scene of the occurrence, which was seven miles from the station. On arrival, they found some 150 men and women assembled, making a tremendous noise, and dancing. When

* *Englishman*, 20th May 1868.

† Cited in Lewis's Bengal Police Guide, p. 205.

the sub-inspector approached them, they all rushed at him with clubs and axes, and struck him and the constables several blows with clubs. The sub-inspector, finding he would be overpowered if he attempted to resist them, desired his men to retire some 100 paces from the crowd, when the mob also retired to their former ground, and commenced shouting and dancing like demons. The sub-inspector then sent to the zemindars of adjoining villages for assistance, and, in the meantime, watched their proceedings. As soon as the zemindars received the message of the sub-inspector, they forthwith came to the spot with assistance, on seeing which the mob made a bolt of it; the police and villagers who had come to their aid, followed, and succeeded in capturing sixteen of the mob. On the sub-inspector going into the hut where the ceremony had been performed, he found the corpses of two men, bearing several wounds on the back of the neck; they were immediately sent in for medical examination. Information of this event reached me at 12 midnight, when I immediately started for the spot, where I arrived at 6 A.M., found the sub-inspector present and making enquiries, and sixteen of the defendants captured. I then went and saw the spot where the Poojah had been going on. I discovered a hut which had evidently been erected for the occasion; the tree to which the deceased had been tied and killed was covered with marks of blood: and I then commenced to ascertain the motive of this unnatural proceeding, when I learnt as follows:—

"That two of the 'Teer' caste had been down to Bengal in charge of some boats; that when they returned, they brought a letter which was addressed to the 'Teer' caste calling on them to become 'Bhugguths;' they were not to kill fish, nor eat them any more. This letter appears to have been circulated among the 'Teer' caste in the Benares, Ghazeepore, and Azimghur districts, and which resulted in the above assemblage, and on which occasion they acted a regular play by five men representing five deities, Ram, Mohabeer, Mohadeo senior, Zetbut, and Mohadeo junior,—that is to say, the three defendants, Bainee, Pirthee Pal, and Bussee, represented the deities Ram, Mohabeer, and Mohadeo junior, and the deceased Shewburt and Ramsawuck, Mohadeo senior, and Zetbut; and, by the orders of Ram, Mohadeo junior and Mohabeer slew Zetbut and Mohadeo senior, Ram having promised to bring them to life again. This appears to be a most curious case, as nothing of the kind has been heard of before. The actors in this affair are a low caste, and next to savages, so that it is difficult to get a proper meaning to this catastrophe. The three actual murderers have been captured, also thirteen others who were present and abetted the crime. The former have confessed to their guilt. The weapons which they used on the occasion have also been discovered. The only article not forthcoming is the letter which was circulated, for which I am making search, and hope, before long, to get hold of it. The chowkeedar and zemindar are much to blame for not having given notice to the police of such an assemblage having got together, and which has ended fatally."

The Garrows have a barbarous custom of offering a human head in some of their religious rites.

Reference is made, in the *Reports of the Calcutta Nizamut Adawlut*,* to the conviction of four Garrows, who murdered two women for the purpose of obtaining their heads, which were required by one of their countrymen for some superstitious ceremony.

In 1839, the late Colonel Jenkins referred to the Nizamut Adawlut a case in which the wife of a Garrow chief, who had adopted one Juggut as her son, having died, it was found that the funeral rites could not be performed for want of a human scalp to bury with her corpse. Juggut, accordingly, came down to the plains, slew the first youth he met, cut off his head, and made off with it.†

Again, in 1850, a party of Garrows entered the house of a man, in the Mymensing district, and cut off his head, which, it appeared, they required to be buried with the daughter of their chief.‡ They were opposed by another person, sleeping in the house. They wounded him so severely that he died three days afterwards.§ The police succeeded in arresting three of the Garrows, one of whom was sentenced to death.

The Dyaks of Borneo also have a practice of offering human heads for the propitiation of malign spirits.

The subject of *Human Sacrifice by Decapitation*—a practice which certainly still exists in this Presidency—is of such great importance that every fact bearing upon it deserves to be collected and carefully weighed. The following details, from the Rev. Mr. Ward's invaluable work on the Customs of the Hindus, will be found to illustrate very clearly the recent cases of *Human Sacrifice* which succeed them. Ward mentions that, at Chitpore, about the year 1788, a decapitated body was found near the image of Chittreshwaree. It, in the opinion of the spectators, had evidently been offered, on the preceding night, to this goddess. One of the Pundits of the College of Fort William assured him that, about the year 1770,

---

* Vol. V., p. 164, as cited in Beaufort's Digest of the Criminal Law.

† Asiatic Journal, 1839.

‡ At the obsequies of a superior Garrow chieftain, a large body of his followers sally forth from their hills, and, having seized upon the first individual of a hostile tribe they meet with, cut off his head, and burn it with the body of their chief.—*Robinson's Assam*, p. 418.

In 1866, I witnessed the nobly picturesque funeral ceremonies of a Kasia of some consequence in the village of Cherra Poonjee. Before the corpse left the house, two goats, with silvered horns, were beheaded with long two-handed swords. It was expected that the decapitation should be effected by a single blow; one of the executioners, who had to repeat his stroke, was violently shouted at by the crowd, and pelted with chips of wood with which the ground was strewed.

§ Police Report, L. P., for 1850, p. 32.

at the village of Soomara, near Gooptipara, he saw the head of a man, with a lamp placed on it, lying in a temple before the image of the goddess Siddheshwaree, and the body lying in the road opposite the temple. He adds that, about seven years previous to the publication of his work, there was found a human body without a head, lying before the temple of the goddess Tara, at the village of Serampore, near Kutwa. In the inside of the temple were different offerings—as ornaments, food, flowers, spirituous liquors, &c. All who saw it knew that a human victim had been slaughtered in the night, and search was made after the murderers, but in vain.

After reading the above facts, we can entertain but little doubt as to the nature and motive of the crime committed in the following instances. In January 1851, a Hindu priest was tried, at Midnapore, for murdering a woman. The woman's son made search for her, but the prisoner drove him away, declaring that he had sacrificed his mother, and would sacrifice him. The neighbours then collected, and deceased's head was found in a room in the prisoner's house where the thakoor was kept, placed before the idol and covered with flowers. The body was in another room. The prisoner stated that he had killed the deceased with a sword; that the thakoor Saligram had appeared to him in a dream, and had ordered him to offer up a human sacrifice; and, in obedience, he seized the woman, who had come to his house, and cut off her head. No satisfactory proof of insanity being given, fanaticism was not admitted as an extenuation of his crime. He was, therefore, sentenced to death.*

In the previous year, three Brahmins of Baraset, near Calcutta, on the Kali Poojah, were sacrificing a goat to that goddess. One of them, after cutting off the head of the goat, deliberately cut off the head of his brother, who was holding the animal, with the sacrificial knife; he then attacked and wounded his nephew. The other persons running off, he escaped; but was arrested some months afterwards, and sentenced to death.†

In June 1854, a case of this kind occurred at Saugor. The prisoner and the deceased were cousins, and had been staying at Bundukpore for some days, worshipping at a celebrated shrine dedicated to Mohadeo. On the day of the occurrence, they went to the 'munder' (as the defendant stated), for the purpose of offering up their heads. Shortly after their entrance, the havildar of the temple, on following them, found the head of the deceased on the sacred stone (*pindee*), the defendant being in the act of cutting his own throat with a sword, and threatening to cut down any one who approached. It was deemed necessary by the Court to inflict such punishment as might deter others from following such an

* Nizamut Adawlut Reports, Vol. IV., part 1, of 1851, p. 24.

† Police Report, L. P., for 1850, p. 63.

example. The prisoner was, therefore, sentenced to imprisonment for life in transportation beyond seas.*

A very extraordinary case of what appears to have been a deliberate human sacrifice, was tried at Seebsaugur, in Assam, in the same year. One Gogoieram, considered by his neighbours as a good-tempered man, having a child ill with fever, said that he was going to the jungles for medicinal herbs and to consult augury as to the fate of his infant. He took with him a neighbour's son, seven or eight years old, who had always appeared to be a favorite of his. He confessed that, after proceeding about 200 yards from his own house, the idea entered his head of killing the boy—he hesitated for a time, and then struck the child a single blow with his *dao*, almost completely severing the head from the trunk—*then, putting his mouth to the gullet, he drank the blood.* After this, cleaning his weapon carefully on the grass, he went home. On inquiry being made for the child, he said that he had gone to fetch firewood. He then took a meal of rice ; and, afterwards, having returned to the place where the body lay, went thence into the jungles to conceal himself. The officer who tried the case came to the conclusion that he deliberately sacrificed the boy to effect the recovery of his own sick child, thinking it would be acceptable to the deotas, or spirits, or the goddess Kali. Many of the tribes in Assam offer up sacrifices of animals for worldly prosperity ; and, in some instances, human beings have been sacrificed to avert sickness or other ills. The medical evidence, that of the neighbours, and even the testimony of the prisoner's mother, all went to prove that the prisoner was, and had always been, of sound mind. He was condemned to death.†

Doubtless, the crime is now less prevalent than it formerly was ; but there are strong reasons for believing that there is scarcely a district in India in which human sacrifice is not still practised, occasionally, as a religious rite.

In the Urdu Guide, published in April 1866, great regret is expressed at having heard that human sacrifices are still practised in some parts of the country.

It was reported in Calcutta, in July 1868, that the occurrence of human sacrifice in India had come to notice of the Secretary of State, who had urged Government to do their utmost to prevent it.

Placing aside the facts involved in the history of Meriah sacrifice, and the indisputable case which forms the conclusion of this Chapter, I do not know that we have absolutely positive proof that human sacrifices have ever been deliberately made in this country within the last ten years.

---

* Nizamut Adawlut Reports, N. W. P., June 1854, p. 762. See also Nizamut Adawlut Reports, Vol. I., p. 13; Vol. III., p. 209; Vol. IV., p. 117.

† Nizamut Adawlut Reports, 23rd Sept. 1854, p. 412.

We have abundance of statements, but many of those require authentication; and, in other cases of undoubted authenticity, the crime has been committed by fanatics, for whose drunken or maniacal acts national custom can scarcely be held responsible. These cases, however, fully show that the practice still lives in the public mind throughout India; and, as a sensible writer on the subject remarked two years ago, "*There is but one step from the popular belief to the fact.*"

In the following paragraphs I have given a series of these reports, from 1839 up to the present year. Although, as I have said, they need further authentication, they are very probably true, and they embody some curious details.

The *Commercial Advertiser* publishes an account of a most horrible *human sacrifice* in the district of Backergunge. A wealthy zemindar had a cause pending for a long time in the Courts. He, at length, gained it, and immediately performed a grand poojah, at which he determined to offer a human sacrifice. One of his own ryots was immediately seized, and immolated. The whole affair has been brought to the knowledge of the magistrate, who has instituted, it is said, a very strict investigation into the matter.*

A Chumar having been found with his throat cut in the house of Balebund Goozer, a Goozer Banian in Marka Sholapore (Bombay Presidency), a report was circulated all through the district that the blood of the murdered Chumar was shed in order to propitiate a demon or rakshas who guarded a treasure which, it was believed, was concealed somewhere about the premises on which the deed was committed.†

A very horrible murder was lately perpetrated in the Chanda district of the Central Provinces. The accused, one Apka Marapa, was supposed by the Deputy Commissioner, who committed him for trial, to have slain his victim for the sake of a rupee, a brass vessel, and a cloth; but Apka Marapa, in his confession, stated that Venkut Ramdoo "was murdered, on the tank of a village called Kondapilly, to appease Mysamer—the power to whom misfortune, affecting the safety of the embankment of the tank, or the prosperity of the crops, is attributed." Apka Marapa also stated that such sacrifices were made every four or five years, and that he himself had assisted at one on a former occasion. The Commissioner believed the confession so far as the motive of the defendant was concerned; and he adds in his report of the case:—"If my views in the present case are correct, it is quite possible that other cases of the same nature may occur in Sironcha, not only without detection, but without even a suspicion of the possibility of their having occurred presenting itself to the minds of the authorities. There would be no public outcry against such a crime. The people who

---

* Allen's Asiatic Journal, 1839.

† *Friend of India*, June 25th, 1868.

knew of the occurrence would regard it as the satisfactory performance of a religious duty likely to bring prosperity to the village, tank, and fields. There would be no danger of any search being made after the victim in most instances, as the murderers would select, as in the present case, a poor man, whom they found at some distance from home, and about whom searching enquiry would not be made by his friends. It is probable that, if the Deputy Commissioner's camp had not been near, the crime which formed the subject of this investigation would not have been reported."

The Chief Commissioner, without ostensibly endorsing these views, considered the matter of sufficient importance to order that an enquiry should be made throughout the Provinces as to whether human sacrifices were still ever resorted to by the people. The result is a confident, if not a conclusive, negative.*

The *Deccan Herald* states that another murder case is under investigation by the Railway magistrate. A boy, thirteen years of age, was the victim; and three marwarrees, one of them a Brahmin, are accused of the perpetration of the crime. The theory of the murder as set forth by the police is, that the accused became impressed with the belief that treasure had been deposited by the late Peishwa in a well near their village, Phoolgaum; and that the boy, their victim, having been born in a peculiar way, possessed the power of discovering it; that the accused enticed the boy to the well after dark and experimented with him in expectation of finding the treasure; and that, being disappointed, to prevent the boy from divulging their important secret, they murdered him by throwing him into the well. The boy's body was certainly found in the well, with all the jewels on it which he had been wearing up to the time he left home; and with no marks of violence on it, but with certain figures in paint on it indicating tha tsome superstitious arts had been practised in connection with it. As the case is still pending, we abstain from any remarks upon the evidence taken by the magistrate. The boy was the only son of his mother, who is a widow. There can be no doubt that the boy has been murdered.†

A native Paper states that a Hindu traveller went into a temple at Nursingpore, and came out mad. Seizing a sword, the lunatic cut off the heads of his wife and children, and placed their heads before the image of the goddess Bhowani. After that he ran amôk through the place, killing or cutting down all who came in his way. In the end he coolly washed his sword in a running stream, fastened it to his waist-belt, and went and hanged himself on the nearest tree.‡

* Calcutta *Englishman*, June 8th 1868.
† *Ibid*, June, 1869.
‡ *Ibid*, February 7th, 1870.

Mr. Reily, head of the detective police in Bengal, told me, in 1866, that, about three years and-a-half previously, he saw a man, who pretended to be mad, standing at the door of his house in Hooghly, brandishing a knife, and declaring that he would kill any one who attempted to enter. It was found that, on the previous day, he had cut off a lad's head, and, after having presented it at the shrine of Kali, burnt it.

Cowell and Woodman (p. 539) cite a curious case, where a father sacrificed his son, because wealth had not accompanied its birth, and afterwards cut his own throat, as a protest against his deity's injustice. *Queen* v. *Bishendharee Kahar*, 7 W. R., Cr., 100.

It seems probable that, in the last two cases, the miserable wretches were either insane or intoxicated.

It is certain that, in our endeavours to discover whether the practice of human sacrifice still lingers in India, we must not expect to find that it prevails anywhere as a steadily-working custom, such as *sati* was, and female infanticide is. If it be practised now, it is only as an extreme measure by which some terrible curse may be averted, or some vast good may be obtained. That human sacrifice has been deliberately practised in Lower Bengal, within the last fifty years, as a means of *preventing famine* and of *checking pestilence*, is almost certain. In his Annals of Rural Bengal, my friend Dr. Hunter shows that the Siva-worship of Lower Bengal is derived from the aboriginal races who, according to Signor Gorresio, held this terrible deity in adoration, appeasing him with human blood. "The first aim of the British Government, on acquiring a province," says Dr. Hunter, "has always been to put down such sacrifices; but, in seasons of scarcity, the priests of Lower Bengal still offer up children to the insatiable demon who terrified the forest tribes three thousand years ago."

"During 1865-66 such sacrifices were had recourse to in order to avert the famine. They were few in number, the police being specially on the alert, and the authorities having got warning by the publicity which the press gave to the two cases that were brought to light. The following are the details of a human sacrifice in 1866, in the Jessore district, one of the oldest settled and most enlightened parts of Bengal: 'A Mahomedan boy, about seven years of age, was found in the scaffold-room adjoining a temple of Kali (the wife of Siva) at Luckipassa, with his neck in the *harcat*, or wooden scaffold, and his neck cut. The tongue was fixed between the teeth, the eyes open, clotted blood on his body, which was quite exposed, and two cuts of a *Khundah* were visible on the neck. The sacrifice, it seems, was not completed, for the object is entirely to sever the head from the body. In a late case at Hooghly, the head was left before the idol decked with flowers."* Dr. Hunter adds that among the

* Calcutta *Englishman*, 19th May 1866.

aboriginal tribes to the south-west of Beerbhoom, he heard vague reports of human sacrifices in the forests, with a view to procuring the early arrival of the rains.

I have been so fortunate as to obtain from Dr. Kenneth McLeod, who was civil surgeon of Jessore at the time, a most interesting note on the above case. I gather from it the following facts. The body of Adee Chokra was brought for examination on the 6th April 1866. He was said to have been sacrificed to the goddess Kali. He was about five years of age, and appeared to have been well developed and nourished. The head was nearly separated from the body by a large gash, at the root of the neck on the right side. About one half of the circumference of the skin of the neck was divided; the edges of the wound were sharp and clean. The vertebral column was divided at *three* distinct points. The appearances were such as to lead to the opinion that the injury had been inflicted with a heavy sharp-cutting instrument with a straight or curved edge; that the boy was, in all probability, suddenly cut by three transverse blows or hasks—the subject standing or lying, most probably the latter. Upon the production of two sacrificial instruments, Dr. McLeod had no difficulty in fixing upon the larger (a *Khunda*) as that most likely to cause the injury, and as corresponding most closely with the sort of weapon he had previously conceived. The body was discovered nearly in the manner described above, in a temple of the goddess Kali, the floor of which was covered with a pool of blood. It is well worthy of remark that information of the murder was first given to the police by the chief priest of the temple (a three-roomed building), who, with two others, was in the temple at the time. He deposed that he heard the cry of a child, exclaimed to one of the other men that some one was being murdered, and told him to go and see what it was, and that, on going into the smaller sacrificing-house, they found the body of the child in the condition described. I shall now give the remainder of the newspaper report cited by Dr. Hunter, it represents the local impression as it existed at the time :—

"The priest of the temple, in order to hide his guilt and concern in the affair, lodged immediate information with the police, and stated that, when he entered the temple in the evening, he heard the cries of a boy, and sent his companion to enquire into the matter, when he found the boy in the aforesaid position, but no others. The mother of the deceased boy suspects some of her enemies; but the authorities suspect the priests, on the ground that it is unlikely that such a sacrifice should have been made without some sort of preparation or communication with the priest of the temple."

Reverting to Dr. McLeod's notes. The body was identified by the boy's mother, who was separated from her husband, one Someeruddy, and was, with her son, living with her brother close to the scene of the tragedy. This occurred about sunset, and it happened that there was a *haut* (market) that evening *immediately* adjoining the temple.

There was, at this time, a strong feud between an indigo factory and a zemindary of that locality. The factory is situated to the east of the *haut*, and the zemindar's cutcherry to the west of the temple. The priests who belonged to the zemindary party asserted that they saw three men leave the temple immediately after the cry, and that two of these were like two employés of the factory. In the details of this story, however, they contradicted each other, and other circumstances rendered it highly improbable. On the other hand, members of the factory party endeavoured to criminate the opposite faction. These charges, on strict investigation, fell to the ground. It afterwards came out that Someeruddy, the father, had been considered insane for two months previous to the murder ; that he had not been at his house for seven days before it, that he was seen taking his son off a maidan on the fatal afternoon, and walking with him in the direction of the *haut*. He was found in his house next morning with spots of blood on his clothes, which he asserted were caused by leech bites. These bites could not be found. He made a statement of where he had been, and what he had been doing on the previous day and night, which was obviously untrue, and was contradicted by other evidence. Suspicion rested strongly upon him. He was sent to the station to be examined as to the soundness of his mind. After careful and repeated examinations, Dr. McLeod came to the conclusion that he was not insane. He was brough tbefore the Assistant Magistrate. The priests adhered to their former statement, and obstinately refused to give more direct evidence. No new evidence could be obtained to implicate him, and he was dismissed.

Whatever may have been the truth in this dark tragedy, it is certain that, fifty years previously, the people of Jessore were not ignorant of the practice of human sacrifice as a means of propitiating the destructive power in seasons of national calamity.

Dr. Robert Tytler has left on record a vivid picture of the moral shock which the first outburst of the great Cholera Epidemic of 1817 produced upon the people of Jessore. The disease commenced its ravages in August, and it was at once discovered that the August of this year had *five* Saturdays. The number *five* being the express property of the destructive *Siva*, a mystical combination was hence detected, the infallibly baneful influence of which it would have been sacrilege to question. On the night of the 29th, a strange commotion spread through the villages adjacent to the station. A number of *Jadoos*, or magicians, were reported to have quitted Morelly with a human head in their possession, which they were, to be directed by the presence of supernatural signs, to leave in a certain and to them unknown village. The people on all sides were ready, by force, to arrest the progress of these nocturnal visitors; for the prophesy foretold that, wherever the head fell, the destroying angel, terminating her sanguinary course, would rest; and the demon of death, thus satisfied, would refrain from further devastation in this part of the country. Dr. Tytler says that, on that night, while walking along the road, endeavouring to allay the agitation and to quiet the apprehensions of the people, the judge and he perceived a faint light issuing from a thick clump of bamboos. Attracted to the spot, they found a hut, which was illuminated, and contained the images of five Hindoo gods, one of which was *Seetillah*—the celebrated and formidable *Oolah Beebee (our Lady of the Flux)*, Avatar of Kali, who, it is believed, is one day to appear, riding upon a horse, for the purpose of slaughtering mankind, and of setting the world on fire. In front of the idols, a female child, about nine years of age, lay upon the ground. "She was evidently stupefied with intoxicating drugs, and in this manner prepared to return responses to such questions as those initiated into the mysteries should think proper to propose." By the light of our present knowledge, we may apprehend that the poor little creature lay, thus prepared, rather as the victim than as the oracle.

At the same time it was reported in the Calcutta Newspapers that "the Sircar of an eminent merchant was, a few nights ago, accosted in his sleep by an elderly, but very fine-looking lady, who introduced herself to him as the dreaded *Oolah Beebee*. On his enquiring what were her commands, she replied—'My lamp wants oil.' This appearing rather enigmatical, the Baboo requested her to be more explicit. She then said, 'I have four dogs, they are hungry, they must be fed with human blood.' So saying, she disappeared. Next day, the story was related to the neighbours, who, with one accord, lost no time in packing up their all and fleeing from their homes."*

The following details of an undoubted case of a human sacrifice, which occurred in 1868, are gathered from the decision of the Judges of the Appellate High Court, which the Hon'ble Elphinstone Jackson, one of the Judges who decided upon the appeal, has most obligingly sent me. Bundal Gere and five others were condemned to suffer death in September 1868, by the Deputy Commissioner of the Sonthal Pergunnas, for having put to death a wandering half-witted Mussulmaun beggar whom they decoyed to the top of a hill and offered up as a human sacrifice to the hill gods. There is no doubt, upon the evidence, that the alleged murder was committed. The dead body was found some days after, with the head severed from the trunk, the arms bound behind the back, the thighs tied with a new cloth round the loins. The body lay upon a large boulder at the summit of the hill. On the stone were marks of poojah having been made there. In fact, from the state in which the body was found, little doubt can remain that the person had been deliberately murdered as a

* Morbus Oryzeus, pp. 27 & 37 of *Notes to the History of the Disease.*

human sacrifice. One of the prisoners admitted to the Assistant Commissioner of Doomka that he and the prisoner Dhurum Sing had deliberately offered up this beggar as a sacrifice, the cause alleged being that Dhurum Singh was suffering from hydrocele, and that his sickness might thereby be allayed. Subsequent enquiry appeared to show that one of the prisoners, Pirthi Sing, had lately gained a civil suit, and that the sacrifice may have been a propitiatory offering consequent on the successful termination of the suit. The Judges of the Appellate Court did not, however, consider that the complicity of Pirthi Sing in the sacrifice was proved. It was stated that the victim was struck twice, the second blow severing his head from his body; the medical evidence confirmed this. The Court confirmed the sentence of death on Bundal Gere and Dhurum Sing, and acquitted the other prisoners. *Vide* APPENDIX D.

CUT THROAT.

By far the larger proportion of murders of this kind which come under judicial and medical investigation in India, are to be traced to feelings of sexual jealousy and injured honor. It would appear, from the details of several cases, that this mode of destruction is often deliberately selected as the punishment of Adultery and Unchastity, and that the wound in the throat is intended to be viewed as an indication or "*Signature*" of the crime for which the deceased has suffered.

By the existing law of Arabia, an adulteress is condemned to have her throat cut by her father or brother, but this is now seldom done. Linschoten said that, if the husbands of the Portuguese women of Goa but once suspect them of adultery, "presently they cut their throats." As will be shown in several parts of this Manual, particular punishments are frequently awarded by the people of India to particular crimes, especially in cases of jealousy. In the present instance, however, too much dependence must not be placed upon circumstantial evidence of this kind, as many cases of murder by cutting the throat are recorded in which the existence of such a motive was not apparent. Still, the following cases show that the question broached above deserves attention and investigation :—

Hurree was tried at Bareilly for the murder of Urjoon. He stated as follows in his confession before the Joint Magistrate :—I strangled Urjoon, my neighbour. I was asleep under a thatch in my enclosure; my wife was asleep in my apartment. At three o'clock, Urjoon leapt over the wall into the enclosure. I was aroused and called out—Who is it ? He gave no answer. I, supposing him to be a thief, endeavoured to seize him ; he sat down in a corner of the wall. I took a hempen rope, and put it as a noose over his neck. I drew it tight, so that the thief fell down, and I quickly got on him, and strangled him by means of the rope. When he was dead, I got afraid, and, taking up the deceased on my shoulders, went out and threw the body in the confines of the adjoining village; and, in throwing it down, I, from rage, cut it with a sword, so that the neck was cut through, nearly severed from the trunk. The Judges of both Courts regarded it as probable that the prisoner detected the deceased in a nocturnal visit to his wife, in prosecution of an intrigue, and that he put him to death, well knowing who he was, and for what purpose he had come.*

This case has great significance, when taken in connection with the two other similar instances cited at pages 353 and 390 of this Manual, in which ***the necks of persons murdered for adultery were hacked, after death***, by the offended parties.

At about the same time, Munrakhund, of Futtehpore, confessed before the Magistrate that, fifteen days previously, he saw one Dabeedeen cohabiting with his wife, but he escaped. Afterwards the man came to his house; a verbal dispute ensued. Dabeedeen poked him with a lattee on the mouth, whereupon he drew him into the vestibule of the house, and, having throttled him, cut his throat with a small blunt hoe or *khoorpee*. He, of his own accord, then told the police that he had killed the man, and produced from an inner apartment of his house, from a quantity of chaff, a bundle which, on being opened, was found to contain the corpse of the deceased. A purse containing 22 rupees was found on the person of the murdered man. The Sessions Judge remarked that, by the prisoner's own account, the act of cutting the man's throat did not follow immediately on the provocation, but first he got him down, planted his knee on his breast, and throttled him.† This last point is of some importance, as bearing upon a question which was raised in a trial which took place in one of the Courts of the N. W. Provinces, as to whether the prisoner had not thrown a man down merely with the intention of cutting off his nose,—the usual punishment of adultery,—without premeditation of murder; but, endangered or enraged by the man's struggles, had cut his throat.‡

Ramsuhaee confessed, before the Joint Magistrate of Allahabad, that, finding a man in the act of committing adultery with his wife, he looked about for some weapon with which to kill him. The adulterer, in the meantime, escaped. Finding a razor, he killed his wife and fled. The throat of the unfortunate woman was cut through, her breasts were

---

* Nizamut Adawlut Reports, N. W. P., 2nd July 1853, p. 812. A singular case was tried at Sylhet in 1857, in which Musst. Najook Bibee, having intrigued with her husband's brother, cut his throat with a dhao as he lay on her bed, pleading that he had tried to force her. The crime appeared to be attributable to jealousy.—*Nizamut Adawlut Reports*, February 13, 1857, p. 145.

† Nizamut Adawlut Reports, N. W. P., 30th June 1853, p. 806.

‡ See also Nizamut Adawlut Reports, N. W. P., January 7th, 1853, p. 32.

sliced open, and the belly was ripped across, so that a fœtus of five months was expelled through the wound from the womb.*

Standing alone, this case would merely be regarded as an instance of wild brutality, the almost accidental result of ill-regulated passions unendurably outraged. It, however, gains a terrible significance when its details are compared with those of another case reported by Mr. Wilkie, then of Dinagepore, several years previously, in which the body of a woman was sent in for examination with her throat frightfully cut, and several gashes on the breasts, and with both the ears cut off—the latter mutilation, when it appears upon the body of a murdered person, being an almost certain evidence that death has been the penalty of adultery. In neither case, then, can the crime be viewed merely as an outburst of blind fury ;—each murderer, doubtless, acted according to a certain form and precedent of ancient tradition.

The other recorded instances of the commission of this crime, for the same cause, are so numerous that a few of them can only be briefly mentioned. A man confessed that he found his wife in adultery, and, in his rage, went to a near neighbour's house for a razor, with which he cut her throat.† A person, suspecting his wife of infidelity, after a short dispute, deliberately took a knife, threw her down upon the ground, and cut her throat.‡ A man waylaid one who had intrigued with his wife, knocked him down, and cut his throat from ear to ear.§ A person acknowledged that he had cut the throat of one who had intrigued with his wife, and four others confessed that they had been present aiding and abetting ; the body, however, was never found,—the prisoners were therefore released.|| Two men cut the throat of their uncle, with a sword, for having abducted their mother, his own sister-in-law.¶ A man, suspecting his wife of intrigue, cut her throat and his own with a sword.**

Chintamoney Thakoor having dishonored the wife of Fakeer Chand

---

* Nizamut Adawlut Reports, N. W. P., August 19th 1853, p. 1016. A case somewhat similar to this occurred in the Moorshedabad District in 1845, where a barber was convicted of murdering his wife in the night by cutting her all over the body with a razor.—*Police Report, L. P.*, 1845, p. 59.

† Nizamut Adawlut Reports, Vol. II., p. 235.

‡ Police Report, L. P., 1846, p. 21.

§ *Ibid*, 1844, p. 19.

|| *Ibid*, 1851, p. 56.

¶ Nizamut Adawlut Reports, N. W. P., September 1st, 1853, p. 1088.

** *Ibid*, Sept. 27th, 1853, p. 1199. It may be scarcely out of place to mention here that there are one or two points which appear to render the moral relations of the crime of homicide on account of Sexual Jealousy in India somewhat different from those which lead to the commission of similar violence in more civilized countries. Thus,—the sense of disgrace and of outraged honor is certainly as strong among these comparatively uncultivated people as it is with any nation in the world. This is shown in the singular fact that the adulteress sometimes urges her husband to sacrifice her life, to redress his honor. A man put his

Nath Jooghi, of Jessore, the injured husband and some of his relatives went to his house at night and killed him with *daos*. "The throat

---

wife to death, at her own request, in consequence of her loss of honor from having been violated by several persons.* This is intelligible enough. Occurring many years ago in Bengal, it illustrates the extraordinary statement of Ramsuhaee, a man of the North-West tried in 1853, the prisoner whose case is narrated above at p. 418, to the effect that an improper intimacy had, within his knowledge and observation, existed for some time previously between a certain man and his wife, "*who had frequently spoken to him (the prisoner) on the subject, and urged him to kill her to save the honor of the family.*" Still there was every reason for believing the prisoner's statement that he found this same man in the act of adultery with his wife, and then put her to death! It may appear singular that so jealous a people should, not unfrequently, be willing to overlook, for a time, the unchastity of their wives—this, however, is probably, in a great measure, owing to the feeling, so common among natives, that it is the exposure which constitutes the disgrace, and in part also to the severity of the punishment generally inflicted by the Courts in nearly all cases of this kind where the guilty parties cannot be proved to have been discovered in the act. Considering how poor, dishonest, and morally degraded the generality of the lower-class natives are, it is worthy of remark that I have scarcely found, in my reading, any instance in which it could be fully proved that a Hindu or Mussulmaun husband connived at his own dishonor with a mercenary motive. An apparent exception to this rule occurred in 1854, in the case of one Oseri, of Bareilly, who, becoming nearly blind, was said to have made over his wife to another man, on condition of receiving food and clothing. They all three lived in one house. The result was that, after frequent disputes, he killed the woman with repeated sword cuts, and then surrendered to the police with the bloody weapon in his hand.—The case which came before the Calcutta Police in May 1868, of a wretch who systematically lived upon the earnings of unfortunate women, and who married a poor creature at Benares and brought her to a brothel, and who beat her to compel her to prostitute herself for the benefit of himself and his mistresses, is no exception to this rule; and it is met by the case of Protab Napit (barber), who, finding that his wife was determined to accompany her aunt to Burdwan and to become a prostitute there, murdered both on the road.† According to Sir John Malcolm, the Sikhs do not punish a man who murders his wife for infidelity. The Chief says, if he were to punish such a husband, all the women in the country would become unfaithful. Ward mentions that, according to the Hindu Scriptures, the merits and demerits of husband and wife are transferable to either in the future state. If a wife perform many meritorious works, and the husband die first, he will enjoy heaven as the fruit of his wife's virtuous deeds; and, if the wife be guilty of many wicked actions, and the husband die first, he will suffer for the sins of his wife.

"An adulterous wife casts the guilt on her negligent husband."—Menu, Chap. VIII., s. 317.

A man who had killed his unfaithful wife declared, at his trial, that, owing to the disgrace which she had brought upon him, "he was dead before, but that now he was alive again, and quite indifferent as to what was done to him."—*Nizamut Adawlut Rep., N. W. P.*, 3rd November 1852, p. 1299.

What must, at first sight, appear to the European mind a very extraordinary case of native *jealousy* was related to me some years since by Mr. J. Blessington Roberts, Coroner of Calcutta:—A prostitute of the commonest kind had a favorite paramour with whom she had agreed that she would not receive her casual acquaintances after a certain hour. The man, knowing that a person was with her later than that hour, and considering therefore that she displayed an undue preference, watched at the door for the unfortunate individual, and cut him down with a tulwar as he went out. It is probable, however, that this crime was due to greed, not to jealousy. Living upon the woman's miserable gains, he feared that this rival would supplant him. The criminal records contain many instances in which prostitutes have been killed by men with whom they have refused to associate any longer.

* Nizamut Adawlut Reports, Vol. I., p. 9.

† Bengal Police Report for 1866, p. 173.

especially was so severely cut, that death must have occurred immediately."*

Wullee was sentenced to death at Chittagong for fracturing his wife's skull with a kodalee, and then cutting her throat with a sickle. He appears to have been jealous of her, but without proved cause. In a dispute she wounded him in the leg with a dhao, upon which he killed her.†

Peeroo Sheik, of Nuddea, cut his wife's throat with a sickle. He accused her of adultery, but the Nizamut Judges held that there "was no ground even for supposing that the woman was guilty."‡

Sheikh Nayer, of Sylhet, cut the throat of his sick wife, who dirtied the house. He pleaded that his wife was intimate with one Sadeer, but failed to establish the fact.§

On the 18th March 1868, it was reported to the Bograh station that a woman had committed suicide by cutting her throat with a sickle. On enquiry, it was ascertained that the deceased, who had an intrigue with her cousin, had been killed by her husband, aided by his relatives. Eye-witnesses were found to testify to the fact. Four men were arrested and sent up for trial, three of whom admitted their guilt before the Magistrate, who committed them to the Court of Sessions.||

Sheikh Chand, of Backergunge, was sentenced to death for cutting his wife's throat. The Judges held that they had no explanation of the cause of the murder, but that of momentary unrestrained passion.¶ There did not appear to be any imputation upon the woman's character: but it is to be greatly doubted whether these crimes are ever committed upon the sudden impulse of mere purposeless anger. See, at the end of this Chapter, *Note on Cases of Murder by Wounding in which no Cause of Provocation is ascertainable.*

In certain cases of cut throat, the fingers are found to be injured, thus furnishing most convincing evidence of the fact that homicide has been committed,—as in the following instances:—

In January 1852, a Mussalmaun was tried at Mymensing for cutting the throat of his stepmother, and separating the head from the body, with a long knife used for killing animals. The evidence of the Civil Surgeon showed that the body presented fifteen other wounds—six on the back, one on the head, three on the right side of the face and chin, one in the bend of the arm, and the rest on the hands. He stated that his mother-in-law (a woman of notoriously ill-temper) denied him food and a fire when he

* Nizamut Adawlut Reports, May 15th, 1855, p. 568.
† *Ibid*, January 5th, 1856, p. 25.
‡ *Ibid*, July 15th, 1856, p. 72.
§ *Ibid*, February 9th, 1857, p. 113.
|| Bengal Police Report for 1868, p. 303.
¶ Nizamut Adawlut Reports, May 26th, 1858, p. 188.

was suffering from ague, and endeavoured to kill him with the knife, which he then turned against herself.*

In the case of a poor child six years old, whose throat was cut from ear to ear and to the spine, by a wretch who stole his ornaments, one slight incised wound was also found on the back of the left hand.†

It happens very much more frequently, however, that, although the characters of the wound are such as to render it a matter of certainty that the individual did not perish by suicide, the hands are perfectly free from any trace of injury whatever. This is often accounted for by the fact that, as in the case of Lord W. Russell, who was murdered by Courvoisier in 1840, the victim receives the first blow while sleeping ;‡ and, should the murderer purpose to repeat it, he refrains from doing so, until hæmorrhage has precluded all power of resistance or movement.

Dahoo Joolaha confessed, upon his trial at Behar in 1852, that, his wife having abused him in the evening, he waited until midnight, and then, deliberately lighting a lamp, cut her throat with the common knife of the house.§

Dr. Woodford has given me the case of a native doctor who was murdered (as proved by foot-prints on the bed-sheet and by other circumcumstances) by a superficial horizontal incision on the right side of the neck, an inch long and only deep enough to divide the external jugular vein, which it did completely. The deceased apparently only had time to turn on his right side before expiring. He was a weak, spare man, about 50 years of age. Dr. Woodford was inclined to think, from the cleanness of the wound, that a scalpel had been used.

In 1855, I examined the exhumed body of a Mussalmaun girl, 16 or 17 years of age. The throat had been severed by enormous wounds, evidently inflicted by repeated chops with a rather blunt instrument (a small but heavy sickle was produced). The vertebræ were completely divided. All that could be clearly ascertained was, that she had gone to rest with her husband, that he had absconded, and that her body was found in the above condition. The hands were uninjured.

The records show that this mode of committing murder is of considerable frequency. When the fingers are uncut, and when the nature of the wound is such as to prove that it could not have been self-inflicted, or the murdered person is so young that all suspicion of suicide must be out of the question, it will be necessary to institute minute inquiries as to whether the deceased was or was not asleep when the fatal blow was struck.

---

* Nizamut Adawlut Reps., Vol. II., part 1, p. 140.

† *Ibid*, N. W. P., 2nd October 1852, p. 1121.

‡ There was, however, a wound on the thumb of Lord W. Russell's right hand, which must have been instinctively raised before the stroke was finished.

§ Nizamut Adawlut Reports, Vol. II., Part 1, for 1852, p. 34.

When it is probable that the deceased was not asleep or insensible when attacked, the absence of wounds on the hands must afford a strong presumption that the murderer was aided by accomplices, as in a case tried at Bhaugulpore in 1853, where it appeared certain that a discharged servant had enticed his late master's son into a field, and there, aided by three other persons, had cut the child's throat, and stripped the body of its ornaments.*

A man, of Rungpore, having been too intimate with a female in the service of the same employer, and she proving with child, he was afraid that, when the intrigue was discovered, he would be punished. He accordingly inveigled her out one night to a place where two of his friends were ready. They seized her, each holding an arm and leg, and the third cut her throat. They then threw the body into a well, which they filled up.†

In a case tried at Moradabad, in 1852, it appeared that a boy, eleven years old, had been murdered by stabs in the throat, apparently inflicted with a knife, which had passed from the right side clean through the throat to the left. The child's great-grandmother declared that she had seen one man holding him down while the other stabbed him, but the evidence of the chief witnesses was discrepant, and the accused were acquitted.‡

A man who was killed by some Santhals in 1856, "had a wound in in the neck which passed through it from side to side, and the left hand was nearly severed at the wrist; but there were no other marks upon the corpse, except a few bruises on the head, as if the deceased had been finished with stones."§

The crime of *killing, by wounding, persons who have first been rendered insensible by drugs or liquor*, is not unusual in this country. Here, of course, the hands will generally not bear marks of wounding.

In 1854, Lukheenarain Das Byragee and Ramdhone Mundul and another persuaded a girl to attire herself in all her finery to the value of rupees 125, pretending they would take her to the house of a rich Baboo, who would keep her. Having intoxicated her, they cut her throat, and took her jewels. They stripped the body, drew the legs by a string up to the neck, put it into a sack, and threw it under a bridge by the highway.‖

* Nizamut Adawlut Reports, Vol. III., Part 1, 1853, p. 152. See also a case in which the throat of a woman was cut by two persons, others holding her.—*Ibid*, p. 177. Also *Reports of the Nizamut Adawlut, N. W. P.*, for August 1854, p. 287.

† *Ibid*, N. W. P., 2nd August 1852, p. 773.

‡ The murderers appear to have been tempted to the crime by the poor child's only ornament, a silver *huslee*, which was worth *one rupee eight annas*. The Sessions Judge remarked that his experience told him that the natives of India will murder for even a less valuable article.—*Nizamut Adawlut Reports, N. W. P.*, 2nd August 1852, p. 773.

§ Nizamut Adawlut Reports, October 15th, 1856, p. 778.

‖ *Ibid*, October 8, 1855, p. 582.

In some valuable notes for which I am indebted to Dr. Woodford, my colleague writes: "The case of the Jewess Leah, who was murdered in Calcutta in 1858 by stab wounds, is of interest, inasmuch as *chloroform was applied to the nostrils before the stabs were inflicted.* This explained the engorged state of the vessels of the brain, which otherwise would probably have been found deficient in blood."

In the following cases, however, a presumption—founded upon the uninjured state of the hands—that the deceased had been held, or had been murdered while sleeping, would probably have been erroneous. In February of the previous year, one Shamchand confessed, on trial, as follows:— "I had given the deceased rupees six to keep. On the day of the occurrence, I called him to my house, and seated him down to smoke. I asked him for the rupees six, and he denied my giving them to him. In a passion, I took a *dhao*, which was in the chupper of the house, and, calling him inside, cut him with it as he put his head inside." The Sub-Assistant Surgeon noted different wounds about the neck, and stated that both carotid arteries were cut, and that the wound was as of a drawing cut. It appeared that the *dhao* was seventeen inches long, and very sharp. When it is recollected that a man must enter the very low doorway of a native hut with his body at a right angle, and his neck craned forward, the possibility of inflicting a fatal cut upon the throat, as it was advanced, before the hands could be raised to protect it, must be self-evident.

In June 1854, Purshad, a barber, was sentenced capitally for the murder of Bishan, one of his own trade. The deceased having gone into a field for the purposes of nature, the prisoner, watching his opportunity, rushed on him, and cut his throat with a razor. Here the unexpected nature of the attack, the position of the assailed, the keenness of the weapon and, probably, the skill of the criminal in its use, would have to be taken into account.*

In 1868, there occurred in Calcutta a case which was, for months, known in the public prints as the "*Amherst Street Murder;*" but in which, although rather strong circumstances of doubt intervened, the evidence, to my mind, was very much more in favor of suicide.

The body of Rose Brown, a healthy young East Indian woman, was found lying in the street, at daybreak, with the throat cut. My friend Dr. Colles found a very deep wound in the neck, beginning, in his opinion, about one hand's-breadth below the angle of the jaw on the left side, and passing across the throat upwards, and ending towards the right side. It divided the great vessels of the neck on the left side, and also the principal cartilage at the top of the windpipe. The vessels on the right side had escaped injury. The wound in the centre had extended to the spinal

* Nizamut Adawlut Reports, N. W. P., June 1854, p. 653.

column, which was slightly marked. The length of the wound was about four or five inches, and the deepest part was about one inch and a half. The wound was quite straight, and this means that it was made by one pass of the knife. About an inch on the right extremity was a little tear or laceration which had been caused by a gap on the edge of the knife, or a stroke over the beads, or a sudden lunge of the head. The knife (produced) has no gap, but the wound could have been caused by it. Dr. Colles mentioned to me a suspicious circumstance, *viz.*, that there were no particular marks of blood on the right hand. "The wound might," Dr. Colles considered, "have been inflicted either by the woman herself, or by the hand of a second person. The inference against suicide is that the wound was lower down the neck" [than is usual in suicide], "and the force required to cut through the cartilage and down to the spinal column was greater than suicides generally show." "The back of the left hand and outside of the left arm and fore-arm were covered with clay and blood." "From the state of the body generally and that of the left arm, I am of opinion that the wound was inflicted while she was in an erect position, and that she almost immediately fell over on her left side." There was grave suspicion against one Madhub Chunder Dutt, who was proved to have been with her that night. The facts in favor of suicide were that Dr. Colles found "no other marks of violence on the body." It appears that there were no decided marks of struggling or scattering of blood on the road. Dr. Colles told me that her hair and dress were not disarranged. To his reasons against the suicidal appearance of the wound, Dr. Colles added, "but, at the same time, a determined suicide might inflict such a wound. I did express my opinion that the wound was probably suicidal, on account of the absence of any wound on the hand, thus showing that the woman had not put up her hand to save her throat."

It was never hinted that the accused had accomplices who held the woman. If she had been held by one or two persons, would not the road and her hair and dress have borne evidences of a violent struggle, and would she not probably have aroused the neighbours by her shrieks before the division of the larynx could have been accomplished? "If," said Dr. Colles, "the wound had been inflicted by a second person, it might have been done from behind." Possibly, but then we have the question, whether the woman could well have been taken so much unawares as to fall dead under such a wound, without time for an instinctive raising of the hands to protect the throat, and also whether so deep and clean a cut could have been inflicted, *at one stroke,* from behind. Under such doubts as these the accused escaped. The knife was a long sailor's knife, moderately sharp.

At page 39 will be found the monition of an Indian Judge upon the importance of reporting upon the condition of the hands in every case of cut throat. I find that, even in many of Casper's cases, the state of the hands is not mentioned. Considering his admirable accuracy, it is probable that, whenever the hands were not alluded to in the reports, they were uninjured. Still, in several of his narratives, we feel that this information would have rendered the histories more complete and satisfactory.

An important question arose in a trial at Jubbulpore, as to *whether death had been caused by a wound on the Throat, or by an injury to the Head.* A young man killed his pregnant wife in the night and disappeared. He afterwards surrendered himself voluntarily. He confessed that, after retiring with his wife, an altercation arose rgarding her unfaithful conduct, when he seized an iron bar called *khurma,* weighing twelve pounds, which lay by, and struck her on the head. She then drew out from a niche in the wall an iron dagger (*kuttar*), and inflicted with it a mortal wound on her own throat. The medical testimony showed that death was caused by either or both of two wounds of a mortal nature; the skull was fractured at the vertex, and beaten in upon the brain, and the throat was so severely cut, or stabbed, that the result must have been quickly fatal. It was held by the Sessions Judge that such a blow or blows as produced the fracture observed must, as was declared by the medical officer, have been followed by instant insensibility, making the subsequent act of suicide imputed clearly impossible, even if there were any coloring of circumstantial probability to sustain it. It could only be inferred that the prisoner, in order to make sure of his object, followed up the blow on the head by the wound in the throat. Under any light in which it could be viewed, he considered that the prisoner's feeble effort to soften the extent of his guilt was, in the face of the clear medical proof, wholly idle.*

The reports show that the question "Can an individual, whose windpipe is cut, speak intelligibly?" is frequently put to the medical witness. The answer appears generally to have been "No; division of the widpipe altogether destroys the power of speech."† It is certain, however, that this assertion requires to be qualified. Undoubtedly, even partial division of the trachea is often attended with loss of speech. Still, where dressings have been carefully applied, and the wound is nearly closed, the divided tube becomes continuous, and whispered speech is possible. Indeed, even where the wound is uncovered, the power of utterance may not be entirely lost. In a case reported by Mr. Davies, of Patna, of a man who was admitted on the 8th of the month with the windpipe nearly cut through, and died on the 15th, having always torn off his dressings, it is mentioned that he "talked incoherently."

---

* Nizamut Adawlut Reports, N. W. P., 5th May 1853, p. 642.

† "When the windpipe is divided, the voice is lost."—Taylor, p. 513.—The above is cited in Baynes's Medical Jurisprudence, p. 66.

Again, in a case of complete division of the throat between the hyoid bone and the thyroid cartilage, Mr. Macansh reported that the patient spoke and was able to make herself understood. Here, however, the vocal apparatus was, probably, nearly uninjured. After the first publication of these remarks, I treated the case of a woman who had cut her throat so extensively, just above the thyroid cartilage, that the arytænoid cartilages were visible. The wound was granulating when I first saw her ; when she closed it, by holding down her head, she could speak audibly in whispers.

Survival after Wounds of the Carotid Arteries.—Dr. Taylor remarks that "there are several cases on record which show that wounds involving the common carotid artery and its branches, as well as the internal jugular vein, do not prevent the individual from exercising voluntary power and running a certain distance."* Mr. D. Tyerman, of Colney Hatch Asylum, has, I believe, been so fortunate as to save life in an instance in which the common carotid was divided. Wounds of the external, and even of the internal, carotid branches, are by no means certainly fatal.† Every Surgeon who reads the following case, will regret that its details are not more full and explicit ; as it stands, it would appear to prove the possibility of survival for some hours after division of the ***common carotid*** artery, even where no surgical means have been adopted, —but this is by no means certain. It appeared that a man was aroused in the night by two thieves, who were in the act of stealing in his house. In struggling with them, one of them cut him in the neck, and they escaped. After receiving the cut, he said that he had seen the prisoners, whom he named, stealing his *goor*, that he had seized one of them, and that the other cut him on the neck with a *dhao*, or knife, and both made their escape. The accused, not having come with the other neighbours, were sent for and confronted with the wounded man, who accused them as above. The man's brother stated that the occurrence happened "*late at night*," and that "*it was then moonlight*." The man *died* "*the following day*." The Civil Surgeon's evidence was as follows :— "I found an irregular deep wound on the neck, apparently caused by a sharp pointed instrument ; the wound, in my opinion, was not caused by the deceased's own hand ; the CAROTID ARTERY *was divided*, and deceased had bled to death. The wound, from its irregular appearance, seemed to have been inflicted during a struggle, such as you mention, between the two parties."

In the Magistrate's Court, the accused pleaded that deceased, when

---

* Op. Cit., p. 309.

† One of the most demonstrative cases of incised wound of the external carotid, in which hæmorrhage was checked by syncope, and where the common carotid was tied with temporary success, has also been given by Mr. Tyerman.—*Med. Times and Gazette*, October 1854, p. 366. For other cases, see Mr. Guthrie's "Commentaries," p. 240.

asked by them to name the persons who wounded him, *gave no answer*. They denied their guilt throughout. One was sentenced to be hanged, the other to transportation for life.

Here the question is—was it the *External* carotid artery or the *Common* carotid that was wounded ? If it was the former, which, however, being merely a branch of the main carotid trunk, is never termed by Surgeons "the Carotid Artery," the statements of the witnesses for the prosecution were *possible*, supposing that the vessel was rather lacerated than cut through by the point of a bluntish weapon like a *dhao*. If the *Common Carotid* artery was the vessel divided, that testimony could only be regarded as just within the extremest limits of possibility. No Surgeon will be prepared to deny that this vessel might become occluded by a temporary clot, if divided by a coarse tearing weapon ; but I can assert, with the utmost confidence, that there is no other known or recorded instance of a person who, after sustaining an incised wound, dividing the Common Carotid Trunk, and remaining without surgical aid, survived long enough to give a distinct account of the transaction, to name his assailants, to have them sent for (irrespective of the distance), and again to accuse them as they stood before him.*

In a case of Mr. Clegg's, a man *lived* half an hour (Taylor, p. 513).

The prisoners should have had the benefit of the doubt, whichever artery was divided.

The Medical Officer does not appear to have been questioned as to the possibility of the statements made by the witnesses for the prosecution.†

* Nizamut Adawlut Reports, 1st December 1854, p. 712. There can be little doubt that the Medical Officer's deposition has been erroneously quoted in the printed report, and that it was the External Carotid which had been divided. Still it is only possible to argue upon such cases as they are placed before us.

† Several remarkable cases of murder by Cutting the Throat will be found in the Nizamut Reports. In 1852, a man of Saharunpore confessed that, having been reproved by his brother for idleness, while they were lying in their beds beside each other, he became so exasperated that he took a sword from the head of the bed and cut him across the neck and shoulder, causing immediate death. He had never been on bad terms with his brother before this.‡ In 1853, one Chutter Singh was sentenced to death, for the murder of five persons—his wife, her grandmother, her mother, and two children of the latter by a European gentleman. The bodies were found lying in a heap in the court-yard of the bungalow with their throats cut. A puppy dog lay on the ground beside them with its head cut off.§ In 1855, a Mussalmaun woman of Beerbhoom, having had a dispute with her husband, cut the throat of her son, about three years old, in such a manner that death must have been instantaneous ; she then inflicted a wound, which caused death two days afterwards, upon the throat of her female infant of nine months. She afterwards cut her own throat—"*superficially*"—as is usual with this class of murderers in nearly all parts of the world. Sentence, Death.‖ In 1853, one Toolsheea, a Mahratta Brahmin of Cawnpore, went to bathe, and was never afterwards seen alive. One Rikhee, one of a class of men called Gungapootras, a set notorious for their evil courses, saying that he had seen the woman

‡ Nizamut Adawlut Reports, N. W. P., 20th September 1852, p. 1037.
§ *Ibid*, 25th February 1853, p. 283.
‖ Nizamut Adawlut Reports, 9th February 1855, p. 181.

Dr. Taylor has laid down the principle that "suicides may graze the ligaments in front of the spinal column, but that they should make deep incisions into the bones, cut off hard bony processes, and divide the intervertebral substance and the vertebral arteries is contrary to all experience and probability." [Page 414.]

The following particulars of a very extreme but clear case have been given to me by Dr. Woodford. A European at Brown's, the confectioner's in Calcutta, was seen walking into the beer *godown* (store) with a cheese-knife in his hand. Search being made, his body was found behind a row of beer casks. The throat was so deeply cut that *the vertebral column bore* TWO *horizontal superficial incisions on its surface.* The knife, inclusive of the handle, was two feet long (blade 16 inches). Dr. Woodford observes that, had there been any suspicion of foul play in this case, or had the knife been missing, few medical men would have been willing to admit the possibility of such a wound having been self-inflicted.

Note on Cases of Murder by Wounding in which no Cause of Provocation is ascertainable.

It will be observed of Sheikh Chand, spoken of at page 421, who was sentenced to death for cutting his wife's throat, and whose Judges remarked that they had no explanation of the cause of the murder, but that of momentary unrestrained passion, that he was a Mahomedan of Backergunge—a class of whom the Magistrate of their district has lately reported,*—"Life is held so cheap amongst the Mussulmauns

---

on her way home, suspicion fell upon him. The police searched his house, his brother's which adjoined it, and another at the back, which it was stated they had bought the day before. The latter premises were of very peculiar construction. They were described by the Joint Magistrate as *Mahratta* buildings, "of which it would be impossible to give a definite description; they were built on no conceivable plan; their rooms (into which the daylight did not penetrate) were dark and diminutive, and almost inaccessible, and they seemed only contrived for the commission of crime, and the concealment of stolen property." The thannadar, accompanied by the prisoners, after proceeding through two low dark cells, which led to a third, found in the last the body of the unfortunate woman, rolled up in a cloth and despoiled of its ornaments, with the throat cut from ear to ear. The prisoners objected to the search of these premises; and, as the police approached the third cell, they managed to blow out the light, and urged that they had no more oil. Between this house and that of Rikhee's brother, there was a low doorway leading to a well, which was within a dark enclosure. By opening the opposite window, a passage could easily be effected from the brother's house, over the well, into the cell in which the corpse was found. There were still visible traces of somebody having been dragged through one window [?] to the other, and it was believed that the woman had been stifled in the brothe.'s house, and finally murdered in the adjoining house of Rikhee.†

* Dr. Mouat's Appendix to the Jail Report, L. P., for 1868, p. 100.

† Nizamut Adawlut Reports, N. W. P., 10th November 1853, p. 1354.

that, on the least provocation, murders are sometimes committed. The Mussulmauns of the district are very easily provoked, and cannot control their passions. The constant use of the dhao in their daily avocations supplies them, unfortunately, with great facilities for committing murder. This fact will explain why murders are so frequent in this district, and committed on such slight provocation."

It is, of course, difficult to form a correct idea of the true nature of the provocation in these cases. We see that an act of frantic violence has been committed, and we are told that the provocation has been of the most trivial kind; but, in societies like this, very serious provocation is likely to be given or to be violently suspected; and I believe that, when the crime has been committed and stands revealed to the law, a spirit of dogged reticence, in which the struggling of something like a rude sentiment of honor and a sense of decency is perceptible, often conceals the provocation. Having seen much of the people, and knowing their power of remaining passive under almost any amount of *pardonable* provocation, I do not believe that these men hack their wives to pieces, with the certainty of being hanged for doing so, merely because "there was a straw in the rice," or because the woman would not talk or bring water or fire; or because, as in the case of Sheikh Chand, of Backergunge, given above, the woman taunted him for not going out with others to cut the rice; or because,—as Somaree, of Tirhoot, who hacked his wife to death with a kodalee, alleged,—the woman kicked the dish which held his food. This case, which is given at p. 346, should here be referred to, as the prisoner added the grave accusation of *infidelity* to his first trivial charge against the unhappy woman.

The following case is evidence of the unreasoning ferocity with which jealousy is capable of possessing these people. In 1856, Pathoo, also a Backergunge man, was sentenced to death for murdering his child-wife by strokes with a *dhao*, weighing thirteen chittacks (26 ounces). There was a wound six inches in length, near the shoulder-joint, sufficient to cause speedy death. The Sessions Judge observed that the prisoner married the deceased when she was an infant, aged four years. "Her father states her age to have been about *eleven* years when she was cruelly murdered by her husband. The only possible motive that I can assign to the conduct of the prisoner is a jealous suspicion on his part of an intrigue between his deceased child-wife and Ashkur. The testimony of the witnesses goes to prove that the deceased was chaste: she was quite a child—it is doubtful whether she had arrived at puberty; and beyond such innocent liberties as are, even in native society, usual and permitted between relations standing in the position that the deceased did to Ashkur (a widower, who married the elder cousin of the deceased), no proof whatever of misconduct on her part can be found on the record." The Court of Appeal observed, "This is a cruel murder of a young wife from an unfounded suspicion of her having an intrigue with a near relation."*

Beenah Baoree, of Chota Nagpore, was sentenced to death for killing his concubine with a sword. His little sons, seven and ten years old, said that he killed the woman, "because she had refused to prepare tobacco." This was, doubtless, the *apparent* cause of his fury. Before the police officers and the Senior Assistant Commissioner, he confessed the murder, assigning jealousy of one Surroop Bhoomij. In the Sessions Court he denied this confession, and said that Hullodhur Chowkedar gave him parched rice to eat and deprived him of his senses. He never had any quarrel with the deceased.†

In some cases of wife-killing by Mussalmauns, regard has been paid to the strictness of the discipline which the men maintain towards the women. In the case of Moolee Mundul, of Rajshahye, who confessed that he had struck his wife, who died from the effects of "two wounds on the head, fracturing the skull, and rupturing or bursting open the sutures which connect the right parietal and the occipital bone," the Sessions Judge observed :—"I do not think that it is a case for capital punishment. The evidence to the fact is not very strong ; the evidence must rest chiefly upon the prisoner's confessions, and, therefore, some little allowance must be made for the provocation which he alleges," [delay in giving him water to drink—abusive language] "for the unhappy state of brutal feeling which exists among the lower class of Mussalmauns, especially regarding the *status* of wives, the degree in which it is regarded as a crime in them to resist or speak disrespectfully to their husbands, and the right of violent correction so commonly believed to exist. I am satisfied that the prisoner never intended to take away the life of the deceased ; and, although I regard the act which he committed as brutal and reckless in the extreme, it appears to me that the considerations I have mentioned above may be sufficient to bar the penalty of death." The Sessions Judge recommended transportation for life, but the Judges of the Court of Appeal considered that justice would be satisfied by a sentence of 14 years' imprisonment."‡

It is certain, however, that there are some of these cases in which no sufficient cause of provocation whatever *appears*. Of this kind was certainly that of Kishtonauth, who deliberately hacked off the head of a little girl of seven, because she did not give him a light for his cheroot,§ and possibly also that of "a son who, irritated at his father for telling him to help himself with food while taking his meal, struck

* Nizamut Adawlut Reports, September 23rd, 1856, p. 593.
† *Ibid*, February 7th, 1855, p. 167.
‡ *Ibid*, February 2nd, 1857, p. 84.
§ *Ibid*, February 29th, 1856, p. 531.

him a blow with a *tanga* on the left side of his neck, and thus killed him." The accused confessed to having committed the crime.*

Kalaram Shah, of Sylhet, was sentenced to death for the wilful murder of his wife, wounding his infant son, and wounding himself. Prisoner confessed before the Darogah, Magistrate, and Judge that, his wife having disregarded his order to bring him water to wash his mouth with, he, seizing a *dhao*, deliberately killed her with it, accidentally wounded his child at the same time, and then attempted to take his own life. The body of the child (of 4) bore *several* wounds, and the woman's head was nearly severed from the body. The prisoner had a fracture of the skull and several severe cuts on the scalp. No further explanation of the crime was elicited.†

On the 17th June 1868, Akbar Alli, of Chittagong, killed his daughter-in-law by knocking out her brains with a *kooralee*. He confessed. The cause of the murder was nothing more than that the deceased, while supplying her husband with *pawn*, accidentally dropped a betel-nut near where the old man was lying down. He struck her two blows on the side of the head, with the back of the hatchet, which caused her death. He was sentenced to be hanged.‡ For further remarks on this subject, *see Hacking with Sword or Bill Hook*, pp. 343-46.

Suicide by Cutting the Throat.

Cases from time to time occur, in which natives inflict wounds upon their own throats, either with a suicidal intention, or with a design to accuse others of the crime. I, when at Howrah, examined the body of a man who, having long suffered from an incurable bowel complaint, was said to have destroyed himself in despair. I found a wound on the throat sufficiently large to account for death, although not involving either carotid : the body was much emaciated, and the bowels showed abundant traces of chronic disease.

In 1839, a woman of Mymensing, when suffering from a paroxysm of pain in her stomach to which she had been for some time subject, took up a sickle and killed her two children, and then endeavoured to cut her own throat.§ Further remarks upon this curious subject will be found in the Chapters on *Suicide* and *Insanity*.

FRACTURES AND DISLOCATIONS.

Was the skull fractured before or after death? Dr. Beatson has mentioned ‖ a case of beating on the head, in which there was an irregular wound on the forehead, and a comminuted fracture of the frontal bone, which was completely crushed in. The body was far advanced in decom-

---

* Police Report, L. P., for 1868, p. 273.

† Nizamut Adawlut Reports, September 18th, 1855, p. 420.

‡ Bengal Police Report for 1868, p. 57.

§ Police Rep., L. P., for 1840, p. 67.

‖ Indian Medical Gazette, 1st April 1866, p. 84.

position, the integuments of the face falling off, and the *os frontis* polished clean by the swarms of maggots, which covered the face and filled the cavity of the skull. Dr. Beatson considered that, if there had been only a wound of the scalp, it would have been difficult to decide as to its having been inflicted during, or having been caused by, the depredations of the maggots; but the existence of the comminuted fracture of the skull was decisive, as Casper's experiments have proved that it is almost impossible to fracture the skull of a dead body by the most powerful blows administered by means of heavy mallets or hammers.

I think that, in these cases, we should only receive Casper's view* with due regard to the form of the weapon and the force with which it is used. Casper says, "In making these experiments, we have usually employed the wooden mallet used to prop up the skull and spinal canal during the process of dissection. In other cases, we have employed hammers and similar weapons. The most powerful blows struck downward upon the body, laid horizontally, were mostly without result, and only after repeated violent blows were we enabled to produce perhaps one or a few fissures in the occipital or parietal bones, or in the temporal bone (squamous portion), and certainly more easily in the latter. We were unable to produce more considerable effects, such as a complete smashing of the skull or fissure of its base, even in one single instance."

Admitting, to a considerable extent, the truth of Casper's argument that the dead skull is less easily fractured than the living one, it is evident that there is scarcely any mode of applying the same degree of force, which the cranial arch could better sustain, than that which a man's arm could impart to a very broad mallet of the kind described. We all know how easy it is to remove the calvarium with the hammer used for that purpose, and there is no reason to believe that the dead skull is proof against comminution by blows from such instruments as a crow-bar, or pick-axe, or the back of a bill-hook.

Allusion has already been made, at p. 340, to certain medico-legal points in connexion with *Injuries to the Head.* A not unfrequent mode of homicide in the North-West, and specially in the Saugor and Nerbudda Territories, is *Pounding the Face with a Heavy Stone.* It appeared in the trial of Hoonah, *rajpoot*, of Saugor, that he attacked a woman, in a much frequented road, and pounded her face with a stone about half a seer (a pound) in weight. Persons attracted by her cries came up, and the murderer was knocked down and secured. They found the woman still alive, but she expired soon afterwards. So dreadful was the assault, that her face was completely smashed in, and portions of the upper and lower jaw (the latter with teeth attached), were found lying separated. The prisoner's naked body was covered with her blood. As the prisoner was

* Forensic Medicine, Vol. I., pp. 244, 5, and 6.

being secured, the woman's gold nose-ring fell from his hand. This the Courts held, with great reason, to be " one of those cases in which, to use the words of an eminent English Judge, it is so difficult to define the invisible line which divides perfect and partial insanity." He was sentenced to imprisonment, in irons, for life.*

Chook Kaie, of Nagode (Saugor), having gone to bring his wife home, probably much against her will, remained some days at her brother's house, and then the pair started on their way homeward. A short time afterwards, the woman ran to a village, saying that thieves had killed her husband. The body was found about seven miles from her brother's house, lying in a nullah, some ten paces off the road. A stone, bearing marks of blood, lay near the corpse. It was shown that the fatal blow, or blows, had completely crushed in the skull from the side of the face, taking effect on the forehead, right eye and nose, to all appearance simultaneously. The woman appears to have given three contradictory statements of the manner in which her husband was killed—that she had been struck by him, and had retaliated by striking him on the head with a stone—that he had been killed by thieves,—and that he had fallen while she was absent getting water. The Sessions Judge remarked that no fall of a mere drunken man, carrying only the force of his own weight, unless it occurred from a considerable height, which was here not pretended to have been the case, could have caused so complete a fracture of the frontal bone and disfigurement of the features; nor would the injury, so received, have been likely to have taken the direction of the injury under comment, which, in itself, led to the almost necessary inference of its having been inflicted with the blood-stained sharp-angled mass of stone produced, which the prisoner must have exerted some strength even to have uplifted. Sentence—transportation for life.†

A young man, of Hoshungabad, in the same territory, having been engaged in a gambling transaction with several persons, they set upon him, some tying his arms and legs, others strangling him with his own turban cloth, and pounding his face and body with stones.‡

A Banda man enticed away a boy of ten or twelve, wearing valuable ornaments, cut his throat, and violently pounded him with a heavy stone.§

In 1852, three persons were sentenced to death, at Bareilly, for murdering a man, by beating him on the face with lattees and an iron coulter. "The bones of the head and face were shattered to pieces, so that even the jaws and teeth were broken into several small pieces.‖

---

* Nizamut Adawlut Reports, N. W. P., 30th March 1852, p. 231.

† *Ibid*, 3rd May 1854, p. 231.

‡ *Ibid*, 28th Jan. 1853, p. 125.

§ *Ibid*, 8th May 1854, p. 495.

‖ *Ibid*, 30th Oct. 1852, p. 1260.

A woman was sentenced to death, at Bareilly, for the murder of a girl of ten, for the sake of her ornaments. The Civil Surgeon found the poor child's face and head "brutally wounded, beaten into a mass by repeated blows."*

A boy, ten or twelve years old, of Bareilly, was found guilty of having enticed away a poor child, nine or ten years old, and of having murdered him for the sake of his ornaments. The child was found in a dry well. The front teeth were broken, the upper lip divided, the inside of the mouth injured. There were fourteen wounds on the cheeks, one cheek bone was fractured, so that part of it came away. There were four wounds on the neck, by two of which the coats of the vessels were exposed. The native doctor who examined the body thought it probable that these injuries must have been inflicted with some partly pointed instrument, such as a tent-peg. The poor child lingered some days, and was said to have stated that the boy and a man were his assailants.†

These cases also occur in Bengal. In 1849, two prisoners were sentenced to imprisonment for life, for having murdered a man in the Bhaugulpore District, by beating him on the head with a stone.‡

In 1853, Omrao, of Sarun, killed his wife by pounding her about the head and face with a stone used for grinding curry, &c. It appeared that he had first cut her about the face, and that part of her under lip had been cut off. He was found to be insane.§

Chogra pleaded guilty of having killed a man, whom he found in adultery with the wife of his late master, by taking up a large stone which was lying at hand, weighing seven and-a-half seers (fifteen pounds) and dashing it on his head, whereby the skull was fractured and death occurred almost instantaneously.‖

Forbes relates the fate of a Gour Brahmin, Cutwal of Poonah, who, being held responsible for the death of thirty-four Telinga Brahmins who had been confined in a close room, was given over by the Peshwa to a furious mob. One of his hands was tied to the end of a turban, the other end being held by some Hallalcores (outcast Hindus); twelve Brahmins of the offended tribe attacked him with large stones. The outcasts, by straitening the turban, kept him at full length running in a circle pursued by his relentless murderers, who, at length, by repeated blows, brought him to the ground and there despatched him by a succession of large stones thrown violently on his head and breast (Vol. I., p. 412).

I once examined the body of an unfortunate policeman, whose frontal

---

* Nizamut Adawlut Reports, N. W. P., 12th Jan. 1853, p. 46.

† *Ibid*, 30th July 1852, p. 750.

‡ Police Reports for 1849, p. 17.

§ Nizamut Adawlut Reports, 18th March 1855, p. 332.

‖ *Ibid*, January 15th, 1857, p. 22.

bone was smashed through the sinuses in various directions, evidently by often-repeated blows.

The *peeree* or *pinrah*, a small but very solid wooden stool used by the natives of Bengal when eating their meals, is frequently snatched up and used with very serious effect. These cases are numerous. One will suffice here. Sheikh Pookeea, of Mymensingh, was found guilty of culpable homicide for having, in an altercation about some kitchen utensils, struck Shoma Sheikh on the head with a *peeree*, inflicting a fracture of the skull, of which he died sixteen days afterwards. The Civil Assistant Surgeon found that the front part of deceased's skull was fractured, and that the anterior lobes of the brain were very much injured, that these injuries were the cause of his death, and that there were also three contusions on the head in addition to the fracture.* For other cases of mortal injury caused by blows inflicted with *pinrahs*, *see* the Section on *Homicide committed by Persons in great Pain*, Chapter on *Insanity*.

I met with a remarkable case of fracture of the skull when at Chittagong. A Kookie brought in the extremely putrid body of his murdered child, a girl five or six years old, whom some person had struck on the head with a club. The scalp had nearly lost all traces of texture, the broken skull moved in it like a smashed cocoanut in a bag. Upon removing the bones of the calvarium, which were broken to pieces and separated at the sutures, I found that, in several very large patches, they exhibited remarkable specimens of that form of nævus which is known as aneurism by anastomosis involving the bone. The parts were sent to the Medical College Museum. This disease had added much to the natural fragility of the bone; but, as the fatal blow must have been very severe, its existence could not have detracted from the assailant's guilt.

In 1855, a man was sentenced to death, at Hoshungabad, for the murder of a person whom he killed while sleeping, with a single stab on the crown of the head with a *kutar*, or dagger.†

A woman, of Azimgurh, confessed that she had murdered a child, *her own nephew*, with a packing needle‡ and a stone pestle. The native doctor deposed that there was a stab over the right eyebrow, which, in its downward passage, had pierced and thrust out the eye. Three of the left ribs had been fractured, and had wounded the spleen. He considered that the iron needle, about seven inches in length, used for sewing up the necks of canvas sacks, was probably the instrument with which

---

* Nizamut Adawlut Reports, April 14th, 1857, p. 503.

† *Ibid*, N. W. P., 29th March 1855, p. 425.

‡ "If death be inflicted with a Packing Needle (*misullah*) it is wilful homicide."—*Harington's Mahomedan Law*, p. 266.

the stab was inflicted, and that the stone pestle would have caused fracture of the ribs, if applied with force.*

The following case is of singular interest in a surgical point of view, and is, as far as I am aware, unique.

In December 1868, Baboo Chunder Mohun Ghose, Second Demonstrator of Anatomy in the Calcutta Medical College, met with a calvarium which is now preserved in the College Museum. An iron headless nail, or "brad," about an inch long, had penetrated the frontal bone in the mesial line, had passed completely through the longitudinal sinus, and had divided the layers of the falx cerebri, between which its point is seen. Consequently its shaft, which does not appear to be corroded, stood in the mid-current of blood of the sinus, precisely as the pier of a bridge does in a river. It appears, latterly, to have caused no inconvenience whatever. The scalp displayed some rather indistinct irregular cicatrices, the edges of the hole in the frontal bone which the butt end of the brad still occupies, are so rounded that it looks like an arterial foramen, and there was not the faintest trace of inflammatory change within. The subject was a native male.

As many huts are blown down every year in Bengal, the nail may have been driven in by an accident of this kind. Or it may be the evidence of a crime resembling that of the Cenci.† *See* a somewhat similar case, by Mr. Piddington, in the Chapter on *Hanging with a view to conceal murder*.

A very singular plea was raised by a prisoner at Cawnpore. A girl eight years old was missing. She had been last seen with one Mussamut Subjadee, her next-door neighbour. This woman admitted that the child had been with her that morning, but that she had brought her back, and left her at her own door. The child's nurse desired Subjadee to open her door. Upon her refusal, the nurse brought the police, who found the door locked on the outside, the woman having gone to a neighbour's house. She was brought, and the door was forced. Nothing was found in the first and second rooms; and, as they approached the third room, Subjadee blew out the *chirag*, and seized the clothes of the child's nurse. The lamp being re-lit, the body of the child was found in the third room, pressed down under a board or door, upon which earth had been heaped. No marks of violence were, at first, discovered

---

* Nizamut Adawlut Reports, N. W. P., 9th September 1853, p. 1145.

† I am indebted to my friend and colleague Dr. J. Phin Smith for a note, from the Italian, of the manner in which Francesco Cenci is said to have been murdered. "Two long nails, like those used in the suffering of Christ, were used. One held a nail over the eye, the other drove it into the brain. The other nail was driven into the throat. The women drew the nails out, and, assisted by the bravos, threw the body over the terrace. It caught the branches of an alder tree. Among the thousand lacerations which the body thus sustained, the marks of the two nails were not observed."

on the body with the exception of a slight abrasion on the temple. In a front *kothree,* forming part of the *burota,* near the entrance door, were found a silver *balee* (the child was found to have seven of these in one ear, and only six in the other) and several fragments of lac bracelet belonging to the prisoner (it is elsewhere said in the report that these belonged to the child, but this appears to be an error), which were considered to have been broken by the grasp of the child's hand. There were slight traces of what might have been a sprinkling of blood (although it was considered that very little could have flowed from the wound, and the earth was found trodden and trampled at that spot). The civil surgeon found a small contused wound on the back of the head. It was hidden by the hair, and had bled so little that it was, at first, overlooked. Beneath this was a very extensive fracture of the skull, with effusion of blood on the brain, which, he considered, must have caused immediate death. He believed it to be the result of a heavy blow from some such instrument as a *lattee.* Certain leading portions of the evidence of the child's nurse were manifestly false. The prisoner declared that, on the day in question, several monkeys had seized and bitten the finger of a niece of one Saadut Khan, and that, when driven from that child, they had come to her house and attacked *her,* that the nurse of the deceased and another had got on the roof of the house and driven the monkeys inside the house, "leaving the deceased with them, and that, probably, they may have killed the child while inside." She immediately locked her door and went away. "*The monkeys killed the child,*" and the nurse, being afraid, hid the body in her (prisoner's) house, but she was not present at the time. A witness confirmed the statement that the child's nurse had awakened him by calling out that the monkeys were attacking a child of Saadut Khan, and he got up and drove them away. After this he heard the prisoner call out that the monkeys were attacking *her,* but he appears to have retired to sleep again. This happened two *gurrees* before the child was sought for by her nurse. One of the Judges of the Superior Court observed that,—"monkeys attacking a child could never cause severe fracture of the skull, such as was here proved to have been the cause of death." It is not mentioned whether the opinion of the medical officer was consulted upon this point. The child's ornaments were not worth more than eight annas, but it was considered that the prisoner had murdered the child on account of a disagreement between her family and that of the nurse. Sentence—imprisonment for life.*

Baboo Bholanauth Chunder says that, at Muttra, the monkeys threw

---

* Nizamut Adawlut Reports, N. W. P., 16th Sept. 1854, p. 364.

an old woman from a terrace as she was looking down at a procession passing below (Vol. II., p. 82).

CRUSHING IN THE THORAX.

Murder is frequently perpetrated in India by *Pressing or Trampling upon the Chest.* The injuries are not, in themselves, of any peculiar surgical interest; but the opinion of the medical witness may be required as to whether they were merely received in a furious struggle, or were deliberately caused by compression of the chest by weights or bamboos.

The reports contain many cases of both kinds.

Bans-dola

Is a practice well known in Bengal, especially in the Northern districts. It is a mode of compressing and rolling the limbs or body between two bamboos with a degree of severity ranging between that which tortures severely, by contusing the muscles, or by rendering respiration difficult, and that which reduces the muscles to a jelly or breaks in the ribs, and crushes the lungs into a disorganized pulp.

In 1840, the *Friend of India* published the following authenticated statement: "A theft took place a short time ago in the district of Dinagepore; the buxee of the thannah proceeded to the spot to investigate, seized a number of the ryots, and in order to make them confess, tortured them. I will mention one man's case, whom one of the ryots, under torture, named as being the purchaser of some of the articles stolen. The man was seized, a bamboo was placed under his shoulders, another across the chest; two men then pressed at the opposite ends of the upper bamboo, and the tongue was forced from his mouth; the brutes, supposing the man was shamming, attempted to force the tongue back, in doing which, some of the man's teeth were fortunately knocked out; had not this occurred, he would have died, as, from the swollen state of the tongue, no nourishment could be given him. Five days after it took place, it came to the notice of an European, who sent the man to the Magistrate; that functionary being absent, the doctor of the station humanely kept him on his own premises, and can speak to the horrid state the poor man was in. The man, to my knowledge, remained fourteen days without being able to present a petition, on accouut of non-attendance of the Magistrate at cutcherry. A number of these ryots also proceeded to the station; but after waiting about twenty days, and finding it impossible to get their petitions heard, and also learning that it may be three or four months before their cases would be decided, they returned to their homes, which will be an encouragement to the police to act in the same manner again."

A correspondent of the *Hurkaru* confirms this account, observing: "The punishment, called in Dinagepore and Rungpore *Bans-dola,* is in common use at some of the thannahs, when required. The sufferer is put on his back on the ground, with arms and legs extended; a bamboo is put before both thighs, and another exactly opposite behind, and they are then tied tightly together at the ends; about four or five inches lower down the thighs, other two are applied as above described, so that the flesh between the superior and inferior bamboos is put on the stretch, the skin being quite tight. This part is beaten with a ruler. The pain is great, and it must be used with much force if any marks be left. When moderately used, a slight general swelling is the result, but it may easily be mistaken for a natural stoutness. The skin is never injured, and, consequently, the torture is seldom discovered. In a certain district, which shall be nameless, a native had it applied to extort a confession; the consequence was, that the thigh mortified, and the man died in the hospital, under the Surgeon, who reported the case to the Magistrate, and the thanadar (or jemadar) was punished by imprisonment, I believe, for six months or a year."

A dacoity having been committed in the Dinapore district, certain persons were taken into custody by the police. When they were brought before the native inspector, Tarini Churn Chatterjee, the inspector struck one of them, Hurree Mistree, one or two blows, and then ordered the constables to subject him to torture in order to compel him to give up the money. He was, accordingly, subjected to frightful torture, the result of which was that he consented to go to his house and produce the money. Accordingly, he was taken to his house, being at the time in a very feeble state, but was unable to produce any money. Whether or no he was again tortured does not seem certain, but at any rate he soon appeared to be in a dying state, whereupon the constables left him, and he died shortly afterwards. The body was examined by the Civil Surgeon, who described it as having been covered from head to foot with bruises. The 4th, 5th, 9th, 10th, and 11th ribs of the right side were broken, and the 8th, 9th, 10th, and 11th ribs were dislocated on both sides of the spine. Both lungs were injured, and the *whole* of the muscles of the back, shoulders and loins, were *reduced to a pulp.* In the opinion of the civil surgeon these injuries were produced by blows, and by a rolling heavy weight. He considered that the ill-treatment must have continued for a considerable time. The evidence of the witnesses went to show that Hurree Mistree was tortured, at intervals, from the time he was arrested, about 4 P.M., up to or nearly up to the time when he died, about 7½ P.M.; that he was beaten and poked by the constables, with their staves, their wooden sandals and their elbows, and that his body was jumped upon. The constables were sentenced to transportation for life, the inspector for seven years.

The following notes of the appearances found in the body of a man supposed to have died from *Bans-dola* were given me by Baboo Koylas Chunder Chatterjee, Sub-Assistant Surgeon of Baraset.

In 1860, corpse of a male, Boshoodeb Poad, sent in March 9. Face, natural in expression ; eyes shut ; no rigidity of the body and extremities ; dark reddish and bluish patches on the face, back, and extremities, except the right lower limb;—left leg and arm swollen. A small punctured wound, an inch deep, just above the left elbow joint. Diffused extravasation of blood in the cellular tissue, under the skin and between the muscles of the left upper and lower limbs. The right arm had a similar appearance, but the extravasation of blood was less. There was no extravasation in front of the chest and abdomen, but it was found on the back, especially along the spine up to the occiput. There was no fracture or dislocation ; no effusion of blood into the spinal canal, or in front of the neck. Some half-coagulated blood in the intestinal canal. Blood spots on the surface of the lungs ; reddish effusion in the pericardium ; heart flabby and empty ; bloody effusion in the pleural cavity; the vessels on the surface of the brain distended. The Sub-Assistant Surgeon gave it as his opinion that death was caused by the irritation of the extensive bruises, inflammation of the intestines, and effusion into the cavities of the chest caused by the pressure, with rolling motion, of some hard substance or substances, such as bamboos.

Question of the amount of Pressure which the arch of the Thorax is capable of bearing.

It is needful that, in the class of injuries noticed above, medical and judicial officers should be able to form some definite idea of the amount of force needful to crush in the chest of an adult. A clue to this is obtainable from recorded cases, in which the *peine forte et dure* was inflicted in England.

It will be remembered that, in this barbarous infliction of *The Press*, it was considered an act of mercy to heap on *suddenly* sufficient weight to extinguish life by crushing in the ribs.

At the Lewies Assizes in 1735, a man had laid upon him, one by one, three hundred-weight,—then fifty pounds more. When he was nearly dead, "having all the agonies of death upon him," the executioner, who weighed about 16 or 17 stone, lay down upon the board which was over him, and killed him in an instant.

In January 1720, William Spiggott, at the Old Bailey, bore four hundred-weight of iron on his body for more than an hour, and, thereafter, was hanged at Tyburn. At the Old Bailey, in January 1721, a highwayman, after enduring the punishment an hour, and having three or four hundred-weight put upon him, at last submitted to plead.

At about the same time, one Haines continued under the Press with 250 pounds for seven minutes, and was released on his submission.

We do not gather from the above facts anything to show under what weight the very strong arch formed by a man's ribs and sternum would be forced in. We, however, see that fatal embarrassment of respiration sets in under a pressure of between 300 and 400 pounds. It is probable that the shock of a body of considerably less weight than this, suddenly cast upon the chest of one lying on his back, would crush in the ribs. It is stated to have been the practice, in some cases, to destroy life by placing a corner of the press-board over the heart.

Enough is here shown to prove that, where it is discovered that most of the ribs on both sides have been fractured, any attempt to show that *moderate* violence occasioned such injury must be set aside.

While writing on this subject, I had some conversation regarding it with Dr. Kenneth McLeod, who mentioned that he had seen such a case in a Lunatic Asylum at Home, many ribs having sustained *double* fracture. Several of these cases have lately occurred in England. One of the latest is that of James Doran, aged fifty-two, who died in the Prestwich Lunatic Asylum early in June 1870. Seven ribs were broken without any corresponding marks of violence. He had been for some time in the Rochdale Union Workhouse, and died in the Asylum on the day of his admission. There was no evidence to show when or how the injuries were inflicted, and the jury found that the man died from natural causes, death being accelerated by injuries, but that there was no evidence to show how the injuries were caused. *The Pall Mall Gazette*, which has been very persistent in calling attention to the many recently recorded cases of this kind, insists that they must have been produced " by heavy quiet pressure, such, for instance, as a heavy man kneeling on the chest." It asks if any other tenable surgical hypothesis can be suggested.* I apprehend that heavy *sudden* pressure,—as where, the patient and a keeper struggling at arm's length, both fall, the keeper uppermost with his knee on the chest,—is far more likely to cause such injury.

It would appear, from a recent newspaper report,† that one of these cases of chest-crushing has occurred in the Colaba Asylum, Bombay. The sufferer was a native, named Gunnoo, who is described as having been so far insane, that he gave absurd answers to questions, was apt to ill-use children, and was addicted to mischievous practices. He was spoken of as a quiet, harmless man, rather silly than mad. He had been

* Brit. Med. Jour., June 18, 1868, p. 635.

† Calcutta *Englishman*, June 13th, 1870.

in the asylum six months, when he became restless, filthy in his habits, and destructive; and the head overseer instructed his subordinates to keep their eye upon him. He was placed in a separate cell with bedding. One day he refused his breakfast and dinner. In the evening he was evidently in a very low state, as beef tea, and sago conjee with brandy were prescribed. While raising him to give him the conjee, the overseer discovered that there was a rib broken. He appears to have died a few minutes subsequently. On examination, it was found that six ribs had recently been fractured, and that there was a rupture of the liver. There were no exterior marks of violence. Dr. Niven gave it as his opinion that "the injuries were inflicted by violent pressure applied by the knees or feet, whether in a struggle with the warders, or with some other insane patient, it was impossible to say.

Dr. Thompson Dickson has lately shown, at the Pathological Society, some "ricketty bones" from an insane patient, aged forty, who had died after an epileptiform seizure, with general paralysis. The bones were very soft and exceedingly fragile. Dr. Dickson referred to cases of fractured ribs in asylums, which have recently engaged public attention, and observed that all the recent cases of broken ribs in lunatic asylums had occurred in patients with general paralysis, and he brought these specimens forward to show how easily bones in such patients may be fractured. In commenting upon this, the Pall Mall Budget alludes to a case of "*twelve smashed ribs and a crushed breast-bone.*"

This pathological question certainly demands further attention and investigation; but, in the meantime, we may feel satisfied that, although the ribs of a Bengali are not exceptionally strong, no justifiable force is sufficient to crush in his chest.

An effectual mode of inflicting this kind of death is mentioned in the *Seir Mutaqherin*. The report ran, and it was generally believed, that Prince Mirza Mehdi, younger brother of Suraj-ud-dowla, "was forced between two of those wooden frames called *taqhtas*, where they conserve shawls and other precious goods, and that, the ropes having been strained hard at one and the same time, he had been squeezed to death."* See also notice of a similar practice in the Chapter on Human Sacrifice, p. 404.

I find three cases, in which it is probable that the chest was crushed in *by one person only*. The civil surgeon of Mymensingh found, in examining the body of one stated to have met his death from beating, having been detected in burglary, that eight ribs on each side were fractured, some in two places. The external bone of the forearm was also fractured. There was no evidence that any but the accused, Sheikh Joomun, had assaulted the deceased. Before the police and Magistrate, he stated that, as deceased was making his escape, he chased him and struck him a blow, and the deceased having fallen on the

* Op. Cit., Vol. II., p. 8.

ground, he assaulted him with his hands and feet. In the Judge's Court he denied the charge, and stated that he only struck him a blow with a stick.*

Unuchia Dosadh, of Behar, was seen in one direction beating and cuffing one Chottrao Gwala, and, afterwards, in another direction, striking him with a *lohangee*, or iron-bound club. There was no proof that any but Unuchia committed the act. There were six external marks of violence, and the right ear was half torn off. "On opening the chest, the ribs, on both sides, were found fractured, with the exception of two or three. The lungs had been pierced on both sides by the broken ends of the ribs, and, on the left side, the vena-cava had been ruptured close to its entrance into the heart." The Judge held that the beating with the *lohangee*, as seen by witnesses, would not account for the fatal injuries. Moreover, the iron rings, with which this weapon was armed, would have left external marks of a different character. Dr. Allen was of opinion that such external injuries must have been caused by repeated blows, and that deceased had probably been stamped upon. The deceased's singular submission under such prolonged maltreatment was, the Judge thought, only to be accounted for, either from his being intoxicated at the time or from the prisoner's being the more powerful and violent man of the two.†

In the third case of this kind, Sheikh Busha, of Mymensingh, was capitally sentenced for murdering his wife. He confessed, but merely admitted that he had struck her once. A woman saw him killing his wife in the jungle. The poor young woman was lying on her back apparently insensible. It was found that there were seven ribs on the left, and eight on the right fractured. The chest was severely bruised. These injuries must have been caused by heavy blows on the chest, and kicking in that region, or stamping on the chest would have produced the injuries.‡

More frequently several persons are engaged in these violent acts.

In 1842, Dr. Beatson, of Shahabad, reported his examination of the bodies of two individuals who had met with violent deaths at the same time :—"Ajrowal Doosaud was covered with bruises about the head and back of his neck, and all the bones of the chest were broken in by kicks or blows. Gopal Aheer was covered with bruises, and had the bones of his chest all broken in ;—these men were killed in a most shameful manner, and by brutal violence."

Seven Hindus were tried in the Court of the 24-Pergunnahs and acquitted in the matter of the death of Jaffer Meer, a Mahomedan. Whoever committed the crime, it appeared certain that death was caused partly by injuires inflicted by clubs and spears, and partly by stamping

---

* Nizamut Adawlut Reports, Dec. 31, 1870, p. 982.

† *Ibid*, Aug. 25, 1856, p. 264.

‡ *Ibid*, Sept. 25, 1855, p. 428.

upon or otherwise violently pressing upon his chest and body. The medical testimony was distinct that the deceased died of the injury to the chest, and that the spear and other wounds were inflicted *before death*. In this case a rather important question of *medical evidence* arose.

"Mr. Montriou, on behalf of prisoner No. 1, urged that the deposition of Dr. Strong could not be taken as conclusive of the violent death of Jaffer Meer; that it was opposed to the science of the present day; and that the state which he represents the body to have exhibited, *viz.*, that of a great quantity of extravasated blood in the left lung, and a large quantity of coagulated blood in the heart, might have arisen from natural causes; moreover, that the opinion regarding the spear wounds to the effect that, if inflicted on the corpse after death, they would not have bled, was incorrect. In support of these views, Mr. Montriou referred to various passages in Taylor's Medical Jurisprudence."

The Court ruled that "the depositions of Dr. Strong are the only medical evidence on the record; had the prisoners wished to impugn the accuracy of Dr. Strong's medical opinion, they should have summoned medical evidence in the Court below for the purpose of contradicting that opinion *on the facts as deposed to by Dr. Strong;* as that has not been done, and as Dr. Strong's evidence is the opinion of a scientific person, resting on his personal observation and on facts within his own knowledge, and is *unopposed by any scientific evidence to a contrary effect*, the Court cannot venture, as it has been urged to do, itself to supply any doctrine laid down in a text book on medical jurisprudence to the particular facts deposed to by Dr. Strong, but accepts that opinion as to the immediate cause of the death of Jaffer Meer."*

Thirteen persons were sentenced to fourteen years' imprisonment at Rungpore, for causing the death of a man whom, it appeared in evidence, they had "pommelled well with fists and clubs, and thrown down under a tree. One prisoner gave him a blow with a thick club on the head, and another used the same club, striking him on the chest in the way in which a pavior uses his rammer." The Civil Surgeon found the chest much flattened, his ribs almost without exception broken; his abdomen bruised; a wound, not of so severe a nature, however, as to account for his death, on the head, and severe bruises on other parts of the body. The sharp edges of the fractured ribs had entered the lungs. In his opinion the injury to the chest was the cause of death; and death, he thought, must have occurred within a short interval. On being informed of the nature of the evidence, as to the nature of the violence and treatment to which deceased had been subjected, he expressed his opinion that the injuries received might have been caused, in the way

---

* Nizamut Adawlut Reports, October 3rd, 1856, p. 759.

stated, though he thought it likely that more violence must have been used than the two blows deposed to as having been inflicted on the chest, to cause the fracture of all the ribs in the manner described. He did not consider it likely that the ribs could have been thus fractured by any blows inflicted while he was standing, or being dragged along before being thrown to the ground, unless some compression from sticks before and behind had been used, which would require much force, and was therefore not so probable. The evidence would seem to preclude the idea of any compression, such as is suggested as a possible cause, having been used; and, had it been, deceased would, doubtless, have mentioned it. He could, therefore, but conclude that the injuries to the chest were inflicted after deceased had been thrown on the ground: probably some of the ribs may have been broken before the last three blows were struck, but there can be little doubt that blows struck with the weapon, and in the way described, would be very likely to break the ribs or to drive them into the lungs as described.*

It was proved that, nine persons of Mymensingh having been drinking together until a late hour, one of them was set upon by the others and killed. The skull was fractured extensively in front; the upper part of the breast-bone was smashed and driven into the chest; five ribs on the left and four on the right were broken, and the cavity of the chest was full of blood.†

Three Chittagong men inflicted the following injuries upon one whom they caught in the act of burglary. Dr. Beatson deposed that death was evidently caused by severe beating. "There were many bruises and scratches. Beneath the scalp there was a quantity of serous effusion with spots of bruising, the brain was congested, and a layer of blood was poured out over its surface. Beneath the integument of the chest, extensive bruises were found; the ribs on the right side, from the 2nd to the 10th, were fractured about three inches from the cartilages; the same ribs on the left side were similarly fractured, and were also fractured posteriorly about three inches from the spine." That these severe injuries were caused by being knelt or trampled on, and that the man must have been most cruelly treated.‡

An intriguer at Rungpore was seized at night, when on the way to his mistress's house, by her relations, and was killed by the following injuries:—Extensive contusions on the back over the right ribs. Three of the lower ribs in front were broken. The spleen was ruptured on the concave side to the extent of about three inches, and about a pound of dark blood was found in the cavity of the abdomen. There was,

---

* Nizamut Adawlut Reports, December 18th, 1856, p. 1082.

† *Ibid*, June 9th, 1857, p. 745.

‡ *Ibid*, March 11th, 1859, p. 43.

moreover, a dislocation of the vertebræ of the neck, which the medical officer was of opinion took place after death, as there was no contusion or extravasation apparent. He considered it probable that the deceased had been lying stomach downwards, and that the contusions were caused by blows of the fist, or feet, or by some one jumping on his back while so lying. The spleen was diseased.*

In a trial at Hooghly it appeared that the three prisoners and deceased were drinking taree together until two in the morning. It was not shown what happened afterwards until the corpse was found. The Civil Assistant Surgeon deposed that he "found the brain in a state of inflammation, probably the effect of over-drinking. The lungs were squeezed to pieces, the undoubted effect of violence. In fact, the deceased was, in some way unknown, squeezed to death." †

In the case of a man of notoriously bad character, who was killed, it was said, on being caught in an act of burglary, it was "discovered that deceased had extensive marks of injury; the extremities were covered with contusions; so was also the scalp. Both bones of the left wrist were fractured. On the left side, nearly every rib was broken, some of them in two or more places; several ribs on the right side were also fractured; the lung on the left side was lacerated by the broken ribs." All this was supposed to have been done by the village chowkeedar, who acknowledged having struck several blows with a spear and lattee.‡

A man of Pubnah had formed a connexion with the younger wife of his neighbour; and, wishing to compel the husband to give her up, applied to the talookdar. The husband was sent for, and ordered to sign an agreement to give up his wife. This he declined to do, and ran home. He was again taken, dragged before the talookdar, severely beaten, and fined 50 rupees. He again escaped, was retaken, and was then subjected to such cruel treatment, that he expired almost immediately upon reaching home. His ribs were broken, and his private parts injured.§

It appeared, in a case tried at Rungpore, that a zemindar's mahout, having begun to fish in a ditch belonging to one Shebah, was opposed by the latter, and a quarrel ensued. Shebah, who was lame, was pushed down, and, upon rising, struck the mahout with a stick; the other then wrested the stick out of his hand, struck him two or three blows with it, and knocked him down. They then both went to the house of the zemindar to settle their dispute,—the mahout, it was said, pushing Shebah as they went along. The medical officer considered that the

---

* Nizamut Adawlut Reports, September 30th, 1856, p. 700.

† *Ibid*, July 11th, 1855, p. 50.

‡ *Ibid*, July 31st, 1587, p. 122.

§ Police Report, L. P., 1844, p. 31.

violence stated by the witnesses was not sufficient to cause the injuries found on Shebah's body after death. It is not certainly known what followed until he was *carried* home, almost dead, by two of the accused. He expired that evening. Mr. Taylor found a contusion on the temple and cheek; the spleen ruptured, four ribs broken, and great extravasation of blood. He considered that the injuries appeared to have been inflicted by continued pressure with a heavy weight, or by stamping on the body, or they might have been inflicted by the heel or palms of the hands, as there was no abrasion or contusion of the skin. The superior Court considered that the deceased was barbarously maltreated after he arrived at the zemindar's house.*

Certain persons, also of Rungpore, having obtained a decree in the Moonsiff's Court against an old and sickly man, named Khurdee, went with the warrant to apprehend him. He escaped on their approach into a neighbour's house; two of the party were ordered to bring him out. After a short time, they came out supporting him by the arms, while his legs were dragged along. In this way he was brought speechless into the outer yard—(*he had made no noise when in the hut*)—where, on being let go, he rolled over, and blood was seen issuing from his mouth. He soon afterwards expired. The prisoners promising to give up the decree, and to pay rupees 10 for the funeral expenses, and to remove the attachment of the property, the wretched relatives concealed the murder, and the body was buried the same evening. But, these promises not being fulfilled, the deceased's son, six days afterwards, complained, when the body was dug up and examined. It was found that the third rib on either side was broken, the soft parts over the whole of the ribs were contused, the lungs were inflated and congested with blood, and a small quantity of blood was also extravasated into the cavity of the chest. The medical officer was of opinion that these injuries were, most probably, caused by heavy pressure, though it was possible, he believed, that they resulted from blows.†

At Chota Nagpore a man was thrown down, and had a heavy stone placed on his breast. His mother removed it; he got up, and was cut down with an axe.‡

Another Chota Nagpore man stated, at his trial, that the darogah extorted his confession by putting a stone on his chest.§

In 1868, a Behar man was called to work on a new well in the Ticarry Zemindaree Cutcherry, but, on his refusal to do so, he was bound hand

* Nizamut Adawlut Reports, 8th Nov. 1853, p. 746.
† *Ibid*, 17th Nov. 1854, p. 608.
‡ *Ibid*, May 30, 1855, p. 642.
§ *Ibid*, Dec. 7, 1855, p. 161.

and foot, and kicked. Ultimately, a heavy stone was placed on his chest; he died in consequence.*

A man, of Saharunpore, was sentenced by the Sessions Judge for having killed his wife, by striking her on the breast, with a heavy stone. The case was thrown out on appeal.†

It is probable that the full truth is seldom revealed in these cases; still the following extract from the decision of a Judge of the High Court, in the case of a Hindu landlord, who, upon addressing irritating and abusive language to certain defaulters among his Mussulmaun ryots, was set upon by them and killed on the spot, appears to show that such injury may be inflicted without premeditation: "It is clearly proved, in this instance, that the prisoner Alee Mahomed seized the deceased by the throat, threw him down, and held him by the throat with both his hands, while he pressed his chest with his knee, and the other prisoners kicked and beat him. The injuries inflicted on the body were fracture of all the ribs on both sides, from the second downwards, and of the sternum, the heart and liver being ruptured by the points of the broken ribs. The throat showed that the deceased was also strangled by pressure of the fingers, and the marks of the nails were visible after death."‡

In the following case the confessions before the magistrate of the prisoners afford some idea of the mechanism of these cases of *pounding;* but, unfortunately, there was no *post-mortem* examination to confirm them. At least three persons of Sylhet, having caught an intriguer, threw him on the ground; some beat him with their hands and feet, and some with bamboos; two of them placed a *moosul,* or wooden pestle, three feet long and five inches thick, generally used for pounding grain, across the deceased's heart, and they sat on each end of the *moosul,* and squeezed him with it, while two others were pushing a stick into his navel. When he was nearly dead, they bound him hand and foot, and carried him away and threw him near his house.§

It would certainly be worth while to inquire, whether the natives have not several modes of inflicting these frightful injuries.

In further illustration of the extreme violence employed in these murders, I shall cite the following details from reports by Dr. Denham, of Behar (two cases), Mr. Mahaffy, of Chumparun, and Dr. Macaush, of East Burdwan.

---

* Bengal Police Reports, 1868, p. 151. The Revd. Mr. ——, of Rupert's Land, stated in a sermon, at which I was present, that, at one of his out-stations, Great Whale River, a native convert, named Mary, having been attacked with fever after delivery, her husband placed her in the hands of two conjurers, who laid her upon her face, and rolled a large stone over her body until she died.

† Nizamut Adawlut Reports, N. W. P., 1st April 1854, p. 362.

‡ Nizamut Adawlut Reports, Vol. II., part 2 of 1852, p. 295.

§ *Ibid*, January 11th, 1856, p. 807.

(1) "A severe punctured wound on the right side of the face; breaking one of the bones of the head" (temporal) "and the lower jaw. Severe bruises on the shoulders and head, five ribs on the right side broken and two on the left. The lungs on both sides greatly congested; a large quantity of blood extravasated within the chest." (February 26th, 1845.)

(2) "A lacerated wound upon the forehead with a fracture of the skull, six ribs on the left side and five upon the right were broken, together with many contused wounds about the body, inflicted with some blunt instrument or instruments." The deceased was a stout muscular man, between 30 and 40 years old. (August, 1844.)

(3) "A wound on the right side of the chest, six inches long and half an inch deep. Another on the same side of the back about three inches long, besides a severe contusion at the lower part of the chest. The breast-bone and all the ribs on the right side of the chest, except the three inferior, were completely broken. One rib on the left side was also broken. A large quantity of blood was found in the cavity of the chest. The aorta being ruptured." (February 12, 1845.)

(4) "The second, third, and fourth ribs of the right side were fractured. The right side of the chest was nearly filled with blood. There was some effusion of blood on the brain. The injury to the chest must have been caused either by violent blows with some heavy instrument, or by some person trampling on the chest." (March, 1844.)

It will be noticed that the first and third of these cases occurred within a month, under the notice of the late Dr. Denham. The frequent repetition of such crimes would appear to depend upon some definite cause, the nature of which demands careful investigation.

The notes on the practice of Compressing the Chest with Bamboos, or with Heavy Weights, and of Trampling on the Body, which will be found in the *Chapter on Torture*, p. 556, should be borne in mind in the investigation of injuries of this kind. It appears highly probable that,—in the case of the old man Khurdee, cited above, in which *the third rib only on either side was broken*, the victim remaining silent while the fatal injuries were being inflicted,—a lattee pressed across the chest was the means employed.

As the medical officer is frequently called upon to examine fractures many days after the alleged period of their infliction, and as the treatment of fracture of the long bones by many of the Bengalee kobirajes is often much above the level of the rest of their surgical practice, his utmost tact and caution will be called for in deciding the probable time at which the injury was received.

Where, as occasionally happens, it is observed that, in addition to other severe injuries, *Both Legs have been broken*,—as happened in the case of a man at Dacca who was stated to have been killed by two persons who caught him in an attempt to ravish their sister;* and in that

---

* Nizamut Adawlut Reports, Vol. III., Part 1, p. 210.

of a wretch, at Bhaugulpore, who attempted to steal mangoes;* or in that of another unfortunate, at Azimgurh, who died in eighteen days after having had both his legs broken by club blows, dealt by thieves who came in the night to steal his mangoes,†—it may fairly become a question whether death has not been inflicted with evidences of premediated cruelty.

In 1848, Dr. Archer, then of Nuddea, reported the case of a man who had suffered *Dislocation of both Elbows* with fracture of the bones, evidently caused by twisting the arms violently, and then beating them with a stick. The joints, Dr. Archer believed, must have been first dislocated, and the bones afterwards broken both above and below the elbow.

The manner in which, often, a crowd of Bengalees fall upon a victim of their displeasure, and beat and tear him to pieces, with sticks, fists, feet, hands, and any weapon which may happen to have been brought or caught up, until the body lies in the midst of them, a mere bloody, featureless, disjointed, broken mass,—is scarcely characteristic of the reputed mildness of the national character. Two examples will suffice. In 1853, a Hindu, carrying on mahajunee business in East Burdwan, went to a village to collect some money. Here a crowd of persons, some of whom were his debtors, seized bamboos and a wooden mallet, and beat him to death. Both arms were broken, the left arm and the left leg were broken by the joints being twisted backwards, the end of the thigh bone protruded at the back of the knee joint, all the vessels of that part were torn, and death must have been caused by hæmorrhage. The nose was also beaten in.‡

In 1854, a man, weak in his right foot and left hand, was attacked by a party, led by a person whose service he had lately quitted, and was beaten to death with clubs. In addition to the *mashed* condition of the left arm, described in the Chapter on TORTURE, Section on *Beating the Joints*, p. 568, the Civil Surgeon found that there were marks of very severe beating over the whole body, but more especially about both legs and the back. There were several incised and contused wounds on the front of both bones of the right leg, and both bones of the right leg were broken to splinters and protruted externally.§

Cases *of injury to the Cervical Vertebræ* are not unfrequently the subjects of judicial enquiry. These may result from hanging, or from strangulation, from twisting the neck, from falls, &c.

---

* Nizamut Adawlut Reports, Vol. II., Part 2, p. 805.

† Nizamut Adawlut Reports, N. W. P., 26th December 1854, p. 853.

‡ Nizamut Adawlut Reports, 10th Dec. 1853, p. 873.

§ Nizamut Adawlut Reports, 5th Aug. 1854, p. 222. In 1866, the Gomashtah of a village in the Tipperah District, who was harassing the ryots, was dragged out of his house by a party of seven men, who "deliberately stamped upon and beat him to death." All were transported for life.—*Bengal Police Report for* 1866, p. 276.

A very strong Cuttack man, quarrelling with another about an ox, took a (nearly solid) bamboo, weighing twelve and-a-half *chittacks*, and struck the back of his opponent's neck, which blow killed him instantly, having, as the native doctor deposed, "broken the first joint of the spine."*

Ramloll Patro Surnokar, of Hooghly, confessed throughout the trial that, being angry with his wife, because she expressed a wish to return to her father's house, he twice twisted her neck, he squeezed her wind-pipe, and, at the same time, pressed down her cheek. The Civil Assistant Surgeon found that the vertebræ of the neck were fractured. He considered that "the fracture had evidently been caused by the head being violently twisted round, which must have caused almost immediate death."†

A Shahabad man having been beaten by several persons, who accused him of theft, appears to have died as they were taking him to the thannah. The medical officer said that death was caused by the severance of an artery in the fore-arm of the deceased by the sharp edge of the bone which had been fractured by the blow of a *lattee*. Some years ago a man who had sustained a simple fracture of the thigh-bone lost his life by injuries to the femoral vein inflicted by the end of the bone, as he was being jolted into the station in a palkee.

A body of armed thieves attacked a village in Behar, on a dark night, made off with ten maunds of grain, leaving a villager dead on his threshing floor. The *post-mortem* examination showed that "the deceased had a punctured wound on the right side, fracturing the rib and piercing the lungs, from which death resulted." The Judges of the Nizamut Adawlut observed that, had the defences of the prisoners been carefully investigated, and had the *post-mortem* examination of the deceased been thoroughly conducted, a right understanding of the merits of the case would, probably, have been obtained. "The Court regret that the Sessions Judge was satisfied with the mere answer of the Assistant Surgeon that death was caused by a *punctured* wound, which, unaccountably, *fractured* a rib, and penetrated to the lungs. Had the Surgeon been questioned as to the internal state of the deceased, and the possibility of the wound having been inflicted after death, the real cause of death would have been more satisfactorily disclosed." The prisoners were acquitted.‡

I cannot perceive the cogency of this objection to the medical evidence. A very sharp bamboo or bluntish spear, used with sufficient force, and striking a rib fully, would *fracture* the rib and *puncture* the lung.

Cases of *Gun-shot Wounds* are not of very rare occurrence in our civil practice. Small shot is sometimes used, but probably not with homicidal intent. For purposes of attack, the Natives of Bengal

* Nizamut Adawlut Reports, August 18, 1856, p. 231.

† *Ibid*, January 19, 1858, p. 41.

‡ *Ibid*, March 25, 1856, p. 621.

generally load with slugs, or roughly cut lumps of lead of greater weight.

In one instance, a man was imprisoned for seven years, for killing another by firing at him a gun loaded with *Seed*, in which it appeared that a single shot had been mixed.*

One Nunhey, of Chunderee (Saugor), confessed that, believing that his brother-in-law had seduced his wife, while yet a virgin, he borrowed a matchlock and practised at a mark to secure a good aim. He approached the man as he lay sleeping on his *charpoy*, and, holding the weapon close to his victim's body, shot him through the heart with two *iron* balls, which were produced in Court.†

In 1853, one Bhowanee, of Furruckabad, was sentenced to transportation for life for *blowing up certain persons with gunpowder*. It appeared that, the prisoner having been betrothed to a girl, the marriage was broken off, and she became engaged to another. Failing to get any redress, he purchased four pice worth,—a quarter seer (half a pound),—of gunpowder, and, entering the girl's house at night, threw it on the *choola* near which she and her mother were sitting. He, as well as they, was severely burned by the explosion. He recovered, but remained much marked with the powder. The two women were so much injured that the younger died five, and the elder fourteen days afterwards.‡

RUPTURE OR WOUNDS OF INTERNAL ORGANS.

Apart from the various other internal injuries, resulting from mechanical violence, observed in all countries, the cases of *Rupture of the Spleen and Liver*, which so frequently occur in India, require distinct comment here. In a country where, owing to the almost universal prevalence of miasmatic poison, the Liver and Spleen of nearly every Native of the lower class may be considered liable to become the seat of chronic enlargement at any period of his life, and where also the practice of beating adults,—especially servants by their masters, and wives by their husbands,—is everywhere prevalent, it is only remarkable that cases of rupture of these viscera are not of almost daily occurrence. A very considerable number of instances of the kind do, from time to time, come under judicial investigation here.

Rupture of the Liver.

The nine years' Medical Reports to the Nizamut contain four cases in which *the Liver* had suffered rupture. It is worthy of remark that three of these occurred under the notice of Dr. Davies, of Patna. In two of

* Nizamut Adawlut Reports, Vol. V., p. 6.
† Nizamut Adawlut Reports, N. W. P., 31st Dec. 1852, p. 1567.
‡ *Ibid*, 13th April 1853, p. 554.

the cases there were also other traces of severe ill-usage ;* in a third, the injury had been caused by the fracture of a rib. Dr. Davies remarked that, in these cases, the injury is sometimes done by a kick or blow ; and often, he had reason to think, by forcing the knee or foot into the right side.

In 1838, Mr. Cornish, a coach-maker in Calcutta, was found guilty of having caused the death of a native saddler whom he had kicked in the side for some fault. The Liver was ruptured.

A Gorait, while employed in an arrest, was set upon by a crowd of persons who beat and ill-used him, until his friends came up and took him home. On the *fifth* day afterwards he went to the Magistrate's Court and complained. His evidence, in which he implicated all the prisoners, was taken, but the Magistrate, not anticipating a fatal result, did not have the deposition formally attested, and ordered him to go to the hospital, where he died the following day. Dr. Collins stated that he "died from external violence resulting in rupture of the liver." The only marks of violence were upon the abdomen. The prisoners pleaded that the deceased died from falling into a ditch when drunk. Dr. Collins held that the deceased was a healthy person, and that the injuries could not have been inflicted by such an accident. A majority of the Judges of the Nizamut Adawlut concurred in acquitting the prisoners, one Judge remarking, "It is very probable the deceased was maltreated and died from such maltreatment, but it is impossible to trust to the evidence as giving a true statement of the occurrence. Had the assault been as described therein, the deceased could scarcely have escaped being killed on the spot." [I do not understand that this applies to the rupture of the liver, but to the character of the attack and the number of the assailants.—N. C.] "I cannot help suspecting that the interval was employed in getting up evidence against the parties accused."†

The following very characteristic cases of rupture of the liver were sent to me in March 1865 by Dr. James Wise, Civil Surgeon of Dacca :—"About mid-day on the 24th September 1864, a great noise was heard in the house of one Potun. On the neighbours going in, they found him beating his wife Neezoo. He was striking her with his fists and kicking her. She was on the ground. Some of the blows fell on her sides and 'bhook' (breasts and upper part of stomach). The neighbours interfered and he desisted ; she remained on the ground and asked for water. Another witness stated that, before death, she complained of pain in her chest and side, and that she died as the sun began to dip, about 6 P.M.

"I examined the body at 7 A.M. on the 27th September ; it was in an

---

* See also a case in which a healthy liver was ruptured by severe blows with a heavy bamboo.—*Nizamut Adawlut Reports*, N. W. P., 12th Jan. 1853, p. 40.

† Nizamut Adawlut Reports, Dec. 21, 1855, p. 951.

advanced stage of putrefaction. No external wound or bruise was visible; there was blood in the vagina and round the labiæ. On opening the abdomen, a large quantity of fluid blood was found in the pelvis and behind the liver; the spleen was congested, but uninjured. The uterus was unimpregnated. The stomach was full of an undigested meal.

"The liver, especially the right lobe, was much enlarged. On the under surface of the left lobe an irregular tear existed, and near it was a smaller one, about an eight-anna piece in size.

"*Case II.*—On Sunday morning, the 1st January 1865, a man named Jafeir, aged twenty-eight, was arrested and taken to the thannah at Putteah. During that night he groaned a great deal, and, on the morning of the 2nd, complained of pain about the liver, and of great thirst. He started that morning for Chittagong, a distance of eight miles. He walked slowly, and the constables struck him with a cane and a tulwar-scabbard. After accomplishing four miles, he was unable to proceed further, and had to be transported to the Sudder Station by boat. He was taken to the Jail Hospital at 6 P.M. He was then very low, complaining of pain in back and chest, and of being too weak to raise himself. He gradually sunk and, at 2 A.M. of the 3rd, he died.

"I examined the body at 7-40 A.M. on the 3rd; no bruises or wounds were visible, and no rib or other bone was broken.

"On opening the chest, the right lung was found adhering to the ribs. Its substance was inflamed, and the pleura covered with fibrine. The left lung was partially congested, but not inflamed. The liver was enormously enlarged, and behind it was a great quantity of dark coagulated blood. On its removal, a large and irregular rupture of the right lobe was found, extending for nearly seven inches in length, from near the gall-bladder across the upper edge of the viscus, towards the broad ligament. It was three-fourths of an inch in depth; and no fibrinous deposit could be detected on its edges. The spleen was enlarged but uninjured.

"How and when did he receive this injury? It must have arisen from some blow inflicted before he reached the thannah on the 1st, or after his departure from it on the 2nd. The opinion I gave was that the groaning and thirst of the night of the 1st arose from pleuro-pneumonia associated probably with an accession of fever. This would explain the pain in the side, &c. It is scarcely credible that a man with a ruptured liver could, twenty-four hours after the receipt of the injury, walk four miles. The constables confessed having struck him. It is, therefore, most likely that the blows inflicted by them caused the rupture on the forenoon of the 2nd. Yet he survived from twelve to eighteen hours afterwards!"

In all cases where the liver becomes so much enlarged as to descend below the ribs, the fragility of its structures is much increased.

Wounds of the liver are by no means necessarily mortal. Mr. Guthrie mentions that he had known three persons who had been wounded [by gun-shot] through the liver, and who suffered little subsequent inconvenience.*

During the Mutiny, two officers recovered from musket-bullet wounds which completely traversed the liver. One of these gentlemen, a personal friend of my own, is at present one of the most active and healthy men in India.

Dr. John Macpherson, now of London, removed a large piece of the liver of a Hindu, who had been wounded by a spear.†

Dr. Taylor considers that wounds of the liver do not prove very rapidly fatal, unless some of the larger trunks are involved. The organ may certainly be torn to a frightful extent without an immediately fatal result ensuing.‡

---

* Commentaries, p. 557. See also Cooper's Lectures, p. 224 (Stabs)—A case of arrow wound of the liver recovered from, by Dr. Goodeve.—*Trans. Med. and Phys. Society*, Vol. V. 1, p. 482.

† This case is quoted in the London Medical Gazette for January 1846.

‡ The following case, not hitherto reported, occurred within my own observation. A stout Brewer's Drayman, about twenty-five years of age, was brought, on a stretcher, to the Surgery of Guy's Hospital, in the summer of 1840, at between 10 and 11 o'clock in the evening. He was found lying in the road, and his horses had taken the dray home without him. His condition was examined by Dr. — Wilson and my friend Mr. Walter Chapman, of Tooting (whose notes of the case, with my own, are now before me), both very careful and accurate observers. There was no mark or evidence of injury; he "was very violent; he swore and endeavoured to strike the bystanders." My notes say that "he walked and moved with the greatest freedom." He was, therefore, considered to be merely intoxicated, and was made over to the police, who took him to the station house. About 6 o'clock the next morning, he was found seated in the water-closet looking very faint and pale; the Surgeon to the station was sent for, but the man was dead before he arrived. A large quantity of blood was found in the peritoneal cavity. The liver *was almost cloven in two* by a vertical fissure, seven or eight inches long and, in some places, nearly three in depth,—which had almost separated its two principal lobes. The edges of this fissure were jagged and irregular, but appeared to have been completely coated with a thick layer of intimately adherent dense coagulum, considerably firmer than the crassamentum of an ordinary clot. Outwardly, the surfaces of this coagulum were not at all irregular, but were smoothly moulded by the pressure of the diaphragm and other surrounding parts. There was no external trace of injury. It was thought probable that he fell from the shaft of his dray, and that the wheel had passed over his body. See somewhat similar cases, Med. Chir. Review for 1831, and Lancet for Dec. 11, 1847.

In the following case also, by Dr. Hunter,* nature's temporarily successful effort to stop bleeding by the deposition of clots was well-marked.

A man who fell from a third storey window. Rupture of Liver. Death on the 10*th day.*—Autopsy, nine hours after death, confined to chest and abdomen. The body was much emaciated, and its surface decidedly jaundiced. Found no lesions in thorax. On opening the abdomen, I found the peritoneal sac filled with a bloody fluid. There were several large clots of blood clinging to the liver, in truth almost completely enveloping that organ. When these clots had been removed, an extensive rupture of the right border involving the entire thickness of the liver, and to the depth from the thick edge of one and-a-half inches on upper, and nearly two and-a-half inches on under surface was discovered. The liver, in the vicinity of the laceration, was connected to the diaphragm by bands of recently organized lymph. Decided efforts towards a spontaneous cure appear to have been made, as a

* Amer. Jour. of Med. Sciences, April 1870.

Ruptures of the liver may heal, at least partially.* In the majority of cases, however, death ensues rapidly where the liver is ruptured by blows.

Rupture of the Kidneys.

Extensive rupture of the Kidney is almost inevitably fatal by hæmorrhage, but life is generally protracted for some hours at least, the effusion being sub-peritoneal. In a man, *æt.* 27, who had fallen on a cask when intoxicated, and who was under treatment in Guy's Hospital for 27 hours, I saw that the left kidney was completely divided transversely into halves, as if cut in two by a blunt knife.†

Dr. Taylor has a similar case (p. 553). Death occurred in between five and six hours. In these cases there cannot be hæmaturia.

I have seen *recovery* from what all who saw the case fully believed to be rather severe rupture of the kidney. A marked case has been given by Mr. Curling.‡ In the most favorable cases, there is hæmaturia, all bleeding occurring into the pelvis.

Rupture of the Spleen.

Cases of *Rupture of the Spleen* are certainly of very frequent occurrence in India, but eleven years' reports contain only thirteen instances. In five of these there were discovered other evidences of severe maltreatment. In two there were traces of injury to the brain; in two others, the spleen had been pierced by the ends of fractured ribs. In the remaining eight instances, the organ appeared to have been ruptured without very extraordinary violence, when in an enlarged and softened condition. In an excellent monograph on "Rupture of the Spleen," Dr. Kenneth McLeod has given§ *seven* cases, which occurred within his own observation, in a year, at Jessore, a very malarious district. Six of these cases occurred among thirty-three cases sent in by the police, for *post-mortem* examination, during the year 1866. I have met with only three instances in my own Indian practice (I ceased to have opportunity of seeing such cases fifteen years ago); two occurred in females struck by their husbands; in these rupture of an enlarged spleen was the only

---

portion of the lacerated hepatic tissue had become united by the fibrin of the extravasated blood. The gall bladder and its duct had escaped injury. I was unable, by a superficial examination, to find any lesions of the coats of the stomach or intestines, save two or three ecchymosed patches. The other abdominal viscera appeared normal. There were no evidences whatever of general peritonitis, as the peritoneum everywhere, except around the liver, presented its characteristic polished surface.

* Case by Dr. Chisholm, Edinburgh Med. and Surg. Journal, Vol. VII. See also Med. Chir. Review, July 1837, p. 270.

† See a case, Med. Chir. Review, July 1837, p. 270, in which rupture of the kidney proved fatal after ten days.

‡ British Medical Journal, May 15th, 1859, p. 441.

§ Ind. Annals, M. S., No. XXII., p. 341.

severe injury discoverable. I find sixteen* other cases in which the rupture of diseased spleens occurred in India, as the result of blows and falls; and many others might, doubtless, be collected. Mr. Heddle, who reported four of these cases,† remarked that :—"In all, the subjects had resided in situations which were remarkably unhealthy; in all, the individuals had been subject to intermittent fevers, either at the time of, or shortly previous to, their decease; and, *in all, that fatal event occurred between the months of August and November*, that is, at the termination of the monsoon, the season during which the native inhabitants of Bombay suffer most severely from fever. The very slight degree of violence which proved sufficient, in all these cases, to produce the serious lesion of the spleen, cannot fail to be remarked; and this fact will explain instances, of not unfrequent occurrence in this country, wherein death, by misadventure, has followed a trifling blow, either accidentally or intentionally inflicted on the abdomen."

Dr. Muir states, in his paper on the Statistics of Unnatural Deaths in the Madras and the other Presidencies,‡ that "in those instances where rupture of the spleen has been the immediate cause of death, that organ is invariably more or less enlarged, sometimes enormously so, as well as soft and friable. A slight blow, such as that produced by a flat open hand, a kick, even a simple push of the person, have, in many cases, caused rupture of the spleen, followed by hæmorrhage into the cavity of the abdomen, and death generally within twelve hours afterwards. In some notoriously malarious districts of the Madras Presidency, enlargement of the spleen is looked upon as a matter of course in almost all natives residing there, and this enlargement of the organ does not appear to be inconsistent with a fair amount of health generally."

Stick and fist blows seldom, if ever, cause rupture of a *healthy* spleen, but the injury may be occasioned by a kick. A case of the kind occurred, at sea, in my father's practice. In the case of a bunniah killed by Mahomedan Punjabees in Delhi, the Sub-Assistant Surgeon who examined the body said that some very hard blows indeed must have been inflicted to rupture the deceased's spleen, which, though larger than usual, showed no trace of recent disease.§

A Midnapore man was assaulted by the hand, being struck on the face and side. He fell upon the ground, and expired before morning. The Sub-Assistant Surgeon found that the body exhibited marks of severe beating about the head and other parts, and that the immediate cause of death was rupture of the spleen, which was in a natural and healthy state. In

---

* Very many other cases might be collected by one specially engaged in investigating this subject.

† Transactions of the Medical and Physical Society of Bombay, Vol. I., p. 304.

‡ Madras Quarterly Journal of Medical Science, July 1868, p. 118.

§ Nizamut Adawlut Reports, N. W. P., 17th Jan. 1852, p. 42.

his opinion, the rupture could only have been caused by the violence which had evidently been used to the deceased.*

Casper relates four cases of rupture of *healthy* spleens,† and Dr. Kenneth McLeod saw, in the Edinburgh Infirmary, a young man who, with other injuries caused by the passage of a waggon-wheel over his abdomen, had the spleen completely divided in two ; he lived several hours in a state of collapse.

Mr. Hutchinson has reported the case of an apparently healthy native, about twenty-five years of age, who died almost immediately after receiving a blow on the left hypochondrium, with a small piece of brick-bat :—"The spleen could scarcely be said to be enlarged." When at Howrah, I examined the body of a married girl of twelve, who had died from rupture of this organ. Her husband had struck her on the side with a very slight bamboo bow used in beating out the seeds of cotton. The spleen was enlarged.

In one report I find it merely stated that "there were several contused marks externally over the region of the spleen." *Care should always be taken to describe the condition of the spleen, as regards the healthy or diseased state of its structure.*

In giving an opinion of the degree of violence required to produce rupture of the spleen and liver, it is important to bear in mind, that cases of *Spontaneous Rupture* of the *Spleen*, in intermittent fever, are upon record.‡

A perfectly well-marked and unmistakable case of spontaneous rupture of

---

* Nizamut Adawlut Reports, N. W. P., Nov. 30, 1855, p. 839.

† Vol. I., pp. 115, 253, 256, 259.

‡ See cases of a Corporal of Artillery and of a Sepoy, by Messrs. Leckie and Greig, as quoted by Dr. Webb,—Pathologica Indica, p. 144. Also American Journal of Medical Science, for April 1845, p. 524, and for October 1842, p. 369 ; and London Med. Gazette, Vol. XXXV., p. 512.

A case of *spontaneous rupture of the spleen* occurring in a native *æt.* 28, suffering from "common continued fever," has been reported by Mr. Z. M. Browne, of Hyderabad, in the Transactions of the Medical and Physical Society of Bombay for 1853-54, p. 318.

In 1856, Professor Möller, of Konigsberg, published a case of what appears to have been spontaneous rupture of the spleen, and analysed *twenty-five* other cases of spontaneous rupture which he had been able to collect. In nine of these cases the amount of the disease which preceded is so meagre, that no conclusion can be drawn as to the ætiology. In six, it occurred in the course of typhus, gastric, yellow and malignant intermittent fever. The remainder seem to have resulted from ordinary intermittent fever, where *the hot stage* appears to be that which most predisposes to the occurrence.—Brit. and For. Med. Chir., Rev., Oct. 1856, p. 540.

"Occasionally, though seldom, enlargement of the spleen proves fatal by rupture, in which case death takes place suddenly, either at the commencement of the cold fit of ague, or by even the slightest exertion of the invalid walking, it may be from his own charpoy to that of his comrade." Dr. C. Finch, in Trans. of the M. and P. S. of Calcutta, Vol. IX., p. 1, page 29.

Dr. T. W. Wilson suggests, with great reason, the probability that, however softened and congested it may be, the spleen never ruptures spontaneously except under the action of muscular pressure—while the patient is turning or moving suddenly.

the spleen occurred in a patient of my own in the Calcutta Medical College Hospital. He was a Danish sailor, only twenty-five years of age, but of herculean build, and lofty stature,—I think the strongest-built man of his age I have ever seen. His ship had arrived at Mutlah, less than a week previously; and he was very ill with the severe intermittent of that locality, one of the peculiar effects of which is (or was then) to bring the lower end of the spleen, to about the size of a goose egg, down below the left ribs, after three or four paroxysms. When I saw him, his case was an ordinary one, but, in a few hours, he began to sink. About a pound of blood was found in the pelvis. It had escaped from two transverse cracks on the surface of the considerably, but not excessively, congested and enlarged spleen. The quantity of blood effused was too small to have been the sole cause of death, which I attributed rather to nervous shock. The impression which the minutest enquiry left upon my mind was, that this was a genuine case of spontaneous rupture of the spleen in intermittent fever.

Dr. A. Porter of Akola (Madras Presidency) has recorded* a case, in which it appears very probable, although it is by no means positively proved, that a rupture, nearly half an inch in length near the hilus of a softened spleen, *was caused by a tetanic spasm* of the diaphragm and abdominal muscles. Dr. Taylor cites cases of *Rupture of the Liver* caused by the muscular effort employed in avoiding a fall from horseback, and by the shock of falling on the feet from a considerable height.†

In the investigation of cases of this kind, it will generally be inquired of the Surgeon—How long can a person live after his spleen has been ruptured? The reply must be—That the period of survival will probably vary much according to the circumstances of each case,—the position and extent of the rupture, the healthy or diseased, the indurated or softened condition of the organ. It would appear that, apart from mere vascular fulness, solid enlargement of the spleen, from organic change in its tissues, generally tends to retard hæmorrhage from its ruptured surfaces. Death may result from rupture of the spleen at any period from a few minutes to several days. For example,—Professor T. W. Wilson favored me with his report of the case of Kanla Dome, who received several blows in a scuffle with a Burkundauz. "*He died immediately.*" There were no external marks of injury. An immense quantity of blood was found effused into the cavity of the peritoneum. The spleen was ruptured in two places on its inner, or concave, surface,—one rupture was about two inches long, the other about an inch. There were coagula in both splits. The spleen weighed 12½ ounces, and was

* Madras Quarterly Journal of M. S., October 1866, p. 403.

† Cruveilhier speaks of rupture of enlarged livers and spleens, in children, resulting from palpation, in the course of a medical examination.

so friable as to yield easily to the finger, and not to bear handling without falling to pieces. The man was in good condition, and had not previously been ill. Dr. Wilson adds, however, that he was a drunkard,—and that this is a cause of softening of the spleen.

Dr. A Porter, Zillah Surgeon, Akola, reports* the case of one who, having met his death while drinking with some companions at a "Kul-lah" shop, was also probably a drunkard. He received a blow from a bamboo over the splenic region, fell down, and "*almost immediately expired.*" No external wound or bruise was visible. "On opening the abdomen a large quantity of sepia-like fluid—changed blood—was found in the pelvis and about the spleen ; of the latter nothing remained except the capsule which, from its size, gave evidence of the spleen having been considerably enlarged when the accident occurred. The rupture extended for some inches along the external surface, near its anterior border. The other organs of the abdomen appeared healthy."

We may contrast these rapidly fatal cases with that recorded by Dr. Chisholm,† of an artilleryman who, in descending a declivity, fell on a large stone. He suffered so little inconvenience at the time, that he was able to work at the forge that evening, and on the following morning. He was then attacked with symptoms which were altogether of a febrile and acutely inflammatory character. He *died nearly five days* after the fall. Upon the posterior convex side of the spleen, there was a rupture through the whole of its substance, at least two inches in length. The edges had a florid appearance in some places, in others something like sphacelus could be perceived. The spleen itself was of very considerable size ; but, in other respects, had no appearance of disease. No mention is made of blood effused into the abdominal cavity. "For a year before, he had been frequently harassed with dangerous attacks of Remittent Fever."

Dr. Duffin has recorded‡ the still more remarkable case of a soldier, *æt.* 21, who was hit on the left side by a piece of shell, on the day of the final attack upon the Redan. He was suffering from "severe pain in the left side, which was augmented by pressure over a circumscribed space, corresponding to a point a little external to the cartilage of the 9th rib, and not more than three inches in circumference ; anxiety of countenance, and accelerated pulse, *but no abrasion on the surface,* no fractured rib, *no swelling or discoloration of the part.*" He was treated for the symptoms, and discharged two days after, at his own request, and to all appearance quite well. He returned to his duty, which "he performed as usual" for two days, when he was re-admitted with symptoms of double pleurisy under which, with pericarditis, he sunk *on the 18th day* after receiving the blow." The peritoneum, throughout its entire extent, was of an

* Madras Quarterly Journal of M. S., October 1866, p. 403.
† Edinburgh Medical and Surgical Journal, Vol. VII.
‡ Dublin Hospital Gazette, Nov. 1, 1855, and American Journal of M. S., April 1856.

almost perfectly black appearance, as well that of the parietes as of the intestines; the omentum was likewise black, but in no other respect did the peritoneum differ from its healthy character. It was still glistening, tense, and elastic. The spleen was about three times its ordinary size, ruptured to the extent of two inches in its long axis, and to a considerable depth in its anterior and external aspect; its substance was infiltrated with congealed and black blood; the vessels were uninjured. There was no fractured rib, no laceration of the parietal peritoneum.

In this case also there is no mention of blood effused into the peritoneal cavity.

In an interesting paper on this subject* Dr. Waring, of Washington, held that, in these cases, the predisposing causes of rupture are, in the great majority of instances, 1st, *Enlargement with Engorgement;* and 2nd, *Hypertrophy* and *Induration* with *brittleness*. So also Dr. K. McLeod points out that these accidents are liable to occur in cases of, 1st, *Simple Engorged Spleen*; 2nd, *Hypertrophied Engorged Spleen*; 3rd, *Small Hard Spleen*; 4th, *Large Hard Spleen.*

Cases present themselves, from time to time, in which persons in whom rupture of the spleen or liver is supposed to have occurred recover,—often with recurring attacks of peritoneal inflammation.† Mr. Marcus G. Hill, who fell in the Mutiny, mentioned to me an instance which occurred at St. George's Hospital, in which Mr. C. Hawkins had reason to believe that a person who had been run over recovered from a rupture of the spleen. This, however, was not proved to have been the case. The strongest evidence which I can discover of the possibility of recovery from wounds of the spleen is that given by Mr. Guthrie, who states that he has "seen accidentally, after death, cicatrices in the spleen corresponding to external marks, indicative of a former wound."‡ This, however, cannot be taken as proof that ruptures of the spleen are otherwise than inevitably mortal.§

* "Report of three cases of Ruptured Spleen; with remarks on the different organic changes which give rise to this, and the different modes in which it may occur."—*Amer. Journal of Med. Science*, October 1856, p. 354.

† Mr. Bennett, of Hailsham, Lancet, 22nd March 1845, and Mr. H. Jackson, of Sheffield, Prov. Med. and Sur. Journal, 10th Dec. 1845; also Guthrie's Commentaries, p. 562.

‡ Commentaries in Surgery, p. 561.

§ *Note on the Operation of Removing the Spleen.*

As these pages may come under the notice of a large proportion of the medical men practising in India, the following practical hint may not be altogether out of place:—

Death from rupture of the spleen is so common an occurrence in this country (few Civil Surgeons, of fourteen years' experience in Bengal, having met with fewer than from eight to twelve cases) that,—in the absence of any certain facts whatever tending to show that a rupture through the capsule of the spleen can be recovered from,—it appears right to submit to the judgment of the profession any course of treatment which may appear to afford a chance of life in such cases. Instances are on record, in which considerable portions of the spleen, protruding through wounds, have been successfully removed. See Fergusson Phil. Trans., Vol. XI, 1737-38, p. 425 (three ounces and-a-half of protruded spleen ligatured and cut off); and McDonnel, in Webb's Pathologia Indica, p. 144,—in which a large portion of the spleen of a native was excised.

Dr. French, then of Nowgong, Assam, reported * the case of a prisoner who, while under treatment for diarrhœa, died suddenly. " The spleen

Mr. Hyatt removed, by ligature, a portion of spleen " about the size of one's hand" which protruded through a tulwar wound, and in which circulation was still going on. He was discharged perfectly well.—*Indian Medical Gazette*, April 1, 1868, p. 85.

There is also on record the case, considered to be authentic by Guthrie and South, in which the Spleen of a man, wounded at Dettingen, was found protruding and covered with dirt,—it was cut off, and the patient recovered. See also a second case, J. and C. Bell's Anat. and Phys., 4th Ed., p. 352 ; and a third by Morgagni, from Fontanus, in which the woman survived five years.

It was clearly proved, by the experiments of Heister and Vallisnieri, that removal of the spleen in the lower animals, dogs, &c., has been recovered from without evidence of any serious derangement of the vital functions. Professor Adelmann, of Berlin, has collated, in the Deutsche Klinik of the 26th April 1856, fifteen cases, in which the spleen has been extirpated successfully, in consequence of various diseases and injuries. Dr. Tanner has given† a *resumé* of nine cases, in which *complete removal* of the spleen was had recourse to in modern times. The measure appears to have been successful in *two* of these cases, Schultz's and Péau's. In the first, the entire spleen protruded through a wound ; in the second, a much hypertrophied spleen with splenic cyst was removed from a lady twenty years of age. These are all the grounds of encouragement which we, at present, have in undertaking this operation. In any other than a set of cases which are, under other treatment, necessarily and invariably mortal, so severe a course as that about to be advocated would scarcely be sanctioned by the above data ; but, here, I consider that the facts adduced justify me in recommending that, in any case where a person having been struck in the situation of the left floating ribs, is found by the Surgeon to be evidently dying from hæmorrhage, an incision should at once be made, a hand introduced into the abdominal cavity, and the spleen extracted and removed, after deligation of its vessels.

The chief objection to this plan is that heavy blows on the abdomen generally occasion severe collapse, and that, in an anemiated person with diseased spleen, such collapse could not, at once, be distinguished from that attending hæmorrhage from a ruptured internal organ. Here it must be remembered that the symptoms resulting from concussion of the solar plexus (where the injury is not followed by almost instant death) are transient, while those of hæmorrhage into the abdominal cavity rapidly increase in intensity. Still I would not advise any surgeon to remove the spleen in a case where he was not confident that the patient was dying from internal hæmorrhage. This could be the only source of very serious fallacy. It might be difficult, at once, to distinguish a case of severe rupture of the left kidney (in which, as is often the case, the evidence of bloody urine was not procurable) from laceration of the spleen ; here, however, the first incision would reveal the presence of a large quantity of blood *behind* the peritoneum; and the operation, carried only thus far, could scarcely hasten the inevitably fatal issue of the case. Dr. Kinloch Kirk has described cases in which the left lobe of the liver, becoming enlarged, is felt in the usual position of an hypertrophied spleen. In the possible event of such an organ becoming ruptured, an error in diagnosis would merely lead to ineffectual interference in a case of mortal injury.

The incision should extend just below the last floating rib, from the anterior edge of the *quadratus lumborum* muscle to rather more than an inch beyond the point of the cartilage of the rib.

After a few expriments upon the dead body, the removal of even an enlarged spleen, through such an opening, will be found to be a matter of little difficulty.

Professor Simon, of Heidelberg, has removed a kidney, by an extra-peritoneal incision, in a case where urinary fistula had been caused by unavoidable injury to the ureter in an operation for the removal of cystoid disease of the ovary. " The patient now enjoys the best health, being employed all day at work, and being able to take long walks." *Deutsche Klinik*, April 9, *and Medical Times and Gazette*, May 21, 1870, p. 570.

* Ind. Annals of M. S., No. XV. of 1862, p. 273.

† Practice of Medicine, Vol. II., p. 150.

was enlarged $8\frac{3}{4}$ inches in its long and 5 in its transverse diameter; was greyish in color, and weighed one pound thirteen and-a-half ounces; its consistence was greatly diminished, and was more friable than it ought to be, presenting a large grumous, pultaceous mass enveloped in its capsule, which was of a firm character. Nearly about the middle of its length, but nearer to the inferior margin than to the superior, and on its inner surface, there was a recent laceration about ten lines long running diagonally, and extending into the substance. This was the cause of death. On the outer surface was a cicatrix of a former rupture, one inch in length, also running diagonally, and around it there was an organized blood-clot of firm consistence, which adhered strongly to the organ and the parietes of the abdomen."

Dr. James Wise has given a case * in which it appears very probable that a sepoy recovered from spontaneous rupture of the spleen.

We must be careful not to mistake for the vestiges of traumatic rupture of the spleen, those wedge-shaped, yellowish, cheesy masses, and those yellow retracted callous cicatrices which result from apoplexy of the spleen, or embolism of its vessels.

It should be borne in mind that Sir James Simpson has described a class of cases in which pregnant and parturient women have suffered from rupture of the spleen. I am not aware that any observation on this point has been made in India.

Rupture of Liver and Spleen.

Three Mussalmauns were convicted, at Mymensingh, of having attacked the house of a woman against whom they had a grudge, and of having conveyed her to their own house, where they assaulted her so severely that she died on the following day. The Civil Assistant Surgeon deposed that death was caused by *rupture of the Liver and Spleen;* that there were contusions all over the body, more especially on the sides of the chest and belly, and that these contusions and ruptures were apparently the result of violence; that he cannot exactly state what might have been the result of those injuries if the spleen and liver had not been ruptured, but that deceased was, from the state of her body, which presented a mass of bruises, dreadfully beaten, and that she might have possibly lived two or three hours, or even longer.†

I was, some time ago, requested by the counsel for the defence to watch, as an act of compassion, the trial of a man accused of having caused the death of a native by kicking him. As there was, besides rupture of the Spleen, rupture of the Kidney, I was obliged to inform my legal friend that, although the spleen may be ruptured by very moderate blows, and *possibly* even by force of muscular contraction in one who, being

---

* Indian Annals of M. S., No. XIX, 1865, p. 329.

† Nizamut Adawlut Reports, Jan. 24, 1859, p. 59.

pushed, endeavours to save himself from falling, the coincidence of splenic with renal rupture carries with it the gravest suspicion of a very violent assault, probably by kicks.

One of the most remarkable cases on record of coincident ***rupture of the Liver*, *Spleen*,** and the ***Kidney*** is narrated by Dr. Fayrer.*

Ram L., *æt.* 25 years, a Hindoo confectioner, was admitted to the Medical College Hospital on the 20th February, with simple Colles's fracture of the left fore-arm and compound dislocation of the right wrist-joint, caused by falling from a tamarind tree, from a height of thirty-five or forty feet. The pulse was very feeble. On the 21st, there was also great depression, and he complained of pain in the hypogastrium. Had passed urine once since the accident. It was uniformly bloody, but contained no clots. On the 22nd, he passed bloody urine again, and the wound began to put on an unhealthy aspect. The pulse became stronger day by day; hæmaturia ceased, pain in the hypogastrium subsided, but slight fever continued. There were no further evidences whatever of any abdominal injury. The urine and secretions were normal, and, but for unfavorable changes which occurred in the arm, all seemed to be doing well. The injury was so severe that, from the first, it was considered doubtful if the limb could be saved. Suppuration spread, and, within a short time, symptoms of tetanus set in. Amputation, at the middle of the fore-arm, was performed on March 4th. He died on March 8th, *sixteen* days after the accident.

Post-Mortem Examination.—Lungs, healthy and crepitant; firm, decolorised clots in the right ventricle passing into the pulmonary artery; left ventricle very much contracted; a small decolorised clot in the aorta. Liver studded with numerous pyæmic patches of whitish-grey softening, each rather smaller than the tip of the little finger, and extending about a quarter of an inch into the substance of the liver. There are a superficial rent on the posterior thick margin of the right lobe and two others on the under-surface. There is also a dark line along the upper and anterior surface, which is apparently another superficial rupture nearly healed. Spleen with two ruptures in its posterior edge, the upper one extending deep into its substance. Left kidney—At its upper end is a very extensive rupture running up into the hilus. The areolar tissue surrounding the vessels at their entrance into the hilus was dense from infiltration of blood. Nearly three-fourths of the kidney, including its upper and nearly all its posterior surface, and a great part of its anterior, is of a pale buff color, and soft and doughy to the touch. The portion so affected is separated from the sound part by a dark-colored wavy line of demarcation, which can be seen extending through the deep as well as the superficial structures on the surface of the incision made obliquely into the anterior surface of the organ. About two ounces of

* Medical Times and Gazette, May 18th, 1867, p. 522.

blood-clots lay on the great omentum, which was folded and wrinkled upwards. Some coagulated blood over the kidney and left side of pelvis. No peritonitis. Cavity of bladder clear and healthy.

Dr. Fayrer remarks that we have here rupture of the spleen, kidney, and liver, without any symptom of any abdominal injury at all, except hæmaturia of a few days' duration. This, which passed away without leaving any further sign of mischief, was attributed to some comparatively trivial injury of the bladder or kidney. Not the least suspicion existed that the abdominal viscera had been so seriously injured.

It is not known whether he struck against anything as he fell, but it is evident that his hands touched the ground first. This appears to show the pre-existence of great and nearly equal fragility in the structures of the liver, spleen, and kidneys.

Legal Decisions.

The following is an extract from a letter from the Hon'ble the Court of Directors, in the Military Department, dated 4th July 1838, published for the information of the Army:—

"The court-martial proceeded to the trial of Ensign Sutherland G. G. Orr, of the 23rd Regt. N. I., on a charge of wilful murder, in having 'struck and kicked with his hands and feet, on the left side of his body, Powel, his servant, and thereby occasioned a rupture of the spleen, whereof he, the said Powel, died at the same place on the same day.'

"8. Of this charge, the court-martial found Ensign Orr to be 'not guilty,' a finding which was 'approved' by the Commander-in-Chief.

"9. It being evident, from the finding of the court-martial on the charge against Lieut. Stokes, that they considered themselves not to be limited to the strict terms of the charge, but to be empowered to find any minor degree of guilt as established by the evidence, we are disposed to view their acquittal of Ensign Orr of the charge of murder as an entire acquittal of all and every degree of guilt as connected with the death of his late servant.

"10. We have, however, observed with much regret, from the evidence adduced on the trial, that Ensign Orr inflicted a blow or blows upon the man, whose death gave rise to the charge against him, and we are of opinion that his conduct was highly reprehensible. We cannot doubt but that this melancholy instance of the death of a fellow-creature so immediately after receiving the blows, will act as a powerful and effectual warning to Ensign Orr, and to the service at large, to abstain hereafter from the unworthy, degrading, and highly reprehensible practice of striking or beating their native servants. Whilst expressing this hope, we desire that Ensign Orr be informed that if, contrary to our expectations, he shall be proved upon any future occasion to have been guilty of such misconduct, whatever may be its degree, he will certainly be dismissed from the Company's service.

"11. We desire that you will publish this despatch in General Orders."

Bysagoo Noshyo, quarrelling with his wife, struck her a blow on the face, and gave her a kick, which ruptured the spleen, so that she died immediately. He repented directly, for he was found with the woman in his arms, succouring her ; and he admitted that he had killed his wife. *Sentence*, one year's rigorous imprisonment.* *Held*, that the husband was guilty of an offence under Sections 319 and 321 of the Penal Code, and not of an offence under Sections 320 and 322.—*Weekly Reporter*, Vol. VIII., No. 7, September 1867, p. 29. See also case of Punchanun Tantee.—Cowell and Woodman, p. 339.

Robert Bruce, an Artilleryman, was tried at the Calcutta Criminal Sessions, 3rd June 1868, for "causing hurt" to a native boy. He kicked the boy, who was suffering from diseased spleen, on the side. Death shortly followed.

His Lordship, addressing the prisoner, observed that he (the prisoner) had no intention, probably, when he kicked the lad, to inflict any serious injury, but still His Lordship considered that the prisoner must have known the dangerous consequences of such an act, especially when inflicted on a native of this country. The sentence of the Court was that he undergo six months' rigorous imprisonment.

From its position, the *Duodenum* is less liable than any other part of the small intestines to be ruptured by external violence, but several cases have been recorded. See one by Mr. Hinder, of the Calcutta Native Hospital, in which a strong Ooriah Bearer having been kicked in the belly about an hour and-a-half after his morning meal, died, from collapse and peritonitis, in about six or eight hours. There was a small rent in the duodenum, through which its contents had escaped into the peritoneal cavity.*

For important Indian cases of, 1st, *Rupture of the Duodenum*, *see* Chapter on SUICIDE, Section on Suicide caused by Pain ; and 2nd, *Rupture of the Pancreas*, *see* Chapter on TORTURE, Section on Binding the Body in Painful Positions, p. 563.

A curious case of rupture of the *Jejunum* has been recorded by Dr. G. E. Seward.† The following are the leading particulars. The Foujdar's report stated that a police Carbaree was sleeping in his own house. His two sons were lying by him. On a sudden he cried out loudly : he felt that two blows had been struck on his abdomen. From that time his abdomen swelled and became painful. He could no longer defecate. He died on the next morning. The people believed his death to have arisen

---

* Ind. Med. Gaz., June 1, 1866, p. 157.

† Bombay Med. and Phys. Trans. No. IV., N. S., for 1857 and 1858, p. 20.

from a natural cause. This, however, being very doubtful, the body was sent in for inspection. A light was burning in the room; the doors were closed; the deceased was strongly impressed with the idea that a man had inflicted those two blows; he was greatly alarmed; he afterwards vomited water, then blood. The *post-mortem* examination was not made until *five days* after death, in the middle of June. It was undertaken with the full anticipation that there was rupture of some abdominal viscus. There was considerable decomposition. Semi-fluid feces were found in the pelvis, but no extravasated blood. About eight inches from the duodenum the jegunum was found "completely rent asunder." The following is from the original:

"*1st.*—The peritoneal coat of the portions of bowel, to the extent of about five inches above and below the rupture, is covered with patches of lymph, easily separable in flakes. No lymph is observed on the mesentery. The general surface is pale, mottled, or striped with dark red in the course of the *veins* (which are gorged with black blood); red, of a lighter hue, coloring the mesenteric border. At the point of disunion, the mesentery is torn to the extent of a quarter of an inch.

"*2nd.*—This portion" [mesentery] "has evidently been the seat of acute disease, as shown by its deep blackish red aspect. The rent, possibly the result of perisaltic motion prior to death, or more probably effected by rough handling of corpse during its carriage, or during forcible protrusion of bowel-contents (by compressed gases) on opening the abdomen.

"*3rd.*—On one side of the rent, redness extends an inch from the line of lesion, and merges suddenly into a deep blackish spot. The serous membrane is irregularly torn, and retracted from the edge of the rent. The muscular tissue is dark, and thickened for one-third of an inch across the bowel at this edge of the tear; and thence a red line extends around the gut at extreme limit of ruptured serous coat. The serous coat of the second portion is also irregularly torn and retracted. Corresponding to the black spot already noticed, is a small, round, shallow, concave depression (an ulcer apparently ?), and seemingly situate on the subserous tissue. In a line with this, on the circumference and towards the free edge of tube, a hole in base of a small triangular flap of serous coat, which would be applied to the side of a tongue of the same coat on the other half. Next again to this, a thickened dark spot in middle coat; and to this, the submucous tissue, if not the mucous coat of one of the valvulæ conniventes, is adherent. Its size is that of a dhall grain. The mucous membrane appears to be unaffected. The valvulæ conniventes of the duodenal portion are stained with yellow bile. The other detached portion of tube is perfectly free from stain, and of the usual color. The contents of the upper part have escaped into the abdomen, the remainder consists of soft fœcal matter of deep brown color, with altered particles of dhall and ooreed; the lower contains grey chyle.

"4*th*.—The retraction of the serous membrane, the thickened everted edges of the rent, exclusive of the thickening, the result of disease, would indicate that the rupture happened during life, or certainly before the tissues had lost their contractibility."

Dr. Seward reported that, "at the plane of rupture, disease had existed, and did exist, at the time when deceased was taken ill, sufficient to permit of the tearing asunder of the bowel by its own action. I am of opinion that death was brought about by a natural cause, namely, the breaking asunder of the bowel weakened by disease."

The above description is not extremely clear, and I think that many will consider that, although the intestinal structures may not have been previously in a healthy condition, the bowel was rent across by a blow.

Ruptures and Wounds of the Heart.

It is well known to medical men that compression of the chest and blows and falls not unfrequently determine rupture of some portion of the heart or thoracic blood-vessels—when those organs are in a perfectly healthy condition ; and that,—when their tissues have undergone fatty or earthy degeneration, or have become aneurismal,—very slight local injuries, the muscular exertion which attends a struggle, mental emotion, sexual excitement, or sudden exposure to vicissitudes of heat or cold, are liable to occasion lesions resulting in sudden death. This is nearly equally the case in Europe and in India.

It appeared, in a trial at Cuttack, that there was "a punctured wound on the upper part of the right side of the chest, which *had wounded the pericardium and large vessels in the vicinity of the heart*, and likewise the upper part of the right lung ;" still it was shown in evidence that, having been stabbed by a knife in the breast, the unfortunate man, "after recovering himself from the shock, pressed his cloth with his hand over his wound, and ran towards his own house, but fell down after proceeding a few paces, and thence crawled along the ground to a house which was close at hand, and there died *within about forty minutes* after receiving the wound.* It is much to be regretted that a fuller surgical report of the facts of this remarkable case is not obtainable.

Professor T. W. Wilson favored me with the details of the following most important case of rupture of the heart, occurring in a scuffle, but evidently from natural causes.

A Hindu of Rampore Beauliah, aged 35, an habitual drunkard, feasted with thirty others during the night of the 23rd July 1850, celebrating the Kalee Poojah, and drinking freely. After this, he and five others went to drink again, at 10 A.M. A quarrel and scuffle ensued; he fell,

* Nizamut Adawlut Reports, Sept. 27, 1855, p. 467.

and it was *supposed* that he received a blow. He never spoke again. There was the trace of a bruise on the head, but no other outward mark of injury. A bloody fluid was issuing from the nose, and there was a strong odour of spirits. The brain was in a high state of congestion, but there was no effusion of blood. The lungs were also much congested; and, in the lower lobe of the left, the vessels had given way, forming a sanguineous apoplexy. The pericardium was found distended with from a pound to a pound and-a-half of fluid blood. This had escaped through a rupture in the right ventricle, close below the semi-lunar valves. The heart was natural in size, but the right ventricle was thin and its muscular tissues soft; there was one tear with a small band joining; below this, were two ragged cracks, like chaps, of no great depth. Dr. Wilson justly argued that this was the natural result,—the vascular system being over distended, the lungs becoming engorged during the heat of a breathless struggle, and the structures of the heart being preternaturally weak.

Dr. Theodore Duka has given* the case, singularly resembling the above (except that, here, the injury was probably caused by direct force upon a diseased heart), of a Mahomedan, *æt.* about 65, reported to have died suddenly after a fall during a scuffle arising from gambling. There were two lacerations of the right ventricle (there was fatty degeneration of the organ); there were no external marks of injury to the chest, but, what is very remarkable, there was also rupture of the pericardium. This rent was situated over the apex of the heart, and was covered by the lung. Its direction was horizontal, and its length about three lines. There was effusion of blood round its edges to the extent of two lines.

In cases of this kind, it is of importance to determine whether the muscular tissue of the heart has become wasted, or has undergone fatty degeneration, since it has been found that direct violence may cause rupture of a healthy heart.†

Mr. Prescott Hewett has described a case, in which the *septum ventriculorum cordis* was found ruptured in a boy aged five, over whose chest a heavy cart wheel had passed.‡ The following somewhat similar case, by Mr. H. J. Carter, of Bombay, deserves notice.

A Parsee, aged about 40 years, temperate and healthy, robust and well formed, was knocked down by the shaft of a four-wheeled vehicle, and survived the accident about eight-and-forty hours. There were several

---

* Ind. Annals of M. S., No. XV., 1862, p. 257.

† As in a case reported in the *Medical Gazette*, in which the stroke of a musket ball, probably glancing sideways, ruptured the right ventricle without tearing the pericardium. Similar lesion has also occurred as the result of falls, and of great mechanical violence, where the structure of the heart has been healthy, and no external trace of injury has been perceptible.—As in the cases reported by Mr. Prescott Hewett, in the 1st vol. of the Transactions of the Pathological Society of London, p. 81.

‡ *Op. Citat.*

outward bruises and excoriations. None of the bones of the chest were fractured, the lungs were much engorged. The cavities of the heart were empty. There was an aperture, large enough to receive a small walnut (about three-quarters of an inch in diameter), close to the apex of the interventricular partition. Its circumference was soft, shreddy, whitish, and lymphy,—in fact, it was evidently a tear; it formed a direct communication between the ventricles, was of recent occurrence, and, in all probability, had been occasioned by a fall, or by force communicated from without.*

The late Dr. James Macrae reports the case† of a European admitted after the battle of Sadoolapore, with *rupture of the septum cordis*, without any wound of the chest or fracture of ribs. He had been struck by a cannon shot immediately over the breast, and under the nipple, on the left side. The chest presented only a very slight bruise, the skin not even being rubbed off. He, however, appeared to be dying; pulse small, frequent, and feeble; surface cold and moist; countenance anxious. Stimulants, opium, &c., were of no use; and, after four days, he died. There were found echymosis under the skin, echymosis of the anterior surface of the heart, and there was rupture of the septum cordis, so that the finger could be passed from one ventricle to the other, through a jagged and ruptured opening.

Dr. Edward Goodeve told me that, in the above case, there was a continuous *bruit* prolonged over both the first and second sound.

Mr. Carter adds the following note by M. Ollivier—That the seat of rupture of the heart from external violence is more frequently in the right than in the left cavities, the reverse of this takes place when the rupture occurs from other causes. Out of eleven cases occurring from external violence, the right cavities were torn in eight, and the left in three; and, in six of these cases, the auricles were ruptured.

It will be seen that, in his remarks on Injuries inflicted by weapons commonly in use, Dr. Hutchinson mentions (page 332) that he has known rupture of the heart result from a *lattee blow*. He kindly sent me the subjoined note of the case at the time. November 24th, 1864.—Body of Munee Lal: *External marks* of injury,—slight contusion on vertex, large lattee wheal diagonally across left breast below, and to the right of left nipple, and reaching to margin of ribs; slight abrasures below right knee. *Internal appearances,*—scalp congested; below contusion no fracture of skull or effusion within.

Brain healthy.

Lungs healthy generally, a few tubercles at apices. Pericardium full of

---

* Trans. of the Bombay Medical and Physical Society for 1845-46, p. 97.

† Report on the Field Hospital of the Army of the Punjab, Ind. Annals Med. Science, April 1857, No. VIII., p. 700.

fluid blood, right ventricle of heart ruptured close to septum, and not far from apex; no fatty degeneration of heart or venels.

Abdominal viscera healthy.

In 1855 Lutchmun Gowalla, being engaged in an affray, received "a blow with a club near the region of the heart, which killed him on the spot." The late Dr. Simpson found "a contused mark across the lower part of the left side of the chest, crossing the position of the heart, apparently from a *lattie blow*; corresponding to this mark there was some extravasation of blood under the skin among the muscles, covering the ribs; a portion of the left lung was bruised, and the apex of the heart ruptured, three-fourths of an inch in length,—the rupture communicating with the left ventricle of the heart. These were the only marks of injury which I observed, and death appears to have taken place immediately on receipt of the blow, because no blood of the ventricle of the heart had escaped through the rupture, the immediate cause of death being the shock to the nervous system paralysing the action of the heart. The blow was not a severe one, as there was neither wound of the integuments nor fracture of the ribs; and, had the blow been in another part of the body, it would not, in all likelihood, have been productive of any bad consequences."*

In a memoir on *Lacerations* of the heart, the results of exteral violence independently of any penetrating wound, Mr. Gamgee† gives the *causes* which produced these lesions in twenty-eight cases. Falls from a height or from a carriage in motion, 9. Passage of a wheel over the chest or other forcible compression of it not accurately defined, 10. Kick from a horse, 4. Bullets fired against the chest from gun or pistol, 4. Blow of unknown kind, 1.

The *Duration of Life* after the accident, is not mentioned in nine out of the twenty-eight cases. In eleven of the remaining nineteen, death was instantaneous; of the other eight, one got up, ran a few steps, and fell dead; one lived half an hour, two lived two hours; one three hours; two four hours; and one fourteen hours.

In forty-two cases of *Wound* of the heart, Dr. Purple‡ gives the following statistics of the *Duration of Life*. Right ventricle, maximum 29 days, minimum died immediately (four cases of positive recovery, in all of which the right ventricle was the part injured), average 9 days. Left ventricle, maximum 66 days, minimum 5 minutes, average 13½ days. Right auricle, maximum 7 days, minimum 2½ days, average 4¾ days. In two cases in which both ventricles were wounded, maximum 6 days, minimum 4 days.

---

* Nizamut Adawlut Reports, Feb. 14th, 1855, p. 220.

† Researches in Pathological Anatomy and Clinical Surgery.

‡ Statistical Observations on Wounds of the Heart, and on their relations to Forensic Medicine, with a table of forty-two recorded cases, New York Journal of Medicine, May 1855, p. 411.

Although it was long believed that cardiac affections were among the rarest diseases of India, it is now well known that they are of by no means unfrequent occurrence here; and subsequent observation has confirmed a statement which I made twenty years since, to the effect that the habits of Europeans in this country greatly dispose them to suffer from fatty degeneration of the cardiac muscular tissue.* In a valuable memoir published in 1855, Mr. C. N. Macnamara mentions that out of twenty-four men of the 1st European Bengal Fusiliers, who died at Dinapore, between February and September 1855, three died from rupture of the great vessels near the heart, the consequence of fatty degeneration.† In one, the descending cava had given way at its junction with the auricle. In the other two cases, the aorta had given way, in one case within, and in the other just without the pericardium.

It was formerly believed, and may still be the popular opinion, that all wounds of the heart produce almost instantaneous death.‡ It is now, however, well known by medical men, that the structures of the heart often sustain severe mechanical injuries which, by certain adaptations of the parts, are prevented from being fatal, often for hours and days, and sometimes even for weeks.§

Life appears generally to be more or less protracted, in cases of injury to the heart, under the following circumstances:—When the injury does not extend beyond the muscular walls; when the wound penetrates the muscular coat obliquely; where it is a mere puncture, or is in the direction of the stronger muscular fibres; or where it is ragged and lacerated, as in the case of gun-shot; where the large blood vessels and the proper arteries and veins of the heart remain intact; where the instrument remains fixed in the wound.

The most remarkable case of survival after injury to the heart or its great vessels on record, is probably one narrated by Mr. William White, then of Rangoon. A soldier was wounded in the storming of the Great

* Practical Treatise on the Management of Diseases of the Heart, &c., in India, 1851, 77.

† Indian Annals of Medical Science, Oct. 1855, 182.

‡ Taylor, 307, 325.

§ From a series of cases collected by M. M. Ollivier and Sanson, cited by Dr. Taylor, it would appear that, out of *twenty-nine* instances of penetrating wounds of the heart, only *two* proved fatal within *forty-eight hours*. In the others, death took place at the varying periods of from four to twenty-eight days, after the receipt of the wound. I cannot but believe that these statistics, although, of course, literally true, are altogether deceptive—*i. e.*, if they are intended to show that, out of twenty-nine persons receiving wounds of the heart, there is any probability whatever that twenty-seven would survive at least forty-eight hours. The probability rather is that not more than two out of the twenty-nine would survive forty-eight minutes. There can scarcely be a doubt that most of the cases collected by these authors were obtained from books, where they were published as rare instances of injury to the Heart:—the rarity of such cases mainly depending upon the period of survival. No medical man would be likely to consider an ordinary case of wound of the Heart,—*i. e.*, one in which the wound was simple, and death almost instantaneous,—as worthy of record.

Pagoda, *on the* 14*th April* 1852. The ball entered a little above the anterior fold of the left axilla, taking an oblique direction to the cavity of the chest. At first he appeared to be doing well, and the wound closed. Subsequently, his health declined with feverish symptoms and evidences of pulmonary disease. A few days before his death, it was noticed that "the action of the heart was weak, but natural, its systole and diastole regular and equal." He died, worn out and emaciated, *on the 24th of June.** The ball appeared to have entered the chest between the third and fourth ribs, passing downwards to the left side. There was a circumscribed empyema, the cavity of which extended from the first to the seventh rib, and contained a pint of pus. A small portion of the cloth of the jacket was lying loose at the orifice of a canal situated about the middle of the lung on its convex aspect—this canal, passing forwards and inwards, stopped short close to the union of the pulmonary veins, where all further traces of the passage of the ball were lost. On raising the Heart, however, a hard and firmly-impacted substance was felt at its apex ; this, on examination, proved to be the ball, in the left ventricle, at its most inferior part, crossed and recrossed by the cordæ tendineæ and carneæ columnæ which firmly secured it in its position. The Heart was perfect in every part. Mr. White considered that the only conclusion which could be arrived at was, that the ball must have perforated a pulmonary vein, and thus passed into the left auricle, and ultimately into the ventricle.† Dr. Burton Brown and I most carefully examined this heart some years afterwards. We could not discover the slightest trace of any route by which the bullet could have entered. Unfortunately, the pulmonary veins have not been preserved.

In cases where the internal viscera are found extensively ruptured, any allusion to the absence of external bruises is generally met by the question :—"Is it possible that a blow or kick might be inflicted on the abdomen, sufficiently severe to rupture one of the viscera or a great blood-vessel, and yet no external mark be left ?" The answer must be in the affirmative. I have met with more than one instance in which the passage of a wheel over the belly, causing rupture of the Liver, Kidneys, or

---

* It appears, in the printed report, that death took place *on the 24th of January*, but this is evidently a typographical error.

† Fournier gives the case of a Soldier, who survived a gun-shot wound of the chest six years, and died from another cause. The ball was found lodged in the right ventricle of the Heart, near its apex, enfolded in a great measure in the pericardium, and resting on the *septum medium.* (Cas Rare ; in Dict. des Sciences Medicales, as quoted by South.)

Dr. Carnochan, of New York, has published the case of a man who lived twelve days after having been wounded in the chest by a Colt's revolver bullet. There was pericarditis. A bullet, one inch in circumference, was found enveloped in a delicate cyst, and embedded to the depth of a quarter of an inch in the muscular tissue of the Septum of the Ventricles. "The wound had entirely cicatrized" [?] ; "there was no outward visible sign of its presence" (Amer. Med. Monthly, April 1855 ; and Ed. Med. Journal for October of that year.) With Dr. White's case, the series is rendered complete by an instance noticed by Plouquet, in which a bullet remained lodged in the right ventricle for years. (South.)

Bladder, has not left the faintest discoverable trace externally. Nearly all writers on wounds have recognized this fact. Morgagni illustrated it by the case of an ecclesiastic, whose skull was fractured by a blow which failed to rend his silken cap.

Injuries to the Abdominal Viscera are doubtless occasionally inflicted by *Bans-dola* and similar modes of compression. In 1847, Dr. Irvine, of Patna, reported the case of a native policeman whose death was evidently occasioned by pressure upon the Liver and Spleen, the convex surface of the former being inflamed, and there being a round gangrenous depression on the right edge of the Spleen. There had been hæmatemesis previous to death. Dr. Irvine considered that these injuries arose from the waist being very tightly bound with some pliable substance.

Blows on the Abdomen producing Concussion of the Solar Plexus.

Native grooms, or syces, are frequently killed by kicks received in the abdomen by horses, and I think especially by ponies. In some cases, death occurs immediately from shock ; in others there is rupture of bowel, with extravasation of its contents into the abdominal cavity and fatal peritonitis.

One of those cases of death occurring suddenly from *a Blow on the abdomen,* from concussion of the solar plexus, independently of discoverable injury to any organ, came under my notice at Chittagong. It was stated that the deceased had been struck with a thick pole on the right loin, and had expired almost instantaneously. No trace of injury or of grave disease could be discovered on the most careful examination. I, therefore, reported that, as blows inflicted upon the front of the abdomen had been known, in several instances, to cause death by a shock to the nervous system, it was probable that, in this case, like force applied to the side of the belly had acted in a similar manner.

In 1849, a case occurred, at Monghyr, in which a boy was said to have been killed by two kicks. The medical officer found that the right lung had been diseased for some time. He could discover no sign of violence, and stated that, in his opinion, fever was the cause of death. The magistrate asked if a kick on the stomach would cause death. He replied that the organs of the abdomen were healthy, but that, if the boy was kicked severely on the stomach, it might cause instantaneous death. The magistrate, therefore, *inferred,* that the second kick, said to have been given by the prisoner to the deceased, fell on the stomach and caused death ; he therefore committed the prisoner, to which course the superintendent of police seems to have objected.*

---

* Police Report, L. P., 1849, p. 15. In the following case, death very probably resulted from this cause, but the fact was not discovered by dissection. A man being angry with his mistress, the widow of his brother, for speaking to a person of whom he was jealous, struck her two slaps, and kicked her violently "under the breast,"—she died immediately.—*Nizamut Adawlut Reports*, N. W. P., 3rd Nov. 1854, p. 532.

The following case of death, after a severe blow on the body, unattended with any discoverable organic lesion, has great medico-legal importance. Two men of Sewan (Sarun) went to the house of one Lowtoo, to press him as a "*begar*." He was preparing to smoke, and his daughter, a child of eight, stood close by him, holding his hookah. He said he would go when he had smoked. One of the men then seized him and beat him with an iron-bound *lattee*, and the other gave him "a violent dig in the ribs" with a long heavy *lattee*; the blow knocked him down over his child, whose neck is said to have been twisted, and who remained insensible from that time till nearly the following morning, when she expired. The above circumstances appear to have been clearly proved, not only by the evidence of five eye-witnesses, but by the account given by the prisoners themselves. Lowtoo was carried inside, and afterwards went, with the support of two persons, to the ticcadar of the village to complain. Returning home, he was ill all night, vomiting violently after drinking water. He expired next day at noon. On the following day, Dr. Fleming found the bodies swollen, from the heat of the weather. He found no marks of injury whatever. The healthy state of the viscera led him to suppose that death might have been caused by some narcotic poison, but he allowed that the contents of the stomach might present the same appearance, though no poison had been administered.*

Danger of Cold Drinks when heated.

No authentic case of death or severe illness from drinking cold water, when heated, has come at all within my own observation; but once, having drunk with avidity a tumblerful of effervescing lemonade in a crowded and over-heated theatre, I experienced sensations which taught me that such cases of fatal shock to the great abdominal ganglia probably do occur. Mr. M'Gavin gives, in a paper "On the Danger of Cold Drinks in Harvest," some facts illustrating the risk of drinking cold water. There had been, a short time previously, several fatal accidents among harvesters in Scotland, owing to the general belief that, if you are ever so hot, water on which the sun has been shining can do you no harm. Here, Dr. M'Gavin argues, is the mistake: "Cold liquids at the freezing point, or a little above, rarely produce dangerous effects, while those ranging from 51 degrees to 53 degrees are, if the body is heated and fatigued, commonly followed by serious results." "The explanation,' says a writer in the *Pall Mall Gazette*, "is just the same as that which answers for the cold bath—the reaction is greater the colder the water. It is very hard, indeed (as most of us know), to get up a reaction after a bath of about 59 degrees. Another reason why very cold drinks do not hurt is because we take less of them at a time. Ices are eaten

* The last sentence is scarcely intelligible, probably owing to a misprint; but it appears to show that no internal organ was ruptured.—*Nizamut Adawlut Reports*, 4th Nov. 1854, p. 542.

by spoonfuls, iced water is drunk by sips [not always so in India], sherry-cobbler by small sucks : thus, in every case, the fluid gets partly heated in the mouth, and also covers a very small extent of mucous membrane. Ice too, after dinner, can do little harm. In South America, a native rarely travels without some Indian corn flour to mix with his water, just as we make a drink for horses. This prevents any evil effects from water drinking ; it also stimulates the action of the gastric juice, as do the lumps of toast in soup, which are not without their hygienic use. When you are tired and hot, then, remember always to drink by small mouthfuls ; you will quench your thirst better, and save all risk to your stomach. Some people are stricken down at once after the cold draught, as if by apoplexy ; others only get a chill, followed by a more or less perfect reaction. It the reaction is normal, all is well ; but if too much blood is drawn to the interior of the body in order to restore the equilibrium between skin and stomach, in three or four days, congestion and inflammation set in of lungs, kidneys, brain, or of the stomach itself, and make you regret you did not drink according to Dr. M'Gavin's rule."

Rupture of the Uterus.

I am indebted to Dr. Wise, Civil Surgeon of Dacca, for the following very rare case in which the *Uterus* was ruptured by a kick. Hoormut was severely beaten by her husband, on the morning of the 27th. She was lying weak and ill, and the same evening she died. The evidence is very contradictory, but the above was the substance of the deposition given by her brother-in-law at the *post-mortem* examination on the 1st March. I found no external mark of injury, but, above the mons veneris, an extravasation of blood among the muscles was observed. An enormous quantity of fluid blood was found effused into the peritoneal cavity. A rupture of the uterus at its fundus was the only internal injury detected ; through this laceration, the membranes of a fœtus between the 2nd and 3rd month protruded. There was no mark of injury in the vagina or cevix uteri. The liver, spleen, and intestines were healthy. The stomach contained a partially digested meal of rice.

Injury to the Testicles.

So many cases are on record, in which this mode of assault was adopted, in several instances with fatal result, that the practice demands a separate paragraph.

This mode of assault is mentioned in Deut. XXIV., v. XI : "When men strive together one with another, and the wife of the one draweth near for to deliver her husband out of the hand of him that smiteth him, and putteth forth her hand, and taketh him by the secrets :

"Then thou shall cut off her hand ; thine eye shall not pity her."

This law becomes clearer when it is understood that such an assault is extremely liable to prove fatal.

The practice of dragging an enemy along by the genitals is rather frequent in India. The consequence sometimes is, that the integument gives way and is torn off.

The ancient Hindu law recognized this mode of assault, but does not appear to have attached any danger to it, ruling that, "If a Sooder hath plucked a brahmin by the hair, or by the beard, or should take hold of a brahmin's neck, or testicles, the magistrate shall cut off both his hands."—(*Halhed*, p. 235.)

A dispute on money matters arising between two traders of Delhi, some indecent language passed, when one seized the other, and dragged him along with such violence that the whole preputial integument was torn away.*

Some peculiar significance is evidently attached to this mode of assault.

A Cossiah woman confessed that she went with her husband to their *pan* garden, when, he having climbed a tree seven or eight cubits high to get a ratan, it broke in his grasp, and he fell to the ground, when she, seeing his helpless condition, seized the opportunity, and with a stick struck him over the nose and face, and completed the murder by squeezing his testicles until he expired. There were two very severe scalp wounds, and the testicles were swollen.

Major Birch, Deputy Commissioner, who tried the case, noted that "this appears to be an operation understood by the Cossiah women, as he recollected that Mr. D. Scott, Commissioner of Assam, informed him that a case had occurred of a European soldier attempting to commit a rape on a Cossiah woman, who effectually frustrated his attempt and severely punished him in this manner.†

In June 1855 a Midnapore woman confessed that her husband returned home one night and found her paramour and another in his house, upon which he was killed by squeezing the scrotum with the hand and strangulation.‡

In the remarkable case of drugging and then murdering a Jain Priest at Bhaugulpore in 1865, one Phoolchand confessed that, when the priest became insensible, Gopaul Singh squeezed his throat, Sunker rode on his chest, Juggernauth held his hands, and Mooseedeen squeezed his private parts with his feet.§

Lutfullah says that "one sound kick on the scrotum" completed a thug's murderous work.

Wyh this violence is added to that of strangulation is not clear. It can scarcely be doubted that it alone has repeatedly killed, probably by nervous shock.

---

* Nizamut Adawlut Reports, N. W. P., September 21, 1854, p. 415.

† Nizamut Adawlut Reports, April 5, 1855, p. 371.

‡ *Ibid*, July 27, 1855, p. 150.

§ Beng. Police Rep. for 1865, p. 35.

Moobrack was capitally sentenced in the Konkun (Bombay Presidency) in 1845 for having murdered a man with whose wife he had an intrigue, by "seizing him by the testicles, which he wrenched in the most violent manner." It was shown that the deceased was a man in rude health, that he was not suffering from any disease, and that, after the violence described "his testicles" [scrotum] "were swollen to the size of a cocoanut."*

It appeared, in a trial at East Burdwan, that one Gosimdas visited the house of a woman with whom he had an intrigue, in which one of the accused, named Tarachand, wished to supplant him. He was seized by several persons, and "tortured in a way to prevent his interfering in future with the wishes of Tarachand." The man died under the ill-treatment to which he was subjected. The evidence of the medical officer proved that he died by violence, the testicles being crushed and the lower part of the body bruised.† See Chapter on TORTURE, *Section* on *Compressing the Testicles*, p. 558.

MUTILATION.

In common with most other primitive nations, the Hindoo and Mussalmaun rulers of India seem to have considered the summary mutilation of a criminal a surer and more economical mode of punishment than the infliction of imprisonment at the expense of the State.

Cutting off the Hands and Feet.

Being dissatisfied with the slow progress of his success in besieging Ormus, Albuquerque intercepted all vessels bringing provisions to the island, cut off the ears, noses, and hands of all the captives, and sent these mutilated unfortunates on shore, desiring them to tell their countrymen that he would serve all others so who might attempt to bring them provisions.

"He" (the King of Achen) "is very cruel to his subordinates, daily cutting off their hands, armes or legges, upon small or no occasions."—*Peyton's Voyage*, 1614.

Dr. James Irving mentions, in his Concise View of the Progress of Military Medical Literature, Edinburgh Medical and Surgical Journal, No. 163, that, in some remarks on amputation made in John Woodall's "Whole Works," 1639, we have one of the first hints as to the expediency and safety of amputation at the ankle—a proceeding to which his attention was first drawn by observing the effects of some Eastern punishments, in which the feet are cut off; and, although he confesses that he should not

* Bellasis' Reports, p. 234.

† Nizamut Adawlut Reports, October 12, 1855, p. 644.

be the first to make the experiment in surgery, yet he wishes to draw attention to the method.

At the Mayor's Court in Calcutta on the 24th October 1749, one Rudoo deposed that, on having a certain proposition put to him, his uncle was exceedingly angry, and said, " Whose ears are to be cut off, or whose hand, for doing a thing of this kind?"

This practice appears to have been quite as prevalent in Bengal under Seraj-ood-dowla and his predecessors as it was, a few years since, in Lahore, under Runjeet Singh.* Ward, the missionary, states that he had been informed that, before the English criminal law was executed at Calcutta, the most bloody scenes were frequently witnessed. " Criminals were brought to the river side, where, with blunt instruments, they cut off the hands of some, the feet of others, and other members of others, and then turned them adrift. Some of these poor wretches fell down on the spot, and lay there until they died; and others, unable to bear the exquisite torture arising from the mangling and amputating of their limbs, plunged into the river, and found a watery grave."

In the 17th and 18th centuries the practice of mutilation was universal in India.

---

* According to Harington, the penalty to be adjudged, under the Mahomedan law, on conviction of the crime of theft, was, for the first offence, amputation of the right hand; and for the second, amputation of the left foot. Also an ancient Danish custom, as will be shown hereafter. Retaliation for offences against the person, not affecting life, was restricted to wounding and maiming in the following instances:—1.—For any member of the body severed at the joint; as a hand, arm, foot, or leg. Also for the fingers and toes, or part of them, if separated at the joint. 2.—For an ear, or part of an ear, cut off. 3.—For the nose, if completely cut away. 4.—For the lips, or either of them. 5.—For the teeth, or any number of them. For an injury to the eye destroying the sight, without forcing the eye from the socket. The retaliation, in this last case, was to be inflicted by holding a hot iron before the corresponding eye of the offender, till sight became extinguished.

Mutilation also had a prominent place among the penalties enjoined by the ancient Hindu law. "With whatever limb," says Menu, "a chief commits the offence, by any means in this world, as if he break a wall with his hand or foot, even that limb shall the king amputate, for the prevention of similar crime."—Chap. viii., s. 334.

Again, "Of robbers, who break a wall or partition, and commit theft in the night, let the prince order the hands to be lopped off, and themselves to be fixed to a sharp stake." " Two fingers of a cut-purse, the thumb and the index, let him cause to be amputated on his first conviction; on the second, one hand and one foot; on the third, he shall suffer death."—Chap. ix., ss. 276-77.

" For stealing more than 50 *panas*, a hand shall be amputated."—s. 324.

" For taking things belonging to priests, &c., the offender shall instantly lose half of one foot."—s. 325.

We have already seen that, according to the Hindu law, if a person of Sudra caste plucked a Brahmin by the hair or by the beard, or seized him by the neck, the Magistrate was to *cut off both his hands*. If a Sudra, through pride, spat upon a Brahmin, his *lips were to be cut off*.

In that Law nearly every imaginable kind of mutilation was adjudged for various offences. Such as, of hand or foot, both hands, one hand and one foot, both hands and both feet, buttock, lips, penis, half the penis, testicles, pudenda, fundament, ears, nose, breaking the teeth, finger or fingers, pulling out the eyes.

In ordinary criminal cases, capital punishment was very seldom inflicted by the Sikhs. The most incorrigible culprits were punished with the loss of a hand, or of nose and ears.

When the Emperor Humayoon took Chunar Ghur, after a spirited defence of six mouths, he cut off the right hands of all the artillerymen who had so long baffled him.

The Rev. J. Long has noted that, about 1770, a fellow was detected, at Moorshedabad, setting fire to a house by throwing the *ticka* of his *hukah* in the *chuppers* (thatch). He was tried, and sentenced to have his left hand and right foot cut off.

This practice, although interdicted by the British Government, still lingers in some of the Native States.*

It has been stated that the late Coorg Rajah, whose daughter received so much kindness from Queen Victoria, was in the habit of keeping those in his presence constantly in an attitude of supplication, and that if their hands dropped, he ordered those members to be struck off. If any complaint was uttered, the offending lips were to be cut away.

The following report appeared in the Calcutta *Englishman* of the 10th October 1868 :—"We are sorry to see the barbarous and cruel practice of cutting off a prisoner's hand, for an offence of which he was found guilty, on the plea that it was the hand which perpetrated the offence, being practised in Cabul. This punishment has always been a favorite one with despots in India and central Asia. We have seen numbers of men in the Punjab and its neighbourhood who had lost their hands under former governments for the offence of killing cows."

The same authority reports on the 22nd of June of that year :—

"We hear from Rajpootana, that, in spite of the prohibition of the Viceroy, and in spite of the efforts of the Political Department, kine-killing is still punished by some of the chiefs by mutilation. Recently some Mahomedans were caught on the frontiers, who declared they had been exiled for this crime. Several of the band had their ears cut, but, as they refused to make any complaints, the matter was allowed to drop."

In June 1870 it was reported in the *Jubbulpore Chronicle* that a thief who had purloined some property of the Maharajah of Gwalior had been sentenced to have his right hand cut off.

While I was bringing out my last edition, a gentleman who had been long residing in Nepal told me that mutilation was, a few years previously, one of the commonest judicial punishments in Katmandu. He had frequently known *Noses* cut off for adultery and public shame, the *Hands* for theft, and the *Testicles* for rape and bestiality. Under the present more enlightened Native Government, mutilation is almost

* In the *Friend of India* of August 23rd, 1855, it is stated, "Mutilation has disappeared altogether in the Punjab."

wholly prohibited by law. A case had, however, occurred, not long previously, in which a woman, formerly of good caste, having repeatedly broken the caste of men of respectablity by intriguing with them, was at length seized, deprived of the end of her nose, and turned out of the country.

A very graphic account of the manner in which ten culprits had their hands cut off in Nepal in 1831 was given by Dr. Bramley at p. 158 of the first volume of the Indian Journal of Medical Science. The skin of the fore-arm having been strongly retracted, the hand was cut off through the wrist-joint. The unfortunate men had to restrain the hæmorrhage by grasping the stumps until their friends came, and, twising some linen in a cord-like shape, bound it with considerable tightness, commencing at the bend of the elbow, carrying it forwards as far as the edge of the stump, and securing it at this point so as to prevent it from becoming loosened. One of these ten men died on the third day, the others recovered, and were robbing again before their stumps were healed.

It appeared in a trial in the Konkan (Bombay Presidency) that Puddoo Bin Bappo had, with his gang, plundered and burnt the lines of a party of the Ghaut Police. The Jemadar of the party, being taken prisoner, joined his hands in supplication, but Puddoo cut them both off with his sword, exclaiming, "Are not these the very hands that beat me with a shoe?"*

A remarkable case of mutilation occurred at Muthra in 1853. Lall Doss was tried for the murder of Luchee by attacking him with a sword, *cutting off his hand,* which he carried off, and inflicting other wounds. Mohun, uncle of the deceased, mentioned, in the course of his evidence on the trial, that, twenty-five years ago, this prisoner also wounded him (the deponent), and *cut off his hand.* The prisoner, since wounding him, had turned *byragee,* and wandered about, but spoke rationally. The prisoner said that "he cut off the hand of Luchee, because the *brother* of Luchee had stolen his book!" "There was not," the Judge held, "the slightest reason to believe that there was any foundation for this story. It seemed to be a pure hallucination of the prisoner, who, under this impression, inflicted on the supposed offender the ancient native punishment for theft,—*viz.*, cutting off his hand."†

A prisoner was convicted of cutting off his wife's hand; but no

---

* Bellasis' Reports, p. 231.

† Nizamut Adawlut Reports, North-Western Provinces, 30th May 1853, p. 712. By the English law, "No criminal is to suffer the punishment of mutilation. If a prisoner is sentenced, in conformity with the futwa of the Law Officer, to lose two limbs, instead of being made to undergo such punishment, he is to be imprisoned and kept to hard labour for fourteen years; and if any prisoner is sentenced to lose one limb, he is, in lieu of such punishment, to be imprisoned and kept in hard labor for seven years."—*Beaufort,* First Ed., 857.

punishment was awarded, in consequence of the prayer of the injured party that her husband should be released.*

I had under treatment a slave girl of Chittagong, who, among other frightful injuries inflicted upon her person with a *dhao* by her master's brother, who had intrigued with her and had become jealous, had one hand cut off through the carpal bones, evidently at a single blow. The surface granulated, and healed rapidly. It had fortunately happened that she had received aid, at the time, from a retired native doctor.

A man severely wounded five persons with a sword and spear, but was apprehended. Two other persons were tried for deliberately cutting off the hands of this prisoner; but they were released and rewarded, as it was shown that they did so with a view to his apprehension and in self-defence.†

Mutilation by cutting off the *Nose and the Right Hand* is still one of the punishments for intrigue practised by the Hindus of Bengal and the North-Western Provinces. So lately as 1850, a man of Baraset, near Calcutta, being jealous of his wife, deliberately cut off her *Nose, Lips, and Right Hand.*‡

It was reported in a trial at Nursingpore, in 1852, that one Lutkun was disfigured by the loss of his *Nose*—an act of retaliatory revenge executed by the relatives of a *brahminee,* whom he seduced. They had also maimed his *Right Arm*, in an attempt to cut it off.§

Blinding.

A reference to the early pages of Indian history will show that the tyrants of the East generally put out the *Eyes* of their brethren, as a safe mode of setting at rest all disputes regarding their succession.

Gholam Kadir Shaik put out one of the eyes of the Emperor Shah Alum with his own hand, and, in his turn, had his eyes torn out of their sockets, and his nose, ears, hands, and feet cut off by Scindia. Ferohsyur deprived of sight Yezziddin and Ali Tebar, princes of the blood royal, and Humayoon, his own younger brother, by having a large red-hot needle drawn across their eyes. In the same manner, the Emperor Ahmed Shah and his

* Nizamut Adawlut Reports, Vol. I., p. 344.

† *Ibid*, Vol. I., p. 310.

‡ Police Report, L. P., 1850.

§ Nizamut Adawlut Reports, N. W. P., 19th March 1852, p. 202.

Such, judging by the words of an ancient Danish ballad, were formerly the punishments of Seduction and Adultery in the north of Europe.

> "They tore away his Eyes so bright,"—
> * * * *
> His Left Foot then and his good Right Hand,
> They hewed them off at the king's command."

Menu says—"Of a man who through violence forcibly contaminates a damsel, let the king instantly order Two Fingers to be amputated, and order him to pay a fine of 600 panas."—Chap. viii., p. 367.

mother, Oodem Bhai, were blinded by order of his rebellious minister, Mir Sheabeddin. This also is said by one authority to have been done to the Emperor Ferohsyur himself. It is added, in the Seir Mutaqherin, that this operation did not deprive him entirely of the light of day.*

Raj Beni Bahadyr had his eyes plucked out for malversation, it was said, but, in reality, because he had too many connections with the English.

In Vol. II., p. 427 of the Nizamut Adawlut Reports is the case of a man who was sentenced to 14 years' imprisonment for putting out his wife's eyes with a hot iron, "the pupils of both eyes having been totally destroyed."

We find, in Macnaghten's Reports, the trial of a man who, having tied the hands and feet of his wife, threw her down, sat upon her breast, and put out her *Eyes* with a heated iron ! †

Gouging is a practice by no means unknown in India. Aleef and Neamutoollah, of Backergunge, were sentenced to 14 years' imprisonment for taking a man, against whom they had enmity, to a deserted homestead, where they threw him down on the ground ; and, one of them sitting on his chest, they destroyed both of his eyes "by means of some internal violence applied by pressure with the finger on the eye-balls." The Civil Surgeon deposed that the tissues of the eyes were destroyed, the sight completely gone, and that the man would be blind for life.‡

Sunjoo Fakeer was sentenced to 16 years' imprisonment at Nuddea under the following circumstances :—His wife, a child of about 12, declared that she, being taken away from his house, he on the road attempted to have connexion with her under a tree in some waste land ; but she, being very young, protested. He then hit her left cheek, tied both her hands with cloth, and bit her thumb; he then tightened a cloth round her neck, and pressed his fingers into both her eyes and blinded her. The report of Dr. Palmer, the Civil Surgeon, showed that the right eye bore the appearance of having been burst by some mechanical injury, and that the effect might have been produced by a finger being thrust in. He subsequently reported that her life was in danger. His successor, Dr. Halls, deposed that

---

* Dr. Fryar describes blinding by a hot needle as a Persian practice. He says of their monarchs: "Their jealousy is so fervent that they keep their sons like captives, till the father's death enlarges the eldest; when the younger brothers, uncles, and nephews on both sides, on the appearance of the rising sun, see their last. As if the blood royal were prophan'd, unless they fled to the hot iron as the only means to expiate for its affinity, which being drawn over the most sensible parts (their eyes) strikes from the rays of their kinsman's diadem such a sparkling lustre, as for ever after makes them irrecoverably blind ; to seek recovery whereof, or any for them, is a treason unpardonable." (p. 347.)

† Vol. II., p. 427. A person being jealous of another, had him seized, cut off his *Nose* and *Chin*, put out his *Eyes* with the hooked point of a *dhao*, and then beat him to death.—*Police Report, L. Provinces*, 1838, p. 71.

‡ Nizamut Adawlut Reports, January 4th, 1856, p. 17.

the girl's sight was completely destroyed, and that her blindness arose from inflammation caused by the insertion of fingers into the orbits.*

According to Sonnerat, if any Brahmin has merited death, his eyes are put out, but he is permitted to live.

In 1853, certain persons were convicted of having assaulted one Phool Mahomed, who, besides other injuries, *had a Peg driven into his Eyes*, in consequence of which total blindness resulted.

In 1852, one Bahwaneedur, of Allahabad, having some time previously put his wife away, on suspicion of misconduct, and having located her in a hut close by his own, since which time there had been constant quarrelling between them,—murdered her. She was found strangled in the hut. Her left *Eye* had been wounded by some sharp instrument, and the Surgeon considered that there must have been a great deal of violence exerted in the destruction of its textures, as if there had been an intent to extract it forcibly. The other eye was also punctured. There were the appearances which would result from suffocation. The deceased seemed to have had a great struggle for life, as shown by bruises on the back.†

These atrocious barbarities are also inflicted even upon *the Children* of the intriguer. At about the same time, a young boy of Bundelkund was found lying dead in a field. The medical officer stated that the skin of the neck was abraded as if by a rope passed twice round it—the *Eyes* were punctured with some sharp-pointed instrument, and the point of the *Nose* was cut off. The person tried for the murder said that one Choonta, who had taken away the child's uncle's wife, offered him seven rupees to kill the child, as the child's father was at enmity with him. The boy's father confirmed this latter statement.‡

It is necessary to observe some caution in giving an opinion upon the condition of the Eyes of persons whose bodies have been for some time exposed in the fields,—as these parts are generally attacked by birds of prey.§ For further remarks on Blinding, see p. 549.

Cutting off the Ears.

It is a common practice, both in Bengal and in the North-West, to cut off the *Ears* of Intriguers.

Allusion is made at p. 533 to the case of a Dinagepore woman who, in addition to various bruises and other injuries, had lost one Ear and a portion of the other; and also to another instance [at p. 419] described by Dr.

* Nizamut Adawlut Reports, November 19, 1857, p. 396.

† *Ibid*, N. W. P., 17th April 1852, p. 326.

‡ *Ibid*, 23rd January 1852, p. 61.

§ Forbes mentions that a person is appointed to watch the Parsee bodies exposed on Malabar Hill to ascertain which of the deceased's eyes the birds of prey first pluck out, as they attach some superstitious idea respecting the happiness or misery of the departed spirit from the circumstance.

Wilkie, who found another Dinagepore woman's throat cut, her breasts gashed, and *both her Ears* cut off. See also p. 390—case of Harkoa.

In February 1854, a man was convicted at Sylhet, upon his own confession, of knocking another down with a heavy club, and then cutting off his Ear. He pleaded that the complainant had enticed away his sister-in-law.*

Ausgur Ali pleaded guilty at the Calcutta Criminal Sessions, June 2nd 1868, of having attacked a woman with whom he had been cohabiting. He mutilated her face in a fearful manner with a knife, and cut one ear completely off. 10 years' penal servitude.

Two men were convicted, at Tipperah, of cutting off the ear and knocking out the front teeth of a person suspected of having carried on an intrigue with the wife of one of them.†

In a second case, also at Tipperah, Mahomed Abbas and Ooda Gazie were sentenced to three years' imprisonment for having slit the ear and knocked out three of the front teeth of Mahomed Danesh by way of "putting a mark on him to recognize him hereafter," he having been caught in the act of entering the former prisoner's house at midnight with improper intentions towards his wife.‡

Ahbed Karrigur, of Backergunge, being jealous of his wife, although she was in a very weak state of health from fever, asthma, and dropsy, took her from place to place to avoid the person whom he suspected. She being too ill to leave the house one morning, his jealousy led him to attribute her reluctance to another cause. He cut off her right ear from the root with a dhao. The shock hastened her death, which occurred almost immediately after she was brought to the dispensary.§

The Nawab Meer Jaffir Ally is said to have been betrayed by one whom he had, in his prosperity, cruelly treated, by causing his ears to be cut off.

This is also not unfrequently the punishment of trespassers and thieves.

A prisoner having cut off the ear of a man, who had burglariously entered his house during the night, was acquitted, as no guilt was considered to attach to the act.‖

Two very young lads, of Agra, were found guilty of having deliberately cut off the ear of a neighbour who would not allow their cattle to remain in his field. An altercation ensued: when they got the man down, one of them assisted in holding him, while the other cut off his ear with a *khoorpa*, or spade.¶

---

* Nizamut Adawlut Reports for February 1854, p. 192.

† *Ibid*, 3rd Nov. 1854, p. 526.

‡ *Ibid*, January 15, 1857, p. 31.

§ *Ibid*, May 1, 1855, p. 476.

‖ *Ibid*, Vol. III, p. 285, as cited by Beaufort.

¶ Nizamut Adawlut Reports, N. W. P., 24th Oct. 1854, p. 604.

A chowkedar was charged by an individual with stealing from his house a sum of money, &c. While the thief was making his escape, a female inmate of the house cut off one of his ears. Upon the arrest of the alleged culprit, he stated that he was intimate with the daughter-in-law of the complainant, who, in a fit of jealousy, cut off his ear. The Sessions Judge, finding clear evidence for conviction, sentenced him to four years' imprisonment.

Cutting off the Lips.

In 1855, a woman and her son, inhabitants of Nowakallee, murdered the wife of the latter. The male prisoner, displeased with the dinner prepared for him by his wife, a girl 14 years old, struck her on the head with a small bamboo twig. She then began abusing him, his mother, and all connected with him. The prisoner, who was peeling some sugar-cane with a *dhao*, went up to the girl and deliberately cut off her *under lip*, saying, "I will cut off your mouth for daring to abuse my mother." The mother and son then laid hold of the unhappy girl, dragged her into the cook-room, and despatched her.*

In 1851, a man was found guilty, at Bopal, of cutting off the *nose* and a portion of the *upper lip* and *cheek* of his wife (sixteen years old), apparently under the influence of groundless jealousy.†

Cutting off the Nose.

Cutting off the *nose* is a common punishment of sexual crime, throughout India. This is evidently a very ancient custom; indeed, we have glimpses of it in Hindu mythology.

Nasuk, on the Godavery, near which there are rock temples, is said to derive its name from Luchman's having cut off the nose of the female Rakhasha Soorpanakha.

In one of the fables of the *Hitopodesa*, a jealous man is described as having bound his wife to a post. A procuress supplies her place; and, while she is in that situation, the suspicious husband cuts off her nose. The bawd protests that her own husband cut off her nose, while the unchaste wife declares that her virtue has rendered her proof against razors. A writer, early in the seventeenth century, tells us that "Chatagun is also reckoned amongst their cities. They are a most subtile and

---

* Police Report, L. P., for 1844, p. 44:—"A once-born man who insults a twice-born man, with gross invectives, ought to have his tongue slit." "If a *Sooder* falsely accuses a *Brahmin*, a *Khetree*, or *a vice* of either of the crimes of *Atee Patuk*, or *Maha Patuk*, or *Anoo Patuck*, the magistrate shall cut out his tongue, and thrust a hot iron of ten fingers' breadth into his mouth." (*Halhed*, p. 208, also p. 214.) "With whatever member a low-born man shall assault or hurt his superior, even that member of his must be slit or cut, more or less, in proportion to the injury."—*Menu*, c. V., s. 270-279. Pope Sixtus the Fifth appears to have subscribed to this retaliative system. Having discovered that a miserable joker had pasquinaded his sister, he sentenced the wretch to lose his hands and his tongue.

† Nizamut Adawlut Reports, Vol. I., p. 859.

wicked people, and are esteemed the worst slaves of all India, for that they are all thieves, and the women whores, although this fault is common through all India, no place excepted. They have a custome, never to dress or seeth meat twice in one pot, but have every time a new one. Whensoever they are found in adulterie, they have their noses cut off, and are thenceforward narrowly looked to, that they keepe not each other's company."*

Coddem Hossein Khan, Governor of Poorania, being displeased with an astrologer, ordered him to be taken to the public market and there to have his nose cut off.

The Nawab Meer Cassim Khan ordered an intriguer's nose to be cut off, and himself to be put upon an ass and carried in that condition all over the town, after which he was banished.†

Hyder Ally and Tippoo Saheb were in the habit of cutting off the noses and ears of those of their English prisoners who were caught when attempting to escape. One was afterwards led round the fort on a jackass, with his face to the tail.‡

Tippo, before Mangalore, cut off the noses and ears of the whole of a sepoy brigade who attempted to prevent an execution.§

The reduction of Khistipoor, a town of Nepal, cost the conqueror so much trouble that, in resentment of the resistance made by the inhabitants, he cut off all the men's noses. After the lapse of 23 years, Colonel Kirkpatrick was reminded of this act of barbarity by observing that a great proportion of the people sent to transport his baggage across the hills were deprived of their noses. To perpetuate this exploit, the Sovereign ordered the name of the place to be changed to Naskatapoor.

Dr. Gibson mentions, in his account of the Province of Guzerat published in the 1st number of the Transactions of the Medical and Physical Society of Bombay, that, among the Doonjas, the crime of sorcery is very common, and that many women may be seen throughout the country whose noses have been cut off, as the punishment of their witchcraft.

The writer of an article on "The Women of Hindustan,"‖ says that he had twice or thrice seen this punishment of unchastity inflicted immediately upon conviction of the crime. It was done with much ceremony by the village barber, who, having first shaved the woman's head, at a signal from the chief of the *panchaiut* (council of five Brahmins) "snips off her nose with a small pair of shears." He adds that the Punjabees used to obliterate all traces of beauty in the person of the delinquent, by the application of oil of vitriol, or some other escharotic acid.

---

* Purchas, Part 2, p. 508.

† Seir Mutaqherin.

‡ James Bristow's Narrative.

§ Forbes, Vol. II., p. 461.

‖ Asiatic Jour., N. S., Vol. XXIX, p. 298.

Removal of the nose is, or was lately, a judicial punishment in Nepal. Hence the skill of native practitioners in the rhinoplastic operation.

It was reported, in June 1856, that a mehter living in the Chandney Chowk, Calcutta, being enraged with his wife, because she refused to bring him water to drink, took a knife and cut off her nose.

Salamut Russooa, of Rajshahye, pleaded guilty of having cut off the nose of his adulterous wife. She had an intrigue with her brother-in-law. Her husband had remonstrated with her over and over again. From her own statement to the Deputy Magistrate, she must have been a woman of the most worthless character. She admitted the intrigue. Waking up in the night, the husband saw the paramour running out of the room. After having subjected his wife to a storm of reproaches, he allowed her to go to sleep, and then committed the assault upon her. He was convicted under section 326 of the Indian Penal Code.*

In June 1858, it was reported in the *Mofussilite* that a naick of the City Police, named Sheikh Kullun, thinking that his wife was unfaithful, threw her down in the street, placed his knee on her chest, and cut off her nose.

Forbes mentions that the female *confidante* of an intrigue between one of the Peshwar's (Ragobah's) officers and one of his concubines was condemned to have her nose cut off, and thus remain an example to the other slaves in the harem.

Many illustrations of the existence of this practice in the Bombay Presidency might be given. Witloo Walud Bappo, of Ahmednuggur, was tried for murder in April 1841. Considering that his wife was an adulteress, he cut her nose and ear with a dagger, and then stabbed her twice in the stomach.†

Puthoo Johra, of Ahmedabad, finding one in the act of adultery with his wife, killed him with his sword, and with the same weapon inflicted a wound on her nose and face.‡

A case in which a man of Bhooj mutilated the nose and upper lip of his sister-in-law is mentioned in the Bombay Dispensary Reports, Vol. II., p. 199.

Macnaghten's Reports contain a very singular case, where a woman had entered into a formal engagement to allow her husband to cut off her nose, hands, and hair in the event of her behaving improperly. She having forfeited her pledge, her husband convened a Punchayet, forced a confession of guilt from the woman and her paramour, read to the assembly his wife's engagement, and, having received their authority to enforce its conditions, deliberately took up a knife and cut off her nose.§

---

* Weekly Reporter, Calcutta High Court, Vol. iv., Nov. 1865, p. 17.

† Bellasis' Reports, p. 141.

‡ *Ibid*, p. 95.

§ Nizamut Adawlut Reports, Vol. I., p. 296.

In 1854, a Rajshahye man confessed that he had abducted the wife of another, dissuading her from returning home by telling her that her husband "would cut off her nose and hair;" enraged at her obstinacy, he murdered her.* Choonna, of Meerut, admitted that he had killed a prostitute, with whom he had cohabited for eight years, by stabbing her in the throat with a *bichooa*, or dagger. They went to a hut near the Ganges, where they drank a bottle of spirit, the prisoner smoked *churrus*, then both slept. Waking in the morning, prisoner said he should cut off her nose and leave her; she said she would then be of no further use, and that he had better kill her, but that he would not escape. He then stabbed her.† One Banee, of Moradabad, when on trial in 1852, for the murder of his wife, stated that, on her refusing to admit his embraces, he took a knife and threatened to stab her in the stomach, and to cut off her nose. She then seized the knife and stabbed herself.‡

A Rajpoot, discovering his uncle's widow with her paramour, cut off their noses with his sword.§

A woman of Tirhoot, having lost her nose, took oath, first, that one Bheeka cut off the part, whilst her husband held her hands; and afterwards that her husband did it, and that she had implicated Bheeka from motives of enmity. The husband was proved to be the real criminal.||

In 1854, Adaree Daiee, of Nuddea, confessed that, waking in the night and finding that his wife had left his side, he took a knife, and discovering her with a man, threw her on the ground, and cut off the tip of her nose "with the view, he alleged, of spoiling her beauty."¶

A rather obscure case, involving a mutilation of this kind, was tried at Sylhet in 1853. Meeaboollah, a discharged Burkandauz, went to the house of a prostitute in the town, and offered to marry her; she objected that she had not seen his house, and they went together for that purpose. She wore her ornaments. She was never again seen alive; but, on the second evening, her body was found, about 200 yards from the prisoner's house, with the throat cut from ear to ear, and the face shockingly mutilated. Her ornaments were gone. One of the persons who first discovered the body declared that, when he saw it, the nose, with a gold ornament in it, was on the face. Yet, two hours afterwards, when the darogah arrived at the spot, the nose and upper lip were wanting, and he reported that they had been eaten off by jackals. The native doctors, who examined the body, deposed, on the contrary, that the nose and lip

---

* Nizamut Adawlut Reports, 30th Nov. 1854, p. 695.

† Nizamut Adawlut Reports, N. W. P., 10th April 1852, p. 288.

‡ *Ibid*, July 23rd 1852, p. 723.

§ Nizamut Adawlut Reports, Vol. I., p. 327.

|| *Ibid*, 16th Dec. 1854, p. 738.

¶ *Ibid*, 9th Nov. 1854, p. 555.

had been cut off by a sharp instrument: but this, the Judge remarked, was not mentioned in their written report, and was open to suspicion.*

Ubdaot Singh, of Etawah, having intrigued with his brother's mistress, concluded the affair by cutting off part of her nose with a sword.†

Mussumat Mandarsee, a woman of Banda, who appeared in court in male attire, was found guilty of having, with the assistance of another woman, thrown down her female cousin, and nearly cut off her nose. The quarrel appears to have arisen upon money matters, with mutual charges of dissolute life.‡

Nujjuff Khan, of Furruckabad, having been intimate with a woman who had begun to receive the addresses of another, enticed her to remain with him, seized her, sat upon her chest, and cut off her nose with a knife.§

One Thakoorpershad, of Goruckpore, suspecting his sister-in-law's servant of intriguing with his mistress, turned him out of the house and service. Catching him afterwards concealed in the woman's house, he, with the assistance of three others (one of whom held the man's feet and one his hands, while the other sat on his chest), cut off the man's nose, and forced water into his mouth with a view to break his caste. The prisoners declared that the man leaped from the upper story of the house, and, falling on an iron pot, his nose was cut off. As is usual in such cases, the prisoners spoke of the man as a thief, not as an intriguer. The Judge observed, that "it is not usual among the natives to punish a thief in this manner; but it is not at all unusual so to punish a person convicted of such criminality as Ramruttun was suspected of."‖

Biting off the Nose and Ears

Is by no means a very rare brutality either in Bengal or Up-country. In eighteen months, I saw two cases, at Howrah, in which part of the nose had been bitten off, and one in which a segment had been taken out of the upper part of the ear, evidently by human teeth.

Lulla, of Moradabad, having been left in the house with his cousin's wife, who had been confined only fifteen days previously, stabbed her fatally in the abdomen with a knife,¶ and then endeavored to bite off her nose.**

* Nizamut Adawlut Reports, 18th March 1853, p. 330.

† *Ibid*, N. W. P., 11th Oct. 1852, p. 1147.

‡ *Ibid*, 20th Oct. 1853, p. 1321.

§ *Ibid*, N. W. P., 21st Sept. 1854, p. 413.

‖ *Ibid*, 11th March 1853, p. 361.

¶ It is mentioned as a custom, in that part of the country, among Hindus, for a woman who has been recently confined, invariably to keep a knife, sword, or other weapon on her bed.

** Nizamut Adawlut Reports, N. W. P., 22nd Sept. 1853, p. 1179.

Injuries inflicted by tearing Ornaments from the Nose and Ears.

The ears and nose are occasionally torn or cut in forcibly removing the rings worn by native women and children.*

Ewaz, of Delhi, was found guilty of having enticed a child to a retired place, and there robbed him, cutting the lobe of his ear to the extent of half an inch, to get one of his ear-rings.†

In a Report of the Coimbatore (Madras Presidency) Dispensary for 1852,‡ Mr. Porteous mentions that he treated within the year "lacerated wounds on eight out and nine in-patients; all these formed cases of criminal process, and *were all inflicted by tearing off the ear-ornaments forcibly*. In only one instance was much deformity caused, the united portions having sloughed away. The divided extremities of the lobe were generally cut even with scissors, and brought together and retained by a couple of pins, and a surface of collodion given around, with speedy and satisfactory results.

A Meerut man was sentenced for having forcibly torn the *nuth* from a woman's nose, as she was walking through the town. The Civil Surgeon, who examined the injury which she had received, confirmed her statement of the occurrence.§

Cutting out the Tongue.

The Emperor Feroshur, considering that a Hindu of distinction, Rajah Sobachand, had been too free of speech, ordered his tongue to be cut out; the man underwent the operation in all its rigor, but "he continued to speak as freely as ever." The author of the Seir Mutaqherin says, that the Vezir Mahmed-Amir-Khan had such a cordial aversion to the descendants of the Prophet, that, hearing by the way a man who sung the words "Aoly, the Saint of God!" he ordered his tongue to be cut off.

The notorious Hurrydass, of Lahore, used to turn back his tongue against the fauces previous to being buried. In investigating cases in which the tongue is said to have been cut out, it is right to bear in mind that tongue-swallowers and impostors who pretended that their tongues were cut out in Barbary, have, from time to time, practised upon public cre-

---

* Three men and a woman were convicted, at Dacca, of having beaten to death a female, who appears to have been a doctress and whom they accused of witchcraft. They also robbed her, forcibly tearing out the rings from her ears and nose, which were found lacerated.—*Nizamut Adawlut Reports*, 17th Jan. 1855, p. 65. It must be borne in mind that the nose-ring (*Nuth*), usually worn in Bengal, is easily removable, but is often forcibly plucked away. The ear-rings (*kurn-oo-phool, balees, &c.*) are frequently soldered, in which case thieves do not hesitate to cut or tear the part.

† Nizamut Adawlut Reports, N. W. P., 25th August 1852, p. 877.

‡ Madras Med. Board Reports for 1855, p. 342.

§ Nizamut Adawlut Reports, N. W. P., 22nd November 1852, p. 1368.

dulity in Europe.* The late Dr. Heathcote told me of a lad, at Seharunpore, who had this trick of "swallowing" the tongue.

Bheem Singh, of Cuttack, confessed before the magistrate that twenty-five men entered the room, where a tyrannical man hated by his ryots was sleeping, and dragged him out by a cord fastened round his neck, striking and reproaching him. They then cut off his ears, his nose, and tongue from the root, and murdered him. Prisoner was sentenced to transportation for life, as an accomplice.† After I left Howrah, in 1855, my successor, Dr. Archer, had under his care a man who had been maltreated in a boat. Among other injuries, part of his tongue had been cut off.

Mutilation of the Membrum Virile.

Macnaghten's Reports contain the trial of a slave girl, apparently not more than twelve years of age, who was found guilty of deliberately cutting off the *Membrum Virile* of a man who had purchased her.‡

Dr. S. Coull Mackenzie has mentioned to me the case of a woman at Howrah who, in a fit of jealousy, thus dismembered her paramour.

In 1852, a youth of eighteen or twenty, was convicted of an attempt to cut off the *Membrum Virile* of a lad of twelve, with a ***hussooah***, or sickle.§

In 1849, a prisoner confessed, at Purneah, that he and his brother had murdered a man on account of his great reputation as a wizard. They made him drunk, and then, tying him with cords, cut off his private parts, and threw him headlong into a well.‖

It would appear that this is the orthodox mode of treating wizards in India, as I find that, in 1830, 159 inhabitants of Dewallee, Konkan, were tried for the murder of a wizard whom they had set upon and killed with sticks. In order to remove the enchantment which he was supposed to possess, nails and wooden pegs were driven through various parts of his body, and his penis was cut off and thrown into the same hole in which he was buried with his face downwards.¶

---

* In a pamphlet describing the practices of thieves and impostors—*The Discoveries of John Poulter, alias, Baxter*, 1703,—we are told that "Gaggers are beggars, some of whom go in a sailor's dress pretending they were Galley slaves, and that their tongues were cut out by the Turks, and their arms were burnt in the Row Galleys. To deceive the world, they cut the strings of their tongues, and swallow it down their throat, and make their arms raw by perpetual blisters; but, if they were taken to the whipping post, the dumb would speak."

Formerly, says a writer in the Monthly Mirror for 1809, men who pretended that their tongues were cut out by the Algerines, got a pretty good livelihood, but this mode of exciting compassion is now out of fashion. See an earlier allusion to these impostors in Malcolm's London.

† Nizamut Adawlut Reports, Sept. 5, 1856, p. 362.

‡ Vol. II., p. 29.

§ Nizamut Adawlut Reports, Vol. II., Part 2, of 1852, p. 130.

‖ Police Reports, L. P., for 1849, p. 19.

¶ Bellasis' Reports, p. 46.

Early in 1853, a woman of Sylhet was found guilty of murdering a child by cutting off his private parts with a clasp knife, and throwing him into a tank.

"A mechanic or servile man," says Menu, "having adulterous connexion with a woman of the twice-born class, shall lose the part offending.*

"If a man, by force, commits adultery with a woman of an equal or inferior caste, against her consent, the magistrate shall confiscate all his possessions, cut off his penis and castrate him, and cause him to be led through the city mounted upon an ass (Hindu Law, Halhed, p. 271.)"

In 1853, a man was sentenced in Calcutta to suffer a year's imprisonment for inflicting a severe wound with a *hussooah*, or sickle, on the *Membrum Virile* of a person who intrigued with his wife.—Mortification and death ensued.†

Dr. Chuckerbutty tells me that, some years since, a person of Tipperah discovering that his brother was intriguing with his wife, emasculated the man and cut off the woman's breasts.

At Tipperah, in 1868, the body of a man, unknown, was found on the banks of the Goomtee River with his private parts cut off, thus leading to the belief that he had been trespassing in some zenanah. Certain persons were apprehended by the police, but discharged by the magistrate.‡

Cases are upon record§ which appear to show that the Natives, when avenging disgrace done to females, often kill in a manner which denotes the nature of their victim's offence.—*Parte in quâ peccatur, in eâ etiam punietur.* A man's body was found, at Rajshahye, with one eye scooped out, and an ear cut off, and the *testes* mangled and partly cut off. In a case at Patna, the body was found horribly mutilated, with the private parts cut and lacerated in such a manner as to warrant the inference that the murder was done out of revenge on the deceased for having disgraced a female.

In 1849, the Sub-Assistant Surgeon of Shahjehanpore reported the case of a Mussalmaun who was treated at the dispensary for a wound extending across the root of the genitals—certain persons attempted to castrate him—one of the testes hung out—but was replaced, and he recovered.

In a report of police cases at Azimghur in 1834-35,‖ Dr. Esdaile notices the case of a Faqueer, who cut off his penis "for the love of God."

---

* Chap. VIII., S. 374.—According to the Hindu Law, as quoted by Ward, a Brahmin having improper intercourse with a virgin, with his own daughter, or with his son's wife, must become an eunuch. Also, if a person defile the bed of his mother-in-law, he must put a red-hot piece of stone or iron into his mouth, and become an eunuch.

† Nizamut Adawlut Reports, Vol. V., p. 551.

‡ Bengal Police Report for 1868, p. 345.

§ Nizamut Adawlut Reports, Vol. IV., pp. 537 and 567.

‖ Ind. Jour. of Medical Science, Vol. II., p. 263.

My friend Dr. Baillie, of the Native Hospital, Calcutta, sent me the following case at the time. "On the morning of the 12th July 1869, whilst engaged with the out-patients, I was called to see a Ḥindu, aged eighteen, who had amputated his penis outside the door, a few minutes before. He was bleeding profusely, but was perfectly rational. After securing the vessels and dressing the wound, I asked him how he came to commit the act; he laughed and said it was to keep him out of trouble, which he was sure to fall into, so long as he retained the member, and to this statement he still adheres. He says he meditated the deed the previous night, and had, only a few minutes before, paid a pice to a barber in the hospital compound for the loan of his razor. His object in coming to the Hospital was to be within reach of aid, and thus avoid a fatal result. He is now nearly well, and, seemingly, very cheerful."

About ten years ago Dr. Baillie sent me notes of the case of a Mahometan boy, *ætat* 11, whose death was caused by a bungling circumcisor. He was stated to have died of cholera, and had been buried when the police disinterred the body. It was found that he had been killed by a deep incision behind the glans. He was a healthy plump boy. The part had been roughly bound up. This was done by a barber.

Lutfullah terms circumcision a "hurtful and sometimes fatal operation."

It is well known in Bengal that little boys, piddling against bushes in gardens and jungles, are liable to have the penis severely lacerated by mongoose (*herpestes* or *ichneumon).*

In addition to similar cases alluded to above, we may cite that of a Mussalmaun who, in some trivial squabble, knocked his mistress down, and, while she was insensible, inflicted severe wounds on her *Pudenda* with a razor.*

EUNUCHS IN INDIA.

The Mahomedan conquest created a large demand for these wretched beings in India. Many were provided in the country, and large numbers were imported within the memory of man. Fryer said that, in Persia, the white eunuchs came from Georgia, the black from Arabia and Africa, Baboo Bholanauth Chunder (Vol. I., p. 80) quotes some authority to the effect that the eunuchs of the zenanas at Moorshedabad come from different places in Abyssinia, from Tigra, Daucali, Nubia, and the Galla country. Some years ago a vessel in the port of Calcutta was discovered to be freighted with a cargo of these wretched beings.

Dr. Chuckerbutty informs me that he has conversed with one who had, himself, gone through this process in Arabia. The dealers there lie in wait for *very young* and promising boys. They take them to some solitary spot where they sweep off *everything*; and, having applied some dressing, leave the victims. Returning some hours afterwards, they take them

* Nizamut Adawlut Reports, Vol. II., Part 1, 1852, p. 215.

away, if they find them alive; complete amputation is the rule.* Sir Thomas Glover, in Purchas (Part 2, p. 1299), says, "Many of the children that the Turkes do buy, they castrate, making all smooth as the backe of the hand (whereof divers doe dye in the cutting), who supply the vses of nature with a silver quill, which they wear in their turbants." Dr. Fryer (p. 393) says of the eunuchs in Persia: "They are gelded so inartificially, or butcherly rather, that all is cut off, nothing of witness being left, but as clear as the skin will permit; and thus they are given over to nature to cicatrize. If they live, it is well; if not, they try others till they do; wherefore a Chyrurgion skilled in this act is of greater value than if he was expert in every other part, and deficient in this.

There was, and may still be, "the *kojah* ward" in the Monghyr Jail, where several of these miserable beings were confined. My friend Dr. Duka showed me two of the survivors when I inspected the Jail in 1861. They had the general appearance of very tall and bony old women. There had been complete amputation. The orifice of the urethra was depressed and guarded by two small folds (*labia*) of integument.

Some very remarkable notes, collected by my friend Dr. H. Ebden, have been published in the Indian Annals of Medical Science for April 1856, which show clearly that there, at present, exists a very extensive system of making and of trading in eunuchs in the States of Rajpootana and, doubtless, also in Delhi and Lucknow. The operation is performed by eunuchs—the base of the genitals is encircled by a tight ligature, and the whole genitalia are swept away by a single stroke. Those who retain the penis are but little valued or trusted. The operation is generally performed at a shrine, with many precautions and with some affectation of religious ceremony. There cannot be a doubt that children are bought and stolen for this infamous trade. Many of the eunuchs are said to be orphans and foundlings, but it is also shown that adults not unfrequently submit voluntarily to the operation. An old Mussalmaun, who had lived for a long time among the eunuchs, stated that he had only heard of one man having died, out of fully a thousand operated upon. Some extraordinary facts, regarding eunuchs in India, will be found in the report of a case tried at Mynpooree in 1852,† which will again be alluded to in the Chapter on Unnatural Crime. I am obliged by my friend, Dr. Hugh Macpherson, with some depositions and copies of reports upon this case, from which I take the following particulars:—Dr. Macpherson reported to the Judge that the Eunuch Bhoora, out of whose murder this inquiry arose, had been deprived of all external organs of

* Camerarius says: "The King of Puna amongst the Indians caused his eunukes or guards of women, not only to have their privie parts cut off, but also their noses and armes," page 189.

† Nizamut Adawlut Reports, N. W. P., 6th November 1852, p. 1314.

generation. The mutilation seemed to have taken place before puberty, for, excepting that the breasts were undeveloped, the body had all the appearance of that of a woman. There was no indication of hair on the chin, although the deceased could not have been less than twenty-five or thirty years of age, while all the limbs were rounded and soft, and the skin fine and delicate. The body was covered with valuable ornaments of the sort usually worn by wealthy native females, on the brow, in the ears and nose, and on the wrists and ankles.

The following are extracts from the deposition of Khurrugjeet, *alias* Pyuzoo, eunuch, or *Hijrah*, taken on the 7th March 1853 :—" I am thirty-five years of age, and my profession is that of dancing. Was made an eunuch at the age of sixteen years. At first Bhung (an intoxicating drug) was administered to me, and then the genitals were mutilated. The respective members were bound up with strong thread, or *dorah*, being bound on. After an hour, the mutilation was effected with a razor, the effects of the drug producing insensibility. A piece of cloth, of the size of the wound produced by the operation, was tied upon it, with a poultice of boiled rice and milk. After this, warm-water fomentations were used in like manner until the wound healed. By using every day the boiled rice, milk, and warm water, the blood was stopped.* The mutilation was performed by a person named Samlee Hijrah, at Koheyree Kei, Muddunpore. About forty or fifty young persons and adults have been mutilated to my knowledge ; none have died under this operation before me. There are three sorts of eunuchs, *viz.*, one born so, and the other two are made so. One called Salundnee, and the other Badamee. The Salundnee Hijrahs are chiefly made beyond the river Jumna, and the Badamee in Chundeyree. There is no fear of life in making the latter sorts of Hijrahs, but" [there is in] "that of Salundnee, for they are made so by cutting literally the members from the root, while the Badamee are made by cutting off the half only.

"Men who are fond of dancing willingly get themselves made eunuchs. The parents never willingly permit or suffer them to be made eunuchs. They, by their own desire, make themselves so, and no stolen boys, but purchased ones, are made eunuchs.† The wound heals after a month. Pouring warm water every day on the wound prevents the urinal orifice from closing up. Eunuchs often live long. There is one in Palee, by name Gubela, 100 years old. Eunuchs are never sick by any other disease than the usual one [ones ?]. I have not heard that any eunuch has become mad, but once we turned a eunuch out of our caste, because he

---

* It is evident that this statement is not accurate in some of its details.

† In India, the divisions of labor are very accurate. Possibly eunuchs do not run the risk of stealing their victims, but the stealers and sellers of children are common in this country There are many varieties of these; the most remarkable were the Megpunnah Thugs who murdered travellers for the purpose of obtaining their children, whom they sold.

ate bread given to him by Bala sweeper. *We* never use any intoxicating drug, opium, gunja, &c., but other Hijrahs do so abundantly."

A writer at Delhi remarked in the *Delhi Gazette*, in September 1865, that, during his sojourn in the interior of the district, he learned that eunuchs are in the habit of kidnapping children of tender age, and emasculating them. Indeed, the number of eunuchs he saw there was greater than in any other district, excepting perhaps the Rajpoot States ; and he considered it to be absolutely necessary that Government should take strict measures for putting a stop to their nefarious practices.

As recently as July 1870, it has been reported that "at a village near Nassick (Bombay), Dr. Birdwood has discovered 350 cases of adult mutilation of such unexampled atrocity as must call for the interference of Government."*

Legal Decisions.

A prisoner convicted of castrating a boy, with his consent, from which operation death ensued, was sentenced, under all the circumstances of the case (the youth and ignorance of the prisoner, the absence of all malice, the express desire of the deceased, and the fact that such operation was not unusual among hermaphrodites), to imprisonment for two years. *Nizamut Adawlut Reports*, Vol. 3, p. 17, as cited by Beaufort. See also Beaufort's Digest, 2nd Ed., para. 3873, for the Mahomedan law relative to the crime of castrating slaves and others.

When a man of full age (*i. e.*, above eighteen years) submits himself to emasculation, performed neither by a skilful hand, nor in the least dangerous way, and dies from the injury, the persons concerned in the act are guilty of culpable homicide not amounting to murder.—Queen *v.* Baboolun Hijrah, 5 W. R., Cr., 7, Cowell and Woodman.

This case was tried at Gya late in 1865 :—"The whole private parts were simply cut off." Death followed in a few hours. Those concerned "were all eunuchs, upon whom a similar operation must have been performed."

Mr. Maine, Inspector-General of Police, N. W. P., has urged that rigorous measures should be adopted in regard to eunuchs in Behar, Oude, and the North-Western Provinces ; and Major Carnell has, I believe, recommended that, with a view to extirpating this atrocious evil, all eunuchs should be registered. Registration of such extraordinary births should be made compulsory under strict penal provisions, and the owning of an unregistered eunuch should be made criminal.

Epicenes in India.

Numerous scattered allusions to a class of persons called "*Hermaphrodites*," attendant upon the Courts and Camps of Native Princes,

* *Indian Daily News*, July 4th, 1870.

appear in our Indian literature. The allusion by St. Paul to those "who are born eunuchs," in contradistinction to those "who *are made* eunuchs by man," occurs repeatedly in Halhed's Hindu Law. Dr. Honigberger mentions (p. 153) that, at Lahore, he had the opportunity of seeing "several ***Hermaphrodites*** who enjoyed the privilege of being admitted to all births and nuptial festivals, to congratulate the parties and get presents, this being, in fact, their sole means of subsistence." Forbes says (Vol. I, p. 359): "Among the followers of an oriental camp, at least of the Mahratta camp, to which we were attached, I must not omit the ***Hermaphrodites;*** there were a great number of them in the different bazars, and I believe all in the capacity of cooks. In mentioning these singular people, I am aware I tread on tender ground; I cannot solve doubts and difficulties, nor shall I enter into particulars respecting them. I shall merely observe that there were a considerable number of human beings called Hermaphrodites in the camp, who were compelled, by way of distinguishing them from other castes, to wear the habit of a female, and the turban of a man. I was called into a private tent, to a meeting between the surgeon-major and several medical gentlemen of the army, to examine some of these people: my visit was short, and the objects disgusting."

In a description of the Court-life of Ali-Verdy-Khan, given in the Seir Mutaqherin, mention is made, among other wits and joculators who amused the Court, of the ***Hermaphrodite*** Mahmood-hijrah. The editor remarks: "He was introduced in the hall, not as a curiosity of the ***Hermaphrodite*** kind (for the species is so common in India as to pass totally unnoticed), but only as a cracker of jokes and sarcasms. There are," he adds, "three sorts of men who bear the name of ***Hijrah,*** or ***Hermaphrodite,*** in India. Those that are naturally so, by having the two sexes full and distinct, one over the other, or one within the other, or only in part, or a confused medley of both. This is the first class. The second, called ***Hijrah*** likewise, and also zenana, or feminine, are a species of young men ***born*** impotent, with tall slender bodies and beardless faces; and, although one would think that such a condition has nothing attracting in itself, yet are there people (and such is the depravity of mankind) that force themselves into it, and bring themselves under the denomination of ***Hijrahs*** by art; this being the third class. These are young men that assimilate themselves to that deplorable appearance, or have been emasculated by their unnatural parents; and this is done by twisting and wringing, and tormenting the part several times a day in a course of several months or even years. All these (who would believe it ?) have female inclinations, and wear a female dress; and there is at Lucknow a whole lane inhabited by these wretches; and this is all that decency allows me to say on that head." (Vol, I., Part 2, p. 687).

Casper has a case (Vol. 3, p. 250) which appears to throw some light upon the manner in which the multiplication of these miserable beings in India was brought about. An unmarried woman swore that, for the last three years, she had never had casual connection with any man, but frequently with the woman Johanna K., who was formed like a man, and this the latter also confessed. Casper gives a full description of J. K., who was a male having hypospadia in an extreme degree, the urethra opening externally immediately after passing through the triangular ligament close to the root of the penis. The child born of this union was very remarkable. "It was mature and healthy, but *its sexual organs were fashioned almost precisely like those of Johanna K.*"

Dr. Taylor alludes (p. 856) to a case of Dr. Lever's, in which a healthy woman had three children, who were the subjects of sexual malformation. Here the point of interest would have been to ascertain the condition of *the father*.

Dr. J. B. Wright, then of Jeypore, describes a class of "naturally born" eunuchs called *Khojas* [*Hijrahs?*] In them "the urine is voided painlessly through a minute aperture just above the symphysis pubis, in the abdominal mesial line. This orifice is, in many cases, surmounted by a small organ similar in appearance and position (?) to the female clitoris or to a miniature penis." Their pelves are described as being very wide. These people are in great request as the custodians of zenanas. It would appear, from the above account, that these persons suffer from congenital deficiency of the anterior wall of the bladder and of the symphysis pubis, with more or less imperfect development of the genitals. In Europe, however, such cases are of very rare occurrence, and it would be difficult to imagine that a class of such unfortunates could be collected, except by a search throughout the whole population of India.

This subject will again be referred to in the Chapter on Unnatural Crime.

It is stated that there is, among the public singers and dancers of this country, a class of *gelded and infibulated women*. I met with a description of these persons, in an English Medical Journal, many years since; but cannot now refer to the authority. This allusion to the subject may, however, lead to further investigation.*

---

* Nearly all the practices of mutilation employed by the natives of India have been known in Europe, and even in England, during the last six or seven centuries.

We are told by Ælian that "Zaleucus, the famous Locrian law-giver, passed a law that any person convicted of adultery should lose both his eyes. The first offender was his own son. The father determined that the law should take its course, but still, pitying the criminal, ordered that one of his own eyes and one of his son's should be put out. He must have copied this view from the ancient Egyptians.

By a constitution of Charlemagne, the malefactor and criminal were to lose an eye for the first fault, for the second the nose was to be cut off, and for the third, the penalty was death.

William the Conqueror took terrible vengeance on thirty-two soldiers of Alençon, by

We are told by Linschoten, (Purchas, Part V., p. 504) that there are those, in the kingdom of Pegu, "that sow vp the privie part of their

---

cutting off their feet and hands, for calling, in derision of his mother's family—"*Hides! La pel! al parmentier!*

In 997, the Norman peasantry rose against Duke Robert, who sent Count Rodolph to disperse them: the Count, having arrested the ringleaders and some others, cut off their hands and feet and thus sent them back to their homes.

William de Owe or Eu, having rebelled against William Rufus, was imprisoned, and had his eyes put out. The same fate befel Robert (Curthose) Duke of Normandy. Henry the First commuted punishment by loss of limbs by a pecuniary fine.

In 1119, Eustace Count of Breteuil, who married Juliana, natural daughter of Henry the First, King of England, holding as a hostage the young son of Raoul of Hareuc, commander of the tower of Ivry, had delivered to the King his two daughters by Juliana. Believing that the King would certainly protect his own grandchildren, he tore out the eyes of the young man and sent them to Raoul. Upon this the King abandoned to the vengence of Raoul his two granddaughters. Raoul, in reprisal, tore out their eyes and cut off their noses.—*Andrew Bell's Historical Sketches of Feudalism.*

The Statutes of Clarendon (Henry II.) ordained that any one arraigned for a capital offence should be sent to the water ordeal, and, if convicted, should lose one of his feet, to which it was added in the Statutes of Northampton (1176) that he should likewise lose his hand, and, abjuring the realm, go out of it within forty days. In this reign theft was punished by loss of the eyes.

According to Holingshed, Henry II., in his attempt on Wales, did justice on the sons of Rice or Rees, and also on the sons and daughters of the noblemen who had been his accomplices, by causing the eyes of the young striplings to be picked out of their heads and their noses to be cut off or slit, and the ears of the young gentlewomen to be stuffed.

By the naval laws of Richard the First, it was ordained that one who drew a knife to strike another, or who drew blood, should lose his hand.

In the sixth of King Henry the Third, many citizens of London, who had taken part in a riot, had their feet and hands cut off by Hubert de Burgh, the Chief Justice.

Even Dr. Baker Brown's operation had a place in English law. Chitty mentions that, by the common law, it belonged to the office of the Marshal to protect the Marshalsea Court from prostitutes, as appears in Fleta lib. 2, c. 5, (3 Inst. 205). They were, on their first trespass, to be warned; on the second to be imprisoned in chains; on the third to have the *tressoria* shaved; but, should they transgress a fourth time, *tunc amputeter eis superlabia, ne de cœtero concupiscant ad libidinem.*

Party-rage ran so high in 1403 that an Act of Parliament was found necessary to declare "pulling out of eyes and cutting out of tongues to be felony."

It will be found, in Chamberlayne's *Angliæ Notitia*, that amputation of the right hand, by a cleaver furnished by the king's yeoman of the kitchen, was long the punishment of striking within the precincts of the King's court. William, Duke of Devonshire, barely escaped it, in the reign of James the Second, by the payment of a fine of ten thousand pounds. At a ceremony of this kind (not carried into effect) upon Sir Edmond Knevit, of Norfolk, Baker, in his Chronicle, describes that the following officers were present: "First, the Serjeant Surgeon, with his instruments pertaining to his office; then the Serjeant of the Wood Yard, with a mallet and a block to lay the hand upon; then the King's Master Cook, with a knife to cut off the hand; then the Serjeant of the Larder to set the knife right on the joint; then the Sergeant Ferrier, with searing irons to sear the veins; then the Serjeant of the Poultry, with a cock" (which, being cleft in twain, was regarded as a soothing application to the bare stump), "which cock shall have his head smitten off upon the same block, and with the same knife; then the Yeoman of the Chandry, with sear clothes; then the Yeoman of the Scullery, with a pan of fire to heat the irons, a chafer of water to cool the ends of the irons, and two forms for all officers to set their stuff on; then the Serjeant of the cellar with wine, ale, and beer; then the Serjeant of the Ewry, with bason, ewre and towels."

daughters, leaving onely passage for vrine ; which, when they marry, pass vnder the surgeon's hand for remedie."*

Several important questions are not unfrequently proposed to medical witnesses, in cases of wounding, with regard to *The Relative Position of the Parties,* when the wound was inflicted.

When at Howrah, I was called upon to attend a thief, who had been seized and wounded. From the position and character of his wounds, on the feet, knees, buttocks, and backs of the hands, I at once suggested my conviction that he had been wounded with a sword while lying on the ground, with his hands and feet raised to protect his body.

QUESTION OF POWER TO INFLICT WOUNDS.

There are several cases in the Reports where it was inquired,—whether prisoners whose hands were contracted by leprosy or by cicatrices were capable of wielding a deadly weapon. This question was generally answered in the affirmative. I find two cases in the Reports, in which blind men were found guilty of killing their wives for infidelity. One of these cases has been already cited at p. 420. The prisoner was completely blind of one eye, the sight of the other was so greatly impaired that he appears to have been incapable of work. He killed the woman by blows on the neck with a sword. Here, of course, it was a matter of importance to ascertain what degree of vision remained. In the other case, the murderer was entirely blind,—according to the evidence of the native doctor and others, he had been so for

---

The loss of the offending hand was formerly the first punishment of an assassin: Damien, Ravilliac, Felton, all suffered this. The practice is still common in Italy. In France, a parricide has his right arm cut off the moment before he is guillotined.

King Jayme el Conquistador, being in a rage with the Bishop of Girona, formerly his confessor, for having given a testimony unfavorable to his interests, had his tongue cut out. Cutting out the tongue was a common Russian punishment in the time of Peter the Great. By ancient forest law, the convicted deer-stealer lost a forefinger or a thumb, and thus became a "poltroon," *(pollice truncatus,)* unfit to carry arms. The cutting off the ears of Prynne, Leighton, and Bastwick, after they had been nailed to the pillory, was an event of direful portent in English history. The slitting of a gentleman's nose by order of the Duke of Monmouth, at Whitehall Stairs, gave origin to the Coventry Act. The punishment of Abelard (Cir. 1120) is well known; and it is scarcely necessary to do more than allude to the refinement of cruelty which has generally accompanied the execution of a traitor in England. Castration was said, not many years ago, to be still the punishment which the law awards to a Negro, who is found guilty of a rape in the Slave States of America.

An Act of 1792 provided for the punishment of persons found guilty of "mutilating or dismembering any slave or slaves" in our West Indian Possessions.

* So also Burton quotes Bembus, who says, in his Venetian History, of the inhabitants of Quiloa in Africa: *Lusitani quorundum civitates adierunt qui natis statim fœminis naturam consuunt, quoad urinæ exitus ne impediatur, easque quum adoleverint sic consutas in matrimonium collocant, ut sponsi prima cura sit conglutinatas puellæ oras ferro interscindere.*

years. He confessed freely that,—his wife having admitted that a criminal intimacy existed between herself and a man for whom she worked, and who, she said, had asked her to live with him, and not to remain with a blind man,—he, at midnight, killed her, while she was sleeping, with a bill or *gurasa*, inflicting no less than nine wounds, one of which completely severed the vessels of the neck. The next morning he told the chowkeedar what he had done.*

In one of the Reports we find it questioned, whether a lad, twelve or thirteen years of age, was physically capable of cleaving the skull of a person of his own age, and of cutting the side of the neck to the spine. This was answered in the negative, upon consideration of the prisoner's slight muscular development, and the lightness of the weapon. Cases of deliberate murder, by children from twelve to fourteen years of age, are, however, not rare in the criminal records of this country.†

In one case, a girl, who appeared not to have reached the age of puberty, and was declared by her parents to be only nine years and a few months old, was found guilty of drowning another child in a rivulet, not a span deep, for the sake of her ornaments.‡

In 1852, a girl "nine years and three months old," was found guilty of murdering her husband's niece, a child of six, by killing her with repeated blows of a heavy stick, scratching her face afterwards with a knife. She was sentenced to imprisonment for life.§

A very remarkable case, in illustration of this question, occurred in Assam, in 1853:—A girl, "a mere child of ten or eleven years," confessed to have taken a recently sharpened *dhao* in both her hands, and to have struck her husband two blows on the head with it. The deceased, who was a strong healthy man, received two wounds on the head, from which the brain protruded, his little finger had also been severed from his right hand. He died on the following day. The weapon produced was a *dhao*, one cubit and eleven fingers in length, including the handle, with a blade, two and-a-half fingers wide, and weighing eleven chittacks, or 22 ounces. The girl was sentenced to ten years' imprisonment.‖

Instances very frequently occur in the records in which mere children are proved to have taken active parts in assisting older criminals in the commission of murderous acts.

In 1852, a woman was convicted, at Akyab, of the murder of her husband. Mr. Mountjoy found three wounds on the head of the deceased,

---

* Nizamut Adawlut Reports, N. W. P., 11th July 1853, p. 840.

† Macnaghten's Reports, Vol. I., pp. 148 and 215; II., pp. 2 and 471.

‡ *Ibid*, Vol. I., p. 213.

§ Nizamut Adawlut Reports, Vol. II, Part 2, of 1852, p. 45.

‖ *Ibid*, Vol. III., Part 2, p. 57. See also the case of a girl, ten or twelve years old, who had certainly not reached the age of puberty, who killed her husband by blows on the head with a *dhao*.—*Ibid*, October 16th 1854, p. 467.

one of which, fracturing the occipital bone, was sufficient to have caused death; the head had also been nearly severed from the body by repeated blows, and the back was one mass of shocking wounds, such as might have been caused by the *dhao* produced, which weighed about two pounds and-a-half. The Commissioner remarked that it might appear surprising, and almost incredible, that a small and apparently weak female, such as the prisoner, should be capable of inflicting the deep and deadly wounds described by the Civil Surgeon. But the women in the villages of Arracan are generally employed in cutting up firewood for domestic use, and they thereby acquire a great facility in using the *dhao*, or long heavy knife. The habit of pounding paddy with a heavy pestle, in a large wooden mortar, also gives them considerable strength in the arm.*

BLOOD MARKS.

Natives, when wounded in affrays, &c., are always careful to bring all the clothes which have become stained with their blood, as evidence of the severity of the injuries which they have received. Indeed, they and the friends who accompany them often appear more anxious to display the bloody clothes than the wounds themselves. It is generally suspected that, in many of these cases, the blood of a fowl is used to enhance appearances. I do not know, however, that such has been proved to be the fact in any instance. This is possibly attributable to a traditionary knowledge of the old Hindu law under which, "If a man of an equal cast, and of equal abilities with another, should strike him with a weapon or anything else in such a manner as that no blood flows from him, the magistrate shall fine him thirty puns of cowries; if a little blood is shed by the stroke, the magistrate shall fine him sixty-four puns of cowries. If the skin is torn so that much blood flows from thence, the magistrate shall fine him one hundred puns of cowries; if both the skin and flesh are torn, and a greater quantity of blood is by such means shed, he shall fine him twenty-four *Ashrufees*" (gold mohurs); "if both the skin and flesh are torn, and a bone is broken, and blood shed, he shall confiscate all his possessions, and banish him the kingdom."†

Since the tests for distinguishing the blood of a human being from that of one of the lower animals,—as those proposed by MM. Barruel, Taddei, and others,—cannot avail in evidence upon criminal cases, it must, of course, rest with the police to show, as far as possible, whence blood-stains, to be subjected to examination, have been derived. The chemical examiner can only be expected to state whether the matter found on a weapon, garment, or other object, is blood or not; and he

* Nizamut Adawlut Beports, Vol. II., Part 1, of 1852, p. 329.

† Halhed, p. 229.

may, in certain cases, also be able to suggest whether the effusion has taken place before or after death.*

It may be worthy of remark that it would appear that, in the generality of cases occurring in the North-West, where the tulwar or other cutting weapon with which a murder has been committed has been missing, it has been at length found in a neighbouring *Well*. In Bengal, the readiest place of concealment is either a *Tank* or the *Thatch* of a hut. In a case, tried in the North-West Provinces, where a person had evidently been killed by sword wounds, it was held by the Sessions Judge to be a strong additional cause of suspicion against certain of the accused parties that no sword was found upon any of them, except one, who was wearing his;—seeing that a murderer always (?) takes the first opportunity of hiding the weapon which he has used.† In some of the recorded cases of wounding in India, it is distinctly stated that the culprit cleaned the bloody weapon after committing the crime. In many other instances, the bill-hook or sickle has been thrown into a tank or buried. In many, however, stains are found upon the blade or handle of a suspicious weapon, and are sent to the chemical examiner for analysis. I find only three instances among the old records of that gentleman's office, in which it was satisfactorily proved that the marks on articles sent for examination were those of blood. In two of these, the stains were found on the blades and within the scabbards of tulwars. It is easy to perceive that stains upon a sheathed weapon would be better preserved and more readily detected than upon almost any other. The following cautions should be observed in sending in weapons and garments supposed to be stained with blood for chemical analysis. In all cases means should be taken for ascertaining the *identity* of the weapon, garment, or other article.‡ A careful inspection of the weapon will sometimes at once lead to the deduction of important evidence. In the case where five persons of one household were found murdered at Baitool, cited at p. 428, one sword was found in an out-of-the-way well; it was notched and bent, and was believed to have been that with which the crime was committed. Another tulwar was found in some brushwood near the house,—it had blood-stains on the *handle*, as if bloody fingers had grasped it, but its blade was clean and within a scabbard;—it was, therefore, concluded that the prisoner had placed it there himself. The article (if dry) should be sent precisely in the condition in which it is found, care

* Mr. Baynes mentions that great weight is attached by the natives of this country to the evidence of blood-stains. A washerman is brought forward, who deposes in the most confident manner that "the stain on that cloth is from blood;" if it has even been imperfectly washed, he is equally positive; if any trace remain, he can tell "it is blood."—*Hints on Medical Jurisprudence*, p. 48.

† Nizamut Adawlut Reports, N. W. P., Sept. 22nd, 1852, p. 1047.

‡ Taylor, Ed. Cit., p. 901.

being merely taken to remove any living insects which may be upon it, or within its crevices or folds; it should first be enveloped in white paper, and then secured in tin. If *wet*, it should be placed or spread upon white paper over a perfectly clean dish or plank, isolated in such a manner that ants and other insects may not approach it, and dried gradually but completely, not in the sun, but in a room where a brisk draught enters. Should the paper receive any stains, it should also be folded and sent in a separate packet.

In India, several insects, and especially the small red ant, speedily fix upon any cloth or other object stained with animal matter, which they rapidly devour, often removing, in a few hours, not only the stains, but the portions of cloth which they occupied. In the case of blood-stains, it is especially necessary to guard against this, as the removal of the fibrinous portion of a stain by insects will always obscure the inquiry as to whether the hæmorrhage occurred before or after death. As a rude test, however, of the difference between recent blood-stains and certain other mineral and vegetable stains, exposure of the surface to red ants may, in some degree, aid investigation. It is probable, however, that the stains of sweet fruits, such as mulberries and oranges, would be equally attacked by insects. Where a suspicious weapon has been found sheathed, care should always be taken to send the scabbard : this should be split open, previous to its despatch, in the presence of the medical officer ; or, in his absence, of the magistrate, who should carefully observe whether the stains within appear to be old or of recent date. To enable the chemical examiner to judge fairly whether the hæmorrhage occurred before or after death, and whether it was arterial or venous, stained garments should be sent *entire*—small strips of stained cloth are rarely sufficient. The principal stains which are liable to be mistaken for blood in this country are, Iron Mould, Citrate of Iron Stains, Fruit Stains, such as those of the Mulberry and Sorel, or Meesta, &c., the marks of Huli Powder (Abir)* and Ochre, and of the Catechu in Pan. In a trial at Futtehpore, the prisoner alleged that certain small, but suspicious, stains on his clothes were from chewing betel. Dr. Warneford, however, examined them chemically, and proved that they were of blood.†

In a case tried before Mr. Baynes, a knife which had been found in the house of a confessing murderer bore two or three dark reddish spots, which everybody supposed to be blood ; no one credited the prisoner who declared that the murder had been committed not with that, but

* The coloring matter of this, as used in Bengal, is the powder of the Cæsalpinia Sappan, which, according to O'Shaughnessy, contains a principle much resembling Hæmatin In Bombay, especially about Kotrah, it is stated that the principal constituent of this powder (that called Goolal) is a dye from the Basunty flower, *Butea Frondosa*.

† Nizamut Adawlut Reports, N. W. P., 8th May 1852, p. 424.

with another weapon. On examination under a microscope, these spots proved to be small masses of some red-colored leaf which had adhered to the blade, and had there become partially decomposed.*

Detection of Blood-stains on a Knife covered with Rust.

M. Daubrawa was requested to ascertain the existence of blood-stains on a knife which was suspected to have been used in the commission of a murder. The knife, having lain a long time in a damp place, was rusted, but certain bright rust-free spots could be distinguished amid the rust. On heating the point of the blade, these spots scaled off, while the rust remained adherent ; on the other hand, on immersing the knife in dilute hydrochloric acid, the bright spots remained untouched, although the rust was readily dissolved. It was probable that these bright spots were blood-stains ; but, as some non-nitrogenous organic acids will produce similar marks, some of the detached scales were heated in a test-tube, and, by the disengagement of ammonia from the hematine of the blood, caused a blue color, on reddened litmus paper. The whole blade was then macerated for a long time in distilled water, which acquired a reddish discoloration ; and, by the aid of a lens, fibrine could be seen adhearing to the blade in the situation of the bright spots. Ammonia, added to the solution, caused no precipitate ; nitric acid gave a white precipitate ; it became turbid by heat ; solution of chlorine at first produced a green tint; this color then disappeared, and white flocculi were deposited. These different fluids having been evaporated to dryness and burnt, and the residue dissolved in hydrochloric acid, demonstrated the presence of iron by its appropriate re-agents.†

Dr. Day, of Geelong, has introduced a simple test, easy of application, for the detection of blood-stains.‡ It consists, in the addition of tincture of guiacum and "ozonised ether" to a weak solution of blood, when a bright blue color is produced. Schönbein first described accurately the existence of two differently active states of oxygen, called ozone and antozone. A molecule of oxygen may, in this view, be looked upon as neutral or passive, and formed by the union of a negative and positive particle. Ozone, as is well known, is supposed to be found in atmospheric air, in certain electrical conditions ; and it may be produced by passing currents repeatedly through a tube containing oxygen. Some inorganic bodies, as the peroxides of mananese, lead, and potash, contain oxygen in the state of ozone ; others, as the peroxides of hydrogen and barium, are supposed to be in an opposite state, and to contain antozone. Ozone has an oxidising influence on guiacum resin and turns it blue, and thus

---

* Op. Cit., p. 48.

† Journal de Chemic Medicate, and American Journal of Medical Science, October 1854, p. 574.

‡ This quotation is from the British Medical Journal, September 5, 1868, p. 255.

differs from antozone, which has no effect on it. Further, antozonides differ from ozonides, in converting red chromic acid into blue perchromic acid. Van Deen, many years ago, drew attention to this subject, but Dr. Day has more fully worked it out. See a paper on Allotropic Oxygen in the *Australian Medical Journal*, May 1867.

When tincture of guiacum is exposed to air or oxygen, it becomes blue; and this change takes place more or less readily, according as more or less ozone is present. "Ozonides," or bodies containing ozone, have a similar effect. Among organic substances, gum, gluten, and unboiled milk render the resin blue. The reaction with the pulp of the raw potatoe is well known. Other bodies, as starch, fibrine, boiled milk, and the red coloring matter of the blood, have no such effect. Boiling prevents the development of this blue color; nor do these bodies recover it when cool. But,—while neither blood nor antozone, when applied separately, have any bluing action on guiacum,—yet, when they are applied *together*, an intense blue is the result. If a drop of blood be mixed with half an ounce of distilled water, and a drop or two of guiacum be added, a cloudy precipitate of the resin is thrown down: and the solution has a faint tint due to the quantity of the tincture used. If now a drop of an ethereal solution of peroxide of hydrogen be added, a blue tint will appear, which will gradually deepen and spread after a few minutes' exposure to the air. This test acts better when very small quantities of blood are used; as otherwise, if the blood is in excess, the solution is red, and gives, with antozone, a purplish or dirty green color. So minute and delicate is the reaction that, in a case where the microscope failed to identify any blood from a stain on a man's trousers, Dr. Day succeeded in obtaining sixty impressions. Water has the effect of destroying the shape of the blood-corpuscle, and so it cannot sometimes be recognised by the microscope; but it in no way interferes with this new chemical test. Its accuracy may be thus shown. A piece of linen was stained with blood in the year 1840 (Guy's *Forensic Medicine*, 3rd ed., p. 316); from this a fibre was taken, containing at its extremity a most minute stain of blood; this was placed on a white slab, and treated first with a drop of tincture of guiacum, and then with a drop of "ozonised ether;" and, although the quantity was so small, and no less than twenty-eight years old, the characteristic blue appeared at once. The writer in the British Medical Journal, to whom I am indebted for this account of Dr. Day's observations, has found the same result in blood obtained from the urine in a case of hæmaturia; and also in blood drawn from different animals. Dr. Taylor, in the *Guy's Hospital Reports*, has shown that red coloring matters, cochineal, kino, catechu, carmine, &c., exert no such influence; and, as far as it is at present known, no other red stain will produce this result. Black currants will cause a stain resembling that of blood more than any other;

but antozone has no effect upon it. Ink-stains will cause a blue with guiacum ; so will rust stains produced by citric or acetic acid on iron ; but then *no* "ozonised ether" need be used, and this at once distinguishes such stains from blood. "Ozonised ether" is a wrong term to use ; for it contains antozone, and not ozone, and to this is due its reaction. Ether which contained an ozonide would blue guiacum resin, whether blood were present or not. The test-solution is the ethereal solution of peroxide of hydrogen, which is an antozonide. The so-called "ozonised essential oils," as oil of turpentine, lavender, &c., really contain antozone ; and to this may be ascribed their use in detecting blood ; for, at first, oil of turpentine was used, instead of the peroxide of hydrogen, but the results were unsatisfactory. If the blood-stain be on dark cloth, the test, as above described, may be used ; but then an impression must be taken off on white blotting paper, otherwise the blue color will not be visible.

The exact nature of the chemical change that takes place is doubtful, but the test is so simple and easy of application, and, above all, so very delicate, that it is likely to become very generally used. This test fails, as other tests have failed before, to show whether the blood-stain is human or not.

Mr. Sorby states,* in a report on the spectroscopic examination of blood-stains, that the one-thousandth of a grain of blood gives a characteristic spectrum ; and that, in urine, a single drop of blood in a pint can be detected by it ! In the case of suspected blood-stains, a few fibres of the fabric are to be soaked in water in a watch-glass, and the solution placed in a cell of barometer-tubing of one-eighth or one-tenth of an inch diameter, and half or three-quarters of an inch long.

In recent stains, two absorption-bands in the green are readily seen in the spectrum.

DEATHS FROM BEATING.†

Besides the kinds of punishment already noticed, various modes of beating are practised by the people of India,—of these the chief are, beating with a Shoe, with a *Kora,* or Whip (an instrument which appears scarcely ever to have been out of the sight of the Mussulmaun potentates of India in olden times), or with a Lathee, or Office Ruler ; the last mentioned is, of course, a formidable weapon ; it is much in use, and very severe beatings (sometimes involving fractures) are often inflicted with it.

It is chosen on account of its weight, and also particularly because its smooth surfaces are as little as possible likely to leave marks.

---

* In a paper on the Process of Detecting Blood in Medico-legal Cases, by Dr. Taylor, Guy's Hosp. Rep., Vol. XV. 1870.

† If a person be killed by successive blows wfth a whip or stick, retaliation for murder is not due, according to the opinion of Aboo Huneefah. Other Mahomedan authorities seem to hold that homicide by these means incurs *Kisas—Harington.*

In 1855, a Moorshedabad man, who was intriguing with a widow, having been caught by her brother, was so severely beaten with fists, and kicked, and beaten with rulers, that he lingered for eighteen days, and then died.*

Four Hindus of Jessore got an enemy down and, having held him firmly by the neck on the ground, beat him severely on all parts of his body with "short round sticks" or "small round staffs." He was able to cry out, and thus obtained assistance. Generally these unfortunates are so completely throttled, gagged, or muzzled, that they are unable to give the alarm. He died in about forty-eight hours. Dr. Palmer found the viscera in a perfectly healthy state; but, from injuries to the abdomen, caused, he considered, by beating with some blunt weapon, there was such hæmorrhage as would inevitably occasion death.†

The fact is that these instruments are used as cooks use their rolling-pins in pounding steaks, and with the same effect upon the muscles.

It would appear, from the Madras Report on Torture, that a belt of thick leather, worn by chuprassies, is often used with much severity in that part of the country. The peons' belts in Bengal are usually made of softer materials. Flogging with switches, as of the bambu or tamarind tree, or with coca-nut fibres or castor-oil rods, or with the stinging ***Bichattee (Trajia Involucrata)***, is a not unfrequent practice; but, in the present day, the latter appears generally to be considered as a punishment for school boys, commonly in use by the masters of the more remote Patshallas, or hedge schools of Bengal. In the last century, however, it was regarded by Burke in a much more serious light.‡

Although not distinguished for pugilistic skill, the Bengali has a mode of ***bruising***, which has great effect upon a prostrate foe, especially when several assailants work together, striking with the ***Elbow and Fist***. This practice of ***Keel Koneh*** beating is especially prevalent in Eastern Bengal.

One or two illustrations of this very common mode of assault will suffice.

Three Mussalmauns of Backurgunge were sentenced to transportation for life, for having, with the assistance of another, beaten a healthy man, aged thirty-two, so severely, that he died on the spot. The Mofussil inquest showed that blood was exuding from the eyes and nose of the deceased, and that contusions were apparent upon the face and neck behind the ears and on other parts of the body. Evidence showed that he was held by

---

* Nizamut Adawlut Reports, August 31, 1855, p. 334.

† *Ibid*, July 29, 1856, p. 129.

‡ "For others, exploring with a searching and inquisitive malice, stimulated by an insatiate rapacity, all the devious paths of nature for whatever is most unfriendly to man, they made rods of a plant highly caustic and poisonous, called *Bechettea*, every wound of which festers and gangrenes, adds double and treble to the present torture, leaves a crust of leprous sores upon the body, and often ends in the destruction of life itself."

the scruff of the neck by one of his assailants, while the other three literally pounded him to death. The blows are said to have been inflicted by the fists and elbows only.*

In the same year, three Hindus of Shahabad, being interrupted by the owner of a field in which they were cutting grass, threw him down, and two of them holding him down by placing their sticks across his throat, the third, with the assistance of another man not before the court, mounted his belly, and struck him with their fists and elbows. The man died on the spot in consequence of external injury caused by the blows.†

In this class of cases the pressure on the neck is sometimes sufficient to cause suffocation. See a case in which an intriguer was caught by the husband and three others. He was thrown down, one sat on his chest, a second squeezed his throat, while the two others beat him. The native doctor declared that there were marks of blows from the knees to the neck, that the throat was swollen, and that "blood was collected or coagulated in it." He considered that death was caused by strangulation.‡

Beating with the heavy leather *Shoes* worn by Mussalmauns, and by the common Hindustanee wooden shoes, is usually considered merely as a sharp punishment involving great disgrace. One of these shoes, wielded by a powerful and enraged man, is, however, a very dangerous weapon, with which fatal injuries must, not unfrequently, have been inflicted.§

In a case tried in 1817, it was proved that a police darogah had caused his *dhanuk* to strike an aged man three or four times with a shoe. It was also stated, but not proved, that the prisoner had struck the deceased on the head with a *mukh*, or pin, as thick as a man's wrist. The man died seven days afterwards. The darogah was, consequently, dismissed from office, and sentenced to a year's imprisonment.

In 1852, one Kadir Buksh, of Tirhoot, having preferred a complaint against persons who had grazed their cattle in his oat field, a punchayet was convened by the gomasthas of the estate. The punchayet found him guilty of false complaint. Upon this, the gomasthas ordered two men to tie his hands and give him twenty blows with a shoe on the back of the neck and head. This they did, after taking off his turban. Upon seeing this, his friends called out *dohaee!*—on which the executioners decamped. He then tried to make his way to the thanna; he was overtaken, and beaten and dragged along, and poked with lattees until he became senseless. He expired early the following morning. Dr. Kinsey found that death had ensued from congestion of the brain, the result of a beating about the head, neck, and back. There was a contusion on the

---

* Nizamut Adawlut Reports, July 4, 1855, p. 6.

† *Ibid*, Oct. 2, 1855, p. 528.

‡ *Ibid*, 14th February, 1856, p. 405.

§ Allusions to "Beating with Slippers" will be found in the Madras Report on Torture Append. C., No. 15, p. clxiv.

chest, apparently from a *lattee* blow, the lungs were also in a state of great congestion, and the heart full of blood. There were no marks about the head; but, from the above appearances, it was, he considered, evident that the man died struggling for breath, in consequence of exhaustion of all nervous energy, resulting from great efforts to free himself.*

In 1849, Dr. Ross, then of Hooghly, reported upon the case of a woman whose death was alleged, as he considered with probability, to have been caused by beating with shoes. He found that blood had been effused into the chest and abdomen, and that inflammation to some extent had supervened. There were marks of very extensive bruises over the chest and abdomen. Otherwise, the body presented no traces of disease.

In 1856, Fukeer Churn Pater, of Cuttack, was found guilty of culpable homicide, for having laid hold of a man by the neck with one hand, and struck him five or six blows with his shoe with the other. He fell groaning on the ground, and was taken home, where he passed the night moaning and suffering great pain, and vomited and voided blood ; and, on the following morning, expired, having been insensible some hours before his death. The native doctor, who held the *post-mortem* examination, deposed that deceased died from blows inflicted with considerable violence, which caused accumulation of blood in the heart, lungs and stomach [?], and that the body exhibited no symptoms of disease or previous illness.†

In 1855, Imdad Allee Khan, of Sarun, was sentenced to four years' imprisonment, for beating a man with a shoe so severely that his spleen was ruptured.‡ Sheikh Kannoo, of Mymensingh, pleaded guilty of having fractured (fatally) the skull of his wife, aged fifteen years, by kicking her with his wooden shoes on.§

The practice of *Beating Thieves and Intriguers to Death* is fearfully common both in Bengal and in the North-West Provinces. There is little to be said with regard to the medico-legal bearings of these cases, except that the blows are inflicted with most unrelenting severity,

---

* Nizamut Adawlut Reports, October 18th, 1853, p. 649. In the same year, certain men of Lohardugga (Chota Nagpore), who were parties in a feud of very long standing, were tried for the murder of one Beegna, their opponent's servant. A witness stated that the deceased and another having been seized by the prisoners, one of the latter ordered that "Mungra should be beaten sixty stripes, and Beegna twenty-five stripes, with a shoe, and one Aubuck began to beat Beegna, upon which Bhoopnath said, 'What, is he your father, that you beat him so gently?' and Bhoopnath himself then began to beat him with a shoe. Beegna then seized Bhoopnath's arm, whereupon Samsoonder got up in a rage and knocked him down, with an iron-bound club." It was said that he died from the effects of this blow, and that his body was thrown into a disused well in Bhoopnath's garden. The case was not considered to be proven.—*Nizamut Adawlut Reports*, Jan. 12th, 1853, p. 52.

† Nizamut Adawlut Reports, May 21, 1856, p. 820.

‡ *Ibid*, Sept. 6, 1856, p. 315.

§ *Ibid*, Sept. 28, 1855, p. 475.

evidently with a conviction that the offender's life is a forfeit, and that mercy is altogether out of the question.*

It is to be trusted that the following are somewhat extreme instances. In 1853, several persons, attendants of the Nawab of Moorshedabad, were tried for the murder of two men, suspected of theft, by torturing and beating them. The cruelties to which these poor wretches were subjected extended over the interval between the 31st of March and the 5th and 6th of April. A list only can be given of the punishments inflicted upon them while they were being hurried about to the different spots, where they declared that the property was secreted, with a vain hope of gaining respite from their sufferings. They were beaten with a *corah*, with a *cutcha beyt* (babool tree) with thorns on it, and a mehter's *jharoo* and a bamboo ; sharp wedges were driven between their fingers, their hands being tied—the feet and hands were tied to separate tent pins. They were tied up to the tent poles with their heads downwards, and beaten with the *beyt*†—one of them had his chest trampled on—and they

---

* See Macnaghten's Reports, Vol. II., pp. 262, 322, and 423; Nizamut Adawlut Reports, Vol. II., Part 1, of 1852, pp. 407, 515, 683; and several other cases in later volumes. Also Nizamut Adawlut Reports, N. W. P., March 10, 1853, pp., 356 and 357, (distinct cases,) &c. Several of the Mahomedan law authorities appear to have sanctioned great severity in the treatment of thieves. According to Harington, it is stated in the Hidayah that, "if a person come in the night to a stranger and carry off his goods by theft, and the owner of the goods follow and slay him, nothing whatever is incurred; the prophet having said, 'Ye may kill in preservation of your property.'" It is to be observed, however, that this is only where the owner cannot recover his property but by killing the thief. The three following cases are cited in the *Humadeeyah*. 1.—If the owner of the house see a thief breaking into it, he may kill the thief, or throw a stone, or shoot an arrow at him. It is not requisite to warn him first according to Aboo Huneefah: though Aboo Yoosuf says that warning should be first given to the thief; and, if he do not then run away, he may be shot. 2.—But if a thief enter your house, and you apprehend him, he may be armed and will attack you; in this case you may shoot him, and it is not necessary to warn him. 3.—Aboo Yoosuf further says, that if an unarmed thief enter a house, and if the owner, though strong enough to seize him, apprehend that he would run away and escape with some of the effects; it is lawful, in such case, to strike or kill the thief. So also the Mosaic Law—"If a thief be found breaking up, and be smitten that he die, there shall be no blood shed for him."—Exodus, xxii, 2.

The ancient Hindu magistrates, probably, had nearly as much difficulty as our own officers have in judging whether one thus treated was a robber or an intriguer. Their law held that "if any man goes to a woman, and forcibly commits adultery with her, and that woman, from bashfulness and modesty, exclaims that thieves attacked her house, then the magistrate shall fine that woman five hundred *puns* of *cowries*" (Halhed, p. 303).

† In the oration already cited, Burke described that—"the ryots were tied two and two by the legs together; and their tormentors, throwing them with their heads downwards over a bar, beat them on the soles of the feet with ratans, until the nails fell from the toes; and then attacking them at their heads, as they hang downwards, as before at their feet, they beat them with sticks and other instruments of blind fury, until the blood gushed out at their eyes, mouths, and noses.—Not thinking that the ordinary whips and cudgels, even so administered, were sufficient, to others (and often also to the same, who had suffered as I have stated) they applied, instead of the ratan and bamboo, whips made of the branches of the *Bale* tree—a tree full of sharp and strong thorns, which tear the skin, and lacerate the flesh far worse than ordinary scourges."

were both severely scorched. The bodies were buried, and were not afterwards found; but it appeared clearly from the evidence of eye-witnesses, among whom was the Nawab's European coachman, that one of the men had his hands and feet torn by tent pins, was burnt all over his left arm and shoulders, and from the knees to the feet. The left hand of the other was broken, the skin of both feet torn off. There were marks of burning on one hand. He was raw from the knee to the foot and, in parts, from the neck to below the waist. The skin was off, and the body much swollen. One of the witnesses described the bodies of the men as being "quite raw and colored from the beating, and the fingers without skin on: the eyes only escaped." Latterly, the tormentors appear to have made attempts to save their victims' lives, by having in a native doctor, who applied poultices, &c. It was stated that the men died of cholera; and they were buried with some show of care. Several of the prisoners were found guilty of culpable homicide and were transported.*

Teprah Fakeer and others, of Rungpore, having caught one who had intrigued with Teprah's wife, was beaten to death. The medical officer deposed that "the cause of death was compression of the brain and injury to the spinal chord, the result of a severe beating on the back, most probably inflicted with a bamboo." He further stated that "the muscles of the back were reduced to a state of pulp, and were infiltrated with blood to below the knee. There was no rupture of the spleen or any other organ." The Judges of the Appellate High Court ruled, that "a person who beats another brutally and continuously so that the back of the victim is reduced to a state of pulp, and yet studiously avoids breaking a limb (the very fact of his taking such a precaution evincing deliberation), is guilty

* Nizamut Adawlut Reports, 5th October 1853, p. 581. Several remarkable cases of murder by *Beating* may be found in the Reports of the Courts of Nizamut Adawlut. Among others, the following:—In 1853, a Cuttack man was openly attacked at his own house by several persons, led on by *his younger brother* with whom he had long been at feud, was violently beaten on the body, had a rope fastened under his arms, by which he was dragged along, while several persons continued to strike at him with bamboo clubs, the marks of which covered his whole body, until at length he received a blow on the head which proved fatal.—(*Nizamut Adawlut Reports*, 5th October 1853, p. 568.) Several persons, natives of the Kossya Hills, were convicted, in Assam, of having beaten to death, with a heavy club, a man whom they believed to be a wizard. They confessed freely, saying that he destroyed their wives and daughters by witchcraft. One of them was his wife's brother—*they found out that he was a sorcerer by breaking an egg!*—(*Nizamut Adawlut Reports*, 11th December 1854, p. 737.) Again, in 1855, three men and a woman from the northern part of the Dacca Division, where a great deal of superstition prevails, went to the hut of a reputed witch, intending, they said, to make her discontinue her enchantments. One of the men threw her down on her charpoy, and pressing her down by rolling her hair round his foot, beat her with his fists, while another, sitting on her loins, beat her in like manner with his fists until they left her dying; they then tore off the ornaments from her nose, ears, and body, and plundered the house. She appears to have been in the habit of prescribing medicines for children, which seems to have given rise to reports of her practising magic.—*Nizamut Adawlut Reports*, 17th January 1855, p. 65.

of murder, or culpable homicide not amounting to murder, according as there may or may not have been grave provocation."*

Medical officers are very frequently called upon to ascertain the cause of death in bodies, regarding which the note "*Reported to have been beaten some days since*" is all the guiding information that can be afforded. In some few of these cases, it will be found that severe injuries, such as fracture of the ribs, &c., &c., have actually been inflicted. In a second class of cases, there will be found traces of internal disease, which will leave the surgeon in some incertitude as to whether their development was, or was not, determined by external injuries. Thus, in two cases occurring within a few months of each other, I found extensive pneumonia in the bodies of persons who were stated to have been beaten severely with *lattees*. In a third class of instances, either with or without the traces of blows, death is found to have occurred from natural causes. In certain cases of this and of the preceding kind, it is often difficult to convince ourselves that our reports should not contain a hint that an intentionally false charge has been preferred. When, however, we recollect that the Bengalee, ill-fed and living in an atmosphere saturated with poisonous miasmata, with vitiated fluids and faulty or actually degenerated organs of secretion and elimination, is liable to have the balance upon which his defective functions act deranged by any unusual vicissitude of pain, or fear, or uncontrollable rage—we shall not be unwilling to admit that a quarrel, a struggle, or a beating, in itself of no very grave severity, may actually determine the onset of fatal cerebral, thoracic, or abdominal disease. Still again, in a fourth class of cases, the appearances discovered may be such as to justify the medical officer in suggesting that the report of beating or other violence appears to have been intentionally false. This step, however, should always be taken with considerable reserve. A few months previously to the publication of my last edition, I reported that a child, whose death was alleged to have resulted from ill-usage, had died of cholera; that the appearances presented by the contents of the stomach and upper bowels were such as to lead me to suspect very strongly that she had taken native remedies for that disease; and that, consequently, there existed clear presumption that those about her must have been well acquainted with the real cause of her death.

The subjoined cases are of considerable practical importance. In one, a young lad while ill, but not dying, from cholera, was cruelly hacked to death; in the other, a girl was beaten and kicked while (as it was considered) sickening for cholera. Fortunately, the offenders made free confession in both cases; otherwise, in the first, detection of the evidences of cholera might have tended at least to embarrass the medical officer in

---

* W. R., Appellate H. C., Vol. V., No. 20, June 1866, p. 78.

forming an opinion as to whether the wounds had or had not been inflicted before death, it being, *primâ facie*, most improbable that any one would have the brutality to murder, in this manner, a child prostrated by cholera; while, in the second, discovery of the evidences of death by cholera, without any traces of beating, would incline to the opinion that the charge of assault was maliciously got up for the purpose of ruining an innocent person.

Jeeno Bibee, of Hooghly, with a *kataree*, or hatchet, murdered her step-son, ten or eleven years of age, who had been suffering two or three days from an attack of cholera, but was, nevertheless, not dying at the time. There was a desperate wound on the throat and cheek. The child and his step-mother often quarrelled, he complaining that she did not give him enough to eat. She confessed freely, before Magistrate and Judge, saying that she scarcely knew what she was about when she committed the act.*

Sheikh Loree Mahomed confessed to the extent of giving his wife, a girl of thirteen years, three blows with the fist, and one kick, because she had not cooked his food. That he left her lying on the ground, and that, on his return in the afternoon, he found her dead. The Sessions Judge remarked:—"The evidence tends to show that the deceased died of cholera or looseness of the bowels" [there does not appear to have been any medical evidence in this case] "after having been beaten by her husband. I find no proof that the beating was the cause of death, nor is it probable that a healthy girl would be so easily deprived of life. An attack of cholera frequently proves fatal in a few hours, and it appears that cholera was then prevalent in the town; the deceased probably neglected to prepare her husband's food from a feeling of illness." The Sessions Judge recommended acquittal, but the higher Court, considering that the death from cholera was not satisfactorily proved, and that the prisoner had confessed that he assaulted her, and that her death followed in the course of the day, convicted the prisoner of culpable homicide.†

Fictitious Marks of Beating.

The late esteemed Dr. Kinloch Kirk sent me the following note, less than a month previous to his death by the mutineers, at Gwalior.

"It is a common practice among the Sikhs, who profess to show the effects upon their persons of blows by such a weapon as a stick, where the charge is perfectly false, to make marks on the skin, by means of repeatedly rubbing over the same place with a bit of kunkur, or a fragment of vitrified brick, till they make a long red mark. This is generally so well done, that even an experienced person may be deceived, unless aware of the trick.

---

* Nizamut Adawlut Reports, August 30, 1856, p. 293.

† *Ibid*, May 29, 1856, p. 859.

The said marks, however, *being in lines radiating towards the right elbow,* if applied by the person himself, and showing very fine red parallel lines where the cuticle has been perforated, may, on careful inspection, generally be readily recognised as indicating friction with some rough substance, and not blows.

"The Sikhs are the only persons I have ever known to practise this trick."

BURNS.

Except as regards those burns which are inflicted as a means of *torture*, to which ample reference is made in the Chapter devoted to that subject, and those which are made by native practitioners, by moxa and charcoal *gool*, by way of counter-irritation in cases of spleen, rheumatism, &c., all that I am aware of as being remarkable in this class of injuries here is, that native children very frequently fall into the fire. There is probably not a village in India where many children may not be seen miserably scarred or with contracted necks or limbs from this cause.

SCALDS—SUN-BURNS.

In India, an excessive degree of sun-burning produces, in certain subjects, especially in thin-skinned Europeans of rufous complexion, a state of parts precisely resembling an extensive scald. This danger is chiefly incurred by those who venture to bathe in tanks, upon which the sun is shining. As they leave the water, their backs are burnt. Their position is that of a hand placed on a mirror upon which a tropical sun is shining. The drummer boys, up-country, are well aware of this danger. About five years ago, a red-haired European, who had been bathing in a tank in Entally, came to the Medical College Hospital with nearly as much vesication upon his back as would have been caused by pouring the contents of a kettle of boiling water over it. His recovery was, however, much quicker, as the injury to the skin was less.

In 1868, the death of a man named Ram Sao, said to have been killed by *lattee* blows, came before the police at Lokemanpore in the Bhaugulpore district. The Civil Surgeon stated decidedly that the beating had not caused death, but was of opinion that death might have been caused by a severe scalding, the marks of which were plainly visible. There was, however, no proof that the man had been scalded, but it appeared that he had been rolling about drunk in the sun, and the medical officer said that death might possibly have resulted from heat-apoplexy, though this would still leave the marks of scalding unaccounted for. There was a long correspondence carried on between the police, judicial and medical authorities, but the question was never cleared up, though the three persons accused were committed under section 304.*

* Bengal Police Report, for 1868, p. 119.

I cite the above as being, possibly, a case of sun-burn. I have certainly not seen such a case in a native, but it is a matter of yearly experience that both Hindus and Mahomedans are liable to die from sun-stroke; and I think that, as a general rule, sinapisms produce vesication much more readily in ill-fed natives than they do in the generality of Europeans. I leave this point for future illustration.*

INJURIES AND DEATH FROM LIGHTNING.

These deaths are very frequent in India, but I do not know that the profession have added anything material to the knowledge of this subject obtained in Europe. The Commissioner of Burdwan reports that, in 1869, *sixty-two* persons were killed by lightning in that district. In the Cuttack district, *twelve* deaths occurred from this cause.

I attended, at Chittagong, a native lad who had been thus stricken down, when working in a garden situated upon a very low hill. The symptoms were those of severe shock to the nervous system,—collapse from which re-action was not very easily obtained.

In 1859, the new barracks at Nursapatam were struck by lightning, and three sepoys were struck down ; they survived the shock, but, for some time, the life of one was doubtful.†

Surgeon F. Carter has reported the very remarkable cases of three sepoys who were struck by lightning, while sleeping on an isolated mountain eminence, during the Hazara campaign. Though they all described the feeling, on being struck, as a sudden shock, as if struck by a bullet, they became instantly insensible, and remained so for some two hours or more. They appeared to be dead, and their deaths were reported to the surgeon. In the morning they were perfectly sensible, did not complain of much pain, and had no alarming symptoms. The details of the severest case will sufficiently display the manner in which the lightning acted upon the bodies, clothes, and bayonets of all three, and upon the cartridge boxes of two. *Sunt Sing.*—The entire back, from the shoulders down to the loins, was charred and bared of skin ; the burn then turned round to the front lower part of the abdomen, left side, and extended down the front and round to the back part of the thigh in a sort of spiral form. The burn was, for

---

* The Negro is believed to be exempt from sun-stroke. Do the *aboriginal* races of India enjoy the same immunity? Dr. Boisliniere, a member of the St. Lewis Medical Society (*Humboldt Medical Archives*), says that the peculiar immunity of the Negro from sun-stroke is, as he believes, owing to the fact of his having, as it were, *two livers*, one interior, the other exterior —his skin. The black pigment deposited there is, in fact, black bile, or the constituents of bile, and this hydrocarbon keeps up that glossy, ebony hue. The Negro never gets bilious ; a large quantity of bile is required to keep him black.

I do not think that this argument will stand, as the last fatal case of sun-stroke, in a native, which has occurred in my practice, was in as black a man as Calcutta produces, except, perhaps, in the Fisher Caste.

† Ind. Med. Gaz., June 1, 1867, p. 152.

the most part, superficial, but there were several considerable-sized patches deeply burnt. His bayonet, which was in its leather case, was marked in several places, chipped as if struck with a harder metal, and having the blue-black appearance as if burnt ; but the leather of the case was torn, but showed no signs of having been burnt ; his leather cartridge case, and tin-swivel, which he also wore, was torn in several places, but showed no signs of having been burnt. The clothes he wore were : 1st, regimental coat, which was rent up the back in several places ; 2nd, two light under-shirts also rent up the back ; 3rd, pyjamas rent down the left thigh. None of these showed any signs of having been burnt, nor was any cloth deficient. The burns were dressed, and the man forwarded to the Field Hospital at Aghee. October 23rd, Camp Aghee.—Re-admitted to regimental hospital tents, much reduced in strength and weight, considerable foul discharge, as might be expected from so large a raw surface, and two large patches of rather deep sloughs in process of separation. No part of the burn has yet began to heal. Ordered tonics, brandy, and morphia at night. To be dressed with calamine ointment. The burn now healed very rapidly, and, under the influence of good food, &c., and scrupulous attention to cleanliness, his health rapidly improved. November 17th.—Perfectly well, with the exception of slight contraction of the left thigh : leave for three months.

The following report of a *post-mortem* examination is by Baboo Odoy Chand Dutt, Sub-Assistant Surgeon of Pooree.* At 4 P.M., on 17th May 1867, I examined the body of Ramo Swame, aged eighteen or twenty, reported to have been killed yesterday evening, by a flash of lightning on the side of a road. There was a small temple opposite to the spot where the deceased fell, but there were no trees in its immediate vicinity. Deceased had no umbrella with him. It was raining hard, and there were thunder and lightning at the time he fell.

The following injuries were found on his body :—

A lacerated wound, three inches long, dividing the skin, and situated transversely behind the right parietal prominence. The epicranial aponeurosis beneath the wound was undivided and entire. Beneath it there was an effusion of dark coagulated blood, extending from the margin of the wound forward, and inward to the middle of the forehead, and about four inches long and two broad. On removing the skin and aponeurosis from the skull cap, the following fractures of the cap, dividing the bones through their entire thickness, were observed :—

1*st*.—A longitudinal fracture, commencing a little above the right frontal prominence, and passing backward over the right parietal prominence to the back of the head. 2*nd*.—An oblique fracture com-

* Ind. Lancet, August 1, 1859, p. 14.

mencing from above the left temporal bone, proceeding backwards and inwards to the posterior end of the sagittal suture; then downwards and outwards to meet the posterior extremity of the fracture first described, and passing beyond it to the extent of an inch and-a-half. *3rd.*—A fracture commencing from the first or longitudinal one over the right parietal prominence, passing inwards and forwards over the top of the skull, to the point of union of the coronal and sagittal sutures. The skin from the lower margin of the scalp wound behind the right ear, down to below the larynx, was of a reddish black color and hardened or leathery. The patch was about an inch broad on the neck, but double that breadth under the chin. A similar burn on the left shoulder, from one to one and-a-half inch in breadth, extending from the posterior edge of the shoulder forwards, and downwards to two inches below the clavicle. The muscles and cellular tissue beneath these patches of burnt and hardened skin were unaffected. There was a similar mark or burn on the anterior and inner part of the right thigh below the groin, four inches in length and one inch in breadth. A similar but slight and smaller mark on the left thigh; a lacerated wound, dividing the skin, situated transversely on the abdomen, two inches below the umbilicus and five inches in length. A penetrating wound of the abdomen, two and-a-half inches long, a little above and parallel to the left Poupart's ligament.—Through this wound about four feet of the small intestines had protruded. They were of a dark red color, and singed and contracted in appearance. Another lacerated wound, four inches in length, dividing the skin and situated below the left Poupart's ligament, parallel to the penetrating wound of the abdomen above described. No other marks of burns or injuries were found on the surface of the body. On opening the skull, the right side of the brain was found to be covered with a thin layer of blood. In other respects, the brain was normal in appearance. The lungs and heart were not altered in any way. The stomach contained a quantity of undigested rice and vegetables. The portion of the bowels inside the abdominal cavity appeared somewhat redder than natural. The liver, spleen, and kidneys were normal in appearance.

Referring the question to my friend Dr. Oldham, of the Geological Survey, whose researches into the history of Ærolites are well known to the scientific world, I am informed by him that there are cases on record in which injuries, which have not proved fatal, have been occasioned by these bodies in falling.

CAUSES OF DEATH AFTER INJURIES.

The always important questions which may arise regarding the *Causes of Death at various periods after the infliction of Injuries,* are often of great interest, and of some complexity in India. It may be taken as a general rule that, wherever individuals suffering from grave and progressive disease of any of the principal viscera are attacked with severe disorder,—whether occurring spontaneously, as in fever or dysentery, or resulting from any mechanical violence or injury, as a beating or a fall,—their lives become seriously imperilled ; the faulty state of their viscera being likely to interfere materially with all reparative processes in their systems.

Twenty-four years ago I went carefully over the whole of the records, at Guy's Hospital, of cases in which Injuries and Surgical Operations, not in themselves of an essentially fatal character, had been followed by death at periods of a few hours or days,—during a period of fifteen years. The results were that, out of 153 such cases which had occurred in the hospital, death had resulted from inflammation of internal organs or secreting surfaces (excluding the liver and spleen) in 143 instances. In the remaining 19, the patients died from other causes, such as tetanus, sloughing, hæmorrhage, suppuration, gangrene, erysipelas, diarrhœa, and total deficiency of reparative action in the wound. In one only, the precise cause of death was not ascertained. Out of these 153 cases, there was marked disease of the spleen, liver, and kidneys in 93 cases. In the 143 cases of death from internal inflammations, there was also superadded marked disease of the spleen, liver, or kidneys, or of all these organs at once, in 90 instances.

In commencing his search for the cause of death in any case, where the operation of violence is suspected, the surgeon must determine to satisfy himself upon three points :—(1)—Whether the injury was, in itself, essentially and necessarily mortal ; (2)—Whether the deceased had previously suffered from organic disease of any important organ ; and (3)—Whether the appearances are such as to lead to a belief that death resulted from the injury or the disease, or from both of these together, each acting upon and aggravating the other.

It is generally well known that, in Europe, intemperate persons, the subjects of organic disease of the abdominal depurative viscera, are, in an unusual degree, liable to suffer from *Uncontrollable Hæmorrhage,* in consequence of comparatively slight operations and injuries, as well as after childbirth and during salivation. I have met with several instances which have convinced me that this predisposition is much increased in India, doubtless in consequence of the operation here of marsh poison as an additional cause of cachæmia. One or two illustrations of this fact will suffice. In 1853, I was called upon to examine the body of a European, who had died under suspicious circumstances. He was a stout and well-made person, about thirty-six years of age. His habits had been notoriously intemperate, and the Magistrate of Howrah had, on that account, removed him from the place of a police constable some time previously. I found several small wounds and scratches on one side of the face and forehead. The most considerable of these was a narrow ragged puncture on the temple, which reached the pericranium, but into which I found that I could not succeed, by the most careful dissection, in tracing any branch of the temporal artery. Still the entire body was so completely blanched, that death must certainly have resulted from hæmorrhage. The liver was enlarged and probably fatty, *the kidneys were mottled in a remarkable degree.* His native servant stated that he had shut himself into his room with a large supply of ardent spirits ; that, on the day preceding his death, he had fallen from his bed on a bottle which, in breaking, had wounded him ; still that they had been afraid to disturb him, and that he had continued to drink spirits and to bleed until he sank. This statement was confirmed by the appearance of the floor and bed, which were almost covered with blood. The fragments of a quart bottle were found by the bedside. I had no hesitation in testifying that, judging by the account of his habits which I had received, and by the state of his organs, he had probably died from hæmorrhage in the manner alleged.

About ten years ago, I was twice called to attend an excessively intemperate European who, on two occasions, barely escaped with life from attacks of most violent and persistent hæmorrhage. Once from a sloughing chancre involving the frœnum, and again from epistaxis. He, however, survived these attacks several years.

It is unnecessary to dwell upon the well-known fact that hepatic and splenic diseases are extremely rife among the lower classes of natives ; and, when we observe the frequency of intemperance among them,* and their continual exposure to great atmospheric vicissitudes, it is not surprising that they should be often afflicted with renal disorders.†

Splenic disease frequently prevents recovery from injuries in this country. We can hardly expect a compound fracture to do well in one of the emaciated subjects of splenic cachexia, when we know that the application of a fly blister over the enlarged spleen would almost inevitably cause gangrene, and that cancrum oris (which is, I think, more properly called malarious sloughing phagedæna) may at any time attack and destroy

---

* A native is never a tippler: when addicted to spirits, he always drinks with a determination to make himself drunk as speedily, and as completely as possible. He can generally state the precise quantity of liquor that will produce this effect,—as half a bottle (perhaps the average dose), a bottle, a bottle and-a-half, or two bottles.

† Dr. Morehead collected 31 cases of Bright's disease in the Jamsetjee Jejeebhoy Hospital, Bombay.—(*Transactions of the Medical and Physical Society of Bombay*, No. X.) ; and Dr. Edward Goodeve was, I believe, one of the first who ascertained that this lesion is not unfrequent among natives in the Bengal Presidency. Dr. Joseph Ewart has published some interesting remarks upon "The Causes, Pathology, and Treatment of Granular Kidney" as observed in the Ajmere Jail.—*Indian Annals of Medical Science*, April, 1855, p. 539. My Native Wards in the Medical College Hospital generally contain one or two cases of *Morbus Brightii.*

him. Sir Ranald Martin's remark that the blood of these unfortunates demonstrates, by its hue, the presence of splenic disease on making the first incision, must have suggested itself to every surgeon in India. The blood of these patients has precisely the appearance of thin claret.

The tendency of this state of the system to render mortal, injuries which would be trivial in persons of sound constitution, was brought forward very clearly in a trial in the Calcutta Supreme Court, in August 1837.

A Mahomedan lady was tried for the murder of a young female child. It appeared that the child was suspended by the hands, and beaten. The hands swelled, and were dressed with chunam and turmeric. The blows were slight. Deceased came to the house about two years previously, being one of the girls who came from the country that was inundated. She had spleen, and fever, and ague, when she came. She used to remain well ten or twenty days, and then got ill, and then well, and this continued to the day of her death. She was subject to purging. She had sores on her hands and body, her feet, back, and head. She had itch on her body, hands, and head.

Mr. O'Brien, after describing the wounds on the body, stated: "I observed during the child's life, when brought to the hospital, that she had enlarged spleen. She smelt of turpentine. I think deceased died from the sloughing ulcers, which brought on the irritation which caused her death. I opened the body for the purpose of examining the spleen ; it was enlarged and indurated, and double its natural size. I saw some worms that had crept out of the body—intestinal worms. I consider the sloughing was produced by the disease of the spleen, and it would not have taken place in a healthy subject ; disease of spleen predisposed to that affection."

"Dr. Raleigh knows the disease of enlargement of the spleen, generally the result of repeated attacks of fever; generally exists in a very disordered constitution, and one greatly reduced by fever, and is accompanied by affections of the bowels. Generally speaking, when a constitution is in this state, the most trivial injury to the skin is followed by rapid sloughing and gangrene; generally speaking, it is the result of external violence, or of blistering. In a subject of that description, such injuries as Belall has described would be likely to produce that effect ; certainly not on ordinarily healthy subjects. The scratch of a pice [pin ?] might have produced sloughing to a great extent."

"Dr. J. R. Martin.—Spleen is almost universally the result of fever. In the Lower Provinces, persons become peculiarly obnoxious to injuries ; so much so, that a leech, a blister, or any other abrasion on the skin or the surface ends in a very unkindly manner. Fatal results might be produced by injuries that with healthy subjects would be quite harmless."

"Verdict—not guilty."

Young and healthy natives generally recover well and quickly from the effects of severe bodily injuries. This has been ascribed to the temperance and simplicity of their mode of life, and to the very sparing quantities of nitrogenous food which they consume.* I have certainly often seen numerous and enormous wounds, on the persons of natives, heal without occasioning a single bad symptom ; and there is generally a quietude and absence of irritability about natives which render them in a remarkable degree capable of preserving that rest and those restrained positions which favor the healing of wounds. Still I have never seen or heard of anything which would lead me to conclude that the people, of Bengal at least, have greater soundness and reparative power of constitution than are to be found generally among healthy Europeans : and I feel convinced that the constitutional vigour of these people has been much over-rated. True, the Bengalee lives upon a plain diet in which a very small proportion of nitrogenous material is contained, but his food is often scanty in quantity, and probably consists of the worst kinds of rice, fish, and lentils ; he works hard, he is badly lodged and badly clothed ; he is greatly exposed to severe vicissitudes of temperature ; he is perhaps an opium-eater or gunjah smoker, and is probably a drunkard, consuming the worst of all spirituous liquors in large quantities ; scurvy very often lurks in his system ; his internal organs have suffered more or less in structure from the above causes. His body is lean and anemiated ; he has been habituated to sexual excess from his boyhood ; and, if the inhabitant of a town, he probably suffered from syphilis and from the use of mercury employed with the most reckless carelessness. This is by no means an unfair description of a considerable proportion of those who seek relief at our dispensaries. In such constitutions, manifestations of great reparative power are scarcely to be looked for. It is very remarkable how distinctly the disorders which are consecutive to injuries and operations in Bengal carry with them the evidences of miasmatic influence. In place of the surgical fever, erysipelas, and tedious suppuration so common after wounds among the diseased and ill-lodged poor of Europe, we have here fever of true intermittent character, gangrene, diarrhœa, and dysentery,† while cases of traumatic tetanus are very much indeed more frequent in India than in Europe, although scarcely so inevitably destructive to life. In city atmospheres in India, persons of all races, and apparently of all

---

* Mr. Baynes says that—" From some peculiarity either in the constitution or mode of life of the natives of this country, wounds not immediately fatal more frequently and more, readily heal than in the European subject : so that, if the constitution survive the first shock, it is apparently in less danger from attacks of fever, inflammation, erysipelas, &c., which, in other climates, are so frequently the secondary causes of death.

† In the records, I find eight cases in which fatal diarrhœa or dysentery supervened in cases of wound, and only one case of erysipelas.

constitutions, are liable to surgical fever, phlebitis, osteo myelitis, and other evidences of blood poisoning after wounds and surgical operations.

In the cases of those who die in hospital from the effects of wounds inflicted with malicious intent, it appears to be generally conceded, as a matter of course, by the judicial authorities, that life has been sacrificed, despite of the employment of the most judicious medical and surgical treatment attainable.* In cases, however, where severe wounds have been evidently mismanaged by native practitioners (as in an instance where, some of the ribs having been cut through, cow-dung was applied and oozed into the pleural cavity),† it is generally inquired whether the patient might not have recovered under proper treatment, and whether his death was not attributable rather to mismanagement than to the injury? This is well answered by Taylor—"The true distinction in all such cases is that, if the death was evidently occasioned by grossly erroneous medical treatment, the original author of the violence will not be answerable; but, if it arise from the want merely of the higher skill which can only be commanded in great towns, he will be responsible, because he has wilfully exposed the deceased to a risk from which he has, practically, no means of escaping." Again, Baron Platt is reported to have observed, in 1845, that,—"If a man inflicted a wound likely to produce death, and the wounded party should fall into the hands of an unskilful practitioner, whereby death was hastened, the aggressor would still be responsible for the result. If the wound had not been likely to produce death, but by unskilful treatment death ensued, then that would not be murder."‡

Howliah Bin Pursapee was tried in 1831, at Dharwar (Bombay Presidency), for murder. There was an old quarrel between prisoner and deceased: meeting at the gate of their village, deceased coughed in a contemptuous manner. Upon this provocation, prisoner drew his sword, inflicted a wound, and made off. The wound was on the fleshy part of the calf, the sinews were cut, the bone exposed, and the wound gaped open very wide. It was shown that an ignorant person had attempted to doctor the wound, and, instead of sewing it up, had kept it open, and, by the application of inflammatory medicines, had so irritated the wound

---

* In one case only do I find it inquired of a sub-assistant surgeon whether every attention was paid to the dressing of a patient's wounds during his stay in hospital, and whether maggots attacked any of his wounds before death. The replies to these questions appear to have been satisfactory.

† The wounds of persons brought in from distant mofussil villages are, of course, generally in a miserable condition: chunam and huldee (lime and turmeric) are favorite applications. In cases of hæmorrhage, large masses of raw cotton, powdered with charcoal dust, are among the least objectionable applications. In a report of the Coimbator Dispensary (Madras Presidency), Mr. Porteous says that nearly all his patients had their wounds either foul, or filled up with charcoal and oil, or jaggery and chunam (treacle and lime), requiring some days ere they would clean.

‡ Op. Citat., p. 274.

that mortification ensued, which was the immediate cause of death. The Sudder Court held that the offence of which the prisoner had been proved guilty was culpable homicide, and not murder, and therefore passed a sentence applicable to the former offence, *viz.*, ten years' imprisonment with hard labor.*

Mr. Baynes observes,—"The culprit must take what may be called the *consequences of his country*. A native of India can, clearly, have no right to complain if he be punished for inflicting a wound which proves mortal, under the comparatively unskilful treatment which it will probably receive, merely because, had it been inflicted within the reach of European skill, it would, most probably, not have proved so ; but, on the other hand, he has a right and claim to all the mitigating considerations which may arise from the fact of *unusual* means having been resorted to in order to its cure ; or from the wounded party neglecting to resort to the *usual* means ; or from the fatal effect being clearly traceable to the state of constitution of the deceased at the time ; and the Court will, in all cases, put to itself the question,—was the amount of injury inflicted apparently sufficient to cause death in a person of ordinary health and vigour ?"†

Where the medical evidence showed that the deceased would not have necessarily died from the effects of the wound, had it not been for the state of his health, and where there was no proof of any intention to take life, the Court held that the prisoner could not be convicted of wilful murder, but passed sentence for culpable homicide. Reports, L. P., 1856, Part I., page 936 ; Reports, W. P., 1856, Part I., page 404. *See para.* 3993. Beaufort's Digest, Second Ed., page 776, para. 3923.

Fagoo, in a gambling quarrel, struck Chedi once on the face with a lattee. Chedi seems either to have been knocked down by the blow, or to have sat down at once on receiving it. The evidence is not consistent on this point. The medical evidence proves that tetanus had supervened upon the wound : that the wound was not, in itself, either severe or dangerous ; and that, even then, it was possible enough that, under proper remedies, he might have recovered. He was, however, taken away in a *dooly* towards his own house, which he never reached, dying on the way in the boat crossing the river, the day after he had been seen and prescribed for. Convicted of culpable homicide, but without any aggravating circumstances calling for heavy punishment.‡

Dr. Kenneth Mackinnon has very justly insisted upon the danger which attends the practice of sending all wounded persons to the sudder sta-

* Bellasis' Reports, p. 60.
† Op. Citat., p. 56.
‡ Nizamut Adawlut Reports, June 7th, 1856, p. 940.

tions—quite irrespectively of the length of the journey and of the severity of the hurt.

TORTURE.

The causes of many of the kinds of bodily injury brought under the notice of medical men in India would be perfectly inexplicable if attention had not been paid to the various modes of Torture practised by the natives.

Seeing that the last vestige of judicial Torture* was not expunged from our own Criminal Code until the year 1771; that, at the commencement of this present year, 1870, it still lingered in four cantons of Switzerland; and that, according to M. Emile Anderoli, it has not long ceased to be known to the Russian police;—it is not surprising that, in ancient times, the absolute rulers of India should have employed this potent means of intimidation and extortion upon their subjects; or that, among a crafty and timid people, the traditions of the practice should be preserved, and not unfrequently acted upon in the present day.†

Very little information can be gathered from books with regard to Torture, as now practised in Bengal. Mr. Taylor mentions‡ that it was formerly a common practice, among zemindars in the neighbourhood of Dacca, to confine their ryots in irons, and to subject them to Torture of different kinds; but that they, in the present day, seldom go beyond the length of imprisoning their ryots, though instances of more severe punishment occasionally occur.

I have been at considerable pains to ascertain the various modes of Torture still known, and had recourse to, in Bengal. Much of the information embodied in the following details has been furnished me, in reply to

---

* The *Peine Forte et Dure.*

† An archer having attempted the life of the Emperor Akbar, the bystanders were anxious that he should be tortured to make him confess the names of his confederates. Akbar, however, refused on the ground that a confession, extorted by such means, would be as likely to involve the innocent as the guilty.

Murshed Kuli Khan, who became Nawab of Bengal in 1718, was, among his other atrocities, remarkable for the severity with which he extorted revenue from the zemindars. We are told that he used to oblige defaulters "to wear leather long drawers, filled with live cats, and to drink buffalo's milk mixed with salt, till they were brought to death's door by diarrhœa." The *chora* (or whip) was also constantly in use. According to Stewart, one of his agents, Nazir Ahmed, used to deliver over the captive zemindars to be tormented with various refinements of cruelty, such as hanging up by the feet, bastinadoing, and setting them in the sun in summer; and by stripping them naked, and sprinkling them frequently with cold water in winter. Another of his people, Synd Reza Khan, ordered a pond to be dug, filled with everything disgusting, to which, in scorn of the Hindus, he gave the name of Bickoont (*Paradise*), and through this detestable pool the defaulters were drawn by a rope tied under their arms. During the seventeenth century, the practice of tying wretches to palm trees with their bodies smeared with honey, to attract the red ants, was by no means unfrequent, especially in Batavia. It will presently be shown that this last-mentioned barbarity is still prevalent in Madras.

‡ A sketch of the Topography and Statistics of Dacca, 1840.

my questions, by several native gentlemen of high character and extensive information.

My original report on this subject appeared in the *Indian Annals of Medical Science* for October 1854, not many days after it became known in Calcutta that the Governor of Madras had directed, in Minutes of consultation dated 9th September 1854, that a strict inquiry should be made into the alleged practice of Torture for the purpose of realizing the revenues of the State in that Presidency.

The following pages contain reference to all the modes of torture mentioned in the Report of the Commissioners appointed for the investigation of these practices. It will be observed that a similarity, almost amounting to identity, exists between the modes of torture practised in this and in the Madras Presidency,—a fact which goes far to prove that these atrocities have been prevalent in every part of India from a period at which the laws or, at least, the national customs were the same throughout the country.

Torture was not prescribed by the ancient Hindu Lawgivers.* The practice was, doubtless, introduced by the Mussalmauns.

Torture was much used by the Mahomedan rulers of India. Thus we read, in the Seir Mutaqherin, that, when Ali Verdi Khan left his conquest, Cuttack, under the Government of his young grandson, a vagabond fakir, called Shah Yahya, became a favorite of the prince, and commenced upon the rich men of the district a plan of extortion so systematic that "his house became a tribunal of inquisition where the business of scourging and torturing went on regularly, so that the cries of the oppressed reached the cupola of Heaven." This, naturally, led to a storm.

Shimshir Khan so tortured Hadji Ahmed, brother of the Nawab Ali Verdi Khan, for the space of sixteen or seventeen days, to oblige him to the discovery of his concealed riches, that the unfortunate prince expired.

We have abundant evidence that this atrocity has now become intimately blended with the customs of all sects and classes of natives throughout India. The poor practise torture upon each other; robbers on their victims, and *vice versâ;* masters upon their servants; zemindars upon their ryots; schoolmasters upon their pupils; husbands upon their wives; and even parents upon their children.†

---

* Branding and pouring hot oil into the ear are sanctioned by Menu, and are repeatedly mentioned by Halhed, but only as *punishments* for detected crime—not as tentative measures in cases of suspicion or as modes of torture.

† "We have instances of torture being freely practised in every relation of domestic life. Servants are thus treated by their masters and fellow-servants, and children by their parents and schoolmasters, for the most trifling offences; the very plays of the populace (and the point of a rude people's Drama is in its satire) excite the laughter of many a rural audience by the exhibition of revenue squeezed out of a defaulter, coin by coin, through the appliance of familiar "provocatives," under the superintendence of a caricatured Tehsildar; it seems a

It is stated, in the Madras Report, that the priests place the *kittee* and *unanthal* (instruments of torture) before the Triputhy Idols, and expose them to the sun, if their votaries are backward in their offerings.* That one of the most common kinds of punishment in the schools is to suspend a boy by the hands, with the fingers joined, to a rope pulled up to a beam; this is inflicted on boys above twelve years of age. Another punishment is to pinion the boys, and cause them to stand in a bending posture with their thumbs on their toes ; another is tying the hands with the knees within the arms, and then thrusting a stick between the arms and knees and rolling the boys over.† I have been informed, by a native christian gentleman, that flogging with the stinging *bichattee* plant and tying portions of this plant upon the body, are punishments in common use by native schoolmasters in Bengal. Again, it is stated in the Report that Indian mothers often make their children (as a punishment) stand in painful positions looking at the sun.‡ The Sub-Judge of Mangalore informed the Committee that, a short time previously, in his own compound, a native tied his child's hands together, and then put some pepper into his eyes, castigation having failed. He understood that this was not at all an uncommon mode with parents of subduing their children, and that not only among the most ignorant classes.§ I was informed by my friend the late Mr. Bedford that, previous to my relieving him at Chittagong, the son of an East Indian of indifferent character employed there, with whom I was also acquainted, came to him with inflamed eyes, declaring that his father had punished him by introducing red pepper into them.

In 1869 the Rev. J. Long, of Calcutta, obtained photographs of a series of pictures of the tortures practised upon boys in the village schools of Bengal. These punishments are described as follows in Mr. Long's introduction to Adam's Reports on Vernacular Education published in 1868.

"A boy is made to bend forward with his face toward the ground; a heavy brick is then placed on his back, and another on his neck ; and, should he let either of them fall within the prescribed period of half an hour or so, he is punished with the cane.

"A boy is condemned to stand for half an hour or an hour on one foot; and, should he shake or quiver, or let down the uplifted leg before the time, he is severely punished.

---

time-honored institution, and we cannot be astonished if the practice is still widely prevalent among the ignorant, uneducated class of native public servants."—*Madras Commissioners' Report*, p. 50. "In one of the satirical processions which take place in Dacca once a year, there is a representation of a Darogah torturing a man in the most indecent manner. Would it have been so if these *things were uncommon?*"—*Dacca News*, December 13, 1856.

* Appendix C. No. 14, Salem, p. cxliii.

† Appendix C. No. 10, Canara, p. cxiv.

‡ Appendix C. No. 14, Salem, p. cxliii.

§ Appendix C. No. 10, Canara, p. cxv.

Mussamut Monea was found guilty at Sarun, in 1855, of having robbed and stripped a girl of five, and of having drowned her in a well.*

In the same year, Mussamut Nuthiab was sentenced to death at Bhaugulpore for having decoyed three little boys into a garden, where she took off their ornaments. Upon the elder remonstrating, she threw him down a well, out of which he was taken dead.†

Adults are not very unfrequently drowned in Wells.

The author of the Seir Mutaqherin has alluded to a practice of conveying young men, in meat doolies, into seraglios, where they were ultimately thrown into wells by the ladies, or, on detection, by their masters

In 1851, a Hindu was sentenced to death, at Purneah, for killing his wife by throwing her into a well. The darogah reported that, upon raising the corpse out of the well, in which there were six feet of water, it exhibited a black mark, as if from the blow of a lattee, on the right side; another on the right fore-arm, as if from drawing a cord; a third, eight fingers in length, from the top of the shoulder to the neck, apparently the brand of a hot iron; a fourth, also of a burn, from the throat, extending over the shoulder, fourteen fingers long.‡

Again, in 1852, a Hindu of Shahabad was sentenced for having murdered a boy four or five years of age, and for having attempted the life of the child's mother, by throwing them into a large well about thirty-five feet deep.§

Doojah, of Shahjehanpore, confessed that, finding his elder brother's wife in criminal connexion with a person named, he pursued her and threw her into a well, where she was drowned.‖

It does not appear that, in falling into these wells, the bodies of the victims generally receive fractures, or other very severe injuries, which might lead to doubt in the Surgeon's mind with regard to the cause of death. There are two kinds of wells,—the *kua*, or well of small diameter; and the wide-mouthed well or bricked reservoir (*indara*). The bodies of those who fall or are thrown into the former, are, of course, more likely to present traces of contusion, &c. Where, however, a dead body or an infant is merely dropped in head foremost, and is not thrown with a forward impulse, no injury beyond those received by

---

* Nizamut Adawlut Reports, 26th June 1855, p. 806.

† *Ibid*, 7th December 1855, p. 866.

‡ *Ibid*, Vol. I. of 1851, p. 1512.

§ *Ibid*, Vol. II., Part 2, of 1852, p. 500.

‖ Nizamut Adawlut Reports, N. W. P., 18th April 1854, p. 424. See also Police Report, L. Provinces, 1844, p. 13 (a reputed witch thrown down a well). *Ibid* for 1849, p. 19 (a wizard treated in like manner).

chillum of a pipe, or *kalika*, called in Bengali (*Kalika puriya dag deoyá*); 2nd, by red-hot charcoal *or a gul* (*Gul puriya dag deoya*); 3rd, by a lighted torch (*Máshal diya porána*); 4th, by red-hot iron (*Loha puriya deon*); 5th, by heated oil (*Garam tel dhaliya deoyá*)—*or pouring hot oil*, or by hot water. It cannot, however, always be ascertained how the burns have been inflicted.

The surgeons' reports, sent into the Nizamut, contain the details of several cases where torture by fire was evidently had recourse to. It is not perfectly clear, in all, by what means the heat was applied, but the following are evidently examples of the 2nd, 3rd, 4th, and 5th modes. I have met with one case of the first kind in my own practice. In a case sent in by Mr. Stanlake Batson, of Shahabad, in 1841, it is mentioned that "the patient had a circular wound on the fore-arm, near the elbow, occasioned by the application of some heated body to the part." The individual at first appeared to be feigning insanity, and accounted for the injury in more than one improbable way; he, at length, stated that the malik of his village aud others alleged against him that his mother was a dain, or witch, and had applied a hot tiklee to his arm to torture him, with a view to compel him to leave the village; although doubtless false, this statement must be taken as representing an existing practice.*

Dr. Archer, when at Howrah, informed me that a case occurred within his observation at Kishenagur, in which a native, finding a man in his house evidently with no good intention, overpowered and bound the intruder; and then, seating himself beside him, lighted a pipe and continued, from time to time, to apply the heated chillum to the unfortunate wretch's flesh, until he had rendered him a very fit subject for surgical care.

In examining cases of this kind, it must be borne in mind that the application of the charcoal *gul* and of a rude but very severe kind of moxa,—both producing circular or oval eschars,—is among the most frequent practices of the native doctors, especially in cases of enlarged spleen and chronic rheumatism, and as an ordinary means of counter-irritation.

A case remarkably illustrative of this point occurred at Mooltaye, in the Saugor territory, in 1851. It was reported to the Tehsildar of the place that a dâk hurkaru,—who had lately come to his home from duty, and for three or four days had been ill with vomiting and purging,—had died the night before; and that, owing to his wife having an intrigue with a person named, and to consequent domestic quarrels, there was suspicion of foul play. Upon viewing the body, this officer found that the belly, hands, and feet were black, as if scorched by fire. The man's mother-in-law confessed that she had poisoned him with white arsenic. He appears

* See also Nizamut Adawlut Reports, Vol. II., Part 1, of 1852, p. 211, and Macnaghten's Reports, Vol. II., p. 56.

to have received medical treatment. The Tehsildar afterwards informed the Sessions Judge that it is customary, thereabouts, to have the part affected with disease or pain burnt with hot iron, and that he supposed this process had been applied in the present instance. If so, the Judge considered it likely that it was done at the instance of the sufferer, or the neighbours ; and it would, of course, be the cue of the prisoner (assuming her guilt) to maintain and encourage the belief that his illness was from natural causes.*

Reference is made, in the Madras Report,† to the prevalence there of cases in which *wounds and marks, with blistering juices, &c., are self-inflicted* for purposes of false accusation. *See* above, p. 286, use of the juice of the Marking Nut. In March 1865, the Assistant Magistrate of Howrah sent me a girl, about ten years old, for my opinion as to how certain marks on her cheeks, arms, and back were caused. She asserted that they were burned with a hot chillum, whereas the accused declared that they had been made with some paint. I found a large circular brown mark on either cheek, each of these marks had a clean and perfectly defined edge. The marks on the arms and back were parallel brown streaks with clean edges ; there was no vesication, but the cuticle was beginning to separate. Such even, clear-edged, symmetrical marks could not have been inflicted with a heated body upon any person who was not in a state of complete insensibility ; and, from their shape, it was evident that they could not have been caused by the application of a chillum. I gave it as my opinion that a fluid irritant had been applied, and that the case had been trumped up.

3rd.—In 1841, Mr. Wilkie, of Dinagepore, reported that a Mussalmaun woman had died from the effects of being burnt with a mashal. He found a circular ulcer, three inches in diameter, on the back ; the whole of the inner sides of both thighs and the pudenda were blistered, as were also both arms and breasts ; there were likewise a patch on the outer part of the right thigh, and an ulcer two inches long on the popliteal space of that limb.

In 1845, a well-known housebreaker, of Purneah, was arrested in the act of committing a burglary; and the brother of the owner of the house, being determined to discover where the rest of the gang had secreted the property, tied up the robber with his feet to one post, and his hands to another immediately opposite ; and then, with the assistance of the chowkedar and another servant, lit a good-sized torch and burnt him from head to foot. The police concealed this atrocity. A few days afterwards, the magistrate received a report from the darogah and mohurir who sent in the thief in a cart, saying that he was ill with fever. The

* Nizamut Adawlut Reports, N. W. P., Feb. 6, 1852, p. 105.
† Appendix C., No. 8, Cuddapah, p. xcvii.

magistrate, going to see him, found "*his flesh literally burnt off his bones.*" He died that night, refusing to say how or by whom he had been thus treated. The darogah and mohurir were sentenced to five years' imprisonment for endeavoring to conceal this atrocity by false report.*

In Captain Meadowes Taylor's "Confessions of a Thug," the narrator says :—" They threw me down, * * * a red-hot pice was pressed upon my forehead ; it was held there as it burnt down to the bone."

This practice of torturing thieves by fire, either is or has been, until lately, very prevalent in Bengal. An active officer of the Force told me that the expression *gurm kuro ! warm him !* was familiar to every policeman under the old regime.

It has lately been ruled, in Calcutta, that causing death by *branding* a thief, without the knowledge that the act was so immediately dangerous that it would, in all probability, cause death or such bodily injury as was likely to cause death, is punishable, under section 304 of the Penal Code, as culpable homicide not amounting to murder.—Queen *v.* Khedun Misser, 7 W. R. Cr., 54—Cowell and Woodman.

In the following case, torture by fire was evidently the preliminary to murder, under the most barbarous circumstances : In September 1845, Mr. Wilkie, of Dinagepore, examined the body of a Mussalmaun woman, in which he found that the lower part of the abdomen, the external genitals, thighs, legs, feet, and palms of the hands had been extensively scorched by fire, before life was extinct. There was a wound above the left ear. This ear and part of the right ear were cut off. Mr. Wilkie considered that she had probably been first stunned, and then burnt. It appears more likely, however, that the fatal blow on the head was inflicted last. Again, in 1844, Mr. Macintyre, of Furreedpore, found on the body of a Mussalmaunee, "a compound fracture of the right leg and violent contusion about the breast and head ; she appeared to have been burnt about the breast and armpits," where the skin was blistered in large patches ; some violence also seemed to have been inflicted about the pudenda. In 1849, Dr. T. W. Wilson, of Rajshahye,

---

* Report of the State of the Police in the Lower Provinces, for 1845, p. 19.

Noted by Gerrard that, in 1635, the French put live matches to the fingers of some English sailors to make them confess, being loaded with timber, and tell to what place they were bound.

"Sir William Bannatyne's soldiers seized a woman, and bound her, and put lighted matches betwixt her fingers for several hours ; the torture and pain made her almost distracted, she lost one of her hands, and in a few hours she died."—*Wodrow's Church of Scotland.*

At a Court-martial held at Spithead, John Berkley and Jonathan Stoker, who belonged to His Majesty's Ship *Weazel*, were sentenced to receive each 104 lashes on their bare backs, for putting a lighted match between the fingers of two men and a boy who belonged to a French vessel.—*Gent's Mag.*, April 1731.

examined the person of a Hindu female, and found a rather trivial burn, apparently occasioned by the application of some heated substance to the skin of the hips, close to the anus, producing blistering and removal of the cuticle.*

Sir Mordaunt Wells sentenced a man to seven years' imprisonment for having thrown his wife down, and having burnt the pudenda with a brand from the fire. It was alleged that they had disputed about dinner, but it is probable that jealousy may be regarded as the cause in nearly all these cases.

In 1852, near Azimgurh, an elderly man of some wealth and of notoriously dissolute habits, was killed in the house of one of his assamees, where he had an intrigue with a married female. The native doctor deposed that he found the body covered with blisters from the application of fire, and the hair of the head and face was burnt off.† Marks of violence were found on the throat, the windpipe had been forcibly compressed by the application of some hard substance, and death by strangulation had resulted.‡

The flame of a torch, or the oil which drops from it, is the manner of torture commonly used by dacoits to compel persons to give up concealed property.§

Tytler mentions‖ that, on entering a village immediately after a dacoity had been committed, he was shown two stakes, with a shallow pit dug beween them, over which they had suspended the master of the house, and had actually roasted him over a slow fire, until he pointed out the place where his little treasure was hid. He persisted so long in concealing it that he died the next day.

In a trial for dacoity, with torturing to death, deceased's son stated that, after the departure of the dacoits, he went out and found his father in agonies on the ground in the court-yard, the upper part of his body being wrapped up with tow to which the dacoits had set fire. His hands had the marks of having been tied together. His father said that the dacoits had pressed him down by placing the *dhakee*, which was near him, upon

* See also the case of a man convicted of wounding the pudenda of his wife, and of having thrown burning fuel upon her, as punishment for unchastity.—*Nizamut Adawlut Returns*, Vol. I. of 1852, p. 762.

† Burning the beard (*Dariporia dhaya*) is also mentioned as a Bengali mode of torture.

‡ Nizamut Adawlut Reports, N. W. P., Jan. 7th, 1853, p. 24.

§ See Macnaghten's Reports, Vol. I., p. 14; Nizamut Adawlut Reports, Vol. III., Part 1 of 1853, p. 51 (with a red-hot stick), and p. 410 (with a torch); of 1854, p. 451 (torch); p. 728 (torch); *Ibid*, p. 742 (torch); Bengal Police Reports, 1838, p. 36 (burning); *Ibid*, 1868 (cotton was placed round a woman and lighted), p. 73; Nizamut Adawlut Reports, August 1851, p. 182 (sprinkling with hot oil); *Ibid*, p. 247 (torch); *Ibid*, December 1854 (oil from a torch), p. 853; *Ibid*, Feb. of same year, p. 259 (torch); Jan. 1852, p. 48, (torch); *Ibid*, Jan. 21, 1857 (match), p. 40; July 22, 1859 (bamboo shavings), p. 213; Nizamut Adawlut Reports, N. W. P., 27th Aug. 1852, p. 907 (hot oil).

‖ Present State of India, Vol. I., p. 108.

his heart ; the old man died from the injuries at noon next day. The prisoners were convicted.*

In his Report for 1848, Mr. Dampier mentions† that, in the district of Nuddea alone, *one hundred and seventy-four* persons were entered, within the year, as having been engaged in dacoitees with torture. In some instances, this barbarity has been carried to fatal lengths, as in the case of an old man of Dinagepore, who was so severely burnt with torches by dacoits, to make him give up his money, that he died nine days afterwards ;‡ and in that of another aged man who was similarly tortured in Nuddea with so much cruelty that he died from lock-jaw four days subsequently.§ The only instance which I find in which any other mode of torture was employed by dacoits, was one in which the woman of the house had her thigh compressed between two pieces of bamboo, called a *chepa,* to enforce her to discover her husband's property. This, however, occurred in Assam—(Kamroop).||

It is rather satisfactory to know that these dacoits, who are so free in torturing others by fire, are not unacquainted with its effects upon their own persons. It came out at a trial at Hooghly, in 1866, that, in a gang commanded by the prisoner Matabdee, " the members, when introduced into the gang, were always subjected to a burning or branding on the thigh *to try their mettle*." The Judge and Dr. Herbert Baillie, the Civil Surgeon, examined the persons of the prisoners who stated this, and of two others, and found the scars of the burning on each in the place indicated.¶

A railway gate-keeper having interrupted six men in taking away some sleepers, was seized and held down over the fire until he fainted.**

A case is mentioned in the Madras Report, in which two peons were punished for burning a suspected person with the end of a cheroot.††

4t*h*.—A man was sent to me for examination by the Magistrate of Howrah, with evident traces of a recent burn on the perineum and buttock and about the anus (there was no internal injury). He declared that a heated iron had been applied by certain persons a day or two previously. I confirmed the probability of his assertion.

In August 1843, a man and his concubine were sentenced, at Nuddea, for burning the pudenda, and also other parts of the body of a Hindu female child, three years old, with a red-hot iron *hata* (*ladle*).‡‡

---

* Nizamut Adawlut of Calcutta, July 9, 1840.

† P. 53.

‡ Police Reports, L. P., 1838, p. 44.

§ Police Report for 1845, p. 57.

|| Police Report, August 1854, p. 218.

¶ Nizamut Adawlut Reports, Sept. 6, 1856, p. 405.

** Bengal Police Rep., 1868, p. 364.

†† Madras Report, Appen. 7, p. lxxxiv.

‡‡ Nizamut Adawlut Returns, Vol. IV., Part 2, p. 279.

In 1853, one Jeebia (Hindu) and others, complained to the Deputy Magistrate of Nowada, accusing certain persons of having burnt her with a hot iron *hussooa* (*sickle*) on her body, and of having made her mother eat cow's flesh, charging them with having bewitched a child. She and others were, in consequence, tried for perjury. The Court, however, decided that there was no direct or positive proof of the falsehood of the above statements.*

In 1840, one Rajee Mundul, from motives of jealousy, burnt his wife on the thigh and other parts of her body with a heated sickle ; she was found dead on the following day, and the prisoner confessed to having burnt her, not thinking that it would cause her death.†

Again, a man was convicted, at Rungpore in 1844, of having burnt his wife (whom he had caught in the act of committing adultery) with a hot iron. Death appears to have resulted.‡

A goldsmith of Cawnpore was sentenced to imprisonment and a heavy fine, in 1853, for having tied his runaway apprentice's arms, stopped his mouth with some cloth, and burnt him in ten or twelve different parts of his body with a heated iron spoon. The boy suffered some time in hospital, and was marked for life.§

Three Hindus of Cuttack were sentenced to imprisonment in irons for seven years, for having, on a false accusation of theft, bound one who served them as a laborer hand and foot, and burnt him in about twenty-seven places with a heated sickle. Witnesses deposed that they saw the man lying bound and insensible in defendants' house, near a fire and two sickles. Dr. Pringle said that, at one time, the wounds were dangerous from suppuration, and that they must have been made by a weapon shaped like the sickle produced in Court.‖

The following is from the Calcutta *Indian Daily News* of November 9, 1868 :

"A native female, residing in Kidderpore, is at present in custody, charged with having, with a pair of heated tongs, burnt the lips of her sister-in-law, a girl of about twelve years of age, simply because the latter had, the day previously, eaten a portion of the other's dinner."

It was stated in the Calcutta Newspapers in May 1868, that Moulvie Abdool Luteef had then before him two cases, in each of which a woman

---

* See case in which an unfortunate ryot of Midnapore was seized, evidently by the orders of his talookdar, and carried to a house where he was tortured by fire, and beaten to death with sticks and shoes.—*Nizamut Adawlut Reports*, Nov. 1853, p. 792.

† Police Report, L. P., for 1840, p. 62.

‡ *Ibid*, for 1844, p. 33.

§ Nizamut Adawlut Reports, N. W. P., 30th September 1853, p. 1217—"If he (a once-born man) mentions the names and classes of twice-born persons with contumely, an iron style, ten fingers long, shall be thrust, red-hot, into his mouth."—*Menu*, v. 271.

‖ Nizamut Adawlut Reports, March 30, 1857, p. 416.

was charged with burning another woman on various parts of her body with a hot iron.

A Mussalmaun, in the Bood-Bood Sub-Division (Burdwan), had a wife and a nika wife. The latter murdered the infant daughter of the former, by drowning her in a tank, after having burnt her body in several places with a hot iron.*

These uses of the hot iron are also well understood in Madras. Shortly before the last edition of this work appeared, a man in Tanjore branded a young boy with a hot sickle for an act of ordinary carelessness; later still, a man of Vallore swung a young girl to the beam of his house by her hands and hair, beat her, and branded her face and arm with a hot knife, because she had taken nine pice from his room.† The head Assistant Magistrate of Tinnevelly reported that there was then "a man in hospital suffering from severe maltreatment, having been half-roasted alive," by villagers, who caught him in an attempt to rob.‡

The following most atrocious case was reported in the *Madras Mail* of the 20th September 1869. At the special sessions of the Tanjore Court, a Mahomedan Kazee, named Abdul Kureem, was tried and convicted of inflicting grievous hurt on his wife. She was found by the medical officer to be suffering from grievous burns on her thighs and abdomen, her body was marked with bruises, and her face with scars. It appears that he had been married for about a year to the poor creature, whom he frequently beat after she had been prematurely confined. He said, "As you persist in saying you will return to your mother's house, I shall burn you." The following is part of her evidence. "He returned home about 10 hours in the evening, and prepared a fire on the hearth. He put the bill-hook into the fire to make it hot. He gagged me with a cloth, and tied me round the body, and put a piece of split bamboo across the back of my neck and tied my hands to it. He tied my legs with a rope. He sat down on my neck and breast, and took away my cloth and burned my body with the bill-hook. Then he untied me, and took me to the well and put me in the water. He had taken out the cloth from my mouth, but he put one hand over my mouth, and the other on my neck. Then he took me back to the house, and ordered me to serve him with the food that was there. I served him. Then he put a rope round a beam, and tied the rope to my hair, and tied my two thumbs together with thread, and kept me so till the next morning. He staid by me. If I cried out loud, he would beat me. Early in the morning he released me. When he staid in the house he staid with me, and when he went out, he locked the door. After two or three days, some females came on a festival day to hear the

---

* Bengal Police Report, 1868, p. 204.
† Appendix C., No. 16, p. clxix.
‡ *Ibid*, cxcvi.

Koran read. My husband said he should lock me up, and go and read the Koran. I asked him if it was right to lock me up when all the women had come. Then he stabbed me with the scissors in the left side of my face. He put me into the room and locked the door. The wound bled. At 9 o'clock in the evening he returned and released me. I said I wanted to go to my mother's house. He said he had already forbidden me to go, and burnt me for saying I would go; and, if I went to my mother's, she would marry me to another, and my body which he had seen, must not be seen by others, and therefore he should stab me. Then he tied me again. My hair was tied to a rope round the beam, and a padlock was attached. Then he went out. When he came in he untied me, and fastened my hair by a rope to the pillar and padlocked it. He took the bill-hook, and said he was going to cut me. I asked him if he thought that, after doing all this, he would go to Makani free from all sin. He said—Where did you get such a tongue? Then he stabbed me with a small knife under my left eye. I said it is not a good time to cut me, the neighbours are stirring, postpone it a while. It was then night. He consented, and he then kicked me on the wound where I had been burnt. He lay down in the passage, and left me tied. After some time I heard him snore. I spoke to him two or three times to see if he was awake. He did not speak. I cut through my hair with an iron nut-cracker I had concealed, and got another cloth, and went out of the house by a back door."

It was reported in the Autumn of 1866 that a native woman had been committed for trial, at Bombay, on a charge of branding a little girl with a red-hot knife.

Torture by Boiling Oil or Water.

In 1777, Peggy was executed at Calcutta for the murder of Susannah, a slave girl, "by scalding her to death with hot water from a kettle."*

There is a case, in Macnaghten's Reports,† in which a Mussalmaun slave girl, between eight and nine years of age, accused her mistress of tying her with a cord, heating some oil, and pouring it on her private parts. The correctness of this statement appears to have been confirmed by the Civil Surgeon.

"A shocking case of torture is now under investigation. A young female has had her right hand almost burnt to a cinder, by an opulent zemindar, whose ryot she happens to be."—Report from *Calcutta,—Allen's Asiatic Journal*, Jan., April, 1840, p. 121.

In 1842, Mr. Kean, of Moorshedabad, reported the case of a Hindu in whom both hands and one foot were so much burned that mortification

---

* Morton's Decisions of the Supreme Court of Judicature, Bengal, p. 260.

† Vol. I., p. 55.

ensued. The injured toes, the fingers of both hands, and a large portion of the right hand were thrown off. Mr. Kean considered that the injury must have resulted from the immersion of the parts in some boiling liquid.

In the same year, the body of a Mussalmaun girl was sent in for inspection to Mr. J. Macrae, at Monghyr. All that could be discovered, was that "the hands and lower parts of the arms were burnt almost to cinders."

In his Report for the first six months of 1842, Mr. Dampier mentions a case in which the police of Thaunah Mirzapore, in the Moorshedabad district, tied together the fingers and toes of a man suspected of dacoity, and drove wedges between them to the greatest extent of tension. He was then laid out on his back in the sun; this not producing the desired effect, his hands and feet were dipped into boiling water, then the ligatures were unloosened and bandages dipped in oil, tied round the fingers of both hands and the toes of the left foot, and lighted. Failing to obtain a confession, they kept him in the Thaunah, without any remedies being applied, until the fingers and toes became gangrenous. These parts ultimately dropped off.*

In 1854, one Nunda Sonar, of Sarun, inflicted this horrible torture *upon his own child.* The boy, aged only about ten years, was found one night by the police lying crying in the street. His body bore marks of beating, and his hands of burning. He stated that his father had beaten him the day before; and that, six months previously, he had, when drunk, tied him up, bound his hands with tow, and then set fire to it; and that, during the six months, he had been confined in the house. The poor child had lost the use of his hands, and his statement was fully corroborated by witnesses.†

A horrible case of murder by torture, in which this barbarity was used, was brought to light in March 1855. Some idols and other property belonging to the Rajah of Pergunnah Jalda in the Maunbhoom district having been stolen, several suspected persons were apprehended by the Rajah's people, and brought to his *gurh*, or petty fortress. They were, one and all, tortured to extort confession. All were beaten and kept in restraint for about three days, being at night all fastened by the feet to one rope. Two, however, being the most suspected, were the most severely treated. Their fingers were tied together and shivers of bamboo were driven between them. This was also done to the toes; boiling oil was then poured on their hands and feet. Having made a kind of pincers, by tying two cross-sticks together, they squeezed therewith the testicles of Sadhoo Churn (who subsequently died) "and so emasculated him."

---

* All the Police Officers were, of course, severely punished for this atrocity.

† Nizamut Adawlut Reports, December 1854, p. 793.

A string with a noose was put on his penis, and, the other end of the string being made fast to a tree, one of the tormentors struck the tense string with a stick. Upon the body of this unfortunate man being examined by the Civil Surgeon, it was found that the hands were fearfully lacerated, as if by stakes or pieces of iron driven through them; besides which, he had marks of having been scalded with boiling oil or water. The medical officer considered that the injuries inflicted on the hands, feet, and private parts of the deceased, were sufficient to cause, and did cause, death.*

I have a note of the case, mentioned to me by a medical officer, of a sonar (goldsmith), of Seharunpore, who was tied down on his charpoy, oiled tow was twisted round his fingers, and set fire to. He was at last strangled.

The following case affords a glimpse of harem-life, in which it is now impossible to distinguish between that which was reported and that which was done. It was alleged that Hosanee Khanum, wife of Dewan Kefaitoollah, of Hooghly, having had a disagreement with one of her maid-servants, ordered her to be thrown into a *deg*, or cauldron, of boiling water, but the vessel tilting over by the weight of the woman, defeated the cruel purpose. She was soon seized and brought back; the mistress then taking a knife cut her throat, so as to cause immediate death. The body of the victim was then secretly removed and buried in the course of the night. Case sent to the Nizamut Adawlut. From *Bhaskur,—India Mail*, 1840. The evidence before the Court was very conflicting. It was stated that, the unfortunate woman, having been detected in stealing and pawning a nose-ring belonging to one of the servants of the house, was repeatedly beaten on Sunday, Monday, and Tuesday with a brick, and the stalk of the leaf of a palm tree, on and about the joints; and, on Tuesday evening, she was beaten, and a stick . . when she told them to do as they pleased, as they would not have an opportunity of doing so the next day. She cut her throat, but did not die. The Khanum consulted what should be done, and four persons were ordered to kill her by stamping on and pressing down her chest, belly, and throat. The evidence of the Assistant Surgeon showed that she must have been beaten for a length of time, and with the endeavor to leave no trace. A woman confessed that she and three others, one of whom was a boy twelve years old, had killed deceased by standing upon her, and that she herself stood upon her belly. Delawur, the boy, confessed that he assisted in killing her by standing on her belly.

The superior Court acquitted the Khanum of murder, but convicted her of causing or countenancing the ill-treatment, and sentenced her to a fine of rupees 1,000, or a year's imprisonment.

The following report appeared in the Calcutta Papers in September

* Nizamut Adawlut Reports, March 2, 1855, p. 315.

1869 :—" A most atrocious case of police torture in Upper Scinde is noticed by the *Sindian.* A person accused of murder was seized by the police; and by the sanction or connivance of a magistrate" [this statement is absolutely incredible], " a confession was extorted from him by resorting to violence of a nature quite equal in atrocity to the torture inflicted on persons in the days of the Spanish Inquisition. The unfortunate victim's legs were muffled with cloth, and, oil having been applied thereto copiously, the police set fire to it. The sufferings of the man may be more easily imagined than described ; and, although he, for some time, held out, the torture had at last its proper effect. The man confessed, or at least made a statement criminating himself, and it was then that the police relaxed their severity ; and struck, not by remorse, but fear, had him carried to the nearest medical officer procurable there, by whose advice the man's leg was amputated, in order to save his life."

In 1846, a wealthy merchant of Arrah, suspecting some of his female servants of theft, *put them to the ordeal of dipping their hands into a vessel of boiling water.**

The same brutality appears to be commonly practised in Madras.

The Judge of Mangalore mentions that, in a case which came judicially before him, a Brahmin woman had burned with hot oil the thigh of another woman whom she suspected of theft.†

The Civil Surgeon of Chingleput received into the jail, in May 1854, a female suffering from two " severe burns, one on the inside of each of her thighs, high up, close to her private parts."‡

The Civil Surgeon of Coimbatore mentions a case, in which a sheristadar, to extort confession, enveloped the limbs of a person in cotton soaked in oil which he set fire to. Death ensued.§

The Collector and Magistrate of Tanjore reports that a man of that district, having lost some small article from his house, " proceeded, as a matter of ordinary routine, to dip the hands of his three wives in boiling cow-dung, to induce them to confess if they had taken it."‖

Pouring hot oil into the ears and nose (tel dhala) is a mode of torture well known in Bengal.¶

The house of a relative of the Julpigoree Raja having been robbed, some of his burkundazes beat or otherwise tortured certain neighbouring

---

* Mr. Dampier's Report, 1846, p. 2.

† Appendix C., No. 12, p. cxxii.

‡ *Ibid,* No. 10, p. cxiii.

§ Appendix C., p. clxxxv.

‖ Appendix C., No. 16, p. clxix.

¶ " Should one, through pride, give instruction to priests concerning their duty, let the king order some hot oil to be dropped into his mouth and ear."—*Menu,* c. v. 272. " If a Sooder listens to the Vedas of the Shaster, then the oil, heated as before, shall be poured into his ears ; and arzeez and wax shall be melted together, and the orifice of the ears shall be stopped up therewith.—*Halhed's Code of Gentoo Laws.*

ryots, till each named another as the robber. One Palanoo was at last seized, and taken to a house and beaten, and a bamboo laid on his belly, as he was extended on the ground, on the ends of which two men stood, from which he became nearly senseless; and then hot oil was sprinkled over his body, and finally poured down, or attempted to be poured down, his throat, and he died. A party in this crime was found guilty of aggravated culpable homicide.*

Torture is also said to be inflicted by *compelling the victim to sit on an iron vessel containing heated sand or oil.* This is termed *tela bhajá*—frying in oil.

Fastening the body to the limb of a tree under which a fire has been kindled, for the purpose of suffocating with the smoke.†

Ordeal by Heat.

"On great occasions let the king cause the party (accused) to hold fire, or to dive under water, &c."

"He whom the blazing fire burns not, whom the water soon forces not up, or who meets with no speedy misfortune, must be held veracious in his testimony on oath."—Menu, c. v., 144 and 115.

In investigating obscure cases of injury by fire in India, it is needful to bear in mind that the Ordeal System is by no means extinct. Of the nine different modes of conducting the ordeal, here, one was by red-hot iron, and another by boiling oil. A full account of these modes of ordeal, as formerly practised in judicial cases, in some measure under the sanction of Government in the Bombay Presidency, will be found in Forbes's Oriental Memoirs, Vol. I., p. 201; and II., p. 25. As lately as 1869, the Government of Madras had to repeat an order prohibiting the *ghee-* (clarified butter) *test*, or *ordeal*, practised in cases of adultery by Brahmins on the Malabar Coast. The Brahmins' memorial states that the "ghee-test" is not compulsory, and that "it is of greater holiness, is certainly no more a torture, and is decidedly less long in healing than the *Vishnoo brand;*" it being "at the worst, a slight burn." Ward mentions that, at Krishnaghur, in 1807, there was a *tapta mukti*, or ordeal by hot clarified butter, tried before 7,000 spectators on a young woman accused by her husband of adultery.

A comparison will show that the plan of the ordeals by fire, as practised by the Hindus and by the English in the reign of Edward the Confessor, was almost identical. Everything was done by the priests, and no one now doubts that, whenever the criminal escaped, they arranged that he should do so. The Brahmins wisely preferred the Balance Ordeal in their own cases, the Saxon priests did not shrink from the fire ordeal; but Gilchrist remarks that "we meet with no example of any champion of the Romish Church who suffered the least injury from

* Nizamut Adawlut Reports, Jan 17, 1856, p. 118.

† Appendix C., p. civ.

the touch of hot iron in that ordeal. But, when any one was so foolhardy as to appeal to it or to that of hot water, with a view to deprive the Church of any of her possessions, *he never failed to burn his fingers* and lose his cause."* George Logothete speaks of a man who, in the thirteenth century, refused to submit to the proof by fire, saying that *he was not a mountebank.* The archbishop pressing him, he declared that he was willing to receive the red-hot iron, provided it was from the prelate's own hand. The latter, too prudent to accept the condition, acknowledged that it was wrong to tempt God. Unquestionably, these ordeals were mere jugglery.† We have several hints of the modes by which the "fire-eaters," whose performances used to be so attractive at our English fairs, contrived to avoid being burnt. Doubtless, tact and dexterity went very far. We know that blacksmiths, glass-makers, plumbers, and practical chemists manipulate hot bodies much more easily than one who has never learnt the act of snuffing a candle with his fingers can. The cuticle is capable of being artificially hardened. We are told, in the *Journal des Scavans* for 1680, that Richardson, a famous mountebank in the reign of Charles II., rubbed his hands and other parts which were to be exposed to the fire with pure spirit of sulphur, "the epidermis being thereby burned and cauterized, the skin, consequently, became hardened and capable of resisting the flame." The great surgeon Ambrose Paré assures us that, after washing the hands in urine and *unguentum aureum*, any one may safely dip them into melted lead; and that, by washing his hands in the juice of onions, he could bear a hot shovel on them, while it melted lead! Camphor and alum were also in high repute. It is said that a *wet* finger may be safely dipped into a pan of boiling sugar, and that hard soap or a soap paste, rubbed over the tongue, will preserve it from being burnt by a hot iron rapidly passed over it.

I think that, in some cases of torture by heat in this country, especially in questions of theft and adultery, an ordeal may have been intended. I only allude to this as affecting the question of malicious intent.

Torture by Cold.

In Bengal, *Exposure to the Inclemency of the Night Air (Nangto karo phala raka) and Sprinkling the Body with Water in Cold Weather (Jhara dhya)* are practices long since employed by the Mussalmauns, inveighed against by Burke, and well known in the present day.

Torture by Cold, understood in Bengal by the expression *Thanda kuro!* (cool him!),—*vide supra*, p. 79. The ancient Hindu law enjoined that "If a pupil commits a fault in the cold season, his master may throw water upon his body."—(Halhed, p. 235.)‡

* History of Ordeals, p. 24.

† Todd says that it was well known in Kotah that those who professed witchcraft "had substances which enabled them to handle balls of hot iron with impunity."—Vol. II., p. 587.

‡ A favorite atrocity of Biren, Duke of Courland, in 1740, was freezing people to death.

Tying the hands behind the back, and hoisting the body up by a rope fastened to the wrists.

The order for this punishment is *lut koy*—make him swing.

This practice is alluded to by Hamilton, who mentions that, in 1709, a native who had incurred the vengeance of the Nawab of Chickacul, "was set in the hot scorching sun three days, with his hands fastened to a stake over his head, and one of his legs tied up till his heel touched his buttock."

A tehseeldar and two chupprassees were convicted, at Saharunpore, of torturing, beating, and starving ten men, with a view, apparently, of obtaining information regarding a robbery. The mode of torture practised was suspension by the arms, which were tied behind the backs of the sufferers to a tree; this cruelty was proved to have been repeated, at intervals, during many days; the Civil Surgeon deposed that one of the persons thus treated died. He, like eight of the nine sufferers, showed marks of ligatures having been bound tightly round his arms; but, in addition, there were marks of burning on the body, the greater part of which was covered with large blisters. This was admitted by the man's companions to have been caused by hot applications and fomentations injudiciously employed, for the purpose of restoring the use of his limbs. Several of the people had temporarily lost the use of one or both of the arms.*

Suspension by the arms or hands is, however, generally accompanied by severe beating, as in the case of a man at Barrackpore who, being suspected of theft, was detained by the police, who tied his arms behind his back by a cloth, to which a rope was attached, by which he was suspended to a bamboo rafter, and then beaten. He was thus left hanging until released by a traveller, on whose approach the police fled. The darogah and several of the police were sentenced to two years' imprisonment.†

In December 1854, three men of Bijnore were sentenced to seven years' imprisonment in irons, for having killed a person whom they charged with stealing a *hooquah*. They tied his arms behind his back, and suspended him from the end of a pole supporting the thatch of a hut, and then beat him with lattees and their fists. He died, in consequence of their ill-usage, a few days afterwards.‡

In the same month, a man of Bareilly was found guilty of having killed a boy whom he employed in his mangoe plantation, by beating him with a lattee after having suspended him to a tree by a rope tied to his hands.§

---

* Decisions of the Nizamut Adawlut, N. W. P., 21st January 1854, p, 54. See instances of the infliction of the same kind of suspension in Madras. Appendix E., p. liii.

† Nizamut Adawlut Reports, 23rd January 1855, p. 103.

‡ Nizamut Adawlut Reports, N. W. P., 1st December 1854, p. 787.

§ *Ibid*, p. 873.

One day in August 1860, the Magistrate of Burdwan, when visiting the female ward of his jail, perceived that the arm of one of the prisoners had been hurt. This led to enquiry, when it appeared that the naib darogah and police of Selimabad thannah had apprehended an old man, aged between 60 and 70, and his wife, aged upwards of 50, upon a charge of receiving and concealing stolen property. They tied the man's hands behind his back and suspended him (it would appear, but is not certain, by them) to the branch of a mangoe tree, with his feet about a cubit and-a-half from the ground, and began to swing him. When he had hung upwards of half an hour, he became senseless. Thinking that he was going to die, they let him down. They hung the woman up by the arms to the roof-pole of the house. The naib beat her with a small stick, and one of the burkundazes beat her with a lattee. She was also beaten with stinging nettles.

One of the witnesses, a child, described the sound "*shup, shup*," which well expresses the noise of striking with wet nettles. She was thus struck on her body and private parts. The burkundaze struck her, while she was hanging, on her right shoulder. Her collar-bone or clavicle broke (this was confirmed by the Civil Surgeon's evidence); she also was beaten until she was senseless.*

This mode of suspension and beating is also commonly employed in Madras. Several instances will be found in the Report.†

In Rutnaghery, Bombay, we hear of hanging a man to a hook, and then whipping him on the bare back; and, when the stripes become visible, sprinkling salt water over it and repeating the operation over and over again.‡

Suspending by the Feet (*Páye rashi diya jhulàna*).

In January last, three men were sentenced at Jounpore for having suspended a man (who appears to have been stealing plantains) to a tree, with his head downwards, and having beaten his feet until the "lower parts of the limbs were literally *pounded* into a confused mass." Death resulted in a few hours.§

It appeared, in a trial at Baitool in 1852, that dacoits had tied a man head and feet to a charpoy which was then placed on end, so that he hung with his head downward.‖

In 1853, certain persons were tried at Mymensing, for suspending a suspected thief by the feet to a beam, and beating him to death.¶

---

* Reports of two trials of torture by the police, held at Burdwan, August, September 1860, by C. F. Bukland, Sessions Judge.

† Report, p. 50. Appendix E., p. xliv, &c.

‡ "Two countrymen were bound together with cords, and hanged up by their thumbs to a tree, there to hang all night."—*Wodrow's Church of Scotland.*

§ Nizamut Adawlut Reports, 24th January 1855, p. 100.

‖ Nizamut Adawlut Reports, N. W. P., 27th August 1852, p. 910.

¶ In Hindu fable, one of the candidates for absorption into Brumhu is represented as hanging, for centuries, with his head downwards.

Suspending by the feet to the bough of tree is mentioned as a torture practised in Bellary.*

Suspending by the Hair.

A Thannadar of Ahmenabad was dismissed for having suspended a prisoner by the hair of his head to a beam, and having ordered him to be beaten, while in that position, with fists and with a kora.†

Just before the Madras Report appeared, a wretch swung a young girl to the beam of his house by her hands and hair, and cruelly beat and burnt her while in that position.‡ *See* the Tanjore case, p. 537.

Lifting by the Moustache

Is mentioned among the tortures in vogue in police cases in Madras,§ also *Lifting by the Ears.*‖

Torture of Witches.

As *suspension* from a tree is an almost invariable feature in the barbarous process, a few notes on this revolting practice may be given here.

The following report appears in Allen's Asiatic Journal for June 1839, p. 91 :—"Teejeeah, an elderly female, residing in a village within the Behar district, was considered by her neighbours to be a sorceress. In consequence of this imputation, she was one day seized by two of the villagers, Narain Roy, and his son, Gunesh Roy, who stripped her, and tied her to a tree; and after beating her unmercifully, with an intention to compel her to confess herself to be a witch, they made her undergo several ordeals, one of which was to put pounded chillies into her eyes, to see whether their smarting would draw tears from her. After this, they suspended her, in a state of nudity, to a tree, and there left her to perish. From this suspension she was released by the humanity of a passer by, who gave information of her condition to her son-in-law. After her release, being ashamed of the exposure she had undergone, and being aware that, if she survived the disgrace, she would be ejected from her caste, combined with the bodily suffering, she, in despair, drowned herself in a tank, where her corpse was discovered floating the following day, and was identified by her son-in-law, who gave intimation of these atrocities to the thanadar of his village, and had the perpetrators of them arrested together with their accomplices."

The following description of the tortures inflicted upon women suspected of witchcraft among the Bheels is from an article published in the East India Army Magazine for October 1854 :—"The sentence of the Bhoopa (witch-finder) having gone forth, twenty or thirty men, the foremost carrying a few grains of the sacred 'ooreed' (a small grain used in divination for the discovery of witches) as a charm against further evil,

---

* Appendix C., p. civ.

† Nizamut Adawlut Reports, N. W. P., 1st March 1855, p. 281.

‡ Appendix C., p. clxix.

§ Report, p. 50.

‖ Appendix C., p. clxv.

approach courteously the unfortunate woman's dwelling. She is seized, if possible before her curse or evil eye can fall on any one present, and over her dim eyes is bound a cloth, containing finely-pounded chillies. Tied hands and feet, she is carried to a neighbouring tree, where a crowd are assembled, to eat and drink at the sick man's or his relative's expense, and to witness or assist in the disgusting ceremony. Two strong ropes, fifteen or twenty feet long, are tied to the woman's ankles, and two others are fastened round her waist: she is then hoisted up to a branch of the tree, and, amidst the yells of the assembly, the ordeal commences. From early morn to sunset, her head hanging downwards, she is swung to and fro with great violence; and, should she that day not confess to having bewitched the sick man, the same brutal work commences next morning, and is continued for three, four or even five days. Generally, however, long before the first day has passed, the burning of the eyes, the cutting of her feet, or the agonies caused by determination of blood to the head, force her to confess that she has coveted a piece of land belonging to the patient, or that she has received some injury or insult at his hands, and that, to procure the one, or revenge the other, she is eating away his heart. She must then request that a particular goat be brought, in the throat of which a vein is opened, and frequently while she is still bandaged and swinging, she drinks every drop of blood which comes from the struggling animal. This is a substitute for the sick man's life, and, the witch's craving for blood being satisfied, a friend now proceeds to ascertain whether the sick man be better. If he reports favorably, the woman is generally released from her tortures, and brought to the patient's room. With a bunch of *neem* leaves she continues for some time making passes over the invalid, particularly his head; a lock of hair is also cut from the crown of the witch's head and buried in the ground, that the last link between her and her former powers may be broken. Her influence is also destroyed by counter-charms of the Bhoopa, and she may be received by her family; but, more frequently, she becomes an outcast, and dies as painful a death as that which she has just escaped. This is not the wildest ordeal through which the Bheel witch can pass. Should, unfortunately, her senses forsake her, the ravings of madness and groanings of pain are considered true evidences of her guilt. Her inability to make the usual confessions is attributed to the secret influence of the devil or her own obstinacy; the angry and intoxicated crowd become greedy for revenge; the senseless body is soon cut to pieces, or a fire is hastily kindled under her head, and the innocent woman is burnt alive."

Todd mentions that Salim Sing, the celebrated Regent of Kotah, was a great persecutor of witches. Throwing them into a pond of water was one of their trials: if they sank, they were innocent; if they unhappily rose to the surface, the league with the powers of darkness was apparent. A grain bag of cayenne pepper tied over the head, if it failed to suffocate, afforded another proof of guilt; though the more humane method of rubbing the eyes with a well-dried capsicum was perhaps the most common, and certainly if they could furnish this demonstration of their innocence, by withholding tears, they might justly be deemed witches. He adds that these *dhakuns,* like the vampires of the German *bardais,* are supposed to operate upon the viscera of their victims, which they destroy by slow degrees with charms and incantations, and hence they are called, in Scinde (where, as Abul Fazil says, they abound), *Jigger-Khor,* or liver-devourers. One look of a *dhakun* suffices to destroy.

The following detail appeared in Cornhill Magazine.* "The women naturally deny the charge [of witchcraft &c.,] vehemently. They are forthwith disrobed and hung, very often head downwards, on to a horizontal bamboo, placed some ten or twelve feet from the ground, on two perpendicular ones planted firmly in the earth. They are then swung slowly, backwards and forwards, while their neighbours, armed with castor-oil rods, stand in rows on either side, and give each a blow as she swings past; and the castor-oil rod is, in willing hands, capable of inflicting very severe punishment. When the victims are half dead from the beating and from suffocation, they are taken down and dragged off to some neighbouring hovel while further tortures are being prepared." . . . . "Fires are lighted and pieces of old iron put in to be heated, and, when all is ready, the unfortunate witches are again brought out, and are oftentimes very cruelly and brutally burnt on their necks and heads with the red-hot irons. Another mode of torture is to cover the face and neck with cotton wool and then set fire to it, or to heat a brass candlestick to a white heat, and compel the accused to carry it about" [?] "until the hand is nearly burnt off. Another plan is to hang the witch from the bamboo above mentioned by the arms, to attach heavy weights to the feet, and to dash them about until the joints are ready to give way. The wretched creatures are kept all this time without food, water and sleep, and are beaten during the intervals of other punishments with the all powerful castor-oil rods. In their agony, the victims very often declare that they really have a compact with a demon, and disclose horrible particulars as to the banquets they share with him; at last it happens that one or perhaps both of the women die under the cruel treatment they have received, and then the assembly is struck with a guilty fear."

Introducing Red Pepper (Lall Mertch) into the Nostrils (naké langkár jhál deon) or Eyes. Burning Lunka Mertch under the Nose (Lunka Mertch dho dya). Covering the Head with a bag. which has contained Red Pepper (Langkâr thaliyate mukha poro) Rubbing Chillies on the Breasts of Females. Introduction of Red Pepper into the Vagina, (Asthana sthane langka deon) or *Urethra.*

These barbarities are very frequently practised, both in this and in the

* P. 414.

Madras Presidency. In June 1853, a man and his mother were sentenced, at Dinagepore, to long terms of imprisonment, for having introduced chillies and ginger into the vagina of the wife of the former, and for burning her with a red-hot *chillum* and *charagdhan* (an earthenware pipe, and a brass stand, about a cubit in length, with a round top, for placing a lamp upon). The Civil Assistant Surgeon stated that the woman had received very severe burns on the thighs and pudenda, causing extensive sloughing and great constitutional disturbance, so much so, as to endanger life; chillies had also been introduced into the vagina, causing severe inflammation and consequent sloughing. The chillies came away after her admission into hospital.

Shortly after the publication of my last edition, the late Mr. Biddle, of Raneegunge, mentioned, in the Calcutta *Englishman*, the case of a poor woman who, *four days after her delivery of twins*, was tortured by the introduction of red-pepper, chillies, and *Maun Kutchu,—Colocasia Indica (Roxb.)*

The late Mr. W. F. Daniel mentioned that, in certain tribes among the Western Africans, whenever a girl shows any very strong indication of sexual feeling before she is betrothed, they at once proceed to produce an obliteration of the vagina by the intense action set up by the forcible introduction of a mass of the *Capsicum frutescens*, or bird pepper.

Throwing dust in the Eyes.—In a highway robbery case, at Dinagepore, the prosecutor, a Brahmin, stated that two men carried him away to a solitary place "flinging dust into his eyes."*

Confinement in a Cell containing Quicklime (*Chuna*)

Is mentioned by Baboo Greesh Chunder Ghose. In a case tried at Backergunge, in 1847, it was alleged that lime had been put into the eyes of a man who was supposed to have met with his death by unfair means. Decomposition had advanced too far to enable Mr. Scanlan to give an opinion upon this point.

When I made an inspection of the jail at Backergunge, in February 1866, I examined a youngish and remarkably strong-loooking native who, having been imprisoned for a long time, put out his eyes with quicklime, doubtless in hope of being released. The corneæ were quite destroyed.

About two years ago, the Reverend James Long told me that, lately, a few miles south of Calcutta, a zemindar had confined one of his ryots in a cell half filled with quicklime.

Blinding with Bhela (Semecarpus Anacardium) *and Chuna.*

Quicklime not being sufficiently corrosive, criminal ingenuity has learnt to quicken its action by mixing with it the intensely acrid juice of the *Marking Nut, vide supra*, p. 286.

---

* Nizamut Adawlut Reports, June 22, 1855, p. 771.

Four Mussalmauns were convicted, at Rungpore, of having, upon a land dispute, beaten Fayradoo in various ways, especially on the arms, with short sticks. One of the assailants told another "to bring *bhela* (a kind of nut, whose juice the washermen use for marking clothes) and lime, and they would settle the rascal." Four men held him down, while two, having beaten the bhela, "dropped the juice into his eyes and, afterwards, put sand and lime into them." They beat him again till they thought he was dead, tied his legs and arms together, slung him to a bamboo, and carried him off to a dry tank where they threw him down after having felt his nostrils to see if he was still breathing, and, on finding that he was, they beat him on the nose. They then went away, saying that he would be eaten by dogs, jackals, or tigers by morning.

The Civil Surgeon "found the man's eyes violently inflamed, threatening entire loss of vision, and the expected result has occurred, the organization of both eyes been completely destroyed."*

The Judge of Mangalore met with a case in which a poor man was totally blinded by having an acrid juice put into his eyes; in another instance, a person who found a boy stealing his cashew nuts, rubbed the acrid juice of that tree into the boy's eyes.†—*See page* 529.

A clergyman informed the Collector and Magistrate of Tanjore that, having missed a cheque from his table, he made inquiry among his servants regarding it. In order to ascertain whether it had been taken by the only child on the establishment, his eyes were filled with red chillies by the other servants, in order to force a confession from him.‡ *See* Chapter on Blinding, p. 483.

The Civil Judge of Salem also mentions, among the general kinds of torture practised by the police in that district, *putting Pepper or Chillies into the Eyes, or into the Urethra or Anus.*§

We read in Mr. Eastwick's "Autobiography of Lutfullah" that the following was one of the tortures practised by the Pindaree plunderers in Malwah: "A horse's grain bag, half filled with ashes and red-pepper in powder, was tied over the sufferer's face, so as to include his mouth and

---

* Nizamut Adawlut Reports, May 18, 1855, p. 586; also November 28, 1856, p. 988, where three others were condemned for the maltreatment of Fayradoo.

The following appeared in the Calcutta Papers in June 1869:—

"A Mussalmaun butcher, in the Dhurrumtollah Bazar, was fined Rs. 20 by Mr. J. B. Roberts, yesterday, for cruelty of a more than usually barbarous character to animals. It appeared that the man had bought a bullock yesterday for the purpose of slaughtering, and after keeping it all the morning in the bazar, the wretched animal, when being taken away in the afternoon, dropped down from heat and exhaustion. Finding other and gentler means of persuasion unavailing, the inhuman brute had recourse to ground chillies, which he rubbed into the eyes of the suffering animal to stimulate it to further exertions. The man's ingenuity in the way of torture was, however, justly punished by the Magistrate."

† Appendix C., No. 10, Canara, p. cxiii.

‡ Appendix C., No. 16, p. cxiii.

§ Appendix C., No. 14, p. cxlv.

nose, the consequence of which was, at first, a most violent fit of sneezing, and if protracted to a quarter of an hour, a horrible death by suffocation."

Tying a horse's nose-bag filled with hot ashes over the head, and violently thumping the back till the victim is forced to inhale the dust, and afterwards denying water, is a (Bombay) practice, of which I have notes from two authorities.

I am informed that *introducing the Arum Colocasia* (*Kachoordata*) *into the ears* (*Kana Kachoordata Daya*) and also *Dhatoora* (*Kana Dhatoora daya*) are modes of torture practised in Bengal.

Tying Bichootee upon the limbs and body appears to be a very common practice in Bengal, to which allusion has already been made. I also hear of "*Besprinkling the Body with Alkoosh water*" (*Alkoosh juldya*). The Alkoosh being described as "a creeper, like Bichootee."

When at Howrah, I examined a man, under whose chin there were a great number of extremely fine, but distinct, cuts or scratches, which had barely entered the cutis. These were said to have been produced by fastening on his neck *a Pounded or Split Bamboo.* This appears to be a well-known mode of torture.

The following appears in the Calcutta *Englishman* for July 29th, 1870 :—

"The *Bangalore Spectator* reports that the Moonsiff of Sholingur and the head Moonshee of the Sub-Collectorate of Arcot have been sent handcuffed to Chittoor for trial, on a charge of torturing a lad whom they suspected of having stolen a gold bracelet from a child. The boy was, according to his own account, cruelly beaten on several occasions, prickly pear thorns were put into his clothes, and he was frequently dipped in wells to extort a confession of his guilt. The accused had offered a large sum to the police to hush up the matter, and consequently the Collector refused to take bail."

We are told that "some part of the boy's body was swollen very much, caused, as he relates, by the introduction of a large prickly pear thorn under the clothes, and dipping him in wells, causing the parts to swell and fester."

In a subsequent issue it has been reported that the defendants have been sentenced by the Sessions Judge of Chittoor to four years' rigorous imprisonment, with a fine of rupees 500 each.

Placing on a Bed of Thorns.—Forbes relates a case of cruelty and extortion which occurred, by order of Scindia, at Tatta. It being determined to make the collector of customs (a Hindu) give up his concealed treasure, a variety of tortures were inflicted upon him. One was a sofa with a platform of light cordage in net-work, covered with a chintz palampore, which concealed a bed of thorns placed under it. The victim, a corpulent Banian, was then stripped of his muslin jama, and ordered to lie down on the couch; the cords bending with his weight, sunk on the bed of thorns; those long and piercing thorns of the *baubul*, or forest *acacia*, which, being placed purposely with their points upwards, lacerated the wretched man, whether in motion or at rest. For two days and nights he bore the torture without revealing the secret. His tormentors, fearing he would die before their purpose was effected, had recourse to another mode of compulsion. When nature was nearly exhausted, they took him from the bed and supported him on the floor, until his infant son, an only child, was brought into the room; and, with him a bag containing a fierce cat, into which they put the child and tied up the mouth of the sack. The agents of cruelty stood over them with bamboos, ready at a signal to beat the bag, and enrage the animal to destroy the child, *vide supra*, pp. 527 *note*, and 530. He produced his treasure, and, on his recovery, he was sent for to Court, invested with a sirpaw, or rope of state, and exalted to a high situation in another province; there to accumulate more wealth, and, at a future period, be again subject to the capricious fiat of a needy despot.*

Introduction of a Ruler, Stick, or other foreign body into the Vagina (Rúle puriya deon, and Lati puriya deon.—Rúldhaya).

It would appear that this mode of torture is not unfrequently inflicted. My opinion was called for in two alleged cases of the kind, at Howrah, during twelve months. In one of these it was alleged that an office ruler was the instrument employed. The woman (a widow) stated that the violence had occasioned severe hæmorrhage and pain: she was certainly anemiated and, for two or three days, there appeared to be great tenderness above the pubes. In the other case, it was asserted that a bamboo stick had been employed. Both women were menstruating at the time, (a very suspicious circumstance). No bruise or laceration could be detected in either case. Very guarded opinions were therefore given.

A wretched woman at Hooghly, when under trial for murdering a child for the sake of her ornaments, alleged that her confession had been extorted by the police, who tortured her by fire and by passing a ruler up the vagina. This was not proved, and she was convicted.†

Mr. Simmons, apothecary at Gowalparah, reported, in 1841, upon the case of a Hindu woman, said to have been ill-treated by her husband, in which he found sloughing of the vagina, extending to the nympha and groin on one side, and to the urethra. The bladder had also become considerably diseased. He was of opinion that these effects had been caused by the thrusting of some sharp instrument into the upper part of the vulva.

One Calachand Darra, of Jessore (married to a young girl who was very unwilling to remain with him), upon his wife's refusing to

---

* Op. Cit., Vol. II., p. 54.

† Nizamut Adawlut Reports, Mar. 13, 1857, p. 304.

sleep with him, strangled her; and afterwards suspended the body by a cord to a tamarind tree, attempting to make it appear that she had destroyed herself. Witnesses who first saw the body observed that the genitals were swollen, marks of injury to the pudenda were also evident when the darogah held the inquest. The native doctor who viewed the body said that there was the appearance of a stick having been forced into the private parts, but he could not examine minutely, as the body was decomposed.*

One Hurree Ram and a relation of his were condemned to death, at Bareilly, in 1852, for the murder of the wife of the former. It appears probable that the unfortunate woman had given her husband cause for jealousy. Cries were heard in the night, when a neighbour, rushing in, found the man transfixing his wife's neck with a spear, while his relation held her head. It was found, upon examining the body, that she had been also stabbed in the pudenda.†

Dwarkanath Mundul, of Chota Nagpore, was sentenced to transportation for life for the murder of his child-wife, only about twelve years old, by striking her on the head with a "*Sumut*" (cudgel or pestle about two cubits long and weighing three seers), and by thrusting the instrument into her private parts. Of this there were four eye-witnesses. The Sub-Assistant Surgeon testified that death was caused by concussion of the brain and by the injury to the private parts.‡

Introduction of similar bodies into the Rectum.

This mode of torture is, undoubtedly, common, and has not unfrequently occasioned death. The following cases will be sufficient in illustration, although others might be cited.

A prisoner, convicted of having beaten a boy and of having thrust a stick besmeared with chillies up his anus, thereby occasioning his death, was sentenced to imprisonment for life in the Alipore Jail.§

In 1842, Dr. T. W. Wilson, then of Mymensing, found on the body of a Mussalmaun woman distinct marks of strangulation and wounds (their character was not described), in the lower bowel, which he considered to be of necessity mortal. An old woman was tried for this crime.

Dr. Dickson, of Behar, examined the body of a Hindu man, into whose rectum it was evident that some blunt body, such as a lattee or bamboo, had been forced, producing great injury to the intestine and effusion of blood into the abdominal cavity.

Dr. Kenneth Mackinnon found the bladder punctured in this manner.

Rather frequent allusion is made to this violence, in cases where other

* Nizamut Adawlut Reports, 31st July 1854, p. 158.
† Nizamut Adawlut Reports, N. W. P., 5th April 1852, p. 268.
‡ Nizamut Adawlut Reports, May 8, 1857, p. 650.
§ *Ibid*, Vol. III., p. 97.

severe injuries have been inflicted. Dr. Denham, of Gyah, examined the body of a Hindu man, in which he found contusion about the face, and fracture of all the ribs on the right, and of four on the left side. There was also great laceration at the verge of the anus, and the cavity of the abdomen contained a very large quantity of extravasated blood.

In 1848, four natives of Purneah were sentenced to seven years' imprisonment for killing a thief, whom they had captured, by forcing a stick into his fundament.*

In the following year some persons of Bograh, suspecting a man of theft, went to his house at night under pretence of smoking with him. After sitting some time, they suddenly seized him, beat him severely, and employed a bamboo in this manner so violently as to cause his death.†

Again, in 1851, a mahajun, of Maldah, having gone to collect advances, his debtor was reported to be from home ; but he was invited to remain and smoke, when two of his debtors appeared, beat, kicked, and knocked him down, a third then placed his feet upon him, and a fourth, with whom he had a suit in the civil court, thrust a split bamboo several times into his person. He died the next day.‡

A most striking case of this kind was reported by Dr. T. W. Wilson, then of Rajshahye, in 1841. In examining the body of a Hindu man, who had died under suspicious circumstances, Dr. Wilson found some outward marks of bruises on the lower part of the chest and upper part of the abdomen. There was extensive peritonitis. This had been occasioned by the presence of the wooden pipe of a native hookah, lying on the right side of the abdominal cavity. About three inches of the lower end of this pipe remained lodged in the rectum, through the coats of which its upper extremity had passed ; the pipe thus introduced was about twelve inches long.

Three Mussalmauns of Allahabad, suspecting a woman of being implicated in a theft, sent for her, on the pretext that she was required at the house of one of them to undergo the ordeal of chewing rice.

---

* Police Report, L. P., 1848, p. 19.

† *Ibid*, 1849, p. 31.

‡ Police Reports, L. P., 1851, p. 24.

See a remarkable instance in which a Moorshedabad man,—who had died under ill usage apparently accompanied with violence of this kind, and whose body proved to have been suspended by his assailants after death,—was found to be the subject of strangulated hernia. The medical evidence appears to have been imperfectly reported. The Civil Surgeon deposed that the body exhibited no external marks of violence ; but, internally, there was a great deal of inflammation in the cavity of the abdomen and scrotum, and in the scrotum there was a great quantity of the small intestines and some dark fluid like blood in color. That the deceased must, at that time, have been afflicted with strangulated hernia, and that the violence received was either directed to the seat of the disease itself, or caused a sudden shock to the system, terminating fatally at once. The printed report, however, which deserves perusal, scarcely admits of a satisfactory explanation of the man's death.—*Nizamut Adawlut Reports*, 20th October 1853, p. 684.

On her asserting her innocence, she was removed to a closet and beaten. Then one of the wretches got on her chest and held her down—another (a lad of *fourteen !)* held her feet, while the third forced a stick into her fundament. Seeing that blood flowed, they brought water and began to wash the marks off the clothes—the boy pounded huldee, which they applied to the wounded parts. They then pounded charcoal which they were going to apply in order to stop the bleeding. She begged them not to do so, when they let her go ; and she went at once to the thannah which was close by. This statement was considered by the Sessions Judge to be fully corroborated by circumstantial evidence. The Civil Surgeon, who examined the woman on the day after the assault, stated that there were severe marks of blows on the back, and that the skin of the fundament was abraded, as if by the introduction of some sharp pointed instrument ; that these injuries could not have been the act of a single individual, but that no permanent injury had resulted or was likely to result.*

At Mymensing, in 1866, one Alleah being engaged in an intrigue with the sister of Lochun was caught by him in the house. Lochun, with the aid of six others, beat him cruelly, and then inserted an iron rod into his body. The unfortunate man died in hospital shortly afterwards.†

Sheikh Pagoreeah, also of Mymensing, was sentenced to death for murdering his wife. He was jealous of the poor woman, and, seeing some pice in her hand, he asked her whence she had got them; she evaded the question, and he tied her hands and feet up, and also put a cord round her neck to prevent her from calling out. He thrust some pice up her body with a *punjun,* or stick used for driving cattle; and, when he found that the deceased was in her last moments, he tightened the chord round her neck and suspended her to a beam of the house, and gave out that she had committed suicide. The Civil Surgeon attributed death to strangulation by a cord, the impression of which remained on the neck. There were several contusions on the body, and there were found ten pice wrapped up in a piece of plantain-leaf and lodged in the rectum near the orifice of the anus.‡

It is an extraordinary fact, showing how thoroughly conversant the people of Bengal are with this brutal mode of punishment, that, in *two* instances within the ten years preceding the publication of the first edition of this book, *young children* were tried for having caused the death of one of their companions in this manner ! One example will suffice. It occurred at Rungpore. "The deceased and the prisoners were children of eight or nine years old. The two latter quarrelled

* Nizamut Adawlut Reports, N. W. P., 22nd November 1853, p. 1412.

† Bengal Police Reports, 1866, p. 265.

‡ Nizamut Adawlut Reports, 4th August, 1867, p. 148.

with another, whom they abused; the deceased interfered, when they seized him, and, throwing him down, forced a small stick into his rectum, from the effects of which he died the following morning.*

General Ramsay informed me that he sent a fresh corpse to Dr. ———, then lately arrived in India. He found him examining the upper parts of the body, quite at a loss to imagine what was the cause of death. It was only on directing his attention to the rectum that he found that a stick which had been introduced into the rectum had been forced through that intestine.

"A most revolting murder took place in the city of Ellishpore (Bombay Presidency). Two little boys of eight or ten years of age, a Mussalmaun and a Hindu, were playing together, when an altercation took place, and the Hindu struck the Mussalmaun upon the head, and slightly cut him. This was seen by his mother, who instantly seized the Hindu boy, dragged him into a secluded garden, where she first tore out the child's eyes with a large needle and then, assisted by her husband, terminated the existence of her unfortunate victim by thrusting an iron spike up its body. The murderers have been tried, convicted, and sentenced to death."—*Allen's Asiatic Journal*, 1839.

The manner in which the king was put to death was so Oriental in its character and so unexampled in the annals of English crime that I have long thought it probable that Gourlay and Matravers, who murdered Edward the Second, must have been Crusaders.

I was informed by Baboo Grischunder Ghose, Deputy Magistrate of Howrah, that there is a practice of torture, in the eastern and southern parts of Bengal, by introducing into the anus *Kachoor, Cuchao, or Ole Danta,* the stalk of the *Arum Colocasia.*

Introducing a Straw or Wire into the Urethra.†

Compressing the Chest between two bamboos—(Buki bans diya dhulâna—or Bans-dola,) or placing a stone or other heavy weight upon the Chest.

The medical reports to the Nizamut contain many cases in which the ribs on both sides were found broken, and the chest completely crushed. I have devoted a chapter to this subject, p. 493. This kind of injury is, doubtless, sometimes caused in affrays by persons jumping or falling upon the body of their victim, but it is well known that compression of the body by bamboos is practised as a torture, and that it is sometimes carried to fatal lengths. In 1844, Dr. Wilkie, of Dinagepore, deposed that he had no hesitation in testifying that two persons had been "firmly held or bound and died from the effects of *Bans-dola*

* Nizamut Adawlut Reports, for 1846, p. 33.

† Madras Report, Appendix C., p. cxlv, and Appendix E., No. 4, p. vi.

(torture of rolling and pressing with bamboos), the violence of the injuries causing death from the shock given to the nervous system."

In 1854, certain policemen, also of Dinagepore, seized a person on suspicion of dacoity. It appeared that he was, in the first instance, beaten by the mohurir, or acting darogah, and his party; and that, on the arrival of the darogah in the early part of night, he was again severely beaten, three times at least, until, at length, he fell senseless, when he was slung to a bamboo, tied hand and foot, and so carried back dead to a cattle-shed. The Civil Assistant Surgeon stated that "death was caused by congestion of blood in the brain from torture by severe pressure, and that simple beating without some such process as *Bans-dola*, would not cause the appearances he found without more decided external marks." The Judge considered it to be clear that the beating was performed skilfully by sharp raps on the joints, and punching and poking with *lattees*, so as not to leave external marks, that the *Bans-dola* torture was inflicted after the deceased fell, and that the object of this was to ascertain whether he was shamming or not. The witnesses were at some distance in the dark, and "*thelathelee*" with lattees, trying to push the deceased up, could not easily be distinguished, under the circumstances, from rolling two lattees fastened together down the thigh and leg.*

It is stated that the people, in that and the neighbouring districts, have a knack of inflicting insupportable suffering, by rolling the limbs in this manner beween two sticks, without producing any traces of contusion or discoloration.

Placing a hand-mill, or other weight on the chest (*Bookar apar Jathadya*).—This last-mentioned punishment may, like *Bans-dola*, account for a certain proportion of the crushed chests which so frequently come under medical investigation. According to a Hindu history of Bengal, quoted by Ward, Kasum Alee Khan put Raja Ram Narayan to death by placing a great weight on his stomach. In 1845, a gomashta of a talookdar, in the Chittagong division, when collecting rents, seized a ryot, and placing heavy weights on his chest, confined him for twenty-four hours; the unfortunate man died from the effects of this treatment.†

The Surgeon of Cuddapah reported to the Madras Commissioners that, a very short time previously, two prisoners had been brought to him stating that they had been tortured—that heavy stones had been placed on their chests, and a long piece of wood over this, and that on either end of the wood a man had seated himself, causing an almost total inability to breathe. His opinion was that what was stated by these men had really taken place.‡

---

* Nizamut Adawlut Reports, 22nd April 1854, p. 508.

† Police Report, L. P., 1845, p. 44.

‡ Appendix C., No. 8, p. xcix.

A like punishment, known as *Badha or Chitkara Jotemara—dancing with thick shoes upon a person lying, bound hand and foot, on the ground,* is also said to be practised in Bengal.

A correspondent of the Bombay Gazette, *vide* note p. 236, states that in Rutnagherry the accused is made to lie on his back, and is trodden on the thighs by a stout person with his shoes on.*

It will be noticed hereafter that death is sometimes produced by compressing the throat in a similar manner between two sticks.

Probably the commonest mode of torture in Madras is by the *Kittee* (in Telugu *Cheerata*). This instrument merely consists of two sticks tied together at one end, between which the fingers are placed, as in a lemon-squeezer (we have seen that an instrument of torture similar to this is used in Assam); or the unfortunate is compelled to interlace his fingers, when their ends are grasped and squeezed, sand being sometimes used to ensure a firmer gripe ; or he is made to place his hand flat on the ground, and a stick, laid horizontally over the back of his fingers, is pressed downwards at either end ; or the fingers are bent forcibly back towards the hand, or the hand upon the fore-arm (a common practice in Bengal, especially among women).† *Compression of the fingers upon or between bamboos, &c.,* is also practised in Bengal (*Angul badha Hathorimara*). Here also *the fingers are tied closely together, and nails or split bamboos are then forced or hammered between them*—(*dus logee kara*). This was one of the tortures against which Burke inveighed in his denunciation of Debi Sing's proceedings in Rungpore and Dinapore.

In Madras, pressure by the *Kittee* is applied in various ways, as to the *Ears*‡ and to the *Breasts of females.*§ *Twisting Women's Breasts* is also mentioned ;|| so also is *plucking at the flesh with large iron pincers.*¶ *Pinching the inner parts of the Thighs* is another practice there.** In Bengal also, *subjecting the victim to the pinching of several persons* (*Chimti Kata*) is spoken of as a well-known mode of torture.

Compressing the Testicles and pricking them with Thorns. (*Holetipadhara.*)

These are modes of torture practised in Bengal. An instance of the first

* In the reign of Louis Le Gross Cir. 1110.—Thomas de Marne, a brigand of rank, when desirous to force a ransom from his captives suspended them by some delicate part of their bodies or placed them on the earth, and, covering them with stones, walked over them.

† Report, p. 48.

‡ *Ibid*, p. 34.

§ Appendix E., No. 22, pp. xxvii and xxix.

|| Appendix C., p. xcii.

¶ *Ibid*, p. civ.

** Page 48.

kind has already been noticed at p. 539, and it would appear, from the Madras Report, that it is employed by the police in that Presidency.*

These parts are frequently injured in affrays, the natives having a brutal habit of seizing and dragging along an unfortunate opponent by the scrotum. In a case reported by Dr. Denham in 1843, in which death had been caused by an immense wound across the loins and other injuries, it is mentioned that "the skin covering the organs of generation was completely removed,"—probably in this manner. *See* also p. 477.

The various kinds of torture by *Beating* practised in India are noticed in the Chapter on that subject, p. 509.

Rubbing the Face upon the Ground.

This is also spoken of as a mode of Torture. I, when at Howrah, had a child sent to me whose face had evidently undergone this severe discipline. The fatal case of a man,—in whom Dr. Murray, of Beerbhoom, found the nose wounded, the lips much torn, the upper jaw fractured, a quantity of mud about the mouth, and two contused wounds on the back of the head,—was probably of this kind.

Binding the Limbs with undue tightness.

Mr. Pagan, of Midnapore, has reported the case of a Mussalmaun woman whose right arm was, upon admission, very much swollen and discolored, from having been bound very tightly with a rope ; indeed the skin had been cut by the rope, and mortification had then set in. The skin near the elbow joint had been also bruised. The left arm had suffered in a less degree. The right arm and hand, however, remained permanently shrunk and powerless.† It appears to be the practice of the police to bring in prisoners with their arms properly secured. Under these circumstances, attempts to escape might, of course, leave suspicious marks on a prisoner's limbs.

Binding the arms backwards with cords so tightly as to impede circulation.‡

Tightening a Cord around the body.—A native gentleman told me that, when travelling, four years ago, in the neighbourhood of Gya, he was attracted by cries to a place by the road side, where he found a person in small authority tying a man round with a rope until he shrieked. He also noticed preparations for the fire test.

---

* Page 50.

† See the trial of a man for binding the arms of his insane daughter with undue severity.—*Nizamut Adawlut Reports*, Vol. II., Part 2, of 1852, p. 475.

‡ *Ibid*, Appendix C., p. cxlvi and cliii.

Twisting a Rope round an entire limb so as to impede circulation.

This appears to be a rather common mode of torture in Madras. The Collector and Magistrate of Salem describes the practice as "tying coir ropes to [around] the muscles of the thighs and arms, and pouring water thereupon to produce extreme tension."* The Commissioners give an extract from the report of the Zillah Surgeon of Canara, describing the condition of a man who had been tortured in this manner. He had two very deep, foul, and extensive ulcers on his wrists and hands, and a great many smaller ones extending from the wrists to near the shoulders in a spiral direction. The constitutional symptoms were very severe. He stated that his wrists had been placed between two pieces of wood which were repeatedly squeezed together with great force, and that a rough rope, charged with powdered chillies and mustard seed, and moistened with a solution of salt, was very tightly bound round his arms. The ropes were kept on until his arms were swollen four times their natural size [?] The safety of the limbs was endangered, and he left the hospital without any prospect of recovering the full use of his hands.†

The Zillah Surgeon of Guntoor also reported the case of a prisoner upon whom, from the wrists to the upper third of either fore-arm, there were distinct marks of tight ligatures. On one wrist, the skin was abraded, and suppuration had followed.‡

The Bull's Hide Torture,

A practice well known in most barbarous nations, was long in use especially in Western India. We read in Purchas of an unfortunate commander who was sent "to a salvage island, called Torza, where hee" [The Khan] "causeth offenders to die, by sewing them, their hands bound, in a new-flayed hide of a buffall, which drying shrinketh so as it puts them, in a little-ease, to a miserable death."§

---

* Appendix C., No. 14, p. cxii.

† Report, p. 8.

‡ *Ibid*, Appendix C., No. 5, Guntoor, p. lxxii.—See also Appendix E., pp. xxi—xxxvi (A rope twisted round one arm from the wrist to the shoulder and the person suspended by it for ten minutes)—and xxxviii.

§ Purchas's expression "*little-ease*" will be recognised by the antiquarian reader as an allusion to cells for the confinement in uneasy positions of unruly apprentices and others, which, in Purchas's time and long subsequently, were to be found in nearly every prison in England from the Tower of London downwards. The following notices of these places are from *Notes and Queries:*

Lingard says that "the cell, Little Ease, was of so small dimensions, and so constructed, that the prisoner could neither stand, sit, nor lie in it at full length. He was compelled to draw himself up in a squatting posture, and so remained during several days."

Randle Holme described a place of similar use at Chester. "It was 'cut into a rock, with a grate door before it.' In it the prisoner could neither stand, sit, kneel, nor lie down, but be all in a ruck or knit together, so, and in such a lamentable condition, that half an hour will tame the stoutest and stubbornest stomach, and will make him desire to be freed from the place."

Forbes describes the *Sheep-Skin Death* as a cruelty sometimes practised by the Mahrattas. The culprit is stripped naked, and, a sheep being killed, the warm skin of the animal is immediately stretched to the utmost, and sewed tight over the prisoner's body ; he is then conducted to the flat roof of the prison, and exposed to the fervour of a tropical sun. The skin, contracting by the heat, draws with it the flesh of the agonizing wretch until putrefaction, hunger, and thirst terminate his suffering.—*Op. Cit.*, p. 55, Vol. II.

In the Memoirs of a Thug, we have mention of a torture by tying up the fingers and hitting them on the ends.

Binding or otherwise constraining the body in painful positions.

A great variety of cruel devices of his kind are in vogue in both Presidencies. Thus—in Bengal—there is *keeping a limb flexed or extended. Making the victim stand on one leg and torturing the lifted leg as often as it is allowed to touch the ground* (*Ek thanga darkarana*). *Binding the arms behind the back and forcing them with a lattee* (*thick stick*) *inserted between the back and arms* (*Pit moradhiya*).

Stocks (Sholadya).

A writer in the *Bengal Hurkaru*, Calcutta, in 1840, says : "I have seen the stocks used in all parts of Bengal ; they are made of two heavy saul timbers, with holes cut to hold legs of different sizes ; so, by way of torture, they put a stout man's legs into the small holes, and a confession quickly follows. I saw a young fellow clapped into the stocks, who was found on the road with a few *lotas* and a cloth, without being able to

---

The Chester Little Ease is described as having been "a hole hewed out in a rock; the breadth and cross from side to side is seventeen inches, from the back to the inside of the great door ; at the top seven inches ; at the shoulders, eight inches ; at the breast nine and-a-half inches; from the top to the bottom, one yard and-a-half, with a device to lessen the height as they are minded to torment the person put in, by drawboards, which shoot over across the two sides to a yard in height or thereabouts." An excavation in the rock, corresponding with this, was recently discovered on the spot.

One Richard Sale, a Quaker, was twice shut up here in 1656, and kept in for about three or four hours. "Being pretty corpulent, he could not be put into that narrow hole, without much violence, so that four men had much ado to thrust him in, and at several times by the crushing of him, the blood gushed out of his mouth and nose. His health, by this frequent barbarity, was much impaired, and his body and legs swelled, so that he languished about two months after this last time of his being put there, and then died in the sixth month, 1657, imputing the cause of his death to the cruelty of his persecution."

There was also a Little Ease in the Jail at Boston in Lincolnshire in 1605, used for the punishment of offences committed in jail. It was, however, larger, as it contained a pair of stocks.

There was another in the Guildhall, London, and there were lately three others, of course long disused, in the neighbourhood of Liverpool. They are described as "small sugar-loaf-shaped buildings." My impression is that the cell in the Tower resembled, in vertical section, an *inverted* sugar-loaf.

account for having them. He confessed, next day, to having robbed his master ; but, when the case came on, the master declared him innocent. The fellow had his heels cocked up in the air for twenty-four hours, and his head and back on the cold damp earth. I have no doubt he would have as readily confessed to having murdered his mother, for the stocks is a system of torture which a man soon gets tired of."

In 1856 a police mohurrir and burkundaz were sentenced to six months' imprisonment for extortion and illegal confinement in having detained a man in the stocks for three days, and only releasing him on the payment of forty-four rupees.*

In Madras, these modes of torture appear to be cunningly proportioned in severity in such a manner as to cause every degree of suffering from considerable annoyance to exquisite torment. Thus there are *Stocks for the Hands and Feet*. Persons are compelled *to remain in a stooping position with a greater or less weight upon the back—to stand on one leg holding the toes, or with the other tied up*. In some cases a log of wood is also placed on the head ;†—*to stand with the muzzle of a musket resting on the great toes*,‡ or to *sit on the haunches with bricks or sharp pointed stones placed in the bends of the knees*.§ One of the most common modes of torture in Madras is the *Anundal* (in Telugu *Gingeri*), —*tying a man down in a bent position with his own cloth or a rope passed over his neck and under his toes*, the head being sometimes brought down to the knees. Often a stone of greater or less weight (sometimes a man)‖ is, at the same time, placed on the back. The whole Report is filled with references to cases in which this torture was employed in various degrees of severity.¶

It appears that, in all the above modes of torture, *Exposure to the Sun* is usually added to the victim's other causes of suffering.

In some of these cases the torture is continued until death results.

The Acting Collector of Nellore reported that a case had recently been reported to him, in which an old man, having been tied up in a burning sun, was attacked with apoplexy, from which, after an interval of some days, he died.**

A case was tried at Patna in 1855, in which a man was taken into a house by two persons, who "tortured and beat him so unmercifully by

* Nizamut Adawlut Reports, September 27, 1856, p. 360.

† Appendix C., p. clxxiv.

‡ *Ibid*, p. clxxiv.

§ *Ibid*.

‖ *Ibid*.

¶ Being carried to final judgment with their heads and legs tied together, is held by the Hindus as one of the punishments of the wicked, anticipatory of the pains of hell.

** Appendix No. 7, Nellore, p. lxxxi.

tying him up, striking him with their fists, kicking him and jumping on his body, that he died within an hour or two." In this case there is mention of the torture of *Gola-lathee*. This consists in bringing the arms over the knees and tying them, and then thrusting a bamboo under the knees and above the arms. Dr. Dicken, the Civil Surgeon, found that there had been such severe injuries inflicted upon the body before death, that he had little or no doubt that death was the consequence of them.*

The details of a very remarkable case of this kind have been published in the *Indian Annals of Medical Science*, by Sub-Assistant Surgeon Suyd Mahomed Jaun, in medical charge of Jhung, Punjab. In December 1854, he was called upon to examine the body of a man, aged fifty, who was stated, in the thannah report, to have been struck with a shoe on the private parts by a burkundaz, from the effects of which blow he died in about eighteen hours. There were no outward traces of violence. On opening the abdomen, about six ounces of bloody serum flowed out. *The Pancreas was vertically lucerated from above downwards at its right extremity through about half its breadth.* A small clot of blood was found close to this wound. The whole organ looked highly congested, with extensive extravasation of blood into its cellular tissue. It appeared that the deceased had been arrested on suspicion by the prisoner, who, in order to exort a confession, placed him on the ground, tied his hands together, and, having forced his knees between his arms, fixed him in this position by passing a long stick under the bends of the knees and over the arms. Then throwing the wretched man on his back, he began to beat him with a shoe on his buttocks and genitals, and kicked him more than once until he fainted; when, being supposed to be dead or

---

* Nizamut Adawlut Reports, September 10, 1855, p. 360. There is still preserved, in the armoury of the Tower of London, an instrument in which this principle of torture was carried to perfection.

In the reign of Henry VIII., Sir William Skevington, Lieutenant of the Tower, immortalised himself by the invention of a new instrument of torture called Skevington's Daughter. In 1604, a Committee was appointed by the House of Commons to enquire into the state of a dungeon called "Little Ease" in the Tower. They found that the place itself was very loathsome and unclean, and not used for a long time either for a prison or other cleanly purpose. They found here an engine of torture designed by Mr. Skevington, some time Lieutenant of the Tower. This instrument appears to have rolled and contracted the body into a ball until the head and feet met together, and forced the blood to ooze from the extremities of the hands and feet, and frequently from the nostrils and month. See *Jardine's Reading on the use of Torture in the Criminal Law of England*, 1837, p. 15.

The following entries appear in a *Diarium Rerum Gestarum in Turri Londinensi*, on the 10th December 1580:

"Thomas Cotamus et Lucas Kirbœus presbyteri, Scauingeri filiam ad unam horam et amplius possi; ex quo prior copiosum sanguinem e naribus emisit."

On the 1st of September 1582, "Johannes Getterus Scauingeri filia cruciatus est."

dying, the victim was released. When he came to his senses, the man complained of a severe pain in the epigastrium, but was able to walk home (about a mile) supported by two persons.

Forbes states that, in Travancore, for debts and non-payment of fines inflicted as a punishment, debtors are confined by the sircar, or chief of the district, who draws a circle round the prisoner, from which he dare not move ; then, gently laying a sharp stone on the crown of his head, demands payment of the sum required : on refusal, he places a flat stone over the other, and ties it firmly on ; additional weights are gradually accumulated, with a repetition of the demand ; until the sharp stone, penetrating the head, either insures payment, or causes a painful death.*

In the Autobiography of Lutfullah we find this described as one of the tortures practised by the Pindarees. The victim "was made to stand pinioned in the sun with a stone of enormous weight on his head, first inserting a gravel stone of the size and shape of a small grape, which gradually forced its way through the skull to the brain."

The same author mentions that a modification of this process was employed in Malwah as a mode of executing robbers. This was "inflicted by putting a man horizontally on one side with his head on a flat stone ; a ball of stone is then put on his upper temple, and the executioner inflicts a fatal blow with a large wooden hammer on the small ball, which smashes the head at once, and the brain is dashed out."

Placing stinging or gnawing Insects upon the Skin.

A common punishment in Bengal is placing *spiders* or a *mole cricket* (*gryllus gryllo-talpa*), called by the natives *ghoorghoora pooka,* on the navel, covered with a shell or earthen pot. It is said that these produce a swelling which is not unlikely to be mistaken by the surgeon for a large furuncle. In a case tried at West Burdwan, in 1855, the prisoner stated that, in consequence of a quarrel he had with him about entering the women's baree of the zemindar, to sell brass articles, without his permission, the zemindar had him beaten and tortured by the application of beetles to his navel.†

On the 14th March 1868 a head constable and two constables of the Government railway police were sentenced to five years' imprisonment and a fine of rupees 200 at the Hooghly Sessions Court, for torturing a servant of the station master at Serampore on suspicion of theft. The evidence went to show that they put the man into a godown and beat him with a cane on the posteriors, and with their batons on various parts of his body ; they also pressed his throat with a bamboo. Russick Lall Bose told

* Op. Cit., Vol. I., p. 253.
† Nizamut Adawlut Reports, Sept. 18, 1855, p. 409.

a gareewan to bring *ghoorghooras ;* he dug two out of the earth on the side of a tank. One was first applied to his navel covered with a *batee*, and then the other.

In Madras, the *Poollay Insect*, the Carpenter Beetle, some burrowing beetle, or the potter's insect, is frequently secured in a cocoanut shell, over the navel, or is fastened on the scrotum or some other sensitive part.*

That old practice of *exposing persons to be gnawed by ants*† was formerly common in Bengal.

Baboo Bholanath Chunder mentions that in Jahn-nugger, near Krishnugger, was a petty landlord who punished his defaulters by putting them into "a house of ants," and that the Nawabs of Moorshedabad used to confine men for arrears of revenue to "a house of bugs."‡ Exposing themselves, in public places, to the attacks of insects is one of the practices of religious mendicants in India.

Ward alludes to a practice of the Hindoos of "hanging their children up alive in trees for the ants and crows before their own doors." He thought that this is done when the child is born with bad omens, or is supposed to be afflicted by some evil spirit.§

---

* Appendix C., pp. cxli and cxlv.

† The Burmese say that, among the trials to which Boodhu was subjected, were smearing him with molasses and letting the flies torment him, and scorching with fire.

‡ Op. Cit., Vol. I., p. 44. The ingenuity of the Inquisitors of Spain did not overlook this mode of torture. William Lithgow, the traveller, thus describes a part of his sufferings when imprisoned and tortured at Malaga early in the seventeenth century: "I was miserably afflicted with the beastly plagues of gnawing vermin which lay crawling in lumps, within, without, and about my body,—yea, hanging in clusters about my beard, my lips, and nostrils, and my eyebrows almost enclosing my sight. And, for a great satisfaction for their merciless minds, the Governor caused Areta, his silver plate keeper, to gather and sweep the vermin upon me twice in eight days, which tormented me to the death being a perpetual punishment; for mine arms being broke, my hands locked and sticking fast to the palms of both hands, by reason of the shrunk sinews, I was unable to lift mine arms to stir my fingers, much less to avoid the filthy vermin; neither could my legs or feet perform it, being impotent in all. Yet I acknowledge the poor infidel (a Turk who was to watch me) some few times, and, when opportunity served, would steal the keys from Areta, and about midnight would enter my room with sticks and burning oil, and sweeping them together in heaps, would burn the greatest part, to my great release, or doubtless I had been miserably eat up, and devoured by them."

§ An ancient atrocity of this kind is thus described in the quaint language of the translator of Camerarius. It is the fate of Mithridates, once the trusted domestic of Artaxerxes: "They take two troughs made of purpose, so even, that the one is neither longer nor broader than the other; and he that is to be punished is layd vpon his back into one of them, and then covered with the other: after, they are both fastened together, yet so, as the feet, hands, and head lie without them, by holes made for that purpose, all the rest of the bodie being covered and hid within. He hath meat given him as much as he will eat, and if he will not eat, they constraine him to eate by force, pricking his eyes with needles; and, when he hath eaten, they give him to drinke honie mingled with milke, and they power thereof not oneley into his mouth, but also upon his face, turning him so that the sunne striketh evermore into his eyes, in so much as his face is continually covered with flies: and for that he doth within these troughs all the needs that a man eating and drinking is forced to doe; with the

There appeared, in *Once a Week*, for May 1866, a very graphic account of an iron apparatus which was unearthed by a flood from below a great tamarind tree, at a cross-road in Jamaica. The following is part of the rather sensational description of this relic. "There could be no doubt of its being made to secure a naked human body alive ; while, in sad testimony of this knowledge, in an open wooden box beneath, lay the bones of the sufferer who once had passed from life to death in its most accursed grasp. Round the knees, hips, and waist, under the arms and around the neck, iron hoops were rivetted close about the different parts of the body ; iron braces crossed these again from the hips right over the centre of the head. Iron bars and plates encircled and supported the legs, and, at the lower extremities, were fixed plates of iron like old-fashioned stirrups, in which the feet might have found rest, had not a finish to the torture—compared to which crucifixion itself must have been mild—been contrived by fixing in each stirrup three sharp-pointed spikes to pierce the soles of the victim's feet. The only support the body could receive, while strength remained, or life endured, was given by a narrow hoop passing from one end of the waist-bar, in front, between the legs, to the bar at the back. Attached to the circular band under the arms, stood out a pair of handcuffs, which prevented the slightest motion in the hands ; and, on the crossing of the hoops over the head, was a strong hook, by which the whole fabric, with the sufferer enclosed, was suspended.

"Quivering in agony, there she swung, the blazing sun striking fiercely on her nakedness, quickly causing a terrible thirst to rage throughout the frame, and, while yet life was strong, the fevered blood to course madly through the swollen veins. Not long before the ants, pondering over the drops of blood, which fell from her spike-pierced feet, would climb in countless myriads up the old tamarind tree, across the branches, and down over the iron bars, to the fountain of this horrid feast ; while mosquitoes and sandflies disputed with these and many other parasites which should suck fastest at the life and strength of a poor human creature, hung up to be eaten thus alive."

The writer supports his terrible theory by a quotation from Bryan Edwards's History of Jamaica, which shows that, in the negro rebellion of 1760, two Coromantyn negroes, who had been concerned in the massacre, were hung alive in irons, and left to perish in that dreadful situation. He, however, adduces no evidence, beyond that of native tradition, in proof that the woman in question or any other woman was ever thus treated.

---

filth and rottennesse of his excrements there engender wormes, which eat into his bodie ; and when they see that the patient is dead, they take off the upper trough, and find his flesh all eaten by this vermin, even to his very entrailes. Mithridates then, after he had languished in this miserie the space of seaventeene dayes, dyed at last with horrible and grievous paine."

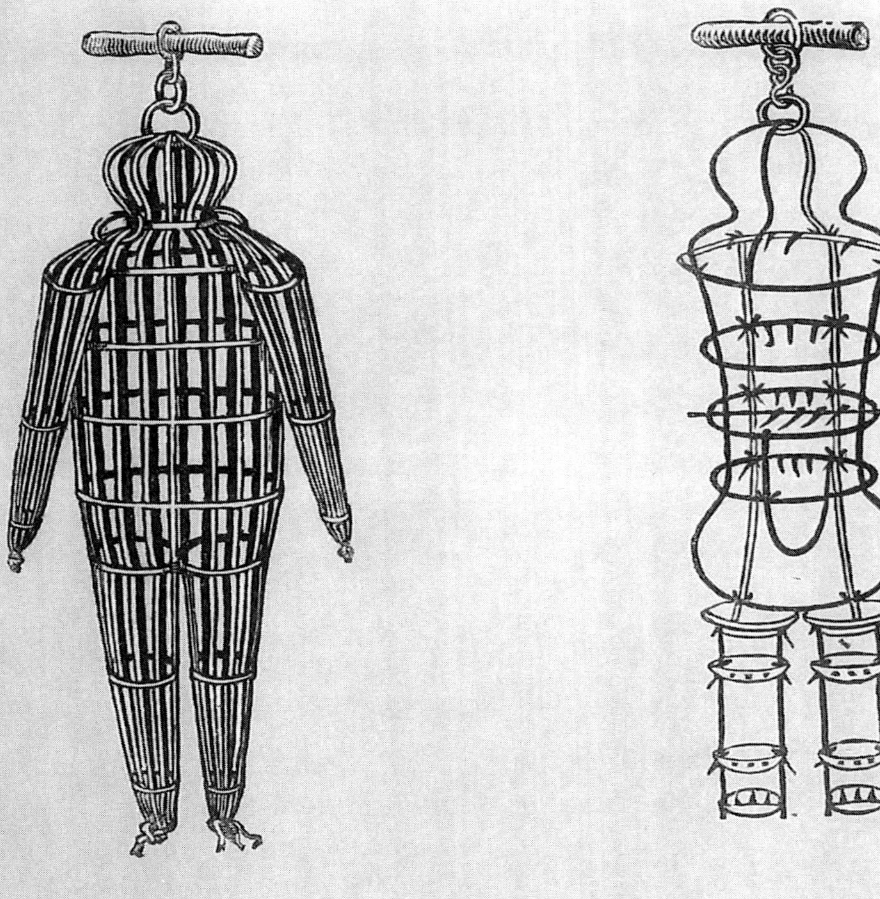

"HANGING IN CHAINS."

Apparatuses used in the East and West Indies.

A very similar relic was sent by the Rev. F. Mazuchelli, from Furreedpore, to the Asiatic Society's museum, in March 1868. It is made of common hoop-iron, and is quite in the human form. Mr. Mazuchelli wrote: "One authority tells me that dacoits when caught years ago, say some sixty or seventy since, between Dacca and Calcutta, were put alive in this cage, and exposed to the air to die of hunger, and as a lesson to others. Another authority tells me that the culprit was hung first and then put into the cage, and the cage hung up to a tree to deter others. But what seems to me the most probable story is, that under the Nizamut (the criminal government) of the Nawab Nazim of Moorshedabad, in the last century, and even afterwards under the English rule, it was the custom to hang persons convicted of murder, at the sudder or chief station of the district, and, after decease, to remove the body in a cage to the native village of the deceased, and there suspend it on a gibbet as a warning to others. Now the cage I have now in my possession, and which I willingly offer to the Society, is that in which, according to report of the people of Whau-Wharazpore, Thana Betka, the corpse of one Goriah Moochee was placed there after execution for a murder, of which he had been convicted."

My own belief is that these are the ordinary apparatuses in which the bodies of dead malefactors, sentenced to be "hanged in chains" were suspended, within my own recollection. A murderer was thus sentenced to be hanged, at Nassick, in 1828. This practice was forbidden in the Court's letter of the 10th February 1835.* Baboo Bholanauth Chunder, who is now only about forty-one years of age, recollects to have seen the skeleton of a highwayman, hanging in chains, at Kurdah, near Calcutta.

On the opposite page, the West Indian and the East Indian apparatuses are accurately represented.

The Collector and Magistrate of Canara has known a prisoner to be put into a nest of red ants as a means of extorting confession.† In 1853, the Zillah Surgeon of Guntoor reported to the Judge that he had examined a prisoner in a criminal case, the whole of whose back was disfigured by the cicatrices of numerous small sores, there was also one sore of great size, near the spine, and there were marks of tight ligatures round both arms. The man stated that he remained tied by the arms to a tree all night, and was severely bitten by large black ants. From the appearance of the sores, they being, for the most part, small, insolated, and rather deep, and from the marks of the cords on his arms, the Surgeon was of opinion that the prisoner's statement was correct.‡

---

* Bellasis' Reports, p. 12.

† Appendix C., No. 10, Canara, p. cviii.

‡ *Ibid*, No. 5, p. lxxi.

Sticking Pins or Thorns under the Nails

Is practised equally in this Presidency and in Madras.*

Keeping under Water.

We have already seen that dipping unfortunates in water or mud until they were nearly suffocated was, long ago, practised by the Mussalmaun rulers in Bengal. *Keeping under water* (*Jaladabana*) is still a Bengali torture. It is also practised in Madras.† The Magistrate and Collector of Tanjore reported that there was still a young girl under treatment by his native doctor for a severe wound received, when she was dropped down a well by a rope fastened round her neck, by a man who wished to force from her information as to what had become of an ornament lost by another child at play.‡ *See* the Arcot case, p. 551.

Filling the mouth with pebbles and striking the chin upwards, with sufficient force to break the teeth (*Darimara*) is spoken of as a Bengali punishment.

Pulling the Hair on both sides (*Chooldhara tana*).

In Bengal this is generally practised upon females. In Madras, there are several contrivances of this kind. Such as *tying two persons closely together by the top-knots, and tying the hair of the head to a donkey's or buffaloe's tail. Plucking out the Beard* (reckoned by the natives a great disgrace) is a common torture in both Presidencies.§ *Twisting the ears; striking two offenders' heads together; placing a person in the sun with his hair loose, and compelling him to turn his head rapidly to and fro.*‖ For notes on the last three practices in Bengal, *see* pp. 530 & 562.

Beating the ankle and other joints with a soft mallet or piece of wood¶

Appears to be a common torture in Madras. A case has already been cited in this Chapter, p. 545, which shows the barbarous manner in which repeated blows are inflicted upon the extremities by natives of this country. In 1854, the Surgeon of Behar thus described one only of the injuries which he found upon the body of a man whom several persons had beaten to death with clubs. "The left arm, from half way down the

---

* A mode of torture, called *soufflee*, was used in Italy towards the end of the sixteenth century. Splinters of cane were driven under the nails. The humane spirit of that age is illustrated by the explanation that this was only employed for aged men and children.

† Report, p. 50.

‡ Appendix C., No. 16, p. clxix; see also p. clvi of the same.

§ Report, p. 48.

‖ Appendix C., p. clxxiv.

¶ *Ibid*, pp. clxxxvii, cxciii.

shoulder to the extremities of the fingers, was one mass of dark-colored pulp. The elbow joint was completely destroyed, and the bones in the neighbourhood shattered to atoms, and the brachial artery was torn in shreds."*

Since September 1851, all medical men in the Madras Presidency have been instructed by the Medical Board to examine, personally, every prisoner on his committal to jail. This order, the Commissioners have no doubt, is punctually carried out. Still their attention has been attracted by the singular absence of almost all medical testimony. This, however, appears to be accounted for by the remark that, "ordinarily, the violence is of a petty kind, although causing acute momentary pain; and even many of the severe kinds of torture invented by native ingenuity leave no mark behind them. Delay is, no doubt, often purposely interposed between the infliction of ill-usage and the delivery of the accused to that custody which is subject to European supervision, and thus marks, when made, become obliterated."

In both Presidencies, native invention has been fertile in the discovery of tortures and modes of ill-treament *which leave no marks*—such as *Exposure to the Sun. Starvation* (*Sokea mara*)—(to this is added, in Madras, the torture of *being prevented from obeying the calls of nature or from Sleeping*). *Slaps and blows with switches. Pinching by several persons* (*Chemti Kata*). *Imprisonment. Running up and down* is a Madras punishment.

In describing the course supposed to be taken in a case of house robbery, the Calcutta *Indian Daily News* of July 22nd, 1870, tells us:—"Three or four servants are 'spotted,' as being most likely to confess something. Once at the thannah, the result is almost certain, if the Chowkeydars are true to their salt. Their duty is to walk the prisoners about, not with apparent aimlessness, but with the purpose of pointing out where the stolen property is hidden. Chowkeydar number one walks them about till, say ten at night, he is relieved, and Chowkeydar number two walks them about till twelve, and so on. Towards morning, the prisoners find that walking for many hours consecutively is not amusing, and also reflect, in their own language, that *il faut dormir*. Then why not sleep? It is quite easy to confess, to point out the nearest hut as the residence of the guilty receiver, and, if one sits six months, at all events one sleeps in gaol. Confession is full accordingly. Those who have experienced this system must heave a sigh of regret for the halcyon days of Chili-vinegar in the eyes, and a thick bamboo pressed down upon the chest and ribs. Hunger and thirst may be borne for a day or two, but to keep a native

---

* Nizamut Adawlut Reports, 5th August 1854, p. 222.

who, like a dog, can sleep at any time, awake for more than eight hours in the twenty-four, is the highest refinement of torture."

Closing the Nostrils till the victim is half suffocated (*Nak tipa-dhara*) and *Tickling* (*Katakatoor dya*) are also mentioned. I even find more than one allusion to the disgusting brutality of *Making Water into the Victim's Mouth* (*Mooka moota dya*). This was done in a case, given in Macnaghten's Reports, where an unfortunate wretch was barbarously put to death by several assailants.

Various *modes of inflicting Degradation and Mental Suffering* are also practised. An enumeration of these may appear foreign to a medical work. Still, as the Surgeon is generally consulted in inquiries of this kind, it is necessary that he should be acquainted with the whole system. Thus, in Madras, persons of respectability are confined with others of low caste; or a Brahmin is made to carry a sweeper on his back, or a necklace of bones or other disgusting and polluting materials is placed round his neck.*

These are evidently modes of vexation adopted by the Mussalmauns, with a knowledge of Hindu customs. It is stated that Seraj-oo-Doulah was betrayed by a fukeer, with whom he took refuge, who had formerly been a merchant, but was degraded by the tyrant by having his head shaved, and the urine of an ass poured upon it.

We have seen (pp. 488-89) that shaving the head is one of the modes in which it has been usual to punish an adulteress in India. Cutting off the hair of the head was the first and lightest part of the punishment to be undergone by a Brahmin woman convicted of adultery (Halhed, p. 275). A Chehteree, committing this crime with a Brahmin woman having no master, was to be fined and to have the hair of his head shaved off with the urine of an ass (*Ibid*, p. 319). The author of the Seir Mutaqherin says that a favorite expression of abuse with Shaocat Jung was a woman's phrase—*sir mondi*,—to be hairless, to have the head shaved, or to be shaved at all, being a great opprobrium among all kinds of women. Camerarius says: "In Greece and wel neere in all the East, to shave the head and the beard was held for a great punishment." "In many places the punishment of fornication was, that the fornicator should have his beard chopt off openly with a keene axe, and so to be sent away; which to him was a mark of infamy." "It was the custome in France that the wife accused and convicted of adultrie by her husband, should be shaven, and that her cloaths should be clipt off round about her, and of a good height; and that she should be carried in that manner throughout the towns and villages, to be seene of everie one." "Let vs add hereunto that which Theuet affirmeth, how yet at this day it is a kind of punishment in the Isle of Candie to cut a man's beard. So, in times

---

* Report, p. 48.

past, among the Indians, the king made him be poled that had committed some great offence, as a marke of extreame reproch."

In 1852, a man deposed, in a trial at Jounpore, that certain Mussalmauns had seized, bound and beaten him, and had thrown him into a pit. One of them had proposed to put bones, goor, and mowa into his mouth, and thus deprive him of his caste, but that they decided to carry him into Oude.*

In this part of the country, it is alleged that respectable persons are confined in privies, or are compelled to clean them out, and that women are exposed to every degree of indignity. Some of the details already given are sufficiently horrible; still, even beyond this, the extent to which this latter atrocity is stated to be practised is such that I should feel unwilling to do more than allude to the subject, unless proved cases could be cited (a result which is rendered difficult by the secrecy which would, of course, be maintained both by the injurers and the injured), were it not that I have reason to believe, on good authority, that the evil probably still exists. I have a note, dated 17th March 1855, from one in whose statements regarding the tortures practised in Bengal, I have never been able to detect an error, in which the following practice is mentioned—"making male and female near relations naked, and putting the male upon the female by force, or violating the person in the presence of the near male relations."† The following extract represents a Burmese atrocity. I cite it because it but faintly represents an incident which my friend Dr. T. W. Wilson assured me that he believed occurred, at about the same time, in Bengal.‡

The subjoined appeared in Allen's Asiatic Journal for October 1840, page 116:—

A letter from Rangoon is as follows:—"A most brutal piece of busi-

---

* Nizamut Adawlut Reports, N. W. P., 25th September 1852, p. 1082.

† More than one case occurs in the Reports of the Courts of Nizamut Adawlut, in which there appeared to be strong reason for believing that the crime of Rape was committed with a cold-blooded intention of bringing disgrace upon the woman's family. In October 1853 a young married woman of Cawnpore was tried for an attempt to murder her infant by throwing herself with the child in her arms into a well. Circumstances came out in evidence which led to the belief that the prisoner had acted under feelings of extreme excitement, caused by the disgraceful conduct of the Zemindars and others who, being enraged at a deposition made by her husband, had revenged themselves upon his wife, by putting upon her a grievous indignity. The men were tried on a charge of rape, and were found guilty by the Sessions Judge of an aggravated and indecent assault. There was, however, so much inconsistency in the statements of the woman and her witnesses, that the Superior Court acquitted the defendants, on appeal.—*Nizamut Adawlut Reports*, N. W. P., 2nd March 1854.

In 1855, a man and his brother, of Rajshahye, were sentenced, on their own confession, for a rape on a respectable widow; the plea was that the master of one of the men suggested the crime in revenge for her having abused him for allowing his horse to injure her paddy crop.—*Nizamut Adawlut Reports*, December 28th, 1855, p. 973.

‡ If more explicitness be needful, it will be found in Roquets' description of the third plate of Hogarth's Rakes' Progress.

ness has taken place upon two respectable Christian females, by order of the Myo-woon of Rangoon. The parties alluded to are Mrs. R—— and her young sister. Mrs. R.'s mother is a Burman, but her father was a Christian, and she was brought up in his faith. Some time after his demise, the mother married a Burman, by whom she had the young sister; the Burman father also died many years ago, and, when this girl came to mature age (about two years ago), she was baptized as a Christian. Now some say, for this act the following brutal punishment was inflicted; and others (which I also believe) affirm that the Myo-woon, having seen the girl during one of their feasting processions, was smitten with her beauty, and demanded her as his concubine. Be that as it may, they were both called up by the Myo-woon and placed in the criminal gaol in the following shocking manner: both feet in the stocks, extended apart as far as could be done; their arms stretched out and lashed down; their clothes stripped off, and their whole persons exposed; lighted lamps placed (here follows a passage that must be suppressed). There they were lying without any hope of relief. The unfortunate females, probably overcome by their intense sufferings, were, after a few days, released, on giving security that they would go to the pagoda and not worship the Stranger's God."

It was alleged that Achumbit of Mooteeharee, owing a grudge to a man for not having invited him to a feast, ordered one Surwan Mallee to outrage the modesty of the man's daughter when she went to bring water from the well. In the midst of the confusion, the woman's child fell from her arms and was trodden upon and killed by Achumbit. He was sent up for trial, but was released.*

A very extraordinary case was tried at Meerut, in October 1854, in which it was clearly proved that one Khoobee Singh having, probably by his own criminal conduct, involved himself seriously with the police, compelled certain persons, his nephew and others, to kill him by striking him with a sword on the back of the neck. Nearly all the witnesses concurred in saying that the chief reason expressed by the unfortunate man, in insisting upon being put to death, was that the Kotwal had accused him of participation in a robbery, and threatened that, if he did not produce the money, he would seize all the women of his family and parade them naked through the bazar, but that, if he died, his family would not be disgraced.†

Among the questions proposed to witnesses in the Madras inquiry was the following:—"The Tehsildar probably does not permit it" [Torture] "in his own presence. But is there an understanding that, if he orders a man to be treated *Cayidah procaurum* (according to custom), or some

---

* Bengal Police Report for 1868, p. 176.

† Nizamut Adawlut Reports, N. W. P., 18th October 1854, p. 573;—see also for 30th August 1853, p. 1048

words to that effect, he is to be subjected to such ill-usage?"* A writer in the *Bombay Gazette*, quoted in the *Bengal Hurkaru*, December 8th, 1859, states that, in Ratnagherry, if the prisoners or witnesses do not state what is wanted by the police officers, they tell the peons under them and others to *explain the matter fully to them*. This expression has a technical meaning; and, when it is used, the men are taken away and tortured. I long believed that there must be certain "cant" phrases by which the several modes of torture are known. For a considerable time, I could gain no information on this subject, or the names of the tortures were merely rendered into Bengali by my informants. The following expressions were, at length, collected for me by a native gentleman whose means of obtaining accurate information were unimpeachable. I may add that his memoranda were sent to me in the middle of March 1854,—some time before the Report of the Madras Commissioners was submitted to Government.

Bhalakaro Bhojhoy. (Make him understand well.)
Jalkhoyak ana. (Bring him after he has drank water.)
Kala ghora niaghoy. (Take him to the black room.)
Jaladoboy. (Keep him under water.)
Khaya ana. (Bring him after he has eaten.)
Patkara ana. (Bring him after he has been well prepared.)
Sava kara ana. (Bring him after he has been well served or respected.)
Lut Koy. (Make him swing.)
Thanda Kuro,—Garam Kuro. (Cool him, or Warm him.)

The subjoined statement, regarding the practices of the old police, was sent to me by a trustworthy native gentleman, too late for insertion in my last edition:—

"The following are some of the methods which are resorted to by the police officers to extort confessions from criminals:—

"*1st*.—When a criminal is apprehended, the police officers, to make him confess, first of all hold out to him hopes of pardon, &c. Should this fail, then they take him to a sequestered place, where they beat and otherwise maltreat him till he confesses.

"*2nd*.—Or they tell him, if he be not the only party concerned in the case in question, to name his accomplices, and what part of the proceeds of the booty he received for his share; and, should he confess all these, he would be converted into a witness. When thus excited, they admit their own guilt, or implicate others.

"*3rd*.—Should the case be of a very aggravated nature, and it is necessary

* Appendix G., No. 1, p. 134.

to obtain the confessions of criminals, the police officers raise in them hopes. If they do not succeed, they take the prisoners in a private place, put some *ghurghooria*, a kind of insect found in marshy places, in their navels, tie their clothes around their waist, and suffer them to bite on unmolested. The prisoner, not able to bear these excruciating tortures any longer, confesses his guilt, and tells the names of his accomplices.

"*4th.*—Should the criminal still remain silent, the police officers take him to a secret spot, and bring out the members of his family or his kept woman, and attempt to dishonor her before his eyes. The prisoner then owns whether he is the only party, or implicates others.

"*5th.*—All those culprits who are arrested by the police are kept apart, so as to bar their hearing each other. The officer then comes to one and says that "such a prisoner has mentioned your name, and affirms that you are perfectly acquainted with the secrets of the affair; so confess, otherwise you will get into a scrape." When thus threatened, the prisoner confesses his guilt, or tells that so and so are the principal actors in the transaction.

"*6th.*—Or the police officers bind prisoners with clothes, so as to leave no marks, and make them stand, having the sun just opposite to their face. When thus intimidated, they also confess.

"*7th.*—Or they put small sticks between the fingers, the ends of which they tie very tightly with a string; and this process is so effective that prisoners, though they be fully aware what would result from their confession, cannot refrain from acknowledging their guilt, and, when real criminals, pointing out the place where they had hidden the booty."

If we combine what we know of the condition of the English peasantry in the reign of Stephen, with that which we read of the agriculturists of Germany when they bent under Tilly's yoke, we obtain some idea of the state into which the rural population of India must inevitably fall under any relaxation of our police system.

John of Salisbury laments, in his Polycraticon, the evils of Stephen's days, when "every rich man made his castles, and held them against the king, and the land was filled with castles. Grievously they oppressed the miserable people of the land with their castle works. When the castles were made, they filled them with devils and evil men; and then they seized every one who was supposed to have any property, man and woman, both by night and by day, and put them in prison for their gold and silver, and punished them with such inexpressible torments as none of the martyrs ever suffered. They hung them by the feet, and smoked them with foul smoke, and they hung them by the thumbs or by the head, and hung fire to their feet. They put knotted cords about their heads, and twisted them till they pierced to the brain. They put some in dungeons, where were adders and snakes, and toads, and so tormented them. Others they placed in a *crucet-house*, that is, in a chest which was shut and narrow and shallow, and they put in sharp stones and pressed people in them, till all their bones were broken. In many of the castles were things very horrible and hateful,—these were '*sachenteges*,' that were as much as two or three men could lift; and they were so contrived that the man was fastened to a beam, with sharp iron about his throat or neck, that he could neither sit nor lie down, nor sleep, but was compelled always to support that weight. Many they tormented with hunger. I cannot tell all the sufferings and all the torments which the wretched people bore during the nineteen years of Stephen's reign."*

Turning from the "*kala or thanda ghur*" of the Norman Baron, we find the author of "Pictures of Life in Germany" opening before us a glimpse of a very similar mode of living which, just five centuries later in the world's history, was established by John Tzerclais in the homesteads of Germany during the Thirty Years' War.

"The plunderers took the flints from their pistols, and forced the peasants' thumbs in their place;† they rubbed the soles of their feet with salt and caused the goats to lick them; they tied their hands behind their backs; they passed a bodkin threaded with horsehair through their tongues, and moved it gently up and down; they bound a knotted cord round the forehead, and twisted it together behind with a stick; they bound two fingers together and rubbed a ramrod up and down till the skin and flesh were burnt to the bones; they forced the victims into the oven, lit the straw behind them, and so they were obliged to creep through the flames, and these were not the most horrible torments."

Indian Laws against Torture.

If a woman, or a person intoxicated, or an idiot, or a sick person, or a child, or a man under violent dread, hath performed any transaction, it is not approved.‡

For the laws prohibiting Torture by the Police, *vide supra*, pp. 79-80.

Where several prisoners were all concerned in a case of Torture, and were prosecuting a common object, each was held guilty as a principal, and not as an abettor of others. *Queen* v. *Tarrinee Churn Chuttopadhya and others*, 7 W. R., Cr., 3.

Exposition of a police officer's powers of arrest and detention of accused persons and witnessess, with a view to the suppression of the practice of Torture. *Queen* v. *Behary Singh and others*, 7 W. R., Cr., 3; Cowell and Woodman, p. 770.

---

* *Chron. Sax.*, A. D. 1137. Wright's England in the Middle Ages.

† Lutfullah says that the Pindaree robbers pounded or pinched the ears of their victims "between the lock of a gun."

‡ Halhed, 315.

ASPHYXIA.

Strangulation.

The practice of Thuggee, although now almost entirely suppressed by the active exertions of Government, could scarcely have been operative for so many centuries throughout the length and breadth of all India without leaving strong traces of its marked atrocities upon the criminal habits of the people.

The fighting Bishop of Bayeux, who preferred the mace to the sword, was scarcely more chary in the shedding of blood than is the Bengalee, when merely prompted by a calm intention to take life for his own advantage, without being goaded on by any urgent promptings of revenge or terror of detection. That is to say, he will rather use his hands or a cloth than his *hussooah*—unless he believes that the latter will be more effectual.

It is considered that Thuggee has prevailed in all parts of India ever since the first irruption of the Mussalmauns. The practice has been clearly described by most of the European travellers who visited this country during the seventeenth century, especially by Thevenot and Dr. John Fryer.*

The first definite and full account of the Indian Stranglers was given, in 1820, by Dr. Richard Crozier Sherwood, a Madras Surgeon,† and the subject

---

* M. Thevenot's description of Thuggee, as practised on the road between Agra and Delhi in 1666, has been frequently cited. Fryer, who came to the country six years later, makes a very distinct allusion to Thuggee, at Surat, in the following passage : "They were fifteen, all of a gang, who used to lurk under hedges in narrow lanes ; and, as they found opportunity, by a device of a weight tied to a cotton bowstring [*i. e.* the string of a bow for beating raw cotton] made of guts (with which they tew cotton) of some length, they used to throw it upon passengers, so that, winding it about their necks, they pulled them from their beasts, and dragging them to the ground, strangled them, and possessed themselves of what they had. One of them was an old man with his two sons, the youngest not fourteen. This being their practice, they were sentenced, according to the *lex talionis*, to be hanged ; wherefore, being delivered to the Cutwal, or Sheriff's men, they led them two miles with ropes about their necks to some wild date trees. In their way thither they were cheerful, and went singing and smoking tobacco, the Banyas giving them sweetmeats. They being as jolly as if going to a wedding ; and the young lad now ready to be tied up, boasted that, though he were not fourteen years of age, he had killed his fifteen men ; wherefore the old man, as he had been the leader of these two, was first made an example for his villany, and then the two striplings were advanced, all as the rest were, half a foot from the ground ; and then, cutting their legs off that the blood might flow from them, they left them miserable spectacles, hanging till they dropped of their own accord."

By the Mussalmaun law, a person strangling another was not liable to suffer death, according to the doctrine of Aboo Huneefah (though he was, in the opinion of the two disciples), unless he be notorious, for committing this offence ; in which case [*i. e.*,e vidently of systematic Thuggee], if he have not shown signs of repentance before he is apprehended, he should be punished with death as an example.—*Harington*, p. 269. So, also, a Strangler confessing his crime, or detected with the usual implements of strangling and stolen property, may be sentenced by the Imam to be beheaded and crucified—p. 328.

† Asiatic Researches, Vol. XIII., p. 250.

was taken up, at about the same time, by Mr. Shakespear, then Superintendent of Police for the Western Provinces. Subsequently, the investigations of General Sleeman led to the exposure of the whole system, and to its almost entire suppression.

The six most recent trials, for Thuggee, in Bengal, which I have succeeded in noting, were held—one at Midnapore in September, 1852*—this, however, was merely supplementary to a trial held in 1838, and ended in the conviction of an aged Thug Jemadar of two murders committed many years previously;—another at Dacca, in May 1854, where a man was found guilty of participation in two acts of thuggee about twenty years previously;† and the third at the same place in December of that year. The crime for which the prisoners were sentenced, was committed fourteen years before. The fourth was tried at Midnapore in August 1855; the prisoner had been denounced as a Thug in 1840.‡ The fifth was the conviction of a Jemadar Thug for crimes committed previously to 1845, which took place at Dacca in 1856.§ The remaining case was decided at Dacca in 1857. The murders had been committed in 1829 or 1830.|| It was stated that, during the year 1854, only two cases of Thuggee occurred in the Punjab.¶

The last conviction for Thuggee in the North-West Provinces, to which I find reference, was on the 11th June 1852, for a crime committed several years previously.

In his Administration Report for 1867, Mr. Mayne, Inspector-General of Police, observed: "I am convinced that no such thing as Thuggee exists now in the North-Western Provinces" (p. 110).

It has, however, already been shown, p. 148 *et seq.*, that the practice of *Thuggee by Poison* is still very generally prevalent throughout all India.

It appears, from the accounts given by the above authorities, that, in Madras, two Phansigars (or stranglers) were considered to be indispensable to effect the murder of every victim, and commonly three were engaged. The most frequent mode of perpetrating the act was by one of them suddenly putting the cloth round the neck of the victim and holding it, while the other end was seized by his accomplice; the ligature, crossed behind the neck, was drawn tight, the two Phansigars pressing the head forwards, while the third villain, crouching in readiness behind the traveller, seized his legs and threw him forward upon the ground. In this situation, he could make little resistance, and the man holding his legs kicked him until life was extinct. They generally buried the body, with its face downwards, in a sandy place or dry water-course, where the soil

---

* Nizamut Adawlut Reports, Vol. II., Part 2, of 1852, p. 581.

† *Ibid*, Vol. IV., p. 621.

‡ *Ibid*, Aug. 17, 1855, p. 303.

§ *Ibid*, June 2, 1856, p. 915.

|| *Ibid*, July 15, 1857, p. 54.

¶ *Friend of India*, 23rd August 1855.

is dug with facility [at present, as we have already seen, by no means a rare mode of concealing the bodies of murdered persons in Bengal]. They often made deep gashes in the bodies, from the shoulders to the hands and to the feet, laying open the abdomen and dividing the tendon of the heel ; wounds were also made between the ribs into the chest ; and sometimes, if the hole was short, the knees were disjointed and the legs turned back upon the body. These precautions were taken to expedite the dissolution of the body, as well as to prevent its inflation which, by raising or causing fissures in the superincumbent sand, might attract jackals and lead to the exposure of the corpse. When the body could not be readily interred, it was tied in a sack and hidden, or was thrown into a tank or well. Forbes states that, during 1808 and 1809, no less than sixty-seven bodies were taken out of wells in the single district of Etawah ; and Baboo Bholanauth Chunder mentions that it was on the discovery of thirty dead bodies in different wells in the Doab, that Thuggee first came to the knowledge of the Calcutta Council in 1810.

The *Megpunnah* Thugs, who murdered poor travellers solely for the purpose of selling their children, almost always threw the bodies of their victims into rivers.

The appearances of Decomposition may possibly be mistaken for those of Strangulation.

On account of the peculiar appearances presented by many bodies in India during the advance of decomposition, there is frequently some danger of the medical officer's assuming that the aspect of the corpse affords presumption of death by Strangulation,* and there certainly do appear to be one or two cases in the records in which it might be questionable whether an error of this kind had not been committed. Where the corpse is found in an attitude which seems to denote that death has come upon it by surprise,—with its arms thrown out and its fingers spread, its lower limbs widely separated and partially drawn up, its head lying back, its neck projecting and turgid with dark fluid blood, the mucous membrane of the larynx of a dirty red colour, the tongue protruded, bloody froth escaping from the mouth and nose, and bloody fluid from the eyes and ears, the eyes starting from the head, the scalp puffy and appearing, when cut into, almost like a bloody sponge,—it is not singular that the idea of Strangulation should first present itself in the surgeon's mind. Standing *alone*, however, these signs go for nothing, when putrefaction has much advanced. They are merely the ordinary

---

* Especially if he bear in memory Shakspear's description of a strangled person :—

" ———His face is black, and full of blood ;
His eyeballs farther out than when he lived,
Staring full ghastly, like a strangled man :
His hair upreared, his nostrils stretch'd with struggling ;
His hands abroad display'd, as one that grasp'd
And tugg'd for life, and was by strength subdued."

KING HENRY VI., PART II., ACT 3.

appearances in a rapidly decomposed full-blooded body, the head and shoulders of which have not been kept raised.

These appearances may be advantageously compared with those observed by Dr. James Anderson in the body of a strong, healthy young man, who was believed to have been strangled by two other muscular able-bodied men. The body was doubled up, the knees drawn up to the chest, there were numerous excoriations on the neck and chin, and deep broad marks round the neck. Ecchymosis was observed in several places under the skin covering the fore part of the chest. The vessels of the head were turgid with blood ; a bloody froth was in the mouth and nostrils, the tongue was protruded, the lungs and right side of the heart filled with fluid black blood, and much ecchymosis was found in the cellular tissue in front of the neck. There was no mark of a rope round the neck, and no water in the trachea or stomach. Death was ascribed to Strangulation.

In 1855, there was tried at Beerbhoom one of those too common cases in which a girl, of between nine and ten years, was killed for the sake of her ornaments. Dr. Sheridan's evidence showed that the body was in such an advanced state of decomposition that minute examination was impossible ; he could not, therefore, give a positive opinion as to the cause of death. From some of the appearances present on examination, however, he thought death had resulted from violence, inasmuch as the tongue protruded very much, the features were much distorted, the eyeballs projected from their sockets, and lividity of the finger nails existed. These appearances, he thought, might have been produced either by external violence to the chest or organs of respiration, or by advanced decomposition. He had examined the deceased's neck and found it was not dislocated ; a large quantity of hair had been pulled out by the roots from the head, but he could not say whether by accident or violence. The prisoner confessed that she gave the girl a blow on the right cheek near the ear, which knocked her down, and then she kicked her on her right side ; she then saw that she was dead, and took the armlet and cloth.

The Sessions Judge remarked that, in the *sooruthal* prepared by the darogah, on the 10th of April, the day after the murder, there is no mention made of the appearances noted by the medical officer,—namely, the protruding of the tongue, distortion of the features, projection of the eyeballs from their sockets, and lividity of the finger-nails, which could scarcely have failed to attract the notice of the darogah had they been present at the time of the inquest, and therefore he (the Judge) was inclined to think those appearances may have been produced by advanced decomposition, as remarked by Dr. Sheridan, particularly as he did not view the body till the second day after the *sooruthal* had been drawn up.*

* Nizamut Adawlut Reports, 6th June 1855, p. 671.

In 1825, Dr. Fuller, of Nuddea, reported his examination of the body of a Mussalmaun woman. The eyes were somewhat protruded and very blood-shot ; the lips swollen and darker than natural ; the tongue slightly protruding between the teeth ; and froth issuing from the nostrils. There was a mark behind the right ear, probably from the pressure of a person's knuckles. There were also three marks, apparently caused by the pressure of the ends of the fingers or knuckles, on the right side of the neck ; a similar mark on the right cheek, and two others on the left cheek, on a line with the lower jaw. Below these, again, there were two similar marks, one very distinct, on the left side of the neck. There were several marks of scratches in front of the right shoulder, above the right breast ; the pectoral muscle under this part was discolored, and blood was extravasated. This, he considered, might have been caused by a blow, or the pressure of a person kneeling on the part. The whole of the integuments of the head, face, neck, and chest were darker than natural, and discolored underneath, particularly the scalp. The brain was suffused by dark blood, the lungs gorged and dark, the bowels of a dusky red color. Hence Dr. Fuller inferred that the woman had met her death from Strangulation.

Did death arise from Strangulation or from some Cerebral Affection ?

This question came prominently forward in a case tried in 1859. A well known Mookhtear, of Mymensingh, was found dead on the bed of a prostitute (the prisoner) in her house in the bazar. It was reported, first, that he died of epilepsy, then of cholera. The case was complicated by the fact that deceased's cousin, who had spent the night with another prostitute in the same house, and those who, with him, removed the deceased to his own house, declared to the darogah that deceased had died in his own house of epilepsy. They were evidently desirous of having no enquiry. The darogah, however, considering that the body presented suspicious appearances, suggested that there should be a *post-mortem* examination. The Civil Surgeon stated that he examined the body twenty-four hours after death, and that death resulted from Strangulation; that there were three marks on the throat, such as would be produced by the nails of the hand ; that these marks, the congestion of the brain and lungs, and the perfectly healthy appearance of all the external organs, left no doubt in his mind that the deceased had been strangled ; and that there were no signs of epilepsy. It appeared that the woman in whose house he died had been the Mookhtear's mistress for three years. That, the night previous, she had strongly urged deceased to give up a mistress with whom he had lately associated. They then smoked *gunja*. A woman, who lived in a house close by, was awake all night, being ill with cholera ; she heard no noise or disturbance in the prisoner's house ; but, just before dawn, she heard a noise of "*hoo! hoo!*" on which the prisoner said, "be quiet." Shortly afterwards the prisoner came out and asked her for fire, and, on her enquiring what had happened, said, she did not know what was the matter with the deceased. Another witness stated that, about day-break, she heard prisoner call deceased and him to get up, and she then heard a gurgling in the throat, and that, when she got up, she saw deceased being carried off in a helpless state ; she did not know whether he was alive or dead. The cousin said that the prisoner called him up early in the morning, being apparently in much alarm at the condition of deceased. He put his hand to the deceased's mouth and found it open, and he heard a slight noise in the throat. He sent the prisoner for a light. He carried deceased off while he was in a helpless state ; he did not ascertain whether he was alive or dead. A Mookhtear, residing in the same house as the deceased, said that, when brought home, the body was still warm, and that the breast moved ; he sent for a kobiraj. In reply to the question whether deceased was liable to epilepsy, he stated that, every two months or so, deceased would lie down, and no one disturbed him on those occasions. Another Mookhtear stated that, once in the preceding year, he and deceased were sleeping together ; deceased made a noise ; he gave him some pushes, when he spat out some phlegm and thanked the witness, saying he had saved him from choking. Prisoner stated, in her defence, that deceased was subject to a disease resembling epilepsy; that his old illness came on in the course of the night ; that she awoke and heard a rattling in his throat, and found he was speechless, at which she at once gave the alarm to his cousin. She held further that it was impossible for a woman like her to have alone murdered the deceased ; that no motive for her doing so had been proved ; that, if the deceased had been murdered, the people of the house would have heard the disturbance, and his cousin would have come to his assistance ; further that the cousin would not have removed the body, but have left it in her house, and have had an enquiry. In the course of his argument, condemning the prisoner, the Sessions Judge held that it would not be difficult for a woman to throttle a man when helpless from intoxication.

Mr. E. A. Samuells, the Judge of the Nizamut Adawlut, remarked : "I am not satisfied in this case that death was the result of Strangulation. It is true that the medical witness deposes that it was; and I do not in the least doubt his skill and perfect good faith in his conclusions from the appearance which the body of the deceased presented ; but I cannot shut my eyes to the fact that the authors of the best works on Medical Jurisprudence find it necessary to caution the medical examiner against mistaking the effects of apoplexy, hysteria, epilepsy, or intoxication for those of manual strangulation, and that, in each of the above diseases, they observed that persons suddenly seized with fatal symptoms may, in their agony, apply their hands to their throats and thus produce marks similar to those which might be expected in cases of strangulation. It is to be observed also that some of the appearances mentioned by the Civil Surgeon are those which occasionally attend decomposition in this country, and which, Dr. Chevers says, have, on two occasions, apparently, been mistaken for appearances resulting from manual strangulation. The Judge urged that the general evidence was in the prisoner's favor. 'It has been suggested,' he wrote, 'that the deceased had been partaking of *gunja*, and may have been so stupefied as to be unable to resist;' but the evidence does not show that he was in any such state of intoxication when he entered her hut with the prisoner. The effects of *gunja*, when taken in moderate quantities, are not such as to produce extreme prostration; and I conceive it most improbable that, if the prisoner had attempted to strangle the deceased with her hands, he should not have been able to throw off and shout for assistance." . . . "There is evidence that he had before been subject to sudden attacks of illness, and it seems not improbable that he may have gone to sleep in a constrained position with his head hanging over the end of the *charpoy*, and that this, combined with the *gunja* which he had taken, may have brought on a fit, during which he applied his hands convulsively to his throat; and which, for want of prompt assistance, terminated fatally. I do not say that it may not have been otherwise, and that the Civil Surgeon may not have been correct in his opinion of the cause of death; but the evidence against the prisoner, under any circumstances, is much too doubtful to admit of a conviction. I acquit the prisoner and direct her immediate release." *

Strangulation to be distinguished from Suicidal Hanging.

It is, of course, a matter of primary importance that the Surgeon should be able to distinguish between Strangulation (which is not often self-inflicted, and which very rarely occurs accidentally,—and then nearly always under circumstances which explain themselves)† and Suicidal Hanging. Our first step, in obtaining this information, is to become acquainted with the modes in which Strangulation is usually effected. The commonest modes of strangling now adopted in India appear to be as follow :—

---

* Carrau's Reports, No. III., 1859, p. 260.

† *Accidental Strangling.*—There is, or was, a stone at Foremark, Derbyshire, of which tradition declares that a man, having stolen a sheep, tied its fore-legs together, and so carried it round his neck. Wishing to rest, he placed the animal on the stone; but the sheep, slipping over on the other side, strangled him. A similar story is told of one John Oxley, who had stolen a deer.—*Notes and Queries*, 2nd series, Vol. I., p. 15.

There is precisely the same legend at Ilfracombe, and it has also been traced in Wales and Normandy.—*Leisure Hour*, May, 1862.

The following is from the Medical Record (New York) for August 1, 1868, p. 262: An Orkney Paper relates a singular case of strangulation in the Island of Stronsay. An old man, named Neil Macpherson, who was carrying on his back a bag, containing 2½ stones of sugar, turned into a stable to rest himself. To lighten his burden, he allowed the bag to rest on the edge of a manger; but, whilst he was momentarily off his guard, it fell to the ground, and the rope by which it was slung over his shoulder tightened round his neck and killed him.

Compressing the Throat with the Hands or with the assistance of the Knee or Foot.

Strangling with the hands appears to be one of the most prevailing modes of killing children, with a view to stealing their ornaments, practised in Bengal. In a good many instances, as we have seen, the throat is cut, or the skull is fractured, or the victim is thrown into a well,—but the last appears to be practised more frequently towards Hindustan, where reservoirs of this kind are more common than in the South.

In very young infants, pressure with the hands is, of course, sufficient to effect the deadly purpose. The following illustrative case is selected from many :—

In 1853, a woman confessed to having squeezed the throat of an infant four months old, which had been left in her charge by its mother; the child was found in the prisoner's arms injured about the neck, which was swollen and scratched, and had apparently been squeezed. The prisoner acknowledged that she was to blame, and that it was her fate to destroy the child,—which died in four hours. The Civil Surgeon declared that death was caused by pressure of some kind applied to the throat. It was decided by the Court that the prisoner had probably intended merely to do such hurt to the child as would seriously alarm the mother.*

In older children, however, a greater amount of power is generally employed. Thus, in 1853, a woman confessed, at Cuttack, that two other women having stripped a child seven years old of her ornaments, and twisted her cloth round her mouth, and tied her hands behind her, she, upon compulsion, laid hold of the left hand of the deceased, while she held her own infant in her left, and one of her companions sat on the deceased's chest, while the other squeezed her throat with both her hands, and she groaned and died.†

See a similar case in Bellasis's (Bombay) Reports, p. 88.

In 1805, one Sona Ghazee confessed that he had killed his mistress by seizing her by the throat, and holding her tight for nearly an hour.‡

Two men of Hurda confessed that they jointly throttled to death with their hands a person who had intrigued with the wife of one of them.§

See a curious case, in which a boy having been strangled, apparently by the pressure of the knee, the accused declared that he had been killed in a bamboo *chepa*, or press, by an evil spirit.‖

---

* Nizamut Adawlut Reports, Vol. III., Part 1, of 1853, p. 222. See also another case, in which a child of five months was throttled by its mother.—*Nizamut Adawlut Reports*, N. W. P., May 6th, 1853, p. 646.

† *Ibid*, Vol. III., Part 1, 1853, p. 227.

‡ Macnaghten's Reports, Vol. I., p. 60.—See also *Ibid*, 139, and Vol. II., p. 355. See also Nizamut Adawlut Reports, N. W. P., April 9th, 1853, p. 519 ; and Nizamut Adawlut Reports, October 11th, 1854, p. 441.

§ Nizamut Adawlut Reports, N. W. P., December 9th, 1853, p. 1467. See also these Reports for July 16th, 1853, p. 866—(Three persons found guilty of throttling a man.)

‖ Nizamut Adawlut Reports, April 15th, 1859, p. 117.

The following case appears to show that a single individual may be capable of inflicting the utmost degree of violence upon the throat of an adult, occasioning instantaneous death. In 1852, a man of thirty-two was convicted of attacking an old woman, seizing her by the hair, dragging her into a house, throwing her down, and stamping upon her throat, and violently wrenching and breaking her neck.*

In 1852, a man of Furruckabad, eighteen years of age, confessed that, having discovered that his wife was unfaithful, he had murdered her by striking her on the face and neck with a *koorpa*. The Civil Surgeon found several incised wounds on the face. The windpipe and soft parts about the throat were also ruptured, and the spine fractured a little below the head.†

I have met with only one suspicious case of fractured cervical vertebræ in this country. The injury was terribly severe, but the body was too much decomposed to admit of an opinion regarding the manner in which it had been inflicted. For cases of fracture of the cervical vertebræ, *see* p. 451.

One Dalla, of Bareilly, confessed, at the thannah, that he murdered a child of six by compressing his neck with his feet. On trial, he declared that the boy was lying close to a wall, when he (prisoner) leapt down from the wall, and his foot fell on the neck of the child, who died.‡ A boy of fourteen was convicted, at Cuttack, as an accomplice in the wilful murder of a child of eleven. He said that he saw a person, whom he named, squeezing deceased's throat with both his big toes.§ A woman of Jounpore confessed that she had killed a child eighteen months old, by placing her foot on its throat.‖

Dr. Duncan Stewart mentioned to me the particulars of a case which he was engaged in investigatiug many years since. An aged woman was found dead on her bed ; suspicion arose ; there was scarcely any external trace of injury, but it was found that one of the wings of the ossified thyroid cartilage had been broken and forced inwards, causing suffocation.

It would not appear, from the records, that those very severe injuries to the neck, such as laceration of the muscles of the throat, rupture of the tracheal rings, &c., &c., occasionally observed in European cases of Strangling, are frequent in similar instances in India. I have more than once found traces of very severe contusion of the muscles of the throat ; and the appearance of coagula in the trachea, in Dr. Leckie's case, p. 589, will be remarked. Still, whether owing to the employment of several accessories in these cases, or the use of long soft cloths which form a part of nearly every native's dress—or to a theoretical acquaintance

---

* Nizamut Adawlut Reports, Vol. II., Part 2, of 1852, p. 935.

† Nizamut Adawlut Reports, N. W. P., December 21st, 1852, p. 1536.

‡ *Ibid*, March 3rd, 1855, p. 298.

§ *Ibid*, October 18th, 1853, p. 660.

‖ *Ibid*, March 29th, 1855, p. 439.

with the practices of the Phansigars which must exist among all classes in India—it is certain that the rule which maintains that "in Strangling, a much greater degree of violence is commonly employed than is necessary to cause destruction,"* will be found to have very numerous exceptions in this country.

Compression of the Throat with Sticks or other Solid Bodies.

It may be inferred from facts given in the Chapters on *Bans-dolla* and *Beating*, that placing a stick across the throat, a rather frequent practice in Bengal, is a means of keeping down and silencing a victim which is had recourse to in various kinds of homicidal assault. Wherever this is done, it is, I believe, fully intended that the victim shall never rise again; and by means of it, in all probability, the *coup de grace* is sometimes given, after much slow torture, in some cases where mere Strangulation would have been deemed too merciful a death.

Intriguers are frequently put to death in this manner.

In 1838, a Hooghly man, after having endeavoured to break off a criminal connexion between a person and his wife, discovered them together in an equivocal posture; on which he threw the lover on the ground, on his back, and then, placing a stick across his throat, strangled him to death. Three days afterwards, he killed his wife, by placing his foot on her throat, and threw her body before the police, who had come to arrest him for the murder of her lover.†

It appeared, in a trial at Cuttack, that one Dusruthy Sreechundun having been in the habit of intriguing with the wives of the villagers, a party of men arranged to kill him. They waylaid him, and threw him down on the ground, one stood on his neck, then a bamboo was placed across his throat; its two ends were pressed down with hands and feet; one stood on his stomach, and the rest held his hands and feet. These prisoners were transported for life.‡

Gour Chand, of Rungpore, having an intrigue with a woman whom her brother made the Bustemee of another man, was, on being caught near the house, tied by the hands and feet to the props of a hut and beaten; he was then given water in which salt had been dissolved, and was untied. They then took him away to a distance, threw him down, and putting one bamboo over, and another under, his neck, and pressing down the ends of the former, strangled him. Two of the prisoners were condemned to death.§

Shaik Bahadoor, of Tirhoot, actuated by jealousy, murdered his wife

---

* Taylor, p. 678.
† Police Reports, L. P., 1838, p. 133.
‡ Nizamut Adawlut Reports, August 3, 1855, p. 253.
§ *Ibid*, February 4, 1856, p. 337.

by putting a lattee across her throat, and standing with a foot on each end of the stick. He escaped.*

In 1848, three persons, of Chumparûn, caught a man in the act of stealing two buffaloes, and tied him to a post, with the alleged intent of taking him to the thannah ; but two of them, being enraged with him on account of previous acts of theft and intrigue, took him into a field, and there strangled him by compressing his neck between two bamboos.†

It appeared, at a trial at Tirhoot, in 1853, that a widow having become pregnant, several of her relatives took her and a woman who lived with her into a remote place, whither two witnesses declared that they were attracted by hearing screams, and saw both the deceased on the ground, each held down by three men, who strangled them by pressing lattees across their throats.‡

A similar crime was committed at Shahjehanpore (N. W. P.) at about the same time. The relations of a young woman, suspecting her of frailty, took her at midnight to the banks of a Nuddee, where a man who had been guarding his field declared that he saw her lying on the ground, and each of two persons named pressing on different ends of a stick placed across her throat.§

In 1841, Mr. Dickson, of Gyah, gave evidence in a case where it was stated that murder had been committed by pressing the man's neck between two lattees. Mr. Dickson thought that a mark found on the throat of the deceased was such as would have been produced by the pressure of a cord, in strangulation ; but, the body being in an advanced state of decomposition, he considered that a mark caused by lattees would not be different from that observed.

In a dispute about date trees at Nuddea, one Gridhur struck Sooruck Khan with a banghy bamboo, stunning him. A companion laid the bamboo across the fallen man's neck applying pressure to it with both his hands. Gridhur thumped the man's abdomen with his fists, and knocked him also on the same part. The medical officer found the head split above the left ear, there was a black mark on the neck ; there was blood in the stomach indicating the application of great violence. He considered that death was caused by the blows on the head.‖

Four Hindus were cutting grass without leave in the field of one Sewdewan Narain. Upon being remonstrated with, two of these threw him down, and placed their sticks across his throat, while the other two mounted his belly, and struck him with their fists and elbows. He died on the spot.¶

* Bengal Police Reports, 1868, p. 184.
† Police Report, L. P., 1848, p. 6.
‡ Nizamut Adawlut Reports, 27th August, 1853, p. 316.
§ *Ibid*, N. W. P., 17th January 1853, p. 63.
‖ Nizamut Adawlut Reports, May 19, 1855, p. 592.
¶ *Ibid*, October 2, 1855, p. 528.

At the trial of certain ryots for the murder of a gomashta at Midnapore, in 1853, two of the prisoners confessed that they and others suddenly seized the deceased, threw him on the ground, beat him, and squeezed his neck between two pieces of stick, which caused his immediate death. One of these sticks was a split bamboo, three feet long, and weighing about three pounds; the other was a close-grained stick, three feet long, weighing about two pounds.*

In 1841, Dr. Duncan, of Chittagong, gave evidence in a case where it appeared probable that death had resulted from compression of the throat with a broad flat stick, but the details are not sufficiently full to lead to any practical inference.

In 1846, the inhabitants of a village in the same district, disturbing a stranger in the act of thieving, killed him by pressing a bamboo on his neck. There were no external marks of violence.†

One of the murderers of a child of five, at Bareilly, confessed that he had pulled at the *Huslee* (silver ring) round the child's neck. Elsewhere he stated that he had filled his victim's mouth with earth, and made compression on the throat with his fingers.‡

A girl of thirteen was discovered strangled in a field. The Civil Surgeon deposed that he found a mark extending round the neck, as if it had been tightly bound with a cord. The front part of the neck was much bruised, and the windpipe and parts within the throat were ruptured. One Mohun appears to have committed the murder for the sake of a silver *Huslee* which the girl wore on her neck. The injuries described certainly appear to have been such as might have been produced by compressing the girl's throat with the narrow edge of her Neck Ring.§

In 1853, two persons were convicted at Behar of strangling a youth of fourteen, for the sake of his ornaments, and of then dismembering and concealing the body. It appeared that one of the prisoners, a powerful man, was seen pressing the deceased upon the ground with the step of a ladder on his throat, while the other prisoner held him by the feet.||

Compressing or Tying the Throat with a Cord, Cloth, or Stalk.

In 1849, Mr. F. Henderson, then of Moorshedabad, examined the body of a Mussalmaun, which was tied, head and knees together. There was

---

* Nizamut Adawlut Reports, Vol. III., Part 2, of 1853, p. 12.
† Police Report, L. P., 1846, p. 3.
‡ Nizamut Adawlut Reports, N. W. P., 3rd March 1853, p. 311.
§ *Ibid*, 13th January 1855, p. 42.
|| *Ibid*, Vol. III., Part 1, of 1853, p. 54.

also a thinner cord passed tightly round the throat, leaving its mark impressed on the skin. The face was livid and swollen ; a little blood had oozed from the nostrils. The general appearance was that of a person who had died from Strangulation or Choking. There were no external wounds or marks of beating.

Again, in 1846, Dr. Greig examined, also at Moorshedabad, the bodies of a woman and girl, in both of which there was a mark round the neck of a thin rope tied tightly in such a manner as to cause death by Strangulation. The rope still remained on the neck of the girl. There appear to have been no other outward traces of violence.* Five convicts of Midnapore Jail went out to work in charge of a burkundauz. They attacked their guard in a lonely spot, tied his feet together, and his hands behind his back, and then strangled him by knotting round his throat old pieces of cloth and "*newar*," which they had used to support their irons. He was a powerful man and appeared to have resisted violently. It was considered that the prisoners, who were much weaker men, attacked him when he had fallen asleep.†

In 1855 a Moorshedabad boy was strangled for the sake of his ornaments. The neck and mouth were tightly bound by the boy's own cloths.‡ A woman of Sylhet, having quarrelled with the mother of a child of six, the poor little boy having told that she had stolen some ghee from them, strangled the child and concealed the body in a tank. The child's mouth was "stuffed up, and his head covered with a cloth."

In July 1854, one Bhowanee was capitally sentenced at Furruckabad for having, as he himself confessed, strangled his sister-in-law, aged fifty-five years, with a flexible twig tow from a *dhak* tree. The twisted stick was found on the neck of the corpse. He was supposed to have been aided by accomplices.§

The stalks of the *Urhur* dhal appear frequently to afford a ready instrument for Strangulation in the North-West.

---

* Strangulation with a cord, Macnaghten's Reports, Vol. I., p. 75.—See also a case in which a Hindu confessed to having strangled a child with a cloth for the sake of his ornaments. —*Ibid*, Vol. I., p. 41. A man of Shahjehanpore was sentenced capitally for murdering a boy seven years old by tying a handkerchief tightly round his neck. He then threw the body into a well.‖ A man of Rajshahye having become jealous, apparently without just cause, of his wife, a girl of thirteen, knocked her down and strangled her with a cord.¶ A lad of thirteen was murdered at Furruckabad for the sake of his ornaments. The body was found in a deep well with a tight cord wound twice round the neck.** A man of Cawnpore confessed that he and four others strangled a person by tying a handkerchief round his neck. The body was found in a well with a *roomal* tied round the neck.††

† Nizamut Adawlut Reports, Novr. 24th, 1854, p. 655.

‡ *Ibid*, Novr. 28th, 1855, p. 833.

§ *Ibid*, N. W. P., for July 1854, p. 105.

‖ Nizamut Adawlut Reports, N. W. P., May 3rd, 1853, p. 634.

¶ *Ibid*, April 6th, 1854, p. 449.

** *Ibid*, March 29th, 1852, p. 226.

†† *Ibid*, Novr. 15th, 1853, p. 1371.

In 1854, a boy of seven was murdered at Shahjehanpore, for the sake of his ornaments. The body was found in a field of *Urhur*, with a stalk bound tightly round the neck.*

A boy of Jounpore was murdered in a precisely similar manner about two months subsequently.†

A case has recently been reported from Madras in which a woman nearly succeeded in strangling herself by means of her long hair.

There is a distinct and very important class of cases in which the victim is ***strangled after having been rendered insensible by Blows on the Head or by other mechanical means.***

In 1841, Dr. Leckie, then of Bhaugulpore, examined the body of one Poorun. There existed extravasation of blood over the left side of the scalp. The left temple was considerably bruised externally, the inner surface of the scalp was generally of a red color, and the blood-vessels were turgid. Marks of compression were observed on the front of the neck, attended with slight extravasation of blood on the left side. The trachea internally was also injected, and contained a few loose clots of blood. Several bruises existed upon both arms, and were further marked by effused blood being found in the cellular tissue. Dr. Leckie was disposed to attribute death to the effects of Strangulation and the injuries above detailed.

The following case, by Mr. Alexander Grant, then of Bhaugulpore, affords a very demonstrative illustration. In 1845, Mr. Grant examined the body of a female, apparently eighteen or nineteen years of age, who was reported to have met with a violent death on the previous evening. The body was fresh, and lay in the cot in which it had been brought. The features were composed, the eyes half open, the lips livid, the jaws firmly closed, and the mouth contained a bloody saliva. The only mark of external violence was a dark horizontal line around the middle of the neck, as if a cord or bow-string had been tightly applied there. The lungs were crepitant, and of a reddish brown color. When cut into, they were found filled with blood and froth. The heart was healthy, and its cavities were filled with dark fluid blood. On making pressure on the lungs, a frothy mucus issued from the nostrils. The abdominal viscera were much congested, but their structures were healthy. The stomach contained a plentiful meal of undigested rice, which gave out no particular smell, as of opium or of alcohol; the mucous coat was injected equally with that of the intestinal canal and the womb. In the vagina was a copious purulent discharge. The bladder was empty. Upon removing the scalp, a broad circular patch of effused blood was observed over the right vertex, and

* Nizamut Adawlut Reports, March 21st, 1854, p. 301.

† *Ibid*, May 6th, p. 478.

a smaller one over the left vertex, while there was a similar patch over the upper and left side of the forehead. There was no fracture of the bones, but the contusions must have been inflicted with some blunt instrument before life was extinct. The vessels of the brain were loaded with dark blood, but there was no great engorgement of this organ, the substance of which was healthy. The absence of any appearance of natural death, the evidence of her having taken a hearty meal a short time previous to death, the line round the neck, the marks of injury on the head, the condition of the lungs and other viscera, appeared to Mr. Grant sufficiently positive proofs of death from violence; and he was disposed to venture the opinion that deceased was first stunned by the blows on the head, and then strangled by the application of a cord round the neck, and pressure by the hand on the mouth and nostrils. He was of opinion that, had not previous insensibility been produced, there would have been some external marks on her body to indicate her struggles. Any doubt as to suicide seemed removed by the contusions on the head, which could not, by any probability, have been self-inflicted, while the evidences of intoxication or narcotism were not present.

The details of the above case carry with them, in the most demonstrative manner, indication of the various points of inquiry which should be thoroughly made out by the Surgeon in every examination of this kind,—*viz.*, the evidences of death by Strangulation—the presence or absence of signs of drugging or intoxication—the existence or non-existence of traces of a struggle for life—and the appearance or non-appearance of injuries to the head sufficient to have caused insensibility.

A Mussalmaun of Dacca having hired a boat, took a prostitute with her property on board, under pretence of taking an excursion. During the night, he made her drunk, strangled her, and threw the body overboard.*

For cases illustrative of the crime of *Strangling persons while under the Influence of Drugs or Intoxicating Liquors*,—See pages 156 *et seq.* and 223 of this Manual.

There occurs, in this country, still another very important and difficult class of instances, *viz.*,—those in which *the individual having been strangled*, whether in a state of insensibility or otherwise, *is suspended by the neck*, either immediately or after the lapse of an interval.

In 1852, a Hindu confessed, at Backergunge, that he and three others had committed the murder, by strangulation, of a man, who had an illicit connexion with his sister, and of a woman who had given her medicine to produce abortion, and had published her disgrace. He avowed that they had thrown the man down, placed a bamboo across his throat,

---

* Police Report, L. P., 1843, p. 40.

and pressed it down with their feet on each side until he died, one of them holding down the feet and legs, and another holding down his head by the hair;—they had afterwards killed the woman in the same way. That, having despatched both, they hung their bodies by ropes upon a mangoe tree (where they were found next morning), that it might be thought that they hanged themselves. When discovered, the body of the man hung with the feet raised above the ground, the woman's feet touched the earth, and were bent or doubled in consequence. When the Civil Surgeon examined the bodies, the circumstances of the case were not known. He appears to have reported that there was a mark all round the neck of each body, and a protrusion of the tongue, as if death had been caused by strangulation. This mark he considered, or at all events was understood to consider, was that of the *rope*, and he was of opinion that, in neither case, was this mark produced before life was quite extinct. If so, it was concluded, the woman must have been too far gone to rally, as her feet rested on the ground. One of the Sudder Judges remarked that the medical officer's opinion, if correct, would belie the confessions, and quoted Dr. Taylor's statement,* that ecchymosed marks may be produced on the neck of a dead body suspended soon after death, and the assertion of Merzdorff that it would be in the highest degree difficult, if not impossible, to determine medically, from an inspection of the body, whether a man had been hanged while living, or whether he had been first suffocated and hanged up immediately after death. He further quoted Beck, on the same subject, who holds (page 628) that the ecchymosed mark is a decided proof of suspension during life, but, at the same time, quotes Orfila as unequivocally stating that, in twelve experiments on the dead body, some immediately after death, some after 6, 8, and 18 hours, the depression made by the cord and the skin under it, as well as the sub-cutaneous cellular tissue, presented precisely the same appearances as they do from suspension before death: from this he inferred that the appearance noted all round the neck was not inconsistent with the statements of the prisoners that they strangled the deceased first, and then suspended them.

It does not appear evident that the medical officer's deposition belied the confessions of the prisoners, nor does any real discrepancy exist between the opinion of Beck, and that held by Orfila, Taylor, Devergie, and Merzdorff. In comparing homicidal cases of strangulation and hanging with the results of experiment, a broad distinction must be drawn between real and apparent death. A person strangled, stunned, suffocated, or poisoned may remain *physiologically* alive for a considerable time, after all outward evidences of life have ceased. Indeed, physiologically,

---

* Page 677, Fifth Edition.

life is not absolutely extinct until the cessation of cadaveric rigidity, often at a period of many hours after the occurrence of apparent death.* It is therefore probable that, all other circumstances being equal, the appearances of vital disturbance produced in the structures of the necks of persons strangled or hanged previous to death, and of bodies suspended at periods from five minutes up to the cessation of rigidity several hours after apparent death, would merely present a series of vascular changes gradually receding from the strongest to the least marked.

In 1853, a Hindu, of Dacca, was found guilty of strangling his wife, and of suspending her body to a mangoe tree at the back of her father's house.†

A man, of Mymensing, having intrigued with a widow, and not giving her sufficient means for her support, she complained to the village Punchayet, who decided that both parties should be beaten. The man was seized by his father and was struck several blows, but the woman managed to escape. The paramour, enraged at having been summoned and beaten before the Punchayet, pursued her with three of his relatives. On coming up with her, they strangled her; and, hanging her body on a tree hard by, reported that she had committed suicide.‡

In the same year, the father and brothers of a girl of Tipperah, finding her in company with a man with whom she was intriguing, seized the man, and, holding him down by the neck, arms, and legs, strangled him. They then hung up the corpse, and reported that he had destroyed himself.§

A man of Serajgunge, having failed to persuade a woman with whom he had an intrigue, to break off the connexion, murdered her. There were several discrepancies in his own confessions, and in the statements of the only eye-witness—a boy of twelve—but it appeared probable that he had first compressed the woman's throat with his hands, until life was nearly extinct, and that he then suspended the body to a tree.‖

In 1854, a man of Jessore, after having brutally injured his young wife, strangled her, and then suspended her body by the neck to a tamarind tree.¶

One of these cases occurred in 1853 at Shahjehanpore in the N. W. Provinces. Some persons having been employed by a spirit-seller to pull down the shop of a rival dealer, knocked down the unfortunate

---

* This distinction is of very great importance, and full validity in a large proportion of medico-legal investigations involving an examination of the body—but any attempt to make use of it in cases of *disputed survivorship* would be evidently irrational and vexatious.

† Nizamut Adawlut Reports, Vol. III., Part 2, of 1853, p. 107.

‡ Police Report, L. P., 1848, p. 33.

§ *Ibid*, p. 37.

‖ Nizamut Adawlut Reports, 22nd August 1854, p. 283.

¶ *Ibid*, July 31st, 1854, p. 158.—Already cited at page 219.

abkar, got on him, pressed his neck, and strangled him, and then suspended him by the neck to a burgol tree close by. The evidence was, however, not thought sufficiently reliable to justify conviction.*

Two men of Bareilly confessed, on apprehension and before the Joint Magistrate, that they laid a plan to murder a person who appears to have intrigued with the wife of one of them. They threw him down, strangled him with a rope, and then suspended his body to a tree.†

One Mohumda, of Dehra Doon, having been too intimate with the wife of a *fakeer*, but failing to persuade her to go to his house, strangled her husband, probably with the woman's assistance, and suspended his body to a beam in the house.‡

A Bogra woman (see p. 594) was found hanging. *Post-mortem* examination showed clearly that strangulation by hand, and not by hanging, was the cause of death.§

Pengah Doe, a chowkeedar of Dacca, being enraged and probably intimidated by the reproaches of a cast-off mistress, clutched her by the throat, and never relaxed his grasp till his victim was dead. He then, assisted by his father, a man of eighty, hung up the body.||

HANGING.

In India, as elsewhere, the Medical Jurist's opinion is especially called for (1) in cases where bodies have been suspended after violent death; (2) in instances of suicide, and of (3) murder by Hanging; and (4) in cases of apparent drowning, &c., where it is questionable whether death has not resulted from homicidal Hanging.

Suspension of Murdered Bodies by the neck.

I. Aware of the great prevalence of suicide by Hanging, the criminals of this country not unfrequently destroy their victims by blows, &c., and suspend them, with a hope that their deaths will be attributed to self-destruction. The foregoing remarks will show that the detection of such cases cannot always be easily accomplished. From time to time, however, collateral circumstances, the revelations of eye-witnesses, or the confessions of the criminals have furished us with nearly demonstrative instances of each description of crime.

The following narrative, by Dr. Beatson, strikingly displays the difficulties with which the investigation of some of these cases are fraught.¶

Body of a man, name unknown, said to have been found suspended in a

---

* Nizamut Adawlut Reports, N. W. P., 21st June 1853, p. 784.
† *Ibid*, 6th July 1852, p. 635.
‡ *Ibid*, 24th November 1852, p. 1371.
§ Bengal Police Report for 1866, p. 248.
|| Nizamut Adawlut Reports, April 1856, p. 658.
¶ Ind. Med. Gaz., April 1, 1866, p. 83.

stranded boat, near the village of Sreenugger. Hindoo, age twenty to thirty; loins clothed with a large dhoty of good cloth, not disordered. The hands and neck are tied together by a halter attached by a noose to the right wrist; from which it passes behind the right hip, between the legs, and in front of the left hip to the left wrist, which is passed between the strands of the cord. It then passes up to the right side of the neck, surrounds it, and forms a running noose with a slip knot. The running end has been divided at some distance from the body by a knife. The feet are also tied together by a cord passing once round the ankles, but not tightly; the right heel being drawn up and nearly released. The body is that of a stout strongly-built man, and well-nourished; the chest and abdomen are covered with hair; putrefaction has far advanced; the head and face are enormously swollen, and covered with flies and maggots; the eyes and tongue protrude, and the cuticle is stripped off in flakes from the trunk. The cavities are distended with gases, rendering the ligature binding the hands and neck, very tense. There are no wounds or injuries on any part of the body, and the skull and ribs are unbroken.

This may have been a case of suspension after death, by other persons, to give the appearance of suicide, of murder by strangulation, or of suicidal hanging. The first is the least probable; it is certain that death was not caused by beating or wounding: and, supposing, the man to have been killed by poison, or to have died from natural causes, it could have served no purpose to suspend him in a manner so suspicious. For the second, the co-operation of several men would have been required; a young and powerful man would not have succumbed without a struggle, of which his body would have borne marks, and the murder could not have been effected at the place where the corpse was found, without some noise having been made. In support of the third supposition, it appears that ligatures, similarly prepared, might be self-applied. The feet being first bound, and the end of the halter attached to a beam, the noose may be drawn over the head and the left wrist thrust through the untwisted strands of the cord. Both hands still remain free to form the last loop, through which the right wrist can be passed, and, on the man casting himself off, all would have been drawn tight. The result of the police investigation was that no noise or struggle had been heard; that no suspicion attached to any one; that no one was missing from the neighbourhood; and that the man was an entire stranger, who had never been seen in it before the discovery of his body.

This case should be compared with one by Dr. Woodford, in which, before throwing himself into a well, a man tied himself by the neck, hands, and feet, in a complete net-work of thin rope—p. 638.

The district of Bogra appears to hold an evil pre-eminence in the special addiction of its inhabitants to the device of suspending the bodies of murdered persons by the neck. In going over the annual Police

Report of that district for 1868, I find that no less than nine such cases were brought to light within that twelvemonth.

In January 1852, the body of one Hossein Buksh was found hanging on a tamarind tree, just outside the garden wall of a person named Sheikh Mohasun, at Hooghly, the defendant in the trial which ensued. It was made out in evidence, with a great clearness, that the deceased, led either by an intention to steal, or by a desire for revenge on account of an illicit connexion which existed between his wife and the prisoner,—made his way, late on the fatal night, into an upper room of the prisoner's house, armed with a hatchet. He struck at and slightly wounded the wife first, and then the prisoner, who, however, struggled with him and, aided by three of his servants, threw him down, and tied his hands with a rope. Nothing further was distinctly known until the body was found hanging, on the following morning, by the darogah, who had come to inspect the premises, upon the prisoner's information that the deceased had entered his house with an intention to steal, and had, after wounding him, run away. Dr. Ross deposed that he saw the body hanging. The rope was tied to a lower and upper branch. [It appears that these two branches were more than three feet apart.] It could not have been adjusted by him in any other manner than by standing on the wall, from which he was too far. [The tree stood off three feet from the wall.] The place where the rope was tied to the two branches was inclining away from the wall, and away shortly from the trunk of the tree; the distanee and the [intervening position of the] trunk of the tree rendered it impossible that the deceased could have tied the ropes himself. The only way that the hanging could have been effected was by others, either on the wall and tree, or on the tree only. There was a quantity of blood between the wall and the tree. Dr. Ross examined the body, and was of opinion that death was caused by his being stunned or stupefied by blows on the head, giving rise to profuse hæmorrhage, and by his being hung by the neck, while in that state of insensibility or stupor, until life was extinct. The marks on the neck showed that he was not lifeless when he was first suspended, but he must have been very near it, as the mark on the neck had not the perfect characteristic parchment-like appearance which invariably exists when death has occurred from hanging exclusively. The lungs and heart also did not exhibit the morbid signs which are the results of Hanging—there was no gorged state of the vessels of the lungs, and the heart was completely empty of blood. There were various marks, scratches, and abrasions on the surface of the body, more particularly on the arms; the outer skin of the right wrist had been scraped off by some means, either by having been tied by a rope, or dragged over a rough surface. The two first fingers of the right hand had been removed some years ago. The remaining stumps of the fingers were permanently bent towards the palm, and prevented the perfect antagonism between the thumb and the remaining fingers, so that he would be more easily overpowered by his assailants, and the same mutilation would prevent him from adjusting the rope with which he was hung with the accuracy observed.* The blanched state of the brain, the tongue, and the gums, went far to prove that he was in too weak a state, from loss of blood, to have hung himself. The weapon which was probably employed was of a bluntish nature (if at all of a cutting character), as the wounds were much contused. †

The proceedings of the Calcutta Coroner's Court in the following very remarkable case were sent to me by the late Mr. Piddington:—

Bhemo, wife of a poor oil-man, had been suffering, for a year or more, from severe spasmodic pains in the stomach (*sool bedna*), probably caused by worms, and had often expressed an intention of destroying herself, a wish to die, &c., if she could find no relief shortly. On the 2nd July 1848, the festival of the *Oolta Ruth*, her husband, on returning from his work, found, as he said, the door fastened, and, on opening it, saw his wife hanging to two of the bamboo cross-beams of the roof. He gave the alarm to the police. On *post-mortem* examination, on the following day, the features were very much swollen, bloody serum issued from the mouth and nostrils. On removing the hair, Dr. Maxton observed blood issuing from a small hole in the scalp. This hole penetrated the right parietal bone, and extended upwards of two inches into the right hemisphere of the brain. It appeared "to have been produced by a gimlet or brad-awl,

* A case which, in some measure, meets this particular point, is cited by Taylor. A woman was found dead in her bed at the Hotel Dieu, with her head hanging out, and with a silk handkerchief carried twice round the neck, and then tied in front. In this instance, in which there could be no doubt of suicidal strangulation, the deceased *had lost four fingers of her right hand*, so that the member had been, from a very early period, of but little service to her; "Nevertheless," remarks Dr. Taylor, "she contrived to tie the cravat round her neck with great firmness and dexterity. It is easy to conceive that, had her body been found in a suspicious locality, a plausible opinion of homicidal strangulation might have been formed from the maimed condition of her hand. This case then," he adds, "will serve to teach us a proper caution in drawing our inferences as to what persons, laboring under any corporeal infirmity, are capable of doing, when they make attempts on their own lives,"—p. 683. See also the case of the Prince de Conde, who, it was alleged, could not have hanged himself on, account of a defect in one hand, which, it was thought, prevented him from tying the knots (p. 669).

† Nizamut Adawlut Reports, Vol. II., Part 1, of 1852, p. 18.—In the following case, there was certainly reason to suspect that the deceased was hung by others, but the decomposed state of the body rendered the proof of this defective. In 1843, Dr. Murray, of Beerbhoom, examined the body of a man, in which he found great swelling of the temple and cheek extending to the ear, and very well marked behind the ear, over a space at least three inches long and about two inches broad. These parts were gorged with blood, which, in some places, was coagulated. The state of the brain was so altered as to preclude an opinion as to whether it had or had not been injured. There was the mark of a rope round the neck. This, Dr. Murray believed, had been produced after death, because the skin was merely corrugated, and, there was no injury to the superficial blood-vessels, soft parts, or windpipe, nor any luxation of the spine. The tongue was [protruded?] between the teeth, but there was no swelling either above or below the mark on the neck, neither was there any congestion in any part of the head, except on those spots first alluded to as bearing marks of violence.

or some sharp-pointed instrument finer than a nail. There was a great extravasation of blood within the cranium." He did not think it possible that such a wound could be self-inflicted, and held it to be "of course more impossible," that, after such a wound, the deceased could hang herself. A wound of this description would induce immediate stupor, and, during that stupor, a person might be hung. There was no pus about the wound, which was, no doubt, perfectly fresh. This mode of destroying life, by perforating the skull, has often been employed in children. He had no sort of doubt that the whole must have been perpetrated by other persons, and that the deceased could not have destroyed herself. There was a dark livid mark, as if produced by a cord, running upwards and backwards, on the neck ; the body was quite fresh, and there was no doubt that the mark of hanging had been produced during life. Heart nearly empty ; lungs and liver very much congested ; the stomach and intestines inflamed, the latter containing worms. He considered that either the wound of the brain or the strangulation by the rope would have caused death.

Nothing whatever could be found to throw any suspicion on any person connected with the deceased. The house-door was public, there were neighbours on both sides, and there was but one entrance to the room. No robbery had been committed. In his charge to the jury, the coroner, adverting to some other instances of mysterious murders, without any apparent motive (one or two of which had also occurred on *Feast Days*), suggested as the only possible means of accounting for them, and for this one, that they may be perpetrated in fulfilment of vows to Kali, as the ancient human sacrifices at Kali Ghat were known to be. Verdict, "wilful murder against some person or persons unknown."

This case may be advantageously placed beside that of the man whose longitudinal sinus was transfixed by a nail, *vide supra*, p. 437.

A man of Sylhet struck his wife with a piece of split bamboo about the body, for eating more than her share of pawn, until she died. He than hanged her body on a tree.*

A man of Dinagepore, who had been in the habit of maltreating his wife, was stated by two witnesses to have shown them her dead body in his house, and then, with their assistance, to have carried it to the jungle and suspended it to a tree. He was acquitted.†

It appeared, in a trial at Moorshedabad, that a person was chased by others into a house, and that, immediately after their departure, he was found suspended by the neck to a beam with his toes touching the ground. The medical officer discovered no marks of violence, but stated that

---

* Police Reports, L. P., 1838, p. 76.

† *Ibid*, 1849, p. 29.

death resulted from strangulated hernia. The prisoners were found guilty of culpable homicide.*

The wife of a man living in the 24-Pergunnahs, having a criminal intrigue with another Hindu, she and her paramour enticed the unfortunate man out of his house at night, killed him or rendered him insensible (it would seem by severe blows), and suspended his body to a tree.†

It appeared, in a trial at Cuttack, that a Hindu, charging another with theft, beat him to death. The man's body was afterwards found suspended, with marks of violence upon it, in such a position as to render it evident that he had not hanged himself.‡

I do not meet with the record of any instance in which a native was *proved* to have been *poisoned and afterwards hanged,* although this crime has been much spoken of (perhaps erroneously), and has been suspected in cases like the following :—In May 1854, Mr. Stuart, of Azimghur, reported that he had examined the body of one Soobhao, chumar, and had found a mark round the neck ; it was, however, only superficial, and he believed that the string was put on after death. The sub-cellular tissues on either side of the neck were perfectly natural. There was, indeed, no sign of strangulation, but the stomach and intestines, especially the inner coat of the former, were much congested and inflamed, as if he had died of poisoning. The stomach contained some dark fluid, which was forwarded to Calcutta for examination, but no poison could be discovered.

I have more than once had opportunity of verifying Dr. Yeolly's observation, that the mucous membrane of the stomach is liable to be found much congested in death from hanging. Doubtless, microscopical examination would enable us to distinguish this from the lesions produced by corrosive poisoning, and from the effects of decomposition.§

---

* Nizamut Adawlut Reports, October 20th, 1853, p. 684, already cited at p. 554,—Note.

† *Ibid*, Novr. 18th, 1835, p. 772.

‡ *Ibid*, June 7th, 1854, p. 697. Many other cases in which *persons who have beaten to death, or otherwise severely injured by blows*, have been hanged.—*Bengal Police Reports*, 1868, pp. 304, 305 (three cases), 307 (three cases, one that of a poor child of nine beaten to death by his father for not bringing his hookah), pp. 309, 310.—*Nizamut Adawlut Reports*, May 1, 1855, p. 473, and April 27, 1857, p. 586.

§ A very singular case occurred at Burdwan in 1851. The wife of a police burkundauz was discovered hanging in a cow-house, but nothing could be elicited from any person. The Civil Surgeon deposed most positively that the deceased did not die, and could not have died, from hanging; but was unable to assign any cause of death. She was a young and healthy woman; the stomach was sent to Calcutta for analysis, but no traces of poison could be discovered. The father of the woman, who was in the house at the time, deposed that she had hanged herself. While the examination of the witnesses at the Magistrate's court was pending, the body of the woman's father was found hanging in an out-house belonging to his son-in-law, the burkundauz. No one could or would say anything about him, except that he was found hanging and quite dead. The Civil Surgeon again deposed that death could not have been caused by hanging or strangulation. No traces of poison were found in the stomach,—and thus the matter remained. The husband had ill-treated his wife. It was conjectured that the man administered some vegetable poison to his wife, and then, with

Suicidal Hanging.

II.—This mode of self-destruction is very prevalent among the natives of Bengal. Of twenty-one cases of suicide in Calcutta, investigated by Dr. Woodford, in his capacity of police surgeon, during the year 1850, ten were effected by hanging.* Dr. Woodford remarked that, in suicide, the passion, or rather the mania, with natives, is in favor of hanging.† See p. 670-71.

In most cases of suicidal hanging, by natives, very few marks of violence are discoverable. The only appearance worthy of remark, which I have noticed in any case of the kind, was an abrasion on the left side of the cheek and forehead, evidently caused by attrition against the perpendicular portion of the cord, which I observed in a young mallee (gardener) who had hanged himself, and which, at first sight, appeared like the trace of a blow.

Dr. Woodford has remarked upon the determined manner in which these people often suspend themselves at no great height above the ground. He has obliged me with the following note on this point :—" Medical men in Europe would be surprised if they could see the Bengalis suspended by the neck, in cases of suicide, with their heels resting on the ground, and standing as it were in a curved position,—that is to say, the neck being only six inches nearer the ground than it would be were the individual standing erect. At times, they hang by throwing themselves from a window-railing, which may not be more than three or four feet from the ground, and not unfrequently from the leg of a bedstead ; in such cases, the head may not be more than a foot from the ground. Bengalis very rarely suspend themselves from any height, from off a chair or stool, as in Europe."

I found one of the Chittagong hill-men hanging by his dhotee, the ends of which he had fixed, standing on tiptoe, to a bar above him. He had then accomplished the act by bending his knees and falling a little to one side.

Murder by Hanging.

III.—The perpetration of this crime is often suspected, but I cannot discover many instances where it has been clearly brought home to prisoners in India. In the following case, however, there can scarcely be a doubt that it was actually committed. In 1826, a married female, from twelve to fourteen years old, but arrived at the age of puberty, was found in her house tied by a rope round her neck to one of

---

the assistance of her father, suspended her corpse; and subsequently, when the case was coming on, fearing that the father might reveal the crime, he treated him in the same manner.—*Police Report*, L. P., 1851, p. 61.

* *Bengal Hurkaru, Medical and Scientific Gazette*, June 14th, 1851. It is not mentioned, however, whether the whole of these cases occurred in natives.

† The Abbe Dubois, whose experience of native customs was principally gained in the Madras Presidency, says that it is the women chiefly who resort to self-slaughter in moments of despair, almost always brought on by the harsh and tyrannical manner in which they are treated. They put an end to their lives by hanging themselves, or plugning into a pond or river.

the beams of the roof, with her feet upon the ground. One Abhursa was seen running from the house shortly before, out of breath, and much flurried. On the neck of the deceased were observed the marks of fingers, and of the nails also having been violently applied; and the witnesses deposed that, from the appearance of the body, they had no doubt a rape had been committed. The prisoner contented himself by a simple denial of the accusation. It was decided, however, that the single circumstance established against the prisoner was insufficient to prove his guilt.*

A woman, residing in the 24-Pergunnahs, was reported to have murdered her husband, with the aid of three men, by hanging him, in revenge for having beaten her and her paramour some days previously.†

A notoriously bad character, of Poorneah, discovering that his wife had intrigued with his nephew while he was in jail, taxed her with her crime, and deliberately hanged her.‡

The following appeared in the Papers in May 1868:—

A most determined execution of Lynch law has just occurred in this district. A Pasee of Shahpore was seized in the neighbouring village of Pusdeora in the act (as the people of the latter village say) of committing theft. He was beaten, knocked down, his arms were tied behind him, and he was then and there hanged, not in some secluded corner, but on a tree in the middle of the village closely surrounded by houses, as we suspend a crow on a fruit-tree *in terrorem*. The Pusdeora people declare that the Shahpore men have been of late perpetrating continual robberies on them, and that this severe example was absolutely necessary. The authorities, however, believe that this was not the true cause of offence, but that there was "a lady in the case." Meanwhile, some twelve persons have been apprehended, of whom some at least will be proved to have been active in the execution.

There are several cases on record in which *persons, having been cruelly beaten or otherwise misused, have been hanged while still living.*

In 1855, Ugnee Dass, of Cuttack, was sentenced to transportation for life, for having beaten his daughter-in-law until she became insensible, and then suspending her by the neck, while still living, that it might be supposed that she had committed suicide. Dr. E. B. Thing deposed: "I examined the body and found severe marks of beating on the whole length of the back and buttocks, and there were likewise marks or blows on the head and forehead; there was also a mark round the neck, such as would be produced by a rope when a person is hanged. There was one distinct mark or blow on the top of the forehead as if occasioned by a blow from a stick, or from being knocked against something; there were other slight bruises on the back of the head. The body was such a

---

* Macnaghten's Reports, Vol. II., p. 460.
† Police Report, L. P., 1840, p. 121.
‡ *Ibid*, 1844, p. 22.

mass of bruises altogether that there was no tracing with what particular weapon or instrument they were inflicted ; there is no doubt they were caused by beating."

In reply to the question, " Did you find any blood collected in any parts of the body, and have you been able to trace the direct cause of death ?" he stated, "Yes, she appeared to have all the symptoms of a person who had been strangled by hanging. There were congestion of the lungs and congestion of the brain. There was no disease apparent."

On being asked, " Could the mark on the neck have been caused by a string or rope being pulled across the neck by another person ?" he replied, "Yes, it might have been caused in that way ? but I don't think it was caused in that way, because the chances are that, had it been thus caused, there would have been other marks, and not one single line, by the party struggling. The line extended obliquely upwards on the side of the neck, but it is possible it may have been caused by a person holding the string, though not likely." *

IV. *Cases of apparent Drowning, &c., where it is questionable whether death has not resulted from Homicidal Hanging.*—Experience of criminal cases in all countries tends to show that the murderer is never satisfied with his work. He can never boldly leave matters to themselves, in defiance of suspicion, but must do something, and generally does it with a marked singularity which attracts attention, and at once fixes the brand of criminality upon his act. He will not bury the body, lest the earth should burst or sink, or the grass should wither, or grow greener there than on other spots,† or lest wild animals should burrow into it, or

* Nizamut Adawlut Reports, Oct. 2, 1855, p. 531. A case which will be found at p. 61 of the same volume may have been of the like description.

† The ideas alluded to here exist in the "Folk Lore" of most nations, and many of them are founded on correct observation. In *Notes and Queries*, 3rd Series, Vol. VI., is a story of one Newton, who was executed in 1821, for highway robbery with violence, but who protested his innocence to the last, and, in his address to the Court soliciting arrest of judgment, said, "I venture to assert that, if I am innocent of the crime for which I suffer, the grass for one generation at least will not cover my grave." The narrator of the history says, in 1853, numerous attempts have, from time to time, been made by some who are still alive, and others who have passed away, to bring grass upon that bare spot. Fresh soil has been frequently spread upon it, and seeds of various kinds have been sown: but not a blade has ever been known to spring from them; and the soil has soon become a smooth, and cold, and stubborn clay. We read in Baker's Chronicles that, "in the second year of King Edward the Sixth, Master Arden, of Kent, having been, by procurement of his wife, murthered in his own house, being dead, his body was carried out and laid upon the ground, in a close hard by, where this is memorable that, for two years after, the ground where his body lay bore no grass, but represented still, as it were, a picture of his body: only in the space between his arms and legs there grew grass, but, where any part of his body touched, none at all." This appears to have been a very popular notion in those times. It is stated, in Dr. Bailey's Life of Fisher, Bishop of Rochester, that "touching the place of his burial in Barking churchyard, it was well observed by divers worthy persons of the nations of Italy, Spain, and France that were then abiding in the realm, and more diligently noted,

tear it up, or lest a train of insects should guide the avengers of blood to it,* or a torrent should descend and lay it bare. The cover of the thickest jungle will not conceal its stench from the birds and animals which will gather round it. Every reservoir, far and near, will be searched for it; weights will not keep it down in water; fish will collect and struggle above it; the next dry season may bring it to light. An eddy† will mark where it lies sunk on the bed of the deepest stream. A fatal blow has been struck,—he cannot throw open his doors courageously, and say,—This man came to rob and wound me, or to outrage my feelings, and I struck him dead in self-defence or in sudden rage;—but he must take the body forth at night and hang it before his door, with the stamp of murder upon it; or he must try to burn it piecemeal in a stove or furnace, although he knows, professionally, that, with such means as are at his disposal, it would take cart-loads of wood to consume a human body,—and that with an odour which must tell the tale to every passer-by. He is not content to strangle his victim, and to cast his body forth where it would be doubtful upon whom suspicion ought to rest—but he must separate it limb from limb, and place each fragment where it must certainly be discovered, and tell its own history. He knows that, when his cow or his goat dies in the fields, the jackals and crows and vultures speedily devour it; he, therefore, exposes his victim, in like manner,—when the wild creatures either avoid it or leave its wounds untouched. He deliberately murders in a manner which would make it appear that death was suicidal, and then hastens to undo his work, and to leave the evidences of murder clear and unmistakeable.

In the following case, although the prisoner was acquitted in the absence of certain proof, there could scarcely be a doubt that murder by hanging had been committed, and that the body had, subsequently, been exposed with an intent to make it appear that death had occurred in some other manner.

In 1824 the body of a married girl, only fourteen years old, was found on the bank of a pond, a short distance from her husband's house, "with the mark of a cord having been fastened round her neck, *and with other*

---

and wrote the course of things, and with less fear and suspicion than any of the King's subjects might or durst to do, that, for the space of seven years after his burial, there grew neither leaf nor grass upon his grave; but the earth still remained as bare as though it had been continually occupied and trodden." The plain fact probably was that these spots were much visited, and were trodden upon so frequently that the clayey surface was not allowed to produce grass.

* See Nizamut Adawlut Reports, Vol. III., Part 1, of 1853, p. 228, already cited at p. 27.

† "A corpse-candle," says Aubrey. "When any Christian is drowned in the river Dee, there will appear, over the water where the corpse is, a light, by which means they do find the body; and it is, therefore, called the Holy Dee."

marks of violence." Her husband, on being first apprehended, declared that his wife had eloped, and that he did not know what had become of her. He afterwards stated that the woman had hung herself in his house, and that he and his father, from fear of being brought into difficulty, concealed the circumstance and removed the body to the place where it was found the following day. It was proved that the deceased had been in the habit of leaving her husband's house and returning to that of her father and mother. This circumstance, it appeared, created great discontent towards her on the part of the husband and his father.* The Judges of the Nizamut were divided in their opinions upon this case ; one of them confirmed the sentence awarded by the law officer of the Court of Circuit, but two others agreed with the Circuit Judge in acquitting the prisoner.†

It is not unfrequently inquired of medical officers in this country whether persons, whose bodies have been discovered in tanks or ponds, have not been hanged previous to submersion. A question of this kind

---

* This is a very frequent cause of quarrels in native families, and has often led to murder. See the case in which a man slaughtered his wife, aged only thirteen years, with a *dhao*, for going to her mother's house in contempt of his orders (N. A. Reports, Vol. III., Part 1, of 1853, page 393) ; and another instance in which the victim was fifteen or sixteen years of age (*Ibid*, p. 64). Also a case of homicide arising from this cause—*Ibid*, October 8th, 1853, p. 652. Two cases of this kind will be found—*Ibid*, August 1856, p. 245, and November of the same year, p. 913. At p. 101 of the same volume will be found the case of a man who, being refused access to his wife by his mother, killed his mother, by cutting her throat with a sola-cutting knife, and wounded his wife. At p. 646 of the same volume is a case in which a wife returning to her mother's house, the husband severely wounded his mother-in-law with a knife, and then wounded his own throat.

These cases are of very frequent occurrence in the N. W. Provinces—see Nizamut Reports of those Provinces, August 28th, 1852, p. 936 ; October 30th, 1852, p. 1269 ; March 5th, 1853, p. 339 ; March 16th, p. 368 ; August 11th, p. 977 ; August 17th, p. 1002 ; September 9th, p. 1155, and 15th, p. 1162 ; December 7th, p. 1145 ; July 1854, p. 99 ; and many other instances. The Abbe Dubois has explained the cause of these tragedies. He describes that, the marriage festival being over, the young wife is taken back to her father's house, which continues to be her principal abode until she has grown up into a state fit to discharge all the duties of matrimony. It is then notified that the girl has become a woman, and is qualified to live with her husband. Then, after completing the ceremonies to which this occasion gives rise, she is conducted in triumph to the house of her father-in-law, where she is detained for a while to accustom her to the society of her husband ; and, after a month or two, her own parents return and take her home with them. The residence of the young woman is thus, for the first and even the second year, divided between the house of her husband and that of her father. This is accounted a mark of good understanding subsisting among them. Its concord is most probably soon dissolved, when the young wife, beaten by her husband, and harassed by her mother-in-law, who treats her as a slave, finds no remedy for ill-usage but in flying to her father's house. She will be recalled by fair promises of kind treatment. They will break their word ; and she will have recourse to the same remedy. But, at last, the children which she brings into the world, and other circumstances, will compel her to do her best, by remaining in her husband's house, with the show of being contented with her lot.

† Macnaghten's Report, Vol. II., p. 350.

was put to me by the Magistrate of Howrah in 1855. Decomposition in water, however, tends greatly to obscure the appearances in such cases.

Murdered by Drowning and afterwards Hanged.

In 1868, Someeruddeen Karigur, of Backergunge, taking umbrage at his wife for some act of disobedience, first beat her, then held her head in water till she was drowned. Her body was afterwards recovered by the aid of two other persons and suspended from a tree to make it appear that she had hanged herself. From the *post-mortem* examination it appeared that the deceased had died from suffocation caused by drowning. The charge of murder having been brought home to the accused, he was sentenced to transportation for life.*

Signs of Death by Hanging.

I have carefully examined the bodies of eight persons who were known to have been strangled by hanging, and about the same number of those found hanging. Not having kept notes of these cases, I can only speak from the strong and distinct impression which they have left upon my mind. Under these circumstances, however, I cannot attempt to decide authoritatively upon the subject; the following remarks are, therefore, merely intended to suggest further investigation in a question of exceeding importance, nearly every detail of which still remains debatable.

It must be premised that all my experience in this subject results from the examination of the bodies of *natives* who have died by Hanging. In these cases, three great drawbacks are frequently operative: (1) there are rarely, in the ill-fed, spare-bodied, and generally more or less anemiated low-class native, that plethora and tendency to active hæmorrhage which so frequently determine the appearance of marked lesions from hanging in the bodies of Europeans; (2) the darkness of the native's skin in great measure conceals those delicate appearances of congestion, ecchymosis, and abrasion in the track of the ligature and elsewhere, which often become useful guides in Europe; (3) the bodies are frequently brought in an advanced state of putrefaction—a condition which nearly or quite destroys every known sign of hanging.

It will be proper to notice the chief evidences of hanging, *seriatim.*

Congestion of the Face and Scalp.

This, a very uncertain sign, will rarely be marked where the subject has not been exceedingly plethoric, and is often not distinguishable—especially (as is generally the case) when the cord has been removed immediately upon discovery of the body, or where attempts have been made to resuscitate. In many instances of hanging, where the noose is

---

* Bengal Police Report, 1868, p. 74.

open, all return of blood by the veins is not prevented; and, in cases where strangulation is complete, supply by the carotids is intercepted, and that by the vertebrals must speedily cease.

Meningeal and Cerebral Congestion and Effusion.

There is, probably, no pathologist in existence who can safely measure the degree of congestion presented by any brain in which neither inflammation nor sanguineous extravasation is present. The meningeal vessels of men and animals, destroyed by hæmorrhage, are not empty; and in all cases of natural death, where the head is not kept raised (which it never is in bodies brought in for inspection here), these veins will be found turgid. It is certainly unsafe to give an opinion, which may involve the life of an accused party, upon the authority of a mere guess. Dr. Taylor observes that the venous congestion of the cerebral vessels is rarely greater in hanging than in other cases of asphyxia. It has often been said of morbid anatomists that they never examine a body in which they do not find "the vascular points in the centra ovalia unusually numerous." Where the entire surface of the brain presents a decided pinkish hue, or blood has actually become extravasated, the evidence is of value; but these appearances are but rarely found as our guides in cases of Hanging. Romer (cited by Taylor) found apoplectic extravasation of blood only once in one hundred and one cases. Sir B. Brodie refers to two cases; Casper did not observe a single instance in one hundred and six cases.*

Assistant Surgeon Lithgow has reported† the case of a European gunner, *ætat* twenty-four years, who attempted to hang himself while intoxicated. He was admitted with very stertorous and difficult breathing and coma. His condition improved on the following day. He could be roused, but there was still stertor, and the urine was bloody. On the morning of the third day, these symptoms continued. That evening he fell back in a convulsive fit, accompanied by increased dyspnœa. He died in an hour and-a-quarter. There were found about three drachms of blood effused between the calvarium and dura mater; it had escaped from a *rupture of the longitudinal sinus*, near its termination posteriorly. The lungs were

---

* The late Dr. Kenneth Mackinnon mentioned to me the particulars of a very singular case, in which there could not be a doubt that, quite unintentionally, stranglers *saved their victim's life by cutting his throat!* In 1835, a man, travelling through Tirhoot, fell in with a gang of Thugs, who strangled him. He became unconscious. Upon recovering his senses, he found that his throat had been cut, and that a fellow-traveller lay strangled to death by his side. Mr. Charles Mackinnon met him on his way to Mozufferpore, attended to the wound in his throat, and recovered him in six weeks. He was able to give a description of the gang which subsequently led to their apprehension. Four of them were sentenced to death. It can scarcely be doubted that the violent measure of cutting the man's throat effectually relieved the vessels of his brain of any undue congestion which the throttling may have produced. The case is also detailed in the Bengal Police Report for 1836, p. 34.

† Bombay Med. and Phys. Trans., No. VIII., N. S., for 1862, Append., p. viii.

congested, the right distinctly apoplectic. The kidneys were much congested. There were several ecchymoses in the mucous membrane of the stomach.

Dr. Woodford has obliged me with the following case in which he considered that extravasation of blood on the brain occurred after death in a person hanged :—"In 1859, I examined a very interesting case, the body of a native woman, named Soudamonee Dossee. I found a strong double rope tied round the neck, with the slip-knot under the left ear. On removing the rope, a dark deep livid mark was observable, taking an upward and backward course ; on the left side of the neck and above the cord, was an irregular and interrupted ecchymosis about two and-a-half inches long, and an inch and-a-half wide. The whole of the anterior part of the scalp had faint traces of ecchymosis; there was a thick clot of extravasated blood, about the size of a rupee, on the surface of the left hemisphere of the brain anteriorly, and an irregular extravasation of blood over the whole upper surface of the right hemisphere of the brain. The thoracic and abdominal viscera were healthy but congested.

"The interesting question to be decided in this case was, were these abnormal appearances the result of injuries sustained before or after the suspension? I was inclined to attribute them to the latter cause, bearing in mind the difficulty of suspending a body after death. My impression proved to be correct. The mother of the young woman, on returning home from her day's labor, found her daughter hanging, and cut her down unassisted ; the body fell heavily forwards with the forehead to the ground, which explained the ecchymosed state of the forehead and extravasation of blood on the brain *after death.* The ecchymosis on the left side of the neck remained unaccounted for; probably it arose from the slipping of the knot, or in a hurried attempt to remove the rope after the body fell."

With great deference to the experienced judgment of my friend and colleague, I think that the question of the occurrence *post mortem* of the effusions of blood described above is debatable. Persons are frequently suspended by the neck after death, and there is nothing to show how long the body had been hanging when it was cut down and met with the accident to which the extravasations are attributed. Dr. Christison (Taylor, p. 380) found that sometimes the appearance of contusions could hardly be produced on a dead body two hours after death ; on other occasions they might be slightly caused after three hours and-a-quarter, but this period is near the extreme limit. Whenever the warmth of the body and the laxity of the muscles are not considerable at the time the blow is inflicted, the appearance of contusions during life cannot be distinctly produced. It is, therefore, only on the trunk that, even in the most favorable state of the body—namely, when warmth is retained and the blood continues altogether liquid—that a mark resembling a contusion on the living body can be produced so late as two hours after death.

Protrusion of the Tongue and Eyes.

These appearances, when they are present, are, of course, merely due to congestion. I have never noticed marked protrusion of the eyes, and have never seen the tongue protruded, except where putrefraction was far advanced.* Where the tongue has been lacerated by the teeth, it affords safer evidence. Dr. Riecke noticed this in several instances.

In a case where it had to be judged whether a woman had been hanged before or after death, the body was swollen in different parts from blows, and stained with blood which was trickling from the ears, nose, and mouth; and there was a quantity of blood on the floor about three feet from the body. The medical officer stated that, when he saw the body, during the *post-mortem* examination, the tongue protruded, and this could not have taken place unless the body was suspended when life was not extinct. Several witnesses declared that the tongue was inside the mouth when they saw the body suspended. The Sessions Judge considered that the fact stated by the medical officer was a very material one. The Judges of the Court of appeal observed: "The deposition of the Civil Surgeon, in consequence of the decomposed state of the body, when he saw it, is far from satisfactory or conclusive; but it would lead to a suspicion that the deceased had been suspended during life, from the protrusion of the tongue. That, however, appears to be by no means an unequivocal sign on that point; for we find, in a note at page 623 of Beek's Medical Jurisprudence, that the same effect has been produced in the dead body by fixing the cord in a particular situation,—*i. e.* above the *os hyoides.* No marks of violence were discovered on the body, except that the neck was broken, which might have been caused by the suspension."†

Dr. Taylor says (p. 654) that the tongue "is enlarged, livid, and either compressed between the teeth, or sometimes protruded.

Dr. Guy says (p. 276): "The same injected and swollen state of the base of the tongue, with or without protrusion, occurs also in death by hanging, and affords a strong probability of suspension during life."

The result of Dr. Beatson's Indian observation‡ is that "the faces of the hanged are invariably calm and undistorted, and protrusion of the eyes and tongue seldom exists except as the result of putrefaction.

After examining several cases of hanging, suicidal and judicial, Dr. R. F. Hutchinson, Civil Surgeon of Patna, has noticed an appearance invariably present in male cases; it would also be present in females were it not for the difference in their dress. It is valuable as indicating suspension during life, and, as far as he can learn, it has not been noticed

---

* Devergie found that there was protrusion of this organ in eleven cases out of twenty-seven.

† Nizamut Adawlut Reports, July 13, 1855, p. 61.

‡ Ind. Med. Gaz., April 1, 1865, p. 83.

by any writers. It is ***the flow of saliva out of the mouth, down the chin, and straight down the chest.*** The appearance is unmistakable and invariable, and ***could not occur in a body hung up after death,*** the secretion of saliva being a living act. Of course this sign is best seen on the naked chest, and, in ninety-nine cases out of a hundred, the chest is exposed, for the suicide hangs himself with his chaddar, and criminals are hung in their dhotees only. Dr. Hutchinson has seen the saliva-line even on a koorta, and, on one occasion, the drip took place through the execution cap.*

Mark of the Cord.

In nearly all cases of hanging, this mark is very distinct; but, unfortunately, it presents nearly the same characters when the body has been suspended shortly after death, as it does after execution or suicide by hanging. It has already been noticed that, in this country, the mark is often attacked by ants. I found it very distinct in a woman who had attempted suicide; the line was perfectly defined, dry and condensed, slightly depressed, much darker than the adjacent skin, and harsh and branny to the touch, but there was no appearance of ecchymosis or exudation of blood from the surface. While the first edition of this sheet was going through the press, I examined what was alleged to be the trace of a thin cord by which a young female was suspended seven days previously. The line was very oblique (corresponding with a noose, the knot of which touched the occiput), and was clearly defined by the separation of the cuticle throughout its entire length, as if by the application of a blistering substance. A guarded opinion was given. I have since seen a similar line on the neck of a man, who stated that he had been suspended for a short time. It has already been noticed that this mark may be found clearly defined, with the cuticle adhering to it, after decomposition has advanced considerably—see page 39. Neither in suicidal hanging, nor after execution, have I been able to detect any ecchymosis in the cutis or in the integuments along the course of this line. I have, however, seen the skin cracked in one or two places with a few points of bloody exudation.

The beads worn by Hindus (*malla*) sometimes leave a very distinct mark on the neck after death, which it is, of course, needful to distinguish from those of hanging or strangling.

I have notes of the evidence of Dr. Maxton, late Police Surgeon, Calcutta, in the case of a plethoric young Mussalmaun woman, in whom it was doubtful whether fatal congestion of the brain was caused by the tightening of an amulet cord round the neck, or by some other cause. The cord, when cut off, was embedded in the muscles of the neck, which was very much swollen (it is not said from decomposition)—("it left a dark livid mark").

---

* Ind. Med. Gaz., August 1, 1867, p. 200.

Ecchymosis of the Muscles.

This is frequently absent in cases when death is known to have resulted from hanging, but I have occasionally met with it. Where the ecchymosis has been found excessive, and out of the way of the cord, as near the chin or towards the clavicles, it has created suspicion of foul play. Still it is possible that, in suicidal hanging, ecchymosis might be produced in any part of the neck by the shock of the fall and over-stretching of the parts. There are certainly many known exceptions to the rule,—still it obtains generally, and particularly in India, that suicides effect their purpose with as little violence as possible.

I have never found any appearance of *injury to the vertebræ or their ligaments* in cases of hanging.

In a very spare but muscular native, judicially hanged at Alipore, whom I examined chiefly for the purpose of observing the state of the carotid artery on the side opposite to the knot, I found a clean strip of the inner coat of the vessel torn up to the distance of rather more than an inch. It appeared evident that this had been done by the rope as it slipped upwards.

Neither have I ever found any portion of the air passage ruptured, considerably displaced, or ecchymosed. The base of the tongue and glottis are usually livid in a marked degree, being almost of a violet hue (some stress should probably be laid upon this appearance, which deserves further investigation). The mucous membrane of the larynx and trachea is generally somewhat congested, but much less so than that of the glottis. The trachea very frequently, but not always, contains a small quantity of pinkish or brownish froth, made up of extremely minute air bubbles. Dr. Taylor thinks that this is only likely to be met with in cases where the obstruction to respiration has been incomplete. It has always appeared to me to be due to a few spasmodic efforts to carry on respiration below a nearly complete impediment. There is an appearance which I have never failed to notice in cases where the individual has been hanged with a rope. This is an exudation of clear mucus from all the muciparous follicles of the larynx and upper part of the trachea. If the tube be slit up at the back and carefully opened, while any fluid that it may contain is allowed to flow downwards, the position of every follicle will be observed to be marked by a semi-globule, nearly as large as the head of a small pin. Hence the surface has nearly the appearance of the clearer kinds of white shagreen used for sword-grips. This appearance was not perceptible in the air-passage of a man who hung himself with a thick cloth. I am not able to state whether it is found after death from other modes of pressure on the neck. I have remarked it five or six times, in unmistakable cases of hanging, and should be glad to learn that it had been further investigated.*

* In a case like that of Governor Wall, in whom the larynx was inflexibly ossified, this appearance could not be expected to exist.

A case, which illustrated, with rather terrible demonstrativeness, the fact that the ***amount of injury done to the structures of the neck in hanging is determined by the distance of the fall***, has lately occurred at Richmond Bridewell, Dublin.* Andrew Carr, a discharged soldier of the 37th Regiment, who had served in India, was executed for murder. "The bolt was drawn, the wretched man fell, and then a horrid spectacle was witnessed. A drop of fourteen feet had been arranged, in deference to the opinion of a learned professor, who prescribed this length as necessary in order to produce instantaneous death by dislocating the neck. The truth of the theory was indeed established, and the experiment proved successful beyond expectation. The body fell to the full extent of the rope, and then, with a sudden snap, the head was wrenched off and flung a distance of several feet to one side of the yard, while the trunk dropped to the other side, a ghastly mass, with the nerves twitching convulsively from the violence of the shock. The fragments of humanity were quickly gathered up and placed in a coffin to await the inquest, which was held at twelve o'clock. Captain Boyd deposed that he became aware of what had happened by the sudden recoil of the rope, and hearing the sound of the body falling into the yard. Every precaution had been taken to execute the sentence as humanely as possible. The rope was sound, and the whole apparatus in perfect order. The height of the drop had been fully discussed, and many considered fourteen feet too great a fall—an opinion in which he concurred himself, believing eight feet enough; but the surgeon of the prison, being anxious to lessen the sufferings of the convict, thought that length necessary to produce instantaneous death. Dr. Humphry Minchin, the prison officer, deposed that all the parts were divided completely across, and the vertebræ fractured, which alone would cause immediate death. He could not account for the decapitation on ordinary principles, for the fall was less in proportion to that of Kilkelly, the last-executed prisoner, in Kilmainham Gaol. Some of the force of the fall is usually expended in tightening the noose, but he feared that, in the present case, the noose was tightened beforehand. The Rev. Mr. Anthony stated that, before the prisoner went on the trap, he heard him complain that the rope was choking him before the time. Other witnesses bore testimony to the humane conduct of the officials. The jury found that the decapitation was the result of accident, for which the prison officials were not to blame, and that Carr was duly executed."

This recalls to my mind the manner in which some of my schoolfellows, who were rabbit-fanciers, used to put the young rabbits out of their misery when they became diseased and "potted," in consequence, as it was considered, of eating too much green meat. The animal being held up by

* *Home News*, August 5, 1870, p. 13.

the hind feet, a strong and quick blow with the ulnar edge of the hand, falling upon the back of the neck, smote the head off.

The uncertain character of the evidences of Asphyxia, as displayed in the thoracic organs, will be noticed under the head of *Drowning*.

In the present state of our knowledge, the most satisfactory evidences of suicidal death by hanging in an able-bodied person are,—the presence of the characteristic oblique line and of one or more of the laryngeal and tracheal lesions noticed above, without any traces of stunning blows on the head, or marks upon the body of violent resistance, or proof of the presence of poison or alcohol in the stomach. Extreme ecchymosis of the muscles of the neck is always suspicious ; and fracture or *lateral* dislocation of the vertebral bones appears to afford certain evidence of homicide.* In addition to these, thoracic and cerebral evidences of Asphyxia, when existing in a very marked degree previous to the commencement of putrefaction, are of considerable, but secondary, importance. Decided traces of cerebral hæmorrhage, when unattended with marks of blows on the head, or with evidences of any greater amount of injury about the neck than the cord would be likely to inflict, although rarely found, afford strong additional evidence of death by hanging.

In all cases where it is alleged that a body has been found hanging, or apparently strangled, with a rope, cloth, &c., around its throat, the police should be expected to send in the ligature with the body, for examination by the medical officer. Should the police find the body putrid with the ligature still on, they should on no account disturb it. Should there be any reason to believe that life has not departed, the loop should be cut through, and the cord or cloth sent in, as removed, not doubled together or unfolded, but coiled in a covered earthen vessel, that the shape which it took upon the neck may be preserved, if possible. Except in sudden emergency, the knot should not be *untied*. Where the ligature has been taken off previous to the arrival of the police, those who have removed it should be expected to produce it. The police officer should also describe clearly, in his *sooruthal*, the manner in which the rope or cloth was attached to the neck, and (in cases of Hanging) how it was found or described to be fixed to the beam, branch, &c. Examination of the cord may often be attended with as important results as inspection of the body,—sometimes even more so. A person may have been strangled by a rope or cloth not sufficiently strong to suspend his body, or a ligature used in strangling—as a handkerchief, or short rope with ends which have evidently not been recently divided—may be produced as the instrument with which hanging was effected. Or a small cord may be produced in a case where

* Devergie, as quoted by Taylor, found the ligaments between the first and second cervical vertebræ ruptured once in fifty-two cases of suicidal hanging. M. Ansiaux found the posterior ligament of the spine ruptured, and the transverse ligament of the atlas stretched in the body of a female who had hanged herself.

the neck presents a broad depression, or *vice versâ*. Or the rope or cloth may be sufficiently long and strong, but may bear evidences of not having been used in suspending a body (that part of the loop of a rope used in hanging which has touched the skin is generally observed to be marked with a brownish line, corresponding with that on the neck, which would probably be found to be caused by imbibition of serum and perspiration, and by the adherence of portions of epidermis).

Observance of the following rules will generally afford us some aid in arriving at a correct conclusion in cases of hanging and strangulation.

The ligature and the mark on the neck should first be carefully examined and compared.

Search should then be made, by external examination and by dissection, for the traces of any injuries, apart from strangulation or hanging, *not apparently self-inflicted,* which may have been sufficient, in themselves, either to destroy life, to cause extreme weakness, or to occasion insensibility,—especially for traces of blows or wounds on the head or chest, or severe bruises on the back or limbs, or evidences of a mortal struggle with a powerful opponent.*

It should then be carefully weighed whether any injuries which may be discovered may not have been *self-inflicted ;* for example, small punctured wounds on the chest or abdomen, or slight or even very considerable wounds on the throat may have been and not improbably have been inflicted with suicidal intent. A considerable incised wound on the throat of a person found hanged would generally afford strong evidence that the individual had destroyed himself, as it would rarely happen that a murderer, failing to accomplish his first purpose, would resort to another mode attended with greater difficulty. To this latter rule, however, the case already cited in which a man was first strangled and then had his throat cut, must be regarded as showing the possibility of an exception.†

The evidences of poisoning, narcotism, or intoxication should then be sought for. Here probability may be our only guide. The deceased may have been in the habit of eating opium, or may have been drugged and then strangled or hanged while in a state of insensibility ; or, being distressed and impatient under the slow and painful operation of an irritant poison, he may have hanged himself. It is, however, very improbable that a criminal, having administered an *irritant* poison, should be unwilling to allow it to work out its effects, and should proceed to hang his victim while living, to strangle him or to destroy him by other vio-

* Formerly criminals in India were *hamstrung* before being hanged. When such execution was hastily done on a march, all chance of the culprits being released by their friends was thus obviated. See a case in which the legs were cut off, p. 576, note.

† See also a case in which a woman's throat was cut, she having first been rendered senseless by strangulation.—Police Report, L. P., 1849, p. 35.

lence.* Taylor cites a case, by Foderé, in which it was discovered that the death of a person found hanging was occasioned by poison. It is not mentioned, however, whether the poison used in this case was narcotic or irritant, or whether the death was believed to result from suicide or murder. Neither is it easy, in a body found hanged, to decide that *death* resulted from poisoning. It is evidently just at the time when the agony produced by the action of a strong irritant poison had become most intense (when all the appearances of inflammatory action would have become fully developed in the stomach), that a person bent upon suicide would be likely to hang himself. The body of a person so poisoned may, however, be suspended after death.

Search should then be made for marks of strangulation; should these be distinct and be attended by bruises, stabs, or incisions on the body, the question lies between suicide and homicide; where, however, there are traces of stunning blows on the head, the case is probably one of homicide.

The body of a person accidentally strangled may, however, present scratches and other marks of attempts to extricate himself; but these are not likely to be very severe, as, in most cases of accidental strangling, consciousness must be destroyed suddenly.

Where distinct evidences of strangulation and hanging are found together, the case must have been homicidal.

SUFFOCATION.

Drugged and Suffocated.

A case involving more than one important medico-legal point with reference to the investigation of death by suffocation, was tried at Moradabad, in 1854. One Mulhooa was tried for the murder of his wife. It appeared that the woman was loose in her conduct, and had been detected by her husband in an intrigue shortly before her death. He took her to her parents; and, on the night of his return home with her, a verbal altercation occurred between the couple. On the following day, the woman died. Nothing whatever was known of the circumstances attending her death,—she and the man were alone. Her husband reported at the thannah that she had died of cholera. As deaths by cholera are not usually reported, the report excited suspicions, which led to the apprehension of the prisoner. In the Judge's Court the man changed his statement, and asserted that his wife died by poisoning by opium; the evidence of the Sub-Assistant Surgeon, who examined the body, was positive that death was not caused by cholera, dysentery, diarrhœa, or poison, and that all the appear-

* Perhaps the only recorded exception to this is found in the well-known case of the Marchioness de Ganges.

ances on the *post-mortem* examination denoted death by suffocation. The Judges of the superior Court remarked that the medical testimony (upon which almost exclusively the prisoner's conviction had been found by the Sessions Judge) could not be considered perfectly conclusive as to the cause of death, though it, doubtless, pointed strongly at extinction of life by suffocation. The Sub-Assistant Surgeon was certain, from the appearances which he observed in examining the body, that death was not caused by cholera, and "strongly suspected" that it was caused by smothering. The internal organs, lungs, stomach, &c., were in a healthy state, but congested. There was no external mark to denote suffocation, which, it was conjectured, might have been effected by pressure over the mouth. It did not appear that the *brain* had been examined at all, which was a rather material omission. The Civil Assistant Surgeon (whose opinion on this evidence was called for by the Court) deposed that, assuming the correctness of the Sub-Assistant Surgeon's description of symptoms, he could attribute death to no other cause than suffocation, but was unable to say "with certainty" that death was so caused. The Judges noticed that, if death were caused by homicidal suffocation at the hands of the prisoner, it would most probably have occurred *at the time* of the ill-treatment, and not after the lapse of a considerable interval; whereas all the witnesses referred the quarrel to the evening before, and the woman's death to the following day. They believed it to be certain that most individuals would have it in their power (unless greatly incapacitated by disease or intoxication, and this young woman was declared to have been in full health and strength) to offer to such a mode of attack a degree of active resistance likely to leave on their persons undoubted evidence of murderous violence having been resorted to. When asked if he found any indication of poisoning either by a mineral or vegetable substance, the Sub-Assistant Surgeon answered (referring to the stomach and its contents) in the negative. He stated his perfect conviction that she did not die from any poison,—"there was no inflammation or ulceration of the coats of the stomach or intestines." It was, however, they remarked, observable that some of the appearances mentioned,—*viz.*, the right cavities of the heart filled with dark fluid blood, the left side empty, lividity of skin, internal organs congested, though healthy in structure,—seemed to be very similar to the *post-mortem* appearances of death from opium as described in Taylor's Medical Jurisprudence.*

The late Dr. Heathcote, who fell in the mutiny, related to me a case, in which, from some appearances of injury about the wrists, ankles, and throat, and a dislocation of one of the toes, with a full stomach, smelling of

* Nizamut Adawlut Reports, N. W. P., 27th May 1854, p. 586. See also an interesting article by Mr. H. J. Carter, of Bombay, on the Remarkable Pulmonary Congestion attending Poisoning by Opium.—*Trans. Medical and Phys. Society of Bombay*, 1848, p. 25.

spirit, and congested lungs, he gave a decided opinion that death had been caused by suffocation after a full meal by persons who had probably dined with him, intoxicated and perhaps drugged him. It was found that he was a *fukeer* who had saved money. Certain other *fukeers*, knowing this, went to him. They had taken food together, he became intoxicated and was held down, while one sat on his head and suffocated him. They then dug up his money from under his *choollah*.

The following case, although it is one of strangulation rather than suffocation, is so similar to the above that it must be inserted here. In 1865, a gang of road poisoners planned the robbery of a *Jain* priest, who was known to be wealthy. They provided themselves with an offering of drugged sweetmeats, of which the priest ate, when he became insensible. One squeezed his throat, another rode on his chest, a third held his hands, and a fourth squeezed his private parts with his feet. The priest trembled convulsively and died.*

In not a few cases, the medical officer, being convinced with regard to the cause of death, *omits to examine the abdominal viscera, especially the intestinal canal.* I could cite more than one instance of this kind, in which the question—was death caused or accelerated by cholera ?—has tended to unsettle the medical evidence and to shield a criminal who could scarcely have hoped to escape punishment under this often-repeated plea.

A case illustrative of this point was tried at Goruckpore, in 1854. It appeared, from the statements of three witnesses to the fact, and of the accused herself, that she kicked a child, aged ten, once in the side or stomach; that she did not lay her hands on the child; and that the child did not fall on receiving the kick. The father of the child deposed that his daughter came home to him at the time stated, and, after telling him that the prisoner had beaten her, fell down and died. The *sooruthal*, bearing the date of the child's death, describes a black mark, or bruise, on the right side, which the witnesses to that document verified in the Foujdaree Court ; though, at the Sessions trial, they professed to think it was only a mark caused by the *dhotee*. The Civil Surgeon, however, stated that there were marks of strangulation on the neck and throat, but no marks of kicks ; that congestion of the brain had been caused by strangulation ; that death from suffocation must have been immediate ; but, if caused by a kick, some internal injury of the spleen or other organ would have been visible, which was not the case; but that, in either case, the deceased would not have been able to get up and walk [?]. It was mentioned by the Superior Court, that it would have been more satisfactory had the Civil Surgeon been interrogated as to the actual appearance of the throat, with reference to the marks of strangulation, as he spoke only of *injuries* about the throat, gullet, and neck. The Judges of both Courts

* Beng. Police Rep., 1865, p. 35.

believed that the child had not been killed by a kick, and that the story of the sudden blow had been trumped up to turn aside the legal inquiries regarding the cause of her violent death.*

Many cases will be found in the criminal records—especially in those of the North-West Provinces, in which death was caused by forcing cloths, earth, &c., into the mouth. In some instances, at least, this would appear to be done with an intention to stifle the victim's cries;—still, where death results from so cruel and reckless a form of violence, it is doubtful whether this plea should be held as mitigatory.

One Ramchurn, of Goruckpore, was found guilty of rape upon a girl of eight. The child, who appeared to understand the obligation of an oath, declared that the prisoner threw her down, and filled her mouth with sand.†

A boy, apparently only twelve years of age, but shrewd and intelligent beyond his years, was convicted of having robbed a child of four of her ornaments, after having filled her mouth with mud, and nearly strangled her. The child was found in a field, with her mouth filled with earth, and with the marks of fingers on her neck. She afterwards said that the prisoner had thus maltreated her.‡

A very young man of Mirzapore was sentenced to death for murdering a boy of twelve for his ornaments, by filling his mouth with mud. The Civil Surgeon deposed that the cause of death was, in his opinion, suffocation and consequent congestion of the brain, produced by the mouth and air-passages of the deceased having been filled with mud, whilst he was alive.§

A lad from thirteen to fifteen years of age was sentenced, at Agra, to transportation for life for having robbed a girl of four, his near relative, of her ornaments, after having filled her mouth with *bhoosa*. The Civil Surgeon deposed that death had been caused by suffocation, consequent upon the mouth of the deceased being filled with *bhoosa*.‖

One Bhageeruttee, of Goruckpore, was sentenced to death for the murder of a boy of nine for his ornaments. He confessed before the Deputy Magistrate that he put a cloth in the child's mouth, and, seizing his throat, had choked him.¶

An old woman of Tirhoot, finding a little girl of six digging up some grain from her field, felled the child with a heavy clod, and then suffocated her by pressing her clothes against her mouth, until she ceased to

---

* Nizamut Adawlut Reports, N. W. P., 23rd November 1854, p. 743.
† *Ibid*, 20th October 1853, p. 1318.
‡ *Ibid*, 24th May 1853, p. 697.
§ *Ibid*, 15th September 1852, p. 999.
‖ *Ibid*, 23rd January 1852, p. 51.
¶ *Ibid*, 11th February 1853, p. 208.

breathe. She then stripped off the clothes and ornaments, and buried the corpse.*

A bustamee of Rajshahye, who lived alone, and had the reputation of possessing some money, was found dead in her house, with a cloth stuffed into her mouth. The murderer could not be discovered.†

The instances are by no means very few in which *drunkards, while lying stertorous on their backs, have been suffocated in the act of vomiting.* One of these was published by Dr. Ormerod, *cir.* 1845. Another occurred to Dr. James Anderson, late Deputy Inspector General of Hospitals, Calcutta, when he was in medical charge of a European regiment.

The following case is given in the Statistical Reports of the Health of the Navy, 1837—43, Part 2, East India Station, p. 54 :—A seaman returned from leave of absence in a state of helpless intoxication ; he was seen by the Assistant Surgeon; but, as he appeared only to require rest, he was sent below to his mess, where he commenced singing. Half an hour afterwards he was found lying on the deck quite dead. Supposing the liquor he had taken while on shore might have been poisoned, the body was carefully examined, when it was found "that, in the act of respiration, the patient, while vomiting, had drawn into the rima glottidis a piece of half-masticated beef, where it remained fixed, and completely prevented the air from passing into the lungs."

The following remarkable case was sent to me in March 1857 by the late Dr. A. Simpson, and his brother-in-law, the late Dr. John Brown :—The body of Seokeah Dosadh, *ætat* about forty years, was sent for examination in consequence of a report that poison had been administered in his food. In the lower lobes of the lungs were observed, on section, numerous round cheesy masses of variable size, from that of a mustard seed to that of a split pea. This deposit was contained within the bronchial tubes, and extended to their termination in the vesicular structure of the lung, which did not seem implicated, as evidenced by its perfect crepitancy. The upper parts of the lungs were healthy. The larynx and trachea contained a similar but thinner fluid in small quantity, and only lining the mucous membrane. The appearance of the matter found in the stomach was similar. Microscopic examination and subsequent enquiry

* Police Report, L. P., 1843, p. 8.

† Police Report, L. P., 1844, p. 21. See also a case detailed in note to p. 150. It will be borne in mind that there are several recorded instances in which suffocation by forcing cloth &c., into the fauces, was suicidal. In addition to those cited by Taylor, p. 702, one of an artillery soldier under treatment in hospital, where he had previously attempted to throw himself out of a window—who destroyed himself by thrusting a Linen Compress into his throat while he was under the close observation of a special attendant—may be mentioned.—Amer. Journal of Medical Science, July 1854, from Prag. Vierteljahrset, 1853, 2 Bd., p. 111.

See also a case given at page 156 of this Manual in which there was reason to believe that two women of Benares were *burked.*

showed that this matter was *suttoo*. It appeared that deceased had taken a hearty meal of *suttoo* at noon, and that, a few hours afterwards, he vomited, and then suddenly was seized with dyspnœa and noisy respiration, and gradually became speechless and insensible, and died within an hour.

It was considered that there was no cause beyond extreme repletion and a sudden fit of vomiting, to account for the sudden entrance of the food into the air-passages ; nor was there, in the history of the case during life, or in the appearances after death, anything to lead to a belief that a narcotic poison had been employed.

Still, I think that, if the full truth could have been ascertained, it would have been found that this unfortunate man was in a drunken sleep when the vomiting began.

Surgeon-Major T. Moorhead, 26th Cameronians, has reported* the case of a private soldier, aged twenty-eight, who was discovered, at night, by the man lying next to him, to be breathing loudly and with great difficulty, as if there were some obstruction about the lower part of the trachea. He was at once removed to the dispensary, where he died in about fifteen minutes. Several small pieces of potato were found in both bronchial tubes, where these sub-divided into small branches. There was great œdema of the glottis, no doubt from the irritation caused by a foreign body. The epiglottis was remarkably large, and so thickened in structure that it probably performed its functions very indifferently. The lungs were greatly engorged with blood. In the stomach were found several small pieces of potato of the same kind as those found in the bronchial tubes. Assistant Surgeon Cunningham verified the nature of the foreign bodies by microscopical examination. The deceased had drunk some beer and also rum in the course of the evening before retiring to rest. He had been sick, and had vomited while in bed.

Dr. Taylor cites a case of this kind (p. 696) in which a man, going to bed intoxicated, was suffocated by a piece of potato-skin adhering over the *rima glottidis*.†

It would scarcely be an exaggeration to assert that a proportion of mankind die suffocated by *the impaction of living fish in their air-passages.* I have met with five recorded cases of this singular accident, of which three have occurred in India within the last few years.

---

* Ind. Med. Gaz., Dec. 1, 1869, p. 264.

† Two cases of death from swallowing the stick which natives use instead of a tooth-brush are recorded, by Surgeon Watson (Ind. Med. Gaz., June 1, 1869, p. 147), and by Surgeon Hutchinson (*Ibid*, July 1, of same year, p. 141). In the former, a piece of willow stick, six inches in length, "was found lodged in the duodenum, one end of it was projecting through the coats of the duodenum into the under-surface of the liver, which was inflamed and suppurating." The second case is of great importance, in this place, as death, in an old woman, was caused by bronchitis and asphyxia, although the stick was "lying quietly in the æsophagus, and resting on the lower margin" [curvature] "of the stomach."

The following is related in "Wanley's Wonders," Edition of 1806, p. 114, Vol. I :—

"A certain priest that was well skilled in swimming and groping for fish had, in a deep place under the banks, caught a perch, which, to hold the better, he put into his mouth, and so swam back to his companions. The perch, with her struggling, slipped so far into his throat, that the miserable priest was strangled by it, notwithstanding all the endeavors his associates could use to the contrary."

In the same manner a warder belonging to the Bagne at Toulon, while fishing in the dock, caught a fish about seven inches long and two broad; and, not knowing where to place it while baiting his hook, held it between his teeth. The fish struggling, slipped its head first into his mouth, and then down his throat, completely filling up the cavity. The man rushed about for aid, but soon dropped dead from suffocation.*

In 1859, Dr. White reported† the case of a strong Madras Bheestee, into whose mouth a fish had jumped while he was bathing. On opening the mouth, the tail of a large cat-fish presented itself with the body firmly fixed within the fauces, and filling up the isthmus completely. It had entered flat, so that the fin of one side was posterior to the velum, and opened out on any attempt being made to withdraw the fish. The operation of œsophagotomy was commenced and abandoned. A piece of cane was made into a probang, and, with it, attempts were made to press the fish downards into the œsophagus. It did pass downwards, when the patient at once ceased to breathe, gave one convulsive struggle, and died to all appearance. The trachea was immediately opened, and respiration was restored. In the course of the night the man coughed up the fish, the fins having become softened by decomposition.

Dr. White states that "this is by no means an uncommon accident in India. Natives bathing and swimming, which they always do with their mouths wide open, in tanks that abound in fish, are not unfrequently brought to hospital dying from suffocation and alarm with a large cat-fish firmly impacted in the fauces. It is a coarse kind of fish, with long bony fins very sharp indeed at their extremities."

In 1865, a native boy about four years old was brought to the Calcutta Medical College Hospital, with a *Coie* fish impacted in his glottis. These fish are very tenacious of life out of water. The poor child appears to have taken up the fish, and to have put its head into his mouth. In its struggles, its head passed the glottis, and all attempts to withdraw it were prevented by the catching of its gill-plates, anchor-wise, below the vocal chords. The child was suffocated.

Another case occurred in Burmah about two years ago.

---

* British Med. Jour., April 11th, 1863, p. 369.

† The Indian Lancet, October 1st, 1859, p. 71.

Punctiform Ecchymosis in the interior of the body as a proof of Death by Suffocation.

In a memoir on this subject,* Dr. Ogston shows that the spots or effusions in question, with a few and partial exceptions, are found to vary in size from a pin-point to a large pin-head, and in number from three or four to thirty or forty in the respective localities. In fifty-two of the cases, the blood-spots occurred on the surface of the lungs; in thirty-one, on the heart ; in twenty-two, on the inner face of the scalp ; in eighteen, on the pericranium ; in fourteen, on the thymus gland ; in nine, on the interior of the pericardium ; in eight, on the root of the aorta; in five, on the liver; in two, on the skin ; and in four, singly, on the spleen, diaphragm, pulmonary artery, and pleura costalis. In only two instances were these ecchymoses seen in upwards of two hundred drowned bodies, and in only one of between forty and fifty hanged persons. Dr. Ogston has never met with them after death by strangulation. On the other hand, he has sought in vain for these blood-spots in nine cases of undoubted death by suffocation—all adults. Without denying the occasional, though rare, occurrence of punctiform ecchymoses after deaths from other causes, or insisting on their necessary presence in every instance of death by suffocation, he concludes that their discovery in considerable numbers, in well-defined shapes, and limited in size, on the heart, lungs, and thymus gland, especially in infants, either with or without other corroborative tests, and in the absence of other obvious morbid conditions, will afford the strongest presumptive evidence, if not absolute proof, of suffocation.

Twenty-nine years ago I observed that, in certain cases of death, attended with suffocative action, ecchymoses are found upon the plane of the descending thoracic aorta, as it becomes visible through the transparent pleura upon raising the left lung.† I said that this lesion " consists in the presence of numerous raised spots of red or purple ecchymoses, varying from one to four lines in diameter, occupying the cells [areolar tissue] immediately in contact with the denser portion of the external coat, and remaining attached to it after the loose filamentary tissue of its sheath has been torn away. These may be presumed to have been effused by some of the numerous vessels which can always be traced to their circumference ; and generally appear to have been so recently deposited, as to lead to the surmise that they are formed either shortly before death, or during the struggle of the last agony. This form of lesion, together with the state of œdema already noticed, is usually found in conjunction with a turgid state of all the capillary vessels supplying the arterial parietes ; and it is observed in cases where death has been attended with

* Brit. Med. Jour., Sept. 26, 1868, p. 332.

† On Acute Aortitis, Guy's Hospital Reports, Vol. VI., 1841, p. 307.

greatly protracted struggle, as in hydrophobia ; or with suffocative action, as where aneurismal or other tumors have compressed portions of the air-passages : it is also frequent in instances of extensive thoracic inflammation, and especially in pleuritis of the asthenic kind. This appearance is not discoverable, either in the aortic sheath below the diaphragm, or upon either of the smaller arterial trunks." *For opinion in a case where it was questioned whether death arose from Strangulation or Suffocation, vide* APPENDIX E.

For cases of *Suffocation by Carbonic Acid Gas*, see page 292.

Dr. Kenneth McLeod has mentioned to me an instance, in which three men, having incautiously gone to sleep in a small brick-room of Raneegunge, in which a charcoal-fire was burning, were suffocated by the fumes.

The following case of *death from Suffocation, probably from a mixture of Sulphuretted Hydrogen and Carbonic Oxide*, was sent to me by the late Mr. Piddington, Coroner of Calcutta:—

"On the 11th of March 1857, the chief officer of the ship *Fiery Cross* ordered the fore-peak of the vessel to be cleaned out. This order was given at half-past ten in the morning, and a man went down to hand up a number of empty boxes and small boat-casks. He appears to have sustained no inconvenience. There was also a considerable quantity of bilge-water, which had accumulated there, and the men were occupied in lowering buckets and baling it out. About four in the afternoon, the third officer, wishing to see how much water remained, lowered a light down, which was not extinguished, and was hauled up burning. He then ordered a lascar to go down and see what water there was; he did so, and immediately fell senseless. Shortly after this, the serang went down, and also fell senseless. The bodies were both hauled up by means of boat-hooks;—the serang yet alive, though insensible ; the lascar seems to have been alive also, but to have died almost immediately.

"*Post-Mortem Examination.*—There were no marks of violence upon the body, but the face and neck looked puffed. The vessels of the brain and ventricles were engorged with blood. The heart was empty, the liver was engorged, and the stomach was full of food.

"My opinion is, deceased died from congestion of the cerebral vessels.

"*To the Coroner.*—The state of the lungs was perfectly natural; there was excessive congestion of the liver; the state of the lungs did not show the usual signs of suffocation from noxious gases ; the only anomalous symptom was that, on opening the vein of the arm, an unusually large quantity of fluid blood flowed, of a dark rich purple color, such as I have before observed in cases of death produced by noxious gases.

"The serang suffered greatly from low fever, and some delirium, but recovered.

"The cause of this accident undoubtedly was the disturbance of the water and mud, causing the evolution of the gases ; and, as the light burned, they were probably Sulphuretted Hydrogen, with perhaps, from their rapid effect, a mixture of Carbonic Oxide."

SMOTHERING.

When at Howrah, in 1854, I was witness of a frightful accident, in which—the front of an upper-roomed brick building, over-filled with bags of linseed, giving way—a perfect torrent of the seed, weighing many tons, buried and smothered about fourteen unfortunate coolies, men, women, and infants at the breast. The only aid I could render was to assist in digging them out *by hand.* This was a most distressing process. When we dug away below, the linseed came down, in tides, and filled up our excavations; when we worked above, we buried the bodies still deeper. This latter plan was, however, found to answer best. All the dead countenances were placid, around each mouth the linseed was wet, apparently from saliva, not mucus. Wherever the bodies were exposed (the men merely wore dhotees), the pit of a linseed was clearly impressed upon every portion of the skin, so that I thought that the first body which we uncovered was deeply pock-marked.

Dr. Kenneth McLeod has published two cases of persons killed by the falling in of high river banks, where they were digging clay.*

1. The body was rather decomposed; face swollen; tongue protruding; head and shoulders were more livid and decomposed than the lower part of the body; skin and hair covered with sand; no wound or bruise anywhere; body robust and well-rounded; scalp infiltrated with sanguineous serum, skull entire, brain not examined; mouth filled with sand and earth; tongue and pharynx plastered with a layer of the same; œsophagus stuffed with mud; larynx contained a large quantity of earthy sand of finer grain; mucous membrane acutely congested, of a bright red color; trachea, bronchi, and larger bronchial tubes filled with still finer and moister sandy matter, which did not penetrate into the smaller bronchial sub-divisions; lungs uniformly and intensely congested; heart flabby, dilated and *empty* (from *post-mortem* causes ?); stomach filled with a recently-eaten meal of rice, &c.; a few streaks of dirt on the mucous membrane near the cardiac orifice.

Dr. McLeod justly terms this a case of "drowning in sand." He hardly anticipated that the spasmodic gasps of asphyxiation could have sucked the sand so far down the air-tubes, and he was somewhat surprised to find a small quantity of it in the stomach. He has examined at least two cases of drowning in muddy water, and found mud in the air-passages and œsophagus; but it is much more difficult to realize the

---

* Ind. Med. Gaz., Dec. 1, 1869, p. 264, and Jan. 1, 1870. p. 13.

passage of dry sand and earth so far, in such quantities and in such circumstances.

In the second case, the suction into the lungs was even stronger, while no swallowing effect seems to have been made.

2. Eyes, ears, nostrils, and mouth filled with coarse sand, which also powdered the skin and filled beneath the nails of the fingers and toes; mouth and pharynx plastered, but not filled with sand; œsophagus powdered with grains of sand; stomach contained none; larynx and trachea about two-thirds filled with wet sand; lining membrane intensely red; bronchi, to third and fourth divisions, contained sand; lungs intensely congested, not gritty on section.

DROWNING.

In Bengal, where a tank adjoins nearly every dwelling, and where passage across the wider rivers, in small and ill-constructed boats and dug-outs, is extremely perilous during a great part of the year, cases of accidental drowning are, of course, frequent. To take a single example;—in the Commissioner's Report for 1869, it was shown that, during those twelve months, in the four districts of Bograh, Dinagepore, Moorshedabad, and Rajshahye, there were *five hundred and eighty-five* deaths from drowning. In the Burdwan division, there were registered, during that period, *nine hundred and ten* accidental deaths from this cause; and, in the Cuttack district, *two hundred and twenty-seven*.

Even in the Hooghly, near Calcutta, it is no rare thing, in the rains, to hear of the loss of a ferry-boat, containing some twenty natives, of whom every soul has perished. The number of children drowned in tanks every year must be almost incalculable.

It appears, at first sight, very singular how many bodies of adult natives are found in tanks, without any strong suspicion of suicide or murder. It is generally believed, by persons of the lower classes, that those who perish in this manner have fallen victims to epilepsy (*mrigi-roga*—commonly expressed *mrigi*) under demoniacal influence. When, however, it is borne in mind that almost every native literally passes a certain definable portion of his life in the tank nearest to his dwelling, and that bathing is going on in every tank, at nearly all hours—before sun-rise, when the water is very cold,—and during the heat of the day, when the rays of the vertical sun are nearly all reflected from the polished surface of the water,—it is scarcely singular that many bathers should die suddenly, from natural causes, where visceral disease has long been steadily progressing, and merely requires some exposure or cause of internal congestion to determine the fatal issue; and that some should drop down in the water and be drowned when under the influence of cramp, of heat syncope, of true heat-asphyxia (*sourdee ghurmee*), of apoplexy excited by heat, or epilepsy, the paroxysm of which is not very unfrequently excited by the glittering appearance of still water.

On the 8th August 1870, Dr. Woodford pointed out to me, in his dead-house, the body of a poor native woman who fell epileptic over a vessel, in which she was preparing a bath for her sick child, and was scalded to death.

It appears to be generally believed that where, as not unfrequently happens persons die suddenly on the margins of reservoirs, and are found lying, with their heads in the water, they have fallen epileptic. This may be the case in certain instances, but it is probable that, when occurring towards mid-day, or in the afternoon, these are generally cases of sun-stroke, or heat-apoplexy. The pathology of this disease has still, in great measure, to be investigated.* Dr. Russell found, in examining the bodies of several men who were struck down by intense heat, that, in all, the brain was healthy, no congestion or accumulation of blood being observable, although there was a small serous effusion in one instance. The lungs, however, were, in all these cases, congested, even to blackness, through their entire extent ; and indeed, so densely loaded, that complete obstruction must have taken place. There was also an accumulation of blood on the right side of the heart, and in the great vessels approaching it. In two cases which I had an opportunity of examining carefully, during the hot season of 1855, I found appearances similar to these, except that *there was no over-distension of the right cavities of the heart.* Had one of these men been found dead in a tank, these evidences of asphyxia might, not unreasonably, have been attributed to drowning. The bodies of persons sinking in the water under such circumstances would, however, be expected to present certain of the signs of drowning in addition to these. The subject is one of great importance, and deserves fuller investigation than it has hitherto received.

Still it rarely happens that the bodies of persons, thus dying, are brought to the Civil Surgeons for examination, except in cases where death has occurred under manifestly suspicious circumstances, as where the corpse is discovered in a well ; or is found in a reservoir with traces of wounding or other violence ; or has been sunk by weights, &c., in an unusual manner ; or, having been for some time missed, is believed to have been unfairly dealt with.

More than one judicial officer, especially Mr. Sconce of Chittagong, and Mr. Alexander of Howrah, has expressed to me surprise and suspicion at the extraordinary number of deaths alleged to have occurred from *mrigi* in persons whose bodies have been found in tanks. The latter gentleman informed me that, when he first went to Chumparun,

* See a very elaborate Memoir on Insolation, or Heat-Apoplexy, published by the late Mr. Marcus Hill in the Indian Annals of Medical Science, for October 1855.

he was astonished at the number of persons reported daily to have died from drowning in different tanks in the district, owing to dizziness or swimming in the head, called "*mrigi.*" The persons so dying *were principally women and female children.* It struck him as suspicious that so many should be carried off daily in this manner. He, therefore, issued positive orders that all the bodies should be brought in for *post-mortem* examination. Upon this, the reports decreased wonderfully. He believed that many of the persons reported to have died in this manner had been made away with. This class of cases assuredly still demands a rigorous inquiry.

Upon this point, the following case is noteworthy. On the 10th August 1868, information was lodged at the Khettal Police Station (Bogra) that a woman, who was subject to fits of epilepsy, was drowned while bathing. The medical officer pronounced that the deceased had died under suspicious circumstances. On enquiry, it oozed out that the woman had been killed by her husband, aided by a relative of his, owing to her having quarrelled with her mother-in-law.*

There is one set of cases, if not of drowning, certainly of immersion, and of choking with mud and water, which are of great and fatal prevalence among the Hindus inhabiting the entire length of the Gangetic valley, but which do not, at present, come within the power of Police interference. I refer to the exposure and destruction of the sick on the banks of the river—or the practice of *Gunga-Jatra*, or *Ghat Murder*, as it has long been generally termed. It is held, in the Agni Purána, that "those who die when half their body is immersed in Gungá water, shall be happy thousands of thousands of ages, and resemble Brahma." Consequently, it is the practice to bring those whose cases are by their ignorant kobirajira declared to be hopeless, to the banks of the river; and, as life appears to ebb, to plunge the lower part of the body into the stream. The effect of this practice, especially at night and in the cold season, is self-evident. On one occasion, while stationed at Howrah, being in the habit of landing at one of the ghats to which the sick are brought, I actually, without lingering for a moment, saw two persons expire in this manner in the course of a single week. A very few years since, it was the practice to fill the mouths of these unfortunates with water until they were stifled.† This murderous habit is strictly a portion of the rite, but it is supposed to have been abandoned by Hindus of the better classes. Among the more ignorant and bigoted, however, it doubtless continues prevalent.

The atrocity of *sacrificing children by exposing them to be drowned,*

---

* Bengal Police Report, 1868, p. 308.

† *Calcutta Review*, December 1848, p. 431, from which most of these particulars are derived. See also Ward's Chapters on "Funeral Rites" and "Public Morals;" and McCosh's Topography of Assam, page 111.

or to be devoured by sharks or alligators as offerings to the goddess Gunga, was formerly prevalent at Hurdwar, Saugor Island, Bansbaryah, Chaugdah, and other places on the Ganges. Full references to this atrocity and to the Regulations which were issued to check it, will be found in Beaufort's Digest* and in the Rev. Mr. Ward's Work.†

Dr. Fayrer tells me of the recent case of a man who was attacked by the bees which swarm in the Marble Rocks near Jubbulpore. He at once leapt into the river, but the insects continued to settle upon his head, whenever he rose from a dive, so pertinaciously that he at last became exhausted, and was drowned. (Q.—Did he not die from sheer nervous exhaustion ?)

The practice of *destroying children by throwing them into wells* is one of considerable prevalence. Its commission is probably determined by the fact that many children are accidentally drowned in these reservoirs, and that the murderers trust, on this account, to evade suspicion.

In 1845, a Behar woman, having long had a quarrel with two other females, inveigled a child of each into a field, where there was a large well. She made them sit down and pick each other's hair, and, finding an opportunity, threw them in. One of them was saved.‡

In June 1853, a Hindu woman was tried at Bhaugulpore, for the murder of her male child, five or six months old. She was seen at night near a well, and something was heard to drop in. Suspicion was excited, and she was questioned, but evaded answering. Early next morning, the well was searched, and the child's body found. The well belonged to one Fukeer Chowkeedar, who was proved to have been on the spot when the body was taken out, but who, for some unexplained reason, reported at the thannah that the child had died a natural death. The woman pleaded guilty, and stated that, *not having milk for her infant,* she threw it into the well. She was proved to be in very indigent circumstances, and not to have had milk for her infant. One of the witnesses to this effect had been the temporary wet-nurse to the deceased, and had given it milk late in the evening of the day of its death. On being sent into the sudder station, the body was found to be too much decomposed to allow of examination. The Civil Surgeon, however, recorded that there were no external marks of violence, and that the skin had not the appearance of that of a drowned person. This ignorant, simple woman's evident poverty, and want of sustenance for her child, were humanely taken as extenuating circumstances, and she was sentenced to imprisonment for life.§

---

* Paras. 3935-6-7.

† Vol. II., p. 122, Third Edition

‡ Police Report, L. Provinces, 1845, p. 13.

§ Nizamut Adawlut Reports, Vol. III., Part 1 of 1853, page 807.

In 1866 (a time of famine) a woman came into Chyebassa, begging, with her two grand-children, aged about eight and nine years. She threw them into a river, and drowned them "simply because they asked her for some food which she had with her." The eldest was drowned.*

In November 1852, a Hindu woman was tried at Shahabad, for drowning her two children—five and two years old, in a well. The bodies of the children having been found, and the darogah knowing the well to be considerably raised from the ground, sent for the prisoner's brother-in-law, who admitted that, on the night before the occurrence, there had been a quarrel between the prisoner and his wife, and that it was supposed that the prisoner had, in a rage, thrown her children down the well. The prisoner at first declared that the children had fallen into the well accidentally ; subsequently, she confessed the deed, stating that, on the morning after her quarrel with her brother-in-law's wife, when she awoke, she felt so aggrieved, that she took the children to the well, and threw them down ! She further declared that she first placed her little girl on the edge of the well, when she fell in, and afterwards her boy, who fell in also, she turning her head away ; and, on being asked why she did this, she said that her fate was broken, and her heart suggested the deed. The evidence of the Civil Surgeon showed that death was caused by drowning. The only circumstance which seemed in any away to explain her act was mentioned by the woman with whom she had quarrelled, who said that her mother had died of eating opium, and that it was supposed that, when her spirit visited (or, as the witness described it, mounted on her,) she was fierce and quarrelsome. Sentence of death was passed.†

* Bengal Police Report, 1866, p. 226.

† Nizamut Adawlut Reports, Vol. II., Part 2, 1852, p. 789.—Crime of this description is by no means rare among the natives, and was formerly much more prevalent than it is at present. It will be found in Beaufort's "Digest," that several instances having occurred in which individuals were convicted of putting their children to death from an impulse of passion, with the intention of revenging themselves for a real or supposed insult or injury offered to them by another person, under the idea that the guilt of shedding the blood of the innocent victim would lie on the head of the person offering such insult or injury ; proclamation was made throughout the Ceded Provinces, declaring that any person who should be capitally convicted of putting to death his or her child or children, or of putting to death any other child or person, in consequence of a real or supposed iusult or injury, should invariably be punished with death (Para. 2893, p. 536, C. O., Nos. 32 and 55 of Vol. I.) The practice, however, has been merely checked. In 1817, a Hindu was found guilty, at Etawah, of bringing his infant daughter before the door of a person who had beaten him, and of wounding her with a kutter (or dagger) and throwing her down as dead "*under the mistaken notion that the guilt of her innocent blood would lie on the head of his enemy.*" (Macnaghten's Reports, Vol. I., p. 340.) In 1853, a Hindu, at Moorshedabad, who had engaged in a violent quarrel after drinking, brought out his child, only twenty-three days old, and killed her by dashing her on the ground, *that his opponent might suffer in consequence.* (Nizamut Adawlut Reports, Vol. III., Part 1, of 1853, p. 521.) Only a few months since, a Hindu, at Shahjehanpore, murdered his wife, a child only eight years old, while she was sleeping, to revenge himself upon his father-in-law. (Nizamut Adawlut Reports, N. W. P., August 1854, p. 222.) In 1845, a woman of Tipperah, whose husband had married a second wife which led to constant

This is a common crime in the North-West Provinces.

In August 1854, a Hindu woman at Jaunpore, drowned her female child, a year and-a-half old, in an indara, apparently to revenge herself upon her husband, who had slapped her face.*

Mussamut Neemia drowned her child three years old in a *kua* tank, without any discoverable motive. The case was very carefully weighed by the Judges of both Courts. No suspicion whatever of insanity existed. About a month previously to the murder, she became the mother of another infant. It was doubted whether she had been the subject of puerperal fever (mania ?) but the relatives stated her to have been in good health at the time, and about her usual work. (She may have been apparently in good bodily health, and yet have suffered from puerperal mania.) She was sentenced to imprisonment for life.†

Mussamut Guadawa, of Jaunpore, having been abused and beaten by her husband, left his house and threw her son, a child of two, into a well, where he was drowned.‡

Shortly afterwards Mussamut Munnee, of Allygurh, having quarrelled with her husband, murdered her daughter, aged two years, by throwing her into a tank.§

In that part of the country also women thus ill-used or offended very frequently throw themselves and their infants into wells. The females are often rescued—the children generally perish.

Mussamut Bisoonee, of Jaunpore, had a quarrel with another woman (the females had been intriguing with each other's husbands), and threw herself into a well with her girl, a month old, in her arms. She was taken out alive, but the child perished. The next day, the other woman also threw herself into a well, but was brought out living.‖

---

disputes, concluded an altercation by returning to her room, and murdering her own child as it lay asleep upon her bosom. (Police Report, L. Provinces, 1845, p. 40.) See also three very remarkable instances of homicide committed upon this principle, by Brahmins, towards the end of last century, in Sir J. Shore's paper "On Some Extraordinary Facts, Customs, and Practices of the Hindus." (Asiatic Researches, Vol. IV., p. 336.) Some mitigation of these crimes may, possibly, be found in the gross ignorance and superstition out of which they spring; but no palliation of this kind can be admitted in the case of a Mussalmaun woman who was sentenced, upon her own confession, at Beerbhoom, in 1851, for murdering her deaf and dumb son, aged six years, by cutting his throat with a *bhattee*, or coarse knife, and throwing him into a tank, with an avowed desire of bringing a false accusation of murder against her paramour, who had abandoned her. (Nizamut Adawlut Reports, Vol. I. of 1851, p. 515.) See also p. 71 of this Manual.

* Nizamut Adawlut Reports, N. W. P., for the above date, p. 298. See also Nizamut Adawlut Reports, Vol. II., p. 375. (A woman in a sudden fit of passion threw her child into a well, where it was drowned.)

† *Ibid*, N. W. P., 9th January 1852, p. 16.

‡ *Ibid*, 16th July 1853, p. 871.

§ *Ibid*, 18th October 1853, p. 1301.

‖ *Ibid*, 10th December 1852, p. 1469.

A remarkable case of suicide and murder occurred at Rungpore in 1854. It appeared that two sisters-in-law, Mussamatans Kaootranee and Panbee, whose husbands ill-treated them, went at midnight to a tank, carrying with them the infant of the former, twelve months old. One or other of them cut the child's throat, both then threw themselves into the water. Panbee was drowned; the other's heart failed her, and she crept out.*

Mussamut Rabee, a Mahratta, of Saugor, exasperated in a dispute with another female about a trifling debt, jumped after dark into a well, with her infant, aged eighteen months, in her arms. She was extricated alive, her infant was drowned.†

Gureebinoa, of Azimgurh, on being abused by her husband for not having his food ready, ran with her infant in her arms to a brick well, and threw herself and child into it. As she fell, the child slipped out of her arms and was drowned, but the villagers hearing her cries, came and rescued her.‡

Mussamut Doorga, of Muttra, enraged at being refused food by her mother, left the house and threw herself and her infant girl into a well. She herself was brought out alive, and apparently uninjured. The child was drowned.§

Mussamut Nawuleea, of Muttra, quarrelled with her husband's brother, and threw herself into a well, where there was deep water, with her infant daughter. She supported herself by swimming, but the infant was drowned.‖

Children are often drowned for the sake of their ornaments.

In 1806, a Brahmin of Allygurh was found guilty, upon his own confession, of murdering two children, by throwing them into a well, after robbing them of their ornaments.¶

---

* Nizamut Adawlut Reports, 28th October 1854, p. 521.

† Nizamut Adawlut Reports, N. W. P., 4th May 1852, p. 392.

‡ *Ibid*, 8th July 1853, p. 829.

§ *Ibid*, 3rd March 1855, p. 302.

‖ *Ibid*, 11th November 1854, p. 694. See also Nizamut Adawlut Reports, Vol. II., p. 55. (A mother convicted of throwing herself and her two children into a well, causing the death of the younger child, apparently under the influence of sudden anger, excited by an altercation with her husband.)

¶ Macnaghten's Reports, Vol. I., p. 102. See also Reports of N. W. P., 25th February 1852, p. 133. (A boy of six robbed and drowned.) *Ibid*, 1st December 1852, p. 1423. (A boy of nine made away with in the same manner.) *Ibid*, 8th October 1853, p. 1282. (A similar case), p. 226, and for July 1854, pp. 11 and 54 (by a boy ten or twelve years of age). In August 1854, *Ibid*, p. 266, a man sentenced for throwing his newly-married wife, a child of eight or nine years, into a well, after having stripped off her clothes and ornaments.—Nizamut Adawlut Reports, Vol. IV., pp. 59, 192, 293.

Mussamut Monea was found guilty at Sarun, in 1855, of having robbed and stripped a girl of five, and of having drowned her in a well.*

In the same year, Mussamut Nuthiab was sentenced to death at Bhaugulpore for having decoyed three little boys into a garden, where she took off their ornaments. Upon the elder remonstrating, she threw him down a well, out of which he was taken dead.†

Adults are not very unfrequently drowned in Wells.

The author of the Seir Mutaqherin has alluded to a practice of conveying young men, in meat doolies, into seraglios, where they were ultimately thrown into wells by the ladies, or, on detection, by their masters

In 1851, a Hindu was sentenced to death, at Purneah, for killing his wife by throwing her into a well. The darogah reported that, upon raising the corpse out of the well, in which there were six feet of water, it exhibited a black mark, as if from the blow of a lattee, on the right side ; another on the right fore-arm, as if from drawing a cord ; a third, eight fingers in length, from the top of the shoulder to the neck, apparently the brand of a hot iron ; a fourth, also of a burn, from the throat, extending over the shoulder, fourteen fingers long.‡

Again, in 1852, a Hindu of Shahabad was sentenced for having murdered a boy four or five years of age, and for having attempted the life of the child's mother, by throwing them into a large well about thirty-five feet deep.§

Doojah, of Shahjehanpore, confessed that, finding his elder brother's wife in criminal connexion with a person named, he pursued her and threw her into a well, where she was drowned.‖

It does not appear that, in falling into these wells, the bodies of the victims generally receive fractures, or other very severe injuries, which might lead to doubt in the Surgeon's mind with regard to the cause of death. There are two kinds of wells,—the *kua*, or well of small diameter; and the wide-mouthed well or bricked reservoir (*indara*). The bodies of those who fall or are thrown into the former, are, of course, more likely to present traces of contusion, &c. Where, however, a dead body or an infant is merely dropped in head foremost, and is not thrown with a forward impulse, no injury beyond those received by

---

* Nizamut Adawlut Reports, 26th June 1855, p. 806.

† *Ibid*, 7th December 1855, p. 866.

‡ *Ibid*, Vol. I. of 1851, p. 1512.

§ *Ibid*, Vol. II., Part 2, of 1852, p. 500.

‖ Nizamut Adawlut Reports, N. W. P., 18th April 1854, p. 424. See also Police Report, L. Provinces, 1844, p. 13 (a reputed witch thrown down a well). *Ibid* for 1849, p. 19 (a wizard treated in like manner).

contact with the water can be expected to result from the perpendicular fall.*

When at Howrah, near Calcutta, I was sent for to see the remains of a European who had fallen head-foremost into a well in the yard of a reputable inn. He had drank rather freely, and left the billiard table where he had been playing at night, making his way to a corner of the compound where the well was. The mouth of the well was about four feet across, and was surrounded by a parapet about a cubit above the ground. He appeared to have stumbled upon this low parapet, and to have struck his forehead upon the sharp edge of the opposite margin of the mouth of the well. He was found almost immediately afterwards, his head and shoulders immersed in the shallow water and the mud. He was brought up quite dead, the stunning blow on the head, and the position of the body having, doubtless, hastened suffocation.

It is singular that, among the many recorded cases which I have read of persons being thrown into wet wells up-country, I have only been able to find one in which it appeared that severe injury was noticed to have resulted from the fall.† Here, a boy having been robbed of his ornaments, and thrown into a well, the witnesses observed a scar on the head, which was considered to be owing to the body having struck against the sides of the well. The Surgeon, however, stated that death was owing to suffocation by drowning, and that he did not observe any external signs of violence.‡

In another case, a boy of eleven, robbed of his ornaments, and thrown into a well, was drawn up severely bruised, and with his arm broken. It is not mentioned, however, whether the well was wet or dry.§

On the other hand, the Reports contain numerous remarkable instances in which persons thrown into wells were preserved almost unhurt.||

---

* Magistrates may compel the owners of tanks or wells adjacent to any public thoroughfare to fence them in such a manner as to prevent danger. Police officers are to ascertain, from time to time, the state of public wells without proprietors, and to report when they are insecure, with a statement of the expense required to make them secure. Beaufort, paras. 3189 and 3195.

† A boy of ten, who was robbed of his ornaments and thrown into a *dry* well, was killed by fracture of the skull.—*Nizamut Adawlut Reports*, N. W. P., September 1st, 1853, p. 1068.

‡ Nizamut Adawlut Reports, N. W. P., October 8th, 1853, p. 1282.

§ *Ibid*, Feby. 21st, 1852, p. 128.

|| See Police Report, L. P., 1848, p. 9. (A boy thrown into a well by a robber, seized a tree growing out of the brick-work of the well, screamed for help, and was rescued.) *Nizamut Adawlut Reports*, N. W. P., September 3rd, 1853, p. 1113. (An old woman robbed of her ornaments and thrown into a well. The water being unequally deep, she escaped.) *Ibid*, October 3rd, of the same year, p. 1228. (A boy of twelve robbed and thrown into a well. The thief threw a heavy stick down at him; this the child accidentally seized, was supported by it, and saved.) *Ibid*, October 3rd, p. 1238. (A hump-backed man, while stooping over the brink of a well, was pushed in from behind. He fell head-foremost. The water was deep, but he got upon the wooden framework or wall which encircled the water and supported the sides, whence he was rescued.) *Ibid*, January 14th, 1854, p. 25. (A girl of twelve, having been robbed of her necklace, was pushed into a well. She sunk, but rising

Drowning by homicidal violence is by no means so rare an occurrence now as it appears to have been in the time of the Mussalmaun law-givers.*

---

again, clung to some shrubs and weeds growing out of the sides of the mud, until she was rescued.) *Ibid*, March 23rd, 1855, p. 381. (A woman of eighty, travelling with two men who carried her property, was told to look into a brick well, where she would see the deity Sheo. She did so, and was thrown in. She fortunately clung to a brick and supported herself in the water, which was eighteen feet deep.) *Ibid*, July 6th, 1852, p. 633. (A feeble woman, stating herself to be aged eighty or a hundred years, robbed of her ornaments, and thrown into a well, supported by clinging to the branch of a tree.) *Ibid*, March 30th, of same year. (A girl of ten was robbed of her ornaments and thrown into a well. The water was ten cubits deep, but the bore being very narrow, "the child struck across it by her shoulders and feet, her back only getting wet." The witnesses, however, stated that, when she was got up, she was insensible, and did not recover till she had been warmed before the fire.) *Ibid*, October 22nd, 1852. (A girl of eight was plundered of her ornaments, had a handkerchief tied round her neck, and was dropped into a well, "but the knot had been unloosed by the water" [?]; "and whether owing to the air in the handkerchief and clothes, or whether the child, in her simplicity, being not aware of her danger of drowning, placed herself on her back, she did not sink, and was brought up, uninjured.) *Ibid*, May 16th, 1854, p. 546. (A woman thrown into a well by her paramour, saved by clinging to a brick. A man threw his mistress and her infant into a well. The woman dropped the child, which was drowned; she clung to the projecting root of a tree four or five feet below the brick, and was rescued.—*Ibid*, March 7, 1856, p. 551.

It is somewhere mentioned of Jung Bahadoor, I believe by Mr. Oliphant, that, aware of a custom which the Nepaulese have of dropping people into wells, he practised the art of falling into those reservoirs with impunity.

* By the Mussalmaun Law, if a person immerse an infant or an adult in water, from which there is no prospect of his escape by swimming,—as, for instance, in the sea,—he is not liable to retaliation for wilful homicide, according to Aboo Haneefah (as no wounding instrument is used); but the two disciples and Shafijee maintain that he is. All agree, however, that it is manslaughter only, if there be not water enough to endanger life, without swimming; or if the person thrown into the water be capable of swimming, and his arms and legs be not bound, nor a weight tied to the body, and the place be such that he may escape by swimming. The same difference of opinion exists between Aboo Haneefah and his disciples, if the person were drowned from being repeatedly immersed in water till he died. Aboo Haneefah held that, homicide by drowning being of rare occurrence, the deterring from it, by capital punishment, was of less consequence than with respect to prevalent offences. See also Beaufort's Digest, para. 3912.

The ordeal of suspected witches by water, by the Rajpoot Bhoomeas, deserves attention in illustration of this subject, The rules, which appear to be carried out with a precision which would have delighted Hopkins the Witch-Finder, are described as follows by a writer in the *East Indian Army Magazine* for October 1854:—"The suspected person is confined up to the neck in one side of a common canvas pack-saddle, and in the other side are sewn up two and-a-half cakes of cow-dung; the whole is now thrown into a deep pool, and, should the unfortunate woman sink, she is sometimes saved; but, if she unfortunately floats, she suffers the fatal penalty of her supposed crime. A still more cruel ordeal is for a man to drag the woman into deep water, where he supports himself by the aid of a strong bamboo, another person on the bank fires an arrow, and, on its leaving the bow, the man leaps on the woman's back and presses her under; if she continues below the water until the arrow is brought back to the archer, she is no witch; but, should her struggles or any accident bring her to the surface before that time, she is considered guilty, and adds one more victim to the number sacrificed to this deadly superstition." This is also a Bengalee mode of ordeal.—*Ward*, Vol. I., ed. of 1822, p. 55.

Allusion has already been made to the frequent commission of deliberate murder by children of tender years.

The following cases of drowning by young girls require more especial notice here:—

In 1810, one Mussamut Odhaneah, a girl only nine years and four months old, was convicted, at Allygurh, of having drowned a child in a nullah not more than a span deep, and for stealing the ornaments worn by the deceased.*

In 1852, a married Hindu girl, of Hooghly, "only twelve or thirteen years old," was left by herself in charge of an infant, a month old. The mother of the infant not returning when she was expected, the girl appears to have carried the child about four miles, and was seen on the way patting it, and endeavoring to soothe it. Its body was afterwards found in a tank, without any traces of blows, having evidently died from drowning. It was thought probable that, in her weariness and despair at the infant's fretfulness, she had thrown it into the tank. The child had not worn any ornaments.†

In 1853, a Hindu woman of seventy and a boy of ten or twelve years were convicted of having stifled a child eight years old in a shallow ditch (probably by placing a hand over his mouth and nose, and sinking him in the water), and of having robbed him of his ornaments. The medical officer found "the lungs distended with air, the blood-vessels gorged, and the right side of the heart full of blood," whence he deduced that the death was a violent one, and was probably caused by suffocation, but the decomposed state of the body prevented certainty. There were no external marks of violence.‡

In 1843, a woman and her paramour were condemned, on their own confession, for the murder of the former's husband, having twisted his cloth round his mouth, and killed or drowned him in a ditch containing three feet of water; the deceased being a weak man.§

Three boys driving their cattle into the Soane for water, saw a person, who was afterwards proved to be a bad character and a thief, lay hold of a traveller in the midst of a piece of dead water, and, tripping him up, hold him under till life was extinct.‖

A Rajshahye man confessed that, having abducted a married woman, he sat down with her on the river side, and she refused to accompany him further—saying that, if he accompanied her to her father's house, the

---

* Macnaghten's Reports, Vol. I., p. 213, previouly cited.

† Nizamut Adawlut Reports, Vol. II., Part 2, of 1852, p. 467.

‡ Nizamut Adawlut Reports, Vol. III., Part 1, of 1853, p. 634. See also similar cases.—Macnaghten's Reports, Vol. I., p. 76; and Nizamut Adawlut Reports, Vol. III., Part 1, p. 197.

§ Nizamut Adawlut Reports, Vol. III., Part 1, p. 192.

‖ Police Report, L. P., for 1843, p. 13.

inmates would not receive her; if she became a *boistumee*, and went with him, he would desert her as soon as his wife was old enough to cohabit with him; and that, if she returned home, her husband would cut off her hair and nose. He was to go by himself,—as for her it was better she should die. That, not being able to persuade her to go on, and, on her saying that he might strike or kill (*mar*) her, he got angry, seized her by the hand, and, dragging her to the river, forced her into the water, in a place where the depth was up to the knees, and with his left hand held her hair, and with the right on the back of her neck kept her head under water till she died. He then lifted up her body, and, finding that she had ceased to breathe, he left the corpse in the water and went home—taking with him her ornaments and the things she had given him.*

A man of Baraset, walking along the banks of the river with a person who had seduced the wife of one of his relatives, dragged him into the water, and held his head under until he was dead.†

A Sylhet man having had intercourse with another's mistress, the injured person waylaid him on the banks of a jheel, and, aided by others, bound him hand and foot, and threw him in.‡

Several persons of Jaunpore were capitally sentenced for murdering two men, one of whom they severely wounded, and then bound and threw into a *nullah*. §

Mussamut Mykeea, of Shahjehanpore, was convicted of the murder of a girl ten years of age, by drowning her, after tying her hands with a rope made of *bukhela* grass, after which she took the silver ornaments from the body.‖

Cases are of rather frequent occurrence in Bengal, in which persons are knocked down either in the shallow water of irrigated or flooded paddy fields, or in the small pools which so abound over the whole country, and die either from the effects of the blow, or from drowning while in a stunned condition. More than one of these cases was brought to me for investigation at Chittagong, but the bodies were so much decomposed, that I could form no opinion from them of the cause of deaths.—Two chuprassies attached to the G. T. Survey, began to catch fish in a hole, about eight feet square, with a foot and-a-half or two feet of water in it; the surface of the water was about the same depth below the level of the ground, and a small bund of the earth thrown out rose about the same height at the edge. The owner of the pool interfered with them. One of them struck the man with a cane stick, the other with his hand, and knocked him into the

* Nizamut Adawlut Reports, 30th November 1854, p. 694.

† *Ibid*, 1850, p. 63.

‡ *Ibid*, 1848, p. 35.

§ Nizamut Adawlut Reports, N. W. P., 5th August 1853, p. 955.

‖ *Ibid*, 24th November 1854, p. 752.

hole. Several very unintelligent witnesses saw the occurrence, and stated that the chuprassies held the old man down with their lattees;—running up, they saw the chuprassies take the man out in a dying state. The Assistant Surveyor considered it impossible for a man to be drowned in the hole by two others holding him down with the canes produced in Court. The medical officer found the body too much decomposed for examination. The only fact proved, therefore, was that the deceased was struck, fell into the pool, and died.*

It was reported, shortly before the publication of my last edition, that a native woman had fallen into a well in Calcutta, and had drawn in and drowned a man who attempted to save her.

The reports of the North-West Provinces are replete with instances in which persons have been *murdered and thrown into wells*, and many have been cited in this Manual. This, we have already seen, was a frequent practice among the Thugs.†

It by no means very rarely happens in this country, that persons are more or less completely *strangled, and then thrown into wells or tanks.* Cases of this kind may, of course, call for very careful discrimination on the part of the medical jurist.

Chyetunno, Christian, and Mussamut Dungun Mallah, of Backergunge, were sentenced for the murder of a girl ten or twelve years old, married about a year previously, to the male prisoner, who had for some time cohabited with the female prisoner, his brother's widow ; each of the prisoners accused the other of throttling the poor child, whose body was found in a hole with shallow water. The mouth was full of blood, blood issued from the nose, and those who observed the body saw black marks on either side of the gullet. The medical officer received the body when it was too putrid for examination.‡

A delicate-looking girl, from thirteen to fifteen years of age, was sentenced at Jaunpore to imprisonment for life, for strangling a young boy, the son of her husband's former mistress. The body was found in a well. There can scarcely be a doubt, judging by the confessions of the prisoner, and another woman, her accomplice, that the boy's neck was compressed. The Civil Surgeon considered that his death was caused by

---

* Nizamut Adawlut Reports, November 3rd, 1854, p. 528.

† See page 56. In addition to the cases in which the bodies of murdered persons were thrown into wells, which were afterwards filled up,—see two others, Nizamut Adawlut Reports, N. W. P., 13th November 1854, p. 711, and Police Report, L. P., 1845, p. 31. Col. Sleeman mentions that, during the scarcity of 1833, the bodies of two hundred people in a village in the Jaunpore district were thrown into one large well, which was then closed. For additional cases of persons murdered, and then thrown into wells, see Nizamut Adawlut Reports, N. W. P., 22nd September 1852, p. 1053 (a person killed by fracture of the skull and thrown into a well); and the 1st November following, p. 1277 (a woman's head being severed, the body cast into a well).

‡ Nizamut Adawlut Reports, October 11th, 1854, p. 441.

drowning; the boy might, he thought, have been thrown into the well before he was quite dead.*

Mukowa, widow, was found guilty, in 1836, at Dharwar (Bombay Presidency), of having, under pretext of affection, enticed a boy of seven to a lonely place, where, for the sake of a few ornaments of trifling value, she murdered him by strangulation, and then threw his body into a well.†

In a country traversed by many large and rapid rivers, into which it is customary to throw the corpses of a large proportion of the poorer inhabitants, it would be expected that the bodies of murdered persons would very frequently be made away with in this manner. Doubtless, there occur many instances of the kind which never come under the notice of the authorities; and several cases are given in the Reports, in which bodies were thus disposed of. The recorded instances are also not unfrequent in which the bodies of murdered persons have been sunk, not only in tanks but in rivers, either by fastening the limbs to some weight at the bottom,‡ or by attaching to them bags of earth or bricks§ (stones not being common in Bengal), or by tying large gurrahs (earthen vessels) round the neck or waist.||

The fact of a body being found sunk in a river with earthen vessels or other weights attached, or secured to a stake, cannot, however, in the absence of other evidences of crime, be considered as proof of homicide. The bodies of the Hindu poor are frequently sunk in this manner.¶

---

* Nizamut Adawlut Reports, N. W. P., January 5th, 1853, p. 15.

† Bellasis' Reports, p. 113.

‡ Nizamut Adawlut Reports, Vol. I. of 1851, p. 661; and Macnaghten's Reports, Vol. II., p. 163.

§ Nizamut Adawlut Reports, Vol. III., Part 1, of 1853, p. 406—and two other instances. Also Calcutta Police Report for 1852, p. 5 (body sunk in a tank). Nizamut Adawlut Reports, N. W. P., for July 1854, p. 107 (body sunk in a well).

|| Case reported by Mr. Hutchinson, of Shahabad, in 1844. A similar case has occurred under my own notice. See also Police Report, L. P., 1838, p. 71 (a man murdered and his body sunk in the river, with pots filled with sand fastened to his waist). *Ibid* for 1845 (the body of a woman believed to have been murdered, found sunk in a tank, with pots of earth fastened to it). Nizamut Adawlut Reports, December 3rd, 1853 (body of a murdered man found floating in the river, the hands and feet tied together with a rope which was twice tied round the neck, reaching to the waist, where it was also tied twice round, and a gurrah attached to it). *Ibid*, March 2, 1855, p. 304 (the skeleton of a murdered man found sunk in a river by means of *koolsees* filled with sand). Nizamut Adawlut Reports, N. W. P., July 23, 1852, p. 727 (a headless body found in a river, the hands and feet bound with ropes, and four large gurrahs attached to sink it).

Body of a man supposed to have been strangled sunk with gurrahs in tank.—*Nizamut Adawlut Reports*, July 5, 1855, p. 11, for other similar cases, *vide supra*, p. 23.

A boy pushes another into a tank, his mother cuts the body with a sickle, and pegs it to the bottom of the tank.—*Bengal Police Report*, 1868, p. 228.

¶ Ward says, that the poor of Bengal "throw the body into the river, or fasten it with a stake and cord by the side of the river, or tie a pan filled with water to the body, and sink it."

A very common practice prevails among criminals in the N. W. Provinces of *sinking bodies of murdered persons enveloped in blankets, cloths, and bags.* It would appear that the corpse is tied up to render its conveyance more easy, and that it is recklessly thrown into the water without removing the covering. This unguarded course, however, frequently leads to detection.*

There are so many exceptions to the rule that the bodies of Mussalmauns are buried, and that those of the poorer Hindus, having been partially consumed or scorched, are thrown into the river, that it would be difficult to point to any circumstances which should give a suspicious character to the discovery of the body of an unknown native, left on the bank or floating upon the surface of an Indian river, unless there were evidences of its limbs having been tied during life. All of the very poorest natives, Mussalmauns as well as Hindus, dwelling on the banks of the large rivers, unhesitatingly commit their dead to the stream, whenever they are unable to incur the expense and trouble of burial or incremation. The strict rule of the Hindu Shastras enjoins that lepers (whose absolution is not performed by their sons), those who die by accident or suicide, and those who, renouncing their families, become mendicants, should not be burnt after death.† Adherence to these rules, especially in the cases of those who commit suicide, or are accidentally killed (who cannot "be thrown into the desert like wood," as the Shastra commands), would lead to the submersion of a great number of suspicious bodies. Fortunately, however, it rarely, if ever, happens that such corpses are brought from the river for medico-legal examination.

Judicial Drowning.

"If a woman causes any person to take poison, or sets fire to any person's house, or murders a man, then the Magistrate, having bound a stone to her neck, shall drown her, upon condition of her not being with child."—*Halhed*, p. 306.

This practice was rather frequently had recourse to by the Mahomedans.

---

* Nizamut Adawlut Reports, N. W. P., 10th February 1862, p. 110—(A man beaten and throttled to death; his body tied up in a sheet and thrown into a tank.) July 20th, 1852, p. 689—(A man strangled, his body carried to the river wrapped in his own *doputtah.*) *Ibid*, February 4th, 1853, p. 153—(A man strangled, his body wrapped in his own blanket with a large stone, and sunk in a *nuddee.*) *Ibid*, May 17th, 1853—(A man killed by injury to the head, his body tied up in a cloth with a view to taking it to the river.) *Ibid*, July 16th, 1853, p. 866—(A man strangled, his clothes rolled tightly round his arms and legs, before throwing the body into the river.) *Ibid*, October 20th, 1853, p. 1311—(A girl hacked to death, the body first buried, then disinterred, wrapped in a sheet and thrown into a tank.) *Ibid*, December 8th, 1853, p. 1451—(A man's throat cut, his body wrapped in a blanket and thrown into a well.) *Ibid*, April 28th, 1854, p. 451—(A man strangled with a cotton rope, his body wrapped up in a blanket and thrown into a well.) *Ibid*, January 8th 1855, p. 21—(A woman strangled or hanged, her body placed in a *pote* and thrown into a well.)

† Calcutta Review, September 1851, p. 223.

The author of the Seir Mutaqherin says that, in 1763, Meer Kassim Khan thus disposed of many of his state prisoners, disaffected grandees of his Court, among whom were two who had been Deputy Governors of Azimabad, Ramnarayan, and Raja Rajbullub. They were, probably, all thrown into the Ganges, with bags of sand or vessels of water fastened to their necks. His translator adds that Juggut Sett, the great banker, and his brother, Raja Seroopchand, were thrown into the river from a tower of the fort of Monghyr, which was long pointed out by the boatmen. The banker's faithful servant, Chunni, insisted on dying with his master.

Suicide by Drowning.

Formerly, suicide was systematically committed in this manner; and although, under the control of our Government, these practices have been greatly checked, still it is probable that no ancient superstitious custom has or ever will become entirely extinct in India.

Dr. Buchanan Hamilton says, that the prejudice against lepers in Bengal is so great, that some of the lower castes, when seized with this disease, cause themselves to be destroyed. They are placed in a boat, and, a bag of sand being tied to their necks, they are carried to the middle of the Ganges, and there thrown overboard. The people thus drowned are perfectly willing, both because they are miserable and helpless, and because they think that the sin to which the disease is attributed will be removed by their dying in the sacred stream ; and they cannot afford to have the forms of expiation (*Prayaschitta*) performed, as is usually done for the Brahmans or wealthy persons that may be afflicted with this disease. The books of law (*Dharmsastra*), he was told, condemn this kind of expiation by drowning, or rather say, that the expiation by ceremony (*Prayaschitta*) is the only one effectual ; but a passage of the Mahabharat is interpreted so as to recommend the drowning, and where perfectly voluntary, it perhaps saves the unfortunate wretch from much worldly suffering.*

The following statement appeared in the *Friend of India* of September 1, 1864, p. 972 :—

" Mujgaon, in Hurdui, has lately been the scene of a most extraordinary tragedy. A man, named Bhujaohad, has, for some time, been suffering under a loathsome disease, and was bed-ridden. So intense were his sufferings that his entreaties to his friends had been unceasing to take him to the Ganges, and sink him in that sacred stream. His prayer appears to have been at last responded to. Three relatives, now in custody, went to the house of the deceased, with a dooly and kahars, placed Bhujja in it, had him conveyed to the banks of the Ganges, and there sank him in due and ancient Hindu form, tying an earthen pot charged with sand to

* Montgomery Martin's E. Bengal, Vol. I., p. 114.

the head, and another to the heels. Bhujja's wife made no objection to his removal from the house; and the kahars, who say the man was alive when committed to the stream, assisted throughout the tragedy without a murmur. The whole matter might have passed quietly into oblivion had not the widow, for some cause or other, divulged the affair to the police a few days ago."

Ward mentions that "a friend of his saw sixteen females drown themselves one morning at Allahabad. Each had a large empty earthen pan slung by a cord over either shoulder ; a Brahmin supported each as she went over the side of the boat, and held her up till she, by turning the pan aside, had filled it, when he let her go and she sunk. While Dr. Robinson resided at the same place, twelve men went in boats to drown themselves in the same spot. Each had a piece of bamboo fastened to his body, at each end of which was suspended a large earthen pan. While these remained empty, they buoyed them up on the surface of the water ; but each man with a cup kept filling the pans from the river, and as soon as they were full, they dragged their victim to the bottom. Ward also relates the instance of a devotee who drowned himself near Nuddea, by sinking himseif in mid-stream with pans fastened to his neck and waist.

If a body be found sunk in this manner in either a *tank* or a *well*, it must be certain that either murder or suicide has been committed. In my last edition, I remarked that I had not met with any instance in which a person seeking self-destruction in one of these reservoirs attached weights to his body. Dr. Woodford has, however, given me one. He writes :—"In 1867, I had occasion to examine the body of a very interesting case, which was that of a native man tied by the neck, hands, and feet, by a complete net-work of thin rope, to which was attached an iron weight of 28lbs. The evidence showed that, after fastening the weight securely to his feet, he must have slipped himself from the edge of the well into the water, where he was found drowned. In such cases the manner in which the rope is tied should be carefully scrutinized. In examining the body of a woman found sunk in a tank with *gurrahs* attached to it, I felt convinced that it was in the last degree improbable that the strong knots with which the rope was tied round her waist could have been fastened by herself.

In the Report already noticed, Dr. Woodford shows that, out of twenty-one suicides which came under his notice in Calcutta, during the year 1850, six were cases of drowning. There are only two cases of accidental drowning noted in Dr. Woodford's table, but this merely represents the small number of bodies recovered. For Statistics of Suicide by Drowning in India, see p. 670.

A few brief additions may be made to the rules for the investigation of cases of supposed drowning, laid down by the European medico-legal authorities, to illustrate the proper mode of inquiring into such cases in India.

Dr. Woodford has favored me with the following very important note ***on the time at which submerged bodies rise in this country*** :—

"On several occasions I have been referred to by medical brethren in the mofussil (country) as to the ***shortest time*** in which it is ***possible*** for a submerged body to rise to the surface of the water in this country. The information has been sought in reference to some important cases of murder depending on the verification of time. The ***shortest time*** I have known, at the hottest season of the year, has been twenty-four hours,—that is to say, when the body has been entirely submerged in deep water, which is a very different thing indeed to a body being found floating close to the edge of a sloping tank in ***shallow water***. In such cases they may rise to the surface in four or five hours, or, should the head be resting on the bank at the extreme edge of the water, the feet will then rise to the surface, and the body float almost as soon as life is extinct."

On the 1st of January 1867, I had the opportunity of noting the precise, yet different, time a certain number of bodies took in rising to the surface of the Hooghly when the thermometer stood at 75° Farht. The steamer *Calcutta*, with some 500 or 600 passengers on board, had just passed the Bank of Bengal on its way to Armenian Ghat, when the vessel grounded; but she let in water with such rapidity that nearly if not all the passengers were panic-stricken, and, though the steamer was sinking in deep water, some plunged into the river, others took to boats which came to the rescue, in such crowds that many tumbled overboard, and some boats capsized altogether, and numbers were drowned.

The accident occurred at 6-30 P.M., and it was computed by the Police that some 30 to 50 passengers had lost their lives; of these only nine bodies were recovered. It is of these nine I purpose giving an account from my note-book, as they all fell into the water at the same time, or within a few minutes of each other. The question, therefore, naturally arises, why they did not rise to the surface at or about the same time ? Some may have been held under by ship chains ; but, from close inquiry, I do not think that could have been the cause in the majority, although it may have happened to some of the number who rose later, but I am disposed to attribute it to the difference of dress, which may, by its different degrees of thickness, have delayed decomposition.

1. Job Simson, East Indian, picked up at the moment of expiring; conveyed to the Howrah Hospital, but arrived dead.

2—R. H. Harris, East Indian ; 3—Edwin Hayes, East Indian; 4—Abdool Rohoman, Native; submerged, 6-30 P.M., 1st ; rose to surface, 9 A.M. on 5th ; 87 hours submerged, or upwards of $3\frac{1}{2}$ days ; thermometer 75° Farht. The three bodies were covered with sand and mud, the hands and feet were soddened, the faces and necks were livid, and the hair on all was perfect.

5. Mrs. Dyer, European, 3 days and 23 hours submerged ; same

morbid appearances as 2, 3, and 4, except that one eye had been eaten by fish.

6. George Smith, European, three days and twenty-three hours submerged; removed from water on the 5th instant, at 5 P.M.; examined by me at 8 A.M. on 6th; similar morbid appearances as 2, 3, 4, and 5, but face and neck decomposing rapidly; hair perfect.

7. Louisa Brown, European, submerged at 6-30 P.M. on the 1st; rose at 8 A.M. on 6th instant; 4½ days or 112 hours.

8. Miss Taylor, European, submerged at 6-30 P.M., 1st; rose at 10 A.M., on 7th instant; 5½ days or 136 hours; identified by the clothes only; much decomposed.

9. ——————, European girl, not identified, submerged at 6-30 P.M. on the 1st; rose at 10 A.M. on the 9th instant; decomposing, yet in a fair state of preservation; hair nearly all off the head, and the cuticle of the scalp peeled easily off.

To these may be added the case of James Augier, a European, who was drowned in the same month, on the 26th January 1867, at 6 A.M., and rose to the surface at 10 A.M. on the 30th; submerged four days and four hours; thermometer 68-70° Farht.; much decomposed; hands soddened, and skin peeled off; the boots had preserved the feet."

Dr. Taylor remarks that, "if, in examining a body taken from water, we discover traces of mortal disease, or marks of external violence sufficient to destroy life, then there is always room for suspicion. Why the body of a person, who has really died from natural causes, should be afterwards thrown into water, it would not be easy to explain; but we can readily appreciate the motive where murderous violence has been used."*

This rule, it will be observed, applies here to bodies found in tanks, lakes, wells, and rivulets, but not to those discovered in the Ganges and its tributaries.

External appearances.—The very characteristic pallid condition of the bodies of Europeans recently drowned is, of course, not recognizable in natives. It might be noticed in persons of high caste and light complexion, but the hue of the low-caste native's skin only appears darker after death. Neither can any discoloration of the lips of these people (short of extreme congestion) be at all received as a guide.

The tongue is generally described as being "swollen and congested, frequently pushed forwards to the internal edges of the lips, sometimes lacerated by the teeth."—Taylor, p. 625. I have not observed very extraordinary congestion of this organ in cases of drowning; it will, doubtless, be most marked in very plethoric subjects. Mr. Bishop† found, in the

* Page 700, 5th Ed.

† Quoted by Dr. Taylor, p. 629.

body of a female, which had been in the water about an hour and-a-half, that " the tongue was neither swollen nor indented, but pallid."

Brain.—Allusion has already been made to the danger of grounding a medico-legal opinion upon observation of the fulness of the cerebral and meningeal veins after death from Asphyxia. Dr. Taylor remarks :—" That a congested state of the cerebral vessels is often met with in the bodies of the drowned, is a fact which cannot be disputed; but the same degree of congestion is observed not only in other cases of Asphyxia, but also in the inspection of bodies where death has proceeded from various causes unconnected with cerebral disturbance."—Fifth Ed., p. 666. In the case of adult females, Mr. Semple *found the cerebral vessels nearly empty.** Apoplexy, the result of mere congestion, is a very rare occurrence in drowning. Dr. Taylor has met with reports of only two cases. A rather obscure case was reported in 1844, by Mr. Macnash, of East Burdwan, in which the body of a healthy female child, found in a tank, presented no trace of external injury, except a slight and apparently accidental scratch on the neck, but internal examination showed that death had been occasioned by apoplexy, as a considerable quantity of blood was found effused in the brain. He considered that suffocation by drowning might have produced this appearance.

In 1834, I assisted in examining the body of a sailor who fell into the sea from the yard-arm vertex downwards. This accident happened, if I remember rightly, in the Mediterranean ; he survived it several weeks, although with severe cerebral symptoms, and died in Haslar Hospital. We found very extensive effusion of blood beneath the arachnoid of both hemispheres.† Injuries of this kind are only liable to occur, in India, in falling from the larger sort of native vessels, and from buildings and trees overhanging rivers and tanks.

Dr. Taylor mentions (pp. 644-45-46) cases in which *the vertebræ of the neck were fractured in drowned persons.* While I was Secretary to the Head of the Medical Department, it happened that there passed through my hands, in one year, regimental reports of two unmistakable cases, in which poor fellows, taking " headers " into shallow water, struck the bottom, and broke their necks.

According to the authority above cited,—" The only characters met with *internally* upon which any confidence can be placed to indicate that the individual has been drowned, are the *presence of water in the stomach,* and the presence of *a mucous froth on the lining membrane of the trachea ;* but, at the same time, the restrictions to the admission of these signs as positive evidence of drowning, may be such as to throw great uncertainty on the correctness of a medico-legal opinion

* Lancet, May 1841, and Op. Citat., p. 682.

† Noticed by Dr. Taylor, p. 644.

founded simply on their existence." The presence of water in the stomach affords strong evidence of drowning,—when it is salt, when it is in very great quantity, or when it is of peculiar color, as in peat bogs, &c., or contains weeds or confervæ. Throughout the greater part of India, the first of these is out of the question. It is well known that, where the power of deglutition is lost, or the drowning person never rises to the surface, water may not enter the stomach. Again, its presence in moderate quantities, without admixture of weeds or mud, can scarcely go for much in persons who are habitually water-drinkers. I find, on comparing five cases of drowning quoted by Dr. Taylor, that in one case the stomach contained three ounces of liquid; in two, half a pint; and in one, about a quart. Dr. Ogston found water in the stomach in five cases out of seven. Usually, the natives do not drink more than a pint of water at a time. Still the discovery of a quart of rather indifferent water in the stomach of one of them would hardly appear singular. It would be very desirable that, in sending in the bodies of persons supposed to have been drowned, the police should state whether the bottom of the reservoir or channel in which the body was found was of mud or sand, and also what kind of vegetation grew on its margin, and within it, whether grass, large aquatic weeds (tank jungle), or green mantling. As most of the bodies dissected in the Calcutta Medical College are procured from the river, examination of these would be likely to throw considerable light upon the question whether water enters the stomach and lungs of a body immersed after death. The late Professor Walker, of the College, informed me that he has never seen water in the stomachs or air-passages of bodies from the river.

According to Dr. Taylor, "water does not readily penetrate into the stomach of a subject which has been thrown in after death; the sides of the œsophagus applying themselves too closely to each other to allow of the passage of the fluid. If putrefaction has advanced to any extent, it is possible that water may enter." We must, at the same time, consider that, with the advance of decomposition, the distension of the internal organs with gases rather favors the expulsion than the ingress of fluids and air.

Water may or may not be present in the lungs of persons drowned; and Dr. Taylor remarks that "there is little doubt that the quantity may become increased after death, because it is now well known that water will penetrate into the lungs, before the access of putrefaction, when the body is thrown in dead."

In 1866, I happened to be present when a native lad, *ætat* about fourteen, was brought out of the tank in Dalhousie Square, Calcutta; so that he received immediate aid. It was, from the first, evident that a great deal of water had entered the bronchial tubes. He became my patient in hospital, and it was strange that no emetic could be got to act. On about the third day, I had to leave, but I understood that he died shortly afterwards of pneumonia.

When at Chittagong, I examined a case, in which the detection of *foreign matters in the air-passages* established a very important point in evidence. The body of a child was discovered in a tank at a considerable distance from his own house, and suspicion was naturally excited that he had been conveyed thither and made away with. Dissection afforded clear evidences of death from drowning ; the fauces, larynx, and trachea contained small portions of green vegetable matter, and the right bronchus was almost completely filled with so large a portion of an aquatic weed, doubled together, that it appeared astonishing how any such body could pass the rima. It was afterwards proved distinctly that no weed of the kind grew in the tank where the body was found. Further inquiry led to the discovery that the boy's body had been found by a woman in a tank near his home, in which the weed lodged in the air-passages grew abundantly. This female had conveyed the corpse to the more distant tank, which belonged to a person against whom she bore a grudge.*

The presence of *mucous froth in the trachea and lungs* is a frequent and important sign, but it is not always present ; it may result from strangulation, apoplexy, narcotic poisoning, and other forms of Asphyxia ; and is liable to disappear after long submersion, or where the subject is allowed to remain exposed to the air for several days before it is examined.† Dr. Casper's observations on the putrefactive process bear with considerable importance upon these forms of Asphyxia. He found that, of all the internal organs, the larynx and trachea are the first to exhibit the changes of decomposition. If the person have not died by Asphyxia or laryngitis, the whole extent of the mucous membrane of the trachea will be found perfectly pale, while the body remains fresh, or exhibits a few green spots upon the abdomen. As soon, however, as this green color begins to spread over the abdomen, but before any change has taken place in any of the other internal organs, the mucous membrane of the larynx and trachea will have become discolored, acquiring a cherry-red color, which gradually, with the progress of decomposition, settles into a dark brown. In many hundred bodies examined, of persons of all ages, and with his attention directed particularly to this point, Dr. Casper declared that he had never found a single exception to the rule here stated.‡

The generality of bodies found in Indian rivers and tanks have

---

* See a case of drowning, by Mr. H. Carter, in which mud was found *throughout* the air-passages.—*Trans. of Medical and Physical Society of Bombay*, No. IX., p. 43, 1842.

† Taylor.

‡ Gerichtliche Leichen. Oeffnungen Zweites Hundert, Berlin, 1853; and Amer. Jour. of Medical Science, July 1854.

suffered, more or less, from the depredations of fishes, &c. I, when at Howrah, examined a putrid corpse which had evidently been sunk in water. I gave it as my opinion that the water in which the body had been lying was of recent collection, as there were no traces of gnawing. It was decided, by two American Coroners, that fish do not begin their depredations upon a body until after decomposition has set in. This may be true as regards bodies drowned in the sea; but I have known bodies, in Indian tanks and rivers, attacked either by fish or water-rats, or aquatic insects, before there was the slightest sign of decomposition.

There are many facts which show that our present knowledge of the *Condition of the Thoracic Organs, and especially of the Heart, in cases of Asphyxia,* is very far too loose and indefinite to guide us safely in forming a decided opinion upon cases involving a suspicion of homicide.

Thinking it right to draw my illustrations, as far as possible, from the pages of our best authority, I shall quote the following contrasted observations cited by Dr. Taylor :—

Case, by Dr. Farquharson, of a woman whose body had been in the water about an hour.—Examined about sixteen hours after death. The trachea and bronchial tubes contained watery froth or frothy mucus. On compressing the lungs a discharge of watery froth took place from the mouth, a small quantity of watery fluid having previously escaped when the body was turned over. *All the parts of the pulmonary tissue were gorged with blood, and were much heavier and of a darker red color than in the normal state; the posterior portions of both lungs were more engorged underneath, or from position; the right cavities of the heart and the coronary veins were filled with dark fluid blood, the left cavities were empty.*

Case, by Mr. Bishop, of a woman whose body had been in the water about an hour and-a-half.—Examination twenty-four hours after death. Mucous froth in considerable quantities was found in the trachea; the vesicles were exceedingly minute in the upper part, but at the lower portion of the tube they were as large as a mustard seed; a small quantity of clear fluid flowed through the bronchial tubes when the lungs were raised. *The lungs were not collapsed: they crepitated on pressure, and were rather bloodless anteriorly; posteriorly they were somewhat gorged with blood, apparently from gravitation. The right side of the heart was very flabby, and contained scarcely any blood.*

Dr. Taylor had justly contrasted these cases "as showing the variable nature of the appearances met with in the drowned." They prove far more than this—they display, most convincingly, the great variability and uncertainty of the signs of Asphyxia, for there can be no doubt that both were genuine instances of Asphyxia by drowning; and yet all recorded observation tends to show the prevalence of a conviction that the essential and invariable characteristic evidence of Asphyxia is the accumulation of blood in the right heart and in the lungs. I believe this opinion to be decidedly erroneous.

The following case first particularly drew my attention to this point.

In going through the wards of a London Hospital, many years since, I found a number of gentlemen endeavoring to restore animation by galvanism, artificial respiration, and other means to a young, strong-looking man, who had been treated too freely with opium in an attack of Delirium Tremens. The heart's action was maintained for a considerable time, but every measure ultimately failed. It was found, upon examination, that the right cavities of the heart were well contracted and almost empty, while the lungs were very extremely engorged with blood, and were studded throughout with a multitude of small apoplectic effusions. Here a tolerably powerful heart had been kept in action by galvanism for a considerable period after natural respiration had ceased, forcibly propelling the blood into the lungs, where it could not be oxygenated, and the effect was certainly an extreme example of Asphyxia, with a nearly empty right heart and engorged lungs. Since meeting with this case, I have looked with particular care to the state of the right heart in examining the bodies of those who have died from Asphyxia, and have found that, while in many of the cases the right auricle and ventricle probably contained more blood than is usual in the generality of instances where death is not attended with any distinct impediment to the circulation, there were certain hearts in which, quite apart from the effects of decomposition, neither cavity was at all remarkably full, and that there were several in which, the auricle being somewhat distended, the ventricle was well contracted, and contained no unusual quantity of blood. I am not, at present, prepared to offer a demonstrative explanation of these three sets of cases, but I believe that these various conditions of the heart are determined as follows :—(1.) Where there occurs a *mechanical* impediment to the passage of blood through the lungs,—either gradually, as in cases of old emphysema or mitral contraction, or suddenly, as in failure of a weakened left ventricle,—the right side of the heart, already more or less dilated and deficient in muscular power, and with an imperfect safety-valve action, yields under the obstruction, and is found over-distended after death. Again, similar over-distension of the right ventricle occurs where death is immediately caused by an influence which suddenly and entirely suspends innervation, as under the full action of carbonic or prussic acid.—(2.) In cases of ordinary mechanical strangulation and suffocation, the heart's action usually continues for longer or shorter period after respiration has ceased.* This has been clearly proved by Sir B. Brodie, and has

* We have scarcely means of judging for how long a time after apparent death the human heart naturally continues to retain a certain amount of nervous and contractile power. We know for how lengthened a period the hearts of certain fishes—especially of the shark and ray species—retain this power after separation from the body; and very strange indeed as it may seem to be, we must not entirely reject, although we may be disposed to qualify, an observation made by Lord Bacon, who says, in his History of Life and Death,—"I

since been confirmed by numerous observations, especially by those of Nysten,* whose experiments have shown that the power of the right side of the heart continues long after the irritability of the left side is extinguished.† The length of time during which unoxygenised blood is thus circulated, and the freedom with which it traverses the lungs, must depend mainly upon the muscular tone of the heart, the completeness of its safety-valve apparatus, and the freedom of the pulmonary vessels. Upon the gradual cessation of the heart's action, the walls of a perfectly healthy

---

remember having seen the heart of one that was bowelled, as suffering for high-treason, that being cast into the fire leaped, at first, at least a foot and-a-half in height, and after by degrees lower and lower, for the space, as I remember, of seven or eight minutes."

It is mentioned, in a pamphlet of the time, that, after the body of Bellingham (who was hanged for the murder of Mr. Percival, in 1812) was dissected—"It was noticed that his heart continued to perform its functions—or, in other words, to be alive—for four hours after he was laid open."

Probably, the most remarkable instance of long-retained muscular irritability of the human heart after death is one observed in the dissecting-room of the Calcutta Medical College on the 1st February 1861, and reported‡ by Mr. J. Macnamara. The body of a Hindu male, about twenty-five years of age, was brought in for dissection from the Police Hospital, where it was believed to have been kept for several hours after death. There was general anasarca, and the liver was cirrhosed. It came to the dissecting-room at about 6 A.M. At about 7 the arteries were injected with an arsenical solution, a pound to six or seven gallons of water. At 11, the prosector opened the thorax and abdomen for the purpose of dissecting the sympathetic nerve. At noon, Mr. Macnamara distinctly saw the heart beating; there was "a regular rhythmical vermicular action of the right auricle and ventricle. The pericardium was open, the heart fully exposed, and lying to the left of its natural position. The heart's action, although regular, was very weak and slow. The left auricle was also in action, but the left ventricle was contracted and rigid, and apparently motionless. The spontaneous contractions continued till about 12-45. The right side of the heart contracted, however, on the application of a stimulus, such as the point of a scalpel, for three-quarters of an hour longer."

Had the contemporaries of Vesalius, in 1564, been acquainted with facts like these, the accident of his having opened the body of a man in whom the heart still beat might have been visited upon that great anatomist with a penalty short of absolute ruin.

* As quoted by Dr. Sieveking.

† Mr. E. R. Bickersteth has found, in experiments on animals, that, in death from the inhalation of chloroform, the respiratory movements cease before the cardiac. That the heart continues its action, uninfluenced by the chloroform, for a period longer or shorter after the cessation of respiration, and that its then failing may be considered as a natural consequence of respiration having ceased, and as independent of the influence of chloroform. That if, after the respiration has ceased, and while the heart is still in action, chloroform continues to be absorbed into the system, its movements become impaired or cease,—the chloroform, in such case, acting directly upon the heart. And that, if artificial respiration be had recourse to, before the cardiac contractions are seriously affected, and be properly maintained for a sufficient period, the respiratory function may be re-established.—*Edinburgh Monthly Journal*, September 1853.

Two Surgeons observed the state of the pulse of a criminal who was executed in the prison at Albany, U. S. The heart did not cease to act until nine minutes and-a-half after suspension. During the fifth minute, there were no less than 128 pulsations.—*Med. Times and Gazette*, 1st July 1854, as quoted by Taylor.

Dr. Fayrer's experiments, in my presence, showed that, in animals killed by cobra-bite, and that in a cobra killed by carbolic acid, the hearts continued to act after respiration ceased.

‡ Indian Lancet, February 15th, 1861, page 53.

right ventricle will, to a greater or less degree, contract, and expel much of its contents, first by the safety-valve, and, further, by the pulmonary artery. Hence, in one of these cases of Asphyxia, the right ventricle should be found either nearly empty, or merely containing a normal quantity of blood ; and this will, I believe, be observed to happen wherever the heart has been sound and powerful, and no other disturbing influence has been in operation. During the hot season of 1855 I examined the bodies of two robust and healthy men, lately arrived from England, who died asphyxiated, from Insolation, or what has been erroneously termed "Heat Apoplexy." Both of these men died evidently suffocated from gradual arrest of pulmonary innervation. I watched one of them until he expired, and the means which I employed—chiefly friction, over the front of the chest, with a mixture of mustard, spirit, and turpentine oil—tended to maintain the action of the heart for some time after the arrest of respiration. I examined both hearts *in situ*—raising and dividing the pericardium, and the yielding wall of the right ventricle with forceps and scissors. *The right cavities were decidedly not over-distended ;* they merely contained small and very loose coagula of yellow fibrine, and a little fluid blood. The lungs, however, were enormously congested. I consider these observations of considerable weight, as they were made with the utmost caution in the recent bodies of two perfectly healthy muscular men dying *gradually* from Asphyxia. Dr. Taylor mentioned, in his Edition of 1854, that, in cases of hanging, where the inspection has been delayed for several days, distension of the right cavities of the heart may not be observed (page 639). He also remarks that, after drowning, "independently of the changes which have taken place in consequence of putrefaction, the right cavities of the heart, and the vessels connected immediately with them, may be found collapsed and generally destitute of blood" (p. 608). He does not, however, explain this latter circumstance. It is mentioned, incidentally, by Drs. Jones and Sieveking, in their Morbid Anatomy, that, in the *post-mortem* examination of the body of a lad who was brought in asphyxiated by drowning to St. Mary's Hospital, and for whom some efforts were made to restore animation, there were found none of the visible signs commonly attributed to drowning, *and there was no congestion of any of the viscera.**

In his admirable review of the medical evidence of Death from Drowning, in relation to the case of W. B. Kirwan, Dr. Taylor remarks that "cases have been met with where the lungs have not been found gorged, and the cavities of the heart empty ; but I cannot call to mind a case where *the lungs have been found engorged as a result of Asphyxia and the cavities of the heart empty.* The absence of the distension from one or both organs would, in general, render it impossible to

* Page 416.

give, upon medical grounds, an affirmative opinion that death had taken place from Asphyxia."* In Mrs. Kirwan's case it was observed that "There was no blood in the right or left cavities of the heart, or in the great vessels, and the lungs appeared much congested." This, however, was thirty-one days after death, when such evidence could not be regarded as satisfactory.

A case showing the vital importance of settling this physiological question definitively occurred in a trial at Mymensing, in 1853.

A man had quarrelled with his two brothers about money matters. His body was found, bound with cords, floating down the stream of a nullah. No one actually saw him murdered; but the evidence tended to render it extremely probable that he was struck, perhaps killed, at all events rendered insensible, and then tied hands and feet together and thrown into the nullah. The Civil Surgeon deposed that "although no marks of violence were observable on the body, owing to the decomposed state in which it reached the station" (it had *floated*), "still the decomposition was more advanced externally than internally."—"From the state of the heart and lungs, death was caused by Drowning and not by fever (though he might have had fever), for the circulation of the blood and respiration must have been in action at the time of his having been immerged in water. The lungs were filled with water and blood, and the *heart also was filled with coagulated blood, which could not have been the case had the body been immerged in the water after death.*" The Sessions Judge held that it was evident, from this statement, that life was not extinct when the man was carried to the river. Mainly noticing the difference between the statement of the Surgeon and the assertions of the chief witness, who declared that the man was dead before he was thrown into the water, the law officer acquitted the prisoners. The Judge considered that the body was thrown into the water before life was extinct, and convicted.†

It is, however, a fact, which will, I am confident, be generally accepted hereafter, that, although in many cases of Asphyxia, the power of the right ventricle is overcome, and its cavity is found gorged after death, there is a set of instances in which, the action of the heart continuing after the cessation of respiration, the right ventricle is found well contracted and nearly empty, the lungs being congested in an extreme degree. Unless this fact be admitted, it may, in certain cases, be found difficult to substantiate our opinion that death has resulted from Asphyxia.‡

The question must not, however, be decided without due consideration

---

* Dublin Quarterly Journal of Medical Science, February 1833, p. 98.

† Nizamut Adawlut Reports, 3rd November 1833, p. 840.

‡ We may fairly imagine the following conversation occurring between a prisoner's counsel and the medical witness in a case of drowning. *Q.*—To what cause, speaking physiologically, do you attribute death in this case? *A.*—To Asphyxia. *Q.*—In what state did

of all the facts which may be brought to bear upon it. Dr. Ogston* found, in fifty-three instances of drowned subjects, that the right cavities were empty in two cases ; merely moist in one case ; containing a little blood in three cases ; nearly full in three ; full in fifteen ; distended with blood in seventeen ; inordinately distended in twelve. Here then we find nine cases out of fifty-three, which, at first sight, appear to countenance the views advanced above. With the exception of one instance, however, where the right cavities were found "nearly full" of blood, eleven and-a-quarter hours after death, these cases afford us no such aid. I have only spoken with regard to the condition of the heart previous to the occurrence of decomposition ; whereas in eight of these nine case, examination was made from four to fifty-six days after death.

Indeed, it is difficult to judge how many of Dr. Ogston's fifty-three cases can be taken into this inquiry. We find that, in thirty, the bodies were examined, at from eleven to seventeen, one-and-a-half hours after death. Here, unfortunately, two distinct sets of cases are inextricably thrown together,—*viz.*, those in which examination was made *during* and *after* the cessation of cadaveric rigidity. All, therefore, that we can deduce from Dr. Ogston's researches in favor of the above view is, that in five out of the thirty cases (one-sixth), the right cavities were not found distended within fifty-five and-a-half hours of death, while Dr. Ogston's experience did not afford any recent case in which these cavities were found empty or containing merely a small quantity of blood. Still the importance of even one apparently exceptional case, like Mr. Bishop's (where, twenty-four hours after death by Drowning, "the right side of the heart was found very flabby and contained scarcely any blood"), must not be overlooked, as indicating the existence of a distinct law, the operation of which is not the less real because it is frequently interrupted. To judge fairly of the state of the heart in cases of Asphyxia, the bodies should be examined previous to the cessation of cadaveric rigidity, and the state of the auricular and ventricular walls,

---

you find the right cavities of the heart ? *A.*—The auricle appeared full. The ventricle was not distended. *Q.*—Would you say that the right ventricle had suffered "a sort of paralysis of its muscular tissue ?" *A.*—No. *Q.*—Does not Dr. Carpenter lay it down, in the first edition of his Manual of Physiology, page 403, as a rule to which he does not state any exception, that, in cases of Asphyxia, "the venous blood accumulates in the pulmonary artery, in consequence of the obstruction of its capillaries ; it distends the right cavities of the heart ; and the accumulation extends to the venous system," &c. ; and that "the right side [of the heart] suffers from over-distension, which produces a sort of paralysis of its muscular tissue ?" Does not Dr. Watson, in Vol. I., Ed. 3, p. 67 of his Lectures say, that, in death from *Apnœa*, "the lungs remain full, the right chambers of the heart distended, and therefore less capable of contracting ?" And are we not also taught by Dr. Alison, in his Outlines of Pathology, p. 30, that, in such cases, we find the left side of the heart "nearly empty ; and the blood accumulated on the right side and in the lungs ?" How, therefore, do you explain your statement, so utterly opposed to the generally received opinion of physiologists, that an individual can die asphyxiated, without a paralyzed and over-distended condition of the right ventricle of the heart ?

* London Medical Gazette, for August 1851, page 290.

and the quantity of blood contained in the cavities should be decided upon while the organ remains *in situ*. The heart should never be raised from the pericardium until the projection or depression of the walls of its right cavities, and the amount of their distension or otherwise with blood have been carefully ascertained.

Again, in cases of Asphyxia, the *Lungs* may be found in almost any condition, from a state of extreme vascular distension attended with rupture of the vessels or pulmonary apoplexy, to one of unusual bloodlessness. Dr. Taylor says, in describing the appearances in cases of Drowning: "The lungs are sometimes found gorged, and at others pale and collapsed" (p. 679, 5th Ed.). In fact, the vascular condition of the lungs in cases of Asphyxia will vary according to the plethora or anemia of the individual's system, the state of his heart, the rapidity or slowness in the operation of the causes which led to death, and a variety of other circumstances.

In thirty out of Dr. Ogston's fifty-three cases, the examination is shown to have been made within seventy-one and-a-half hours after death. Of these thirty cases, the lungs were found sparingly congested in four, congested in twelve, and highly congested in fourteen. Hence it is sufficiently clear that Asphyxia by Drowning is not essentially characterised by extraordinary engorgement of the pulmonary vessels.

Sir Thomas Watson has an important observation on this point.* He remarks that the gorged conditions of the pulmonary arteries and venous system generally, which constitute the anatomical characters of death by *apnœa*, are even more constantly visible in the dead body when *apnœa* has been gradually produced, than after sudden suffocation; simply, he believes, because they are more *permanent*. After sudden death, however caused, the blood seldom coagulates; and the venous turgescence, consequent upon rapid *apnœa*, although great at first, has time to subside, and disappears before the body is examined.

He must also bear in mind that, in a large proportion of those who die from sudden *apnœa*, the heart and its vessels are perfectly healthy, and, by force of the unimpaired *elasticity* of their tissues, contract to the utmost upon their contents after death.

Credit is due to the late Mr. Henry Piddington, Coroner of Calcutta, for an early and practical recognition of these principles. Upon the appearance of my last edition, he sent me the proceedings in the case of a prostitute who was strangled, probably by hand. Dr. Woodford found that there was marked cerebral congestion. The organs of the chest and abdomen were in a healthy state, the vessels of the lungs were not congested, and the heart was in a natural condition. [Dr. Woodford informs me that he had previously observed this in several cases.]

* Lectures on the Principles and Practice of Physic, 4th Ed., Vol. I., p. 70.

Mr. Piddington remarked that the fact of the heart and lungs being found in a natural state rendered the case very remarkable. In five out of six cases mentioned by Beck, pp. 648 to 650, 7th edition, engorgement of the heart or lungs or of both appears; one only is quoted by Dr. Paris as presenting the organs in a natural state. Theoretically, we may account for the non-congested state of these organs by considering that an apoplectic condition of the brain simulating death is immediately produced by strangulation. The murderer leaves his victim as dead, although there yet remains a minute spark of life which, for a time, keeps up a languid circulation, but does not enable the sufferer to rally, and he finally dies of apoplexy and stupor.

Mr. Piddington was not a medical man, but he is well remembered as a proficient in several branches of physical science, and it is evident that, in this physiological question, his clear discriminative judgment led him, beyond the teaching of books, to an appreciation of the truth.

When, taking these facts into account, it is borne in mind how large a proportion of natural deaths result from Asphyxia, and is remembered that we shall probably not meet with one case in ten thousand in which, after natural death unattended with hæmorrhage or exhausting discharges, abundance of blood will not be found in the left auricle and in the posterior parts of the lungs, we shall be cautious in relying upon the condition of the heart and pulmonary vessels *alone* in forming our opinion, where the life of a suspected party is at stake.*

In the last edition of his work, Dr. Taylor has added his own high authority to the above principles (p. 628).

Dr. Woodford has kindly given me the following striking illustration of the difficulties which beset medico-legal investigation in these cases.

Some years ago he made a *post-mortem* examination of the body of a European sailor at the Police dead-house. He found the clothes saturated with water. Sanious froth was around the nostrils; the hands were somewhat soddened, but the boots, which were wet, had preserved the feet.

---

* See Dr. Taylor's remarks "On the Medical Evidence of Death from Drowning, in relation to the case of W. B. Kirwan." (Dublin Quarterly Journal of Medical Science, for February 1853, p. 94). In this case it was found, *thirty-one days after death*, that "the lungs were healthy" [and "collapsed"], "but congested posteriorly, interiorly," &c.; this congestion was assigned to engorgement of blood during life ["the minute vessels gorged with blood"]. "The heart was healthy, and empty both at the right and left side, as were also the large vessels connected with it." In the newspaper report of this case, the medical man who examined the body was made to assert that the condition of the lungs afforded sufficient evidence of violence, as he had never seen such congestion of the organs, except where death had been attended with a violent struggle. As this rash statement is not quoted by Dr. Taylor, it was probably not made. Still the jury appears to have decided, mainly upon the medical evidence, that this was a case of violent death. One fact may certainly be taken for granted, in cases of this description,—that, when the process of decomposition has once fairly set in, no vascular change in the lungs, short of apoplexy, can be taken as evidence that Asphyxia by Strangulation or Drowning was the cause of death.

It was twenty-four hours after death, and decomposition was advancing rapidly. The skin was vesicated, and the body was covered with particles of sand. The vessels of the brain and the right side of the heart were engorged with blood. The lungs and other viscera were highly congested. He certified that deceased died from submersion in water. The Coroner returned the certificate for explanation, as the Police reported that deceased had died in the Police lock-up from Apoplexy. Dr. Woodford's certificate had been forwarded *before* receipt of the Police Report—a course which he has since been careful not to repeat. The clear explanation was that the body had been carried from the lock-up to the dead-house, a very small godown (store-room) with open windows only three feet from the ground. It was placed on a table under a window, on the west side; rain had fallen all night in torrents, and the wind blew from the west. Dr. Woodford found the body on a table *in the centre* of the room. The clothes were, as we have seen, saturated; and the body was covered with particles of sand. (Dr. Woodford observes that, in Bengal, drowned bodies, which have not been disturbed, are invariably covered with particles of fine sand, the banks and rivers being full of it.) Thus all the usual external appearances of drowning presented themselves, and the internal morbid appearances were simulated by those of apoplectic death. The sand had been driven on to the body by the rain from the loose plaster at the upper part of the window cornice.

BURYING ALIVE (*Samadh*).

We have many references to this practice, not only among the ancient Jews, Goths, and Peruvians, but also, in more recent times, among the Monastic orders of Europe. Partial Burial was inflicted, as a punishment, by the Musslamaun rulers of India;* and it has been generally reported that, in comparatively recent times, a native female buried one of her slave girls alive. Terry witnessed one of these cases when he accompanied Sir Thomas Roe to the Court of the Great Mogul. One of the Emperor's women having been too intimate with an eunuch, "the king presently gave command that a round hole should be made in the earth, and that her

* Sir Thomas Roe, who visited the court of the great Mogul in 1614, mentions that one of Nourmahal's women, being detected in an intrigue, was set up to the arm-pits in the earth close rammed about her, with her feet tied to a stake, so to continue three days and two nights without any sustenance, her head and arms bare, exposed to the violent heat of the sun. If she died not in that time, she was to be pardoned. This is probably the case related by the Chaplain to the Embassy, which will be cited immediately. The translator of the Seir Mutaqherin speaks of "*making a garden of men*" as a Persian cruelty—"burying a couple of hundred of living men in the ground, some in an inverted position, with only their thighs and legs out, and some with only their heads and arms, all the while exposed to a raging sun." By the Mussalmaun Law, if a person be put alive into a grave, and kept there until he dies, according to Imam Mahomed, the murderer is liable to suffer death in retribution; but, in the opinion of Aboo Haneefah, judgment is given for the price of blood only payable by the Aakilah, because the homicide is not committed with a wound.

body should be put into that hole, where she should stand with her head only above ground, and the earth to be put in again unto her close round about her, that so she might stand in the parching sun, until the extreme hot beams thereof did kill her; in which torment she lived one whole day and the night following, and almost till the next noon, crying out most lamentably, while she was able to speak—Ah, my head, my head! Which horrid execution, or rather murder, was acted near our house; where the eunuch, by the command of the same king, was brought very near the place where this poor creature was thus buried alive, and there in her sight, cut all into pieces" (p. 407).

Until a few years since, *the practice of Burying Lepers Alive* appears to have been common in Bengal, among both the Mussalmauns and the Hindus. Accounts of trials for this atrocity in the year 1810 and 1820 will be be found in Macnaghten's Reports.*

Cases still occur in the North-West Provinces.

In 1852, three Zemindars, Brahmins, were convicted, at Seharunpore, of burying their uncle, a leper, while still alive. He had become reduced to a loathsome condition by the fearful ravages of the disease; and, for eight nights and days, lay moaning and crying outside his house, into which he could not be brought by reason of the putrid state of his sores, and their having generated maggots. All this time, he supplicated his nephews to put an end to his miserable existence. They hesitated and questioned for some time; his entreaties and imprecations were, however, more than they could bear, and they decided, as they afterwards confessed, on taking the consequences, and burying him alive. They took him down to a *nullah* at dusk, dug a hole, and thus disposed of the body. They stated that the chest was just warm, but no more. He was, to use their own expression, beyond death when they consigned him to his grave.†

In the following year, two Mussalmauns were sentenced to imprisonment and fine, at Moradabad, for having buried their leprous brother alive, at his own request. He had been afflicted with leprosy ten or fifteen years, his hands had dropped off, the sores on his body were full of worms, and the smell proceeding from him was intensely offensive. He entreated his brothers to bury him alive, and threatened to haunt them in the next world if they refused to accede to his request.‡

---

* Vol. I., p. 218; and II., p. 18; and Vol. III., p. 139, See also Reports of Cases in which Lepers were voluntarily buried alive or drowned, in 1814 and 1816, Vol. I., pp. 229 and 292.

† Nizamut Adawlut Reports, N. W. P., 31st December 1852, p. 1560.

Jacqueline, Countess of Henault, enraged at the obstinacy of Albert Begllirick in defending the castle of Schoonpowen, buried him alive, at night, under one of the platforms of the castle.

By the naval laws of Richard the First, he that killed a man on ship-board was tied to the body and thrown into the sea. If he killed one on land, he was *to be buried with his victim.*

‡ Nizamut Adawlut Reports, N. W. P., 14th October 1853, p. 1288.

The following report brings this practice down to a recent date :—

The North-West Provinces Police Report for 1866 describes a case of *samadh*, which occurred in that year in the Jounpore district. The crime, however, in that instance, was perpetrated "with a difference." The victim, a leper, Purein Singh, was placed in a hole seven feet deep, and there *burnt to death*. The excavated earth was then piled over his remains. The Report of the District Superintendent of Police explains this variation of treatment by the Hindoo superstition, that, if the leprous member of a family be *burnt* to death, the *whole family* will be safe from the dreadful disease. In this Jounpore case, it was said that Purein Singh encountered his terrible death quite voluntarily. Nevertheless, seven aiders and abettors were committed to the Sessions under sections 302 and 306 of the Penal Code.

In April 1868 it was made known that this barbarous rite, of which there are also vestiges in Cashmere, was still prevalent in some of the Rajpootana States. On the 2nd of that month, the Governor-General's Agent for these States remarks that "the better he becomes acquainted with the province entrusted to his political supervision, the more he perceives that the state of society in all the southern and western portion of it is beyond measure backward and rude. Not only do we know but little of what transpires, but the Chiefs themselves have neither information nor power of control in their own territories. Three *samadhs* are reported as having occurred during the past year ; and a record is also given of nine cases extending over six years, with reference to which several depositions were taken. These seem all to have occurred in the Serohi and Marwar States, and were confined entirely to lepers who, when wasted with disease, prefer death to an existence in which life is a burden, and their very persons objects of loathing to themselves and their relatives. The circumstances are all very similar. A poor suffering wretch—influenced perhaps by priests—by relatives glad to get rid of him—and by consciousness of his own noxious condition, expresses a desire to bury himself alive. The relatives for two or three days remonstrate and endeavour to dissuade ; but he is firm ; some of the nearest relatives then get up a procession, dig a pit, the doomed man voluntarily enters it, his friends heap up and beat down the soil, and the whole of the villagers witness the sacrifice. A few days subsequently, the mob visits the afflicted house—opium water is drunk, and the taint is removed. The rite, inhuman as it is, seems to have been long practised ; nothing is hidden or denied—those concerned saying, that it is the established custom of the country. Past offences of this character can scarcely be punished, but there is not the least doubt that the abolition of *samadh* will be as readily and generally accepted as the forbiddance of *suttee*. The rulers of Marwar and Serohi have been addressed on the subject, and both have now proclaimed any connivance in the rite a criminal offence punishable with ten years' imprisonment. The Rao of Serohi, however, points out that no communication on this subject was ever received by him before February last, and that the rite was practised even during the time the British Government administered the State."*

A Hindu is liable to punishment for aiding and abetting in the suicide of a leper.—Const. No. 985. Beaufort, para. 3928.

We are told that, in many of these cases, the persons who dig the pit and cover up the unfortunate wretch are themselves lepers.

Every one in India has heard of certain impostors who pretend that they have the power of remaining completely buried underground for months without detriment. Dr. Honigberger has given an account of one of these people, named Haridas, at p. 128 *et seq.* of his book. We occasionally discover traces of the existence of this practice elsewhere.

In 1868, it was reported from Purneah that, in a village called Peermokam, at the commencement of the Mahomedan fast, a weaver undertook to remain buried during the whole period of the fast. A hole was dug, in which he seated himself; a bamboo roof was made over his head, on which earth was piled to the height of about three feet. When taken out, the unfortunate man was, of course, dead.

The following case was subsequently reported :—

"Two curious instances of fanaticism are reported from Singapore. A Mahomedan priest, who also practised the curing of diseases by charms, in which he was not always successful, determined to increase his sanctity by a temporary departure to a better world. For this purpose, he dug for himself a small cave underground, into which he retired with a candle and a copy of the Koran, and requested his friends to cover the top of the cave with boards and earth, which they accordingly did. He had taken the precaution to put a hollow bamboo through the covering, and through the bamboo a smaller stick, by which he could get air and communicate with his friends. After carefully covering him in, his friends retired till the next morning, when they pulled up the small stick from the bamboo and their signal was answered. On the next morning, however, and on two subsequent mornings no answer was returned, and the cave having been opened, the fanatic was found dead. A few days afterwards, a Malay priest was about to follow his example, and large crowds had assembled to witness the ceremony, but the Police interfered and prevented his committing an act of self-destruction."

Fearful as these errors are, they possibly find their parallels in Great Britain in the present day. It is said to be a common practice, in the remote northern parts of Scotland, for the friends of one in whom the death agony is much protracted, to remove the support from his head, with a view to expedite dissolution. There cannot be a doubt that, almost within the memory of persons now living, the Irish peasantry

* Calcutta *Englishman*, 25th April 1868.

considered themselves perfectly justified in putting a victim of hydrophobia "out of his misery," by smothering him under a feather bed!*

Formerly, *the widows of the Yogees, the caste of Hindu weavers, were not unfrequently buried alive with their deceased husbands.*

Several of the old voyagers to India noticed this practice. Thus we read in Purchas:† "When a great man dyeth, all the women of his house, both his wife and slaves, with whom he hath had carnal copulation, burn themselves together with him. Amongst the baser sort, I have seen (saith Master Frederike) the dead man carried to the place of buriall, and there set upright; the woman coming before him on her knees, casteth her arms about his necke, while a mason maketh a wall round about them; and, when the wall is as high as their neckes, one coming behind the woman, strangleth her, the workman presently finishing the wall over them; and this is their burial.

"Gasparo Baldy, further affirmeth, that not farre from the citie of Saint Thomas is the towne Casta; where the wife is not burned (as at Negapatam), but a great grave being made for the desceased husband, they place the living wife by the dead corpse, and their nearest kindred cast earth upon them both, and stampe thereon."

Dr. Fryer says:‡ "At Hubly in this kingdom [Carnatic] are a caste called Linguits, who are buried upright, whose wives, when they have a mind to accompany their husbands into another world, are set in the same pit with them, covered up to the shoulders with mold; who, after ceremonies performed, have their necks wrung round, and the pit filled up with earth immediately."

In the Parliamentary Blue Book on the burning of Hindu widows, dated 25th March 1830, the report from Tipperah (p. 27) states that, in that district, "female immolation, by means of burying alive, appears to be very prevalent. This custom is peculiar to the *Joogy*, or Weaver, caste; and more than half of the sacrifices which occurred during this year (1825) were done by these means." There were six cases in 1824, and eight in 1825. It is shown, at p. 130 of this Report, that "it has been ascertained from the Pundits of the Sudder Dewanny Adawlut, and other authorities, that this practice, which chiefly prevails in the district of Tipperah, has no sanction whatever from the Shaster."

At page 146 of his *Thesaurus Craniorum*, Dr. Joseph Barnard Davis figures the skull of a Hindu woman who was buried alive with her deceased husband in the sands of Juggernauth, near the Great Temple, June 1826.

Ward found, on inquiring among the Hindus employed at Serampore,

---

* Cases have been several times reported in Ireland, the last as lately as 1861, but it has not been proved, in any instance that I am aware of, that this atrocity has been actually perpetrated.

† Vol. V., pages 556, 557.

‡ A New Account of East India and Persia, p. 153.

that almost every one of them had seen widows thus buried alive. He describes that a large and deep grave is dug near the Ganges, and, after certain preparatory ceremonies, the widow descends into it, and takes the dead body on her lap and encircles it with her arms. The earth is thrown in by degrees, and two persons descend into the grave, pressing it firm with their feet around her. The earth keeps rising ; still she makes no remonstrance or effort to escape. At length it reaches to her head, and then, in haste, the rest of the earth is thrown upon her and trodden down.

In a very similar account of this ceremony given in the Oriental Annual for 1836, it is stated that it frequently happens that the woman is so stupefied by opium as to be scarcely conscious of what she is about, but goes through the necessary forms with mere mechanical insensibility.*

A very singular crime gave rise to a trial at Sylhet, in March 1853. A gomashta, having given offence to two young Hindus, was inveigled by them into their house, at night ; and, with the assistance of their father and younger brother, was murdered. Two of the neighbours, hearing groans in the prisoners' house, asked what was the matter ; but, receiving no reply, went to the house, when one of the prisoners came out and struck the light down, while his mother set fire to part of the buildings. On entering and searching the house, the neighbours discovered a grave, or hole, described as about one *hath* (or cubit) broad, two long, and two deep, which was covered over with a mat. Under the mat was a board, with five or six bamboos laid upon it, and under the board was the body of the unfortunate gomashta, lying amidst mud and water, which half filled the grave. The Sessions Judge considered it probable that the four prisoners tumbled the deceased into the grave, and then, putting the board over him (for the board very exactly fitted the grave), stood upon it till he was suffocated. No outward marks were observable on the body, and it was too decomposed to be examined internally by the Surgeon, who, however, from its appearance, was of opinion that the deceased did not die a natural death, but might have been suffocated.†

SUICIDE.

For Suicide by *Cutting the Throat,* see p. 432 ; by *Strangulation,* pp. 582-89 ; by *Hanging,* p. 599 ; by *Suffocation,* p. 617, note ; by *Drowning,* pp. 629 and 637 ; by *Burial,* p. 654.

Dr. Muir, of Madras, has collected statistics which show that, in India (Bengal Presidency and British Burmah), the proportion of Suicides in a

* The crimes of Sati and Burying Alive are legislated for in Reg. XVII of 1829. See Mr. Parry Davis's Police Regulations and Acts, p. 156.

† Nizamut Adawlut Reports, Vol. III., Part 1, of 1853, p. 309. See also an atrocious case, where a wretch, at Durrung (Assam), confessed to have twisted the neck of his infant daughter, to have thrown her on the ground, and then to have *buried her alive.—Nizamut Adawlut Reports,* Vol. IV. of 1854, p. 561.

population of fifty-five millions is 1 in 25,300, against 1 in 15,200 in England.*

Dr. Woodford tells me that he has "found Suicide stand at 1 to 2,000 of the population in Calcutta."

Such statistics, however, are shaken by the fact that we have strong reason to fear that our power of discriminating between cases of Suicide and Murder in India is, at present, very limited.

Upon this most important question the Report from Bogra, in the Bengal Police Report for 1868, may be read with great advantage. We are told, at page 302, that—

The District Superintendent, under the impression that a majority of the inquests held under section 161, Criminal Procedure Code, failed in eliciting the true cause of death, directed that all bodies, distance and weather permitting, should be sent into head-quarters for examination. This order, seconded by the very careful *post-mortems* of the Civil Surgeon, followed up by the vigorous investigations of the Police, and prompt and painstaking proceedings on the part of the Magistrates, resulted in the arrest of seventy-seven individuals, charged with the murder of thirty-seven persons, whose decease had been attributed by the village Munduls and Chowkeedars to Suicide, snake-bite (cobra), or drowning, or had been altogether concealed. Of these seventy-seven offenders, sixty-three were committed by Magistrates for trial before the Sessions, which Court convicted fifty-three. The above facts are unusually suggestive and startling, for it appears that the *same* District Superintendent, influenced by *similar* suspicion, when in charge of the Pubna District, and in the teeth of every obstacle thrown in the way of his Police by zemindaree agents, village Chowkeedars, and even by the villagers themselves, detected the falsity of fifteen reported Suicides, in ten of which a charge of murder or culpable homicide was established before the lower Courts. The attention of all officers has been drawn to this subject in a Circular Memorandum from the office of the Inspector-General of Police.

Among the various causes of Suicide in India, those on account of (1) *Revenge* or for *Accusation*, (2) for *Religion*, and (3) in consequence of *Physical Suffering* are very remarkable. (4) Suicides on account of *Grief and Shame* are not unfrequent.

(1) *Suicides for Revenge or Accusation.*

The practice of *Chandi*, or self-immolation, was rather frequent among the ancient Rajpoots. Thus, when the Raja Brindabun Das levied a war-subsidy of the Brahmins, some of the wealthiest, having expostulated in vain, poniarded themselves in his presence, pouring maledictions on his head, with their last breath.

* Smith's Annals of Indian Administration, for 1866-67.

Thus cursed, he laboured under a ban of excommunications even amongst his personal friends; and his liege lord, Madhu Sing, of Ambir, in order to expiate his indirect share in his guilt, recalled his troops and distributed twenty thousand rupees to the Brahmins of his own capital.*

Yet again, vengeance still more dire was believed to be called down when the Suicide added to his own the blood of those dearest to him. Legend tells that Oodi Sing, of Joda, having determined to possess himself of a Brahmin's daughter, her father seeing that there was no other course by which he could save her from pollution but by her death, he resolved to make it one of vengeance and horror. He dug a sacrificial pit, and, having slain his daughter, cut her into fragments, mingling therewith pieces of flesh from his own person, made the *homa*, or burnt sacrifice, to *Aya-Mata*, and, as the smoke and flames ascended, he pronounced an imprecation on the Raja : "Let peace be a stranger to him, and, in three *pahars* (a watch of the day about three hours), three days, and three years, let me have revenge." Then exclaiming, "My future dwelling is the *Dabi Baori*," he sprung into the flaming pit. The horrid tale was related to the Raja, whose imagination was haunted by the shade of the Brahmin, and he expired at the assigned period a prey to unceasing remorse.† Todd also says of the Charuns, the bards of the Rajpoots, a body held sacred by those people, that, whenever they guarded caravans, the most desperate outlaw seldom dared to commit any outrage upon their charge. If not strong enough to defend their convoy by sword and shield, they would threaten the robbers with the *Chandi*, and proceed by degrees from a gash in the flesh to a death-wound ; or, if one victim was insufficient, a whole body of women and children was sacrificed, for whose blood the marauder was declared responsible hereafter.‡ The explanation of these crimes throws light upon the motive which actuated a Patna woman, in 1848, to murder her own little daughter, and having concealed the body on the premises of her enemy, to accuse him of the crime—*vide supra*, p. 71 and note,§ and p. 629.

---

* Todd, Vol. II., p. 401.

† *Ibid*, p. 35.

‡ *Ibid*, p. 167.

§ Two or three similar instances were communicated by Lord Teignmouth to the Asiatic Society.|| In 1793, a Brahmin, named Baloo Paundeh, was convicted of the murder of his daughter. He stated that, twelve years before the murder, he and another man were joint tenants of a spot of ground, when his partner relinquished his share. Subsequently his partner claimed a share in the ground. It was referred to arbitration, and a decision even pronounced in favor of Baloo. He was ploughing the land when he was interrupted by his opponent. His words were : "I became angry and enraged at his forbidding me, and bringing my own little daughter, Apurnya, who was only a year and-a-half old, to the said field, I killed her with my sword."

Two Brahmins, petty land-holders, believing that one Goury had entered their house, and

|| Quoted by Forbes O. M., Vol. I., p. 493.

In the trial at Dhoolia (Bombay Presidency) of Myputsing Bin Heerasing, a sepoy, for putting an end to his brother, who was wounded when the police were apprehending them as deserters, the Sudder Court remarked : "Among natives, the sacrifice of oneself, or of a relation, or even of any human being, is believed to bring down vengeance on those by whose act such sacrifice is precipitated." *

Besides the cases alluded to above, instances of Suicide by Burial,† by Poison, and in other ways by persons sitting *Dhurna* (literally starvation, sitting at an enemy's door, and dying by want), with a hope to bring down a curse upon those whose doors they had vainly beset, begging for the payment of debts or for a gift, were formerly not unfrequent in India. I have seen it mentioned that, about forty-five years since, ten lepers of Benares burnt themselves, and ninety others threw themselves into wells, to revenge themselves upon some one who had offended them.

I am informed that, in the inveterate feuds which prevail among rival families and villages Up-country, it is still by no means a very rare thing for an aged person to allow himself to be taken, a willing victim, into his opponent's land, where his people murder him, and charge his crime upon their adversaries. We have some very early notices of this one most prevalent. but, to our European notions, most irrational, mode of revenge. Father Martin wrote, in 1709 :—"There is an old practice which, doubtless, will surprise you, but it is certain those Indians observe the law of retaliation very strictly. If there happens to be a quarrel, and one of the parties pulls his own eye out, or is guilty of Suicide, the other party must inflict the like punishment upon himself or upon one of his relations. The women carry this barbarous custom still further ; when any affront is put upon them, or reproachful word used, they will go and

carried off forty rupees, conducted their mother to a rivulet, where they called out aloud to the people of the village that, although they would overlook the assault as an act which could not be remedied, the forty rupees must be returned. To this no answer was received, nor is there a certainty that it was heard by any person. One of the sons immediately drew his tulwar, and at one stroke severed his mother's head from her body, with the express view as entertained and avowed by both parent and son that the mother's spirit, excited by the beating of a large drum, during forty days, might for ever haunt, torment, and pursue to death Goury and the others concerned with him. The last words which the mother pronounced were that she would "blast the said Goury and those connected with him."

Thus it probably was that, in 1852 or 1853, a Brahmin was condemned in the Nizamut Adawlut Court, N. W. P., for slaying (by hacking her neck) his pregnant wife, that her blood might be upon certain persons who had offended him—*vide supra*, p. 273.

* Bellasis' Reports, p. 190.

† See a case of Suicide and Murder, tried in 1825, in which a fukeer, having failed to receive contributions from a shopkeeper in Zillah Agra, adjourned to a tope without the town, and sat *Dhurna* for some days; when he allowed himself to be buried alive by his companions—*Macnaghten's Reports*, Vol. II., p. 409. See also Asiatic Researches, Vol. IV., p. 49. Baboo Ramchunder Mitter tells me that those who sat *Dhurna* sometimes endeavored to excite fear by striking their own chests with stones, until the stones crumbled to pieces. Regulation VII. of 1820 renders the offence of sitting *Dhurna* punishable by fine or imprisonment.

break their heads against the door of the offending person, who is obliged to inflict precisely the same punishment upon herself. If one woman poison herself, by drinking the juice of a venomous herb or plant, the other female, who was the cause of it, is obliged to do the same; and, should she fail in it, the rest would set fire to her house, run away with her cattle, and be perpetually tormenting her till such time as she had made such satisfaction."

Forbes states* that no security is deemed so binding or sacred as that of a Bhaut, because, on failure of the obligation, he proceeds to the house of the offending party, and in his presence, destroys either himself or one of his family, imprecating the most fearful vengeance of the gods on the head of him who had compelled them to shed their blood. This is deemed a dire catastrophe, as the Hindus are taught to believe that the Bhaut's life, to which a superstitious veneration is attached, over and above their common honor of bloodshed, will be demanded from the aggressor by an offended deity; it is, therefore, very uncommon for an obligation to be broken where a Bhaut stands security.

These barbarities are closely allied to the old Hindu practice of erecting a *Koor*. A circular pile of wood was prepared ready for conflagration; upon this sometimes a cow, and sometimes an old woman, was placed, and the whole was consumed together. The object of this practice was to intimidate the officers of Government or others from importunate demands, as the effect of the sacrifice was supposed to involve great sin in the person whose conduct forced the constructor of the *Koor* to this expedient. Sir J. Shore, who was one of the first to describe this practice,† mentions that an instance occurred in the Benares district, in 1788. Three Brahmins held lands in partnership with others, but the public assessment was unequally imposed upon them, as their partners paid less, while they were charged with more than their due proportion; they, therefore, refused to pay any part of the revenues whatever, and erected a *Koor*, as they declared, to intimidate the Government officers from making any undue demands upon them. An old woman had suffered herself to be placed on the pile; but the timely interposition of authority prevented the completion of the sacrifice; the woman, who was nearly blind, was summoned to appear before the English Superintendent, but absolutely refused, declaring that she would throw herself into the first well rather than submit. The summons was not enforced. This was mentioned by Sir J. Shore as the only instance of setting up a *Koor* which had occurred for many years previous to 1788, although the practice was said to

---

* Op. Cit., Vol. I., p. 377.

† On some Extraordinary Facts, Customs, and Practices of the Hindus, Asiatic Researches, Vol. IV., p. 335.

have been frequent formerly; but it was expressly asserted to have been limited to a very small portion of that province.*

But, in India, such evil practices as these are always liable to crop up from time to time. In his Report of Police cases, at Azimghur, in 1835, already cited, Dr. Esdaile accounted for five out of six cases of Suicide, which had come under his notice, as follows:—"Opium was taken by one woman after a family quarrel; two others threw themselves into wells, from the same cause; a faqueer set fire to himself to warm the charity of the devout, but *overdid* himself; and a Brahmin threw himself down a well, that his ghost might haunt his neighbour."

Dr. Day, of Madras, told me of a man, at Singapore, who cut his throat at his neighbour's door, intending to get him hanged, but cut too deep and died. This custom has a wide range Eastward. We are told† that the Chinese have a book entitled *Si-Yeem*, that is to say, "The Washing of the Pit," a work on medical jurisprudence, very celebrated all over the empire, and which should be in the hands of all Chinese Magistrates. It is impossible to read the *Si-Yeem* without being convinced that the number of attempts against life in that country is very considerable, and especially that Suicide is very common. The extreme readiness with

---

* A reference to Beaufort's Digest of the Criminal Law of the Presidency of Fort William‡ will show with how much difficulty the Brahmins, and especially those of Benares, were restrained by our Government, towards the latter part of the last century, from committing acts of frantic violence in opposition to legal authority. With a view to intimidate the native servants of Government, they erected these *Koors;* threatend to cut their wives and children in pieces, and even did, in some cases, carry their threat into effect; lacerated their own bodies more or less slightly with knives or razors ; and threatened to throw themselves into wells, or to swallow poison. In some few instances, these men destroyed themselves to bring upon their opponents the curse which attaches to the slayer of a Brahmin ; but these cases were the exception. One of these extreme instances, however, occurred in Tirhoot so recently as the year 1843. Two men were candidates for the Mohuntship of a "Muth," or Hindu Temple, at Hajeepore. One of them, Beeran Doss, came to the thannah and desired the Darogah to come quickly, as Pursora, his opponent, had shut himself into one of the temples and set fire to the place. The Darogah found the temple in flames, and forcing open the door dragged out the deceased, most severely scorched and quite insensible. On throwing some cold water on his face, he revived for a few moments, and made use of his last breath to accuse Beeram Doss and two others of having beaten him, thrown him down, got on his chest, forced poison down his throat, and dragged him into the temple, which they then closed and set on fire. The Civil Surgeon found no poison in the viscera, and declared that the man died by exhaustion, and not from any other cause. The door, when the police came, was fastened on the *inside*, which could only have been done by the deceased, and it appeared that he had a quarrel with Beeram Doss and the two others, in which he was struck and otherwise insulted, and he snatched up some fire, rushed into the temple, shut himself in, and set fire to the cloth roof.§

† Ten Thousand Wonderful Things, by Edmund Fillingham King, M.A., 2nd Series, p. 254.

‡ Paras. 3939, 3943, 4, 5, 6, 7, 8, 9, Second Ed.

§ Police Report, L. P., for 1843, p. 8. According to Stewart, it was anciently a custom among the Hindus that, when a Raja was thrice defeated or taken prisoner, he was considered unworthy to reign, and burnt himself on a funeral pile.

which the Chinese are induced to kill themselves is almost inconceivable; some mere trifle, a word almost, is sufficient to cause them to hang themselves, or throw themselves to the bottom of a well—the two favorite modes of Suicide. In other countries, if a man wishes to wreak his vengeance on an enemy, he tries to kill him; in China, on the contrary, he kills himself. This anomaly depends upon various causes, of which these are the principal:—In the first place, Chinese law throws the responsibility of a Suicide on those who may be supposed to be the cause or occasion of it. It follows, therefore, that if you wish to be revenged on an enemy, you have only to kill yourself to be sure of getting him into horrible trouble, for he falls immediately into the hands of *justice*, and will certainly be tortured and ruined, if not deprived of life. The family of the Suicide also usually obtains, in these cases, considerable damages; so that it is by no means a rare case for an unfortunate man to commit Suicide in the house of a rich one, from a morbid idea of family affection. In killing his enemy, on the contrary, the murderer exposes his own relatives and friends to injury, disgraces them, reduces them to poverty, and deprives himself of funeral honors—a great point for a Chinese, and concerning which he is extremely anxious. It is to be remarked also, that public opinion, so far from disapproving of Suicide, honors and glorifies it. The conduct of a man who destroys his own life, to avenge himself on an enemy, whom he has no other way of reaching, is regarded as heroic and magnanimous.

(2) *Suicide as a Religious Rite.*

It is almost needless to mention that *Suicide* has always been held by the Hindu religion to be one of the most acceptable rites that can be offered to their sanguinary deities. According to the *Ayen Akbery*, there were five kinds of Suicide held to be meritorious in the Hindu,—*viz.*, Starving; Covering himself with cow-dung, and setting it on fire, consuming himself therein; Burying himself in snow; Immersing himself in the water at the extremity of Bengal, where the Ganges discharges itself into the sea through a thousand channels, enumerating his sins and praying till the alligators come and devour him; or Cutting his Throat at Allahabad, at the confluence of the Ganges and Jumna. To these might be added the custom which formerly prevailed at the Mahadeo Hills, where men threw themselves from a perpendicular height of four or five hundred feet, and were dashed to pieces on the rocks below—to fulfil the vows of their mothers;* Drowning at Hurdwar, Allahabad, and Saugor; the horrible practice of dying under the wheels of Juggurnath's car; perishing in the cold of the Himalayahs; and the custom of Sati.

---

* Sleeman's Rambles and Recollections, Vol. I., p. 132.

On the 7th July 1864, the editor of the *Friend of India* mentions that, a few days previously, he had seen, near Serampore, two persons crushed to death, and another frightfully lacerated, having thrown themselves under the wheels of a car during the Ruth Jatra festival. It was afterwards stated that this occurrence was accidental. The fact and its explanation must stand on record together.

Sati.

A lengthened history of this practice, which is so fully described in most popular descriptions of India, would be out of place here. Its great prevalence at the beginning of the present century may be judged of by the facts that, in the year 1803, it was ascertained that two hundred and seventy-five wives were burned with their dead husbands within thirty miles of Calcutta; and that, in 1804, one hundred and fifteen *satis* were performed near the city itself.

As lately as February 1866, it was reported that, on the 7th of that month, at midnight, a young man and his wife, Brahmins, had immolated themselves under the walls of the Allahabad Fort. They came from the Oude districts, with hundreds of others, to worship at the confluence of the Ganges and Jumna. A large pile was erected, and they burnt themselves upon it in the presence of a crowd.* It is added that the soil where the bodies were burnt was removed, and was thrown into the river at the confluence, or near it.

The practice of Sati appeared to have been nearly or quite extinguished, in Bengal and the North-Western Provinces, when it was announced, in 1863, that a case had occurred in the Monghyr District, and that the offenders had been prosecuted to conviction.†

A case of true Sati occurred near Sheolee, in the Cawnpore District, in 1868; and, as lately as March 1870, a Brahmin's widow is reported to have burnt herself at Shahabad. Sati still occurs, and may possibly even be prevalent in several of the Native States in India. Cases of Sati occurred at Benares in 1852,‡ and at Shahjehanpore in 1854.§

Masculine Sati.

"The most effectual blowing up, or rather the most expeditious case of masculine Sati, we have heard of for some time, is that of the Rajah of Mandavie, and eight of his adherents, who have involuntarily put an end to their existence by the instrumentality of a quantity of fireworks which exploded about their persons. We have heard no particulars of this affair, further than that by some such occurrence as this, during

* The North-West Gazette.

† Beng. Police Rep. for 1863, p. 9.

‡ Nizamut Adawlut Reports, N. W. P., 30th June 1852.

§ *Ibid*, 1st April 1854, p. 358, and 26th September, p. 433.

some such rejoicings, such a catastrophe has taken place."—*Bombay Gazette*, 23rd November 1839.

This is scarcely worth noting except that there is a practice of male *Sati* or *Koor*. This was probably a mere accident, such as Froissart describes as having occurred in the French Court, King Charles the Sixth being one of the sufferers.

"*Indian Opinion* contains a curious case of male *Sati*, reminding us of the so-called Gymnosophists of Alexander's time. On the morning of the 3rd November last, in the Lahore District, a fanatic, of the name of Ummer Singh, was seen to go out with a pot of water in his hand, and fire in the other, and, when spoken to, would not answer. He went to a field in the midst of a vast jungle, and collected dried branches of trees, brushwood, and grass. When the tree-heap was sufficient, he performed his oblations, combed his hair, took off his clothes, and lit the funeral pile, on the summit of which he placed himself and became Suttee."*

Allied to this was the act, described by Forbes,† of a Hindu visionary who, taking his wife and four children for a walk on the beach at Back-Bay, in the environs of Bombay, informed his wife that he had received an invitation from the deity to go to heaven and to take his family with him, and then deliberately drowned them.

Other Brahmins, described by the same author, devoted themselves to death by eating until they expired with the surfeit.

(3) *Suicides in Consequence of Physical Suffering.*

Tytler mentions that, among women and sick or old persons in Bengal, the crime of Suicide is very frequent, and he attributes its prevalence to the influence of such doctrines as that laid down in the following striking passages from the Shasters :—

"A mansion with bones for its rafters and beams, with nerves for its cords, with muscles and blood for mortar, with skin for its outward covering, filled with no sweet perfumes, but loaded with fœces and urine,—a mansion infested with sickness and sorrow, the seat of malady, haunted with the quality of darkness, incapable of standing long,—such a mansion of the vital soul let its occupier always cheerfully quit."

The natives of Bengal not unfrequently destroy themselves in despair when the subjects of incurable maladies. Formerly these suicides of the diseased and the aged were publicly effected with all the formalities of a religious rite,—the self-devoted individuals being burned alive, throwing themselves into pits filled with ignited materials, being drowned in the Ganges, or crushed to death at Juggernath.‡

---

* *Friend of India*, November 29th, 1866.

† *Op. Cit.*, Vol. I., p. 491.

‡ Many interesting particulars relative to the commission of Suicide by persons who were diseased, poor, or despised, will be found in Ward's work, Vol. II., 3rd edition, pp. 116 and 121. See pages 432, 637, and 654 of this Manual.

In Professor T. W. Wilson's Memoir on the Painful Affections of the Stomach termed by the natives of Bengal "*peetsool*" or "*sool-badna*" (Indian Annals of Medical Science, October 1854), the author mentions that so obstinate is this *peetsool* considered by the natives, that it is attributed to a weapon in the hands of Siva, who inflicts the blow, but cannot remove the disease; the sufferer, in consequence, often despairs and seeks relief by suicide.* The same number of the Annals also contains a very remarkable case by Dr. J. W. Madge, of the Madras Horse Brigade, in which a native horse-keeper hanged himself about eleven hours after receiving a very severe kick on the abdomen, which caused great depression and excruciating pain. In addition to other injuries, it was discovered that the duodenum was entirely divided across (except one small strip) as if by a sharp instrument, and the edges everted to the extent of half an inch at each end.

In a trial at Mynpoorie, the accused stated that his wife, eleven or twelve years of age, committed suicide by cutting herself across the abdomen with a *husya*, "because of the pains in the belly which she had long endured;" the circumstances of the case rendered this statement improbable. Two assessors, Thakoors, acquitted him, remarking that "*women often threw themselves into wells when suffering pain.*" The third, a Vakeel, convicted him of wilful murder.†

A case has already been cited (at p. 632) in which a woman, when suffering from a paroxysm of pain in the stomach, to which she had been for some time subject, took up a sickle and killed her two children, and then endeavored to cut her own throat.

The following report appeared in the Calcutta *Indian Daily News* of the 24th June 1868:—"A native woman, residing at Garden-Reach, having for several months been suffering from a disease of the bowels which caused her intense pain, entreated her relatives to take her to the Ganges, and thus put an end to her. Failing this, she committed suicide by hanging."

Dr. Woodford has long considered that the pain, low spirits, and weak health produced by the presence of *lumbrici* in the intestines in the rice-eating poor of Bengal combine as a cause of suicide. He has kindly given me a note to this effect. A case of this kind occurring in the Calcutta Coroner's Court, as long ago as 1848, will be found at p. 596;

---

* I had an interesting conversation fourteen years ago with Mr. W. J. Ellis, then of Pubna, who considered that *sool badna* depends upon excessive fish-eating, especially of Hilsa fish. It prevails among all classes of natives, from the richest to the poorest. It had almost disappeared from the Pubna jail since the use of Hilsa had been discontinued. He thought that, at any time, he could find a hundred cases in Pubna. He had never discovered any satisfactory explanation by *post-mortem* examination. He had seen several cases in which the patients had destroyed themselves.

† Nizamut Adawlut Reports, N. W. P., 31st May 1853, p. 719.

and I have before me the report upon an inquest held in the same Court on the 5th August 1869 upon a poor creature who hanged herself, in which Dr. Woodford states :—"There were a good many worms. She was from four to five months in the family-way. I have noticed in my experience that persons troubled with worms suffer much from depression of spirits and melancholy."

See also page 432, for two cases in which persons, the subjects of severe bowel-complaints, cut their throats for the purpose of terminating their sufferings.

(4) *Suicide on Account of Grief or Shame.*

The following appeared in 1868 :—

It is reported that, whilst an assistant master of the Poona High School was dying of brain fever, his wife threw herself into a well, and perished two hours before her husband's death. Upon this case, the *Indo-prokash* remarked that "the approaching separation of her beloved consort, whom she loved so well on earth, to be followed by a wretched life of perpetual seclusion, misery, and degradation, and the thought of her being persecuted, instead of being sympathized with and consoled by her relatives in her bereavement, must have emboldened the poor girl to encounter the terrors of a watery grave."*

In some statistical observations on suicide in India, which will be found below, Dr. Muir, of Madras, comments as follows, with an incorrect pen, but with clear judgment, upon the fact that, while twice as many males as females voluntarily put an end to their own lives in England, the proportion is exactly reversed in this country :—

"The position of a wife in India is very different from what it is in England. Having no social status, or if any, a very degraded one, regarded by their husbands more as a servant than as a companion; absolutely passive in everything, and subject to the will and caprice of the lords of their destiny, the Hindu wife is commonly treated with contempt, severity, and cruelty.

"A Hindu marries not so much to gain the affection and sympathy of one who will share with him the trials, and assist him in his struggles with the world, as to have possession of one who will bear children and be subservient to his rule and passions. Mutual confidence, kindness, or concord are, therefore, rarely found to exist amongst them.

"The undivided family of a Hindu (numbering many members of different degrees of relationship) may have many of the advantages ascribed to it, but it is unquestionably a fruitful source of the most serious family quarrels.

---

* *Friend of India*, April 2, 1868. Capt. Meadows Taylor has admirably described the position of an Indian widow in Tara.

"The young wife thrown into such a family, invariably at a very tender age, is too frequently treated in such a harsh and domineering manner, as to drive her to despair, when she resorts to self-destruction as the only effectual means of relieving her from a miserable existence.

"These family discords, as well as the loose and immoral lives too often led by the husbands, are not only the most common cause of suicide of young women, but also account for the larger number of females than males putting an end to their lives."

As in the case of homicide, *vide* p. 429, so also in suicide, we shall not always be safe in admitting that the desperate act has really been prompted by the trivial cause which is alleged. Thus we find in the Annual Report of the Chota Nagpore district, for 1869, the Commissioner mentions that the people have an "unhappy propensity to resent the slightest insult or imputation by putting an end to their own existence." One woman poisoned herself, because her husband reproved her for being untidy, and another because she was asked to feed her own child. We have here the *alleged causes* of the rash acts, but I cannot believe that, in reality, the whole history of human nature presents a single instance of *motiveless* self-murder, except where insanity has been the cause.

A case singularly illustrative of certain remarkable sentiments and customs entertained by the Rajpoots, was tried at Kaira (Bombay Presidency) in 1829. Nurrotumpooree Byragee told the wife of Narron Nuthoo, Rajpoot, that her husband was an illegitimate son. The stigma thus cast in his character was so great in the eyes of the wife, who was also a Rajpoot, as to induce her to forsake him *and to commit suicide*. The Rajpoot, therefore, to revenge this injury, "abandoned his house for hostile purposes" against the other, as understood by the term *Baharwattee*. In leaving, he uttered threats of revenge, and shortly afterwards various acts of depredation and destruction of property were committed on persons residing in and about the menaced person's village. On the commission of each of these acts, a Jhansa letter was found placarded near the spot to the following effect: "Nurrotumpooree, come and redress the injury you have done me, or I vow I will plunder, burn, and murder in your name, and the guilt shall be upon your head." This crime being then greatly upon the increase in the Kaira Zillah, and a severe example being needful, Narron Rajpoot was sentenced to five years' imprisonment with hard labor.*

Forbes mentions† that suicide was a crime generally practised, when he was stationed at Dhuboy, by the higher class of Hindu widows, who, being interdicted from re-marriage, were led into imprudences. Their bodies were often found in the public wells of the city and villages in

* Bellasis' Reports, p. 21.

† *Op. Cit.*, Vol. II., p. 6.

the Pergunna, but none of the Brahmins in the Panchaut, nor any Hindu officer took the smallest trouble to prevent these occurrences. They became, at last, so frequent that he had affixed to the market-place and city gates an order that the body of any female found in a well or tank within the district should be exposed naked for twenty-four hours before it was taken to the funeral pile. No more suicides were committed, "or," he adds with great caution, "they were carefully concealed from my knowledge." Here the worthy Magistrate was, unknowingly, indebted to his classical reading for a precedent in the case of the virgins of Miletum, countrywomen of Thales, among whom an endemic of suicidal mania was at once quelled by the edict which Forbes repeated at Dhuboy.

Modes of Committing Suicide in India.

In the table above alluded to, Dr. Woodford shows that, in twenty-one cases, suicide was committed in the following modes:—Hanging, 10; Drowning, 6; Arsenic, 3; Cut-Throat, 1; by a Narcotic Poison, supposed to be Opium, 1.

Dr. Muir, of Madras,* has formed the following conclusions upon very extensive data:—"In India, of the various methods of committing suicide, drowning occupies the first position, and after it comes hanging. In England, hanging occupies the first position, then follows poisoning, cut-throat, and lastly drowning. In India, men resort to drowning and hanging as a means of self-destruction in about equal numbers, while six out of seven women who commit suicide prefer the water. In England four times as many males as females destroy themselves by hanging, and four times as many males as females by cut-throat, whilst the number of males and females who commit suicide by drowning and by poison is about equal. The number of suicides by lethal weapons is exceedingly small compared with that which exists in England. The most common causes of suicide in India are, according to Dr. Muir, jealousy, family discord, destitution, and physical suffering. Jealousy, with all the bitter feelings which it engenders, is the cause of a large number of female suicides."

The Report of the Inspector-General of Police for the Madras Presidency in 1869 gives confirmation to the above views. Among the entire population of that Presidency, 566 males and 829 females committed suicide. A large majority of suicides were from drowning; 259 males and 145 females hanged themselves; 18 males and 29 females died by poison; and 22 males and 4 females used weapons.

It appears elsewhere† that out of forty-nine Suicides upon whom inquests were held in Madras, in the two years, 1861 and 1862, there were, from drowning, 42; from hanging, 6; and from stabbing, 1.

---

* *Op. Citat.*

† Madras Med. Quart. Jour., April 1, 1863, p. 340.

Dr. Beatson found* that, in forty-one cases of suicide in which he had to investigate the cause of death, at Dacca, in the year 1865, twenty-one were Mussalmauns, twenty Hindus; twenty-seven were females, fourteen males. In thirty-eight cases, including all the females, the method of self-destruction chosen was hanging. The remainder were one, a Mussalmaun, by gun-shot wound ; one, a Mussalmaun, by drowning ; one, a Hindu, by poisoning by opium.

LAW.

The Indian Law regarding Suicide is laid down in the Indian Penal Code, Chap. XVI., section 300, except. 5; and sections 305, 306, 309.

The crime of attempting to commit Suicide was, previous to the year 1860, punishable under the provisions of Section 19, Reg. XIX. of 1807 ; see Nizamut Adawlut Reports, Vol. III., Part 1, of 1833, p. 842.

RAPE.

Instances of this crime appear to be of great frequency in India, and there is also reason to believe that persons are, by no means rarely, charged falsely with its commission.

In the investigation of cases of Rape, difficulty may sometimes arise with regard to the question of *Puberty*.

Cohabitation in marriage certainly takes place much earlier in India than in other countries; and, consequently, the development of puberty is frequently hastened; but it appears very doubtful whether menstruation naturally occurs much sooner in life in India than in Europe. Dr. Webb's Pathologia Indica contains some important remarks on this subject by Baboo Modusoodun Gupta, who shows that, according to Sushruta, "the menstrual discharge begins after the *twelfth*, and ceases after the fiftieth year." Angira, one of the Hindu law-givers, says, that girls are called Rajaswala (or females with menses) after the tenth year. Atri and Kasyapa (Hindu sages) state that, if an unmarried girl discharges the menstrual fluid at her father's house, the father incurs a guilt similar to that of destroying a fœtus, and the daughter becomes *Brisalee*, or degraded in rank. It appears that this doctrine is generally acted upon throughout the Hindu community. According to the Baboo's observation, the females of this country generally arrive at the age of puberty after the twelfth year, when they are fit for all the purposes of marriage. He thinks that Menu very judiciously fixed the time of marriage of females at twelve with men of thirty. Most of the females of this country begin to menstruate after the twelfth year, or at the beginning of the thirteenth, and the function continues till the fortieth and, in some cases, to the forty-fifth. Menstruation at ten years is very

* Ind. Med. Gaz., April 1st, 1866, p. 83.

uncommon; it probably does not occur in more than one or two instances out of a hundred females. It is perhaps equally rare for it to be delayed beyond the thirteenth year. It is the custom of the country, in their early marriages, to send the girl at perhaps nine years, occasionally, to the house of her husband; but, if the husband be so distant that this cannot be done, menstruation is generally delayed till the thirteenth year. He believes that the catamenia appear sooner or later according to the mode of living of the females, and the sexual excitement to which they may be subjected, as he finds that the first menstruation of girls in good circumstances generally takes place when they are eleven years old, even in some cases at ten years. He never observed a female in indigent circumstances to menstruate earlier than the age of twelve years. He has been informed by several women that, when the menstrual flux begins as early as in the eleventh or twelfth year, it does not, in many cases, recur for a year after this first appearance; but, after that period, the secretion again takes its natural course. It may, therefore, be fairly questioned whether or not this, which is supposed by them to be a first appearance, may not be rather a first copulation, and the result of a ruptured hymen.*

Dr. Roberton concludes that "the age for the earliest commencement of menstruation, either in India or England, may be taken at *nine* years."

"Although the *average* age of puberty in India is earlier than it is in England, we may doubt if puberty does actually appear at an earlier period of life in the one country than in the other."

"The remarkable difference between the establishment of puberty in Europe and India, consists in the far greater proportion of Hindus who arrive at puberty at the ages of twelve, thirteen, and fourteen."†

When at Howrah, I examined the body of a poor girl, stated to be only twelve years old, who had lived for nearly two years with her husband, a man between twenty and thirty years of age. Her general appearance was that of a well-grown child of eleven or twelve—there were none of the outward signs of puberty. The uterus was that of a child. The vagina, however, was considerably developed.

I have seen the particulars of a case given by Dr. W. A. Green, then of Dacca, in which he had to perform craniotomy. The patient was a Hindu girl of *twelve* in labor with her first child. The head was impacted, and she died undelivered.‡ Dr. Chuckerbutty informs me that

---

* Op. Citat, p. 277.

† *Ibid*, p. 127.

‡ Dr. Stoakley, of Northampton, Co. Virginia, relates the case of a negro girl, *thirteen* years of age, who brought forth a healthy child of ordinary size, after a natural labor of a remarkably easy character.—*Philadelphia Med. Examiner*, April 1855, and *Med. Chir. Rev.* for October of that year.

he knows an unquestionable case (he knew the child-mother from infancy) in which a girl became a mother at *ten*.

He says that they are frequently mothers at twelve and thirteen.

In European girls born in India a tendency to early puberty has been rather frequently observed. Dr. R. F. Hutchinson kindly sent me two cases,* in which European girls born and brought up in India menstruated so early that they might have been mothers when *eleven years and seven months* old.

Dr. Fayrer has given the ages at which twenty-seven girls, in the Calcutta European Female Orphan Asylum, began to menstruate.† They were all of pure European lineage. The earliest age was at *twelve years* and *two months* in a girl born in India. Of the whole number

Four	commenced	between	12 and 13	years of age.
Eight	,,	,,	13 and 14	,,
Nine	,,	,,	14 and 15	,,
Five	,,	,,	15 and 16	,,
One	,,	,,	16 and 17	,,

According to the Abbe Dubois, who resided in the Madras Presidency, Hindu girls, although married at a very early age, remain at their parents' houses until the first appearance of menstruation, when, after certain ceremonies, they are sent to their husbands.

Mahomedan Law regarding the Age of Puberty.

A girl is allowed, in law, to have attained the age of majority when the signs of puberty appear.—*Macnaghten's Mohummudan Law, Sloan's Edition*, p. 256. If a girl exhibit certain signs of womanhood at the age of nine, ten, eleven or up to fourteen years old, she is, in the language of the law, denominated *baligha bilulamut*, or adult by puberty. Should she exhibit none of those signs up to her fourteenth year, yet, on her attaining the age of fifteen years, she will be deemed an adult, and, in the language of the law, will be termed *baligha bissin*, or adult by majority. It was held that a girl of eleven, if an adult by puberty, is at liberty to contract marriage with a person either her equal or inferior in condition, without the consent of her mother or other guardian. Such marriage is available in law—p. 266.

Roberton mentions the case of a Factory Girl, who became pregnant in her eleventh year.

According to Taylor, the earliest age at which impregnation has been known to occur is *nine* years.

In consultation with Dr. Baillie, he mentioned the case of the daughter of a native gentleman, in Calcutta, who was delivered of a child at the age of *eleven* years. Some native graduates present said that her age was about eleven years and five months. Baboo Kanny Lall Dey says that it is not unusual to see girls of *twelve* who are parents.

* Ind. Med. Gaz., Dec. 1, 1868, p. 277.

† Ind. Annals of Med. Science, No. 26, for March 1870, p. 142.

An assertion either by male or female of their having attained the age of puberty, after they are twelve, or thirteen, or fourteen years old, should be credited and received as conclusive—p. 267.

The earliest period of puberty, with respect to a girl, is nine years—p. 228.

For a very full discussion of this question see the case of Khatteejah Bibi, which came before Mr. Justice Norman; Ordinary Original Civil Jurisdiction; Calcutta, May 16th, 1860.

I am indebted to Moulvie Thumeez Khan, Khan Bahadur, for the following valuable note on Mahomedan practice as founded on Mahomedan law:—

Under the age of *seven* years, intercourse with a female is distinctly and wholly interdicted.

After the *seventh*, and from that to the *ninth* year of her age, cohabitation with a wife is admissible, provided that she be steady and robust, and exhibits unequivocal signs of advancing pubescence.

The practice, as it obtains amongst Mahomedans in Bengal and Upper India, is that a man has intercourse with his wife only when she is about to menstruate for the first time.

It is stated that Mahomed married Ayesha when she was only *seven* years of age, and that she was considered nubile at *nine*.

According to Aboo Haneefa, a male cannot be considered to have arrived at the age of puberty, until he has completed his *eighteenth* year, unless he is proved to have indulged in or to be capable of sexual intercourse. Yoosuf and Moohumaud say the *fifteenth* year.*

In English law, an infant *under the age of fourteen years* is presumed to be unable to commit a Rape; nor is evidence admissible against him to show that, in point of fact, he has attained the full state of puberty, and was capable of committing the crime.†

I find cases in which lads of *fifteen* and *sixteen* years were convicted of Rape. There is an instance on record, in which a boy, *thirteen* or *fourteen* years of age, was found guilty of the crime, and sentenced, in consideration of his youth, to three years' imprisonment.‡ And another, in which a boy of the same age was imprisoned for two years with labor for attempt at Rape on a child of ten, doubt existing as to the consummation of the crime.§ One, in which a lad of *fourteen* was sentenced to five years' imprisonment for Rape on a girl of about the same age.‖ And another, where a boy only *ten* years old was convicted by the futwa

---

* Index to Macnaghten's Reports, Vol. I.

† Roscoe and Archbold, as cited by Beaufort, p. 576.

‡ Nizamut Adawlut Reports, Vol. III., p. 147.

§ *Ibid*, June 10, 1856, p. 962.

‖ Nizamut Adawlut Reports, N. W. P., 4th December 1852, p. 1452.

of rape on a girl, three years of age; the Court sentenced him, as for a misdemeanor, to imprisonment for one year.*

Except as it may affect *responsibility*, I do not think that the plea of early youth has much validity in India.

Mr. John Mayne observes:† "By the English law there is an invincible presumption as to the impossibility of a Rape being committed by a boy under fourteen. Here, probably, an earlier date would be fixed, and possibly the Court might follow some of the American Judges in treating physical capacity as a matter capable of proof and to be proved, independently of any arbitrary presumption (1 Bishop, sec. 466).

It is, however, always a matter of great difficulty to obtain a correct answer with regard to a native's age. Singular questions sometimes arise in the Courts upon this point. A lad calling himself twelve year sof age, but who appeared to be about fourteen or fifteen, was convicted of rape on a child of nine; and, with reference to his extreme youth, was sentenced to only three years' imprisonment with labor in irons.‡ A prisoner tried at Bundlekund for Rape on a child of seven, represented his age to be eleven years; although, in the opinion of the Sessions Judge and of the jury, he must have been about eighteen years old.§

In the case of females, however, it will be generally inquired of the Medical witness, not how old the girl is, but whether he considers that she has reached the age or condition of puberty.

According to the English law, the unlawful and carnal knowledge of a girl *under the age of ten years* is punishable by penal servitude for life; and, if the girl is *above the age of ten, and under the age of twelve years*, is punishable by penal servitude for three years; and, in

---

* Nizamut Adawlut Reports, N. W. P., Vol. III., p. 87; and Beaufort, para. 3018.

† Commentaries on the I. P. C., p. 243.

‡ Nizamut Adawlut Reports, N. W. P., 21st October 1853, p. 1326.

§ *Ibid*, 5th May 1854, p. 474. A man of Banda, who confessed to the murder of his wife, declared, on trial, that he was twelve years of age; although, in the Judge's opinion and in that of the jury, it was clear that he was not less than thirty. He had, moreover, thick mustachios and a bushy beard!—*Ibid*, 9th September 1853, p. 1155. A prisoner convicted, at Allahabad, of murder and robbery, was recommended by the Sessions Judge to a mitigated punishment on account of his youth, he appearing to be only sixteen years old. At the thannah, the prisoner stated that his age was twenty-six. The Judges of the Superior Court observed, that the Sessions Judge had not conformed to the Circular Order No. 105 of the 4th December 1811, which directs that, whenever a Judge may have reason to believe that a prisoner has stated his age inaccurately, he should specify on the record of the trial his opinion as to the *apparent* age of the prisoner. It is not sufficient to say (as the Sessions Judge had done in the present case) that the prisoner is not "of mature age." He was therefore called upon to supply this defect. He reported that, having again had the prisoner brought before him, "his apparent age was twenty." Sentence of death was passed.—Nizamut Adawlut Reports, N. W. P., 1st December 1852, p. 1423. Another question of the same kind arose in a trial at Bareilly in the same year—*Ibid*, 30th July, p. 750. See also a very remarkable case involving a question of this kind—*Ibid*, 30th September 1852, p. 1095.

these cases, it is immaterial whether the act was done with or without the consent of the female.*

Under the 9 Geo. IV., Chapter 74, for the East Indies, section 65,† it was enacted that "If any person shall unlawfully and carnally know and abuse any girl *under the age of eight* years, every such offender shall be guilty of felony, and being convicted thereof, shall suffer death as a felon; and if any person shall unlawfully and carnally abuse any girl *above the age of eight years and under the age of ten*, any such offender shall be guilty of a misdeameanour, and being convicted thereof, shall be liable to be imprisoned for such term as the Court shall award." Here it will be observed that the Indian Act gave a less age by two years than the English Act. The spirit of the Indian Act did not, however, appear to be adhered to in the Courts of this Country. It was held that the consent of a girl of the age of *eight* years was immaterial; and the prisoner was convicted on a charge of "illicit carnal knowledge of the prosecutor's daughter."‡ It was also decided, in a conviction for Rape upon the person of a girl "aged about *ten* years," that the offence is Rape, with or without the consent of the child, if she is "under age."§

The rule practically carried out in the Courts of this country would appear to have generally been that consent on the part of the female, *when under puberty*, cannot be received as any mitigation of the crime.

It is certain that some married girls of nine and upwards live with their husbands.|| It may not be considered that this arrangement takes

---

* Roscoe and Archbold, as cited by Beaufort, p. 577.

† As quoted by Hough, p. 448.

‡ Nizamut Adawlut Reports, Vol. II., p. 452.

§ Nizamut Adawlut Reports, Vol. II., Part 1, of 1852, p. 544. In another case where the girl was *ten* years old, the higher Court of the N. W. P. decided that "the acquiescence of the girl was, with reference to her immature age, immaterial in law."—Nizamut Adawlut Reports, N. W. P., 8th December 1854, p. 813. Some time previously the Sessions Judge of Chittagong held that, in the case of a girl of *ten*, the consent of a child of so tender an age could not extenuate the prisoner's guilt.—Nizamut Adawlut Reports, 25th November 1853, p. 791. See also a similar opinion in the cases of children of *nine*.—*Ibid*, Vol. I., of 1851, p. 471; and Nizamut Adawlut Reports, N. W. P., 21st October 1853, p. 1326; and in that of a girl aged from *seven to nine* years, p. 880.

|| See Baboo Modusodun Gupto's statement, cited above; also the case of a Rajpoot, who murdered his mother-in-law, in consequence of the latter's objecting to the consummation of his nuptials with her daughter, "a girl about seven years of age" to whom he had been betrothed (Macnaghten's Reports, Vol. I., p. 92). Instance of a girl "some nine years of age" who lived with her husband (Nizamut Adawlut Reports, Vol. II., Part 2, 1852, p. 45). Case of a girl "ten or twelve years old, who cohabited with her husband, but unwillingly. (Nizamut Adawlut Reports, 24th Feb., 1855, p. 253). Also a case of Rape on a married girl whose age "did not exceed thirteen years," and who it appeared had not reached puberty, but who had "lived with her husband for some time," and "had been in cohabitation with him."—Reports, Vol. IV. of 1854, p. 657. On the other hand, we meet with rather frequent cases, especially Up-country, in which it is positively asserted that girls of *twelve* and upwards have been married for some time, but have not cohabited with their husbands. See Nizamut Adawlut Reports, N. W. P., 4th January, 1854, p. 14

place *with the consent* of these unhappy children—indeed we have some very strong evidences to the contrary ; still, while such a custom exists in the country, the rule, although not less strictly enforced in the cases of unmarried children, should be and indeed is somewhat more cautiously dispensed in the cases of those who are known to have lived in their husbands' houses, whatever their ages may be.

The *Present Law of India*, as it affects age, is that a man is said to commit "rape" when he has sexual intercourse with a woman, with or without her consent, when she is under *ten* years of age.—*I. P. C.*, sect. 375.

We find Mr. W. Dorin, one of the Judges of the Nizamut, holding, in 1826, that "the English doctrine regarding the assent of children being immaterial, he was against adopting it in this country, where females came to maturity so early."*

Some extraordinary pleas occasionally arise out of the *Question of Consent* in these cases. A wretch of Budaon, when under examination for Rape upon *a child six years old, but to appearance only four*, repeatedly declared that the poor infant seduced him into the commission of the act.† Again, in a trial at Shahjehanpore, the prisoner, an adult, admitted his guilt, pleading that the girl, who appeared to be only *six* years old, of her own accord came to him and consented to the act.‡

A Mugh lad of seventeen having committed Rape on a girl about eight years old, admitted the act, but said that it was with her consent, and that he had had previous intercourse with her. This was disproved by the state of her person,—swelling, hæmorrhage, and destruction of the hymen.§

I have taken the details of sixty-six trials for Rape from the printed Reports of the Nizamut.‖ In only fourteen of these cases did the accused escape sentence by the superior Court.

(a girl about twelve years of age, who had been raped, declared that, though married a year previously, she had never cohabited with her husband : this was confirmed by the evidence of her husband, her mother, and grandmother. The Medical Officer gave it as his opinion that the girl was a virgin prior to the rape). Also *Ibid*, March 16th, 1854, (a girl calling herself *twelve*, but thought by the jury to be *fourteen*, having had similar violence committed upon her, deposed that she had been married for a year, had lived with her husband in the same house, but had not been carnally known by him. The husband deposed that he had been married to the girl a year ; and that, during the last three or four months, she had lived with him ; they slept separately. The Civil Surgeon found such injuries as led him to the opinion that Rape had been committed on her person. The High Court observed that the near approach to maturity of the girl might be thought to cast doubt on the statement that consummation had not occurred during a year's union with her husband, still there appeared to be no reason to question the truth of her charge).

* Macnaghten's Reports, Vol. II., p. 452.

† Nizamut Adawlut Reports, N. W. P., 14th June 1853, p. 767.

‡ *Ibid*, 30th December 1832, p. 1553.

§ Nizamut Adawlut Reports, May 30, 1856, p. 869.

‖ That is, of the Calcutta Court, up to April 1854, including thirteen cases reported in Vol. I. of the Decisions of the Nizamut Adawlut of the N. W. P.

In these sixty-six cases, the ages of the females are stated as follow :—*Four years*, 1; *six*, 2; between *six and seven*, 1; *seven*, 5; *seven and eight*, 2; *eight*, 1; *nine*, 3; *nine and ten*, 4; *ten*, 8; *ten and eleven*, 2; *eleven*, 1; *twelve and thirteen*, 1; *thirteen*, 5; young girl, age not mentioned, 1; *fourteen*, 1; *fifteen*, 1; *fifteen and sixteen*, 1; *sixteen*, 2; *adult women*, 19; *widows*, 5.

It will be observed that in thirty, or nearly one-half of these cases, the females were under the age of twelve.

More recently, a wretch was sentenced at Delhi to twelve years' imprisonment for a Rape and aggravated assault upon a woman seventy years of age ! * Another monster was found guilty, at Bareilly, of a Rape upon an infant apparently not more than three or four years of age, and *still suckled by her mother !* †

A writer from Saugor, early in July 1870, mentioned that a blind man, charged with committing Rape upon a child of three years, had been lately convicted by the Commissioner, and sentenced to four years' rigorous imprisonment.

In a large proportion of the cases of the younger children, it was very clearly proved that rather severe injury had been received. It is mentioned in several of the recorded cases that the vagina was lacerated. In a case where a girl of twelve was raped (not included in the above sixty-six cases), the Civil Surgeon deposed that there was a rupture of the lower part of the vagina to the extent of half an inch.‡ In another case, a poor infant of six years, but apparently much younger, was found by the medical officer to have suffered rupture of the hymen and laceration of the perineum and vagina.§ In one instance only does the violence of the assault appear to have proved fatal, in a girl of ten, who made a declaration that she had been violated by two persons. The medical particulars of this case are not given.‖

In another case (not counted with the above) it appeared, in a trial at Bareilly, that a girl eight or nine years old was violated by a man of twenty-five. The girl did not mention the occurrence to her mother until the evening, when notice was given to the police. A *dhaee* examined the girl, and stated that a Rape had been committed on her person. She was sent to the thannah, from thence to the dispensary, where the native doctor examined her, whence she returned home and died. The length of the interval between the assault and the girl's death, does not appear in the printed report. It was positively asserted that the deceased,

---

* Nizamut Adawlut Reports, N. W. P., June 1854, p. 371; see case in which this atrocity was committed upon a woman of sixty-four.—*Lond. Med. Gazette*, January 1850, p. 38.

† Nizamut Adawlut Reports, N. W. P., 1st February 1853, p. 141.

‡ *Ibid*, 10th March 1855, p. 336.

§ *Ibid*, 3rd March, 1855, p. 375.

‖ *Ibid*, Vol. I., p. 542.

although betrothed, had not cohabited. The Civil Surgeon examined the body and stated that, in his opinion, Rape had been committed on her person, and that diarrhœa had preceded death; that such ailment may have been caused by fright and alarm, but that he could not state distinctly that this resulted or was brought on by the injury of Rape, as other things may have assisted the alarm, and he did not know exactly what took place between the injury and death. The Courts held that there was not sufficient evidence to connect the death of the deceased with the violence perpetrated on her person, and acquitted the prisoner of murder—but found him guilty of Rape.*

The existence of a *Purulent Discharge* in the female is only mentioned in one case that I have met with. A man was accused of violating a child of ten. The Civil Surgeon deposed that he could not state positively that a Rape had been committed, but that the discharge was not natural. There was a slight white discharge from the vagina, and slight swelling of the external parts of generation. These appearances might have resulted from such a cause as the violence alleged; the discharge might have been the result of other causes besides violation or its attempt. The higher Court observed that it was a material omission in the Sessions Judge not to interrogate the Civil Surgeon particularly whether the girl was or was not still a virgin. Neither does it appear to have been inquired whether the accused suffered from Gonorrhœa or Syphilis.† I have treated several cases of *Idiopathic Infantile Vaginitis* (Taylor, p. 996) in India. Cases of *Noma Pudendi* occur in India, but by no means so frequently as might be expected, when it is considered how common *cancrum oris* (malarious phagedena) is in the damp districts of Lower Bengal.

The question has been mooted, in England, whether Rape, attended with Completion (*i. e.* Complete Penetration) can be perpetrated on a child of *Ten* by an adult man.‡ The question is of some practical moment, and a careful investigation of some of the cases presented to the notice of medical officers in this country might assist in elucidating it.

Still it is greatly to be regretted that a merely physiological question of this kind should, both in England and in India, have tended to screen atrocious criminals from the full punishment due to their guilt. Thus Taylor cites a case in which the evidence left no doubt that the crime had been committed on the person of a girl about ten years old. The Surgeon stated that there were considerable marks of violence about the pudendum, but *Completion* (*i. e.* penetration) was, in his opinion, physically impossible on a child under ten years of age. Upon this evidence,

---

* Nizamut Adawlut Reports, N. W. P., 26th November 1852, p. 1385.

† *Ibid*, 26th March 1855, p. 384. This important point has been fully discussed and weighed by Taylor, p. 244.

‡ Taylor, pp. 641-42. See also an important case, Nizamut Adawlut Reports, N. W. P., Vol. II. (1852), p. 1218.

the charge of felony was abandoned.* So, in this country, a lad, apparently about fourteen or fifteen years of age, was tried for a Rape on a girl of nine. He admitted the act, but asserted that it was with the child's consent. A woman, witness to the *sooruthal*, deposed that connexion had taken place. "The Civil Surgeon's deposition was to the effect that a Rape was *attempted*; but, *from the tender age of the child*, he did not consider it could forcibly have been *effected*."† The prisoner was, however, convicted. In the case of a man tried for Rape on a child of three or four, the Civil Surgeon deposed that, on examination of the girl, "he found specks of blood and laceration, from which he concluded that Rape had been *attempted*." The prisoner was convicted of "an attempt at rape;" but, the case being one of unusual atrocity, he was sentenced to ten years' imprisonment with hard labor in irons,—the usual punishment, on conviction for Rape, being imprisonment for seven years.‡ Again, in a trial at Azimgurh, a lad of eighteen was convicted "of an *attempt* at Rape, the medical evidence not sustaining the *completed* offence." The Civil Surgeon was of opinion that *a Rape was not effected*, but he spoke to the *rupture of the hymen*, and to *injury*, from forcible connexion, *having been inflicted on the vagina*. In consideration of his youth and the "slight injuries" sustained, he was sentenced to the mitigated punishment of three years' imprisonment.§ It is difficult to perceive under what circumstances the crime could have been held, in the above cases, to be not "Rape," but an "attempt to commit Rape," when it is an established principle of the English law that "a sufficient degree of penetration to constitute Rape, in law, may take place without necessarily rupturing the hymen"—"the degree of penetration being quite immaterial;"‖ and while it has been maintained, in India, that proof of penetration of the vulva, without rupture of the hymen, is sufficient to substantiate a charge of Rape.¶

On the other hand, I find, in the Nizamut Adawlut Reports of the North-Western Provinces, a case in which a person, apparently about eighteen years of age, was tried for Rape on a child of seven. The evidence of the midwife and of the Civil Surgeon went distinctly to show that the crime had been *Completed*."** A second, in which the Civil Surgeon deposed that such marks of severe injury existed upon the person of a child of eight, as to lead to the opinion that "Rape had been *committed* by violence."†† And another, where the sufferer was a child

---

* Page 991.

† Nizamut Adawlut Reports, N. W. P., 21st October 1853, p. 1326.

‡ *Ibid*, 1st February 1853, p. 141.

§ *Ibid*, 7th March 1855, p. 317.

‖ Taylor, p. 991.

¶ Nizamut Adawlut Reports, Vol. II., of 1852, Part 1, p. 548, and Vol. IV., p. 20.

** Nizamut Adawlut Reports, N. W. P., 5th May 1854, p. 474.

†† *Ibid*, 11th February 1853, p. 206.

of about four years, in which the prisoner was convicted of Rape and sentenced to seven years' imprisonment, it being in the opinion of the superior Court "clear from the evidence of the Civil Surgeon that the offence was *Complete*."* Also, in the case of a child aged about six, but apparently younger, the accused was convicted of Rape, the Civil Surgeon deposing that the lacerations inflicted were very extensive, and that a Rape had been "*perpetrated to the extent possible on an infant*."† It is merely frivolous to argue, as a point of law, even that *complete vaginal penetration* is impossible in any infant, however young, when it is certain, from numerous recorded instances, that such penetration has been effected in children of all ages: the fact that this penetration has, in very young girls, only been effected by severe laceration of the parts should, most assuredly, not be held as a mitigation of the atrocity.‡

The existing Indian law rules that "Penetration is sufficient to constitute the sexual intercourse necessary to the offence of Rape"—I. P. C., sec. 375.

It has been decided in England that any introduction of the male organ within the vulva constitutes penetration.§

Dr. Guy resolves the question as follows :—"The least possible introduction of the male organ within the vulva, even short of the rupture of the hymen, and without the emission of semen, constitutes Rape, provided it be done forcibly and against the will of the female (p. 37).

In cases of alleged Rape, the Medical Officer's opinion will, not unfrequently, be required as to *the manner in which the criminal may have prevented his victim from offering valid resistance, and from crying loudly*. In several of the recorded cases, it appears to have been clear that the females were either held by accomplices (3) or had their hands tied, or placed under them (3). In a very large proportion of the cases (12) it was declared that the females' cries were stifled by wrapping a cloth across their mouths. In one case a woman of twenty stated that the accused stuffed his *ungowcha* into her mouth; a girl of nine was similarly

---

* Nizamut Adawlut Reports, 10th May 1852, p. 431.

† *Ibid*, 23rd March 1855, p. 374.

‡ In a case tried at Cuttack, the medical officer deposed that the sufferer, a child aged about nine years, "had lost all traces of virginity."—Nizamut Adawlut Reports, 24th October 1854, p. 487. In another case, of a girl of nine, the Civil Surgeon of Agra deposed that he "saw the child on the morning of the 28th November, on the fourth day after the occurrence, and perceived no signs of violence whatever, which he considered must have remained visible if the injuries described by the two women had existed on the 25th. He, however, said that the girl was not a virgin; and that, if she had on any previous occasion had connexion with a man, marks of violence would not have remained. It was admitted that she had once visited her husband's house. Here we have also the opinion of an experienced Surgeon of the possibility of the act in a girl of nine.

§ Archbold as cited by Guy.

gagged. This has also been done in Bombay; a man of Ahmednugger committed Rape upon a child of nine, "having stuffed a cloth into her mouth."*

A girl of eight said that the defendant stifled her cries by compressing her cheeks with his fingers; and, in another instance, it appears that a poor child's mouth had been filled with sand.

A singularly brutal case occurred in the Dinagepore district in 1868. A woman, having gone to the haut, did not return at night. Her husband and relations, going to look for her, found her body in a jungle, naked, with several wounds on it, and with a small lattee pushed down the throat. A man, named Boolchand, who was seen returning with deceased from the haut, was suspected, and confessed that he and others took the deceased into the jungle, where one man committed Rape; another, on going to follow his example, was struck by the woman, which so enraged him that he took Boolchand's stick, and, after striking the woman several blows with it, struck it down her throat; they then stripped her and threw the clothes into the river.† I have seen two cases of Rape, in each of which there was a mark of rather severe *biting* on the cheek. In a case, which I have also cited in the Section on *Blinding* (Chapter on *Mutilation*), p. 484, a poor girl of twelve, who was forced by her husband, said that he bit her left cheek, tied both her hands with cloth, and bit her thumb; he then tightened a cloth round her neck, and pressed his fingers into both her eyes and blinded her.‡

The class of cases which is likely to occasion the medical officer most uncertainty in this country, is that in which, although the great body of the evidence tends to establish the fact that girls past the age of puberty, and accustomed to sexual intercourse, have been violated, some of the statements of the prosecutrices and their friends are not susceptible of confirmation by medical evidence. In many of these instances, it appears highly probable that much additional coloring is given to the facts, with a motive which is self-evident. This mixture of falsehood with truth, however, calls for the utmost vigilance on the part of the medical officer in a large proportion of his medico-legal investigations.§

Cases occur from time to time, in which it cannot be doubted that a charge of Rape has been trumped up for the purpose of bringing the accused into trouble ||,—thus :

---

* Bellasis' Rep., p. 13.

†. Bengal Police Rep., for 1868, p. 293.

‡ Nizamut Adawlut Reports, November 19, 1857, p. 396.

§ See a case especially illustrative of the difficulties involved in these inquiries.—*Nizamut Adawlut Reports*, 17th October 1853, p. 663.

|| "Men know well, in many a shyre, how often that many folk endyght Prestys of Rape at the sessyons, and, as there ys sometyme a Rape commytted indede, so ys there ever a Rape surmysed were the women never so willing, and often time where there was nothing done at all. Ye se not many sessyons pass but, in one shyre or other, this pageant is played over."—*Sir Thomas Moore's Supplycacyon of Beggars.*

At the Calcutta Supreme Court, 11th February 1862, Henry M ——was tried upon a charge of Rape. The defence was that the charge was trumped up by one Manuck Sing, zemindar of the village in which the prosecutrix and her witnesses lived, in revenge for several disputes which had arisen between him and the railway authorities on account of the latter having made roads through his property, for the conveyance of bricks to the line. The evidence for the prosecution was full of improbabilities, and there was discrepancy between the statement of the prosecutrix and that of her witnesses in many important particulars. The jury, without a moment's hesitation, returned a verdict of not guilty.*

The crime of Adultery is punished, both socially and legally,† with so much severity in this country that, in many cases, there has been strong reason to believe that (when the law punished both parties alike) women, detected in its commission, have charged their paramours with Rape.‡

Wherever it was possible, the opinion of a medical officer was obtained by the judicial authorities in cases of this kind; but it frequently happened that the reports of native midwives, or of other and probably less

---

* *Englishman*, 12th February 1862.

† Under the Indian Penal Code (section 497), Adultery is punished with imprisonment of either description for a term which may extend to five years, or with fine, or both. In such case, the wife is not punishable as an abettor.

Old Laws.

Any person committing Adultery—"Penalty"—Imprisonment with hard labor for any period not exceeding seven years, and two years in lieu of stripes, Regulation XVII of 1817, section 6; Regulation II of 1834, section 1. See cases in which both parties were convicted, and sentenced to imprisonment.—*Nizamut Adawlut Reports* (N. W. P.), February 7th, 1853, p. 185; June 1854, p. 649; October 26th, 1844, p. 623.

A person accused of Rape was punished for Adultery by the Nizamut Adawlut of Calcutta in 1824. A bearer was sentenced to imprisonment for Adultery with a woman in Calcutta.—*Nizamut Adawlut Reports*, December 23rd, 1854, p. 802.

By the ancient Mussalmaun Law, it was held that, if a person found a man with his wife or female slave, and the wife or slave be assenting to the whoredom, both parties might be slain. There appears, however, to have been reservation to the effect that killing was only justifiable where the slayer was not able to prevent the criminals from effecting their purpose. "Zena" (which included adultery, fornication, rape, and incest) was punishable by the law only upon the evidence of four men, eye-witnesses to the fact, or upon the confession of the offender four times repeated! Under which circumstances, the punishment awarded—stoning to death—was probably seldom inflicted.

By the Hindu law of Menu, an Adulteress of high rank was to be devoured by dogs in a public place, and the Adulterer to be burned to death on an iron bed. A mechanic or servile man, having connexion with a woman of twice-born class, was to lose the part offending—c. viii., s. 371-2-4. It is mentioned in the *Ayen Akbery* that, where the man is inferior, he shall, in all cases, be put to death, and the woman shall have her nose and ears cut off.—Gladwin's Trans., v. 3, p. 211. It appears, however, to have been ruled by Menu that, where the parties were of equal rank, the man was not to be punished for Adultery if the woman consented.

‡ Macnaghten's Reports, Vol. II., pp. 317, 926, 1254; Nizamut Adawlut Reports, Vol. II., Part 2, p. 495; Vol. III., Part 2, p. 39; Vol. IV., p. 427, Nizamut Adawlut Reports, (N. W. P.), for August 1854, p. 300.

intelligent females had to be taken. Considering, however, the extreme care and strict fidelity (rather than the high degree of medical knowledge) required in investigating the generality of cases of this description, it must be evident that much caution should be observed in receiving the opinions of native women upon them, and that it would be safe to expect from these females so much explicitness of detail as to render the reports of their evidence available of submission to competent medical authority.

The native midwife is always of low caste. The Hindu midwives, in Bengal, are Chumarins, the skinner caste. They are often quick-witted, but are barbarously ignorant. In Calcutta, in June 1862, a midwife is said to have declared that she had practised since she was eleven years old.

These *dhaees* often give their statements with great confidence and fullness. In a case where a man had found his daughter, aged nine, lying senseless in a field, and with blood flowing from her private parts, and had her examined by a midwife at the thannah, this woman deposed "that connexion had been violently made, the hymen broken, and the act consummated." She also declared that the girl had not arrived at the age of puberty, and that "she was too immature to have any sensual desire." The Sessions Judge remarked that it appeared that the deposition of the Civil Assistant Surgeon had not been taken on oath. The statement of that officer was, he thought, inconclusive for the prosecution, and, it being of a negative kind, his appearance on trial was not considered necessary or expedient, with reference to the distance of his station from that of the trial. He agreed with the majority of the jury in finding the prisoner guilty. The Judges of the superior Court remarked that the evidence of the Civil Assistant Surgeon, which the Sessions Judge regarded as inconclusive, could not, in justice to the prisoner, be denied weight. He examined the girl, at the latest, four days from the event (the *dhaee* examined her on the day after). He stated that "there were no signs of inflammation, nor any evidences to show that violence had been committed; the hymen was, however, absent. He added his opinion that it was *possible* that no signs of external violence should remain five days after the crime, but that would depend on the amount of violence used. The Court held it to be, if not altogether impossible, yet in the highest degree improbable, that, had the marks of violence described by the midwife existed on the 19th, no trace should remain on the 22nd. The Court also considered the midwife's earliest statement to be inconsistent with the assumption of Rape having been *fully committed* on a virgin child of the immature age of eight or nine. It spoke of little or nothing more than that the girl had recently lost her virginity; slight partial laceration was alluded to, but not swelling or bleeding of the parts, which were additions made in the subsequent examinations of this witness. Further, there was no proof (except the father's statement, not made in his earliest charge) that the girl's marriage had not been consummated. The Court ordered the prisoner's acquittal and release.*

One Kewal was tried, at Delhi, on the accusation of a girl of ten, for an attempt to commit a Rape. Two midwives, who examined the person of the child, deposed that an attempt to commit a Rape on the child had evidently been made, but that the act had not been consummated. The superior Court called upon the Sessions Judge to report whether the Civil Surgeon was examined as to the completion of the offence, and, if not, why the evidence of that officer was not taken on a point in regard to which it would have been of the highest value. The Joint Magistrate explained that there was no Civil Surgeon stationed on the spot, and that it was only in extraordinary cases, requiring particularly great professional knowledge to elucidate them, that the sufferers were sent to the Civil Surgeon at Delhi. He did not consider the rules regarding the examination of European medical officers applicable to this case. The evidence of the experienced women, called *dhaees*, whom he employed, he considered preferable to that of the Native Doctor stationed there. Unless there were an order existing (which he was not aware of there being, applicable to that district), making it necessary to expose the body of a female suffering from Rape to a person of the other sex, he should always think it best to avoid doing so [!] The female herself, if possessed of any modesty, would generally object to such a course as well as her friends; and forcibly to do so, while no direct order applicable to a case occurring so far from Delhi existed, might subject the Government officer so acting to an accusation of illegal or at least oppressive conduct. The superior Court considered that the explanation given by the Joint Magistrate for dispensing with the evidence of the Civil Surgeon was satisfactory. The Court do not appear to have taken into consideration that officer's most questionable opinion that, in cases of Rape, examination by midwives is always preferable to that by persons of the other sex.†

In a large proportion of cases, investigations cannot be made by the medical officer, until the lapse of a considerable period from the time at which the offence is alleged to have been committed. Where this delay is believed to have been owing to design or carelessness, or no steps have been taken to obtain the testimony of midwives or medical opinion, the complaint is generally‡ (not always)§ disallowed.

In some instances, this delay, whether unavoidable or intentional, is so great, as to render it impossible that the medical officer should give more

---

* Nizamut Adawlut Reports, N. W. P., 20th April 1854, p. 431.

† *Ibid*, 14th February 1833, p. 235.

‡ Reports, Vol. I. of 1851, p. 536; Vol. II., Part 2, of 1852, p. 87; Vol. IV., p. 250. Selected Cases, Feb. 26, 1858, p. 78.

§ A case in which the Rape was committed on the 21st August, complaint made at the thannah on the 28th, and then only by the husband's son, a boy of nine or ten years. *Conviction.* Nizamut Adawlut Reports, Dec. 31, 1855, p. 994.

than a negative opinion. In other instances, however, as in certain cases of young children and of unmarried girls, an approximative opinion may, not unfrequently, be formed, even many days after the commission of the offence. Thus, in two cases of full-grown girls, finding the hymen injured, but not in process of contraction,—I have been enabled to state my belief in the truth of the allegation that penetration had probably occurred, for the first time, a fortnight or three weeks previously.

As in England, evidences of *Emission* are not required here to establish the crime of Rape. I find only one case in which the question of the presence of spermatazoa was referred to the Chemical Examiner. Here the medical officer of Umritsur transmitted a portion of wadded *rezae* (coverlet), suspiciously marked, to Mr. Siddons, but zoosperms could not be detected.

As the crime of Rape is often committed with brutal violence on young children in this country, *blood-stains* are frequently noticed on the clothes of both parties.

There are many cases in the criminal records of this Presidency, in which the ravisher sought more or less successfully to destroy the life of his victim. A man of Bhaugulpore, having committed a Rape, and being alarmed at the threats of the female to have him punished, attempted to kill her, by cutting her throat, and then tried to escape.*

A Sylhet man committed a Rape on a girl of ten, cut her throat, and was sentenced to death.†

A girl was found in the fields, at Sarun, with her throat cut; it was supposed that the murderer had first ravished her, and then murdered her.‡

In a trial at Bareilly, a man confessed that he had enticed away his master's daughter-in-law: three others accompanied them, two had criminal connexion with her, and, upon her refusing the third, she was thrown down, and killed with a sword.§ A lad of Benares, who stated himself to be eighteen, but who appeared to be fourteen or fifteen years old, confessed at the thannah and Magistrate's Court, that he had carnal knowledge of a child of seven, had caused her death by so doing, and had stolen her ornaments. The body was found concealed in a room, much decomposed, with a stone on the chest, and a cloth wrapped round the neck. Dr. Leckie, on removing the cloth, found that the whole of the soft parts of the neck had been destroyed, from which he inferred that it had been compressed, and that Strangulation was the probable cause of death.‖ See also a case by Dr. O'Dwyer at p. 694.

---

* Police Report, L. P., 1849, p. 18.

† *Ibid*, 1845, p. 37.

‡ *Ibid*, for 1850, p. 6.

§ Nizamut Adawlut Reports, N. W. P., 30th October 1852, p. 1258.

‖ *Ibid*, 14th June 1853, p. 793.

Where women have died soon after having been raped by several men, death has been attributed to nervous exhaustion. Upon this point I was obliged, in 1867, with a remarkable fact by that excellent physiologist, Dr. J. Barnard Davis. He wrote: "When Mr. Lawson first wrote to me on the subject, he spoke of Marquesan women having boasted of having received embraces from a large number of men in one night at their feasts. I think he said above a hundred, or at all events not many less than a hundred. I made the objection that it was impossible for the woman to bear it and live, and again impossible on the score of time, allowing ten minutes for each act. In eight hours, the number could not exceed fifty. He has now sent me an attested statement of what he and others have observed, and speaks of instances in which five, ten, fifteen, twenty, thirty, up to a hundred acts have occurred in succession. He names one case, in which he heard a parcel of boys, next morning, count over and *name* a hundred and three men who, during the night, had had intercourse with *one* woman, for there was but one woman of the party, and he cuts down the time to five minutes each." Dr. Davis justly adds, "All this, no doubt, is voluntary, and all the effects of violence" [in ordinary cases of Rape by many persons] "have to be deducted."

We find several instances where women of this country have killed those who attempted to ravish them. In 1845, a woman of Monghyr was acquitted of murder by the Nizamut, she having inflicted the wound on the deceased which led to his death, when he was attempting to violate her person.* The readers of Indian History will be familiar with the instance which occurred in 1696, when Soobha Singh, a rebel, having overrun Bengal, killed the Raja of Burdwan, and taken his daughter prisoner, attempted the honor of the latter, when the spirited girl stabbed him to death with a knife which she had concealed, and then pierced her own heart.

It appears in the Seir Mutaqherin that it was universally reported that Sooja-oo-dowla received a dangerous stab from a noble young Rohilla lady, whose honor he attempted, and who was immediately dispatched by his eunuchs. Akber, when he assailed the honor of a princess of Meywar, the wife of Pirthi Raj, was compelled, at the dagger's point, to revoke an edict of infamy which he had issued against her race. Honorable mention has already been made in these pages† of the courage with which the Queen of Ganore, when taken captive in her last stronghold, defeated her enemy in the moment of triumph and maintained her own virtue.

The Hindu mistress of Baz Bahadur poisoned herself when the importunities of her captor, Adam Khan, became dangerously violent.

---

* Police Reports, L. P., 1845, p. 15.

† *Vide supra*, p. 298.

*

The Nizamut Adawlut Reports, Vol. I., p. 1, contain the case of a man who put his wife to death, at her own request, in consequence of her loss of honor from having been violated by several persons.

Fatal Injuries Inflicted in the First Act of Connexion.

Mr. Verelst wrote, in 1772,* "Women in the East are transferred with little ceremony; and, whether they be wives or concubines, the men seldom await their consent. When Colonel Clive defeated Surajah-oo-dowlah, Meer Jaffer sent to offer the Colonel some hundred of Surajah's women who were taken in the camp. Were our laws of Rape (girls under ten years of age are incapable of consenting under our law) and rules of evidence enforced, one-half of the males would incur the penalty of death."

There is a very important set of cases which, it is to be trusted, are almost peculiar to this country, examples of which sometimes come under the investigation of medical officers. These are instances in which *Fatal Injuries are inflicted on the Persons of Young Girls in the First Act of Connexion.*

In 1847, there was a trial, at Bancoorah, in which Mr. Cheek, the Civil Surgeon, was questioned whether he thought it possible that a man, having connexion with a girl eleven years of age, could, *without unusual or extraneous force*, have produced rupture of the perineum from the vagina to near the anus; also, whether a wound of eliptical or diamond shape, large enough to admit three fingers, could have been caused by the simple act of coition. He replied, that he had never seen a case of the kind, but had every reason to believe that rupture of the perineum might occur from a man having connexion with a child of that age. He considered, however, that the mere act of coition would not produce a wound of the shape described above. He thought that, if a rupture of the perineum had taken place from coition, it would have been in a straight line from the vagina towards the anus. (It would appear that the body was not seen by Mr. Cheek.) He considered that a mere rupture of the vagina to the anus is not sufficient to cause death, although the injury is of a very severe nature. In cases of midwifery, such accidents do occur, and are not necessarily followed by death. With regard to the probability of the girl in question having died from the hæmorrhage attending such a rupture, he considered that there is a great difference in various constitutions. In one case, death might be caused by a loss of blood, which would not be fatal in another.

There cannot be a doubt that, in many cases, *unusual and extraneous force is employed.*

---

* View of the Rise and Progress of the English Government in Bengal, p. 141.

Dr. Taylor gives (p. 993) a case of Casper's of a child only ten years of age, whose vagina had been dilated by the mother, at first with two fingers, afterwards with four, and finally by means of a long stone introduced into it, in order to fit her for intercourse with men! The hymen was not destroyed, but there were lacerations in it, the mucous membrane was reddened and painful to the touch, and there was a mucous discharge from it.

In his description of Burmah, Purchas says:* "Gasper Balby and Got. Arthus tell of another custome of their virgins, if that name may bee given them, for, say they: '*Virgines in hoe regno omnino nullas reperire licet; puellæ enim omnes statim a pueritia sua medicamentum quoddam vsurpant, quo muliebria distenduntar et aperta contenentur; idque propter globulos quos in virgis viri gestant, illis enim admittendis virgines arctiores nullo modo sufficerunt.*'"

I was imformed by an eminent Missionary, thoroughly conversant with the customs of the natives in the neighbourhood of Calcutta, that he was assured that means are commonly employed, even by the parents, to render immature girls *aptæ viris* by mechanical means, especially by the use of the fruit of the plantain!†

I was informed by the late Dr. Heathcote that an old Bengalee man, at Akyab, actually *burnt* the private parts of his wife, a girl of ten, to enlarge the opening!

Dr. S. C. Mackenzie informs me that he was told by a servant that the bawds who train up girls to prostitution insert a piece of *sola* (the soft and spongy stem of Æschynomene paludosa, from which "rice paper" is made, and which supplies the place of corks in native pharmacy) as large as the vagina will contain, and then make the unfortunate sit in water: a dilating action similar to that of a sponge-tent is the consequence. They gradually increase the size of the plug.

Moulvie Tumeez Khan, Khan Bahadur, has sent me a note to the same effect precisely. This barbarity is, of course, only practised by the most depraved. He has ascertained that the process is repeated daily for months before the object is attained.

There is a remarkable passage in the ancient Hindu law which may be liable to various constructions, but which was, I believe, intended to act as a check upon this particular atrocity. In the 19th Chapter of Halhed's Code on Adultery, the 5th section is "of thrusting a finger into the *pudendum* of an unmarried girl."

---

* Op. Cit., Vol. V., p. 504.

† Native friends assure me that this atrocity cannot be common; and I am confident that it is not. As I have stated in my Introduction, one of the greatest errors which can be committed in forming an opinion of national character, is to assume that a *criminal practice* which, from time to time, makes its appearance among a people, is a *national custom.*

The punishments vary according to the respective castes of the parties. There are six paragraphs, of which it will be sufficient to quote three.

"If a man, either by violence, or by permission, thrusts his finger into the *pudendum* of an unmarried girl of a superior caste, the Magistrate shall confiscate all his possession, and put him to death."

"If one unmarried girl, by thrusting her finger, &c., should make a passage, the Magistrate shall fine her two hundred *puns* of cowries, and give her ten lashes with a whip."

"If a married woman by thrusting her fingers, &c., should make a passage, the Magistrate shall cut off the hair of that woman's head ; and, if she thus thrust her finger a second time, he shall cut off two of her fingers, and cause her to be exposed through the whole city mounted on an ass."—(pp. 277-78.)*

Our criminal reports contain several instances, in addition to those given above, in which such unnatural mechanical force was undoubtedly used.

In 1853, a wretch, of Bancoorah, was found guilty and sentenced to fourteen years' imprisonment, upon a charge of having committed a Rape upon a girl about ten or eleven years of age, married, but living apart from her husband. There was every reason to believe the statements of the child, that "he took a small lattee, or stick, which was in her hand, and, after using it, '*ad deobstruendam viam,*' to considerable effusion of blood, succeeded in completing his purpose." The injury inflicted does not appear to have been dangerous.†

In 1868, Sookoor Mahomed was found guilty, at Sylhet, of the "culpable homicide of his wife, who was at an age unfit for sexual intercourse, and was wounded from the effects of violence used in a forcible violation of her person by her husband." Unfortunately the medical evidence is not given. The Judge of the Court of appeal remarked that "although the deceased is said by the witnesses to have been eleven or twelve years old, and had nearly attained the age of puberty, there is not only the cruel violence of the act, from which death ensued, but the medical evidence shows that the unfortunate victim was, for some time previously, subjected to unnatural practices.‡

The following case also appears to me to come within this category. Sobanee Doss, also of Sylhet, was offended with his wife, a girl of thirteen or fourteen, for going without him to a feast given by a neighbour. It was proved, by the evidence of eye-witnesses, that he tied her hands together,

---

* Tennant (Vol. I., p. 171) views these rules as parallel with those of the Levitical Code, and considers that they are intended to punish those acts by which "the tokens of virginity" may be destroyed. While they had this operation, it is also clear that they met, in the fullest possible manner, the crime which is the object of the present enquiry.

† Nizamut Adawlut Reports, N. W. P., 30th November 1853, p. 327.

‡ Nizamut Adawlut Reports, May 31st, 1858, p. 199. There may be a doubt regarding the meaning of this expression, but I believe that it refers to the extraneous force in question.

and afterwards beat her with a small bamboo. The girl died that night. The evidence of the Civil Surgeon proved that "a stick or some blunt instrument had been repeatedly thrust into the vagina and anus, causing the perforation both of the bowels and womb; while the *perineum*, or space between the two parts, had been so perforated as to render the whole of those parts nearly one large ragged cavity, and from it two loops of the bowels, each a foot long, had escaped." The Judge considered that, as the neighbours say they did not hear any noise that night, and as it may be reasonably supposed that so dreadful an outrage would have been attended with heart-rending screams, it can only be supposed that deceased was gagged or had by some means been rendered insensible before the crime was perpetrated.

The Museum of the Calcutta Medical College contains a preparation, sent by Mr. G. Evans,* displaying the uterus, vagina, and greater portion of the external parts of generation of a young Mahomedan female, showing laceration of the perineum, and a considerable portion of the vaginal sheath, the effects of violence done to the parts in the first act of copulation, by which a violent hæmorrhage, to the destruction of the child (barely twelve years old), was occasioned. The uterus and parts concerned were diminutive and undeveloped, as might naturally be expected at that tender age, and before the process of menstruation had been established. The coagula at the bottom of the bottle were removed from the vagina after death. The sudden and unlooked-for death of the child, on the first night of her marriage, and the unaccountable quantity of blood found beneath the bed, and upon her linen, led to the suspicion of unfair means having been resorted to for her destruction. The body having, accordingly, been exhumed to ascertain the cause of her death, the perineum and vagina were found ruptured in the manner described, and as is represented in the preparation. But, as a judicial inquiry elicited no facts or circumstances tending to show that any unlawful means had been made use of by the husband to effect his purpose, and his generative organs presenting nothing unusual to account for the appearances, while the immediate cause of her death was satisfactorily explained by loss of blood from the vagina, Dr. Webb believed that this might be considered a case of extreme preternatural weakness or laxity of the genital system of the female, and one of very rare occurrence; for the common practice of Eastern nations, in forcing sexual intercourse upon children, of even earlier years than the subject of the present inquiry, would not appear to be attended with similar disastrous consequences.

This offence was made punishable under the Mahomedan law, when death was the result of the first attempt at connexion—see Skipwith, para. 952, where is cited the case of a prisoner convicted of killing his

* The following description is by Dr. Webb—Pathologia Indica, p. 285.

wife, a girl of eleven years, in his attempt to consummate marriage, and sentenced to fourteen years' imprisonment with hard labor. It is added, that the Civil Surgeon recorded his opinion that the violence had been occasioned by the introduction of some hard instrument. (Nizamut Adawlut Reports, Vol. VI., p. 29.)*

---

* From this and many other facts, it is evident that the ancient law-givers of this country, in providing for the early marriage of females, were careful to protect them against too early cohabitation. The practice of sending immature children to their husbands' houses, which at present obtains, is evidently as much an infraction of the law of the land, as it is a violation of the law of nature.

The practice of early marriage or betrothal has been usual in nearly all unsettled countries, and was common even in England up to the beginning of the eighteenth century. The following examples may be cited from a multitude of others: Isabel, daughter of Philip the Fair, King of France, married Edward the Second of England, in her 12th year, January 1308. Her second child was born when she was seventeen years old. Her eldest daughter was married at fifteen; her second was married in her ninth year to a child of four.

It is mentioned in Abaldini's description of England in 1551, given in Raumer's History of the sixteenth and seventeenth centuries, that "the people in general are tolerably tall of stature, the nobles in great part little, which comes from the prevalent customs of marrying rich damsels under age." It is interesting to contrast this with the observation of another stranger made in 1835: "The *Paysans* of France and the *Contadini* of Italy are, physically, far superior to their degenerate masters; while the nobility and gentry of England differ from the peasantry, in limb and feature, as the racer differs from the dray-horse, or the grey-hound from the cur."

The Civil Law enjoined fourteen and twelve as the nuptial ages for males and females respectively.

"Lordings, since I twelve years was of age * * * * * *
Husbands at the Church-door I have had five."

Such abuses are quite possible, and, when established, are very hard to put down. The following is copied *verbatim* from the *Times* of January 25th, 1867 :—

"The Rescue Society proposes the establishment of a home for young fallen girls from ten to sixteen years of age, of which there is a most urgent need, the Society having to refuse applicants almost daily of this tender age."

Maurice Lord Berkeley (23rd Edward I.) was contracted in marriage at eight years of age, and was a father at fourteen.

When Richard II. married Isabel of France, she was only eight years old. Froissart says that the King was told that his bride was "over young, and that this five or six years she shall not be able to keep him company; thereto he answered and saith, that she shall grow right well in age."

The delicacy of Henry the Seventh's constitution has been attributed to the (alleged) fact that his mother, Lady Margaret Beaufort, was married when only nine years old, and that she was only ten when Henry was born.

Elizabeth Hardwick, afterwards Countess of Shrewsbury, married (Cir. 1533) before she was fourteen; her daughter Grace married, in 1567- 8, at the age of twelve. Audrey, the eldest daughter of the Earl of Southampton, was betrothed to the eldest son of the Earl of Northumberland, but died in her fourteenth year. Her younger sister, Elizabeth, was afterwards married to Lord Percy, in her fifteenth year—this was in 1662.

On the 26th April 1714, a petition was laid before the House of Lords by Mrs. Mary Forrester, Maid of Honor to the late Queen (Anne), and now to H. R. Highness the Princess of Wales, setting forth that, about thirteen years ago, when she was but twelve years of age, she had been married to Sir George Downing, then about fifteen; that Sir George going then to travel, he did, upon his return, show his dislike to the match, which had prevented their cohabitation, therefore they prayed that they might be separated and at liberty to marry

In his ruling upon the case of Sookoor Mahomed, cited at p. 690, the Judge of the Nizamut Adawlut, Mr. D. J. Money, observed: "In a similar case of Bawool Saha, tried by this Court, on the 4th October 1843 (see Nizamut Adawlut Reports), the opinion of the Mahomedan law officer was called for before sentence was passed. He declared that the defence was punishable under the Mahomedan law, provided the husband had not previously had actual connexion with his wife, and the Court sentenced the prisoner to fourteen years' imprisonment with hard labor. Dr. Chevers, in his work on medical jurisprudence, has a note upon this case, see page 482 "(now 692)," where he states that 'from this and other facts, it is evident that the ancient law-givers of this country, in providing for the early marriage of females, were careful to protect them against too early cohabitation. The practice of sending immature children to their husband's houses, which at present obtains, is evidently as much an infracture of the law of the land as it is a violation of the law of nature.' It is impossible to doubt that such cases must often occur, although the marital right may throw a shield over them, and prevent disclosure or discovery. It is one of the consequences of the pernicious system of early marriages which, when followed by early cohabitation is, as Dr. Chevers justly remarks, opposed as much to the law of the land as to the law of nature. Whatever may be the popular opinion on this subject, the unnatural practice has not the sanction of law, and some restriction might be imposed, by legislative enactment, upon the parent to prevent his surrendering his child, at too early an age, to what can only be called the prostitution of marriage. I do not see by what right a girl of tender years is to be delivered over to a husband's custody and the rites of marriage before she is fit for their consummation."

In a case tried in 1857, at Jessore, where a wretch hacked his wife, a child of eleven, nearly to pieces, with a *dao*, because she refused to have connexion with him, the Sessions Judge, Mr. E. Jenkins, observed: It is an abominable, cruel, heartless custom among the lower classes in this part of the country, to allow betrothed girls to go to their husbands, though of too young an age to cohabit with them. It occasions endless misery, and necessarily often brings on premature death to the wife, whose parents, regardless of consequences, seem to think their duty is discharged

---

again. Several of the Lords, and especially the Bishops, spoke against allowing a divorce; and the matter was put off till the 3rd of May, when it was, upon debate, carried by 50 against 48 to reject the petition, all the Bishops being against a divorce, lest it should weaken the obligation of marriage.—*The Annals of King George, Year the First*, 1716.

The whole Peerage might be gone through with similar results. Immature children were always separated for a few years. Still the practice certainly often led to disgracefully early unions.

when making over, be her age however tender, to the husband on demand, their betrothed daughter.*

These considerations probably led the framers of our Indian Penal Code to adapt the law of Rape so far to the circumstances of the country that it now stands as follows :

"Section 375. A man is said to commit 'rape' who, except in the cases hereinafter excepted, has sexual intercourse with a woman under circumstances falling under either of the five following descriptions."

* * * * * * * * * * * *

"Fifthly—with or without her consent when she is under ten years of age."

* * * * * * * *

"*Exception.*—Sexual intercourse by a man with his own wife, not being under ten years of age, is not rape."

It is to be feared that this reservation, benevolent as it is, does not fully meet the evil now in question. It will be noticed that, in two of the cases of this description the unhappy little victims were about *twelve* years of age, and there cannot be a doubt that, as long as the wife is, in fact, *a child*, this danger is incurred. Early in the present year the following report reached India :—

"At the Liverpool Assizes, last week, Mr. Justice Willes, in sentencing to twelve months' imprisonment a man named Thompson, who had assaulted a young girl in his employment, with intent, said it was the duty of persons who had girls of tender years in their service to protect them and watch over their morality ; but the prisoner, instead of doing this, had attempted to destroy the poor girl's character. He hoped that, in cases where girls between twelve and fourteen years of age were assaulted, the question as to their consent would attract public attention, and that largely. He had had to try a great many cases of this kind, especially where girls were servants, and where the masters, instead of protecting the poor children under their charge, had attempted to corrupt them. He hoped that what the present Bishop of Winchester had so often attempted, though unsuccessfully—to have the law which applied to girls of twelve years of age extended to girls of fourteen—would yet be accomplished ; and that the assaulting of such little ones would be an offence against the law without any question of consent. He felt very strongly the necessity for further protection for girls of tender years ; and it was quite absurd to suppose that a law which applied to girls of twelve should not apply to girls of fourteen, as girls were children up to fully the age of fourteen."

I find, among the reports of medical officers filed by the Nizamut, a case, by Dr. O'Dwyer, of Chittagong, which appears to have a very

* Nizamut Adawlut Reports, February 25, 1857, p. 209.

important bearing upon this question. Here, the body of a child was found submerged in a tank, with a laceration throughout the entire length of the vagina, sufficient, in itself, to cause death; but the medical witness believed *that the body had been thrown into the water before life was extinct; he found some swelling about the neck, and he believed the child to have been strangled.* The case admits of doubt, still it is probable that this girl, having been accidentally injured, was at once put out of the way.

A rather similar crime was committed in the neighbouring district of Dacca. A Hindu had been married about four years to a girl not arrived at the age of puberty, but she continued to reside at her father's house, until just before the fatal event, when the prisoner conveyed her to his own house. He stated that she repeatedly refused to yield to his wishes; that he seized her by the shoulders, and accomplished his purpose by force. On getting up, he found that she was dead. Being frightened at the consequences, he carried the body into the cow-shed, and, tying a rope round the neck, suspended the body to the roof, with the hope of making it appear that she had committed suicide. This was denied by the evidence of his family, and marks of hanging were not discovered. In the mofussil evidence, rupture of the upper and lower vagina are alluded to, but this was not confirmed in the Civil Surgeon's evidence. The only external marks found on the body were the swollen state of the features and face, and the oozing of blood from the ears and nose; and these marks, coupled with the history of the case, served to confirm the medical officer in the opinion that the girl had been smothered or suffocated as by violent pressure, such as the weight of the man's body upon her, and stopping her mouth to prevent her screaming (prisoner was charged, in the indictment, with binding clothes over her mouth).—Sentence, imprisonment for ten years with labor in irons.*

It appeared, in a trial at Jessore, that a Hindu confessed that he had strangled a young girl to whom he was married, who was unwilling to remain with him, and who had refused to sleep with him. He afterwards suspended the body by the neck, trying to make it appear that she had destroyed herself. The darogah stated that marks of strangulation and of injury to the pudenda were apparent. The native doctor deposed that there were marks of a rope round the neck, and the appearance of a stick having been forced into the private parts. The Judge of the superior Court considered that there was strong presumption that the prisoner had used the girl in a cruel and brutal manner before he took her life.†

While we have valid grounds for believing that, in some of these cases,

---

* Nizamut Adawlut Reports, January, March, 1858, p. 5.

† *Ibid*, 31st July 1854, p. 158.

a predisposition to rupture of the immature parts is induced by previous mechanical dilatation, and that, in others, rupture is caused by unnatural mechanical force employed at the time, it is only due to those who labor under such accusation to admit that serious injury may be sustained, even by adult females, in the first act. Mr. Spencer Wells relates* the case of a woman *aged twenty-six,* who had been a servant, and had "*always enjoyed good health until her marriage.*" She suffered great pain at the consummation of marriage, and bled a great deal. On the second night she suffered still more. Considerable swelling of the labia came on, and she had great pain and a sensation of weight and dragging in the perineum. After a day or two, she began to notice that some of the fœces passed by the vagina. Latterly the whole of the fœcal matter passed by the vagina, none by the anus. At first, her account was doubted, and it was thought that she had sustained this injury in a previous delivery. It is enough to say that this question was fully investigated, and clearly decided in the negative by positive anatomical evidence. It at first appeared "that the whole recto-vaginal septum had been torn away, but closer examination showed that it had merely been pushed upwards, that portion corresponding to the posterior segment of the hymen having been torn through." She was completely cured by operation.†

It is to be feared that the existence of a severe law, while it may possibly act as a restraint upon the brutality of some men, in other instances leads to the commission of murder ; or to the concealment, until too late, of serious injuries, where, otherwise, timely assistance might be sought for and obtained.

In the following cases *the nature and extent of the injuries are clearly described.* In a case tried at Tipperah, where a "robust young man" was convicted of Rape "on a very intelligent child eight or nine years of age," the child "was found by the neighbours in a very exhausted state, and with her clothes saturated with blood." The girl, answering satisfactorily the questions put to her by the Sessions Judge relative to the binding nature of a solemn affirmation, was examined, and described the violence done her very clearly. From her account the act would appear to have been completed.

The medical officer, Mr. Davis, described the parts of generation as

---

* Med. Times and Gazette, January 21, 1860, p. 61.

† The following case of *Spontaneous Rupture of the Vagina,* which must be almost unique, has been cited in the New York *Medical Record,* December 1st, 1868, p. 440:—Dr. M. A. Pullen brought a case of rupture of the vagina before the St. Louis Medical Society. It had been supposed to be uterine hæmorrhage which the use of the tampon had arrested. Upon examination with a speculum, it was found that the hæmorrhage had resulted from a rupture in the wall of the vagina, extending from the right side, near the os uteri, into the posterior cul-de-sac. The lady attributed the accident to a sudden effect, while much excited, in lifting her infant, which had received a serious fall. He proposed keeping the adges of the rent in apposition by the introduction of sutures.

injured to the following extent, but it is to be observed that he examined the child some days after the occurrence took place. He said that the internal right labium bore marks of injury, and that there was a recently-healed laceration at the posterior part of the vagina. He doubted, however, whether the act, to the attempt to commit which these injuries were probably attributable, had been completed, as the generative organs were in an undeveloped state."*

Bhella Gazi, of Tipperah, was convicted of culpable homicide for having caused the death of his wife, an immature girl probably eleven years old. The husband was a robust man twenty years of age. Although they had been married two or three years, no cohabitation, using the term as descriptive of the connexion between man and wife, had taken place up to the fatal night. She was proved to have been the subject of such serious chronic disease of the lungs, stomach, and intestines that she must have shortly died. On the night in question, her mother-in-law and aunt are stated to have insisted upon her sleeping with her husband. Towards midnight, after screaming loudly, she rushed forth into the courtyard, where she fell prostrate. Her clothes and person were deeply stained with blood, and she was in a state of complete exhaustion. She was taken to her mother's house, where she died on the sixth day, having been unable to utter a word. After mentioning the internal disease alluded to above, Baboo Ramkinnoo Dutt, the medical officer, stated that, "on examining the internal organs of generation, he found the vagina freely open from its orifice to the neck of the uterus, two inches and-a-half in depth." [length ?] "The mucous membrane of the inner surface of that part, close to the neck of the uterus, was very much excoriated, ulcerated, and inflamed, which state of things must have created severe gnawing pains and much irritation. These injuries I consider to have been caused either by forcible penetration by a piece of wood or iron, or by immoderate" [by this expression the Judge of the Court and Nizamut Adawlut understood 'excessive violence in the act,' which, doubtless, was the Baboo's meaning] "intercourse for which the deceased was not yet fit." From the above appearances, I infer that the deceased had a severe attack of diarrhœa complicated with inflammation of the lungs. She also suffered from forcible cohabitation, which, together with the above maladies, caused her death.†

Mr. W. Colles, then of Pubna, has related‡ the case of a girl, apparently about eight years old, who said that, on the previous day, a man had forcible connexion with her, causing her most intolerable pain and much loss of blood. There were no marks of violence externally, but the orifice of the vagina was lacerated in its entire circumference, and the

* Nizamut Adawlut Reports, May 4, 1855, p. 509.
† *Ibid*, June 5, 1868, p. 223.
‡ Med. Times and Gazette, June 2, 1860, p. 560.

perineum was nearly torn through. Symptoms of general peritonitis set in, and she died on the seventh day. ***Post-mortem examination.***—On placing the left hand beneath the uterus, and gently passing the blunt end of a paper-cutter into the vagina from without, the paper-cutter reached the hand within the pelvis without meeting the slightest impediment. Hence fatal peritonitis. The entire track of the vagina was in a state of gangrene. Its posterior wall had been torn through, at its line of junction with the uterus, to the extent of an inch, and the edges of the rent were thin and jagged. The culprit, to all appearance a feeble emaciated man of twenty-three, confessed his guilt.

Mr. Hinder, of the Native Hospital, Calcutta, gives* the case of a Mussalmaun girl, of delicate appearance, about eleven years of age, whom he treated with success for a recto-vaginal fistula, about an inch long, said to be the result of forcible sexual intercourse.

A difficult and complicated case, in which the issue bore upon the nature and extent of the injury sustained by the pudenda, was tried in 1864. The ruling was : " ***Held*** to be improbable, and physically impossible, that a girl of tender age should be killed by any violence in Rape, and not show any external signs of violence." Queen *v.* Banee Madhub Mookerjee, 1 W. R., Cr., 29 ; Cowell and Woodman, p. 640.

It was held by the Judicial Commissioner that a girl, fourteen years old, had been enticed away for the prisoner's purposes ; that he had sexual intercourse with her; and that she died of the effects of that intercourse a few hours afterwards. Two midwives stated that the girl had her loins broken from having had connexion with a man, but a third declared that she had died from cholera. Cholera was raging in the village at that time, and many people were dying of it daily. Several witnesses stated that, at the time of her death, she was evacuating and vomiting. The same witnesses say that there was no blood upon her clothes, which were admitted to be the same as those she had on when she went the evening before. The Judge of the Appellate High Court inferred from the evidence that she was speechless from first to last. The following are the Judge's remarks upon the medical evidence, which it appears was given by a native apothecary (a class who, at that time, were not taught Medical Jurisprudence in College). " The native doctor who examined the corpse found the entrance to the vagina torn open, and a quantity of blood extravasated in the pelvis. He found also extensive inflammation of the intestines and kidneys. He considered that death had resulted from the girl's having had connexion with a man before arriving at puberty. Now I am naturally unwilling to interfere in a matter of medical testimony, but the native dector's evidence appears to me not only improbable, but actually incredible. All our medical jurisprudence books,

* Ind. Med. Gaz., June 1, 1866, p. 156.

Taylor, Chevers, and others, agree on this point, that, when a Rape is committed on a child of tender age, the most palpable outward signs of the offence remain. Had Acharjia been treated as she is said to have stated, her private parts would have been inflamed and wounded, and her clothes (the same, be it remembered, as those in which she was carried off) must have been bloody and otherwise stained; for a young girl not arrived at the age of puberty to have been raped, and not to show any external signs of it, is a physical impossibility. Again, it is admitted that the injuries found by the native doctor might have been caused by a fall. It is admitted, moreover (and this is a very important point), that they might have been caused by the midwives' own examination, which is made with the hands. My own opinion is that they were so caused, and that the thrusting the hand into the person of a young immature child was quite sufficient to account for the rupture of the entrance of the vagina. In any case, I entirely disbelieve that they were caused by a man having had connexion with her. The medical evidence shows that the girl had inflammation of the intestines and diarrhœa ; it is proved that cholera was raging ; it is proved also that, at the time of death, Acharjia was evacuating and vomiting. Taking all this evidence into consideration, I hold this to have been the cause of her death (for the injury to the womb, however caused, could not have killed her in less than twelve hours), and the charge against the prisoner is altogether false."

The papers having been laid before another Judge, the opinion of that authority on the medical evidence was as follows : "The medical testimony of the native apothecary is very unsatisfactory, and throws much doubt and uncertainty on the cause of the death of the girl. The girl was fourteen years old (see evidence of her guardian, Musst. Bowdee) ; native girls are mothers at eleven years. The Judicial Commissioner infers that the girl consented to have sexual intercourse with the prisoner. Under such circumstances, it is highly improbable that the girl should be killed by any violence used by the prisoner in the act of coition, and yet that the pudenda should have no marks of violence ; but such is the statement of the native apothecary. I cannot believe that the prisoner had connexion with the deceased, who, in my opinion, died a natural death. The injury to the womb noticed by the native apothecary may have been caused, as admitted by him in his examination, by the manual examination of the native midwives, who appear, with an exception, to have played into the hands of the Inspector. I fully concur in acquitting the prisoner."

Unfortunately, the medical evidence of the native apothecary is not given in full in the report which I cite. I here give all that the *Weekly Reporter* gives. We have, in this report, no allusion by him to that "injury to the womb" of which both of the Judges speak. The Judges strongly insist that a child of tender age cannot be killed in rape without "marks of violence on the pudenda" or "external signs of violence." The native apothecary is not shown to have asserted that there were no external marks of violence, but a much better surgeon did so in a very similar case. See Colles's case, p. 697. The narrator, a very able authority, says, "on examining the genital organs, *I observed no marks of violence externally*; but on separating the labia, the orifice of the vagina was seen lacerated in its entire circumference, and the perineum was nearly torn through." In a plain way, the native apothecary described a state of parts which appears to have very nearly resembled that in Colles's case. He says that he found the entrance to the vagina torn open, *i. e.*, there was rupture of the perineum; and a quantity of blood extravasated in the pelvis. The private parts would not have been found "inflamed" in a case where death occurred speedily from hæmorrhage, as it quite possibly did in this case, and as it certainly did in the Nyhatty case given below in this page.

I do not deny that there must generally be, in immature children raped to death, rupture of the perineum; but it seems possible that this may be absent where mechanical dilatation has previously been employed, in which case the posterior wall of the vagina might be torn to a fatal extent.

Many other cases of fatal injury, thus received, are on record.

In 1849, a man of Sylhet was sentenced to two years' imprisonment for causing the death of his wife, a child of tender years, by forcibly having connexion with her.*

The *Englishman* of the 28th May 1857 notices the case of a man named Nughoon, who was made over to the Sessions, Dinagepore, for occasioning the death of his wife, aged eight or nine, by making a forcible attempt on her person. Death resulted from the consequent hæmorrhage.

In 1866, one Bissorunjun Mookerjee absconded after committing a Rape on a young girl at Nyhatty, "who died within an hour afterwards."†

In 1868, a Nowacolly man had forcible sexual connexion with his wife, who was only eleven years old, and killed her in the act.‡ In the same year, a man of Hooghly caused the death of his wife, a little girl between nine and ten years of age, by having forcible connexion with her.§

Again, in the same year, the dead body of a girl was found in a lake in the Monghyr district. It was ascertained that she had been enticed away by the accused to a lonely place, where, in his endeavour to rape her, he used her so roughly that she died.‖

Several natives have been prosecuted for ***Rape upon their Wives, where the latter have been under ten years of age.***

The following appeared in the Bengal *Hurkaru* of March 1st, 1862 :—

* Police Rep., L., P., for the above year, p. 35.

† Bengal Police Rep., for 1866, p. 5.

‡ *Ibid*, for 1868, p. 66.

§ *Ibid*, p. 230.

‖ *Ibid*, p. 133. So frequent is this result of the crime in question in India that it is held that "the dying declaration of a deceased person is admissible in evidence in a charge of Rape"—Queen *v.* Bissorunjun Mookerjee, 6 W. R., Cr., 72; Cowell and Woodman, p. 274.

"A native girl under ten years of age charged her husband, before the Calcutta Police, with Rape, stating that she was living with her parents, but that her husband and a woman entered into a house where the offence was committed, by giving her some sweetmeats drugged for the purpose."

I have also a note that Kallah Kahar was to be tried at the Calcutta Criminal Sessions in March 1861, for a Rape on his own wife, a child under ten.

In 1859, the subject of Rape on Children was very fully reviewed in a discussion, the leaders of which were Sir W. Wilde and Mr. Kesteven (Taylor, pp. 994-5-6). One of the main questions raised was *whether rupture of the perineum can or cannot be effected in Rape on a child.* The prevailing opinion appears to have been that such injury could not be so caused. Mr. Kesteven wrote: "I cannot believe that a sufficiently persistent and rigid erection of the penis could be maintained long enough for the commission of such injury, in spite of the resistance of a child of ten years of age." Dr. Taylor holds (p. 995) that facts which he has recorded show that this opinion is erroneous. I do not think that, practically and legally, this question is one of much importance. The medical witness finds injuries, and declares that they are the result of mechanical force. The law holds that *penetration* is Rape. Recorded facts prove that criminals have, with such intent, used extraneous force as by the fingers, by a stick, and even by a hot iron. Having thus atrociously facilitated their purpose, we have every reason to believe that the act has been *completed* according to the legal definition. It can signify little (except as adding to the guilt of the prisoner where extensive laceration has been inflicted) by what precise mechanical means the act has been effected.

Such injuries being present, it will not generally be incumbent upon the medical man to decide whether they were inflicted by the accused or by some miscreant who has been employed in trumping up the case. In noticing the facts on this point, which I gave in my last edition, Sir W. Wilde mentions* that an Army Medical Officer, long resident in India, informed him that he detected the following imposture: "A procuress brought a girl into the Officers' Barracks, Fort William, Calcutta; but the person to whom she was presented, objected to the girl on account of her youth. The bawd, having been disappointed of her fee, in revenge, injured the child, so as to cause very considerable hæmorrhage from the genital organs. The girl was seen by an Assistant Surgeon in the Fort, and the circumstances of the case having been reported to the police authorities, it was discovered to be a conspiracy against the officer to obtain money. The old wretch was severely punished, and the child soon recovered."

---

* Medical Times and Gazette, May 21, 1859, p. 519.

The question of the power of a man, when unaided, to commit Rape upon a healthy woman in her full senses, has always been a difficulty with Medical Jurists. It is discussed, at page 1009, by Dr. Taylor, who appears to incline to the opinion that "inability to resist from terror, or from an overpowering feeling of helplessness, as well as horror at her situation, may lead a woman to succumb, without offering that degree of resistance which is generally expected from a woman so situated."

A stout built Kyeng (hill-man), of Arracan, met two women on a lonely road; producing a small knife, he desired them to accompany him into the jungle. After going some distance, he told one of them to stop. The other, a married woman thirty years of age, the mother of seven children, ran off and hid herself, but was discovered by the prisoner, who, seizing her by the hair of the head, bore her off to the bank of a small stream, and there had forcible connexion with her. After accomplishing his purpose, prisoner again threatened her with his knife, and ran off with part of her garment, and some bundles of false hair. His confession before the Magistrate "was complete." Sentence—five years' imprisonment with labor in irons.*

Kunah Sheikh, of Gowalparah, Assam, lay in wait for a woman on the road, dragged her into the jungle, and effected his purpose. Three witnesses deposed that, having heard the prosecutrix calling out that the prisoner was taking her caste, and going to the spot, two of them saw the woman in a nearly naked state, and the prisoner running off. She had all the appearance of having been assaulted, but they cannot say whether the Rape was perpetrated. Sentence—seven years' imprisonment with labor in irons.†

Fadil Gazee, of Jessore, a tall and powerful man, seeing a married girl of sixteen standing at her door, accosted her, apparently under the pretence of asking for a *soot nullee*, and wished to worm out of her if she was alone; finding that she was, he put his arms round her, forcibly drew her into the house, flung her down, and, gagging her mouth with her right hand, effected a criminal connexion with her. Before her mouth was well gagged, she managed to yell out for assistance, and her cries brought her mother and a neighbour, who found him in the act. He then got up, hastily offered to give her a rupee if she would say nothing more of the matter, and ran off. Two other neighbours heard her cries, saw him make off, and found her in much distress. The matter was reported at the Thannah the following morning. Sentence as in the previous case.‡

It was proved, in a trial at Tipperah, that one Pauchcowri, a Hindu, assisted by three Mussalmauns, waylaid and committed a Rape upon

---

* Nizamut Adawlut Reports, February 1, 1855, p. 145.

† *Ibid*, September 26, 1855, p. 441.

‡ *Ibid*, August 2, 1856, p. 164.

the wife of a Hindu fisherman. The committing officer reported that the fisher class are regarded superciliously in the neighbourhood of Noacolly, and the women are frequently the subject of impertinence which would not be ventured on in instances of females of a better caste. He added, "The idea that the Rape of a fisherwoman is a less heinous offence than the Rape of [a woman of] any other caste is erroneous." The Sessions Judge remarked, "I am certainly disposed to regard her as a decent and modest woman." . . . "The circumstances of her humble position in life, and liability to insult consequent on her carrying fish to market for sale, strengthen rather than lessen her title to protection." "It is an undoubted fact, in this part of the country at least, that the wives of men of low caste, and following pursuits calling them much from home, such as beggars, fishermen, and others, are regarded as fair subjects for insult, and are the general victims in cases of violation."*

This case displays the working of the old leaven of the caste system, under which the Brahmins were subject only to the most moderate punishments, and the common people were treated with less consideration than the beasts of the field. Thus while, generally, the ancient Hindu law visited the crime of adultery with the heaviest penalties, it was ordained that a Brahmin guilty of the crime "shall not be deprived of life, but the hair of his head shall be cut off" (Halhed, p. 274). Again, "if a man commits adultery with an unmarried girl of inferior caste, If it was done by violence, the Magistrate shall take a small fine from him" (*Ibid*, p. 277).

According to the Mahomedan law, a man's confession of *Whoredom with a Lunatic Woman*, subjected him to *Hudd*. A remarkable trial, upon a question of this kind, occurred in Ohio, U. S., in 1853. In the sixth section of the Act for the punishment of crimes, *Curren's Revised Statutes*, p. 184, it is provided that "if any male person, seventeen years old and upward, shall have carnal knowledge of any woman, other than his wife, such woman being *Insane*, he knowing her to be such, every person so offending shall be deemed guilty of a misdemeanor; and, upon conviction thereof, shall be imprisoned in the penitentiary, and kept at hard labor not more than ten, or less than three, years." In this case it was held, for the defendant, that the female, *being an Idiot, had no will*; and, therefore, that *a Rape could not be committed on her person against her will.* It was further claimed that the word "Insane" did not include the Idiotic; and hence that the defendant could be convicted of neither of the charges embraced in the indictment. Mr. Justice Nash ruled that a female Idiot, or an Insane female, is the subject of Rape; and hence, of an assault with the intent to commit that crime; and that a male person, of a proper age, who shall have carnal knowledge of a female

* Nizamut Adawlut Reports, June 9, 1858, p. 227.

Idiot, knowing her to be such, is guilty, under the sixth Section, of having carnal knowledge of an Insane woman, knowing her to be such.*

The Indian law fully meets this difficulty. In regard to Rape it rejects the expression "against her will," and substitutes for it the phrase "without her consent." Section 90, I. P. C., rules that "a consent is not such a consent as is intended by any section of this Code." . . . . "If the consent is given by a person who, from unsoundness of mind, or intoxication, is unable to understand the nature and consequence of that to which he gives his consent; or, unless the contrary appears from the context, if the consent is given by a person who is under twelve years of age."

A very full commentary upon the bearing which this clause of the Indian law has upon cases of Rape upon Idiotic women is given by Mr. John Mayne, at pp. 60 and 241, Fifth Edition of his Commentaries on the Indian Penal Code.

Question of Virginity.

In a few instances, the medical officer may be called upon to decide whether a female is or is not a virgin. When at Chittagong, I was consulted in a case of this kind. A slave or lower servant in a Mussalmaun's family had disappeared. It was suspected that the missing man had intrigued with his master's daughter, and had been made away with by her friends. I was, therefore, called upon to state whether this woman (apparently about twenty years of age) had been accustomed to intercourse. I found the vagina remarkably narrow,† but there was no hymen. I reported that the woman's person did not present the chief sign of virginity, but that the absence of this might have been consequent upon disease, or many other causes apart from sexual intercourse. I was, however, decidedly of opinion that she had not been habituated to sexual intercourse.‡

Rape by Females on Males.§

In 1864, Mr. Gaffney, then House-Surgeon to the Calcutta Medical College Hospital, gave me the following note: A Hindu, aged *nine*, brought to hospital suffering from gonorrhœa, paraphymosis, and retention of urine. On being questioned, he stated that he contracted the gonorrhœa by urinating in the same place with a man who was diseased; under coercion he confessed that he got it in the usual manner, having been led into evil society by a boy a little older than himself.

In May 1870, Mr. Edwin Sanders, now House-Surgeon to this Hospital, pointed out to me, in his dispensary, a Caubul man, who appeared to be

---

* American Journal of Medical Science, April 1854, p. 532.

† Native women are very much in the habit of employing local astringents.

‡ See a remarkable case involving the question of virginity in a native woman of Bombay.—Taylor, p. 1003.

§ *Vide* Taylor, p. 1017.

in a very wretched state of mind, believing that he was the subject of syphilis, thus contracted, at the age of *two!*

Dr. S. Coull Mackenzie, the predecessor of the above-named gentlemen, treated a case of syphilitic phymosis in a Mussalmaun boy of *ten*, who was with difficulty brought to confess, at the hospital, that a servant had taken him to a prostitute's house in the bazar, where he had connexion with a woman.

Dr. Mackenzie informs me that Dr. Maclagan mentions, in his lectures, that debauched women have an idea that they can rid themselves of venereal disease by having connexion with a child. Mr. Gaffney also tells me that, in Ireland, there is an idea that a woman is cured of gonorrhœa by connexion with a chaste person of the other sex: to ensure this, a child is usually the victim. He has seen a case of syphilis, in a boy of *nine*, supposed to have been so contracted.

A case which appears to partake of this character was tried at Chota Nagpore in 1855.

Dwarkanath Rowanee at once confessed, apparently without having had time for reflection, that his little son came to him crying, and said "that person" had come to the house. About three days previously, his son had told him that one Nowan frequented the house. He found Nowan and his wife in the act of adultery, and killed them both with an axe. Nowan's grandfather and other witnesses stated that he was about twelve or thirteen years of age, and incapable of sexual intercourse. In the *sooruthal* he is stated to have been thirteen to fourteen.*

UNNATURAL CRIME.

The works of the older travellers nearly all contain reference to the enormous prevalence of this crime among the "Moors" of India.†

A section of the chapter on Adultery in Halhed's Hindu Law (p. 280) relates to "the carnal conjunction of a man with any beast." Reference is made by Ward to other similar Hindu laws. "If any person have unnatural connexion with a cow, he must repeat the *prajapatya* atonement (a fast commutable by a fine)" (Vol. III., p. 153). Sodomy also called for an atonmeent. The Hindu mythology attributes this crime to some of their deities. Thus the father of Rishyu Shringu cohabited with a deer, and his son had deer's horns‡—a crime much imputed, at least formerly, to Fakeers professing celibacy. Linschoten says: "The men of Pegue, Aua, Iangoma, and Brama weare balls in their yards, which they put in, the skinne being cut, and weare for every child one, till they have three

* Nizamut Adawlut Reports, February 8, 1855, p. 171.

† See Tavernier's Voyage, English Translation of 1678, p. 54; Fryer's New Account of East India and Persia, 1698, p. 97; and Wilcocke's Translation of Staverinus's Voyages, 1798, Vol. I., p. 456.

‡ Ward, 3rd Edition, Vol. II., p. 179.

and may take them out at pleasure: the least as bigge as any wallnut: the biggest as bigge as a little henne's egge. They were invented to prevent Sodomie, which they use more than any people in the world. Abusing the male sexe, causeth the women also to weare scant clothes, that, as they goe, their thigh is seene bare, to provoke men to lust."*

It is stated that this crime is held in light estimation by the Seikhs. Dr. S. Coull Mackenzie informs me that he has learnt that, in the Punjaub, men suffering from gonorrhœa consider that unnatural connexion with a goat is a cure. The same gentleman was informed by an officer, who was with the Nepaul Field Force in the Mutiny, that many ponies had to be killed, the Goorkahs being addicted to that vice.

Sodomy by a Hindu, N. A. R., October 4, 1855, p. 560.

A remarkable case occurred in Benares, in which it appeared that a Hindu lad, having formed an infamous connexion with a Mussalmaun of notorious character, his parents tried every means to induce him to give it up; and, when all other effects had failed, had arsenic administered to the whole of the Mussalmaun's family. Two persons died in consequence, but he against whom the plot was formed, escaped.†

Dr. Clemenger told me, ten years ago, that, in Lahore, the catamites may be at once distinguished in the streets, by their sallow countenances and lustreless eyes. They generally walk in pairs, hand in hand, swinging their arms. I suggested that this aspect of countenance might be the effect of intemperance in liquor or of the use of bhang or opium. He considered that it was clearly distinguishable from the traces which are left by these habits.

Stavorinus mentions some revolting and probably exaggerated instances of the commission of this crime with the Lower Animals, by Mussalmauns. The same iniquity is alluded to by Terry. It cannot be doubted that such atrocities are frequent in the present day. A gentleman of the highest veracity assured me that a late Judge of Hooghly once mentioned to him that, when about to sentence a native to imprisonment on proof of his having committed this crime *in corpore capellæ,* he intimated his decision to the native jury, who hinted that, if so much severity was to be employed against so prevalent a crime, the prisons of Bengal would not be large enough to hold the culprits. Convictions for this crime are however rare; I only find one case in the Records—of Unnatural Crime with a Cow—at Dinagepore.‡

A writer in the Calcutta Review§ states that there were, in 1855, in Lucknow, at least a hundred houses of ill-fame, registered and taxed, which are tenanted by *Men* only. I have clearly cited a statement, made by the translator of the Seir Mutaqherin in 1789, to the effect that there was then

* Purchas, Vol. V., p. 503.

† Nizamut Adawlut Reports (N. W. P.), May 12, 1853.

‡ Police Report, L. P., 1845, p. 23.

§ For September 1855, p. 128.

a street in Lucknow wholly occupied by eunuchs practising this crime. There cannot be a doubt that, previous to its occupation by our Government, male and female children were stolen from every part of India to meet the atrocious demands of that modern Sodom.

Facts came to light in 1852, which prove that there exists, Up-country, a very extensive and abominable trade of unnatural prostitution regularly carried on by eunuchs. Dr. Ebden's paper, already referred to (p. 496), will show how extensively this moral pest has spread in the States of Rajpootana; and a case, tried at Mynpoorie in 1852,—in which one Ali Buksh, quarrelling with an eunuch named Bhoorah, who had lived with him as a prostitute for nearly two years, nearly severed the unfortunate wretch's head from his body,—led to the exposure of the practices of a class of eunuchs, dressed as women, whom they are said to resemble also in shape, who are believed to have vested rights to contributions at weddings, &c., in certain villages allotted to one or more of them under a sort of acknowledged internal government. They have, in fact, a King, according to some, resident at Delhi; others say at Furruckabad.* I have already cited (p. 496) some important documents relative to this case given me by my friend Dr. Hugh Macpherson. From these I have collected the following particulars. Out of the one hundred eunuchs then in the Mynpoory District, fifteen confessed to the Acting Joint Magistrate that they either had been, or were then, guilty of Sodomy. Their Vuzeer stated that there were, at that time, about two or three hundred thousand of these people in the Company's dominions in Hindustan, and also a large body in Bombay. These people never live alone, but in general form a party of five or six living in one house, presided over by the eldest eunuch, whom they call their "Gooroo," who receives part of their earnings, which they profess to obtain by dancing and singing at births and marriages. Dr. Macpherson gave it as his opinion that prostitution of the body in Sodomy, for several years before or about the period of puberty, would unquestionably cause impotence. The native doctors both said that such is the effect notoriously produced by it, and that the wretched creatures who are reduced to this state in their boyhood are, at last, anxious to get rid of the external signs of that manhood which they have forfeited. He adds that native doctor Hingun Khan called his attention to a peculiar effeminacy in the voice of a still unmutilated man who was sent to him for examination, and who had gone to the house of Bhoorah that he might undergo mutilation;—this state of the voice being characteristic of people of such degraded habits, and by which he could at any time readily recognise them. It is well known (*khoola—open*) to every class of natives that almost all, if not all eunuchs, who have female attire and dance at nautches, habitually prostitute them-

* Nizamut Adawlut Reports (N. W. P.), 6th November 1852, p. 1314.

selves unnaturally; and that, wherever there is a house containing nautching eunuchs, the inmates are as avowedly prostitutes as are the public women in any bazar. The native doctor directed Dr. Macpherson's notice to the important difference between the "*Khojas*" (eunuchs employed to guard zenanas, and others who, though equally mutilated, and this always as children or in their boyhood, invariably wear men's clothes, and live a reproachless life), and the "Hijeras," who form the subject of the present observations.

It is to be feared that, especially in the larger Mahomedan towns, Up-country, these practices are so common as scarcely to be regarded as criminal by the ignorant. Thus we find two prisoners, convicted of the crime on their own confession, relying upon the plea that "it was their Occupation."* Again, a wretch who was tried at Delhi pleaded guilty to the charge, evidently apprehending that the penalty of the law can only be incurred when the crime is accompanied by violence. He thought to exculpate himself by averring that the boy, aged thirteen, submitted willingly, in consideration of a payment of five annas. He further urged, in his defence, that this was not the first time he had committed this crime with the same boy.†

Dr. J. Wilson Johnstone, writing from Loodiana, gives an important note of the *Physical Evidences of Sodomy*,‡ which he speaks of as being rife in the large cities of India and common in the State jails. (Only two cases came to my notice during twenty-five months in which I officiated as Inspector-General of Jails, Bengal.) From considerable experience Dr. Johnstone has come to rely exclusively upon diagnosis as afforded by the condition of the mucous membrane. Penetration seldom reaches beyond an inch, and the force expends itself on the semi-lunar folds which, in the empty gut, droop on either side. One arc of the lower anal mucous fold occupies the superior and upper left, a second the inferior lower and right angle of the rectum, and hangs down in a central crescent; the foreign agent impinges against this loose centre, stretches its point of attachment at one or other of the angles, and, in every case of clear penetrative contact (provided the gut has not been distended by polypi, as is not unfrequent in children, or by systematic sodomy when the mucous membrane loses its *rugæ* and the sphincters their contractible power), rupture will be found cutting horizontally onwards, at the left superior or right inferior angle. He has never observed any other portion of the mucous membrane ruptured by a specific act of sodomy. The shape of the wound is characteristic, and it cannot be produced by any *hard* substance. A true sodomy wound is triangular; the base external, with the sides of the triangle retreating into the fundament. Wounds wilfully

* Nizamut Adawlut Reports, Vol. II., p. 49.

† *Ibid*, 15th September, p. 1158.

‡ Indian Medical Gazette, August 1st, 1866, p. 213.

made will be found on the upper and lower surfaces, not on the angles; generally, on the upper and right aspect of the rectal mucous membrane, evidently made by the left hand, and of a notchy, patchy character. (It is noteworthy that about 70 per cent. of Punjaubees, so far as Dr. Johnstone has noticed, are left-handed in minor operations, and it is often useful, in elucidating evidence, to hand the prisoner a needle to thread.) He does not enter into specific proof, as rectal chancre and condylomata, but adds that over 50 per cent. of our prisoners, if narrowly examined, would be found diseased. For an opinion given in a case of alleged Sodomy, see Appendix F.

Ancient Laws.

By the ancient Mahomedan law, the justification of homicide by the party upon whom this crime is attempted is expressly stated, in the Nukshbundeeyah and Humadeeyah, as follows: "A man uses force to commit Sodomy on a boy (*umrud*, literally a beardless youth), who is unable to resist and prevent him, except by killing him.—The homicide in this case is justifiable." Cases are mentioned by Stavorinus and Fryer, where the victims courageously took the lives of their assailants; their conduct brought them the commendation and protection of the public. In the older writers, the crime of Bestiality is specified, as between a man and a quadruped, or a woman and an ape. By two authorities, the discretion of the Cazee, in punishing, for determent, the offences of Bestiality and Sodomy, is stated to extend to death, by ordering the offender to be burnt, or thrown from a high place, or by causing a wall to fall upon him. Scourging or confining in a place of bad odour are also cited as authorized modes of punishment; which castration and excision are declared not to be. Some authorities held that Sodomy should meet the same specific punishment as whoredom, and Shafiee's opinion was that, in pursuance of a tradition from the prophet, both parties should suffer death. In the Tubeen, the perpetration of this crime, with a man's own wife, or with a female slave, is declared liable to *Tazeer*.*

Sodomy was included under the general head of "Zena," or whoredom: and, to constitute legal proof of a crime of this nature, it required the evidence of four respectable male witnesses, or the confession of the guilty person four times repeated before the Cazee, he (the Cazee) declining to receive the confession, and sending the confessing person away the first, second, and third time! (Macnaghten's Reports, Vol. I., p. 382). The punishment for such atrocity appears, however, to have been sufficiently provided for in Regulation XVII of 1817.†

---

* Op. Citat, pp. 256-326.

† The following notes convey nearly all the points involved in the trials recorded in the Reports of the Courts of Bengal and the N. W. P., that can be of importance in a medico-legal point of view. Upon a boy of ten; the injuries threatened life; Macnaghten, Vol. I., 234.

Existing Law.

See Indian Penal Code, Chapter XVI., Section 377, Explan.; and Mayne's Commentary, 5th edition, pages 243, 255, and 257.

PREGNANCY.*

In cases where females are sentenced to death in India, it appears to be customary to call for the opinion of the Civil Surgeon as to whether they are "Quick with Child," or not—apart from any plea of Pregnancy. In native women, the change of color in the areolæ of the breasts, and the appearance of the brown line from the pubes to the umbilicus, described as characteristic of pregnancy by Dr. Montgomery (but only regarded, in the present day, as "minor signs"), cannot, of course, be looked for.

Dr. Graily Hewitt says that *perfect* evidence of Pregnancy is not obtainable until after the third month, unless in those very rare cases where the fœtal heart may be heard just at the end of this time. The

---

The prosecutor, a man aged twenty-one, of good constitution, alleged violence against the prisoner, an old man above sixty-five. Acquittal.—Vol. I. of 1851, p. 1599. A child of five. Seventeen days were lost before the Civil Surgeon saw the child; he could only depose to cicatrization externally, and to some inflammation within; but considered that some forcible penetration must have occurred to produce these appearances.—Reports of N. W. P., Vol. I., p. 444; *Idem*, p. 465. A boy of twelve accused of forcibly committing the offence upon one two years his senior; a medical opinion not taken. Acquittal.—*Idem*, p. 558. One Khurukgir, of Bareilly, made a report at the thannah, that four persons named had forcibly committed Sodomy on his person. Upon examining the informer, the Civil Surgeon reported that "no recent injury had been received by him, but that there were signs of old-standing injury on his person, which could be relied on, as showing that he was addicted to the practice of Sodomy." The superior Court convicted three of the assailants, and acquitted their accuser.—Nizamut Adawlut Reports, N. W. P., 5th February, 1851, p. 178. On a child of three or four years. Injury alleged; a Surgeon's opinion not given.—Nizamut Adawlut Reports, Vol. IV. of 1853, p. 27.

* The practice of assembling Juries of Matrons was long prevalent in India. In the case of Peggy, in Calcutta, in 1777, it was decided by the Court that, as a Christian, the woman was entitled to a jury of Christian women. They returned their verdict that she was not with child, and she was accordingly executed (Morton's Reports, p. 260). This irrational practice came to a termination upon the case of Mukawa in 1836 (Bellasis' Reports, p. 113). This woman, having been sentenced to death, was declared by a jury of matrons (natives) to be in the fifth month of her pregnancy. This report induced the Bombay Adawlut to obtain a commutation of her sentence to one of imprisonment for life. Nine months passed; the Civil Surgeon reported that "the prisoner Mukowa was not pregnant, and that the appearances which might have led to a contrary belief were caused by excessive obesity of the abdomen." Hence arose the question whether it was not competent to the Right Hon'ble the Governor in Council to cancel the commuted sentence of imprisonment for life and revert to the original sentence of death. This point was, of course, ruled in the negative, and the Court decided that, in future, such examination should be entrusted to a medical officer of skill and experience; and that, whenever a capital sentence shall be passed upon a woman in a state of pregnancy, the execution of the same shall be deferred until forty days after her delivery.

evidence obtainable before this date only enables us to conclude that Pregnancy is ***probable***. The ***certain*** signs of Pregnancy are : the active movements of the child unequivocally felt by another; the presence of the child *in utero* ascertained by ballottement, and the sounds produced by the pulsations of the fœtal heart.

The only case, bearing upon this question, which I have met with, is one in which a woman, sentenced for poisoning her husband, simulated Pregnancy, and deceived the Sub-Assistant Surgeon who examined her.*

Casper gives a case, in which a woman, who almost certainly had never been pregnant, was sentenced to eight years' penal servitude, having pleaded guilty of the intentional murder of her new-born child, the truth having been discovered only after she had been confined in jail for almost three years (Vol. III., p. 390).

An even still more extraordinary case has lately been reported.† In November 1868, the following evidences of judicial error were brought to light by an appeal before the Imperial Court of Nancy. Adéle Bernard, a girl twenty-two years of age, was brought to trial on a charge of infanticide. The prosecution alleged that, in October 1868, she clandestinely gave birth to a child, and threw it into a pigsty, where it was eaten. This allegation was confirmed by her own confession both before the examining Magistrate and in open Court. Moreover, a midwife and a parochial Surgeon certified that, immediately after her arrest, they found traces of recent delivery. On this evidence, the Correctional Tribunal sentenced her to six months' imprisonment for the concealment of the birth of a child who was not proved to have been born alive. She went to prison accordingly; and, about a month later, in December, she was delivered of a fine healthy child, perfectly formed. The time allowed for her appeal against a sentence, which circumstances appeared to show was manifestly unjustifiable, had then expired, but the public prosecutor lodged an appeal on her behalf. When interrogated by the President of the Appeal Court, she said that she had been induced to make a false confession by her mother and the midwife, who impressed on her that, if she told the truth, she would get off easily; whereas, if she persisted in denying the accusation, she would certainly be condemned to fifteen or twenty years' imprisonment with hard labor. Some medical evidence was produced before the Court of Appeal to show the bare possibility of a superfœtation. But the Court rejected this hypothesis, held that she had been compelled by intimidation to make a confession for which there was no foundation, and reversed the verdict against her.

---

* Police Report, L. P., 1846, p. 42.

† Med. Times and Gazette, February 6th, 1869, p. 159.

Law.

When a prisoner was pregnant, the sentence of death passed upon her was ordered not to be carried out till such time after her delivery as is usual in such cases. Queen *v.* Mussamut Ghurbhurnee, W. R., 11th January 1854, Cr., 1.

A few months later we find it ruled, in the case of the Queen *v.* Tepoo, W. R., 16th May 1864, and 3rd June 1865, p. 15, that "a woman, being quick with child, is exempt from capital punishment."

The Judges observed : "The prisoner is quick with child, and such a state is always held to be a bar to eventual capital punishment. Following the usual precedents, therefore, we commute the sentence of death to that of transportation for life."

CRIMINAL ABORTION.

In a country like India, where true morality is almost unknown, but where the laws of society exercise the most rigorous and vigilant control imaginable over the conduct of females, and where six-sevenths of the widows, whatever their age or position in life may be, are absolutely debarred from re-marriage, and are compelled to rely upon the uncertain support of their relatives, it is scarcely surprising that great crimes should be frequently practised to conceal the results of immorality,* and that the procuring of Criminal Abortion should, especially, be an act of almost daily commission, and should have become a trade among certain of the lower midwives, or *dhaees*.†

It is stated by Dr. Montgomerie that the Malay women of Singapore are much in the habit of causing Abortion when a large family is likely to prove troublesome.

Ward, the Missionary, described the crime of destroying illegitimate children in the womb as prevalent to a shocking degree in Bengal. In the family of a single Koolin Brahmin, whose daughters never lived with their husbands, it was common for each daughter to destroy a child in the womb annually ; this crime he found also to be very prevalent among widows, so numerous in this country. The pundit who gave him this

---

* The following note appeared in my edition of 1856. The Chief Magistrate's Report on the State of the Town of Calcutta, for 1852-53, contains a most striking illustration of the folly of the present system, among the Hindus, of preventing the re-marriage of widows. Calcutta, with a population of about 416,000, supports 12,419 women of ill-fame, avowed and shameless (London, with its 2,000,000 inhabitants, is said by Lord Shaftesbury to contain not more than 7,000 or 8,000). Of these unfortunates, no less than 10,461 are Hindus. We learn from Dr. Payne's first report of the working of the Contagious Diseases Act in Calcutta, published on the 1st of April 1870, that there were then, *registered* as prostitutes in this City, 7,939 Hindus, 1,162 Mahomedans, 56 Eurasians, 15 Poles, 7 Italians, 5 Englishwomen, 4 Germans, 3 Russians, and 1 Jewess.

† According to Burckhardt, the practice of Abortion is frequent at Mecca, and the seed of the Mecca Balsam tree (*Balsamodendron Gileadense*) is the drug commonly used.

information, supposed that 10,000 children were thus murdered, in the province of Bengal, every month ! ! When Mr. Ward expressed his doubts of this extraordinary and shocking circumstance, the pundit appealed to the fact of many females being tried for this offence in the Courts of Justice, in every zillah in Bengal. He said the fact was so notorious that every child in the country knew of it ; and that the crime had acquired an appropriate name—*Petphela, viz.*, thrown from the belly ; *pet phelanee* is also a term of abuse which one woman often gives to another. It was a fact too, he was assured, that many women died after taking the drugs intended to destroy the child. A Koolin Brahmin assured him, that he had heard more than fifty women, daughters of Koolins, confess these murders. To remove his doubts, he mentioned an instance which took place in the village where he was born, where the woman was removed in the night to an adjoining village, till she had taken medicines, and destroyed the fœtus. Her paramour and his friends were about to be seized, on a charge of murder, when the woman returned home, having recovered from the indisposition occasioned by the medicines she had taken. On making further inquiry into this subject, a friend, upon whose authority he could implicitly rely, assured him that a very respectable and learned Brahmin, who certainly was not willing to charge his countrymen with more vices than they possessed, told him, it was supposed that *a thousand of these abortions took place in Calcutta every month !!* This statement Mr. Ward considered was doubtless over-colored.* The same Brahmin affirmed that he did not believe that there was a single Hindu, male or female, in the large cities of Bengal, who did not violate the laws of chastity.

Mr. Ward was a very careful inquirer, and if, as is most probable, much of the depravity described above existed in Bengal forty years ago, there can scarcely be a doubt that it prevails without any abatement at the present moment.

A considerable number of cases are brought before the notice of medical officers, in which it is stated that Abortion or Premature Confinement has been produced by violent ill-usage, blows, kicks, &c. As these charges are usually preferred by natives against persons with whom they are at bitter feud, and as the evidences of violence are not often very apparent, the medical officer needs do little more than inquire closely and report with caution. The proof of such violence must generally rest with the police.

The real cases are, however, only too numerous.

The majority of cases of this class which demand medical investigation, are those in which the death of both mother and child has resulted

* The Infanticides were, in eleven years prior to 1844, in the United Kingdom, 8,000, or 727 yearly ; the returns were still considered *incomplete.*—Hough's Precedents in Military Law, page 478.

from swallowing drugs, or from the employment of local irritants and mechanical means to cause the expulsion of the fœtus.

Baboo Kanny Lall Dey informs me that, during the period he has been acting as Additional Chemical Examiner, *i. e.* from 1867 up to the present time, there have been *forty-eight* cases of Criminal Abortion sent to their office for report. Out of the various substances sent for analysis he has identified the following articles :—

(1) Arsenic.
(2) Amalgum of Tin, Sulphate of Soda, Silicate of Potash (in one packet).
(3) Sulphate of Copper.
(4) Wood Charcoal.
(5) Capsicum Seeds.
(6) Upang, or "*Achyranthes Aspera.*"
(7) Chitta, "*Plumbago Zeylanica.*"
(8) Lall Chitra, "*Plumbago Rosea.*"
(9) Root of "*Nerium Oleander,*" 6 inches long, tipped with Assafœtida.
(10) Opium.
(11) A powder containing Black Pepper, burnt Sulphate of Copper and Cantharides.
(12) Assafœtida.

Dr. Webb gives the following as some of the methods practised to produce Abortion in India (communicated to him by an intelligent student of the Calcutta Medical College) :—

"Assafœtida, *Lall Chitra* root, Ginger, Garlic, Long Pepper.	Mixed and made into pulp, to be taken internally. After an hour, shampooing of the belly and lower part of abdomen, as well also introducing eight inches length of *Lall Chitra* branch, so as to enter into the mouth of the womb, produce Abortion.

"Tamarind pulp, Jabakkhar Nabon Salt, (Nitrate of Potass) mixed and taken, as well as *lall chitra* branch introduced, produce Abortion.

"Arairaj tree bark [?], black pepper-corns 25, produce Abortion.

"Goluckpore pice [metallic copper], bahoo leaf [bamboo leaves], used for the after-consequences.

"Wookra root [?], black pepper-corns boiled together are used as the above for the space of three days.

"Expressed juice of Boori Gooa Pan, half a drachm, to be repeated every third hour to produce Abortion." [Baboo Kanny Lall Dey tells me that this (*Dipteracanthus dejectus*) is used only in the after-treatment.]

"Assafœtida softened with water was anointed in the region of the navel, and at the same time hot milk was given internally, as hot as could be taken, and a large quantity, in a case of threatened Abortion ; this hastened the expulsion of the fœtus, and the remedy is used for the production of Abortion also."*

---

* Pathologica Indica, p. 281.

In a Madras case of Abortion, one of the witnesses said that *he smelt Assafœtida in the house.* Upon this Dr. Shortt mentions that Assafœtida frequently enters into the composition of native formulas for the production of abortion, and he quotes the above note by Dr. Webb. He, however, adds, that this drug is in every-day use among natives in child-bed, either alone or in combination with other drugs, to keep cold out of the system by its warm stimulant effect. It is believed to be a prophylactic of tetanus and to assist the lochial discharge.

Just as these sheets were going to press, Baboo Kanny Lall Dey kindly handed me the subjoined document, which contains *a description of the various modes of procuring Abortion in use near Calcutta.* He has obtained these facts by paying a woman, who is perfectly conversant with the practice. I speak confidently of these statements as *facts,* because I find them to be perfectly in accordance with nearly all that I had previously learnt on the subject.

"Besides *Lal Chitra,* which is commonly known as being used for criminal Abortion, the following different methods are also resorted to :—

"*(A). Unripe Pine-apple.*—A green, unripe one, only half grown, is used. It is decorticated, and the pulpy mass of a whole one is administered to the woman with a small quantity of salt. It is efficacious only during the earlier months of pregnancy; and, after the third month, its action is very doubtful. But, if administered to suitable cases, the uterus begins to contract within twelve hours, when slight hæmorrhage occurs also. Its action then increases, and, within the course of twenty-four hours the ovum is expelled. Occasionally the woman's life is jeopardized by flooding, but, as a rule, there is not much danger to be apprehended.

"*(B). Akundo (Calotropis Hamiltonii).*—This is used both internally and externally. A small quantity of the milky juice is made into a pillular mass by mixing it with a little wheat flour, and this the woman is made to swallow. At the same time a piece of rag is steeped in this juice ; it is then folded round a piece of stick nine fingers' breadth, or six inches long, and is thus rendered firm and suitable for introducing per vaginam. This is then carefully introduced, and only a portion to the extent of $1\frac{1}{2}$ fingers' breadth is left outside. This plan is useful in all stages of pregnancy, and there is not much danger either to the mother or the fœtus, which latter may, in fact, be born alive if the step is taken at an advanced stage.

"*(C). Lunka Seej (Euphorbium nivulia).*—This is said to be far more efficacious than all the rest.

"A twig about nine fingers' breadth long, and of appropriate size, is selected, and well anointed with good assafœtida (that known by the name of "Mooltanee Hingh" is always preferred) ; and as the twig itself is soft, and consequently difficult to introduce per vaginum, it is rendered stiff and fit for use by putting in its centre a thin bamboo stick. Nothing internally is needed, but the simple application of this stick so prepared is capable of effecting the object within twelve hours. This method is useful at all periods of pregnancy. The fœtus is never delivered alive, but there is said to be no great danger to the woman.

"Occasionally, to make assurance doubly sure, the milky juice of this plant is also administered internally in the shape of a pill made with rice flour.

"This last plan of administering the juice internally is now and then used alone, but is not at all reliable. It is no use at all after the third month of gestation; the step is, however, adopted more frequently for another purpose, for, when once it is administered in this way, the woman becomes incapable of conceiving ever afterwards.

"*(D). Apang* (*Achyranthes Aspera*—the root is commonly used by the natives as a tooth-brush).—This is also employed in a similar way with the *Lunka Seej*. A twig, nine fingers' breadth long, is well covered with assafœtida, and applied per vaginam. The fœtus is expelled in from eight to twelve hours. It is certain in its action, and may be used at any period of gestation, and the child is not necessarily born dead. There is no danger to the mother at all.

"*(E). Shet Koroobee* (*Oleander*).—A piece of root, nine fingers' breadth long, is smeared with assafœtida. The woman gets a shivering fit shortly after the introduction of the stick per vaginam; and, if it be applied in the evening, the fœtus is always expelled during the night. The method may be resorted to at any time during any period of pregnancy, and there is no inherent danger either to the woman or fœtus." [The Baboo obtained one of these prepared roots, which I have examined.—N. C.]

"*(F).* Occasionally a common broomstick is wrapped round with a piece of rag, and its surface is then smeared with assafœtida, and this is then applied per vaginam. It proves efficacious, but is very dangerous, as the broom, if not properly secured, slips upwards and penetrates the uterine walls.

"*(G).* Another, though not a very efficacious plan, is to make the woman swallow a mixture of caustic lime, turmeric powder, and water. This is boiled and made a paste of and swallowed while yet warm. It is useless after the third month; but it is not at all dangerous to the mother.

"*(H). Sujna Bark* (*Moringa Pterigosperma*).—A piece of the bark, about half an ounce in weight, is pounded with twenty-one black peppercorns, made into a paste, and swallowed. This is a very dangerous means, as the woman, as a rule, dies with the fœtus.

"In all the cases where the application of the substance per vaginam is required, a good amount of tact and skill is needed on the part of the applier. If much obstruction is met with at the os uteri or in the cervical canal, a little 'Choоa' (inspissated dregs of the various species of atta, as of roses, sandal, chumpa, jasmin, &c.) is applied to the part on a pellet of cotton, and this is said to bring on dilatation of the os uteri.

"*Lal Chitra* need scarcely be mentioned here, as it is almost universally known amongst the Profession, although it is very certain in its action; producing shivering almost immediately after the application, followed by Abortion in two or three hours; and, although it may be used at all periods of pregnancy, still the fœtus is always expelled lifeless, and the woman is in great danger."

Abortive Medicines Administered by the Mouth.

A careful investigation into the *Internal* means employed for procuring Abortion among the natives is much needed.

Some apparently very harmless vegetable preparations are strongly (probably erroneously) believed to have great efficacy as abortives.

Goor.—Many years ago, Baboo Koylas Chunder Chatterjea, Sub-Assistant Surgeon of Baraset, informed me that the idea that old *Goor* (treacle) is an abortive is prevalent. A case illustrative of this belief was lately recorded by Baboo Indoo Bhusan Mookerjea, Sub-Assistant Surgeon of Humeerpore.*

Doolia, aged about forty-five years, the mother of twelve children, and a widow for the last nine months, was sent in suffering from uterine hæmorrhage consequent on the induction of criminal abortion at about the third month of gestation by a native medicine, which is said by the *hakeems* to be generally resorted to in the neighbourhood of Humeerpore for the purpose in question. She stated that the medicine administered to her was prepared according to the following recipe:—

Green Capsules of common Cotton (freed from seeds and cotton)	8 ozs.
Garlic	$\frac{1}{2}$ oz.
Treacle (long kept)	1 ,,
Water...	2 pints,

boiled down to half the quantity, and strained, and the decoction thus prepared taken in equal doses, three times a day. In taking the medicine, the first day she vomited thrice, and had four or five loose stools, but felt nothing like pain in the uterus. In the course of the succeeding four days, during which the drug, prepared daily, was taken, there was merely looseness of her bowels unattended with vomiting. On the sixth day uterine pains and hœmorrhage supervened; and the expulsion of the embryo soon followed. The hæmorrhage was checked, and she seemed for a time to improve, but died of puerperal fever, with intense pelvic peritonitis, in about a month.

Dr. Waring mentions of the rather pungent seeds of the *Carica Papaya* (*papaw tree*), that a belief in their powerfully emmenagogue

---

* Ind. Med. Gaz., January 1, 1869, p. 14.

properties prevails amongst all classes of women in Southern India,—so much so that they assert that, if a pregnant woman partake of them, even in moderate quantities, Abortion will be the probable result. This popular belief is noticed in many of the reports received from India. In these it is also stated that the milky juice of the plant is applied locally to the os uteri with the view of inducing abortion. Dr. Waring adds that facts in support of the alleged emmenagogue properties of the *papaw* are still wanting.

Pine-apple.—The belief that the pleasant *Anaras* is an active abortive, even when eaten by pregnant cattle, is so general, that Moulvie Tumeez Khan Khan Bahadoor tells me that he tried the experiment of feeding gravid cows and goats upon this fruit, but without effect. A note which I have from Baboo Koylas Chunder Chatterjee renders this matter plain. He said that acid fruits are regarded as abortives—see a notice of the *tamarind* pulp (a most intense and very unwholesome acid when fresh) at p. 714. He knew a case in which a woman aborted at an advanced stage of pregnancy by eating (with that intention) about *two pounds* of ripe pine-apple. This fruit is rendered unwholesome by the presence of a very strong fibre which acts as a mechanical irritant on the bowels. I had under my own care an English lady who died of dysentery, after having aborted, at about the fifth month of pregnancy. The cause of her illness appeared to be the ravenous eating of raw pine-apple.

In July 1852, the Deputy Commissioner of Jubbulpore despatched a fluid, obtained by Dr. A. Wilkinson, from the stomach of a Brahmin woman, who had asserted, in her dying declaration, that she suffered from the effects of Arsenic administered to her by her paramour to produce Abortion. Dr. Wilkinson pronounced his belief that the matter found in the stomach contained *Arsenic;* this was confirmed by the Chemical Examiner's analysis.*

In a case which occurred at Tipperah in 1848, the prisoners are reported to have administered to a woman, who was pregnant by one of them, a mixture of *red sulphuret of arsenic, white oxide of arsenic, blue*

---

* In 1848, a Tipperah man gave his mistress poison, with the view, as he said, of procuring Abortion, but which caused her death in a few hours. The poison had previously been used by him to kill rats, so that he was well aware of its effects.—Police Report, Lower Provinces, 1848, p. 37. Mr. Brown, of Weston-on-Trent, reported the case of a young woman, twenty-four years of age, who was supposed to have died of peritonitis after premature delivery. It was found that she had been the subject of ulceration of the stomach produced by the action of arsenic (probably taken to induce abortion), which was detected in that organ by chemical analysis (Association Journal, October 7, 1850). Mr. Carter, of Newbury, referred to Dr. Taylor the case of a female, aged twenty-two years, who took a large dose of arsenic when she had passed the fifth month of pregnancy. She died in less than seven hours, purged and vomiting, but did not abort. See also Taylor, p. 782.

vitriol and vermillion, for the purpose, as they said, of producing abortion ; the woman died in consequence.*

Baboo Kanny Lall Dey has lately sent me particulars of a powder, which a woman of Furreedpore said had been given to her by her paramour with intent to procure Abortion. Fortunately, she did not take any of it. Dr. Bholanath Bose, the Civil Surgeon, ascertained very satisfactorily that it contained powder of *blistering flies*, *blue vitriol*, and *black pepper*.

In a case tried at Furruckabad, it was stated that the dose which had caused a woman three months gone to abort was five pills and some *soda* and *carrot seeds*.†

In the paper cited above, Baboo Indoo Bhushun Mookerjee mentions that *carrot seeds*, in ounce doses, and plaster *mortar* from a wall some forty or fifty years old, are said, in the neighbourhood of Humeerpore, to be sometimes taken by natives for this purpose.

In 1851, a Hindu was tried, at Backergunge, for administering the juice of some jungle plant to his sister-in-law, seven months gone in pregnancy, in consequence of which she was taken ill and passed some congealed blood. She died in fifty to sixty hours from the effects of this medicine, having previously acknowledged the illicit intercourse between herself and the prisoner, and the fact of his having given her the medicine alluded to, to procure miscarriage. The body was so much decomposed that the Sub-Assistant Surgeon who examined it could merely state that the woman's death was caused by Abortion of a fœtus about seven months old, the after-birth having remained attached to the womb. He could not pronounce that the substance (fluid ?) said to have been administered by the prisoner would cause miscarriage. The prisoner was acquitted. The Judge of the higher Court remarked that the examination of the medical officer had not been sufficiently close. He should have been questioned regarding the properties of the *asclepias gigantea*, and its effect upon the system, when given in large quantities. It is, he believed, an irritant and an active purgative, and is injurious to the system, according to the quantity or frequency with which it is administered.

There can be no doubt that the acrid milky juice of the *Mudar* may act fatally to both mother and child in such cases, by its powerful emetic and cathartic operation.

Dr. O'Shaughnessy has shown that the *lall chitra* is sometimes given internally to occasion abortion:—On this point, *vide supra*, pp. 116 and 252.

---

* Police Report, Lower Provinces, 1848, p. 3. The Police Report of that year makes allusion to four other deaths caused by giving drugs to procure abortion, occurring in Tipperah.

† Nizamut Adawlut Reports, July 8th, 1853, p. 822.

Use of Mechanical Means and Local Irritants.

It is probable that the native abortionists employ a variety of *mechanical means* and of *local irritants* to effect their destructive object. It is believed that the introduction of *Arsenic* is practised, but I have not been able to meet with an instance of the kind.*

Mr. Edgeworth, Commissioner and Superintendent of the Trans-Sutlej States, communicated, in 1855, to the Medical Board some interesting particulars which he had collected in criminal trials regarding the drugs used to produce Abortion by the village midwives about Jullundhur. That most commonly in use appears to be the stem of the *Trianthema pentandra,* called *Bis-kopra* and *Itsit.* This is usually looked upon as an innocent pot-herb. In most cases of which he has heard, the stalk was employed locally; but in one instance it was given with other drugs as a bolus. Another substance, used for this purpose, is the *Mynphul,*—fruit of the *Ranolia dumetorum.* In addition to these, *Cloves, Nutmeg,* and *Saffron, Fenugreek,* and *Sal Ammoniac* are used. A mixture of these seven ingredients was successfully employed in a case tried by him. In another case, a mixture of *Mynphul, Gugger Bel* (*Cuscuta Reflexa*—the branches), and *Malkungni* (*Celastrus Paniculata*) had been given by the mouth.

Professor T. W. Wilson informed me that a by no means unusual mode of procuring miscarriage among the native women of Calcutta is by placing a lighted wick in a *lotah* (brass water-vessel) and applying the mouth of the pot over the hypogastric region, after the manner of a large cupping-glass. Traction is made upon the vessel while it is firmly adherent, and probably a partial separation of the placenta, or, possibly, very severe injury to the uterine parietes, is the result. Probably this means and *pressure* are generally employed at advanced terms of pregnancy.

Dr. Woodford informs me that his impression is that the introduction

---

* In 1849, the Chemical Examiner received, from the Magistrate of the 24-Pergunnahs, a packet of substances which, it appears, were believed to have been used in procuring abortion. Dr. O'Shaughnessy detected *fused litharge, realgar, alum,* and some harmless substances, the whole being commonly used by native women for removing hair from the axillæ and pubes. He thought that, doubtless, some of the substances might, if applied within the orifice of the womb, cause such irritation as would lead to abortion; but, under the above circumstances, their possession could scarcely be deemed a proof of criminal practices. I have made some inquiry relative to the arsenical composition used by natives as a depilatory. The late Baboo Dyalchurn Bysack, my assistant in the Ooterparah Hospital, informed me that it is composed of hurtal (orpiment) and lime. Some persons mix these in equal parts, others use an excess of orpiment or of lime. These are made into a paste of the consistence of thick honey, which is applied lukewarm over the parts, and is allowed to remain from 5 to 7 minutes. The surface is then washed clean with cold water, when the hair is either removed with the paste, or is easily plucked out without pain. This practice is most frequent among the lower classes and women of ill-fame.

of the *Sujna*, or Horse-Radish root, is used in Bengal for this purpose, but not so frequently as the *Lall Chitra* is.

The Hon'ble H. Vincent Bayley, Judge of the Calcutta High Court, informed me some years ago that, in his judicial experience, the commonest mode of causing Abortion in Bengal is by the *Root of the Tamarind Tree*.

Some remarks will be found at p. 252, on the use of the *Root of the White Oleander* as an abortive.

In a trial at East Burdwan, in 1859, it appeared that the death of a pregnant woman had been caused, without the occurrence of Abortion, by drugs administered by the mouth and by local mechanical injury. A piece of root, which was found in her house in a basket, wrapped up in a piece of bloody cloth, was sent to the Chemical Examiner, who describes it as *Saith Kurubee* (Oleander) a poisonous root used by natives to procure Abortion.*

Dr. Waring (p. 60) cites a notice by Dr. J. Newton, of the fact that the bruised nut of the intensely corrosive *marking nut* (*Semecarpus Anacardium*) applied locally to the os uteri, is one of the means in use amongst native women in Madras for procuring Abortion.

The most frequent, and probably most destructive, mode of causing Abortion among the Bengalees is by the introduction into the uterine cavity of a large portion of the root of the *Lall Chitra*, or Plumbago Rosea.

In a case where death was caused at Hooghly, in 1843, by administering means to cause Abortion, there could be no doubt, from the report of the Civil Surgeon, that the deceased had died from inflammation of the womb, caused by the introduction, through the vagina, of a piece of stick called *Cheeta*, but there was not sufficient evidence against the three persons accused.†

In a case tried at Tipperah, in 1856, it appeared that a married woman living apart from her husband, having become pregnant, was taken into the house of a female abortionist, where *Lall Chitra* was used, and where she took some pills containing a portion of *crude mercury* in a state of minute subdivision, and small pieces of a drug called *Surbojala*, which, Dr. Davis observed, "the natives are known to use for the purpose of procuring Abortion, as well as to prevent impregnation."‡

The Hon'ble H. V. Bayley enquired of me, some years ago, regarding the action of *Surbojala* as an abortive. It is said to be prepared from the root of a common jungle tree of a very acrid nature, and to be commonly used in the neighbourhood of Nowakolly for this nefarious purpose. I

---

* Nizamut Adawlut Reports, September 19th, 1859, p. 266.

† Police Reports, L. P., 1853, p. 69.

‡ Nizamut Adawlut Reports, September 15th, 1856, p. 449.

cannot identify it, as it is probably a local name, perhaps for a species of plumbago, as Baboo Kanny Lall Dey explains the meaning of the word to be burning (*jala*) all over (*surbo*) ;—so also *Lall Chitra* is sometimes called *agni chitta,* "fire" chitta. It is not *Surbo Jaya,* the inert *Canna Indica.*

In 1844, it was reported to the Joint Magistrate of Bancoorah, that the relations of a pregnant woman intended to administer drugs to her to procure Abortion. A burkundauz was sent to inquire into the matter. He found the woman very ill, having been recently delivered. She stated that two persons had given her drugs. These individuals were sent in with her paramour. There was, however, no proof forthcoming against them. After her death, it was found that a stick (a piece of which remained in the womb,) had been forced up the uterus, and that inflammation, arising from its presence, caused her death.*

It was reported, in the case of a professional abortionist, convicted at Tipperah, in 1845, that her medicine was *a pill of the Cheeta tree,* and that she also passed into the vagina a stick of the creeper called *Moaheeanee.*†

In his report of 1850, already noticed, Dr. Woodford refers to a case in which he found a portion about four inches long of *Chitra* root "in the gangrenous uterus, with a piece of string, or loosely twisted jute. In a note which Dr. Woodford has kindly written for me he adds: "We thus learn the mode of application, that is, to excite a certain amount of irritation and inflammation and then to remove the root attached by the string, which had here been accidentally broken in the withdrawal."‡

In May 1854, the body of a Hindu woman, who had died under suspicious circumstances, was brought to my hospital, at Howrah, in a very advanced stage of decomposition. The Native Doctor informed me that, when placed in the dead-house, it appeared in a natural condition. I, however, found the womb inverted between the thighs of the corpse, evidently by the gaseous distension within ;§ and, lying beside it, and

---

* Police Reports, L. P., for 1854, p. 64.

† *Ibid,* for 1845, p. 40.

‡ See also a similar case by Dwarkanauth Dass Basu, Pathologica Indica, p. 333. The woman died of peritonitis a few hours after her admission to the hospital. In the uterus a piece of *Lall Chitra* stick was found, the uterus was in a state of ulceration from the contact of this foreign body, the vagina was inflamed and ulcerated. The peritonitis was said to have come on four days previous to her admission to the Medical College Hospital.

§ In a notice of this case, published in Vol. XXI., p. 193, of his excellent "Abstract," my friend, the late Dr. Ranking, remarked:—"We are not disposed to accept Dr. Chevers's explanation that the contents of the uterus were expelled by the accumulation of gas in the intestines." The Editor did not state the reasons for his dissent, but spoke of my case as *similar* to one by Dr. Mayer, of Warzburg, cited in the preceding volume of the Abstract, p. 193. In this latter case, the child was extruded from the uterus of the mother fifty-four hours after death; when there was "found no absolute evidence of death." The reviewer holds that, here, in all probability, the child was expelled by the "mere *rigor mortis* of the uterus." In my

evidently having recently escaped from its cavity, the body of a fœtus of about four months, greatly decomposed, and a portion of the *Lall Chitra* root, seven and-a-half inches long and rather thicker than a common writing quill. This had been scraped,* and was thickly coated with adhesive inflammatory deposit.

I find two other records of Abortion cases in India, observed by Surgeons not acquainted with my case, where this remarkable *post-mortem* accident occurred.

In April 1866, Surgeon Major F. L. Clementson examined, at the Berhampore Dispensary (Madras Presidency), the body of a woman which presented the appearances which are usual when decomposition has been going on for several hours; the fœtor was horrible; the features were so swelled and distorted, that it would not have been easy for those who knew them best to recognise them ; the greater part of the body was, besides being greatly swollen, covered with bullæ.

On the dead-house table was a fœtus of from four to five months old, connected by the funis with the placenta, which was still retained in the vagina. When the body was laid on the table, the fœtus was in utero, but had been expelled by the force of the gases of decomposition. In removing the intestines, "the end of a stick, which had in some way escaped wounding the bowels, was found lying close along the front of the spine and reaching nearly as high as the diaphragm. On tracing it downwards, it was found to have passed through the posterior wall of the uterus at its lower third ; its end was in the upper part of the vagina. The uterus was about six or seven inches long from cervix to fundus, the walls and substance throughout were intensely inflamed, as were the appendages, connecting membranes, and cellular tissue about these parts, which were, moreover, greatly infiltrated. The stick was wound round

---

case, this explanation was quite inadmissible. The body was brought to my hospital frightfully swollen by putrefaction, long after the cessation of the *rigor mortis;* and, subsequently to its being deposited there, the uterus was inverted, and the fœtus was expelled,—the abdomen being enormously distended by gas. This appears also to have occurred in the body of a woman whose case became the subject of a trial at Tirhoot in 1853. A widow, having become pregnant, disappeared, and was reported to have been murdered by her relations. Her body was sent to the Civil Assistant Surgeon, after disinterment, in a very advanced state of putrefaction. "The womb, with a portion of the small intestines, had been forced by the progress of putrefaction (gases in the abdomen) through the external organs of generation, and a small portion of the remains of these [protruded parts?] alone was visible." The right side of the abdominal parietes had burst, so as to give exit to the gases of putrefaction. "From the absence of the uterine organs, he was unable to state if the deceased was pregnant; but, had she been so far advanced as to be unable, from her size, to conceal it, *the womb would not have been protruded out of her body;* therefore, if she had been pregnant, it must have been of short duration." The above cases appear strongly to oppose the conclusion here arrived at by the Medical Officer.

* Dr. O'Shaughnessy mentions that the *Plumbagin* exists principally in the *bark* of the root. It is to be feared, however, that this scraping is merely intended to increase the irritating effects of the blistering substance.

with cloth, which no doubt was, at the time of its introduction into the vagina and uterus, covered with some irritating substance. It appeared that the woman had borne a good character, but her husband had been away from her for three years.*

It is remarkable, in the above case, that the uterus does not appear to have been inverted, and we are left in doubt as to the time at which the fœtus was expelled.

On the 8th of June (it will be noticed that all these three cases occurred in the hottest season) Dr. Hutchinson, of Patna, examined the body of a woman who was said to have taken opium, to avoid the disgrace of an illegitimate pregnancy. Decomposition was well advanced, the stomach was strongly charged with opium. Between her thighs lay the inverted uterus with its inverted fundus filled up with distended intestine, and what was its cavity, fully exposed, and quite dry. No placental scar was apparent. In front of the uterus lay an entire ovum of between five and six months ; placental end lying next to and touching the uterus. The membranes were entire, but dry outside ; not a drop of blood or liquor amnii had escaped to stain the charpoy on which she died, and on which she was brought in. This strange and silent parturition had occurred on the road, unknown to the police, or the bearers who were carrying the body ; no vital energies caused it, but simply the irresistible pressure of intestines distended by putrefaction.

Dr. Hutchinson argues:—" There are cases on record of the contracting uterus completing a delivery interrupted by the death of the woman ; but here there was no contracted uterus, but, on the contrary, a dilated and inverted organ. Moreover, there could not have been contraction, for the woman had died of a poisonous dose of opium, and it is not likely that a contracted organ would have been wholly inverted." " What proofs are there that this was a *post* and not a *pre mortem* delivery. In the first place, the police *Kyfeut*, usually so minute, was entirely silent on the subject of the parturition; if the fœtus had been present when the body left the thanna, it would have formed the subject of a distinct notice. Secondly, had it occurred during life, all the parts would not have been in the position in which they were found ; the fœtus and placenta would certainly have been detached, and there would have been stains on the bed either from the liquor amnii or the placental blood ; inversion of the uterus during life could only have resulted from a retained placenta, which there was not ; and, supposing there had been, the placenta would have been adherent, or at least detached from the fœtus. All these indications were wanting. Thirdly, had the birth and inversion taken place during life, death following soon after, the placental scar must have been apparent, whereas there was

---

* Madras Quart. Jour of M. S., Vol. X. for 1866, p. 181.

not the slightest indication of one. A dead and bloodless placenta was simply pushed off from a dead and bloodless uterus."*

In August 1854, I examined the body of a Mussalmaunee, dead three days, who was alleged to have died in consequence of the employment of means to produce Abortion. I found that this had been effected by the introduction of a portion of *Lall Chitra* root, about four inches and-a-half long, and rather more than half as thick as a common cedar pencil. The contents of the uterus, which must have been of the fourth or fifth month, had been expelled, but this irritating substance remained lodged in its cavity. The lining of the uterus, still coated with decidua, had a seared appearance, almost as if molten lead had been poured over it, and the root was completely draped with a thick shreddy inflammatory deposit. Decomposition had advanced considerably, but the mucous membrane of the stomach, as well as that of the first portion of the duodenum, was of a deep lake color, while the rest of the intestinal tract was pale. This, however, appeared to result merely from a state of high congestion. The stomach contained rather more than an ounce of sanguinolent fluid, exactly resembling strawberry cream in appearance. There were solid fœces in the rectum. Thinking that the powder of *Lall Chitra* might also have been given, I sent the stomach to the Chemical Examiner, but nothing suspicious could be detected.

It appeared, in a trial at Mymensing, that a widow, having entered upon a disreputable course of life, and becoming pregnant, she and one of her paramours had recourse to a woman of the bearer caste, who was "acquainted with medicine," to procure Abortion. This hag furnished "a twig of a creeping plant," which she procured on the bank of the river. This was introduced into the womb : it immediately began to cause pain, but she was entreated by her paramour to bear it for the sake of preserving their reputation. On the following day, she began to complain of severe pain in her stomach, saying that it was owing to some medicine which had been given her for the purpose of procuring Abortion. Her death occurred three days after this. The Civil Surgeon deposed that death was caused by miscarriage ; that the womb was enlarged ; that there was no fœtus in the womb ; it must have been thrown away, and death ensued from hæmorrhage ; that there was a large sore [?] on the surface of the womb, to which the fœtus had been attached, with effusion of blood in and around it ; that the miscarriage must have been caused by the introduction of a stick of a highly irritating nature into the womb, such as the piece of stick shown to him in Court, which was found in the womb. That it was called *akhulmendee* (Lawsonia inermis?), and is universally used by the natives for procuring Abortion by introducing it into the womb. The hag admitted, before the darogah, that she had furnished the medicine to be applied to the

* Indian Med. Gazette, Aug. 1, 1867, p. 200.

deceased's person to cause Abortion ; and, when the darogah asked her to show him the twig, she procured a twig from the jungle, saying that this was what she gave. This twig was produced in Court, together with the piece of stick which was discovered in the deceased's womb—they were of the same kind.*

It might be imagined that a mode of procuring Abortion more violent and cruel than the above could scarcely be imagined. A series of still more deplorable, if not more atrocious, cases is, however, on record. To these Mr. Clementson's case, given at p. 723, belongs.

In 1845, Dr. J. Macpherson, then medical officer of Howrah, examined the body of a Hindu female,† about twenty-five years of age, in an advanced stage of decomposition. She was said to have been recently delivered, and, on her death-bed, to have accused the man with whom she cohabited of having caused Abortion. The intestines within the pelvis were found to be in a state of acute inflammation, with shreds of lymph freely effused ; and, floating among them, and lying transversely, was found a piece of stick, about 5½ inches long, of about the thickness of a small quill, and with one end slightly sharpened. [Doubtless this was a portion of the *Lall Chitra* root.] On examining the uterus, its fundus was discovered to have been perforated by the stick, a small hole, large enough to admit of its passage, remaining pervious. The contents of the uterus had been recently evacuated, its coats were dilated to one-half more than the usual size, and the spot to which the placenta had been adherent was plainly recognizable. No laceration of the os uteri was discoverable: and it was not known what had become of the fœtus. As one end of the stick had the look of having been broken off, it may have originally been much longer, and have been broken off by the violence employed in introducing it. The evidence went to show that no one but the man with whom she cohabited could have had access to her, and it is not to be supposed that she could, of herself, have used sufficient force to pierce the walls of the uterus. Its passing so directly through the axis of the uterus must have been accidental. It appeared that death occurred in about eighteen hours after the receipt of the injury.‡

One Omao Chung, of Sylhet, was sentenced to imprisonment for having, apparently in league with a professional abortionist, killed a woman who was with child by him. The Civil Surgeon deposed that he found in the vagina a root of *Lall Chitra* about ten inches long, which had pierced the further part of the womb, and had caused much inflammation. It appears that this treatment was followed by death in three days.§

---

* Nizamut Adawlut Reports, August 2nd, 1854, p. 188.

† Singularly enough, her name appears, by the report, to have been *Chittra*.

‡ Indian Journal of Medical and Physical Science, April 1845; London Medical Gazette, Vol. XXXVI., p. 102; and Taylor, p. 780.

§ Nizamut Adawlut Reports, December 22nd, 1853, p. 963; and December 22nd, 1854, p. 792.

In 1855, Mr. M. Shircore reported the case of a Hindu woman, about thirty years of age, who was brought to the Medical College Hospital, collapsed and dying, with tympanitis and great abdominal tenderness. She stated that she had miscarried, at between the fourth and fifth month, six or eight days previously ; but distinctly denied having received any injury whatever sufficient to cause Abortion, which she alleged had occurred spontaneously. There were found extensive traces of peritonitis. An abscess was found in the left lumbar region over the psoas muscle, within which was lodged a thin pointed slip of bamboo, about six inches long. There was a gangrenous appearance of the os tincæ, and the lining of the uterus was coated with a dark grumous thin mucus, but the condition of the organ appeared otherwise but little altered, and it displayed no opening whatever through which the bamboo could have been thrust, nor the slightest mark of recent cicatrization. A large ragged ulcer was, however, found in the rectum, at least nine inches above the anus, communicating directly with the cavity of the abscess ; and through this, no doubt, the stick had passed.*

Moulvie Tumeez Khan Bahadur informs me that, about the year 1844-45, he examined a case in which a slip of the petiole of the cocoanut was driven through the *cul de sac* of the vagina, missing the os uteri, into the left iliac fossa behind the peritoneum. It had caused death by suppuration, gangrene, and general peritonitis. The uterus showed that delivery had recently taken place. It was found that a midwife had done this mischief.

Twelve years ago Moulvie Tumeez Khan Bahadur discovered the following appearances in the body of a woman, apparently aged between twenty-five and thirty years, which he was dissecting :—The body was extremely emaciated; the only appearances of disease were as follow:—The whole of the pelvic viscera, with the exception of the bladder, *which was quite healthy*, had been agglutinated together by old peritoneal adhesions. Now, the whole of the pelvic organs appeared to be in a sloughing condition. The uterus did not present any appearance of delivery. Its interior was gangrenous, and its posterior wall was nearly destroyed by sloughing. Between the uterus and rectum, or lower part of the sygmoid flexure of the colon, and opposite to the left sacro-iliac synchondrosis, was a great sloughing cavity, in which lay a stick of the size of an ordinary pen-holder. It appears to be a stalk of the *plumbago rosea*. At one end, about half an inch of the twig is bare, the remainder of its length is smoothly coated with layer upon layer of phosphatic deposit to that extent that it now forms a spindle-shaped body of about the

---

* Op. Citat., for October, 1845, p. 583. In 1847, Dr. Murray, of Beerbhoom, reported, in a criminal case, that he found the womb of a Brahminee woman ruptured ; that it and the abdomen were so much inflamed as probably to have caused death ; and that Abortion had previously taken place. It is to be regretted that further particulars of so remarkable a case are not given.

thickness of the little finger. At one end the laminated structure of the concretion is very well marked; at the other end, the woody structure of the twig appears closely infiltrated with calcareous matter. It is evident that the irritating body was thrust through the *cul de sac* of the vagina into the peritoneal cavity. Lying here, it produced local peritonitis, by which the agglutination of the pelvic viscera shut it completely off from the general cavity of the peritoneum. Remaining thus encysted, it became coated with lime salts as encysted bullets frequently are. This process of deposition served, in some measure, to protect the walls of the *sac* from the acridity of the *plumbagin;* but *the whole* of the stick did not become covered with this protective coating; and thus, the calculus and the exposed portion of its nucleus continuing to act as a foreign body, the woman's powers became exhausted under this constant irritation, until death by gangrene terminated the struggle. See also Mr. Broughton's case, p. 742.

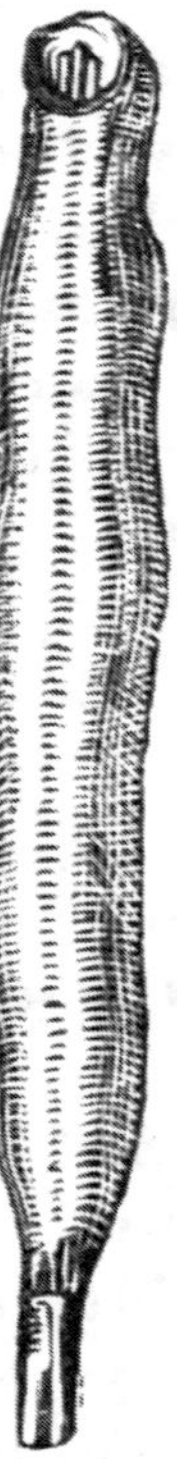

Size reduced one half.

From several recorded cases, it would appear that the *dhaees*, in some instances at least, merely furnish the instrument by which Abortion is to be caused, which is employed by the woman's friends, her paramour, or even by *herself;* hence, doubtless, the great severity of the injuries inflicted in the above cases.

The printed reports of the Calcutta Nizamut, up to the end of April 1854, contain reports of only fourteen cases of trials for procuring Abortion. In twelve of these instances, the death of the unhappy women resulted. But few of these cases embody much information that is valuable in a medico-legal point of view. Many of them, however, show that there is a class of native women who are professed abortionists. A woman was sentenced at Humeerpore, in 1824, upon her own confession, for causing the death of a pregnant female. This hag had been brought from a distance to effect the crime, which had evidently been preceded by others in which she was an agent, she having practised the art, and that not secretly, but as an avowed and successful profession.* At Tipperah, a woman was convicted, in 1845, of having caused death by administering drugs to procure Abortion. It was supposed that this was her regular trade; her charge in each case being *five rupees*.† The Hon'ble H. Vincent Bayley told me of a hag, at Midnapore, who kept an Abortion-shop, had a collection of little bottles of drugs, and grew *Lall Chitra* in her garden! I am informed by Mr. Edgeworth that, about Jullundhur, (Trans-Sutlej States), certain hags make a regular trade by procuring abortion. He is of opinion that, although death frequently results from the means which they employ, these women are not professional poisoners.

One Mussamut Proba, of Sylhet, was sentenced to imprisonment for

* Macnaghten's Reports, Vol. II., p. 335.

† Police Report, L. P., 1845, p. 40.

having produced the miscarriage of a woman who was with child by her husband's brother: death ensued. It appeared that deceased consented to give *ten annas* (little more than a shilling) to the prisoner, who was spoken of as skilful in her art. A root appears to have been the destructive agent employed.*

The reported cases show that several members of a family, as the brothers, the mother, and other female relations of the woman, and the friends of the seducer, by no means rarely become parties to the crime, in their anxiety to conceal the disgrace, or to avert its punishment; that the deaths of both mother and child often result from the administration of drugs, solely by the mouth, without the employment of local means; and that the criminals are apt to plead that they employed means with a view only to restore arrested catamenial function, as in the following case :—

In 1852, three persons were tried, at Cuttack, for the wilful murder of a woman, by means applied, with her own consent, to cause abortion. A man who resided in the deceased's house, and who stated that he was a hundred years old, testified that he had seen one of the prisoners (who evidently followed the profession of midwife, but denied the fact) sit on the deceased's bed with another woman, both on the day of her death and on the day previous, and that he saw her give and apply medicines, internally and externally, to the deceased, who did not afterwards risefrom her bed. The midwife admitted to the Police that, understanding that the deceased's monthly cousres had stopped, she, upon being repeatedly requested to prescribe something for their return, procured some assafœtida and aloes, and prepared two *buttees*, or rolls of cloth twisted round a small stick, and gave them to the deceased, telling her to apply them, one at a time. She stated before the Magistrate that she gave the woman a *pootlee*, or roll of cloth with salt on it, to apply to her private parts (probably the bag of dried and heated salt often used in the treatment of amenorrhœal cases), and also, though in somewhat a confused manner, admitted administering assafœtida and aloes, but disclaimed giving her the *buttees*. The medical officer deposed positively to the fact of the deceased having been recently delivered of a fœtus of about four months, and that her death was caused by injuries thereby occasioned in the womb. The Judge of the higher Court decided that, though the operation was performed with the consent of the deceased, and the death of the woman was not intended, yet, as the act was unlawful, and was attended with probable serious danger, the killing amounted, according to English law, to murder: according to Mahomedan law it is a punishable offence, but it does not come within the five denominations of homicide distinguished in

* Nizamut Adawlut Reports, October 26th, 1854, p. 505.

that law. The prisoners were sentenced to seven years' imprisonment, with labor.*

A thorough development of the intimate history and "physiology" of crime in every district of India is a most useful and interesting work which still remains to be performed, principally by Magistrates, Officers of the Police, and Civil Surgeons,—especially, I think, by the latter, because they generally remain long in their districts. The result of a valuable attempt to obtain such information appears in Appendix No. 1 to Dr. Mouat's Jail Report for 1869: "*Nomenclature and Signification of Castes and Classes of Criminals, with a Sketch of the Chief Crimes committed in the Districts of the Lower Provinces of the Bengal Presidency.*" This report, although at present a mere sketch of the subject, will be found an admirable foundation to work upon. I searched it with great eagerness for information regarding the crime of Abortion, for which certain districts have long been notorious; but I find only three valid allusions to the subject. In the report on Sylhet, one of the very worst districts in this respect, the crime is not even named. It is stated that, in Moorshedabad, the crime of causing miscarriage is principally committed by *Kybertos*. The men and women of this class deal principally in cocoons, and therefore more frequently come in contact with strangers, who come to their women as customers rather than to women of other classes. The evil consequences of this contact of women with men manifest themselves in conceptions and pregnancies. Severance, loss of caste, and other social considerations, induce the *widows* to get rid of their burden privately by means of miscarriage. In Burdwan, we are told that the Sadgops (Hindu cultivators, sellers of vegetables, &c.) head the list in the offence of procuring abortion. Nothing can well be slighter than the above hints; still this is the kind of knowledge of which we stand in need.

The criminal records embody abundant evidence of the fact that the crime now in question is especially prevalent in the Tipperah and Sylhet districts. Out of 27 abortion cases which came before the Calcutta Court of Nizamut Adawlut in the years 1855-57-58-59, *nine* were from Tipperah and *nine* from Sylhet. In a trial held at the latter place in 1855, the Sessions Judge observed: "The crime of procuring abortion is unhappily very prevalent in this district.†

In a trial for homicide, in an attempt to procure abortion, held at Tipperah in 1856, the Sessions Judge observed: "This is a crime most offensively prevalent in this district." In a second case, tried in the same year, the Judge remarked: "The crime of causing abortion is prevalent in this

* Nizamut Adawlut Reports, Vol. II., Part 2, of 1852, p. 910; see also another case in which it was pleaded that medicine was only given for the purpose of restoring the woman's monthly courses, Vol. IV. of 1854, p. 495.

† *Ibid*, June 1, 1855, p. 655.

district, and can only be effectually checked, when established, by serious punishment."

In another case tried in 1857, the Judges of the Court of appeal observed that, "judging only of the cases brought to light in the Tipperah zillah, the crime of procuring abortion would appear to be on the increase."

Dr. Mouat gives a report from Brahman Barria, a subdivision of Tipperah, in which it is remarked: "The crime of causing miscarriage is general in this quarter; but, unfortunately, there can scarcely be any conviction, owing to want of direct proof. Illegal connexions are common, and, when they result in pregnancy, the parties have merely to seek the aid of old women, one or two of whom are to be found in almost every village, who supply noxious drugs. These women subsist by this nefarious trade, but cannot be detected" [?]* "In spite of all manner of precaution, numerous cases come to the notice of the Court; but it is powerless, for no good proof can be found. Besides, this offence being cognizable only by the Sessions Court, the magisterial authorities require the most satisfactory evidence in order to make commitments."

The law has, however, from time to time, succeeded in unearthing these venomous reptiles.

In 1855, Mussamut Radhee, *alias* Rotoori Matab, of Sylhet, confessed that she prepared and administered some medicine to the deceased with a view of procuring abortion, *for which she received four rupees*, and it was in evidence that the deceased died shortly of having had an abortion.†

In 1856, Chandram Paul, of Sylhet, was found guilty of the culpable homicide of a woman by administering medicine to produce abortion. It appeared that the woman's paramour requested him to provide the drugs needful to procure abortion. He did so, and *was paid four annas.* These drugs failing, he pointed out a plant, and told the paramour to take some of the leaves and the roots, which he did, and applied the leaves to the deceased's head and passed the root into her vagina, which caused abortion, from the effects of which she died about ten or eleven days afterwards. The prisoner admitted having given drugs on previous occasions to two other persons to procure abortion. The Civil Surgeon examined the drugs found in the prisoner's house, and deposed that these drugs are generally used to procure abortion.‡

In 1857, Mussamut Pearee confessed that "she gave medicine, not once,

---

* I have noted *ten* instances in which professional abortionists have been convicted in the Tipperah Court: one in 1845 (Police Report for that year, p. 40); two, early in 1856 (Nizamut Adawlut Reports, for that year, Feb. 28, p. 515); and another in the same year (*Ibid*, September 15, p. 440); four in 1857 (*Ibid*, pp. 162, 309, and 447); two in 1858 (*Ibid* April 15, p. 121).

† Nizamut Adawlut Reports, Nov. 8, 1855, p. 780.

‡ *Ibid*, Feb. 15, 1856, p. 434.

but twice, to the deceased, to cause abortion, and that the second dose had the effect; that the woman lived four days after it was administered." The Sessions Judge observed: "That, taking all the circumstances into consideration, the known frequency of the offence, the facility with which detection is eluded, the fearful trifling with life, and the fatal result in this case, I would recommend that the prisoner be sentenced to fourteen years' imprisonment, with labor suited to her sex." The Judges of the Court of appeal remarked: "There is a peculiar circumstance in this case which induces us to confirm the sentence,—*viz.*, that the prisoner was in the habit of keeping drugs of the exclusive character of those used in procuring abortion; and it is a legitimate presumption, therefore, that she was ready at all times to afford the means of perpetrating the like grave offence. With a view, therefore, to deter others from similar practices, we inflict the severe sentence proposed."*

In another case, tried at Sylhet in 1857, the Sessions Judge remarked that the crime of abortion was unhappily very prevalent in that district, and noticed the necessity of inflicting severe punishment on parties convicted of it. Prisoner Boohun admitted that she knowingly administered drugs to procure abortion, and added that she had frequently administered the same to other women without any fatal effect.†

It would appear that, in Madras (see p. 470), Bombay (see p. 742), and Bengal, men and women of the *Barber caste* are occasionally concerned in these criminal practices.

In 1856, Bolienath, of Sylhet, confessed to the effect that he had an intimacy with the deceased, and that she was four months gone with child by him; that he, in order to cause abortion, procured some drugs from Ootun, a Barber, and administered them to her, which caused vomiting and burning pains over the body; that, on the following day, the prisoner got some drugs from one Shamnath, and, on administering them to her, she had a miscarriage, of which she died.‡

In 1857, a Tipperah woman (Hindu), having become pregnant by her own nephew, had recourse to one Mussamat Joyshooda, *alias* Kooshee (a large proportion of these abortionists have *aliáses*), of the Barber caste, and gave her *two rupees* to procure abortion, which was done so effectually that she died the following day.§ When she heard of her victim's death, the hag had the conscience to return the two rupees blood-money, but was sentenced to seven years' transportation.

Among "those trades and professions most useful to the Magistrate," Mr. Tytler (Vol. I., p. 120) gave the first place to the *Barber*. He

* Nizamut Adawlut Reports, February 10, 1857, p. 124.
† *Ibid*, April 30, 1857, p. 603.
‡ *Ibid*, September 25, 1856, p. 619.
§ *Ibid*, February 14, 1857, p. 162.

says : "The Barbers are described in the Shasters as being '*the most cunning amongst men, even as the jackal is amongst beasts.*' They have, as formerly in Europe, the double profession of barber and surgeon."

There cannot be a doubt that, as a general rule, those immediately concerned in the crime of abortion, even when the life of the mother is destroyed, confess with much more readiness than we observe in cases of ordinary homicide. Even the professional abortionists show far more willingness to reveal their profession than dacoits and road-poisoners do. In a trial held at Moorshedabad in 1855, the Judge urged that severity is needful as a check to this crime, which *is considered in this country as a light offence.**

It would be well if the abortionists could be rooted out of India by transportation; but, even were it possible to effect such a clearance, worse effects would follow, as their vile art would be taken up by less experienced and still ruder practitioners, who would slay more than the existing miscreants do. The only effectual cure for this evil would be a removal of the present restrictions upon widow re-marriage.

It is probable that the always credible report of "*died by snake-bite*" covers many atrocities of this kind. This was attempted, but failed, in a case tried at Tipperah in 1857.†

Are drugs occasionally given with the intention of killing the mother as well as the child?

This is a difficult question, but cases from time to time occur in which I consider that it might be properly entertained.

In 1858, Allabux, of Purneah, was sentenced to death for murdering the widow of his brother while in a state of pregnancy. He confessed, in a very circumstantial manner, that he administered drugs for the purpose of causing abortion. These failing, he and others took her to a river bank and murdered her by cutting her throat. "Husnah with one hand put a cloth in her mouth, and with the other pressed her head down; and Halol, with the knife, got on her bosom. Enait and Khedjerbux held her arms. Halol told me to come, and said, '*Let us all do this, that no one may tell against another!*' So all seized her, and Halol, placing the knife at her throat, said, 'All of you press my hand.' We all put our hands on his, and he pressed the knife in. Hassin turned to the other side, and they cut her throat on that side too."‡

Cases have already been cited in which Arsenic was given, in deadly doses, with the alleged intention that it should act as an abortive, to pregnant women—*vide supra*, pp. 116 and 718.

All things considered, I suspect that, in some of these cases, those con-

---

* Nizamut Adawlut Reports, May 29, 1855, p. 620.

† *Ibid*, February 14, 1857, p. 162.

‡ *Ibid*, June 15, 1858, p. 238.

cerned do not care much to measure the strength of the means by which abortion is effected. If the disgraced women dies, all the better ;—they are released, at once, from a stigma and from a burthen.

Writing in 1815, Mr. Tytler, who had been Assistant Judge in the 24-Pergunnahs (South of Calcutta), said : " How often do we see the father murder his daughter, on discovering the intrigue, or the daughter murder the child ! Such intrigues are only disgraceful when the story becomes public ; and, as the publicity throws a stigma on the whole family, any member, by getting rid of the obnoxious person, thinks he does a meritorious action. Thus one murder is not always sufficient." (Vol. I., p. 220.)

In a case tried at Tipperah in 1857, it appeared that a young and healthy Hindu widow became pregnant by her sister's husband. Her father and mother had recourse to one Mussamut Joymallah, who gave her *a piece of a root called chitta and some arsenic,* which they mixed and administered to the deceased. No result following, they, four days afterwards, applied to the prisoner Mussamut Dyonee, who supplied them with a minute pill of *mercury,* which was given to the deceased to swallow, and subsequently applied a piece of the *Lall Chitra* root (called by the hag "*bun polia*") to the vagina, the speedy results of which were a flow of blood and expulsion of the fœtus. The deceased died on the fourth day after this cruel operation. Dr. Davis found a portion of *Lall Chitra* root in the neck of the womb.

In this case the administration of Arsenic, although in a small quantity, appears to me a very suspicious circumstance ; and, in addition to this, we find that the *Lall Chitra root* was left for four days in the womb (a measure which the hag must have known to be certainly fatal). I think there can scarcely be a doubt that the murder of the mother was intended.*

Dr. Taylor has laid down the principle that medicinal substances rarely answer the purpose of inducing abortion ; and that, when this result is obtained, it is generally at the expense of the life of the mother. He adds that mineral poisons have been ignorantly employed for this nefarious object, such as arsenic, corrosive sublimate, sulphate of copper, muriate of iron, and other irritants (p. 782).

It, of course, rests with the Judge to decide whether an act of this kind is done in ignorance, or with homicidal intent ; but, under any circumstances, the act of giving a woman any *known poison,* in sufficient quantity to kill her or to endanger her life, for the purpose of making her abort, must always carry with it violent suspicion of homicidal malice.

The following may be taken as an example of the cruel, if not intentionally murderous, recklessness with which this crime is sometimes perpetrated :—

---

* Nizamut Adawlut Reports, December 5, 1857, p. 447.

Bhyrubchunder Surmah, of Tipperah, entertained for eight years a connexion with a widow, with the full knowledge and sanction of her brother, in whose house she lived. The brother was, consequently, excluded from the village *Sumaj*. It is asserted that she escaped pregnancy in consequence of this long intercourse, until latterly.* When the fact became evident, Bhyrubchunder desired the brother not to be uneasy, but to leave the matter to him. He came to the house accompanied by two females, considered adepts in the act of procuring abortion. One of them gave some drugs. The effect of these not being speedily apparent, the other inserted *chitta* root. The consequence was great disturbance of the system, but the fœtus was not expelled. Some four-and-twenty hours later, Bhyrubchunder had recourse himself to manual violence. He appears to have "inserted his hand into the unfortunate woman's womb with such disregard of consequences as actually to break through the fundus, admitting the hand into the abdomen." He is stated to have thus succeeded in extracting the fœtus (the woman being in the fourth month of gestation). She died on the second day.†

It is worthy of remark that, in this country, *women not unfrequently induce premature confinement when they have nearly advanced to their full period*, and when the child is viable.‡ This is a crime which the medical jurists of Europe appear scarcely to have taken into account. In this country, its commission is, doubtless, generally attributable to a desire on the part of the criminals to anticipate discovery even by a week or two. In other instances, the cause may be attributed to gross ignorance or to miscalculation. It is to be feared that there is yet another set of cases in which delivery is hastened with a determination that the infant shall die in the birth.

In his *Statistics of Unnatural Deaths in the Madras and other Presidencies*, Dr. Muir observes: "The most violent mechanical and medicinal measures are resorted to, to destroy the child before or after it is born, and a class of women exist everywhere who are at all times ready and willing to effect the desired purpose."

A Mussalmaun woman was sentenced to perpetual imprisonment, at Bareilly, in 1851, for having been accessory to the death of her illegitimate child. She stated that she had been delivered prematurely, in consequence

---

* In a case tried at Midnapore in 1858, a widow had been married by the form of *Kuntee buddul*, or interchange of necklaces, the custom among the class called Bustom, upon an understanding that her family *had taken means to cause her barrenness.* When she became pregnant by her husband, his father compelled her to take abortives, which caused her death. (Nizamut Adawlut Reports of July 6th of the above year, p. 297.) I have heard it repeatedly asserted that, whenever illicit connexions occur between Europeans and the women of Assam, they are unfertile. For a note on the use of the *Lunka Seej* and *Surbujala*, for the purpose of preventing conception, see pp. 715 and 721.

† Nizamut Adawlut Reports, Feb. 28, 1856, p. 515.

‡ See a remarkable case, Nizamut Adawlut Reports, Vol. III., p. 269.

of means employed to procure abortion, and that the child, when it began to cry, was choked ; she could not say by whom. The witnesses concurred in stating that she had nearly reached her full time. A native doctor saw the body about ten days after death, and stated, perhaps somewhat rashly, that he supposed, from its appearance, that it had been born alive.*

In January 1854, one Mussamut Petai and her paramour were sentenced, at Cuttack, the first to death, the other to seven years' imprisonment, on their own confession, for having murdered the fruit of their illicit intercourse, a male infant born at the seventh month (the mother having taken medicine to procure abortion), by squeezing its neck.†

The Reports for 1854 contain a remarkable but very perplexed case, in which it, however, appeared very probable that a woman, having arrived at the full period of pregnancy, went to a midwife to have labor induced by artificial means ; that this was effected "*by pressure;*" and that the child was afterwards thrown into a well, with the secundines attached. The Sessions Judge found the mother and the nurse guilty, but they were acquitted by the higher Court.‡

The thannadar of Gohunna (Rohtuck) having heard a report that Mussamut Keesar, a widow, had caused abortion, obtained leave from the Magistrate to investigate the case. The woman, when examined by midwives, exhibited evident signs of recent parturition ; and, at last, admitted that she had been pregnant by her sister's husband, and had had a miscarriage. Search was made, which resulted in the discovery of a *placenta*, buried in the house : this the midwives declared to be the appendage of a child which had gone through the full period of utero-gestation ; whereupon the prisoner freely confessed that the child had been born alive, and was buried by her to conceal her shame. The native doctor examined the body superficially; the head was split, and the eyes and ears filled with earth. He did not open the body, and could not state positively whether the child was born alive or not ; but, judging from its perfect structure, he was of opinion that it was born alive at the full period.§

Two women of Sarun were committed on a charge of procuring abortion, and it would seem, from the admissions made by one of them, that they really tried and intended to commit this crime. It was, however, stated most clearly by the Civil Surgeon that "abortion" did not take place ; that the child was born at the full time, perfectly formed, healthy and strong, but that it died afterwards, either from accident or violence of some kind applied to it." It appeared that the woman, having become

---

* Nizamut Adawlut Reports, N. W. P., Vol. I., p. 152.
† Nizamut Adawlut Reports, Vol. IV., p. 1.
‡ *Ibid*, p. 495.
§ Nizamut Adawlut Reports, N. W. P., March 16th, 1854, p. 273.

pregnant in the absence of her husband, and being annoyed by the remarks, &c., made on the subject, consented to take some drugs, and also to allow the women to apply *pressure* to her abdomen, in order to destroy or remove the fætus in her womb. A witness deposed to having seen one of the prisoners rubbing the woman's stomach, and she confessed that she had taken drugs to procure abortion. It is not shown, in the printed report, upon what demonstrative evidence the Civil Surgeon proved that the woman had not "aborted" (or rather had not been prematurely delivered) by mechanical means; nor is it easy to conceive upon what grounds such a positive conviction could have been arrived at. The Judges of both Courts concurred in deciding, apparently upon the medical evidence, that the crime was not completed, but that the attempt involved criminality.*

It was stated in the *Pioneer*, in September 1867, that a strong check having been placed by our law upon the actual murder of infant children in Rajpootana, it has now become usual to consult an astrologer in the earliest months of pregnancy; and, if it be decided that the child is a girl, to proceed to abortion.

The adoption of proper measures for the check of this atrocity appears always to have been a question of great difficulty, and the action which we have taken appears to have vacillated between non-intervention and over-inquisitiveness.

The notorious prevalence of this practice appears to have led, formerly, to much undue interference on the part of the Police. It was, therefore, ordered that "Police officers inquiring into any charges of Abortion unattended by death, unless expressly ordered to do so by the Magistrates, shall be liable to fine and dismissal."†

It cannot be doubted that, but for a rule of this kind, much inquisitorial tyranny and false accusation might be practised. A strong illustration of this came before me in 1850. On being requested to examine some matters alleged to have been used to procure Abortion, I found them to consist of a scrap of plantain leaf, and a leaf of the jack-tree (*artocarpus integrifolia*) smeared with office ink in such quantities that I dissolved it off, and used it at the commencement of my letter, reporting that a fraud had been attempted.

The *Dacca Prokash* for September 15, 1865, has an article on the difficulty of checking the crime of criminal abortion, which arises from the want of jurisdiction of the Police. The Police will not even receive information regarding that crime, much less interfere with the perpetration of it. Information must be given to the Magistrate; but this rule is

---

* Nizamut Adawlut Reports, October 24th, 1853, p. 702.

† Regulation XXII. of 1816, Section 22; C. O., No. 303, December 31st, 1824; Regulation XXII. of 1817, Sections 12, 13. See an important case bearing upon this point—Macnaghten, Vol. I., p. 349.

tantamount to a prohibition, on account of the many objections, well-grounded or imaginary, which deter people from resorting to a Magistrate for such a purpose.

Writing in 1861, Dr. Shortt mentions that the following rule was then in force in Madras:—

"The Police shall be strictly prohibited from adopting any measures whatever against females, accused or suspected of having procured their own miscarriage, unless there shall have been actually found a fœtus fully formed, without which no charge of causing miscarriage, by whomsoever preferred, shall be entertained." Proceedings of Fouzdaree Adawlut, dated 15th July 1847.

Doubtless, over-diligence on the part of the Police and others in merely suspicious cases of this kind tends to aggravate the evil which it is intended to check. When in the Sylhet district in 1866, I had the advantage of a very interesting conversation on this subject with the Hon'ble Elphinstone Jackson, Judge of the Calcutta High Court. Mr. Jackson mentioned to me a case in which, a policeman having reported that a woman, who ought not to have been so, was pregnant, criminal abortion was had recourse to, it appearing to the culprits to be the most feasible mode of invalidating the charge. Mr. Jackson found that a very respectable and sensible zemindar, with a view to prevent the crime of procuring abortion, invariably reported instances of illegitimate pregnancy occurring in his place. The zemindar was told, "Your precaution has the greatest possible tendency to force people, by intimidation, into attempting the crime which you are anxious to prevent."

A case which strongly displayed the danger of the interference objected to by Mr. Elphinstone Jackson occurred at Midnapore in 1857. The following is an abstract from the remarks of the Sessions Judge:—On the 14th July last, one Modon Mullick informed Sakir Meer, the phareedar of Brindabun Chuck, that Jutee Bewah was three or four months gone with child. The phareedar proceeded to the male prisoner's abode at Brindabun Chuck, and demanded the production of the woman. He then reported to the darogah their refusal to comply with his order, and his own suspicion that they intended to make the woman abort. The darogah, on this, issued an order to Boro Mudoo Singh, burkundaz of pharee Shumgunge, and Jadhoo Kotal, to bring the principal men of the village to him. Boro Mudoo Singh swears that he never saw this order; Jadhoo Kotal appears alone to have executed it, and to have taken six persons, including the male prisoners, on the 22nd of July, to the darogah, before whom they executed an agreement to produce the woman in four days; but nothing of all this was reported to the Magistrate. On the 28th July, Sakir Meer again brought the matter to the notice of the darogah, who issued another order to Boro Mudoo Singh, the burkundaz, to find the woman. He seems to have overlooked that his first order was executed by Jadhoo Kotal alone, and that the burkundaz had taken no notice of it. On the 4th August, after a further lapse of eight days, the burkundaz reported his having heard from Kanto Dullye, prisoner No. 6, that Jutee had died, and that her body had been thrown into the river, by order of the principal men of the village. All these proceedings were, no doubt, illegal and against expressed injunctions. The darogah should immediately have taken orders from the Magistrate how to proceed, but he made no report whatever until the 6th August. On that day, the darogah arrived at the village of Brindabun Chuck, and found the four prisoners in the custody of the burkundaz. The female prisoner (who kept a stock of drugs for the practice of abortion) admitted having administered medicine to the deceased, and the others to having thrown her body into the river.

These wretched people, distressed and thoroughly alarmed by inefficient Police pressure, and having nearly three weeks allowed them to arrange matters in, were goaded into the adoption of that fatal measure which it was the object of the Police enquiry to prevent.

Criminal Abortion in Madras.

Dr. John Shortt has published two cases, with observations, which throw some light upon the practice of Criminal Abortion as it prevails in the *Madras Presidency*.* He observes :—" So long as early marriages and the objection to the re-marriage of widows continue to exist under the toleration of caste, fœticide will continue rampant in Southern India. The moral iniquity of this crime is considered unequal to the inflexibility of caste, or to the attendant disgrace thus entailed on the family. To cloak the failings of erring women, trampled down by caste ties and prejudices, relatives and connexions either assist or connive at criminal abortion, which appears to have no place either in their religion or morals. The guilty individual, to avoid the exposure of the birth of a child, and the consequent expulsion from caste, which, in every instance, is rigorously carried out by her own family and friends, is glad to have recourse to any measure that would save her from such consequences."

Dr. Shortt remarks upon the use of *Plumbago Zeylandica*, or *chittra moolum*, that " it is a universal remedy in dysmenorrhœa, and equally so as a means of producing abortion ; there is, perhaps, scarcely a village in India where the use of this drug, as such, is not known. Its action is that of a powerful irritant ; it is not only had recourse to as an internal remedy, but is more frequently applied externally." The following case from this paper is very interesting, as showing the manner in which some women escape with life after having aborted from the *lall chittra* treatment :—

* Fœticide, Madras Quart. Jour. of Med. Science, July 1861, p. 262.

Rungam, female, *ætat* seventeen, Gentoo caste, 23rd May 1861, complains of distension and pain in the breasts and region of the uterus. Is scarcely able to walk; countenance pale and expressive of pain and debility; eyes sunk; pulse excited, 98; tongue thickly furred; skin hot and dry; urine scanty, high-colored, and scalding; bowels confined; breasts hard and knotty, pressure causing a ready flow of milk. The external organs of generation and vagina were found moist and relaxed, os uteri open and admitting three fingers, lips tumefied and gaping, lochial discharge present. Os uteri and uterine region extremely tender and painful to the touch. With some reluctance at first, and slight prevarication subsequently, the patient gave the following account of herself:—She was married when five years old, and in her ninth year became a widow. Five days previously to her admission, a plug made of some medicine, the composition of which she does not know, was introduced into the vagina by a Barber woman, and retained there for two days, without producing any effect, except some smarting. On the third morning, an old woman of the "Vellaichee" caste was called in. She brought the leaves and root of "*chittra moolum*" (*Plumbago Zeylandica*) in equal quantities, which were made into a mass, and a bolus of about half a pullum (half an ounce) in weight was given her to take *internally*, which she did. About six hours after, on going to a tank to wash some clothes, she felt some pain in the abdomen, soon followed by some discharge per vaginam, which was at first blood, but was afterwards of a pale color. She was troubled by pains until the next morning, when she was delivered of a premature fœtus, which she believes she had carried for about five and-a-half months. She continued to improve under treatment for metritis, and was discharged cured on the 5th June.

Baboo Koylas Chunder Chatterjea informed me that he has met with instances in which women escaped after *Lall Chitra* Abortion, but with the gravest consequences,—peritonitis, hœmorrhage, and discharge continued for months.

The following important information, regarding the drugs used as abortives in the Madras Presidency, has been contributed by Second Dresser Mooneesawmy*:—Moothee, *ætat* thirty-six, caste Pariah, a widow, and mother of seven children, was sent to undergo medical examination when in custody on a charge of criminal Abortion. There were evidences of recent delivery. There was "felt a hard substance, lying flat in the bottom of the uterus, shaped like the letter V, with its angle directed forwards. This, on extraction, was found to be a piece of stick, the mid rib of a cocoanut-leaflet, five inches in length, a quarter of an inch in circumference, with a piece of white rag wrapped round it at one end, and partially broken in the middle. She admitted that, having been frequently annoyed

* Madras Quart. Jour. of Med. Science, January 1st, 1863, p. 205.

by her relations as to her unchastity, she determined to cause Abortion, and had recourse to the acrid juice of milk hedge, *Euphorbia Tirucalli,* in which was soaked the rag, which being wrapped round the stick, was introduced into the uterus by herself (?) She afterwards admitted that, after the failure of *Chittra moolum* and *Garlic,* which she said were commonly used by the natives to procure Abortion, she had recourse to milk hedge. Three or four hours after the introduction of the prepared stick, she experienced a burning sensation and heat in the uterus ; subsequently she became feverish and somewhat delirious ; about nine hours afterwards she gave birth to a still-born fœtus of about six months. This was brought to the dispensary.

The writer adds that this *Euphorbia Tirucalli,* known as *Kullipaul* in Tamil, is considered by the natives as most powerful in its effects, from the acrid properties of its juice. He is also told by some native doctors that several other species of *Euphorbia,* such as *E. Antiquorum* (*Sathara-cally*) and *E. Tortilis* (*Theeroogoocully*) have also the same effects.

Criminal Abortion in Bombay.

For a case in which death was probably caused by Abortion, induced by acrid vegetable purgatives or emetics, aided by direct pressure on the womb, see Bellasis' Reports, p. 99. This case is of great legal importance, as ruling the course to be pursued where a Roman Catholic priest refuses to disclose a death-bed confession, without a dispensation from his Bishop. Dr. H. J. Carter remarked, in 1859,* that the fact that Abortion is produced in Bombay by the introduction of instruments into the uterus is well known. In examining a woman who had been delivered of a seven months' fœtus, he found in the vagina a bamboo stick, six inches long, and one-eighth of an inch broad, which projected into the womb. It was armed, at one end, by a dossil of cotton. He considered that it might have been so inserted by the woman herself, but, being so high up, it could not be withdrawn by her alone. It had fallen into such a transverse position, that it was impossible for a person unacquainted with the relation of the parts to remove it without considerable violence, which, he supposed, with the difficulty in reaching it, was the reason why it was left there.

He gives another case, also of Abortion at the seventh month, in which the nurse of the Midwifery Hospital removed from the vagina a stick about four inches long, bound round throughout with cotton and thread, and coated at one end with *red lead.* There was also brought before the Magistrate a bundle containing three or four other sticks of the same kind, similarly bound round with cotton, &c., which had been found in the woman's house. In a third case the instrument produced, as that with which the Abortion was effected, was a straight piece of a small branch

---

* Bombay Med. and Phys. Trans., No. 4, N. S., Appendix, p. ix.

of *oleander*, about the size of the piece of bamboo mentioned in the first case, but without any arming of lint, and with one end (on which were stains of blood) just as it had been broken off from the continuation of the branch.

Mr. F. Broughton, Civil Surgeon of Kolapore, relates* the case of a Barber's widow, aged fifty, the mother of seven children, who, having "lost her husband, her teeth, and her income," formed an intimacy with a neighbouring goldsmith, of which pregnancy was the unexpected and undesired result. Measures were adopted, and a five months' fœtus, was expelled. Slight hœmorrhage, but considerable pain, followed. Symptoms of peritonitis set in, and she was sent to hospital, at a distance of fifteen miles, arriving almost in *articulo mortis*, on the tenth day after delivery. *Post-mortem* examination revealed general and most intense acute peritonitis. Upon lifting up the inflamed and adherent bowels, some difficulty was experienced in exposing the uterus, and the hand came in contact with a rod which, passing through its fundus, projected three inches into the bowels, which were lacerated and hanging upon its extremity. The other and broken end occasioned an abrasion of the internal membrane, which, at one spot, had proceeded to ulceration. To this was attributed the intense pain experienced in the uterus. This organ was firm and tolerably contracted, and would appear to have been more passive under such fearful injury than the intestines were. Still the bowels were said to have acted. The instrument was a stick or twig, similar to that generally used by natives for cleaning their teeth.

Mr. Broughton states that Abortion is frequently produced in that part of India, by the introduction of long skewers into the uterus. These rods are not intended to rupture the membranes, or injure the fœtus, but are tipped with cotton, and smeared with *euphorbium*, *lead*, or *mercury*. Such irritants, carefully introduced, readily excite uterine action, the fœtus is soon expelled, and the mother does not seem, as a general rule, to suffer any permanent injury. It has occurred to him to see many such cases, extending over a lengthened period, but this was the first which had terminated fatally. He adds,—"I am inclined to attribute the result in this case to accident, the stick probably breaking off in consequence of some convulsive movement of the patient; otherwise we must suppose most cruel violence on the part of the operator. There is yet another way in which it may be accounted for. The instrument may have been clumsily introduced, either by the woman herself, or by others, and broken off, and the perforation may have been caused by the contraction of the uterus upon its point after the birth. I am inclined to the latter supposition, and the more especially as the unfortunate woman concealed

---

* Bombay Med. and Phys. Trans., No. 3, N. S., Appendix, p. vi.

the fact of mechanical means having been resorted to, although she admitted having taken medicines, with a view to the production of abortion."

Laws.

The laws prohibitory of Criminal Abortion in India are laid down in Sections 312 to 316 of the Indian Penal Code.

The older laws will be found in Beaufort's Digest of the Criminal Law, Second Edition, paras. 3951-52 ; 3989, 3990.

DELIVERY.

Several important questions bearing upon this subject arise, from time to time, in the Judicial Courts of India.

Dr. Tanner has related the case of a lady, *ætat* forty-two, pregnant for the first time, in which the fact was established that "a woman may conceive, may go to the full term of gestation, and may be in labor ten hours, without having any suspicion that she is pregnant."

Upon the publication of this, Dr. Shortt, then stationed at Chingleput, Madras, forwarded to the Obstetrical Society of London a somewhat similar case, the chief features of which are as follow :—

A. B., *ætat* forty, European, married in 1844, in India, where she has been residing for the last eleven years, has had two children, the last nine years before. She had been at first actively treated by the speculum and caustic, for inflammation of the womb ; and had likewise taken much medicine, with the idea of removing what was considered to be a dropsy of the abdomen. She was in entire ignorance of her pregnancy. The escape of a watery fluid for two days was considered as evidence of rupture of the ovarian cyst. At the end of two days, severe pains set in, for which she was directed by a surgeon to be placed in a warm hip-bath. Opiates were given. While in the hip-bath, however, delivery of a living mature child occurred, to the great surprise of the patient and her friends.*

Much unnecessary surprise has been expressed at the rapidity with which the women of India, in common with those of most other impoverished and barbarous races, appear to recover from their confinements, and go about their ordinary avocations. This, however, can scarcely be regarded as a national usage. According to Ward, the woman begins to attend to her family business about twenty-one days after delivery—several of the intermediate days being occupied in stated ceremonies. This appears to be the custom among those Hindus who are tolerably well off. According to Baboo Modusoodun Gupto, the Hindu women take a stimulating powder made of hot spices for six days after delivery. This gentleman

* Tanner on the Signs and Diseases of Pregnancy, 2nd ed., p. 42.

states that all women, except Brahminees, remain impure a month after delivery—being excluded from the rest of the family during that time in a separate hut. Brahminee women for twenty-one days. Baboo Prosonocoomar Tagore, however, says that Brahminee women remain impure for eleven days only.* According to Ward, if the child be a son, the mother remains unclean twenty-one days ; if a daughter, a month.

It is very different, however, with the majority of the poorer women, whom necessity compels to return as soon as possible to their domestic drudgery. Ward says that poor women, in the northern parts of Bengal, are known to attend to the business of their families the day after delivery. He was informed that, sometimes, a mother is delivered while at work in the field, when she carries the child home in her arms, and returns to her work there the next day. These deplorable facts, however, have many parallels even in England, especially in cases where the unhappy female conceals the fact of her delivery. They result from the extreme wretchedness, not from the unusual robustness or constitutional vigor of the people ; and the consequence is shown in the dangers which beset the recovery of native women from confinement, and in the rapidity with which old age and infirmity invariably come upon these unfortunates. One of the most pitiable facts in the entire history of campaigning is that, given in the "Recollections of the Rifleman Harris," of an Irishwoman, named M'Guire, "a ghastly picture of illness, misery, and fatigue," who, in the terrible retreat to Corunna, stepped forth from the crowd, and lay down upon the snow, brought forth an infant, and was then seen in the rear of the party hurrying after them, carrying in her arms the babe she had just given birth to. She and her husband managed to carry the infant to the end of the retreat, and to embark. Harris afterwards saw the boy a strong and healthy lad.

Many old writers on the North American Indians speak of that which they regarded as their power of rapid recovery from child-bearing. Of the Indians of Brazil, a writer, quoted by Purchas, says :—"The women, when they are delivered, doe presently goe and wash themselves in the rivers." Another authority says :—"Ordinarily their travail is not so extreme as in our parts of the world, they being of a more hardie nature ; for, on the third day after childe-birth, I have seene the mother with the infant, upon a small occasion, in cold weather, in a boat upon the sea."†

A recent writer, in describing the fine race of fisher-people, of Danish origin, who inhabit the Lowland coasts of Scotland,—Newhaven, &c.,—says that he has been told by an able and intelligent medical man, that the women are so strong that, after child-birth, they are about again in three or four days. Native women generally leave the midwifery

---

* Pathologica Indica, p. 336.

† *Op. Cit.*, Vol. IV., pp. 1291 and 1868.

wards of the Calcutta Medical College Hospital on the eighth day after delivery. According to Baboo M. Gupto :—" In two, three, four, or five days" [after delivery] " the mother generally gets fever, that is fatal without proper treatment." He adds that three or four women out of twenty die of fever and tetanus, in from six to ten days after parturition.* I have long been decidedly of opinion that much of the ill-health from which European ladies in India suffer arises from imprudence in getting up and driving out some seven to ten days after their confinement. The recumbent position ought to be strictly preserved for from fifteen to twenty days.

The following instance of considerable exertion in a native woman after delivery, although remarkable, might be paralleled by numberless instances which have occurred in England. A Brahminee widow, being pregnant by a relative, went five miles from her home. Early next morning, she started to return, and had travelled two miles, when she was overtaken by labor pains, and was delivered of a male child, born at the full period of gestation. She left the child in the dry bed of the stream, and made her way back to the house she was visiting. She pleaded, at her trial for exposure of the infant, that she was in bad health at the time, and that bewilderment and pain so affected her senses as to make her unaware of what she was doing. The Judge held that the fact of her having come from her home, on foot, the day before, and being able to proceed so far as the nullah just before delivery, and to retrace her steps, unassisted, just after that event, was inconsistent with the idea of a weakly state of body, or with the existence of a tertian fever, which she alleged she had long suffered from.†

The midwives of this country are occasionally called upon to testify regarding the evidences of delivery, and give their professional opinions with the utmost confidence. A widow of Banda was tried, in 1853, upon a precedent which is to be found in the Decisions of the Sudder Nizamut Adawlut for December 1842, page 1541, in which the concealment of the birth of a new-born child is declared criminal and punishable by law. Six midwives deposed to the prisoner having been found, on the discovery of the dead body of the child, " with her breasts in such a state of lactation, as indicated that she had been lately delivered of a child, the milk exuding from them being of that stage and kind which is unfit for the immediate nutrition of the infant.‡ One of these midwives also deposed that her private parts were emitting blood. Their general

* Pathologica Indica, p. 336.

† Nizamut Adawlut Reports, N. W. P., July 16th, 1852, p. 683.

‡ See a case in which Mr. M. Adam decided a medico-legal question by finding Colostrum Granules in the milk of a woman four or five weeks after delivery.—*Monthly Journal of Medical Science*, May 1853, p. 474.

statements showed that the prisoner, at first, refused to have her person examined, and only submitted on compulsion."*

This question of ***Compulsory Examination*** is beset with some difficulty. In cases involving very grave criminal charges, and especially in those of infanticide, examination becomes a matter of legal necessity. Women in India are generally much opposed to this ordeal, and occasionally give the medical man considerable trouble. In one case, the woman was so troublesome, that I was obliged to send for the Magistrate, upon whose assurance that, if she did not permit an examination, her complaint would be dismissed, she at length submitted. In this case, certain parties had been accused of employing brutal violence. The symptoms appeared to be very serious, and I considered it to be a matter of absolute necessity that the real amount of injury inflicted should be ascertained without delay. In cases where women have accused persons of having beaten them, &c., whereby abortion was occasioned, I have, after failing to persuade the women to submit to examination, reported their obstinacy to the Magistrate, who has dismissed the charge.

In a case where it was to become a question whether a certain woman had or had not ever brought forth a son, at the full period of child-bearing, I gave an opinion to the following effect,—That it is possible, although I had never seen or heard of such a case, that a virgin woman might present appearances which would create a doubt in the minds of experts as to whether she had not been a mother. On the other hand, having, fifteen years ago, published a work on Medical Jurisprudence, I have ever since had this and the like questions almost constantly before me, but I have never seen a case, and, what I consider of more weight, have never heard of, or, in my extensive reading, read a case in which a woman, who had been delivered at the full period, did not present any appearance whatever which would be recognised by experts as evidence of child-bearing or delivery. The most remarkable attempt to adduce such a case is that made by the late Dr. Montgomery (on Pregnancy, 2nd edition, p. 582), and cited by Dr. Guy in the third edition of his Forensic Medicine, p. 64 ; but this case entirely falls short of proof, seeing that " the lady never carried her children beyond the end of the eighth month." I added that I would not place implicit confidence in any one of the recognised signs of delivery, but I should rely upon the aggregate of these signs, or, to use Casper's words, in "the totality of these traces."

Montgomery lays great stress (p. 582) upon the case of Aimée Perdriat, but the evidence of this woman's delivery was only strongly circumstantial; and the entire absence, at the end of a month after her presumed delivery at the full term, of any signs whatever of such delivery, consti-

* Nizamut Adawlut Reports, N. W. P., December 26th, 1853, p. 1554.

tuted positive evidence that she had not been so delivered, and necessitated her acquittal.

In some cases of alleged abortion or delivery, the practice, common among native women, of suckling their children for several years may lead to some uncertainty.* Pregnancy frequently occurs during lactation among women of all races and classes in India. A native woman complained that she had been beaten by a certain person, and had aborted in consequence; her statement could not be regarded as less probable on account of the fact that she was suckling a strong child between three or four years old. She, however, refused to submit to examination, and collateral circumstances rendered it probable that the charge was false.

I do not find that any accurate statistics have been collected which would show *the average duration of the lochial discharge*—a point of considerable importance in questions of delivery. Taylor says merely that it "continues from a week to a fortnight, or even longer." Dr. Duncan Stewart has informed me that, in this country, it is not to be looked for after a fortnight or three weeks; my own far more limited experience would show that it is often present at a month or five weeks after delivery. Professor Wilson, Dr. Stewart's successor, has remarked that the lochia, or rather a sanguineous discharge, frequently *recur* at about a month after delivery. Dr. Wilson has observed the period of duration of the lochial discharge to be exceedingly various among women of all classes in this country. It is said occasionally to last from three weeks to a month in Europe, but he thinks this is less frequently the case in native women; and that, in natives, the discharge

---

* Ward says that a Hindu woman suckles her child, if she have only one, till it is five or six years old; and that it is not uncommon to see such children standing and drawing the mother's breast. Dr. De Crespigny mentions that, at Rutnagherry (Bombay Presidency), children are kept at the breast, often until they are three and four years of age, with a view to prevent pregnancy. Some years ago, a woman, born and brought up in India, but apparently of pure European blood, was admitted to my ward suffering from unmistakable evidences of starvation. This was due to her obstinate pertinacity in suckling a strong active girl of five. She ultimately sunk. Dr. Waring mentions that nothing is more calculated to excite surprise in the mind of a medical man, newly arrived in Burmah, than to witness the lengthened period to which lactation is carried, with apparent impunity, at least as far as the infant is concerned. No certain period is fixed, the general rule being to suckle one child, until the mother is several months advanced in pregnancy with her next; but even this rule is not strictly adhered to. He has, in more than one instance, seen two children—one a sturdy young urchin of five or six years old, and the other an infant of as many months—engaged in drawing sustenance from the mother at the same time. Three years is by no means an uncommon time at which to wean a child, but instances have come under his notice, of which notes were made at the time, in which lactation was prolonged to four years and six months, to five years, and to six years respectively; the last-mentioned varied the amusement of sucking by an occasional whiff of a cigar! This prolonged lactation does not appear to affect the child in any way—a finer set of children cannot be seen; but it tells wonderfully upon the constitution and outward appearance of the mother.—*Medical Notes on the Burmese*—Indian Annals of Medical Science, No. 1, October 1853, p. 97.

continues bloody for a shorter period than with Europeans. Here *very frequently* among Europeans and Eurasians, less frequently among natives, it has occurred to him to observe a return of the *red* lochial discharge about a month after confinement. Sometimes the discharge had continued more or less to this time, and then became bloody ; in other cases it had disappeared. So frequently has he observed this, that he is never surprised by it, and women themselves have sometimes spoken of the circumstance as the first return of the menstrual discharge after confinement, stating that it returned once after delivery, and then disappeared during lactation. He thinks it quite possible that this return of the red lochia at this period may depend on the greater amount of exercise which is then taken, and may not result from a menstrual molimen.

A few hundred accurate observations upon this question would be of considerable value.

The following case, involving the question of delivery, illustrates the extraordinary craft and audacity with which the natives of India often plan and effect their criminal designs. One Mussamut Janoo, a midwife of Hissar, being employed to attend a woman in her confinement, persuaded the unfortunate creature that the child of which she had been delivered was a monster with two heads, not fit to be looked at ; she afterwards said that it was dead, and that she would take it away and bury it. She accordingly went away. Next morning, the midwife's services being required, she was sent for. She excused herself from going, under pretence that she had herself just been delivered of a child. This improbable story excited suspicion, and the police were called in. She declared that the child was her own. This she also maintained at the trial. It, however, appeared, from the evidence of midwives who examined her shortly after the discovery of the child in her house, and also by the deposition of the Civil Surgeon, that she exhibited no signs of recent confinement. Several of the neighbours who were constantly in the habit of seeing her, deposed that she had not exhibited any outward signs of pregnancy. She did not attempt to prove how she had disposed of the body of the child, which she alleged died immediately after its birth. She was sentenced to imprisonment for seven years.*

The question of *Medical Responsibility in the Induction of Premature Labor* will be found ably discussed, in all its bearings, in Dr. Taylor's work.† A valuable paper on the Induction *of Premature Delivery as a Prophylactic Resource in Midwifery*, by Dr. T. Gaillard Thomas,‡ should also be consulted. It now appears to be generally held by medical jurists

---

* Nizamut Adawlut Reports, N. W. P., 26th April 1853, p. 588.

† Page 792.

‡ New York Medical Journal, February 1870; and Half-yearly Abstract of the Medical Sciences for January to June of the same year, p. 303.

that the induction of Abortion, at an early stage of pregnancy, is justifiable, where it is decided, upon sufficient grounds and competent authority, that delivery is not likely to take place naturally, or without seriously endangering the life of the woman; and there is a most important class of cases in which the induction of premature labor, as clearly distinguished from abortion, is to be resorted to after the child has become viable. The following cases deserve notice as displaying the results of an adherence to the opposite opinion in cases of extremity. A miserably deformed girl of seventeen underwent the Cæsarean operation by M. Lebleu, at the Dunkirk Hospital. She and her child both survived. Ten years subsequently, she informed M. Lebleu that she was three months *enceinte*, and earnestly desired that Abortion should be effected—a proceeding which she had been given to understand was common in Paris, whither she threatened to go, in the event of Dr. Lebleu's refusal. He replied that he was quite aware of the nature of all such proceedings, but that neither he nor any one in the world had the right to take the life of a fœtus in utero, which was as much deserving of care as herself, and that she must submit to a second Cæsarean section. She reluctantly consented, submitted to the operation, and died from hæmorrhage the following day.* There are cases on record, in which the Cæsarean section was successfully performed *twice*.† In the first of these, the woman died five days after a third operation. There is another, in which the mother and child were both saved by Mr. Stoltz (Lancet, December 8th, 1855). M. Stoltz considers that the second operation is not so dangerous as the first, as adhesions are usually formed which facilitate recovery. In a third case a woman twice suffered rupture of the uterus, and was twice relieved by the Cæsarean section.‡ A woman underwent this operation *thrice* with success.§ And, in still another instance, Dr. Michaelis, of Kiel, has reported a case in which he performed the operation for a *fourth* time successfully upon the same woman.‖ On the other hand, Dr. Goodman (cited by Taylor) has collected an account of thirty-eight of these operations performed in England since 1733. Out of this number, only three mothers recovered. In eighteen cases the children were extracted living. It would appear, however, that, in a considerable proportion of these cases, the women were dying when the operation was performed. The volume of Ranking's Retrospect, already cited, contains the details of fifteen of these

---

* Gaz. des Hôp.; and Ranking's Abstract, Vol. XXI., p. 196.

† Dr. Meriner's case—*Ibid*, p. 195.

‡ Ranking's Abstract, Vol. XXI., p. 196.

§ Brit. and Foreign Med. Rev., July 1836, p. 270, cited by Taylor.

‖ Plaff's *Mittheilungen*. Heft. vii-viii., 1836, and India Journal of Medical and Physical Science, Vol. III., for 1838, p. 442,—where it is suggested that, in cases of hopeless deformity of the pelvis, the Fallopian tubes should be divided during the Cæsarean operation;—not, however, an altogether safe proceeding, or one which would certainly prevent the occurrence of tubal pregnancy.

operations performed upon eleven females (*i. e.*, four of the women underwent the operation twice); the results were seven recoveries and eight deaths: none of these eleven women could be regarded as being in a dying state when the operation was performed.

Where we have to decide between the steps of inducing the expulsion of the fœtus at a more or less early period, calculated according to the nature and extent of the deformity or disease and the history and present condition of the patient, or of waiting to perform the Cæsarean section at the full period, we should, I think, unhesitatingly adopt the former course.

INFANTICIDE.

The murder of female children—whether by the direct employment of homicidal means, or by the more inhuman and not less certain measures of exposure, privation, and neglect—has, for ages, been the chief and most characteristic crime of six-sevenths of the inhabitants of British India. Throughout that portion of the country usually known as Central India, and especially in Rajputana, in Cutch Bhooj, in the province of Agra and in Khondistan, the destruction of female children has prevailed in all historic times. Bengal Proper, or the Delta of the Ganges, appears now to be comparatively free from this scourge, but the Bengalees were only prevented by a stringent law from thinning their surplus population by throwing their children to the alligators at the mouths of the Ganges.* It has lately been suggested in a native paper that, in Koolin families, female children are systematically neglected, and that few grow up. For note on the prevalence of criminal abortion among Koolin Brahmins, see page 712. Polyandry still obtains among the Kasias,—Hill-people near Sylhet. Wherever this custom prevails, as among the Khonds and in the Neilgherry Hills, it points demonstratively to the practice of Female Infanticide. Beyond all this, the wilful neglect of female children operates destructively in every town and village throughout the length and breadth of India. By the Hindu, the advent of a female child is superstitiously regarded as a curse, and is practically viewed as a tax and a misfortune. The daughter—so welcome in the English peasant's homestead, so fondly greeted as the crowning honor and presiding grace of every European family of gentle blood—is viewed, alike by the Hindustani Rayut and the Rajput Thakoor, as a certain presage either of poverty or of shame hereafter. The daughter of the Hindu must always be dependent upon others for her support;† she must be suitably married, and a

---

* See Beaufort, p. 535, para. 2889.

† "In infancy, her father should guard her; in youth, her husband should guard her; and in old age, her children should guard her; for, at no time, is a woman fit to be trusted with liberty."—*Hitopodesa.* This is an almost literal quotation from Menu, who adds—"By a girl, or by a young woman, or by a woman advanced in years, nothing must be done, even in her own dwelling-place, according to her mere pleasure."—C. v., S. 147.

crime will be involved in the postponement of her nuptials beyond the age of childhood.* At her husband's death, she must trust wholly to the support of others; and her conduct must be watched with unceasing vigilance, lest shame, with all its direst accompaniments, feud, revenge, and murder, should be entailed upon her house.†

The results of this condition of things may be set forth in a single paragraph. It is clearly established that, in every country in Europe,

---

* "He who takes to wife a damsel of full age, shall not give a nuptial present to her father; since the father lost his dominion over her by detaining her at a time when she might have been a parent.—*Menu*, Chap. ix., S. 93.

It was reported in one of the native papers in May 1868 that a girl thirteen or fourteen years old had hanged herself. It was suggested that she had probably done so in disappointment at not being married.

† A multitude of painful instances might be cited in illustration of the deadly certainty with which the people of this country punish offences against the chastity of their women. Ward mentions that a Rajput of Loodhiana, having been induced by the tears of his wife to spare the life of a daughter born to him, the daughter grew up and had arrived at the age of thirteen, but had not been demanded in marriage by any one. He began to apprehend the danger of her bringing disgrace upon the family, and resolved to prevent it by putting the girl to death. Shortly after forming this atrocious resolve, he either overheard, or pretended to have overheard, some of his neighbours speaking of his daughter in a way that tended to increase his fears, when, becoming outrageous, he rushed upon the poor girl and cut her head off. A Hindu of Mynpoorie seduced the daughter of a Brahmin who had a previous feud with his family. The injured father, finding that his daughter was pregnant, brought her out of the house at night, when all were asleep, and killed her by two sword cuts;—then, rushing with a relation of his into the seducer's house, they killed him and his father, and hacked three others very severely. They were arrested near the spot with the bloody swords in their hands. They exclaimed that they had killed their enemies, and made no attempt to escape or to resist.—Nizamut Adawlut Reports, N. W. P., July 1st, 1852, p. 613. One Badee, of Futtehpore, having learned that his niece, a Brahminee girl, aged about nineteen or twenty years, had intrigued with a Sonar, at once seized the woman's hair, dragged her to the house of the seducer's uncle, and there with a bill, or *gurasa*, killed her with two blows on the neck, and remained near the body of his victim till apprehended by the Police.—*Ibid*, December 22nd, 1853, p. 1538. Neither are such instances of retribution by any means rare in Bengal. It appeared, in a trial at East Burdwan, that a servant in the employ of one Puresh Mullicki, having contracted an intimacy with his master's sister, who was a widow, was discharged for his presumption in aspiring to the favor of one so infinitely his superior. She followed him to his house, and a *nika* marriage was the result, to the unmitigated and undisguised disgust of the woman's family. About twenty days after the consummation of the marriage, the brother, with several of his people, burst, at midnight, into the house of the unfortunate couple. The brother desired one of his party to kill the woman, who was immediately seized and literally hewn to pieces with an axe.—Nizamut Adawlut Reports, November 17th, 1854, p. 604. A host of examples, already cited in these pages, must be taken as proof that there is but little relenting in the calm, vindictive, unsparing nature of the even-tempered, soft-mannered Bengalee. Instances of implacable, unwearying hatred, might be cited, from the pages of the criminal reports of Bengal, which would scarcely be paralleled by any records of Italian vengeance. One will suffice here. In 1846, a Hooghly man confessed that he had murdered a person with whom he was at bitter enmity. He displayed in his statement the utmost hatred against him, declared that the deceased had turned him out of his situation, and then stripped him of all his property; and described how, *day after day, for four months*, he had traced his victim until he met with the opportunity of making away with him!—Police Reports, L. P., 1846, p. 72.

there is an excess of females. The census of 1851 showed that, throughout Great Britain and Ireland, the number of males then amounted to only 48·2 of the inhabitants. The first census of the North-West Provinces of India, in 1863, gave 53·4 as the percentage of males in a population of 30,271,885; while the official census of Mysore, for 1852, showed that, in a population of 3,410,382, the number of adult males exceeded that of females by nearly ten per cent., while the excess of male infants was sixteen per cent.!

Invaluable aid is afforded to those engaged in investigating the subject of Female Infanticide Up-Country in the statistical researches of Mr. Allan O. Hume, C.B., which will be found at page 7 *et seq.* of Appendix C. to Mr. Plowden's General Report of the Census of the North-West Provinces in 1865. The following are a few only of the important results at which Mr. Hume has arrived. He shows that, in the Thakoor caste, 52,763 strong, there was a total of 10,695 *male*, and of only 5,865 *female* children. He writes—"We find that the high percentage of the Thakoors is almost solely due to the abnormal deficiency of female children. They have only two less boys per thousand than, as an average, we might expect to find; but, instead of 153 girls, they have only 111. Out of every thousand of the Thakoor population, there are at least 42 girls, below the age of 12, missing. Amongst the Aheers, again, the high percentage observable is *due partly* to a deficiency of girls, but principally to a superabundance of boys. They are a healthy, out-door living race, and they beget more children, and, I think, more males. Accordingly we find that they have 16 more *boys* and only 9 less *girls* per thousand than the normal average. On the other hand, the Bunneeas and Kaets, while they have about the same number of girls per thousand as the Aheers, have 45 less boys. A sedentary race, they probably beget less children and less males, and those they have are less healthy; with all their care (and they are generally fond of their children), they can only rear 177 boys and 143 girls, while the Aheers (some of whose tribes do certainly murder their girls) bring up 222 boys and 144 girls in every 1,000 of their race." Mr. Hume shows that there "is a yearly loss, or murder of 6½ per cent. more of Thakoor, and 2¼ per cent. of Aheer female infants, than of those of other Hindus." "Amongst all Hindus, and in a less degree amongst Mahomedans (*and I trust this may be particularly noticed*), the mothers and other female relatives take much less care of the female than of the male infants."

Among the Rajputs, it appears to be customary to destroy the infant immediately upon its birth. Sir John Shore found that the mothers of the Rajkumar infants simply starved them to death. Mr. Duncan states that "they killed their infant daughters, or allowed them to die, by denying them all sustenance from their birth."* Mr. Shakespear says that

* See the earlier laws for the control of this atrocity, Beaufort, p. 536, para. 2892.

"the infant is often strangled. Among the Rajputs in the Allahabad territory, the juice of the Mudar plant (*asclepias gigantea*) is usually administered. In the Gwalior districts, the new-born infant is ordinarily put to death by administering poison in the shape of a tobacco leaf, or that of the dhatoora plant ; but this object is said sometimes to be effected by violence." In the other Rajput States, opium is generally employed.* The report on Infanticide in the Agra district, published shortly before the appearance of my last edition, contains several allusions to the practice of poisoning infants with tobacco powder. In the "Punjab Papers on the Crime of Infanticide," Mr. (now Sir Robert) Montgomery mentions, in addition to the atrocities cited at p. 284 of this Report, that, during Hindu ascendancy, when Infanticide was considered no crime, the child was destroyed immediately after birth, by filling its mouth with cow-dung, or by immersing the head in cow's milk, or by drawing the secundines and umbilical cord over the face.

Dr. Kenneth McLeod has mentioned this last to me as a more recent practice. The father, sitting at his door, awaiting the event, is told by the midwife that a daughter has been born to him. His reply in the negative to the enquiry, "Shall the child be made clean?" is the signal for its destruction by this mode of suffocation.

Mr. Thomas Bacon says that, at Benares, female children were either formally sacrificed by the Brahmins in the temple of Ganesha, or they were destroyed in private "by what the Hindus call *drinking milk.* No sooner had the sex of the infant been ascertained, than a cauldron of warm milk was brought into the apartment where the mother lay, and, after prayers for the child's return in the form of a son, the little innocent was immersed in the milk, and held down until life became extinct, when it was carried to the Ganges, and thrown into the stream."

In May 1868, the *Deccan Herald* reports that a wretched creature, named Gunga, a Hindu, had been detected in burying the body of a newly-born infant, *whilst still alive*, beneath a heap of stones, near the Pilot Bunder, Bombay. In June 1870, a Mussulmaun widow of Bombay committed precisely the same crime.

In the Goojerat district, the practice, according to Sir R. Montgomery, is to bury the infant alive. The body is placed in an earthen pot, the top of which is covered with a thick paste of dough. In the Khangar district, the juice of the Mudar is administered ; or death is brought about by causing injury to the navel. According to the late Colonel Macpherson, the female infants of the Khonds are destroyed by exposure in the jungle ravines immediately after their birth.

We have, at present, no means of ascertaining the rates of natural mortality which prevail among native infants in the various districts of

---

* Calcutta Review, Vol I., p. 385.

India. It is, however, nearly certain that but a very small proportion of those born arrive at maturity.*

It appears that, except in those districts where Government employ agents for the express purpose of suppressing Infanticide, cases of systematic child-murder rarely come under investigation in Indian Courts, and the few which are tried are principally those in which the crime is perpetrated with a view to the concealment of illegitimate births.

I find only ten trials for Infanticide among the printed Reports of the higher Courts during a period of four years.†

In reading over the above passages, which remain nearly as they appeared in my edition of 1855, and considering the facts which have, within the last few months, come to light, evidencing the monstrous prevalence of Female Infanticide in India at the present moment, I am glad to find that I did not assume the conclusion that our legislation had swept the country of this social curse. Then, and almost ever since, however, there have been well-wishing philanthropists who have flattered themselves and others with the notion that we had fully succeeded in "stamping out" this evil. Thus I find, under date of the 23rd August 1855, a public journal, of the highest local authority, pronouncing, in a review of "Crime in the Punjaub," that "Mutilation has gone altogether; of Thuggee, only two cases occurred in 1854. *Infanticide has disappeared.*" So also I find an able official writer, whose opinion in this matter may not unfairly be taken as the opinion of many generally well-informed people in India two years ago, committing himself, so recently as 1868, to the assertion that "Thuggee in 1840, Suttee in 1847, Human Sacrifice of Merria, and Infanticide of Western and Central India in 1852, successively succumbed to Indian administration."

A curious and instructive chapter might be written on the "*Stamping out*" of crime in India. At present, the fact is that the flame of Sati, although practically well-nigh quenched, has still a never-dying spark; Road-poisoning lives as the representative of Thuggee; Human Sacrifice is a crime of to-day; and it is now perfectly clear that whatever was done twenty years ago for the suppression of Indian Infanticide must now be done, more validly, again.

The main facts of the movement at present in operation for the suppression of Female Infanticide are so fully before the public that they may

---

* Stewart mentions that it is related of Raja Maun Sing, who died in the Dekkan in 1615, that his Seraglio consisted of fifteen hundred women, by each of whom he had two or three children, all of whom died before their father, except his successor, Raja Bhao Sing. Admitting the probability that the Raja actually lost one hundred children, we may judge what rate of mortality must prevail in the bamboo huts and mud hovels of India, when death is so rife in the palace nurseries.

† Those of the Calcutta Court, from the commencement of 1851 up to April 1854, and those contained in the Reports of the Nizamut Adawlut of the N. W. Provinces.

be noticed with great brevity. Early in 1870, the Hon'ble Mr. Strachey introduced, in the Viceregal Legislative Council, a *Bill for the Prevention of Female Infanticide in India.* The Honorable Gentleman's remarks form an exhaustive history of the practice in mordern times. The following extract from his speech fully illustrates the present position of this question :—

"In 1846, the Jullundur Doab was annexed to the British Crown. He" [Mr. Raikes] "found the practice equally prevalent there. It was practised as frequently ; and other tribes, besides the Rajpoots, used to practise it. A meeting of the influential classes of the Rajpoot community, who boasted of being descendants of the Gooroo Nannuk, was held, and measures adopted to meet the evil. From that time till the mutiny, Mr. Unwin assumed that nothing had been done to mitigate it in Northern India. In 1856, an officer was appointed especially to investigate these facts. Mr. Moore was the officer selected. He personally visited and made himself acquainted with the facts that, in 26 out of 308 villages, in which the crime had been known to prevail, not a single girl under six years of age existed. In another batch of 38 villages which he visited, he found not a single girl ; he found marriage very rare, and in some instances unknown to have taken place within the recollection of the existing generation. In one instance there was not a single girl above six years of age, and there no marriages had taken place for a period of eighty years. In many parts of the Benares Division he also found that marriages had not taken place within the memory of the present generation. He says,—'Not only are there no girls to be found in their houses now, but there never have been, nor has any such event as the marriage of a daughter taken place for more than 200 years.' Mr. Unwin, in Mynpoory, found the same results. In 30 villages, he only found 37 daughters and 329 boys of the same age. And in 11 villages of that number, there were no daughters at all. Shortly after this, the mutiny broke out, in 1857, and, as may have been expected, the subject was lost sight of for some time. But on the restoration of order, the matter again attracted the attention of Government, who, on setting on foot enquiries, found that the custom was fearfully prevalent in Oude in particular, and measures to repress the evil were actively set on foot by Sir Charles Wingfield, with the cordial help of the Talookdars of the Province. Although, undoubtedly, in many parts of the country, a great deal has been done to check the crime, I fear there can be no doubt that the practice is, at the present time, as prevalent as ever. Only a year ago the Lieutenant-Governor of the North-Western Provinces, in conducting his investigations, expressed his opinion that care should be taken in making conclusions ; and I may say that the conclusions which were arrived at were mainly those I have just now given to the Council. He examined a group of 10 villages inhabited by Rajpoots, in 7 of which he found 104 boys, and only one girl ; and the people admitted that for ten years there had not been a single marriage. And in another group of 27 villages, he found that in 22 there were 284 boys and 23 girls. In 10 of these villages, marriage was unknown for a century. In another group of 16 villages, he found 4 only in which marriage existed; and in 9 other villages, he found 71 boys and only 7 girls. I need not continue these terrible illustrations of the prevalence of the crime. They are given on the highest authority, and the results would be actually incredible, if they were vouched for upon a less unimpeachable authority.* The causes which have led to the prevalence of this terrible crime, have already been generally shown in the passage of Mr. Thomason's Report, which I have just laid before the Council. I will read this passage from Mr. Raikes's book, which I think states very fairly what the real cause of this matter is. Mr. Raikes says,—and I need hardly say that there has been no higher authority in this country than Mr. Raikes, in one of the first and most successful offices he held,—to his practical mind, the most tangible, as well as the most powerful motive for the atrocity, appeared to be the system so generally prevalent of exorbitant marriage expenditure. His opinion, however, differed from that of Mr. Robinson as to the best mode of dealing with this evil. He was disposed to look more favorably upon the sumptuary measures which resulted from self-legislation, than in those originating in, and deriving their authority from, Government enactments. There is a necessity of marrying a daughter to a man of higher, or at least equal, means, among the high rank of Rajpoots, and the alternative personal degradation. The father of the marriageable daughter is looked upon with suspicion, with insult, and with reproach by the Hindus. Although this is not practically true of the higher ranks of Rajpoots, still there can be no doubt, I think, that these feelings of family honor have been at the root of this great evil. This is followed by the natural consequence that most extraordinary and ruinous expenditure has been incurred by the people at the marriage of their daughters, and this has been admitted on all hands to be one of the greatest incentives or causes of the crime. The marriage expenses are sometimes so enormous, that the marriage of a daughter brings ruin upon the whole family, and, owing to this circumstance, the Rajpoot father prefers his daughter to perish, rather than that he should be placed

---

* Lutfullah gives a striking illustration of the almost utter destruction of the females of a Hindu race to which this practice may lead, when he mentions that he found in Kach *twelve thousand Jarajas, of whom but thirty-seven were females.* He does not account for this, except upon the ground of Infanticide, but there was probably at work here an evil to which marked allusion was lately made in the *Delhi Gazette,—viz.*, the introduction of a system of concubinage with slave girls from families of lower caste. The writer points to an existing fact of great significance, that, among Thakoors in affluence, when a son is born the wife is frequently discarded, in the fear that the next issue may be a girl.

under the necessity of incurring expenditure for her dower.* After all, perhaps the real great reason of the prevalence of the crime at the present moment is custom—immemorial custom—which among Hindus is to be looked upon as transcendental law. And there can be no doubt that these people are given to murder their children, generation after generation, to a great extent, simply because their forefathers have done so before them ; and they do it, really, without any idea that there is anything criminal in the practice. As to the remedies to be applied to this great evil, we have fortunately no reason to doubt that they can be applied, because we have ample and actual experience to show us that the crime can be dealt with. The measures that have been taken have been of all kinds. The first kind of measures are those which aim at the removal of the causes which lead to the crime, and especially to prevent all that expenditure consequent upon a marriage. The second class of measures have been those of a coercive and practically preventive character. The first class of measures rests with the people themselves to apply ; the other, on the action of the Government. Both classes of measures, taken together, have been extremely successful, and the officer who has met with the greatest amount of success in inducing the Rajpoots to agree to limit their marriage expenses, was Mr. Raikes, at Mynpoory ; and there can be no

---

* A great deal has been written regarding the lavish costliness of Hindu marriages as bearing upon the question of Female Infanticide, but I have preserved the following report, as illustrating more forcibly than anything else that I have heard, the irrationality of this practice ; it is from the *Times of India*, December 13, 1866 :—

"At the sitting of the Insolvent Debtors Court recently, Pandoorunk Trimbuck, a man belonging to the Sepoy caste, applied for his discharge. His debts were Rs. 1,336-13-10, and his assets *nil*. The learned Commissioner (Sir Charles Sargent) asked for some explanations in reference to an item of Rs. 1,500 in the schedule for money expended on the marriage of the insolvent's daughter. His (insolvent's) income appeared to be Rs. 900 a-year only, and thus he had spent nearly two years' earnings on the wedding ceremony. The insolvent said his daughter had become of a marriageable age, that he had found it very difficult to find a husband for her, and therefore he had to spend a large sum of money on the ceremony; out of the money he had to present the husband with clothes and some cash. His Lordship granted the order for discharge."

The following appeared in the Calcutta *Englishman* of June 10th, 1870 :—"We read in the *Allyghur Gazette* how Moonshee Pyare Lall, moved with compassion for the thousands of female babes who are murdered by their parents to avoid the expenses contingent on their marriage, started from Calcutta in 1864, and travelled far and wide throughout the Upper Provinces, convening public meetings at three hundred different places, and by his earnest eloquence prevailing upon his hearers to prescribe a certain limit to expenditure at weddings. In at least sixty of these towns the standard agreed upon has been steadily maintained, and in many others a great improvement has been observed. Sir William Muir had good reason to say that Moonshee Pyare Lall 'deserves the thanks of the Government, and of the whole country.'"

In the investigation into the prevalence of Infanticide in the Punjab, which commenced in 1851, it was shown that one chief gave his daughter seventeen lacs of rupees, another expended ten lacs, a third gave a lac to his niece, married to a poor brahmin from the plains. "It is a question," said Herbert Edwards, "between the father's wealth and the daughter's life ; and the life is taken, and the wealth retained."

doubt that the measures which he initiated there, and which were afterwards followed up by his successor, have met with the greatest success in Oude and elsewhere. There can be no doubt that strong feelings exist among the people themselves in regard to the extravagance of the marriage expenses. And this has been found by experience to have been removed to some extent by bringing a small amount of pressure to bear upon them to limit the amount.* Still, there can be no doubt that the measures which have been most successful have been those of an actual coercing character. These measures, on this side of India, it will be recollected, were advocated by the gentlemen I have named ; and I can give an illustration of the success of them in a few facts. In the Mynpoory district, in 1842, there had been no Rajpoot Chohan girl living in the district. Nine years afterwards, in 1851, there were found to be 88 alive ; and in 1855, the number had risen to 250 girls. In the same year, in the Agra district, the measures taken by Mr. Gubbins gave in a very few years double the number of females then alive ; and the same thing may be proved everywhere where coercive measures have been taken. The measures have been of a very simple character. They consist mainly in the introduction, in the first instance, of a monthly system of registration of the births and deaths in suspected localities, and in the constant system of periodical inspection and examination of the children born. And it has been found, in practice, that this measure practically effects the saving of lives of children when they are just born. Experience has proved, in the most unmistakable way, that it is in the power of the Government to eradicate this frightful crime. Authorities in all parts of the country, without exception, have given their most decided opinion that it is not right, that it is not politic, that the measures taken for the prevention of crime should not be taken in a much more systematic way than anything which has been hitherto done

* The following sketch of Mr. Raikes's proceedings in Mynpoory appears in the *Indian Daily News* of June 30, 1870 :—" On the 12th November 1851, the Rajah and the chief Thakoors of his tribe met Mr. Raikes in conclave, and affixed their signatures to a set of rules having the abolition of the crime for their object. On the 5th December following, deputations of the chief Rajpoot clans in the districts of Mynpoory, Etawah, Agra, Furruckabad, and Puttialee met the Commissioner of the Agra Division, and solemnly adopted the resolutions of the meeting of the 12th November. The agreement was signed by 360 Chiefs, Thakoors, and headmen of villages, representing clans having marriage alliances with the Rajpoots of Oudh, Gwalior, Kerowlie, Jeypore, &c. Amongst the signatures were those of the Rajahs of Mynpoory, Rampore, and Pertabnair. The Mynpoory resolutions might well serve as a model in similar arrangements. They fixed the dower of a marriageable daughter at Rs. 500 for Rajahs and Talookdars ; Rs. 250 for Zemindars ; Rs. 100 for 'others in easy circumstances,' and *one rupee* 'for all other decent people.' If a girl's father chose to give more, well and good, but a persistence in a demand for more on the part of the youth's father, was to be followed by his being 'put out of our brotherhood.' The 'insolence of Brahmins and Bhats and Barbers,' as being 'a cause of needless profusion,' was to become a subject of complaint to the Magistrate. Lastly 'a moderate number of persons only' were to be invited to weddings."

in rooting out this evil. Legislation is absolutely required, I think. I need not now enter into the details of the Bill which I propose to introduce. It is sufficient now for me to say that the Bill proposes to give the Local Governments power to do that which has already been done in many parts of the country; and I may add that the Bill which I propose to introduce has been already sent to the Local Governments and Administrations, and that it has been substantially approved of by all of them. I think, my Lord, that the Council will agree with me when I say that a higher flight for legislation can hardly be mentioned. I think that the British Government has borne too long with this abomination, and I think that the time has come when the British Government should show to the world that it has finally resolved that these things shall cease. I have not for my part the slightest doubt that it is in our power to make an opportunity for interference."

A very remarkable illustration of the efficiency of judiciously-managed Police supervision in checking this crime is given in the Punjab Police Report for 1868.* The village of Raipoor, in the Umritsur district, had become so notorious for the commission of this crime that, in September, 1867, there were only eight girls to one hundred boys. A police force was quartered upon them for two years; and, in the next year, thirteen girls, of whom ten are alive, were born to nine boys.

The Act for the suppression of Infanticide is now in operation, and it was announced, early in August 1870, that the preventive measures prescribed therein would at once be carried into effect in six Pergunnahs in the Zillahs of Bustee and Jounpore respectively.

Mahometan Infanticide.

Mr. Strachey alludes to the fact that, in some parts of the country, the crime of Infanticide is common among the Mahomedans. The Mussalmauns of old, and especially the Jhats and the ancient Chiefs of Bhurtpore, were not untainted with this crime. It was shown by Major Lake, Commissioner of Goordaspore, in the Punjaub, that this wide-spread evil, which extended among certain tribes in the districts of Umballa, Ferozepore, Jullunder, Hooshearpore, Lahore, Mooltan, Jhelum, and Leia, was maintained by several of the Mussalmaun tribes; and the higher the rank, the more certain were the female branches of destruction. A writer in the *Allyghur Institute Gazette*, of the 26th June 1868, observes that the wild tribes of Arabia are considered to have been the first who were guilty of Infanticide, and that this crime is traced as far back as before the birth of Mahomet. This was attributed to the dread of shame which

---

* As cited in the Calcutta *Englishman*, Feb. 24, 1870.

the relations would undergo, if the girls fell into the enemy's power, and led the defeated party to slay their wives and daughters with their own hands. The birth of a daughter in Arabia, where provisions were often scarce, was suggestive of poverty; and this led the people to destroy their female offspring. He attributes the commission of this crime in India to ignorance and prejudice, to an idea that it is a humiliation to the parents that any man should have the power of styling himself their daughter's husband, to inability to endow their daughters with suitable dowries and to meet the expenses of marriage festivals. "Others," he adds, "from reasons unknown, consider it improper that their daughters should, after marriage, settle down near their parents, but they should live at a distance; and thus they argue: 'If we must be separated in any case, it is better to be separated by the great divider of friends—Death—before the affection with which they shall have inspired us shall have made the separation painful to both parties.'"

Exposure of Young Infants.

This barbarity, which is not, in all cases, to be mistaken for Infanticide, is of great frequency among the natives, and appears to be a practice of very ancient standing. Tavernier says:—"When a woman is brought to bed, and the child will not take the teat, they carry it out of the village, and putting it in a linen cloth, which they fasten by the four corners to the boughs of a tree, they there leave it, from morning till evening. By this means, the poor infant is exposed to be tormented by the crows, insomuch that there are some who have their eyes picked out of their heads; which is the reason that, in *Bengalla*, you shall see so many of these idolaters that have but one eye, and some that have lost both." [!] "In the evening, they fetch the child away, to try whether he will suck the next night; and, if he still refuse the teat, they carry him to the same place next morning, which they do for three days together; after which, if the infant after that refuses to suck, they believe him to be a devil, and throw him into the Ganges. Sometimes some charitable people among the English, Hollanders, and Portugals, compassionating the misfortune of those children, will take them away from the tree, and give them good education."

Ward has given, without any reference to Tavernier's account, the following details regarding the custom of exposing infants in the northern districts of Bengal:—"If an infant refuse the mother's breast, and decline in health, it is said to be under the influence of some malignant spirit. Such a child is sometimes put into a basket and hung up in a tree where this evil spirit is supposed to reside. It is generally destroyed by ants or birds of prey; but sometimes perishes by neglect, though fed and clothed daily. If it should not be dead at the expiration of three days, the mother receives it home again, and nurses it; but this seldom happens.

The late Mr. Thomas, a missionary, once saved and restored to its mother, an infant which had fallen out of a basket at Bholahatee, near Malda, at the moment a jackal was running away with it. As this gentleman and Mr. Carey were afterwards passing under the same tree, they found a basket hanging in the branches containing the skeleton of another infant, who had been devoured by ants."*

Writing in 1839,† Mr. Thomas Bacon states that "it has been ascertained that, in some districts, the inhuman parents have buried their living children up to the throat in the earth, leaving the head exposed to the attacks of the wild beasts and birds of prey."

It appeared in a trial at Backergunge, in 1855, that a babe of a few days old was found by the Reverend Mr. Page in a basket, suspended from a tree. The prisoners (Hindus) were the parents, and they pleaded the general custom of the country. The Sessions Judge remarked: "It seems that the exposure of infants, who become afflicted with peculiar fits, within the first few days from their birth, is a very common custom in parts of this district. The belief seems to be that, if the child is to be restored at all, it will be restored by the spirit by whom the child is possessed, if delivered over to its entire mercy. I should think that the child is, on such occasions, utterly adandoned by its parents ; but, in the present case, the parents affirm that they fed the child. Whether they did so or not, it is impossible to say; but, in the absence of proof to the contrary, the prisoners are entitled to the benefit of the doubt."

The Judges of the Nizamut Adawlut remarked that the graveness of the charge—namely, that the prisoners had exposed their infant, in a basket strung up to a branch of a tree, and *had left it there to die*—was not proved. On the contrary, the parents declared, and the truth of their declaration was borne out by the custom of that part of the country, that they had so placed the child in the hope of preserving its life, and were not neglectful of its wants and requirements, the superstition of their class leading them to believe that the spirit which had smitten their child with disease would restore it to health, if left to its mercy. As the child was suffering from disease, and its death, three days afterwards, was not shown by the evidence to have been connected with the exposure, a point of which the Sessions Judge took no notice, they acquitted the prisoners of all offence against the law, and directed their release.‡

In May 1854, a case occurred at Cuttack, which appears to illustrate in a singular manner the superstitious ideas of the Ooriahs. The prisoner's wife having given birth to *three* female children, the first two living, the third dead, he selected the weaker of the two living children,

* Ward, Vol. II., 3rd Edition, p. 123.

† The Oriental Annual, p. 99.

‡ Nizamut Adawlut Reports, May 4, 1855, p. 498.

and deposited it naked in a jungle, among thorns, placing it in such a manner that the birds of prey might readily dispose of it. His alleged motive was the belief that the birth of three children at once was of evil omen to the zemindar, the Government, and the country, and the fear of expulsion from his village, should the portentous occurrence become known. The infant was found alive, but died soon afterwards. On consideration of the peculiar circumstances of the case, he was sentenced to fourteen years' imprisonment, with labor in irons.*

In 1822, a Mussalmaun woman was tried, at Rajshahye, for abandoning her full-grown male child in the jungle, with its navel-string uncut. It was found alive, but it expired in a few hours. She was sentenced to imprisonment for life.

Mussamut Muntornee was sentenced at Patna, in 1855, to three years' imprisonment for exposing her new-born infant in a castor-oil plant field.†

Gunga, a widow, was tried for Infanticide at Ahmedabad in November 1838. Some persons, walking across an open spot of ground, heard the feeble cries of a child, which they found covered over with loose sand. It appeared recently born, and was not at all injured. The child was fed with milk for two days at the Foujdar's. The prisoner was met at the Magistrate's Kutcherry. She acknowledged the child to be hers, and it was given to her; it "was then in perfect health," but it died the following day. The jury who examined the body were of opinion that the child had died, not from the exposure, which appeared to have been momentary, but from being deprived of its mother's milk, through the neglect of the prisoner, so shortly after its birth. One Judge convicted her of murder and another of culpable homicide. The Hon'ble Chief Judge acquitted her.‡

The following case involved considerably more than mere exposure. Mussamut Lukhia, of Patna, was tried for wilful murder of her female infant by exposure after birth. She threw it down a dry well ten or twelve feet deep. It was taken up alive, and every attempt was made by the village people to restore it, but it died that night. The Court of Nizamut Adawlut found that she was aware that death would be the result of her inhuman act, and sentenced her capitally.§

The printed Reports are replete with these sad cases; many need not be cited here, as points of medico-legal difficulty are seldom involved in such inquiries.

As an illustration of this class of cases, may be mentioned that of a woman tried at Cuttack, in 1851, for exposing her illegitimate infant in

---

* Nizamut Adawlut Reports, Vol. IV., p. 341.

† *Id.*, April 13, 1855, p. 384.

‡ Bellasis' Reports, p. 125.

§ Nizamut Adawlut Reports, Sept. 12, 1866, p. 422.

a dry water-course. Her defence was that she placed the child, at midnight, shortly after its birth, at its father's door, and that some one there must have removed the child to the nullah. The Sessions Judge decided that, with reference to the circumstances of the case, and the custom which so commonly prevails in this country, among females situated like the prisoner,—*viz.*, that of placing their illegitimate offspring at the doors of their reputed fathers, in order to make them support themselves and their children,—he did not consider the prisoner's statement improbable. The child survived. Sentence, six months' imprisonment.*

It will be observed how large a number of cases of Infanticide occur in Orissa. In one of these trials, the Sessions Judge remarked upon the prevalence in Cuttack of the offence of murdering new-born children, the fruits of illicit intercourse, or *of exposing them with the intent to destroy them.* It will be borne in mind that this latter mode of Infanticide is that practised by the Khonds, who, although inhabiting the Hill tracts of Orissa, are, save in this particular, entirely apart from the Hindu Ooriahs in customs and in religion.

The custom of leaving illegitimate children at their fathers' doors also prevails in the N. W. Provinces.

Starvation.

This mode of Infanticide has already been noticed (p. 752), and will again be alluded to under the remarks on Infanticide by *Suffocation* (p. 768). A recent writer in the *Delhi Gazette* says: "The system adopted to get rid of legitimate children (girls) is by Starvation, which is an easy process; the mother of the child has various modes of checking the nourishment for the child; when she succeeds in doing so, may I ask how is the law to be applied? I hear that *dhoob* grass, if moistened, pounded, and applied, has such a tendency; and, on the other hand, if suspicion prompts the Magistrate to remove the child from her mother, and to consign it to the care of a nurse of an inferior caste, he will be encroaching on the rights of caste."

Throat Cut.

A woman, of Sarun, having borne a female child which her paramour refused to maintain, left it, in the presence of witnesses, on the bed upon which he was sleeping. On the following day, it was found in some grass jungle, with its throat cut. It eventually died. He was sentenced to seven years' imprisonment.†

In 1848, Dr. Irvine, of Patna, examined the body of an infant (the

---

* Vol. I. of 1851, p. 1129.

† Nizamut Adawlut Reports, Vol. IV., p. 22.

state of whose thorax proved that it had lived) whose head had been severed from its body.

Drowning.

In 1851, one Mussamut Toolsee was sentenced to perpetual imprisonment, at Cuttack, for having placed her illegitimate male infant in an earthen vessel, and sunk it in a river. "She said that the child was born alive and cried; and that, about an hour and-a-half afterwards, when it had ceased to cry, and she did not know whether it was alive or dead, she carried it away and threw it into the river."* Drowning in milk, *vide supra*, p. 753.

Poisoning.

Allusion has already been made to the use in these cases of *Tobacco* (*vide supra*, p. 240), *Datura*, *Mudar*, and *Opium*. Dr. Cutcliffe tells me that, within his experience, the following poisons were used for killing infants in the neighbourhood of Seharunpore: *Arsenic*, *Opium*, *Mudar*. Upon its being discovered that *Datura seeds* were used, the practice of using this poison was dropped.

Opium, *vide supra*, pp. 229 and 232.—Among the practices of the Rajpoots were those of fixing a small piece of opium on the roof of the infant's mouth, or of compelling the mother to rub her nipples with opium, and thus to suckle her child to death. We are told that Pootna came to Krishna, disguised as a nurse with poison on her nipples, but the young Hercules tugged so lustily that she fell dead. Writing at Allahabad, in 1819, Dr. Robert Tytler alludes (in his treatise on *Morbus Oryzæus*) to the "abominable custom of Hindustanee *daees* of rubbing narcotic drugs of every procurable kind upon their nipples, with the intention of lulling the child to sleep, in order that the unprincipled nurse may be relieved from the fatigue of duty which she has voluntarily undertaken to perform." A writer from England says: "The secrets of the *zenana* are never revealed, and who shall say how many female infants—aye and male infants too—are put away and never again heard of. It is a well-known fact that opium is largely used in all *zenanas*, and more especially by mothers, to keep their infants 'quiet;'—no wonder that they are kept so effectually."

Mudar.—More than one allusion has been made above to the use of the milky juice of the *Calotropis Hamiltonii* in Infanticide (pp. 285, 753).

Dr. Burton Brown cites a case from the Nizamut Adawlut Reports, N. W. P., Vol. VII., p. 133, in which a man named Lulloo murdered his own infant daughter according to the old custom of his tribe, when unable to afford a suitable dowry, by pouring the milk of the *mudar* down its throat.

---

* Vol I. of 1851, p. 1127.

Sub-Assistant Surgeon Meer Ushru Ally tells me that, in a Thakoor village, near Agra, the female children are still killed by *mudar* juice.

Mr. McReddie's researches into this subject, at Hurdui, have been cited at p. 285. Writing to the Deputy Commissioner of that district in May 1867, Mr. McReddie mentioned that he believed that, in six cases of infants brought to him for examination since 1866, death was due to this poison. The stomachs were sent to the Chemical Examiner to Government, but no poison could be detected.

Injury to the Head.

Mussamut Bundanneeah, a widow, having brought forth a female infant, the result of illicit intercourse with her late husband's brother, threw the child, just after its birth, into a dry well, which was stated to be fifteen cubits in depth. Strange to say, the child was not immediately destroyed by the fall, and its cries attracted the attention of the neighbours, who took it out. It survived a day and a night. The Civil Surgeon found no external traces of injury, but considered, from the effusion of blood from the nose, that some concussion of the brain was probably produced by the fall.* In 1851, a Mussalmaun and his paramour (the widow of his brother) were sentenced to transportation for life for murdering their new-born child by fracturing its skull.†

A widow, of Seonee, being delivered of an infant,—the fruit, as she asserted, of a casual intercourse with a sepoy in the jungle,—concealed the birth, and buried the child within the enclosure of her house.‡ The Sub-Assistant Surgeon stated that, after examination of the body, and the application of tests, he was convinced that the child (of full term) had been born alive, and that death had been caused by violence done to the head, the skin of which was swelled, and a large extravasation of blood beneath it, especially the left parietal bone, which was fractured in two places. The Sessions Judge held that there was "nothing satisfactory to his mind in the medical evidence. Nothing to show that fracture of bones (soft as those of an infant just born must be) might not have occurred *after* death, in the process of burying [?] or at the time of birth, during a difficult unprofessional delivery; while it was apparent that the common offices to new-born infants had been here omitted."§

---

* Nizamut Adawlut Reports, N. W. P., December 21st, 1852, p. 1524.

† *Ibid*, Vol. I. of 1851, p. 364.

‡ Allusion has already been made (p. 25) to the fact that, in Madras, but not in Bengal, it is usual with Hindus to bury first-born infants, of some castes, temporarily within the precincts of their houses. My friend Dr. J. Phin Smith has kindly given me a translation from the Italian of Pietro della Valle, who visited Western India in 1663, and who found that, at Cambay, the bodies of Gentoo children under two years are not burned but buried, and he saw there, at the burning-place, near the sea, several put under ground.

§ Nizamut Adawlut Report, N. W. P., December 24th, 1852, p. 1541.

The following cases of *Injury to the Head in Parturition* deserve attention, as involving points of great practical moment. Sub-Assistant Surgeon Bindabun Chatterjee has reported* the case of a Hindu female, aged thirty-two, who was delivered in the Lying-in Ward of the Medical College Hospital, Calcutta, of her *second* child ; the presentation was natural, the labor not unnaturally tedious. The child was born dead, in consequence of a rupture of the scalp and escape of the substance of the brain, which occurred during the second stage. On examination afterwards, the scalp was found much attenuated, and a rupture had taken place posteriorly. The line of rupture was even and horizontal, about the level of the upper part of the occipital bone, and two lines running forward in a straight direction from the extremity of the horizontal line. The rupture was symmetrical ; the lambdoidal suture was also ruptured ; *the child was small, and not of the full term.* When at Howrah, I was requested by the husband of a lady, married about eight months previously, to prescribe for her, as she was suffering from inward uneasiness which might, at first sight, have appeared to be the result of dysentery. Suspecting the real cause, however, I requested him to procure a strong dose of morphia on his way home, and prepared to follow him. Upon reaching the house, which was at a considerable distance from mine, I found that my patient, a slender lady of eighteen or nineteen, born in India of French parents, pregnant for the first time, had suddenly been delivered, while in the erect position, the child falling head foremost upon a marble floor. The placenta was still attached. The infant was apparently between the seventh and eighth month, and cried lustily. I could find no mark of injury. Having done all that was necessary, I left the house ; but was hastily recalled in about an hour, and found the child dying. The face and scalp were now pallid, and a large bruise had become apparent on the forehead and vertex,—the part which had come in contact with the pavement. It will be at once perceived how many points of great medico-legal importance these two cases involve.

Unconscious Delivery.

Although many cases of difficult parturition occur in India, the relaxing character of the climate, while it may, in enfeebled subjects, tend to produce inertia of the uterus, generally renders labor easier, if not speedier, than it is in more bracing climates.

One of the most remarkable cases of nearly unconscious delivery on record is given by Dr. George Smith, Residency Surgeon, Hyderabad, Deccan.†

During the night preceding her delivery, at the full term, Mrs. —— had felt quite well ; she rose several times to attend to her sick child.

* Indian Annals of Medical Science, for October 1854, p. 469.

† *Id.*, No. 7, April 1857, p. 629.

About $5\frac{1}{2}$ A.M. she walked from her house to the bungalow in which she was confined. She lay down upon the cot, and experienced a *very* slight sensation, as if her bowels were about to be relieved—a feeling as if something had touched her body followed, and caused her to ask the ayah to lift the bed-clothes ; when, to the surprise and alarm of both, the child was found fully extruded. Dr. Smith found the child born and lying below the bed-clothes, close to the body of its mother; the cord was entire, and the placenta within the vagina. Mrs. —— was awake when the child was born, and yet so little was her notice attracted by her feelings that the delivery took place unconsciously. Had she been standing, or seated on her night-chair, the result would probably have been instantly fatal to the child. Had she been asleep, the child, Dr. Smith was satisfied, would have been suffocated. This was her second child; her first was born with the usual pains, after a labor extending over six hours. Dr. Smith had the utmost confidence in the patient's statements, having made searching inquiries into the case. The child, a female, was a little, but not much, undersized.

Dr. Herbert Baillie was, some years ago, called to see a married European lady in Calcutta, whom he found seated on the commode, with a full-term fœtus and its secundines in the pan.

The following is probably the most remarkable recorded instance of *unconscious delivery during sleep.* Dr. Wendell Case, of Chicago, attended a *primipara,* a well-developed brunette from the south of France. Her husband said that she had been feeling badly all day, and was near the period of her confinement, but rather attributed her illness to over-fatigue on the day previous. She had some severe pains in the lumbar region, and slight nausea. The os uteri was dilated to three-fourths the size of a large dollar. The labor pains did not return, and she fell into a profound sleep, during which the head of the child was fully expelled. In a moment the body was delivered, and in less than twenty minutes, the secundines had passed off, and the uterus contracted with scarcely any pain. She said she had dreamed something was the matter with her, and awoke with a fright, probably the instant the body was expelled. She has been confined twice since, Dr. Case learns, with the usual amount of labor-pains.

Suffocation and Strangling.

In 1822, a widow was sentenced, upon her own confession, at Bundelkund, to perpetual imprisonment, for having destroyed her bastard child, at its birth, by stuffing a cloth into its mouth and burying it in a ditch; she pleaded extreme poverty as an excuse for her crime.*

A case is mentioned in the Bengal Police Report for 1868 (p. 163), in

* Macnaghten's Reports, Vol. II., p. 161.

which the body of a newly-born child was found on the bank of a tank in the city of Doomraon, the mouth being stuffed with mud.

Dr. Cutcliffe informs me that, in his own experience, Infanticide by plugging the fauces with *rooe* (raw cotton) was practised in the neighbourhood of Saharunpore. The children having been thus skilfully suffocated, Dr. Cutcliffe reported that he found the bodies *quite healthy and well-nourished* and without sufficient lesions to account for natural death from disease. Hence he considered that there were suspicions of foul play. Warned by this, they first starved their children to emaciation, and then smothered them.

In 1841, Dr. Pagan, of Midnapore, and Dr. J. S. Smith, of Madras, reported the examination of the body of a full-grown perfect child, with the cord and after-birth attached, the former not having been tied. The face, head, and sides of the neck were livid and swollen; the muscles and soft parts of the neck were bruised and contained some extravasated blood; the lungs floated in water, and were not diseased, but were somewhat engorged with blood ; the wind-pipe was uninjured ; the body was somewhat decomposed. The witnesses concurred in the opinion that the above injuries had been inflicted during life, and that they could not have occurred in delivery, or in burying the body.*

One Mussamut Soomarea, of Azimgurh, had been married two years, and had lived with her husband about a year, during which period she was frequently in the habit of passing some time at her father's house, where she formed an illicit intimacy, and became pregnant. On discovering this, her father sent her back to her husband, but she shortly afterwards returned to her father, who refused to receive her into his house. Her paramour then made her over to a woman in the neighbourhood. Finding that her labor was at hand, and her father absent, she went to his house, where she was delivered, privately, of a male child, which she destroyed, about an hour after its birth, by compressing its windpipe. The native doctor who made an examination of the body deposed, with much confidence, that the child was matured, that it was borne alive, and existed for some time afterwards, and that death was caused by compression of the throat with the hand shortly after its birth.†

The body of a female infant, with the navel-string uncut, was found in the town of Kurbal (Mynpoory). One Mussamut Miseea confessed to the Police that, having become pregnant nine months before, in her husband's absence, she was delivered of a child, and killed it by squeezing

* See also the case of a widow of Patna, found guilty of twisting the neck of her illegitimate child, a few days old, in despair at being turned out of doors by her relatives, and being refused all aid by the father of the child.—*Nizamut Adawlut Reports*, Vol. II., Part 1, of 1852, p. 852.

† Nizamut Adawlut Reports, N. W. P., September 30th, 1852, p. 1102.

its throat. At trial, she denied her confessions, and said her child was born dead seven months after conception, and that, having no one to bury it, she threw it into the pond. Two of the assessors, a zemindar and a Brahmin, acquitted her, the first remarking that a seven months' child, born in such cold weather, would probably have died; the second, that it was clearly a seven months' child, since so much blood flowed ! The third, a vakeel, convicted. The infant bore no marks of violence, so far as the examination of the Civil Surgeon went. He did not, however, suspect violent death, being under an impression, from the mere fact of the navel-string being uncut, that the child was born dead. The Judge held that the slight pressure on the throat of a child necessary to cause death need have left no mark ; but, if otherwise, such marks would hardly be visible after two days and nights' immersion of the body in water. With regard to the navel-string being uncut, that would, he considered, be equally the case with a child born dead, or a child murdered as soon as born.*

---

* Nizamut Adawlut Reports, N. W. P., January 28th, 1853, p. 123. It is evidently a matter of no small importance that medical men in this country should be well acquainted with *the manner in which the umbilical cord is divided and dressed by native women.* Such information is especially called for in cases like the following. A female mendicant of weak intellect, at Jaunpore, gave birth to a female infant, which she left in some straw, where she had slept, and went begging. The child was found dead. The Civil Surgeon examined the child's body, and could find no apparent cause of death. He considered it was probably the result of neglect, as the navel-string had not been severed, the after-birth being still attached. The child had breathed, but death probably took place very shortly after its birth. Nizamut Adawlut Reports, N. W. P., February 18th, 1853, p. 256. Professor T. W. Wilson kindly furnished me with some interesting notes on the manner in which the *Dhaees* of this part of Bengal treat the umbilical cord. He finds that the nurse usually divides the cord, near its insertion to the umbilicus, with a piece of bamboo, sharpened into the form of a rude knife. Sometimes the richer classes get a silver instrument, made like a spatula, for the purpose. Only one ligature, of strong thread, is used ; it is applied next the child, no ligature is applied to the placental end of the cord. The thumb, heated over fire, is repeatedly placed on the navel. [This continues to be done for many days, and may not unfrequently interfere with the process of healing ; in a case which came partly under my own notice, the child's death was attributed (perhaps unfairly) to this practice.] If there is any discharge, the end of the cord is then dressed with burnt rags. Generally the fœtal end of the cord is left hanging without any dressing. Dr. Wilson understands that the separation of the placenta is generally hastened by placing a quantity of hair in the woman's mouth,—this causes an effort to vomit, which brings away the after-birth. It is also said that raw rice, mixed with oil and swallowed, assists the discharge of the placenta.

Dr. Wilson finds that the *Dhaees* divide the cord *before the placenta comes away.* There is, probably, a difference in this practice in different parts of the country ; and this should be taken into account in medico-legal investigations upon this point. Ward says that, at the moment of birth, various religious ceremonies are performed, which occupy about two hours, and that then the umbilical cord is cut. This is probably the custom among the richer Hindus. Mr. Hodgson states that, among the Bodo and Dhimals, the mother herself cuts the navel-string, so soon as she has recovered sufficient strength. In a paper on the native practice of midwifery at Bombay,—published in the Transactions of the Medical and Physical Society of that city, for 1853 and 1854, p. 338,—it is mentioned that, after delivery, a binder is applied, and the expulsion of the placenta anxiously looked for, as *the cord is not*

Mussamut Syneeal was convicted, at Shahjehanpore, of having murdered her female illegitimate child by strangling it with a strip of cloth. She stated that she was binding the cloth on her infant's head; and, being intoxicated by some spirit which she had taken shortly after the birth of the child to relieve a severe internal pain, she did not know if she had bound its head or its foot. The evidence went wholly to disprove her plea of intoxication.*

Mussamut Imamee, of Jaunpore, was convicted of the wilful murder of her male illegitimate child by pressing his neck and strangling him. She placed the corpse in an earthen vessel, and buried it in a corner of her house.†

Infanticide in Madras.

Writing in July 1868,‡ Dr. Muir says: "In the Town of Madras alone, forty-seven new-born children and fœtuses were reported to have been found during the past three years. These new-born children are commonly found in cess-pools, tanks, ditches, drains, or even on the road-side, under circumstances which have left no doubt that they were cast away to conceal the fact of their death. In most of these cases, there are the usual indications of the child having been born alive, and the navel-cord has most commonly not been tied. They are, moreover, unwashed, and present no indications of the ordinary care being taken of them which is bestowed on children born dead, when women are surrounded with the assistance which they ought to have. In some instances, there is unmistakable evidence of violence; the mouth is stuffed with cloths, tightened cords are found round the neck, thus leaving no doubt that the children have been murdered. Yet in very few instances have the police been able to find out the mother or the person who destroyed the child."

It is scarcely necessary to say that *the average weight of new-born native children in Bengal* is probably very much indeed below that of European

---

divided until the after-birth comes away. Before the cord is divided, the blood in it is either pressed in the direction of the placenta, or of the child, accordingly as the child is lively or otherwise. After cutting the cord, it is dressed with salt and turmeric, and suspended from the neck, and the child is not bathed until the cord falls off. Mr. Waring mentions that the Burmese tie the cord in the English manner, and divide it by a see-saw motion with a piece of bamboo split up the middle, forming a most rude pair of scissors. I have heard that, in some parts of Bengal, the lower orders divide the cord by rubbing it on the broken edge of an earthern pot. It appears certain that a ragged state of the end of the cord is not an evidence of neglect in this country. Dr. Wilson is informed that the practice of the Mussalmaun *Dhaees* is very similar to that of the Hindus.

* Nizamut Adawlut Reports, N. W. P., 15th March 1853, p. 366.

† *Ibid*, July 30th, 1853, p. 937.

‡ Statistics of unnatural deaths in the Madras and other Presidencies, Madras Quar. Jour. of Med. Science for the above date, p. 110.

children at birth. A few accurate statistics upon this subject would also be of great value.

Having paid considerable attention to the study of the abnormal conditions of the fœtal circulation, and the results of my researches having tended to subvert the validity of more than one of the tests of live birth generally insisted upon,* I shall venture to devote one or two pages to this important subject.

Previous to 1846, it was generally considered that (1) the discovery of contraction of the whole diameter of the *Ductus Arteriosus* would, even after decomposition had obscured the state of the lungs and of other organs, stand as decided evidence that the child had lived for a considerable period ; that (2) closure of the *Foramen Ovale* might be taken as a certain proof that life had been prolonged for, at least, several days ; and (3) that an uncontracted state of the Arterial Duct, Foramen Ovale, and Ductus Venosus afforded strong evidence that respiration had not occurred.

In my researches on the morbid conditions of the pulmonary artery,† I succeeded in showing that these opinions were erroneous,—inasmuch as (1) *the Arterial Duct may become closed either before or in a very few hours after birth;* (2) *that a child may be born with the Foramen Ovale closed;* and that (3) *the Arterial Duct and Foramen Ovale may be found pervious, even in adult age, without any other discoverable error in the vascular system.* I may now add (4) that *the Fœtal Thoracic Openings and the Ductus Venosus may be found quite uncontracted several days after birth.*

(1). *The Arterial Duct may become closed either before or in a very few hours after birth.*—In October 1846, the body of a female child was discovered buried in waste ground near Ayr, enveloped in a woollen bag. It was in a state of putrefaction, with desquamation of the cuticle. It weighed five pounds, and was twenty inches in length. The scalp was covered with hair, and the nails were full-grown ; a large portion of the brain, which had been reduced to a pulpy state, had escaped through the openings of the skull. Its mouth and nostrils were stuffed with flax. The umbilicus was in the centre of the body, the cord was cut close to the abdomen, and left without ligature. There was an extensive ecchymosis all over the fore part of the neck, and an effusion of blood on the exterior of the trachea. The heart and lungs weighed one ounce ; the lungs were collapsed ; the right was considerably decomposed and sunk when put into water. The left was of a red color and firm in texture, and floated on the surface when immersed in a vessel filled with water ; but, on pressure, there was no crepitation. The right side of the

* See Taylor, p. 400, *et seq.*
† Published in the London Medical Gazette, between July 1846 and September 1851.

heart was filled with coagulated blood; the *Foramen Ovale was partly open*, and the *Ductus Arteriosus* impervious. The liver was large and of a leaden hue; the *Ductus Venosus* almost obliterated; meconium was found in abundance in the lower bowels. Strong circumstantial evidence was adduced to prove that this infant came into the world shortly before six o'clock A.M., and that its body was deposited in the spot where it was subsequently discovered between 10 and 11 o'clock A.M. Admitting that this child was born alive, there was the strongest reason to believe that it did not survive its birth *ten minutes*.

In January 1847, I laid before the Pathological Society of London the heart of a fœtus, born at seven months and-a-half, which died *fifteen minutes* after birth, in consequence of hæmorrhage from the umbilical cord. The *arterial duct* was nearly closed, being merely capable of admitting the shank of a large pin. The tissues of the duct had altogether an appearance of having undergone a gradual process of contraction. The heart and lungs were normal.

In commenting upon this case, Dr. Taylor remarks that, according to Bernt's rule, the medical inference might have been that the child had lived a week. In bringing these two cases together, it is certainly worthy of remark that, in the first as well as in the second, hæmorrhage from the navel might have gone far towards determining the early contraction of the arterial duct. This important question will require further investigation.* However, these cases form such marked exceptions to the rule which obtained previous to their publication, that no Medical Jurist can hereafter venture to declare that a child must have lived several days, merely upon the evidence afforded by a closed state of the arterial duct.

(2). *A child may be born with the Foramen Ovale closed.*—In 1847, my friend Mr. Ebenezer Smith kindly allowed me an early examination of the heart and lungs of a child which appeared healthy at its birth, but soon afterwards became livid, and died convulsed in about twenty-one *hours*. The *Foramen Ovale was completely closed by a firm membrane*. The Arterial Duct was wide, and the right cavities capacious, but the left cavities of the heart were extremely contracted, almost to obliteration, and the mitral valve was merely rudimentary.† I brought this case forward at the time, with the remark that it is impossible to deny that, in the heart of a child which has died within the uterus, and has been expelled in a putrid condition, the Foramen Ovale may be found completely and permanently

---

* It will be very important to observe whether the fœtal passages are contracted in children expelled dead in cases of placenta prævia.

† Mr. Smith has published the full details of this case in the first volume of the Transactions of the Pathological Society of London. A similar case is related by Vieussens, and another by Dr. Williams; but Mr. Smith's is the only completely detailed instance of the kind on record.

closed; but that, in such cases as the above, it would probably be always possible to determine, by an examination of the heart and its appendages, that the closure of the Foramen had occurred at some period or other antecedent to birth. Still, it must be remembered that, in investigating a case of supposed Infanticide, the medical man's attention is at once directed to the state of the Foramen Ovale, and it would not be surprising if, upon discovering that the auricular septum was complete, he should rest satisfied,—seeing that even so good an anatomist as Vieussens does not appear to have considered it necessary to remark any other appearance in the heart where he found the Foramen closed thirty hours after birth, except that the pulmonary artery was extraordinarily dilated.

(3). *The Arterial Duct and Foramen Ovale may be found pervious, even in adult age, without any other discoverable error in the vascular system.*—In October 1837, the body of a woman, aged thirty-two, the mother of eight children, who had died of phthisis of only three months' duration, was examined by Mr. Molloy and myself at Guy's Hospital. The heart was small and pale, but perfectly well formed, except that the *Foramen Ovale* was sufficiently wide to admit the little finger, and that the *Arterial Duct* allowed a large-sized probe to be passed from the aorta into the pulmonary artery, but was guarded on its pulmonary side, by a growth of minute elastic vegetations which, acting completely as a valve in that direction, showed that the permanence of the duct could not have depended, at least during the latter years of life, upon pulmonary obstruction.

(4). *The Arterial Duct, Foramen Ovale, and Canalis Venosus may be found uncontracted several days after Birth.*—In March 1854 Mr. Lee read before the Pathological Society the particulars of the case of a child, in which jaundice commenced immediately after birth. Six days after the separation of the funis (in which process there was nothing abnormal), slight hæmorrhage made its appearance. The blood was thin and serous, scarcely discoloring the linen, and, when dry, not stiffening it. The bleeding continued for two days, it then stopped, but the child soon afterwards sank. *The Umbilical Vein, one Umbilical Artery, the Ductus Venosus, the Ductus Arteriosus, and the Foramen Ovale were all found open.* There was no appearance of inflammation in the structures of the umbilical vein. The blood was without coagula, and appeared entirely deficient in fibrin.* There is a large class of these cases, in which children are destroyed, from six or eight to eighteen days after birth, by irrepressible hæmorrhage from the umbilical vein. These infants are usually jaundiced, and an excessive degree of cholemia is, of course, adverse to the closure of any of the fœtal communications. Mr. Shircore, of Calcutta, mentioned to me the particulars of a case in which there appeared to be every reason to believe that the Umbi-

* Association Journal, April 7th, 1854, p. 307.

lical Vein and a considerable portion of the Canalis Venosus remained permanently open in a child three or four years old ; that is to say, there was a fistulous-looking opening at the umbilicus, into which a probe could be passed directly backwards for some inches. The parents disliking the appearance of this opening, although it caused no inconvenience, Mr. Shircore readily succeeded in closing its orifice.

INSANITY.

The opinions of medical men in India are often called for in cases of real or apparent mental aberration of the most involved and difficult nature. If it be sometimes found impossible to bring about unanimity of opinion in three or four of the most eminent men, whose lives have been devoted to the study of Insanity in England, with regard to the sanity or unsoundness of mind of an educated fellow-countryman,* how much more trying must the task be to a young Civil Surgeon, upon whose fiat depends the life or death of a native, probably from some remote and almost unknown part of the district, in whose mind a perfect chaos of absurd superstitions stands in the place of imagination and religion, and whose every turn of thought and expression is strange and foreign; in whom every attempt to question excites an effort to deceive, and in whom the faculties of cunning and simulation exist in their fullest and most active development? Notwithstanding these difficulties, the printed reports of our Courts show very clearly that dangerous and untenable opinions are rarely given by medical officers in cases of this description.

The chief sets of cases which it appears necessary to mention here are the following :—

Criminal Responsibility of Persons of Weak Intellect.

Lallchand Kyebart was tried at Backergunge, in 1855, for the murder of his wife, who was from thirty to thirty-two years of age, the mother of two grown-up sons by the prisoner, and by all accounts a chaste woman.

He hacked her to death with a heavy *dao,* as she lay on her bed at about $4\frac{1}{2}$ o'clock in the morning. The substance of the prisoner's defence, before the police, is as follows :—" That he was sleeping in the yard of his northern house, and his wife, daughter, and little son in the northern house; that he struck his wife, while she was asleep, five or six blows with a *dao;* that she staggered into the court-yard, and fell on prisoner's

* As shown in the case of the unfortunate Buranelli, who was hanged upon a sentence which appears to have rested upon the opinion of two medical men, who only saw him once, two months after the perpetration of the fâtal deed; while Drs. Connolly, Winslow, and Baly, and two Surgeons, expressed it as their solemn and matured opinion that the prisoner was insane at the time he committed the crime.

bed. I cannot say how many blows I inflicted on my wife in the court-yard. I first struck her on the breast. For seven or eight years I have been suffering from hypochondria; sometimes I remain well, sometimes I get bad, and my mind becomes disturbed. Since I have been thus affected, I fancy my wife is attached to some man. My nephew Kanai, and others of my own caste, used to come to my house and eat *pan* and smoke tobacco. This aroused suspicion in my mind. On the night I wounded her, my wife said to me, since Soorjoomonee has given you medicine, you can't bear to look at anybody; go to her house and remain there. I got angry, and I wounded her. The prisoner then began to talk somewhat incoherently; after a short interval he stated that, at the time he wounded his wife with the *dao*, then produced, his wife seized it, and then, in pulling it away from her, the third finger of his right hand and the thumb of his left hand were very slightly wounded."

Before the Deputy Magistrate, his confession was,—"The date I cannot remember. One night, my wife, Shonye, my daughter Kishoree, and my little son slept in the northern house. I slept in the court-yard of that house. Towards the morning, I got up, brought a *dao* from the house, and struck my wife five or six blows with the said weapon, and then came out in the yard; the *dao* fell down in the house and remained there; afterwards I gave my wife some water to drink; she died afterwards. When I wounded her, my wife was not fast asleep. The night I wounded her, I wanted to go and sleep with my wife. She said, 'Go and remain in the house of her who has given you medicine:' I was then seized with a fit, and did not know what I was doing, and I wounded her. I told everybody before this that my mind was in a bad state, and asked them to tie me up. A year ago, Joogul Dass came to my house, and, in my presence, ate *pan* with my wife and talked to her; he is a man of a loose character, and has ruined two or three men in the village. I could not bear this. Last Bysack, Soorjoomonee, Rokunna, and Parbuttee gave me some medicine; they would not let my wife see the medicine. I think Soorjoomonee gave me the medicine by the advice of Joogul Dass, who visits her house. Since I took the medicine, I have not felt in my right senses."

In the Judge's Court, the prisoner denied the crime, on being arraigned. He first refused to plead, began to make faces, and to shriek out "Bhola." After talking to him a little, he pleaded not guilty. The medical officer, who sat in Court with the Judge and heard the witnesses give their evidence, deposed that the prisoner was sane. He suffered a great deal from spasmodic contractions of the muscles of the neck, which is a painful disease, and which may have made him cross and irritable; but that he did not consider his mind to be affected. The answers of the prisoner to questions put to him by the Judge personally and by the medical officer, through one of the officers of the Court, were coherent and perfectly intelligible. His demeanour was also that of a man in possession of his senses. The medical officer deposed that the prisoner was in the habit of making noises and wry faces when he saw him coming to the hospital. After full consideration of his case, the medical officer was clearly of opinion that the prisoner was sane, and that he was a malingerer; his general health was good. To the above the Judge added his own opinion, from a close watching of the prisoner's demeanour during the two days the trial occupied. He was fully alive to any points that told in his favor; he always shrieked out at the right moment; if any witnesses deposed to his eccentricity, a shriek immediately followed; at other times, he was quite quiet. Before taking his second defence, the Judge had a long conversation with him. There was much method in his way of answering. When he was asked whether he confessed before the Deputy Magistrate, he answered—"They copied the Thannah confession." The Judge added, "I must say that I consider him sane, and always to have been so." The native doctor and others at the jail deposed that he was quiet and inoffensive; that he shrieked out in the night now and then; but this, the Judge observed, he did to keep up the character he had, since his apprehension, assumed of being demented. The Judge concludes: "In my opinion the prisoner was perfectly sane when he committed the murder. The witnesses depose that the prisoner was eccentric, but not that he was so insane as to be an irresponsible agent. It is my painful duty to recommend that sentence of death may be passed upon the prisoner." The Judges of the Nizamut Adawlut observed: "Notwithstanding the strong opinion of the Sessions Judge and of the medical officer, there is, in our opinion, reason to believe, from the evidence, that the prisoner had an insane tendency, such as, although insufficient to justify an acquittal on account of insanity, warrants a less punishment than a capital sentence. The evidence proves that, for years, the prisoner had been violent in his manner, and had discontinued his usual employment; and there is such absence of motive for the crime (unless what the prisoner stated before the Magistrate that his wife would not let him come to her bed) that it is presumable that the prisoner was [mentally] affected at the time. It has been held (page 1532 of Nizamut Decisions for 1851) that a prisoner may not be entitled to be acquitted under Act IV. of 1849, on the ground of insanity; and yet that there may be circumstances to render it proper that he should be exempted from capital punishment. A decision to this effect is to be found at page 354 of the Nizamut Reports for 1854, and there are several others of the same nature. In accordance with the principles therein declared, we sentence the prisoner to imprisonment for life with labor, at the discretion of the Magistrate, in the zillah jail where his case is known, and whence, if necessary, he can readily be removed to the insane hospital." *

* Nizamut Adawlut Reports, October 29, 1855, p. 684.

Eshory Dassee, of Sylhet, killed her own infant daughter, eighteen months old, with a *dao*. The darogah questioned the prisoner, who confessed and stated that she had not been in a sound state of health for two or three months, and that her daughter used to annoy her by crying, and she killed her in consequence. Her husband, who took her and the dead body to the thannah, said that she had been insane during the past two months. The Civil Surgeon deposed that she was not insane, but was of a very low scale of intellect. The Judges of the Nizamut Adawlut observed: "The act of murder in this case is confessed to by the prisoner, and so clearly established that the only question left for our consideration is whether, as recommended by the Sessions Judge, the state of the prisoner's mind at the time of the act calls for any mitigation of punishment according to former practice of this Court, and should prevent capital sentence. It does not certainly appear, from the evidence which has been taken on this point, that the prisoner is actually insane. Her husband, in his statement from the first, deposes that she is in such a state of mind, especially from an illness which she had shortly before the occurrence, as to be unconscious of her acts. The other witnesses, the neighbours, and the chowkeedar, without going quite so far as the husband, depose to her having been at times '*behosh*' after the above illness; and all very distinctly state that she was always in so stolid and imbecile a state of mind as to make them consider her to be foolish. The Civil Assistant Surgeon, without being able to testify as to any actual insanity, deposes to the prisoner's being of a very low order of intellect. Under all these circumstances, referring to the precedent of this Court in the case of Soary Chue Oung and Moonghoo, where the prisoner was found guilty of murder, but shown to be of a low order of intellect, and sentenced only to imprisonment for life, and to other precedents in like cases, we think that the present case is one in which it would be unsafe to pass capital sentence, and it is accordingly ordered that the prisoner be imprisoned for life in the Alipore jail, with labor suitable to her sex."*

Mental Aberration resulting from the use of Hemp and Opium.

From very early periods, these two poisons have been made to supply the place of fermented liquors, by some of those who profess to be the strictest abstainers among both Hindus and Mahomedans. Bernier (1655) describes the Rajputs as great takers of opium, and he sometimes wondered at the quantity he has seen them take. They accustom themselves to it from their youth. *On the day of battle they double the dose; this drug animating them, and making them insensible of danger;* insomuch that they cast themselves into the combat like so many furious beasts, not knowing what it is to run away, but dying at the feet of the

* Nizamut Adawlut Reports, September 30, 1856, p. 718.

Raja, when he stands to it." Dr. Fryer (1672) says: "Opium is often eaten in large quantity by the Rashpoots, Queteries, and Patans, when they fight, which makes them run upon any enterprise with a raging resolution to dye or be victorious." Again, "The plant of which *Bang* is made, grows like our Hemp, the juice of whose seed, ground in a bowl like mustard seed, and mixed with any other liquor, is that they equivocate with their prophet instead of the grape."

Forbes says:* "The Hindus, as well as the Mahomedans, are forbidden the use of wine and spirituous liquors; and I believe most of the highest classes attend strictly to the prohibition. The lower classes are less abstemious; but rich and poor, especially officers in the army and soldiers, are addicted to the use of opium, which they take in large quantities, and enjoy the pleasing delirium it occasions. In battle, it inspires a false courage, and sometimes produces a phrenzy which lasts only for a short time; leaving those who swallow this poisonous drug in a state of languor and imbecility until a renewal of the dose revives the spirits; but its frequent use enfeebles the constitution, and shortens the lives of its deluded victims. Opium is used to a better purpose by the Halcarras, who are a set of people employed as messengers, spies, and letter-carriers. An Halcarra takes a letter, wraps it up in some secret fold of his shabby garment, and with a little opium, some rice, and a small pot to draw water from the wells of the charitable, he undertakes a journey of several hundred miles and receives his reward on delivering the letter."

Captain Meadows Taylor mentions, in his "Confessions of a Thug," that it is customary to drug horses with opium, on forced marches, to ensure their bottom. On the subject of Opium-eating and Smoking in India, *vide supra*, p. 226.

Late in their miserable career, the gunjah-smoker and the opium-eater become utterly shattered alike in mind and body; the opium-eater sinks into the condition of a hopeless driveller; the gunjah-smoker and bang-drinker often remain chronically inebriated, and are sometimes excited to acts of frantic violence; but these states may be readily distinguished from true Insanity.

A few days' tranquillity will generally be alone sufficient to restore one who has been over-excited by gunjah to his usual state of mind.

Still, in a very considerable proportion of cases admitted to the Native Lunatic Asyla of this Presidency, mental aberration is clearly traceable to the habitual use of Indian Hemp and Opium.

Baboo Kanny Lall Dey has published a tabulated abstract of the statistical returns of the five Bengal Asyla for the five years, 1863—1867, from which it appears that, out of a total of 2,283 new admissions, there were, among those patients in whom the cause of mental aberration could be

* Oriental Memoirs, Vol. I., p. 64; see also p. 329.

assigned, the following numbers attributable to the use of *Gunjah*, 878; *Opium*, 33; *Datura*, 1. The same evil influence is operative in the North-Western Provinces. Out of 655 lunatics admitted to the Bareilly and Benares Asyla in 1869, 198 cases were attributed to excessive indulgence in intoxicating drugs and spirits.

A thorough analysis of this class of cases appears to be much needed, with a view to show how far the use of these intoxicants leads to the establishment of confirmed mania. A very large proportion of the cases treated in our native asyla are instances of Acute Mania, of which, in these provinces, the use of Gunjah and Bhang is a frequent cause.

It appears probable that a considerable proportion of the cases in question entered in the returns are instances of mere temporary intoxication by these narcotics. Thus, in his report for 1867, the Superintendent of the Patna Asylum remarks :—" Rarely, if ever, is the strict order requiring personal examination by a Magistrate carried out, and the consequence is that many a man, reeling about the bazar intoxicated with gunjah or spirit, finds himself, on coming to his senses, an inmate of a *pagul-khana* (Lunatic Asylum). Again, in his report for 1868, the same officer remarks:— " In this station, as the jail is no longer under the Civil Surgeon, suspected insanes are at once sent to the asylum; and, therefore, in these local cases, no medical certificate accompanies. I do not feel at liberty to reject such cases, although I know that they are mostly mere gunjah-smokers, and always give them a fair trial, yet I do not think that they should be inmates of an asylum while under observation, nor is it fair to send them to a jail. I would, therefore, propose an outside ward, in which cases under observation might be located, and from whence, if necessary, they might be transferred to the asylum." On the other hand, in his report for 1863, the Superintendent of the Dacca Asylum states that his statistics " do not include cases of temporary insanity from intoxication with gunjah and narcotic drugs. Such cases are found out during the period of observation in the Jail Hospital, and certificates of insanity for admission into the asylum are given only in well-marked cases of insanity." Still his report for that year shows that, out of 322 admitted, insanity was traced to gunjah in 164 cases, and to opium in 8.

The following valuable remarks by Dr. Hutchinson, of Patna, appear in his Annual Asylum Report for 1868 :—" Seeing that so many of the cases admitted to our asylums result from over-indulgence in gunjah or bhang, and are not really cases of insanity, I find some difficulty in classing them, and accordingly ventnre to suggest that all such cases be included under the head of *cannabism;* they are easy of recognition, and the following characteristics will assist in determining them :—In a recent case, the conjunctivæ are congested, the pupils generally contracted, and the countenance wears a peculiar *leery* look, which, once seen, is unmistakable. The pulse may or may not be accelerated, and there is a marked unsteadiness in the gait, with great volubility or continued indulgence in laughter or song. If the muscular system is greatly excited, there is a tendency even to rush wildy onwards in a straight line, unmindful of intervening obstacles, and, consequently, severe bruises, especially about the shins, are often met with. These are indications to be met with in a novice, and I cannot find that there are any unpleasant after-consequences in coming out of the debauch, which, on the whole, seems to be a happy and merry state of intoxication. One woman, describing her sensations, said that she felt as if her spirit wished to pass upwards through the skull, and that her body longed to mount upwards as well.

"Bhang-drinking, as opposed to gunjah-smoking, seems to induce pleasant reveries, like those produced by morphia when sleep is resisted. It is enormously indulged in, far more than gunjah, but is easily overlooked, owing to the absence of excitement. In the confirmed gunjah-smoker, there is greater stupidity and less excitement, a kind of maudlin intoxication with conjunctivæ markedly red. Two tests at once betray the *habitué:* by frequently rubbing up the gunjah and tobacco in the left palm with the right thumb, a corn is produced *on the outside of the last phalanx;* and, if you place before him a *chelum* said to be charged with gunjah, he will inhale the smoke with one long prolonged whiff, which would at once bring on coughing in the non-initiated. A confirmed gunjah-smoker has frequently dark purple lips, but the corn and inhalation will always reveal him."

In his report for 1867, Dr. Wise, of Dacca, observes that "indulgence in gunjah is always associated with other vices, such as spirit-drinking and debauchery. The outbreak of mental disease cannot, except in a few cases, be referred to this narcotic alone. The return is more correctly a record of the number of gunjah-smokers among the lunatics." So also in his report for 1864, Dr. Stewart, of Cuttack, observes that the habit of gunjah-smoking is almost invariably accompanied by dissipation.

Professor Polli, of Milan, remarks* that experience has proved that infusions of coffee, tea, and cocoa always increase the action of hashish; so that, if it is wished to accelerate or augment its effect, it should be taken or administered in an aqueous infusion of one or other of these vegetable substances.

Lemon-juice and vinegar, and consequently citric, malic, acetic, and tartaric acids, in aqueous solution, more or less diluted, arrest the effects of hashish in a person who has taken it, and thus are competent to serve as real antidotes.

---

* Med. Press and Circular, Dec. 22, 1869.

Running Amok.

Some observations, made by a writer, in 1798,* bear so importantly upon this subject that they deserve to be quoted here. "The Indian who runs a *muck* [Amok, Amok,—Kill, Kill !] is always first driven to desperation by some outrage, and always first revenges himself upon those who have done him wrong. They are generally slaves, who indeed are most subject to insults, and least able to obtain legal redress. It has been usual to attribute *mucks* to the consequences of the use of opium ; but the words of Mr. Stavorinus, who says that they are occasioned 'by the swallowing of the opium, or *by other means*,' seem to confirm the opinion entertained by Marsden, that this should probably rank with the many errors that mankind have been led into by travellers addicted to the marvellous. That these furious quarrels and sanguinary attacks do actually and frequently take place in some parts of the East, cannot be controverted ; but it is not equally evident that they proceed from any intoxication, except that of their unruly passions ; and many *mucks* might, upon scrutiny, be found to be of the nature of one, which Mr. Marsden particularizes, of a slave who probably never indulged in the use of opium in his life, a man of strong feelings, driven by excess of injury to domestic rebellion ; or that related in Lieutenant Cook's voyage in the *Endeavour*, of a free inhabitant of Batavia, whose brain was fired more by the maddening fury of jealousy, than by any adventitious intoxication. It is true that the Malays, when bent upon any daring enterprize, fortify themselves with a little opium, in order to become insensible of the danger, as the people of another nation are said to take a dram ; but it must be observed, that *the resolution for the act precedes, and is not the effect of, the intoxication.* They take the same precaution, previous to being led to public execution ; but, on these occasions, show greater signs of stupidity than of frenzy." Upon the whole, this writer believed that "it may reasonably be concluded that the sanguinary achievements for which the Malays have been famous, or rather infamous, are more justly derived from the natural ferocity of their disposition than from the qualities of any drug whatever."

In a highly valuable Report on Singapore, sent in to the Medical Board in 1843, Dr. Oxley, Senior Surgeon of the Straits Settlements, has given a very useful account of the practice of *Running Amok.* He considers that what has been so often written of the revengeful spirit of the Malays is much exaggerated. Polite in the extreme, according to their own ideas, they never indulge in abuse one towards the other ; the only reply to any deviation from this rule is the Kris, for which they will watch their opportunity, and most certainly not afford their

---

* Mr. Wilcocke—Notes to a translation of Stavorinus' Voyage to the East Indies, Vol. I., p. 293.

adversary any advantage it is in their power to deprive him of. This is their code of honor; and, being fully aware of it amongst themselves, provocation is seldom given, and satisfaction is seldom required. When goaded, however, to the necessity, they become perfectly reckless; and, should discovery attend the deed, they attempt no refutation, but sell their lives at the utmost cost they can to the captors. Too often has Dr. Oxley known the officers of police compelled to shoot them on these occasions. Such is one species of "Amok," and how offences of this description are to be dealt with, admits of little doubt; but there is another variety of the "*Orang Beramok*," vastly different, and by no means the least frequent, which requires discrimination on the part of the Medical Jurist, to prevent irresponsible persons suffering the penalty of the injured law. For instance, a man sitting quietly amongst his friends and relatives will, without provocation, suddenly start up, weapon in hand, and slay all within his reach. Dr. Oxley has known as many as eight killed and wounded by a very feeble individual in this manner. Next day, when interrogated whether he was not sorry for the act he had committed, no one could be more contrite. When asked, "Why then did you do it?" The answer has invariably been—"The devil entered into me, my eyes were darkened, I did not know what I was about." Dr. Oxley has received this same reply on at least twenty different occasions. On examination of these monomanics, he has generally found them laboring under some gastric disease, or troublesome ulcer, and these fearful ebullitions break out upon some exacerbation of the disorder. Those about them have generally said that they appeared moping and melancholy a few days before the outbreak. He considers that, among the Malays, monomania almost invariably takes this terrible form. The Bugis, whether from revenge or disease, are by far the most addicted to Amok. He thinks that three-fourths of all the cases he has seen have been by persons of this nation. The Boyans, who come from Pulo Babian, an island south of Java, are the most quiet and peaceable of all the Malay tribes. He has never heard of any instance of Amok amongst them. Dr. Oxley does not appear to attribute this practice to the use of intoxicating drugs, although he draws a very painful picture of the miserable effects of opium-smoking in Singapore.

The practice of Running Amok is also prevalent among the Mughs of Arracan. The following cases, occurring among this people, are remarkable in their obscurity, which is increased by the circumstance that it is not mentioned, in either instance, whether the prisoners were addicted to the use of intoxicating drugs. In 1857, Gnamroo had started with the intention of joining his brother at Thandeng, but his wife objected; he went a little distance from the house, when she persuaded him to return. On his way back, he met a man who was cutting bamboos with a dao. Gnamroo took the weapon, and, upon being told not to do so, attacked the owner, and with one blow cut his arm off. He then followed his wife, cut her arm off, and inflicted other wounds. Both of these attacks were fatal. He then attacked a woman with a child five or six years old. He wounded them severely, when, the handle of the weapon breaking, he was secured. When on trial before the Judge, prisoner acknowledged to his mofussil and foujdary confessions as having been made by his own free will. He said he thought he was bewitched, and did not know what would happen to him ; he wanted to go to another village, his wife and others forbade him ; he then, in anger, took the *dao*, and with it wounded the different persons. His sanity was nowhere questioned. Sentence,—Death.*

On the 22nd September 1857, Moung-wot-kai seized a *dao*, killed four persons, and wounded four others, one of whom subsequently died. The prosecutor said that the prisoner was a good man until he lost his wife ; that, since last August, he had appeared not sane, but never quarrelled with any person. Those whom he attacked were the family in whose house he lived. The woman of the house, his own sister, who was one of the sufferers and died in hospital, said that they had had no quarrel ; he had no reason for doing what he did. She said he had been ailing for two or three months, and was silly ; nevertheless, she said he did his work well, the same as the others. The Civil Surgeon had excellent opportunities of examining and watching the prisoner, who had no fits of Insanity. He had every reason to consider him sane, though a low animal of morose disposition, and that he had run "a muck," which Mughs, like Malays, frequently do. In his confession to the Magistrate, the prisoner said he was suddenly seized with a frenzy when he first cut "Kia-oung" and his sister, that he then went out flourishing his sword, or *dao*, and wounded the others. The doing this, he said, gave him pleasure. He said he had been ailing, and must have been mad. No evidence of a quarrel or cause for this crime could be adduced.

The Judges of the Court of Nizamut Adawlut remarked as follows :—

Mr. *D. J. Money*.—"The charges against the prisoner are clearly established upon the fullest and strongest evidence. He has been found guilty of the wilful murder of four persons, and of wounding as many more with intent to murder. The case is a horrible one. The prisoner ran a muck, as it is called, under the possession of something like a satanic influence. He says himself he was seized with a frenzy, and the atrocious act gave him pleasure ; that he had been ailing, and must have been mad. There was no motive for the murders. He acted upon a sudden, and, from his own account, an irresistible impulse. The case is rendered difficult by the opinion pronounced by the Civil Surgeon regarding the prisoner's mental condition. The medical evidence shows that the

* Nizamut Adawlut Reports, October 12, 1857, p. 281.

prisoner had evinced no symptoms of Insanity since the fatal acts were committed. There is no evidence on the record to prove that he was insane before or at the time of their commission. The Civil Surgeon, however, considers him 'a low animal' of morose disposition; and the Officiating Commissioner, on the ground of his being *of a low order of intellect*, and with reference to the decision of this Court of the 30th September 1856, in the case of Eshory Dassee (*vide supra*, p. 777), recommends that the capital punishment should be remitted, and that the prisoner should be sentenced to imprisonment for life in banishment.

"I cannot assent to this recommendation. There is no question, I admit, in the whole range of Criminal Jurisprudence, more difficult to decide than the question of the responsibility which attaches to the commission of a sudden motiveless murder. In most cases, the Court is relieved from the difficulty by the medical evidence; but when such evidence shows, as the result of careful enquiry, that no symptoms of Insanity have been traceable since the commission of the act, and leaves it to be inferred that the prisoner was sane,—that is, conscious of right and wrong, and of the consequences of the act when he committed it; while, on the other hand, there is the glaring Insanity of the act itself, and the statement of the prosecutor that the prisoner was mad some years before,—I confess it requires a most careful examination of the case, and the utmost caution in weighing the medical evidence, in order to arrive at a safe and just conclusion. With reference, however, to the prisoner being 'a low animal,' or of a low order of intellect, it would, I think, be as dangerous as it would be unjust, in the consideration of such a question, to admit of degrees of Insanity, and to allow the extent of the mental and moral consciousness to be the measure of the punishment. The criminal, in every such case, must be either *out of his mind*, and *wholly irresponsible*, or he had the power to resist the homicidal impulse, and did not, and is answerable for the consequences. The Court can admit of no middle ground in judging of the criminality of the act, and the responsibility attached to it. In the *latter* case, the prisoner would justly suffer the extreme penalty of the law; in the *former*, being irresponsible, he should be acquitted, and confined as a madman, until he is pronounced to be sane, and it would be safe to let him loose.

"From the well-known case of Macnaghten tried in the House of Lords, 1843, Taylor, in his work on Medical Jurisprudence (p. 854, Fifth Ed.), deduces the inference that a *complete* possession of reason is not held to be essential to constitute the legal responsibility of an offender; and a little further on, referring to Jameson's Lectures on Insanity, he stated 'that most lunatics have an abstract knowledge that right is right, and wrong, wrong;' but, in true Insanity, the voluntary power to control thought and actions is impaired, limited, or overruled by insane motives. A lunatic may have the power of *distinguishing* right from wrong, but it is contended, from a close observation of the Insane, that he has not the power of *choosing* right from wrong. A criminal is punishable, not merely because he has the power of distinguishing right from wrong, but because he voluntarily does the wrong, having the power to choose the right.

"Was the prisoner in this case sufficiently sane to be criminally responsible? There is no evidence to prove that he was mad. He was not suffering from any particular delusion of mind. In judging, therefore, of the crime, as the result of homicidal mania, it would be a dangerous doctrine to judge only of the Insanity of the prisoner from the Insanity of the act. Under this reasoning, and upon such ground, almost every crime might be palliated or excused. Absence of motive alone is not a safe criterion. There must be other evidences of Insanity before a criminal can be pronounced irresponsible. See Taylor upon this point, in his work cited above. The sentence passed by this Court, in the case cited by the Officiating Commissioner, was *transportation for life*, on the ground of the prisoner possessing a *low intellect*.

"The sentence now recommended is based upon this precedent. If I could be persuaded that *low intellect* was a mental condition which gave the possessor invariably *less control* over his actions than a higher degree of intellect, irrespective of moral feeling, I might come to the conclusion that he was necessarily *less responsible;* but still there would be *some* responsibility; and, if *responsible at all*, the law must take its course. But as, in judging of the act, I do not think the punishment should depend upon the degree of Insanity, so also I would not allow the responsibility of the act to be affected by a higher or lower order of intellect. I think the prisoner in this case, whatever his intellect was, had the power to control the homicidal impulse; and as, instead of resisting it, he indulged in it, because it gave him pleasure, he justly deserves the extreme penalty of the law. I would sentence him, therefore, to suffer death."

Mr. *J. H. Patton.*—"I have no hesitation in giving my assent to the death-sentence proposed to be passed on the prisoner. He has been guilty of four foul murders, and as many more woundings with intent to kill, and all he pleads in defence is that he was seized with an irresistible impulse to destroy life; and that the act gave him pleasure. That he knew what he was about, there can be no doubt, as otherwise he could not describe the sensations he felt in committing the deeds; and if, with that knowledge, he transgressed the highest command of God and man, he is unquestionably a fit subject for the infliction of the extreme penalty of the law. I would sentence him to be hanged."*

Forbes says of the Moplahs (Vol. I., p. 259):—"The Moplahs engaged in commerce, and, enjoying intercourse with other people, are tolerably

* Nizamut Adawlut Reports, January, 27th 1858, p. 10.

courteous and orderly. Those in the interior, who are too proud to work or engage in agricultural pursuits, are generally an idle, worthless race, parading about the country with a broadsword, or murdering time in the swing. These are of a most turbulent, revengeful spirit, prone to mischief, especially against the Nairs, whom they consider as infidels, proud and haughty as themselves. When intoxicated with *bhang* or opium, they frequently run a muck, and, in a dreadful state of frenzy, kill every person they meet, until they are overpowered and destroyed."

The following is not by any means a singular case in India :—A respectable up-country Hindu, who had been for some years settled in the employ of a zemindar near Chittagong, upon receiving some abuse from his wife and her mother, took down a heavy tulwar from the wall, and literally hacked the former in pieces, and then ran at the latter, who, however, escaped with a severe wound into the elbow-joint. He then pursued another woman, who was passing at the time, and succeeded in wounding her, by thrusting his sword under the door of her house, which she had closed upon him. I found him to be a very healthy-looking and well-mannered man of fifty ; he was perfectly rational, but I learned that he was in the habit of eating nine ruttees ($13\frac{1}{2}$ grains) of opium daily. He appears, however, not to have been guilty of any unusual excess in this way before the crime was committed. As it was necessary to ascertain whether he was, in reality, addicted to opium-eating, I kept him without the drug for four or five days, when he displayed that peculiar nervous agitation, which is so characteristic in opium-eaters deprived of their usual stimulus. He was then allowed a daily supply, but his strength continued to fail until after his trial and sentence to death, when he was attacked with remittent fever, which assumed an almost typhous character, very unusual in that jail, and destroyed him in a few days.

It appears probable that, had not this man's nervous system been greatly shattered by the vice of opium-eating, the abuse which he received would not have excited a blind and indiscriminating impulse to kill in his apparently otherwise calm and rational mind.

The following very singular case was tried at Chota Nagpore in 1857 :—Nundo Rowanee, Burkundaz, met two women in the village of Jhuria, and, without saying a word, suddenly attacked them with a sword, killing one, and wounding the other severely. The son of one of them running out had a hand struck off, and subsequently died ; two other men were also wounded. Prisoner said that he had been attacked by robbers who had also wounded the villagers. Again, that the latter had got up the case. There was no evidence to confirm these statements. Three witnesses, also burkundazes, stated that the prisoner was in the habit of taking gunjah, but he never appears to have been excited to acts of violence by the drug. It was held impossible to discover from the record the motive which actuated him. It was equally impossible from the record to attribute to the prisoner malicious intent or malignant design towards the individuals whom he attacked, as he had only been a few days at Jhuria, and had no cause of quarrel with, and indeed was unknown to most of the sufferers. There was no proof that he was, at the time, intoxicated with *gunjah*. These were deemed extenuating circumstances, and he was sentenced to transportation for life.*

I can offer only a partial demonstration of the fact, but I am convinced that a very large proportion of the murders by hacking to pieces, which have already been referred to in this Report as prevalent in India, are committed under the influence of intoxicating drugs, which, without doing more than add to and maintain furious excitement, enable the otherwise timid savage to carry out his ruthless purpose. In looking over the Nizamut Reports, I have been struck by the frequency with which medical opinion has been called for to decide upon the evidently disordered and unsettled state of mind of these criminals. In a few such cases it has been decided that the prisoners were Insane; in others, attempts to feign Insanity were detected; while, in a third class, there were, at first, marked evidences of something nearly approaching to Insanity, which gradually disappeared in the course of a week or two. The following example may be selected from many. In 1845, Dr. Wilkie, then of Dinagepore, examined the dead body of a woman, and the persons of a boy† and of a second woman who had been wounded with some cutting instrument. The first woman must have died immediately, the boy recovered; the other woman was so severely injured by sword-cuts, that it was at one time apprehended that she would be maimed for life. The Mussalmaun who was tried for this outrage appeared to Dr. Wilkie, on his admission to jail, to be suffering from mental derangement. There were suffusion of the eyes, much cerebral excitement, and fever. All these symptoms, however, subsided within a week, and Dr. Wilkie then considered him sane. In reply to the question whether, if temporary Insanity was produced by fever and nervous excitement (as stated by the witnesses in this case), would it probably be likely to recur, or could such a person be set at large without danger to the community? Dr. Wilkie said that, as this man's temporary Insanity was induced by no appreciable motive or cause, he was inclined to believe that it must be owing to some peculiarity in the brain and nervous system; he therefore was afraid that mental derangement might recur, and that, consequently, his release was not advisable.

* Nizamut Adawlut Reports, May 12, 1857, p. 652.

† It is one of the marked features of these cases of wounding, where jealousy is the cause, that a child often shares the punishment of its unfortunate mother.—Nizamut Adawlut Report, Sept. 1855, p. 420. See also a case (Nizamut Adawlut Reports of the N. W. Provinces for July 1854, p. 124), in which one Nokeh was convicted of murdering his wife and infant two years old, with a heavy chopper (*gundasa*). He merely stated that he had had a trifling dispute with his wife.

The cause upon which this person's mental excitement depended was evidently *physical*, and I have observed a precisely similar condition in one who, having become over-excited by the use of gunjah, was tied and beaten by those about him in the brutal manner generally adopted by natives, with a view to drive away the devils by which they believe the Insane to be possessed. We need a very careful investigation of this class of cases. It would, of course, materially alter the complexion of a violent act, apparently committed in sudden rage, if it were discovered that the culprit had previously drugged himself with the deliberate purpose of maintaining his barbarous impulse.

I am indebted to my friend Dr. W. W. Hunter, LL.D., for the following note :—

In 1790, the Collector of Beerbhoom reported of *Pachwai*, a pernicious fermented rice liquor, that "to its cheapness I ascribe the numerous robberies and other depredations almost daily experienced, it being a notorious fact, on the records of the Criminal Court, that the perpetrators of these crimes first work themselves up to the perpetrating of them by this kind of liquor, and by smoking the herb called bhang."

The following instances in which it appeared that *the criminals were nerved with Wine or Spirits or Opium* previous to carrying out their sanguinary purpose, are worthy of notice (*vide supra, p.* 226). The great importance of ascertaining whether or not such criminals have thus prepared themselves is self-evident, as it decides the question of deliberation.

It appeared, in a trial at Allahabad, that one Chotooa, having endeavoured to persuade a prostitute who was under his master's protection to carry on an intrigue with him, she replied derisively, that "she would ride on an elephant, not on an ass." He then left her house and went to a neighbouring spirit-shop, where he drank two pice worth of spirits, and returned with a sword, which he probably took from his own house on the way ;—seizing the unfortunate woman by the hair, he hacked at her until her body was disfigured by twenty wounds, and the deadly weapon was bent out of shape.*

In a case already cited, which occurred at Budaon, where a man killed five persons, his relatives, by cutting their throats with a sword, it appeared that an open bottle of port wine was found on the table of a room in which the prisoner slept. It was believed by the Sessions Judge that the murderer had taken what wine was consumed to give himself nerve for the deed; or, if vengeance supplied that, to give himself heart to inflict a wound which was found on his own person.†

The following importantly illustrative case occurred in the Punjab, and was reported in *Indian Public Opinion*.‡ "A Poorbea, formerly a sepoy

* Nizamut Adawlut Reports, N. W. P., October 27th, 1852, p. 1246.

† *Ibid*, February 25th, 1853, p. 823.

‡ May 22nd, 1868.

in the service of Runjeet Singh, ran a muck, wounding a woman and two children severely, and killing a child. He then attacked a young man, who, although seriously wounded in the head and neck, ran away bleeding to the police station, where he gave information, which was at once attended to. A number of policemen moved towards the indicated spot, where they found the Poorbea armed with a straw-chopper, with which he at once proceeded to attack them. Providentially, as the scuffle was about to begin, the blade of the chopper, which the miscreant had taken good care to sharpen beforehand, flew off, thus rendering the capture of its owner a comparatively easy matter. The Poorbea was then placed in confinement, in which he died in the course of the day, poisoned by the excessive quantity of opium which he had taken in order to work himself up into a state of fury."

"From subsequent enquiries it appeared that this Poorbea, some time ago, had mortgaged his house to his nephew for Rs. 300, who then sued for the amount and obtained a decree,—the defendant not appearing, as he was too proud to defend himself against a junior member of his family, of which he considered himself the head. At all events, the nephew then sued for execution of decree, got the house sold by auction, when he bought it in. This seems to have preyed on the mind of his uncle, who yesterday morning, after making an unsuccessful search for his nephew, with the view, probably, of murdering him, entered his nephew's house, where he wounded that relative's wife and two children, and killed one. He then ran amuck and attacked the young man whose information led to his capture."

It is a matter of popular notoriety, both in Bengal and in the North-Western Provinces, that *persons intoxicated with gunjah are liable to commit acts of homicidal violence;* hence we find several cases in the Reports, in which prisoners made the plea of intoxication by gunjah as a mitigation of their crimes: thus—

A man of Jessore, having been irritated by abuse from a woman who had lived with him for some years, killed her by striking her over the head with a *kooralee.* In his foujdaree confession, he alleged that he had eaten gunjah during the night, but could not state if he was laboring under the effects of it at the time. To a certain degree, this assertion was supported by the evidence of two witnesses, who found him, shortly after the murder, lying down in some thatching grass with his teeth clenched, and stupefied. The Judges considered that the crime was committed in the heat of blood, and passed sentence accordingly.* One Nund Lall, of Jubbulpore, when on trial for hacking his wife to death with a sword, stated that, labouring under an attack of fever, he asked his wife for some water; upon her not replying, and he having taken

* Nizamut Adawlut Reports, November 25th, 1851, p. 668.

gunjah, a fight took place, upon which he killed her with the sword. This plea was, however, fully disproved by the evidence of witnesses, who represented him as not exhibiting any trace of either illness or intoxication on their arrival at the scene of the murder.*

Three sepoys went over from Bhurtpore to witness the religious ceremonies at Goburdhun. Suddenly, and, as far as could be ascertained, without any provocation, one of them, named Rambuksh, drew his sword, slew one of his comrades by striking his head from his body, and then, rushing forward, decapitated three harmless women entirely strangers to him. He was not arrested until his left forearm had been cut off. He pleaded that he was not aware of what he had done; and, in defence, stated that he had taken *bhang*, and was beside himself. His comrades, who had known him for five or six years, stated that he was a quiet, inoffensive man, and was not intoxicated at the time of committing this act, nor was he ever suspected of being Insane. Before the Magistrate he had said that the man whom he killed had threatened to strike him. He was sentenced to death.†

One Ruttee, of Nursingpore, who had intrigued with another man's mistress, was tried and found guilty of having killed the woman in a jungle, dismembering the body, and robbing it of its ornaments. In his foujdaree confession, he said that he killed his victim under gunjah,—"*Gunjah peeka mara.*"‡

Bhagram Gogori being left alone in the homestead with his young sister-in-law, entered her apartment, and beat her until she became insensible. He then set fire to the seven huts inhabited by the family. They and all the property which they contained were destroyed. The family returning in alarm, he struck those who approached with a lattee, and killed one individual by smashing his skull. A criminal intercourse between the prisoner and his sister-in-law was suspected. He appears to have been previously of a quiet good temper. He said that, feeling unwell, he had inhaled *gunjah*, and was so completely under its influence, that he could not tell whether he committed the crimes or not. Sentence, transportation for life.§

One Madar Buksh, of Mirzapore, hacked his wife to pieces, inflicting twenty-two wounds with a sword, probably under the influence of jealousy. He confessed the crime, saying that he suspected the woman of infidelity, and that, before his return home, on the fatal night, a man gave him a pill to eat: it was *majum*, or *bhang*, and was very powerful. The person

---

* Nizamut Adawlut Reports, N. W. P., 14th January 1854, p. 29.

† *Ibid*, May 23rd, 1854, p. 575.

‡ *Ibid*, November 29th, 1853, p. 1420.

§ Nizamut Adawlut Reports, October 4th, 1855, p. 554.

named denied altogether that he had given the pill to the prisoner. The Judge thought it not improbable that intoxication was resorted to, purposely to gain heart for the deed which was meditated.*

It will been seen, from the foregoing details, that instances of *Running Amok* are scarcely less prevalent in this presidency than in Singapore.

In some of these cases, the crime appears to have been committed upon some grounds of provocation, as in that of the Up-country man at Chittagong, which I have already given, and in the following instances :—A Dacca man invited four boys to dine with him. The dinner not being ready, he sat down to smoke, when one of the lads snatched his hookah out of his hand. Upon this, he seized a piece of wood, struck two of the boys on the head with it and killed them ; he then chased the other two into a house where he killed two other persons. He was sentenced to death.†

A man of Behar had words with his brother, about the division of some property, and, suddenly drawing his sword, wounded him. He then ran into the females' apartments, and there killed his sister, his uncle's wife, and his brother's wife. Thence he rushed into a house opposite, and, wounding the wife of the owner, took to the roof, where he defended himself with his sword for some time, but at last gave himself up to the Government vakeel, to whom alone he said he would surrender. His nephew, a few days before, had informed the jemadar that his uncle was insane ; but, on the jemadar going to him, he did not find anything apparently the matter with him.‡

One Mudhoo Pandah, a Brahmin, of Cuttack, having been prohibited by a bawd from cohabiting with a common prostitute in her house, entered the house armed with a sword, killed the bawd and one of her women, and injured three others, hacking them in a frightful manner.§

Ram Singh, havildar in the Kumaon Battalion, stationed at Dehra Doon, being seated in the orderly-room with the other native officers of the regiment, where they were writing their daily report, suddenly rose and struck one Nardeb, acting havildar, three blows from behind with a kookree. Nardeb died on the spot. The prisoner then rushed about and wounded two sepoys of the corps. At the urgent appeal of the other sepoys he threw down his weapon and surrendered. It was alleged that the

* Nizamut Adawlut Reports, N. W. P., April 22nd, 1854, p. 436. See also a case in which one Kumla, a burkundauze, of Boolundshuhur, killed, without any evidence of sufficient provocation, two boatmen who were ferrying him across the river. The Sessions Judge believed that, having been at a religious festival at Belown, the prisoner had probably indulged in *bhang*, or some intoxicating liquor—and, being temporarily excited, was irritated by the slowness of the men. He was sentenced to death.—*Ibid*, July 16th, 1853, p. 853.

† Police Report, L. P., 1846, p. 47.

‡ *Ibid*, 1848, p. 12.

§ Nizamut Adawlut Reports, October 25th, 1853, p. 710.

deceased had debauched the prisoner's wife, and thus dishonored his house. After his arrest, prisoner said—"I have killed one, another yet remains."*

Kullooa, of Allyghur, confessed, when apprehended, that he had killed his wife with a sword (cutting her almost to pieces), because he suspected her of an intrigue with his brother; the immediate cause of his committing the act being, that she had mixed some excrement in water which she gave him to drink. He also wounded his nephew very severely, merely, he said, because he happened to be in the way at the time, and that, had any other person come in his way, he should have attacked him also.†

The following case is from the *Indian Mirror* of May 21st, 1869 :—

On Monday evening, between seven and eight o'clock, a Mahomedan khalassie, an Up-country man, ran *amok* in a narrow lane, [at Howrah, near Calcutta] and, before he was arrested, had cut down no less than eleven persons,—four men, three women, and four children. The man, Sahawut Ally, it appears, was very jealous, and not without cause, of his wife. He assigns her misconduct as the cause of the fury which possessed him, and, finding he could get no redress for his grievances from the Howrah authorities, he appears to have determined to revenge himself upon mankind in general. He seized a Hoseinee tulwar, and, rushing out into the narrow lane in which his house is situated, he cut down every soul he met ; and, as it was some little time before two constables came up, and after a struggle succeeded in mastering him, the list of his victims is unfortunately very heavy :—

Suneechar Bibee, seriously wounded.
Chundra Bibee, do.
Bilmonia Bibee, do.
Rungeeah (a girl of 12), dead.
Edia (an infant of 6 months), dead.
Dhunoman (a boy of 10), seriously wounded.
Shaikh Islam, do.
Shaikh Wuzeer, cut on the arm.
Shaikh Jokhan, do.
Shaikh Muckdoom Buksh, severe cut on the right hand.
Muckoaman (a girl of 12), cut on the forehead.

A few of these instances where people run *amok* appear to be cases of real insanity. One of these is alluded to in the Cuttack Lunatic Asylum Report for 1865. A man's mind became unsettled by fright, a tiger having sprung at him while he was herding cattle in the jungle. He escaped, but became more and more excited, until he got a tulwar and ran

---

* Nizamut Adawlut Reports, N. W. P., December 2nd, 1852, p. 1428.

† *Ibid*, December 2nd, 1852, p. 1431.

through his village shouting, "Tiger! Tiger!" and cut down all he met with. He was reported to have killed three men.

Oomer Wullud Auwud was one of a party of Arabs travelling from Bombay to Poonah. At about midnight the party were disturbed by the prisoner, who, in a paroxysm of insanity, without the slightest provocation, seized a sword, killed two men, and wounded three others. His insanity was clearly established.*

These two cases, especially the Cuttack one, much resemble that of King Charles the Sixth of France. Froissart tells us that the king's impatience to march on his expedition against Bretagne threw him into a fever, but, despite of all remonstrance, he set forth, notwithstanding the heat of the August weather and his own indisposition. The way being dusty, the king rode apart from his escort, followed by two pages, one carrying his lance, the other his helmet. His distress from the heat was increased by his wearing a jerkin of thick velvet and a heavy cap of scarlet cloth. As he rode past a forest, a tall and ghastly man rushed out upon him, and, seizing his bridle, cried, "Stop, king! you are going where you are betrayed!"—and as suddenly disappeared. While the king was still agitated by this incident, they arrived at a sandy plain, where one of the pages, being overpowered by the heat, fell asleep and let the lance fall clashing against the helmet borne by his companion. The king, roused by the clang of arms, was seized with sudden frenzy, and, imagining himself beset with enemies, rode fiercely with drawn sword among his attendants, and must have killed several if they had not fled. His sword breaking, he was at last secured. He remained in a state of mania for some months, and then recovered his senses only to lose them again permanently in a scene of extreme horror and personal danger to himself, which occurred in his court two years afterwards.

A very remarkable case of *Running Amok*, in which no motive could be discovered, was tried at Moradabad. It appeared that, a number of persons being assembled at about mid-day within the enclosure of the cutcherry of Amroah, one Bhow seized the sword of a burkundauz and rushed round the building, cutting at every person whom he met. He, in this way, wounded no less than fifteen persons,—chuprassees, prisoners, mohurrirs, and witnesses, with none of whom he had any enmity: three of them, however, endeavoured to stop him. He was seized, with some difficulty, by two men, one of whom wounded him with a bayonet. The Sessions Judge postponed the trial three months; the medical officer was thus enabled to watch the prisoner for five months, and deposed that he considered him to be sane; that the only peculiarity he ever observed in him was a disinclination to enter into conversation; that he usually sat in a silent and sullen manner, as he was sitting in Court at the time of his

---

* Bellasis' Reports, p. 23.

(witness) being examined ; that nothing had ever passed which would lead him to suppose that the prisoner, in so sitting silent and sullen, was acting a part ; and that, as far as he had opportunities of judging (and he saw the prisoner within half an hour of the assault), he was capable of knowing that, in wounding the persons in question, he was commiting acts forbidden by the law of the land. [The superior Court observed that the Sessions Judge should not have questioned the medical officer as to whether the prisoner was or was not responsible for his actions. This was a point for legal decision on the evidence.]

The prisoner, on being examined by the Magistrate, deposed that the Deity had made him use the sword; that the Deity likewise wounded him; that a *taweez* found on his person was made, two years previously, to give him bravery ; and that he had had an addition made to this *taweez* lately. He afterwards said that he wished to kill the Magistrate, and again, that he intended to kill that officer's Sheristadar. On trial, he denied everything. Various witnesses, living in the same village with the prisoner, and in those adjacent, and, amongst them, his own brother, deposed to his sanity ; the brother added, however, that he was in the habit of absenting himself occasionally four or five days without cause : another brother deposed to his not being sane. Certain prisoners stated that, on being first admitted to the jail, the prisoner did not appear to be sane, but that, after some time, he became so. It was shown that, previous to running *Amok*, the prisoner had taken off his upper clothing and girded up his loins, as though about to wrestle. One of the witnesses deposed that he saw the prisoner cut a tree with his sword. The Judges concurred in believing that the prisoner was perfectly sane at the time he committed the crimes, and sentenced him to imprisonment for life in transportation. It does not appear to have become a matter of inquiry whether the man was in the habit of smoking hemp, or was under the influence of drugs when this outbreak occurred.*

In the following cases it appears that sane persons ran *amok*, and there is nothing to show that they were under the influence of intoxication when they did so.

Kadir Shaha, of Cuttack, having an enmity against a man, gave him a fatal stab in the breast with a knife; he then went into the house where his own brother (who was involved in the same dispute) was asleep, with his two children, and wounded all three with his knife; he than ran out into the road in a state of nudity, with a *pharsa* in his hand, and cut down or hacked about some small trees between his own and the deceased's house. He acknowledged these crimes, but he and some of his witnesses alleged that he had, two or three days before the murder, been suffering from a complaint called *har phootie*, which, literally translated, signifies pustules

* Nizamut Adawlut Reports, N. W. P., 1st May 1852, p. 383.

of the bones, but which is an eruption of small pustules on the skin, which disordered his mind. The inference to be drawn from the deposition of the Civil Surgeon is, that such disease would not cause mental aberration amounting to insanity. He was sentenced to death.*

In the *Queen* v. *Bishonath Bunneea,* it was proved that the prisoner killed the deceased Pochai and wounded three other persons.

The evidence in this case was very fully and plainly laid before the jury, who found that the prisoner was not insane at the time, and that there was no evidence to show that he had ever before been out of his senses. That he had been perfectly sane ever since, was unquestionable. The Judges of the Appellate High Court observed that this was "one of those cases in which a quiet, peaceable man, by all accounts, suddenly, and without the least motive or provocation, runs a muck against all around him. He may have been sane immediately before and immediately after, and there may be no evidence whatever to show that he was insane at the moment of his attack ; still it is impossible to avoid the conviction that the man's mind was not in its normal state, and that this case is very different from ordinary cases of deliberate murder. We think that, under all the circumstances of the case, we are justified in remitting the capital sentence, and in awarding one of transportation for life."†

The most singular feature in this class of cases, is the impulse which, almost invariably, urges the prisoners, after having satiated their vengeance, to continue their havoc upon unoffending persons. It is evident that no peculiar opinions of religion, or custom, or class can prevail in these cases ; for we find the crime perpetrated, under precisely similar circumstances, by the Up-country Rajpoot, the Bengalee, the Ooriah, the Mugh of Arrakan, and the Malay of Singapore. All that these men can be said to have in common is, that their natures are revengeful, that they live under a tropical sun, and are habituated to excess in the use of intoxicating drugs. Carefully sifted, it is probable that the generality of these cases would be found to be dependent upon the last-mentioned fact.

I find, in the printed Reports, several cases of trial for *Murder,* both in Bengal and Up-country, *committed by known Gunjah Smokers and Opium Eaters.* In 1853, a Mussulmaun was tried, at Backergunge, for murdering his wife by frequent blows with a pole armed at one end with a flat piece of iron. His mother and all the neighbours said that the prisoner had not been in his right mind for eight or ten days previous to the murder. He was, however, quite capable of giving his own defence, and was sufficiently in his right mind to plead Insanity, and to assert that jealousy had unsettled his mind. The confessions, before the darogah and before the Magistrate, were so nearly similar that a translation of either of them

* Nizamut Adawlut Reports, September 27, 1855, p. 467.

† Weekly Reporter, October 1867, Vol. III., Criminal, p. 53.

would suffice.* This man remained, for two years, in the Dacca Lunatic Asylum. Dr. Green stated that, upon the man's admission there, he thought him quite insane. He suffered from cholera and dysentery about eight months subsequent to the murder, after which he began to answer, when addressed (which he did not do at first), and left off his previous mad actions, and, for some months previous to his discharge, behaved himself quietly and rationally. Dr. Green therefore recommended him for release. Dr. Green understood that he was a *Gunjah Smoker*, and thought it probable that he was subject to fits of madness before admission into the Asylum. The prisoner was acquitted.†

In 1852, a native policeman was tried at Moorshedabad, for the murder of another burkundauz, his companion, with whom he appears to have had no previous quarrel. A man who was in his custody stated that the prisoner and deceased were sleeping in a thannah, when the prisoner suddenly called out that he (prisoner) had been bitten by a snake. The witness saw a snake pass by his bed near to the charpaee of the prisoner, who cut it into pieces with a sword; after which, at his request, the witness prepared tobacco for the prisoner to smoke, and returned to bed. Before he was asleep, he heard deceased give an alarm that he was murdered, and, getting up, saw the prisoner strike deceased with a sword. The deceased died from his wounds fifteen days subsequently. Dr. Keane examined the prisoner, and reported him to be sane. The Judges decided that it was in evidence that the prisoner was addicted to smoking *Gunjah*, and that, shortly before the murder was committed, a chillum of tobacco had been prepared for him. Whether there was *Gunjah* or other stupefying drug in the tobacco was not known, but that he was probably under the influence of this drug at the time, and that the sight and effort of killing the snake may have added to his excitement. In the absence of any ascertainable motive for the act, it was regarded as committed in a temporary fit of insanity, arising from excessive smoking of gunjah. The prisoner was therefore sentenced to be imprisoned in transportation for life.‡

One Baba Ramdoss, an aged *byragee* of Saugor, without any ascertainable reason, attacked a young child, which was lying sick, with a knotted stick and beat it to death, fracturing its skull. It appeared, from

---

* Shakespear's test of Insanity, insisted upon by Sir H. Halford :—

"——————— Ecstacy!
My pulse as your's doth temperately keep time,
And makes as healthful music. It is not madness
That I have uttered : bring me to the test,
And *I the matter will re-word, which madness*
Would gambol from!"—HAMLET, ACT iii., SCENE 4.

† Nizamut Adawlut Reports, Vol. IV., p. 258.

‡ *Ibid*, Vol. II., Part 2, p. 676.

the evidence of the *Kotwar*, that the *byragee* was in the habit of using intoxicating drugs, and it was stated that, when the stick was taken away from him, he appeared to be infuriated. The prisoner was placed under the observation of the Civil Surgeon, who deposed that the man's intellect had become considerably clouded by continued indulgence in intoxicating drugs ; and that, indeed, he was almost an imbecile. He was sentenced to imprisonment for life in irons.*

The following case of murder by an opium-eater is important, as showing that the law does not permit men's vices to excuse their crimes :—

Kristo Dass was tried at Seebsaugor, Assam, for having killed a boy, seven or eight years of age, by chopping his neck with a dao while he lay asleep. He confessed that he went to the house and asked a woman there for betel-nut, but did not get it ; that, when sitting by the child's bed, he was seized with the desire to kill deceased, but had no ill-will against him ; besides, ten or twelve years before, he was seized with a similar desire to kill his wife, and wounded her. Before the Magistrate, he added that, his mind being troubled at being denied the betel, he lost control over himself. Several witnesses deposed that he was an opium-eater. After stating the above circumstances, the Deputy Commissioner observed, " The only question that arises is, in the absence of any ostensible motive for the atrocious and bloodthirsty murder of a helpless and sleeping child,—could he have been in sound mind at the time ? It has been clearly proved by the evidence of his neighbours that, both before and after the deed, he was, to all appearance, of sound mind; although it is also shown by the evidence that, some eleven years ago, he made a similar onslaught on his wife, but failed to effect his purpose of murder, and that he was greatly addicted to opium. The medical officer, who saw him frequently while in prison, could trace no symptom of insanity," [Dr. Wallis deposed that he was always morose and sullen, and seldom spoke ; he always sat for hours without changing his position, he cooked his own meals, and otherwise conducted himself like a sane man] " but describes him as of the most morose and sullen disposition, and also a great opium-eater. He considers, from the phrenological development of the prisoner and his uniform morose and sullen conduct, combined with the long-continued use of opium, that he would be easily excited to fits of frenzy, at which time he would consider him as a dangerous character, and unaccountable for his actions. It appears that prisoner had taken opium a very short time before the deed. It is possible that a state of mind, such as described by the medical officer, may have been induced by the abrupt departure of the witness Mussamut Leepai without giving him *tamul*. I do not think that he can be held as not accountable for his actions ; I therefore convict him of wilful murder."

---

* Nizamut Adawlut Reports, N. W. P., February 2nd, 1854, p. 98.

The Judges of the Court of Nizamut Adawlut observed, "The one point in the Civil Surgeon's deposition is that, under a certain combination of circumstances, the prisoner might be excited to frenzy, which would make him a dangerous lunatic, and unaccountable for his acts. But there is no evidence whatever to show that the prisoner was under such frenzy when he committed this murder; indeed, the whole purport of the evidence of those who had seen him shortly before, including those with whom he lived, was that he was on that day, and had been many years continuously, of sound mind, in the sense before stated, as that in which the question of prisoner's responsibility has to be considered. Most of the witnesses state that the prisoner, some ten or twelve years back, wounded and hacked his wife without any motive under a sudden impulse, and two state that he, for about a year afterwards, used to move about as mad (*puglanee*), and threaten children. Prisoner himself states that he acted under a morbid impulse to kill. We cannot admit that such a fact, or anything that has been above cited from the evidence, should bar a capital punishment, nor is the entire absence of motive any such bar (*vide* Nizamut Adawlut Reports, Vol. I., pp. 82, 100; Vol. II., Part 2, 1852, p. 945; Vol. V., Part 1, p. 246). We therefore sentence the prisoner capitally."*

Drugging with Datura.—We have seen (pp. 204 and 208) that, apart from the numerous cases of Thuggee by Poison which occur in India, it is probable that Datura is occasionally employed by designing persons as a means of controlling the actions of those against whom they entertain nefarious designs. It is a matter of common report, although I have not been able to obtain much perfectly indisputable evidence of the existence of such a custom, that slow poisoning by Datura is practised by unprincipled natives upon aged and weak-minded relatives and others, whom, on account of their wealth, or for other reasons, they are anxious to reduce to a state of utter helplessness and imbecility. Cases of this description would, of course, demand the physician's utmost caution and acumen.

The following remarkable case was reported, in 1853, by Baboo Buddenchunder Chowdry, of Hooghly:—"Bhuttacharjee, a student, a resident of Umbika, in East Burdwan, passed his early days in the enjoyment of gay and pleasant company, his chief engagement being music, singing, &c. He, like his companions, was in the habit of smoking hemp in repeated chillums till intoxication was produced. On the 31st of December 1848, while under the effect of the drug, a cousin of his took advantage of his state, and adminstered to him some Datura seeds, to deepen and prolong the inebriation, perhaps to serve some evil motive arising from family disputes then existing between them. The deed being imme-

* Nizamut Adawlut Reports, March 26, 1857, p. 392.

diately brought to light, he was carried out of the inner apartments in a senseless state, and treated with some soothing medicines and a cold bath. From that time, he passed restless nights; his ideas were confused, thoughts roving,—all indicating mental derangement. The finest music and songs, in which he had once taken the greatest pleasure, were disliked; nothing could comfort him, he showed some liking for solitude, laughed at one time and became violently furious at another, tearing and biting the pillows and cloths, and frequently attempted to injure any person who ventured to go near him. He was brought here in irons, and showed every symptom of violence, biting the irons, spitting, grinning, barking, howling, and shouting. The success which had attended the treatment adopted in some of my former cases induced me to try it also in the present instance. I accordingly had the patient's head shaved, and directed him to be put in a *gumla* of warm water, and several *kulsees* of cold water, from the drain of a terrace, to be poured over his head twice a day, morning and evening; two drops of croton oil, with a little sugar, to be swallowed every morning until he could be easily prevailed upon to take other medicines, and a grain of morphia to be repeated every night at intervals of two hours, until he should fall asleep. During the first week, the state of the patient was almost stationary; but, at the end of that time, there were evident marks of improvement, his mind began to regain its reasoning power, and he commenced sleeping some nights without the opiate."*

Investigation of Crimes alleged to have been committed in the Delirium of Fever, under the Irritation of Severe Pain, and by Persons otherwise in Ill-health, &c.—Allusion has been already made, in the account of Dr. Wilkie's case, p. 787, and at p. 421, to instances in which the alleged fact of the crime being committed under the delirium of fever was pleaded in mitigation. In 1814, a man killed his wife, at Moradabad, by striking her on the neck with a sword, nearly severing her head from her body. He soon afterwards made a confused and incoherent confession, stating that he had been ill with fever for ten days, and that he had killed his wife because she had refused to bring him some water. Before the Magistrate, his confession was more clear and circumstantial. His wife, he said, had several times absconded from him, and was in the habit of sleeping at the houses of other people; that she behaved disobediently to him on all occasions, but especially so on the day of her death, when he asked her to do something and she refused; that, being afflicted at the time with a fever and ague, which affected his senses, and being greatly irritated at her insulting behaviour, he seized a sword, and struck her on

* See a remarkable case in which a man of Gorruckpore was convicted of drugging a whole household with Datura, under pretence of curing a member of the family who was insane.—Nizamut Adawlut Reports, N. W. P., April 22nd, 1854, p. 441.

the back of the neck. The Judges, being of opinion that the prisoner was under the influence of a paroxysm of fever at the time of his committing the homicide, directed that he should be immediately released.*

In March 1854, a man was sentenced to six months' imprisonment for having thrown a billet of light wood at his wife (who was inattentive to his request to light a fire for him), when he was suffering from fever, and ruptured her spleen, which was diseased.†

One Dataram was tried at Delhi for the murder of his mother and cousin, and for wounding, with intent to murder, his two brothers, with a sword. It was obscurely shown that there had been a family quarrel about the prisoner's wife, with whose behaviour, apparently in connection with one of his brothers, he would seem to have been dissatisfied. Amongst the principal witnesses were his two brothers, the man whom he attempted to kill, and his aunt, the mother of the little girl, his cousin, whom he murdered. These, on the other hand, deposed that he had been suffering from fever, and that, in the delirium of fever, he had used his sword against the members of his own family, with whom he had no quarrel whatever. The witnesses at the thannah confession of the prisoner declared that he was in the full possession of his senses at the time he appeared before them; the plea of delirium was not advanced until afterwards. The Civil Surgeon deposed that he was decidedly of sound mind, and that, having had him under his observation from within a few days after the perpetration of the crime up to the time of trial, he did not think it likely that he had been delirious simply from fever, and had, in consequence, been impelled to murder his mother and cousin. He did not think it probable that a man in the delirium of fever would commit a murder which he would not have committed if he had been in health; because a patient, laboring under fever, and delirious at the same time, is almost always so debilitated that he cannot get up or walk steadily; and, if he had the desire to commit murder, he could not have the necessary degree of physical strength or cunning to effect it. This man got up in the night, took a sword, and nearly severed from her body the head of his cousin, a little girl eight or nine years of age, and inflicted one other wound on her person. He then murdered his mother, wounding her in six places with the same sword, and, after rushing from the house, wounded his two brothers, and was immediately apprehended. [It must be noted here, however, that, taking into account the various acute disorders of the brain, which might be characterised, in non-medical evidence, as "Fever" and "Delirium," it would not be safe to attempt to establish it as a general rule that persons actually

* Macnaghten, Vol. I., p. 301.

† Nizamut Adawlut Reports, Vol. IV., p. 345.

so affected could neither will nor execute deeds of frantic violence.] The plea of Delirium was not credited. Sentence—Death.*

The practical questions involved in these cases are: *1st*,—Whether it is to be considered that the mental and bodily distress attending upon Fever may be such as to justify the commission of homicide upon comparatively slight causes of irritation? *2nd*,—Whether it is to be concluded that murder may be committed, either with or without additional causes of excitement, in the delirium attending the Fevers of this or of other countries? And *3rd*,—Whether it can be proved that the individual was actually laboring under the delirium of Fever at the time when he inflicted the injury?

(1.) Every one who has suffered from the Fever of this country must retain a vivid recollection of the great mental distress and irritability which accompanied the attack; still it would assuredly be dangerous to establish the precedent that homicide, inflicted upon slight causes of irritation by persons suffering from Fever, but who are not absolutely delirious, is excusable.

(2.) A person who is actually delirious in Fever cannot, of course, be held responsible for his actions. It is not generally considered by medical men, in this or in other countries, that persons suffering from Fever are dangerous to others. In our jails and in the hospital wards at home, such patients lie beside other sick; and, although it occasionally happens that a fever patient rises from his bed, in the height of delirium, and becomes unruly, even this is not very frequent; and instances of dangerous violence *to others* are extremely rare. The violence committed by delirious persons probably bears with it, in all cases, the manifest evidences of irrationality and delusion; and is scarcely, if at all, remembered by the patients when the attack passes off. The plea of delirium, as an excuse for undue retaliation upon a *real* offence, the nature of which the individual clearly recollects, must therefore be received with great caution and suspicion. There is, however, an unfortunate class of cases, in which excess, exposure, undue mental excitement, slight or commencing inflammation of the membranes of the brain, or ordinary Fever, acting upon a constitution in which Insanity is lurking, may lead to frightful violence, even while the evidences of bodily and even of mental disorder are very far indeed short of those displayed in ordinary febrile delirium. In a case where there was reason to believe that nearly the whole of the above causes were operative, my patient answered questions correctly, and appeared to have considerable power of self-control; but his ideas were truculent, and he so frequently alluded to spearing and stabbing, that I thought it right to place all weapons out of his way, and to take measures for coercing him, if necessary,—which, however, was fortunately not the case.

---

* Nizamut Adawlut Reports, N. W. P., August 19th, 1853, p. 1014.

In cases of this kind, however, the physical cause of mental aberration will remain, for some days at least, after the violence has been committed. The evidences of Insanity may be temporary and of short duration, but those of arachnitis or brain fever will only pass off under treatment.

(3.) Should it happen that an act of homicidal violence has been committed in the delirium of Fever, it will be necessary, and can rarely be difficult to prove, that the Fever has continued subsequently to that act, and the characteristic features of the disease should distinguish it, in the judgment of any medical man, from the excitement remaining after intemperance or drugging, and from that agitation which may be expected to exist, for a short time, in a weak, timid, or remorseful culprit, whose passions have lately been excited to the commission of a great outrage.

There are one or two remarkable cases in the Records in which *the circumstance of the accused being in great pain, at or about the time at which he committed the violence, has been regarded as mitigatory.* In 1822, a man,—who had been long suffering under the tortures of rheumatism,* and was unable to move about, having asked his wife for some water to drink, which she refused to give, at the same time making use of very gross and improper language towards him,—was provoked to such a degree that he took up a *pinrah* (a wooden stool on which the lower class of natives sit) and threw it at her ; it struck her on the head and killed her. They appeared to have lived happily before this affair occurred. It was decided that there did not seem to have been an intention to kill. The prisoner was crippled with rheumatism at the time, and still remained in a sickly state ; the act, however, was rather a savage one. He was sentenced to five years' imprisonment.†

In 1851, a similar case occurred at Rajshahye, in which a man was tried for killing a girl, six or seven years old, who had teazed him, by fracturing her skull with a piece of wood or board used as a stool for sitting on, and commonly called a "*pinrah*." It was proved that the prisoner had, for four or five years previously, been laboring under severe gnawing pains in the interior and lower part of the abdomen (probably the *peet shool* so well described by Dr. T. W. Wilson), which Mr. Bedford, the Civil Surgeon, was satisfied were not feigned. His relations all deposed that, since the pain came on, he had done no business, and that he was in the habit of applying or pressing the *pinrah* to his stomach when the pain was excessive. Mr. Bedford considered that, on a periodical exacerbation of disease, in a state of intense irritability, the prisoner might lose his self-command, and be guilty of an act which, at

* The pain in the chronic rheumatism of this country is generally neuralgic in its character.

† Macnaghten, Vol. II., p. 155.

another time, he would not have committed. He was sentenced to seven years' imprisonment.*

I find other cases in the Nizamut Adawlut Reports in which this *peet shool*, or *peet bedna*, was made a plea for homicidal acts. In the more remarkable of these, Sheikh Buxee was tried at Dacca for having entered the house where his son's wife and her mother were cooking, and inflicted several wounds (afterwards fatal) on the mother with a *sein* (hatchet used for cutting date-trees). The daughter, who was pregnant, interposing, received a bad cut on her arm. The prisoner was laboring under a painful disease. He had desired the elder woman to cook fish for him at a time when he was free from severe pains in the stomach which prevented him from eating and drinking. She did not attend to this at the time, but offered him food in the evening when the pain had returned, and he could not eat. The old woman had also vexed him greatly by having a singing party in the house and making merry when he was suffering acute pain. He added, in the Sessions Court, that the pain in his stomach was sometimes so acute that he knew not what he did when suffering from it. Although the witnesses agreed in stating that the prisoner was subject to pains of an agonizing nature, this statement was not confirmed by the testimony of the medical officer, who deposed that "the prisoner does not bear the appearance of a man suffering from any serious internal evil, but partakes of his food regularly. He may be subject to a slight colic." The Judge of the Nizamut held that "colic pains might produce a frenzy of mind that would deprive a person momentarily of a control over his actions ; and, under their influence, where provocation was given, he might not be able to resist a homicidal impulse. But there is no reliable evidence to show that the prisoner was in this condition, or in such condition as to make him, under the circumstances, an object of mercy." "He appears to be of a morose, irascible temperament, easily provoked, and possessing no control over his passions when roused. He had no reasonable cause for the outrage he committed, and the act was as deliberate as it was cruel. The extenuating plea put forward by him I utterly disregard as operating in his favor. I would convict him of wilful murder, and sentence him to death."†

In 1856, Bukshoollah, of Backergunge, sent his brother-in-law to fetch an unripe cocoanut, as he felt thirsty. There being some delay, he became impatient, and kept asking his wife when the man would come. It appears that the wife put him off by saying that the messenger was coming. He then told her to bring him some water ; and, when she was about to give it to him, he seized her by the hair, and with a sickle cut her throat. She died three days afterwards. The Sessions Judge observed :—" The

* Nizamut Adawlut Reports, Vol. I. of 1851, p. 1155.
† *Ibid*, June 10, 1858, p. 231.

medical officer deliberately deposes to the perfect sanity of the prisoner. In this opinion I fully concur. I have talked to the prisoner, and have carefully watched him, and I must say that I consider him to be in the perfect possession of his senses, and consequently a responsible agent. His demeanour in Court was quiet and subdued ; his answers were coherent and much to the point. Before the darogah, the prisoner stated that he wounded his wife when under the influence of a disease called the '*batick-rog*,' a kind of hypochondria. Six witnesses depose that, for some ten days before the occurrence of the murder, the prisoner was suffering from the aforesaid disease, and was in the habit of abusing people, but was not violent."

"This plea of temporary insanity is set up by every prisoner since the superior Court, in the case of *Government* v. *Lallchund Kyeburt* (*vide supra*, p. 774), deemed it proper to sentence the prisoner in that case to imprisonment for life in the zillah jail. In the present case, the most has been made by the witnesses of some bodily ailment, to make it appear that the intellect of the prisoner was temporarily affected by disease ; but the mere effect of bodily disease irritating his temper cannot be regarded as forming any sufficient ground for mitigation of punishment in a crime of this nature." It also appeared that he wounded in the hand and kicked off a young girl who attempted to interfere in behalf of the deceased ; and, in his confession before the darogah, he admitted that he was irritated, because there was delay in bringing the cocoanut, and because his wife did not go to hasten the man who had been sent to fetch it. He was sentenced capitally.* See a very similar case at page 825.

Simbhoo was tried at Chota Nagpore for having killed his wife, from whom he had been separated for some years, by striking her on the head with a club, and throwing her into a pond. For a year previously he had had palsy, and neglected his ordinary work, but had been of sound mind. He freely confessed, saying that he killed his wife through anger, because she had forsaken him, and continued to live in the same village ; but he alleged in his defence that he was not rightly sensible at the time. The jury found him not guilty. They remarked that he had neglected his business for a year ; and, from his demeanour in Court, they consider that his confessions, besides which there was no proof of his guilt, should not be received. The Judge observed :—"I cannot concur in this verdict. Before this Court the prisoner's outward demeanour has been that of a weak-minded person, but he was throughout attentive to the proceedings, of which attention his defence is a marked proof." "As to the infirmity of mind, the witnesses, his fellow-villagers, all say that the prisoner's intellect was not impaired. The prisoner is apparently affected by that

---

* Nizamut Adawlut Reports, July 22, 1856, p. 113.

form of paralysis called shaking palsy, and, as one so smitten is an object that excites compassion, to this feeling, not easily resisted, the jury has yielded; but I am perfectly satisfied that the prisoner was, at the time of the murder, and is now, a responsible agent. Whether the moral effect of a capital sentence will in this case be advantageous is doubtful; but, leaving this to the consideration of the higher Court, it is my duty to recommend that a sentence of death be passed upon the prisoner."

The Judges of the Nizamut considered that his wife's conduct must have led him to take her life in a fit of momentary anger. They thought it very probable that his mental faculties were weakened by the bodily disease under which he suffered. Taking the whole circumstances of the case into consideration, they felt that no good could be effected by sentencing a criminal, such as the prisoner, capitally; and, therefore, though convicting him of the wilful murder of the deceased, sentenced him to imprisonment for life.*

The Plea of Intoxication.—In cases of homicide and wounding, a plea of intoxication is not admitted by the Mahomedan law to bar exemplary punishment. Under special circumstances, it was considered a ground of mitigation by the Nizamut,† who, however, exercised great reserve in admitting drunkenness as a palliation in the worst cases.

That of Chumroo Choorawala may be taken as an example. This criminal was an habitual drunkard, who, shortly after marrying a woman who had a daughter seven years old, began to live upon bad terms with his wife. It appeared that their disputes arose from the fact that, having obtained money from her on the pretext of getting ornaments made for her, he spent it upon himself. On the evening before the murder, he beat his wife so severely that she ran away from him. He brought her back, and then went to a grog-shop, where he got drunk. The Judge considered that he probably drank in the night, for there was no doubt that he was in a state of intoxication when he committed the murder very early on the following morning. He slept in the room with his wife and step-daughter; and, rising at about gun-fire, he ordered his wife to prepare a *chillum*, while he went to the next room to procure fire. As soon as he returned, and without saying a word to his wife, he took from the matted wall a small knife, and, sitting on his wife's *charpoy*, he dug the weapon deep into her neck, face, and chest. His step-child, seeing this, ran out into the verandah, and began to scream. He rushed after the child, cut her throat, and, throwing down her dead body, hastened off, pursued by three eye-witnesses to the latter portion of this horrible scene. He told them to keep off, saying that he

* Nizamut Adawlut Reports, October 5, 1855, p. 571.

† Macnaghten, Vol. I., Index; Nizamut Adawlut Reports, Novr. 27, 1855, p. 832.

would be his own accuser to the Police. He accordingly gave himself up at the thannah. It was considered that, at this time, he was in liquor ; he then admitted the deed, but denied it altogether when he became sober. Before the Magistrate he said he was drunk, and did not know how the murder happened. The Sessions Judge and one of the Judges of the Court of Appeal considered that the crime was without malice, and committed in the drunken excitement of the moment. Two other Judges, however, passed sentence of death upon him, holding that both law officers (mofussil and sudder) had given a *futwa* of *kissas*, and the Mahomedan law which they (the Judges) had to follow does not admit the plea of intoxication to bar a capital sentence. There are cases reported (see Index to Nizamut Adawlut Reports, Vol. V., heading Intoxication) in which that plea has been allowed to bar such a sentence from consideration of extenuating circumstances ; but, in this case, the Judges could discern no extenuating circumstances. Whatever may have been the prisoner's state over-night, he must be held responsible for his acts on the following morning. Some of the witnesses stated that he had been drinking over-night, but there was no evidence to establish that he was overcome with drink even then.*

"In a case of murder committed in a drunken squabble, it was held that voluntary drunkenness, though it does not palliate any offence, may be taken into account as throwing light on the question of intention.—*Queen* v. *Ram Sahoy Bhai*, W. R., 1864, Cr., 24 ; Cowell and Woodman, p. 537.

Law.

For the Indian laws, as affecting crimes committed while in a state of Intoxication, *vide* Sections 85 and 86 of the Indian Penal Code; and Mayne's Commentaries, 5th Ed., pp. 56-7-8.

Drunkenness in the Army.—Article 17 of the Articles of War directs that—

"Any Officer who shall be drunk when on or for duty, or on parade, or on the line of march, shall, on conviction thereof before a General Court Martial, be cashiered."

The Military law makes no reservation with regard to the *cause* of intoxication. Captain Simmons† says:—"It is held that the offence of being drunk on duty is complete when an officer or soldier is found drunk, whether under the influence of liquor, opium, or other intoxicating drug or thing." Major Hough adds that "It matters not what the quantity taken may be; if ever so little, and the soldier be drunk, he is punishable."‡

---

* Nizamut Adawlut Reports, Novr. 27, 1855, p. 830.

† Page 283, as quoted by Hough, p. 208.

‡ *Ibid.*

It is, however, doubtless open to the judgment of every Court to receive circumstances in mitigation of such charges as grounds for recommendation to mercy.

A line of defence not unfrequently adhered to in trials for drunkenness, especially in tropical countries, is that the accused have previously suffered from injury to the head, or from sun-stroke or brain fever, the result of exposure to the intense heat of the climate ; and that, consequently, they have become liable to intoxication after taking exceedingly small or moderate quantities of wine or spirit.* I am aware that many strict officers entirely ignore the validity of this plea—maintaining that men thus circumstanced, knowing that the welfare of the service and their own characters are at stake, should altogether abstain. On the other hand, facts are, from time to time, observed which render it questionable whether certain of these unfortunate cases should not, on medical grounds, meet with a more lenient judgment : thus—

It will be generally admitted that persons who have suffered from severe injuries to the head, *coup de soliel,* or arachnitis, are frequently left extremely susceptible to the operation of all causes of cerebral excitement, and especially to that by alcoholic drinks. To this principle may, undoubtedly, be added the fact that there is a set of cases in which the patient suffers from a morbid and irresistible propensity for alcoholic liquors. I have adduced some important observations upon this "*Oinomania*" in the subjoined note and in the Appendix.† The occurrence of this abnormal condition does not appear to be very frequent. Still the facts adduced by Dr. Guislain and others deserve the careful attention of every naval and military surgeon. Beyond this, there is, I am confident,

---

* Dr. Taylor says that, "In those cases where the head has received any physical injury, as it often happens with soldiers and sailors, drunkenness, even when existing to a slight extent, produces sometimes a fit of temporary insanity, leaving the mind clear when the drunken fit is over. The law makes no distinction between this state and ordinary drunkenness, although juries occasionally show, by their verdicts, that some difference ought to be made." (See cases in Alison, 653.)

† "Drunkenness," says Dr. Guislain, "may present itself as an essential affection,—that is, it may be a true morbid impulse, and constitute a monomania, in all the force of the term. I first saw this affection in a music-master who, every year, or sometimes every two years, abruptly quitted his studies to abandon himself to excessive drinking. He was, at these times, in a state of continual drunkenness, lasting to three or four months, until it disappeared, as it were, suddenly. Then this man became averse to every excess, drank nothing but water, and avoided with extreme care everything that might compromise his health or his dignity. In one of these periods of lucidity, feeling the approach of his disease, he destroyed himself. It is therefore important to distinguish *Mania Ebriosa* from the maniacal exaltation which is the sequela of habitual drunkenness. It cannot be confounded with the love of drink, which is a vice of manners. It differs entirely from these conditions; for what characterises this affection is a morbid inclination, its appearance under the form of monomania, and its periodical attacks, the frequency of the pulse, and the marked debility of the intelligence during the entire periods of the disease."—Dr. Guislain's work on Insanity, Pschycological Journal, April 1854, p. 269.—See also APPENDIX G.

a set of cases in which a morbid appetite for alcoholic drinks occurs as a symptom of cerebral disorder. I have had under my own treatment two cases in which this was distinctly observed. Both patients were men between 30 and 40 years of age, one a military officer, the other a civil engineer; one had resided in India for several years, the other but for a short time; both—and I was particular in ascertaining this point—were habitually moderate in their potations; one had suffered, some years previously, from an extensive wound upon the vertex, the other from cerebral symptoms which were evidently severe, but of which there was no record. I was acquainted with both;—in their usual state, they were quiet and apparently little excitable. Both were attacked, in consequence of undue exposure to the sun, during the hot season, with symptoms of cerebral excitement closely bordering upon acute mania; and in both also the incessant and peremptory desire for beer was the most troublesome symptom. Both patients were sent to England. One of them has returned to India, apparently in good bodily and mental health. I am not aware of the ultimate issue of the other's case. These were evidently marked, though not extreme, cases of Dipsomania—*dependent upon a physical cause.*

These cases are not given here as precedents—the point requires further attention; still I know that they are not solitary instances, and the very important medico-legal question which they involve should not be overlooked.

It cannot, for a moment, be questioned that an officer who is liable to be drunk on duty is wholly unfit to remain in the effective arm of the service; where, however, it can be made apparent, upon clear and satisfactory medical evidence, that the individual, by no fault or culpability of his own, has become the subject of a diseased craving for alcoholic stimulants, it may be fairly held that a lenient sentence, placing him upon half-pay, or upon the non-effective list, will fully meet all the exigencies of the case.*

It would be wrong to omit here a caution which I have occasionally had to observe—in criminal cases, where the plea of Insanity is likely to be made—with regard to *the necessity for reserve in attempting, previous to trial or examination by the Magistrate, to cure or remove the cause of excitement, whether it be the result of Drugging, Cerebral Disorder evidently dependent upon organic causes, or Acute Mania.* Upon committing an act of frantic violence, a native of this country, having undergone examination at the thannah and at the Magistrate's Court, is generally placed, as soon as possible, in the jail under the observation

---

* By G. O. of the Govr. Genl., 13th June 1846, Officers applying for transfer to the Invalids were required to produce medical evidence that their disqualification "has not been occasioned by Intemperance, or other Irregular Habits."

of the Civil Surgeon. Here it, of course, becomes the duty of the latter at once to endeavour to distinguish how much of any disorder of the intellectual faculties which the culprit may present is dependent upon *physical*, and how much upon *mental* causes. He has either been brought in, very shortly after the deed of violence, heated, panting, and almost wild with rage or terror ; or pale, tremulous, prostrated, and horror-stricken ;—or, where the act has been done at a distance, he has been hurried in on foot, from thaunah to thannah, perhaps a distance of from thirty to fifty miles, exposed to the scorching mid-day sun, and to the night cold, roughly treated, and, in short, the subject of nearly all those causes which would most tend to unsettle, for a time, the steadiest intellect ;—he, in fact, appears before the medical officer more like a wild beast just dragged from the jungle, than the quiet-mannered, common-place native that he ordinarily is. These circumstances being carefully looked to and discriminated, the medical officer may,—upon observing that his eyes are inflamed, his head hot, his tongue foul, and his pulse excited, and, upon learning that he is sleepless at night,—feel disposed to exercise the remedial portion of his art, and to prescribe purgatives, nauseants, sedatives, low diet, and cold affusion. I allude especially to this point, as I have seen such a course inconsiderately adopted, under such circumstances, by men of experience and judgment ; and have felt myself bound to counsel against it. In these cases,—unless the physician be convinced, either that treatment is necessary to save the individual's life (which will very rarely indeed happen), or that the experiment of treatment will aid him in forming or confirming his diagnosis (a dangerous course which can only be undertaken by those who possess unusual tact in the investigation of such cases),—it is always safer and fairer towards the subject of our scrutiny to leave his case untreated, under the most careful watching. In fact, with regard to food, lodging, dress, opportunities of ablution, &c., he should be permitted to remain, as far as the fact of his being in a jail will admit of, as nearly as possible under the circumstances to which he has been accustomed. Indeed, if it can be clearly proved that he has been in the habit of drinking spirits or of using drugs, these should be allowed him, in moderate quantities, with very cautious observation of their effects. Under these circumstances, it may fairly be expected that the effects of intoxication, whether by *sharab* or *gunja*, will gradually pass off, and that all unwonted excitement, the result of terror or ill-usage, will be calmed down ; but cerebral irritation, depending upon actual vascular changes, will not be removed ; fever will run its course (and may be allowed to do so until the medical man has fully recognised its presence, and has judged whether it did or did not probably exist previous to the crime), and true mania will probably remain unaffected, except in character and degree. It appears to be generally stated, by those medical men who conduct asyla near large towns, where recent cases are brought in at once, that instances of acute mania are remarkably common, and are, in a very large proportion of cases, highly remediable. It is only *after the Trial* that the physician can be justified in *treating* the criminal lunatic : it can never be an act of justice nor of humanity to place one who has committed a maniacal act *sane* before a jury who are to try him for Murder. I confidently believe that there are some who have been hanged in consequence of this *nimia diligentia medicorum.*

There is no country in which the line between *Outrageous Fanaticism and Religious Monomania* is so indistinct as we find it to be in India. Whether the religious impostor is knave or madman, or a compound of both ; or whether superstitious enthusiasm, acting upon a weak mind and oriental imagination, may not occasionally prompt the rarely very scrupulous native to the commission of wild atrocities, are questions of no small difficulty, which can only be decided by weighing carefully the facts of each case as it occurs. Eccentricity, especially when displayed in the *quasi* religious beggars of India, will rarely be viewed as Insanity in the present day. In any other country than India, the wretches called Aghorpunts would be regarded and treated as dangerous maniacs. Here, however, all such persons would be held responsible for their crimes.

The following account of them is given in Moore's Hindu Pantheon :— "Not only do the Hindus, even the Brahmins, eat flesh ; but they eat, one sect at least, human flesh. They do not, I conclude, kill human subjects to eat," (Lutfullah says that the people in the Ghirnar Mountains have a mistaken idea that these devotees are cannibals, and devour man's flesh if they can get hold of a single unarmed person ; but that this is not credible) "but they eat such as they find in or about the Ganges, and perhaps other rivers. The name of the sect is *Paramahansa,* and I have received authentic information of individuals of this sect being not very unusually seen about Benares floating down the river on" (?) "and *feeding on a corpse.* Nor is this a low, despicable tribe, but, on the contrary, esteemed, by themselves at least, as a very high one, and my information stated that the human brain is judged by these epicurean cannibals as the most delicious morsel of their unsocial banquet."

A modern writer thus depicts these wretches in colors which I am informed, on other and good authority, are not unduly heightened:—"The most loathsome sight at the ghats are the Aghorpunt fukeers (Anglice, Ogres), practical philosophers, who affect to disbelieve that there is any difference between things, and who avow that any difference depends upon the imagination. A cuff or a kick is as immaterial to them as a blessing. They go about *in puris naturalibus,* with a fresh human skull in their hands (off which they have previously eaten the putrid flesh, and from which afterwards they have, with their fingers, scooped out the brain and eyes), into which is poured whatsoever is given them to drink. They pretend to be indifferent whether it be ardent spirits, or milk, or foul water. Their food is the first thing that offers, whether it be a putrid corpse, cooked food, or ordure. With matted hair, blood-red eyes, and body covered with filth and vermin, the Aghorpunt is an object of terror and disgust to everybody. He looks rather a wolf, ready to destroy and then devour his prey, than a human being. I once saw a wretch of this fraternity eating the head of a putrid corpse ; and, as I passed by, he howled and pointed to me, and then scooped out the eyes and ate them before me !"

Colonel Tod met with a tribe of these Aghori near Mount Aboo. They not only existed on the sacred hill, but amidst the impenetrable recesses of the other mounts dedicated to the Jain faith in the Saura Peninsula. One of the Deora Chiefs told Colonel Tod that, when conveying the body of his brother to the pile, one of these monsters, crossing the path of the funeral processions, begged to have the corpse, saying it would make excellent *chatni*.*

These wretches, although not very numerous, are spread over the whole country. Mr. McCosh mentions that, during his residence at Goalpara, two men of this caste were caught gnawing the flesh from a human bone, and were taken up by the police. They were sent to him by the Magistrate for his opinion as to their sanity. One of them was not exactly *compos mentis*, but the other was of sound mind, and told Mr. McCosh that he had been in the habit of eating human flesh for many years. This author accounts for the abominable practices of these cannibals in a very clear manner,—*viz.*, that their object in walking about the bazars picking a putrid thigh-bone, is to extort money from the inhabitants, who preferred paying them a few pice to get rid of the annoyance ; and it was formerly even considered justifiable to shoot them like wild beasts whenever they were found.†

Mention has already been made of wild crimes committed by religious mendicants and impostors.‡ To these may be added an instance in which one Lall Doss Byragee, having lived in the Mountain Koilee Doogree, near Bhudruk, for about a month, with two other Byragees, reported that the goddess Kallee had eaten his two companions. A search was made; the two bodies were found on the mountain with large stones heaped on them ; two clubs were in the hut, and a blood-stained axe was afterwards found near the spot. The prisoner confessed

---

* "Travels in Western India."

† Topography of Assam, p. 87.

‡ See cases in which a Byragee killed a child by striking it on the head with a club, p. 796 ; one in which a fanatic twice cut off the right hands of unoffending persons, p. 482 ; and another in which a Brahmin slaughtered his pregnant wife to bring her blood upon one who had offended him, p. 388 (Note).

to the police that he murdered them both by blows of the clubs and also of the axe, and the wounds showed that both were used; but, before the Magistrate and Judge, he confessed only to have murdered them both with the clubs. He said that, eight days previously, the other two Byragees had bewitched him, as his eyes grew red and he lost his appetite, and that, therefore, he killed them. He also said that the deities Kalee, Nursing, and Juggernauth killed them. He warned a witness, who was up the mountain, to leave the place, as the god Nursing was angry. The Sessions Judge considered that the belief of the prisoner in witchcraft, and his conviction that his gods delight in blood, seem to have led to the commission of the two murders. He agreed with the law officer that he was guilty of the wilful murder of the two men ; and, thinking that it would be a dangerous doctrine to hold that fanaticism excuses the crime of murder, he recommended that the sentence of death might be passed. The higher Court, not being satisfied with regard to the evidence relative to the state of the prisoner's mind, directed that enquiry should be made on this point. The Judge again reported that the prisoner continued to confess, as before, that he struck the fatal blows, yet it was some god who killed them. Dr. Collier said that he was the subject of a homicidal mania caused by religious delusion ; and other witnesses spoke to his silence and moroseness and filth while in jail. This, it was considered, was not surprising in a man who had lived alone like a complete savage in the woods and mountains for years. The Magistrate wrote that his violence was at once checked by fear, and that "he was less sane than most Byragees, all of whom are more or less mad." The prisoner then remembered the origin of the quarrel, which was some matter of religion. "He is a violent and dangerous lunatic. The law officer has changed his *futwa*, and declares him liable to punishment by *deeut* instead of *kissas*." The Judges of the Nizamut Adawlut observed :—"It appears to us that, at the time of the commission of the murders, the prisoner was of unsound mind, so as to excuse him according to law. The medical evidence is to the effect that the prisoner labors under partial insanity in the form of homicidal mania caused by religious delusion ; that he does not seem to have a proper idea of the magnitude of his crime ; and that the mania comes on suddenly. We consider, from all the circumstances of the case, that the murders were committed by the prisoner under the influence of the mania, and the evidence as to his state since his apprehension warrants this conclusion. We therefore acquit him, and direct, according to Section 3, Act IV of 1849, that he be kept in safe custody, pending the pleasure of the Government, with whom the local authorities will communicate in regular course."*

---

* Nizamut Adawlut Reports, 13th September 1856, p. 429.

A chowkeedar, when on his way to Manjheecurun Police station, in Behar, came upon the body of a murdered man ; the skull was laid bare and beaten in, and the whole body was a mass of bruises. Five hundred yards farther on, he came upon a fakir, with blood on his hands and clothes, in the act of robbing a traveller. With other assistance he was overpowered and taken to the station. He turned out to be the murderer. At the time he was considered insane, he confessed exactly what he had done ; how he got off his pony, and climbed up into a tree ; how he shouted and gesticulated and scared away passers-by ; and how he caught his victim, and killed him with his own *lattee*. He at once appended the traveller's ear-rings to his own ears ; and, while resisting capture, he kept on eating *suttoo* and spitting it into the faces of all who came near him. After watching him for some two months, the Civil Surgeon pronounced him sane, or rather not legally insane, so he was committed to the Sessions. By direction of the Judge, the Assistant Superintendent of Police visited the villages where the fakir was known, with a view to gain further evidence. Before the Assistant, the villagers testified to the man's insanity ; before the Judge, to his sanity. He was transported for life.*

Ram Singh, a devotee of the Brahmacharee class, suddenly rushed upon an unoffending girl of fourteen, thrust her into the river, and flung himself in upon her. The girl was drowned, and her body was not discovered. The medical officer, having had the murderer for some time under observation, stated that, in his opinion, the prisoner was sane ; that he had remarked nothing during the interval which led him to think that he had been subject to temporary insanity, or that he had been in the habit of taking intoxicating drugs in large quantities. The prisoner stated at the thannah that he had taken *bhang*, but on trial said, in a wild and wandering manner, that he never took *bhang*, and knew not what had occurred. The Sessions Judge remarked that madness amongst *fakirs*, from their solitary habits, and their being accustomed to take intoxicating drugs, and perhaps from the very idiosyncrasy which led to their adopting the character, is very common. In the face, however, of the medical officer's evidence, he was constrained to think him sane. He was sentenced to imprisonment for life.†

This was probably an instance of murder *under the influence of gunjah*. We have abundant evidence of the fact that *byragees* and *fakirs* keep themselves almost constantly under *the influence of hemp*,— the excuse of the former being that this mode of intoxication abstracts their thoughts from the objects of sense, and assists their absorption into

---

* Bengal Police Report for 1866, p. 133.

† Nizamut Adawlut Reports, N. W. P., September 12th, 1854, p. 353.

the deity.* There is certainly, apart from their dress and other disfigurements, a peculiar gauntness of person, and a wild expression of countenance, in the generality of religious mendicants, which mark them, in common with a majority of the Mehter, Moochee, and Chumar classes, as habitual consumers of hemp and other intoxicating drugs. The face of an habitual *gunjah-smoker* can scarcely be mistaken. The expression of his countenance forcibly carries with it the idea that reason has been partially unseated.

In September 1855, one Sreenibas was tried, at Hazareebaugh, for killing an unmarried girl, ten years old (towards whom ill-will on his part was neither ascribed nor was probable), with a *tangee*, or axe. The girl's father deposed that he saw his daughter pursued by the prisoner, who cut her down, and she died on the spot. On being seized, the prisoner said, "Oh ho! I have killed your daughter to-day, kill you me." He considered the prisoner to be a respectable man, having no quarrel with him himself. The prisoner confessed that, having eaten and drank, he was sitting in the house, when suddenly a voice on the wind said to him, "Your uncles have taken your sister Aunie to bury her in the forest, go you there :—" wherefore, taking the axe in his hand, he went to the forest, and, after a little, being inspired, he heard a spirit voice in the wind say, "Cut off the heads of your brethren, or else take off any one's head." Then, as he went homewards, he met the girl coming with water from the pond to her home; and, being possessed, he, with that very axe, struck her two or three blows. She fell and died. After a little, he was seized by his own father and others, who took away

---

* "Har," says Todd (Vol. I., p. 72), "is the patron of all who love war and strong drink, and is especially the ojbect of the Rajpoot warrior's devotion: accordingly, blood and wine form the chief oblations to the great god of the Indus. The Goséns, the peculiar priests of Har, or Bâl, the sun, all indulge in intoxicating drugs, herbs, and drinks. Seated on their lion, leopard, or deer skins, their bodies covered with ashes, their hair matted and braided, with iron tongs to feed the penitential fires, their savage appearance makes them fit organs for the commands of the god of blood and slaughter."

Royle mentions that one of the popular names of *Gunjah* in the Arabic is *the Grass of Fakirs—vide supra*, p. 219.

According to Ward, "A great number of the Hindu modern saints live in a state of perpetual intoxication, and call this stupefaction, which arises from smoking intoxicating herbs, fixing the mind on God." "Now and then a poor wretch is seen naked, covered with ashes, and his hair clotted with dirt, whose vacant, brutish looks, indicate that he is approaching a state of complete abstraction, and that he may soon hope to enter into this perfect state,—*viz.*, to live in a world of wonders,—without a single passion left to be affected by them. Yet even this abstraction, or contempt of the world, if it can deserve such a name, is brought on by shunning the presence of man, and continually smoking intoxicating herbs." The same author describes that, in a pantomimical entertainment popular among the Bengalees, the *Maun-Bhanjan*, Krishna is represented as assuming the form of a mendicant yogee, his body covered with ashes, and his eyes inflamed with intoxicating drugs. We have already seen that Siva is described as being commonly under the influence of datura and gunjah; and that the latter is Mohadeb's favorite drug.

his axe and bound him. He confessed to them, and asked them to save him. Now also he was making confession voluntarily. The prisoner's father deposed that prisoner was once out of his mind when his mother died ; since then he had been sometimes well, and at other times he was idle. Another of those who witnessed the fatal act and took him into custody deposed to the same effect, and stated that he was a quiet man. Major Hannyngton, who tried the case, decided that the prisoner was evidently of sound mind, not only when under trial, but at the time of the murder. His prior insanity, he considered, was not well made out, but it gave a color to the story of an imaginary demoniac possession. The belief of a Hindu respecting such incursions cannot be measured by our own belief in them, but he was not disposed to view such cases with leniency. The immolation of a victim to a sanguinary demon is, he was persuaded, the real motive in many such instances, and the supposed merit of such an action is held to be cheaply purchased by any punishment incurred. The crime is, however, not so frequent as to require its repression by taking life for life ; but, of minor punishments, the highest is most applicable. He therefore recommended that the prisoner should be sentenced to be transported for life with hard labor in irons. The Sudder Court concurred in this verdict.

Allusion has been already made, at page 409, to the case of a Hindu priest who, according to his own declaration, cut off the head of a woman in obedience to the command of the Thakoor (deity) Saligram. The medical officer testified his belief that the prisoner was not in his right senses, and was an irresponsible agent, and added that his opinion was grounded on the prisoner's personal appearance and the circumstance of his persisting in declaring that, in taking the woman's life, he was only acting in conformity with the orders of the Thakoor, whom he was bound to obey ; indicating thereby that he was laboring under some extraordinary delusion. All other evidence, however, went to show that the prisoner was in his right senses. The plea that he was prompted by a vision of the Deity was urged after the murder had been committed. The Sessions Judge, therefore, recommended a sentence of death. The Judges of the Nizamut observed that the medical officer had not been examined by the Sessions Judge with sufficient care and particularity in this case. The legal test of Insanity in the Courts of this country, they remarked, is laid down in Section 1, Act IV. of 1849 : "No person can be acquitted for unsoundness of mind, unless it can be proved that, by reason of unsoundness of mind, not wilfully caused by himself, he was *unconscious* and *incapable of knowing, in doing the act, that he was doing an act forbidden by the law of the land.*" The medical officer should, they were of opinion, have been examined as to whether, and on what precise grounds, he considered the prisoner to have been, *at the time when he took the life of the woman,* within the description above set forth. "The witnesses to the prisoner's habitual state of mind should have been examined in the presence of the medical officer, and he should have been invited to propose any questions on his own part. He should then have been carefully questioned as to the number of times he had himself seen the prisoner, the nature of his conversations with him, and all the circumstances from which, apart from the prisoner's real or professed religious delusions, he was led to regard him as of unsound mind. The questions should have been expressed so as to elicit an opinion of the medical officer, after his having had the advantage of hearing the statements of the members of the prisoner's family, his neighbours, and other parties, as to the state of the prisoner's mind both *previously to* and *at the time of the murder*, and subsequently *up to the time of the trial.* The Sessions Judge ought not to have referred, as he has done in his report, to the medical officer having visited the prisoner only twice, and for short intervals, without directly questioning that gentleman upon the point." They therefore directed that the trial must be re-opened, the witnesses to the state of the prisoner's mind being again closely re-examined in the presence of the medical officer, together with that officer himself, as above explained, and the prisoner being called on for a fresh defence, and the law officer for a fresh *futwa.* Consequently, the Sessions Judge reported that, in compliance with the above instructions, the whole of the witnesses for the prosecution, together with other neighbours, religious followers of the prisoner, who had known him for some years past, had been examined in the presence of the Civil Assistant Surgeon, who had himself questioned them. That officer had also watched and examined the prisoner in jail; every opportunity had been afforded him to arrive at a correct judgment, and the result was his conviction that the prisoner was not, and never had been, of unsound mind. The Sessions Judge fully concurred in the medical officer's opinion. The evidence as to the habits and manner of the prisoner for the preceding ten years, up to that present time, was clear, consistent, and corroborative of his sanity; and, as the medical officer remarked, the only possible reason for suspecting the soundness of the prisoner's mind, was the fact of his committing murder without good apparent cause. Some of the witnesses, however, stated that the true motive of the prisoner's act was revenge, excited by deceased's intriguing conduct with his wife. Both Courts concurred in finding the prisoner guilty of wilful murder, and in sentencing him to death.*

The valuable teaching of the above case is self-evident. Doubtless the minds of natives are not free from tendency to Religious Monomania. Indeed, constant brooding upon the laws and fables of a wild and bloody superstition†

---

* Nizamut Adawlut Reports, Vol. IV. of 1851, p. 24.

† The revelations of gross superstition in this country are often so ridiculous and unnatural that, even those tolerably well acquainted with the native modes of thought and expression are liable to be startled, and to question whether these wild fancies are not the

must, unquestionably, sometimes unhinge the narrow intellects of these wretched fanatics. Still, where the crime assumes the character of any

ravings of Monomania. It therefore appears to be very desirable that judicial and medical officers should have some insight into the opinions of the natives regarding Sorcery, Incantations, and other kinds of *Jaddho*. For instance, it was certainly not *Insanity* which prompted certain of the good folk of Edinburgh to testify, in 1670, that they had beheld the walking-staff of Major Weir, the Wizard, solemnly pacing, all alone, down the Bow, at high noon, upon its master's errands ; or which led the men of Boston to declare, at about the same time, that a woman tore from the back of a spectre an invisible sheet, which then immediately became visible before a room full of spectators. Neither is the Bengalee to be considered mad when he protests that his enemy insensibly drew all the blood out of his body while seated beside him, or withered his mango trees by shooting charmed arrows into them ;—nor is the Hindustanee to be regarded as a maniac, because he declares that he has eaten a cock which crows in his belly, that a Gond witch has placed a devil in him, which has devoured his liver ; or that she has turned the juice of his sugarcanes into blood ! Much curious and instructive information upon the subject of Witchcraft in India will be found in the following Works:—*In Bengal:* Ward, Vol. I., Ed. of 1852, p. 210. Police Reports, Lower Provinces, 1838, p. 14. *Ibid* for 1843, p. 19. *Ibid* for 1844, p. 9. *Ibid* for 1849, p. 19. N. A. R., May 11, 1855, p. 540. September 30, 1856, p. 720. In the *North-West Provinces:* Sleeman's Rambles and Recollections of an Indian Official, Vol. I., p. 89. Nizamut Adawlut Reports, N. W. P., January 13th, 1855, p. 39. Among the *Bheels :* East India Army Magazine, October 1854, p. 530. The *Koles:* Lieut. Tickell, Journal of the Asiatic Society, Vol. IX., p. 709. The *Bodos* and *Dhimáls :* Mr. Hodgson. *Ibid*, Vol. XVIII., p. 732. The *Assamese :* McCosh's Topography of Assam, p. 23. *Chota Nagpore*, *Kumaon*, and *among the Garrows :* Beaufort, paras. 2888 and 2933. Nizamut Adawlut Reports, November 28th, 1854, p. 682. In *the Central Provinces:* " Once in a Way," p. 47. On the Magic practised by the *Pana Vrastha Brahmans*, and still in use among the *Hindus :* the Abbe Dubois, Chap. xxxvi., p. 341. In the *Bombay* Presidency : Forbes, Vol. 2, pp. 13, 14, 111. Bellasis' Reports, pp. 5 and 201 ; (*Bheels*), 45. In *Guzerat :* Mr. Gibson, Trans. of the Med. and Physical Society of Bombay, Vol. I., p. 27. By the ancient Mahomedan law, Sorcerers, proved to have done serious injury by their sorcery, might be put to death or imprisoned, according to the circumstances of the case. Numerous very remarkable coincidences will be found between the superstitions regarding Witches formerly entertained in the North of Europe, and those now prevalent in Bengal. For example, the meddler in the arts of Physic and Alchemy is generally reputed as a Wizard ; the Ordeals for Witchcraft have been identically the same in both quarters of the world, and many of the minuter details of superstition have singularly corresponded. Thus Ward mentions that, " in Bengal, a person sometimes takes a bamboo, which has been used to keep down a dead body during its incremation, and, making a bow and arrow with it, repeats incantations over it. He then makes an image of his enemy with clay, and lets fly the arrow into this image. The person whose image is thus pierced is said to be immediately seized with a pain in the breast," (Vol. I., p. 100, Ed. of 1822). In his work on the Customs of the Mussalmauns in India (Madras Presidency), Dr. Herklotts has a chapter (1, p. 345) on those means of incantation by which the death of an enemy may be caused. One plan is to read the chapter *tubut* backwards,—*i. e.*, every word spelt backwards,—morning and evening daily, for twenty-one days, at each period forty-one times.

(So also in England—

" He who'd read her aright must say her
Backwards, like a witch's prayer.")

" Or with some earth taken out of a grave, or the earth of the Hindu *musan* (place where Hindus burn their dead), he is to make a doll about a span long, more or less ; and repeating the *soora-e-ullum-turkyf*, with the name of its accompanying demon, or the *tubut* reversed, or the *chayhul qaf*, over twenty-one small thin wooden pegs ; and, repeating it three times over each peg, he is to strike them into different parts of the body of the image ; such as one into the crown of the head, one into the forehead, two into the two eyes, two

one of a set of barbarous practices, which it has long been the steady purpose of our law-givers to extirpate from the land ; and especially where, as in the case of Human Sacrifice, the perpetrator cannot deny that, even upon his own explanation of his motives, he has committed the act with a direct view to his own advantage (see page 399), it is evident that a plea of Insanity must not be met with any yielding of misplaced compassion.

The following case is given by Dr. A. Fleming in his report of the Moydapore (Moorshedabad) Asylum for 1863. Jutta Singh, Fukeer, was brought up under a charge of killing a child with a sword, dangerously wounding another child and a woman, and stabbing a bullock. The man was tried in the Magistrate's Court, and he was sent to the Sessions. The Magistrate did not consider that there was anything in the case to show Insanity, and the man did not attempt to feign madness. The Sessions Judge formed a different opinion, and ordered an enquiry into his mental condition. Dr. Fleming did not hesitate to state that the man had been and was still insane. He was quite rational on nearly all subjects, but, when questioned regarding the murder of the child and the assaults, he stated that a voice from heaven had ordered him to do what he had done. He admitted that he was in the habit of using gunjah ; he seemed perfectly indifferent as to the consequences, and did not wish to be considered insane. He remained in the Asylum and became a good workman, but was incoherent at times, and no one who watched him attentively could doubt that he was a lunatic.

Allusion has already been made to the cruelty with which Insane persons are usually treated by the natives of this country, with an idea that blows, stripes, starvation, and bonds will drive the evil spirits out of their possession. A case of great importance, arising out of this practice, was tried at Cawnpore in 1853. It appeared that one Girdharee had, for some months, been placed under restraint by his father and other near relatives, in consequence of his extravagant conduct, caused, as they considered, by disordered intellect. It was also shown by the villagers that he had, for a short time before the murder, been regarded by them

---

into the two upper arms, two into the two arm-pits, two into the two palms of the hands, two into the two nipples, two into the two sides of the body, one into the navel, two into the two thighs, and two into the two soles of the feet. The image is then to be shrouded in the manner of a human corpse, conveyed to the cemetery, and buried in the name of the enemy, who (it is believed) will positively die."

There is a story, in Madras, of a robbery in an officer's house, where a cunning man, being called in, buried an image of the supposed thief, with a nail stuck into each joint, in the charitable expectation that the culprit would be tormented with rheumatism up to the point of confession. So also, in Lodge's Illustrations of British History, Vol. II., p. 460, among the "Reasons and Conjectures which caused many to suppose that his Honour [the Earl of Derby, who died in 1594,] was Bewitched," we find that—"There was found in my Lord's chamber, by one Mr. Hansall, an image of wax with a hair drawn through the belly thereof, as he reported upon his oath."

as subject to fits of derangement. Contriving to escape, he rushed with a drawn sword into a shrine where some women were making their offerings, and killed one of the females by several wounds, any one of which would have caused death. He then laid down the sword and went to his own house. It could not be shown that he had any cause for malice against this woman; but it appeared, from his statement made on the day on which the act was done, that, exasperated at the restraint to which he had been subjected, and enraged at the taunts which had been cast upon him, he had resolved to commit some violence which might bring his relatives into disgrace, and free himself from their guardianship. He appears then to have denied that he was insane. His statement made in the foujdaree, four days afterwards, showed a connected recollection of all that had passed before, at, and after the murder. On trial, he made a full confession, but pleaded that he was mad at the time when the act was perpetrated; that he had been confined and loaded with irons, which was his reason for committing the murderous assault. The jury, giving the prisoner the benefit of the above evidence, returned a special verdict that he was insane when the act was committed. The Sessions Judge was convinced that the man was not mad when under trial, and the Magistrate "appeared to have satisfied himself of his sanity before committing him." While admitting that the prisoner's intellect might have been disordered, the Judge did not arrive at the conclusion that he was suffering under such unsoundness of mind as would render him "incapable of knowing at the time of doing the act, that he was doing an act forbidden by the law of the land;" on the contrary, he was inclined to believe, from the prisoner's appearances and manner, that there was more of cunning than of insanity about him. He was, in the Judge's opinion, undoubtedly not a subject for a capital sentence; but that officer did not think that the evidence showed him to have been the subject of such unsoundness of mind as to make him irresponsibile for such an act as murder. He therefore recommended a sentence of imprisonment for life. The Judge of the superior Court held that, whatever may have been the prisoner's mental delusions (on which point, he remarked, the information to be extracted from the examination at the trial was very defective), there could be no doubt that he had sufficient reason, with respect to the fatal act, to render him a responsible agent, and as one capable of distinguishing right from wrong. He therefore convicted the prisoner, but, in compliance with the recommendation of the Sessions Judge, and with reference to the circumstances of the case, sentenced him to imprisonment for life with light labor."* It does not appear, in the printed report, that a medical opinion was taken in this case.

* Nizamut Adawlut Reports, N. W. P., July 20th, 1853, p. 896.

The above facts will have sufficiently shown that, in the examination of important cases, what may appear to the European observer as absolutely irrational *Singularity of Conduct* on the part of a native, is not to be viewed as Insanity, except upon a full consideration of the customs and modes of thinking of the natives, as well as of the minute details of the particular cases under scrutiny.

One of the most important Regulations on this subject directed that "*All Insane persons, apprehended by the Police, shall be sent to the Division Hospital with a full report upon their cases.*"* In the absence of such information, the medical officer's means of forming a correct opinion are dangerously and unnecessarily narrowed. I was, on one occasion, very strongly convinced of the importance of this rule. Having been merely requested to examine a prisoner, and to report upon the state of his mind, I visited and conversed with him more than once, and could discover no evidence of Insanity whatever, except that afforded by the circumstances of his crime, as known by common rumour. He was reported to have attempted an imposition, by forgery, in a manner, to all appearance, so unskilful and purposeless, that I could not bring myself to believe that a person of his education and intelligence would have so acted, except under an insane delusion. Before reporting to this effect, however, I requested permission to examine the forged documents, and inquired fully into the particulars of the case. I then at once perceived that the crime, although clumsily managed, bore with it evidences of deliberation and reason; and that rashness and want of principle were probably the leading defects of the prisoner's mind.

Although all human desires probably tend towards nearly the same objects, the purposes of a native are wont to be effected by trains of thought and action so utterly dissimilar to those by which our own are wrought out, that we must not always expect to be able to follow him in his mental operations, or allow ourselves to charge him with Madness, when his singularity or his craft takes his conduct somewhat beyond the scrutiny of our reason.

As the cause was, I believe, long since decided, and as every particular of the trial appeared in the newspapers of the time, I feel at liberty to detail the following illustrative case. A Calcutta Brahmin, possessing considerable property, having brought his health into a desperate condition by spirit-drinking, determined to leave the bulk of his property to a friend, to the exclusion of the members of his own family. He appears to have been keenly aware of the fact that an act of caprice on the part of one generally known to have destroyed himself by intemperance, might easily be interpreted as an evidence of Insanity or Fatuity; he therefore (for it is necessary to say that he appears never to have acted under coercion)

* Skipwith, 490.

took careful measures for carrying out his purpose. He removed to a house on the other side of the river, where, without any attempt at secrecy, he could remain apart from his own family,—requested that I would attend him (although evidently by no means a believer in the efficacy of English medical treatment), and, shortly afterwards, called in two or three of the most eminent solicitors in Calcutta to make his will. This was done, after my written opinion had been obtained by those gentlemen to the effect that, although I could not, from what I had seen of him, undertake to declare that he was of sane and disposing mind, I had seen nothing that could lead me to think to the contrary. He died in about a month after this ; and, upon the production of his will, the fact that he, a bigoted and by no means unusually enlightened native, had devised considerable sums to one or two of our religious charities, and to one of his legal advisers, leaving the bulk of his property to a comparative stranger, to the prejudice of his near relations, must have appeared, to many who had not watched his proceedings, to be the act of one who was either mad or besotted. His was, however, merely the reasonable craft of a native, which had been practised before, under like circumstances. Knowing that his relations would attempt to overthrow the will, and trusting no one, he, doubtless, considered that he rendered the matter secure by binding up certain powerful interests with that of his principal legatee. Hence, it was not difficult to perceive the rationality with which a Brahmin left his money to those Christian charities which were, in all probability, next to his relations, the especial objects of his aversion.

This very important question has probably never been more strongly illustrated than in the long-agitated inquiry into the state of mind of Dyce Sombre. In the course of this investigation it was stated, on the one hand, that this individual latterly acted with the most outrageous and revolting indecency ; that, among other instances of such conduct, he would receive visitors and others in his apartment in a state of nudity, or having only a shirt on, and would exhibit himself out of his apartment in the same state, acting as if unconscious of any impropriety. That he labored under the insane delusion that his wife was habitually unchaste, and that she was frequently guilty of adultery with different persons. That he had threatened to cut off her nose. That he kept a mistress in India, and often admitted Englishmen into her apartments while she was therein, and was unveiled—that being a practice wholly at variance with the habits and feelings of oriental countries with respect to women. That he had falsely alleged that his wife had been unchaste before as well as after marriage ; that she had been abetted in her unchastity by her father and mother ; that she had been an opera-dancer, and that she had concealed the fact. That he would not suffer her to be out of his sight for a moment,—for fear, as he said, that she should commit some act of adultery in his absence. That, at other times, he behaved with the greatest affection towards her, and expressed regret for his misconduct. That he talked of being visited by two spirits, one of a benevolent, the other of a malign character ; one desiring him to murder his wife, and the other forbidding it, and telling him that he would be happy with her at last. That he declared his sister, the Baroness Solaroli, to be illegitimate. That he was suspicious that his food had been poisoned.—On the other part, it was responded that in none of these opinions or actions was there anything that could be regarded as evidencing Insanity in an individual born and educated in India. It was shown that Mr. Sombre resided with the Begum Sumroo from early childhood, and lived with her down to the period of her death, save only during the time when, as a boy, he resided with the Rev. Mr. Fisher, to whose habits and manners he then, temporarily, conformed ; that such residence produced no permanent change in his habits and feelings, which were essentially those of a native of India, in the condition of life to which he belonged ; that, in regard to his habits and conduct, there was no change at any time prior to his decease. That, although he had to some extent acquired an English education, so as to be in a measure acquainted with the manners and habits of Europeans, yet he was strongly imbued with the feelings peculiar to the natives of oriental countries, with respect to the treatment, demeanour, and conduct of women ; and retained such feelings, amounting occasionally to fits of uncontrollable passion and jealousy, to the time of his death ; and that he was naturally of an irritable and suspicious temperament. That the indecencies which had been charged against him, as proofs of Insanity, were really to be referred to his early habits and his Indian notions of dress ; and that occasionally, while resident in the Upper Provinces, he had appeared in his dwelling-house, and in places of public resort, in a state of nudity, or without any article of clothing except a "*lungotee*," fastened round his loins and hips. That he was always of a jealous disposition, and frequently complained of the usages of English society, [certainly most abhorrent to the prejudices of a native of India,] which compelled him to allow his wife to go into company where she received the attentions of other men. That his distrust of General Ventura arose from the General having expressed himself in terms of strong admiration of Mrs. Dyce Sombre.* A refer-

* "One is never asked how his wife does. Such an inquiry would be considered impertinent, and be felt by the husband as an insult. It is still more requisite that, when one visits his friends, he should never show any desire to see the wife, or even speak to her if they meet, unless they be near relations." "What idea can he" (the Native of India) "form of Europeans, when he sees them bring their females to mix in their intemperance, and beholds women shamelessly laugh, play, and toy with men, and even join them, without blushing, in the dance ; he whose wife dares not sit down in his presence, and who has never known or imagined that persons of that sex, with the exception of the common girls and prostitutes, could take it in their heads to amble and caper."—Description of the Character, Manners, and Customs of the People of India, by the Abbe Dubois, published 1817, pp. 188-194.

ence to page 487 *et seq.* will show that, however much brutality it might evidence, there was, in a man of this description, nothing whatever irrational in Mr. Sombre's threat of cutting off his wife's nose as the punishment of her supposed unchastity ; neither was there anything remarkable in the fact that a native of India, living in Calcutta, and anxious to imitate the customs of Englishmen, should have thought it unnecessary to seclude his kept mistress, as he would probably have done a purdah female of respectability united to him in marriage. That there was nothing whatever unusual in the use, by a native of India, of the expression "Nautch Girl," or public dancing-girl, to an Englishwoman, whom he accused of light conduct. That the natives of India were habitually superstitious, and had faith in the intervention of spirits and supernatural agency in human affairs. That he was really doubtful with regard to his father's marriage with his mother, and, consequently, as to the legitimacy of his sisters ; that it was the custom of married Hindu ladies of rank to keep slave girls in the zenanas; that the cohabitation of their husbands with these girls did not involve any violation of the strictest notions of propriety ; and that the children of these slave girls were usually brought up with those of their mistress, and that they acknowledged each other as brothers and sisters. That the destruction of human life, by the mixture of fatal ingredients with food, was a common occurrence among the natives of India ; that the upper classes were habitually apprehensive of such a death, and, in case of temporary illness, commonly attributed it to poison given to kill or injure them; that Mr. Sombre was, at an early age, led to believe that his life was in danger, more especially by the Begum, who frequently warned him to take precautions against divers individuals, and advised him not to eat anything that might be given him by any person, even by the husbands of his sisters.*

---

* "The old Rajah, Bikramajeet, died in June 1834; and, though his death had been some time expected, he no sooner breathed his last, than charges of (*deeuaee*) slow poison, were got up as usual in the zenana."—Sleeman's Rambles and Recollections, Vol. I., p. 183.

From the earliest mythologic period, we find the page of Indian history full of reports, if not of facts, similar to the above.

There is a legend in the Mackenzie MSS., to the effect that Caudava-rayen sovereign of the Vaunier, who ruled in the fort of Tiruividai Churam, in the Arcot district, was, at the instigation of his enemies, poisoned in a cake by his mistress Cupáchi, the leader of a band of dancing-girls.

Rao Maun, of Serohi, was poisoned in one of the Jain temples on Mount Aboo. A spot is still pointed out where it is said that the marble is stained by the poison he voided.—Tod's Travels in Western India.

The father of Padma, the Saloombra Chief of Oodipoor, is said to have been taken off by poison. Pirthi Raj, of Mewar, was poisoned by his brother-in-law of Aboo, whom he had punished for maltreating his sister, and afterwards confided in. The Emperor Akber, wishing to destroy Raja Maun of Ambir, had prepared a *majoom*, or confection, a part of which contained poison; but, caught in his own snare, he presented the innoxious portion to the Rajpoot, and ate that drugged with death himself. Others say that Akber was poisoned

It was alleged also that, up to the year 1843, Mr. Sombre had never expressed any respect or gratitude to the East India Company; but that, on the contrary, he had often bitterly complained of their conduct to him. This was met by the statement that, previous to his leaving India, in 1838, he had declared that it was his intention, in accordance with what he knew to have been the desire of the Begum, to bequeath the bulk of the property which he had acquired from her to the East India Company, for the purpose of founding a college for the upper classes of natives. The not dissimilar act of the Calcutta Brahmin, whose case has been given above, illustrates the fact that the giving or bequeathing of property by a native is by no means a certain evidence of friendship on the part of the donor or testator towards the recipient.

The reports contain various cases which, out of India, would be regarded as undoubted instances of *Homicidal Monomania*,—as, for instance, that of a woman of Purnea, who confessed that, her sister-in-law having come to her house and accused her of theft, and being exceedingly indignant, and under the influence of an evil spirit, she, as soon as her relative left the house, cut the throat of her own infant, only fifteen days old, from ear to ear; and then, being seized with remorse, began to cry loudly, by which means the act which she had committed was first discovered.* Or that of a Hindu, at Allahabad, who, finding a neighbour cutting grass in his field, and inattentive to remonstrance, returned home in anger, and, forming an intention to murder his own child, a girl of two, drove the inmates of his house out of doors, shut the door, and cut off his daughter's head with a *koolhari*, or axe.† In neither of these cases was there any evidence of insanity about the criminals, whose atrocity was precisely that already described at page 627 of this Manual.

Insanity is not unfrequently feigned by natives of this country.

---

by his son Jehangeere, as Bajazet was by his son Selim. Juswunt Sing of Marwar, and Jey Sing of Amber, were both poisoned by command of the Emperor Arungzeb. Mahomed is said to have been poisoned by a Jewess. Some historians report that the life of the Emperor Ferozeshur, when in prison, was attempted by poison. Ghazi-eddin Khan was poisoned by the ladies of his seraglio and his brother, Selabet Jung; and it was believed that the death of Raja Assiri Sing, which occurred at about the same time, was due to a like cause. Some reports state that Prince Mirza Mehdi, younger brother of Suraj-u-dowlah, was destroyed by poison.

It was more than suspected that Prince Fakir-ood-deen, heir-apparent of Delhi, was killed by poison in 1850. (Kaye.)

The following appeared not very long since in the *Pall Mall Gazette*:—"The Nawab of Bhawulpore, son of that Bhawul Khan who helped us at the siege of Mooltan, and got £10,000 a year from Lord Dalhousie for his pains, has just been poisoned, they say." * * * "The Nawab had plenty of energy, and was cautious withal; he used to try all his food on his dogs, and had all his water brought from a distance in sealed vessels under the special charge of a favorite."

* Macnaghten, Vol. I., p. 258.

† *Ibid*, p. 370.

Notwithstanding the extraordinary tact, powers of imitation and simulation, and unwearied patience in carrying out nefarious purposes which mark the native character, there can rarely occur any cases in this country where such simulation ought to baffle the scrutiny of a medical man accustomed to watch the insane. In fact, it appears to be a very safe general rule that no one can pass himself off as insane to a medical man, who observes carefully, unless he has studied the subject of insanity more closely than the physician has done. This is scarcely likely to happen in India. Cases of some difficulty do, however, occur here from time to time. Dr. Kenneth Mackinnon favored me with the very interesting case of a Rajah, the lineal descendant of Seetah, the celebrated heroine of the Ramayanah, who feigned insanity. Dr. Mackinnon was offered large bribes in this case; and, as he steadily pronounced the Rajah to be an impostor, he was accused by the Rajah's people of having taken them from the opposite party. His decision, however, proved correct; for, when the Rajah found that the Courts were acting upon Dr. Mackinnon's opinion, he threw off the cloak of imposture, and resumed the transaction of his own affairs.

One Sheodutta was tried at Banda for the murder of a Police duffadar (who had taken him into custody), by striking him on the head from behind with a heavy *lattee*. Subsequently to the commitment of his case to the Sessions, the prisoner's brother represented that he had, for some time previously, been insane, and had committed the deed in a fit of madness. The Judge therefore directed that the prisoner should be examined by the Civil Surgeon, to ascertain the state of his mind. This officer reported that the man was of sound mind, and quite rational in all he did; that he had had frequent opportunities of examining Sheodutta, and of putting such questions to him as he thought requisite, and that he had noticed no insanity; that, though his demeanour when answering questions was peculiar, his actions seemed perfectly rational, and he believed him to be quite capable of judging right from wrong. While the Judge was reading over the above deposition for the information of the jury and the prisoner, the latter gradually approached a thick walking-stick lying on the Judge's table. Upon the medical officer snatching the stick away, the prisoner made a dash for his own formidable *lattee*, which was in a corner of the room. He was stopped by a chuprassee, whom he struck violently before he could be secured. He had remained perfectly calm until the Judge began reading the Surgeon's deposition. There was no other evidence of insanity. He was sentenced to death.*

Kenkaroo Noshya, of Rungpore, confessed, upon being apprehended on suspicion of having murdered his wife, that, being seized when working

* Nizamut Adawlut Reports, N. W. P., November 2nd, 1852, p. 1282.

in the fields with an attack of ***batick rog*** (that is, literally, flatulency, considered in this case to be "a kind of hypochondria"), to which he had been liable for about a year, and which he implied made him ignorant of what he did when under its influence, he went home and cut his wife's throat. The prisoner's mother attempted to make out that he used to have attacks of this disease occasionally, during which he used to beat her and his brother; and when, on recovery, he observed their sulkiness, and was told the cause, he said he knew nothing about it. None of the other witnesses had ever seen him under the influence of this disease; they were only told by his mother that the prisoner beat her when he had the disease. They stated that he was exceedingly passionate, getting into a violent rage when anything annoyed him; that he went about alone, did not like talking, &c.; they called him a "*pagul*," or half a "*pagul*," or *boura*. When in jail, he was seized, or pretended to be seized, with an attack of the disease, and was sent to the hospital, where he remained thirty-two days. The Civil Surgeon considered the prisoner's madness to be feigned. He was violent at first, but, upon being tied and kept upon low diet, and threatened with punishment if he made a disturbance, he very soon became quiet. On the first day of trial, when required to plead, he did so at once. On the second day, when asked what he had to say in defence, he would not speak, made circles in the air with his hand, and other gesticulations, stopping suddenly and becoming quiet; and, after each stoppage, casting a rapid glance at the law officer and the Judge, which said plainly, "What do you think of that?" After being once or twice told that an answer was required, he gave it slowly and hesitatingly, as if apparently the act of recollection required an effort. The Judge considered that, as stated by the Civil Surgeon, he was certainly a man of a very low grade of intellect; but that there was no reason whatever to believe that he then was, or had been at any time, in such a state as to be incapable of judging between right and wrong. This authority sentenced him to imprisonment for life with labor and irons. The Judges of the higher Court held that the medical evidence, and the facts on record, left no doubt in their minds as to the perfect sanity of the prisoner; and that the mere effect of bodily disease, in irritating his temper, could not be regarded as forming any sufficient ground for mitigation of punishment in a crime of that nature; they therefore sentenced him to death.*

Durponarain confessed fully and circumstantially, both in the mofussil and fouzdaree, that he had taken part in the murder of a prostitute by cutting her throat. The murder, as he described it, was preconcerted, and was effected in the most deliberate manner, partly with the object of bringing the woman's neighbours into trouble, and also to secure their victim's property. The Sessions Judge observed :—"The law officer has found him

---

* Nizamut Adawlut Reports, November 17th, 1854, p. 611.

guilty, and he believes that he was of sound mind when he committed the murder ; but he declares that he is not liable to any punishment till a competent professional man shall pronounce him to be sane. He will then be liable to a sentence of death for the murder of which his *futwa* convicts him." "Whether he was mad or not, I was compelled, as there was another prisoner committed with him, to proceed with the trial. The witnesses named for the prosecution, being many of them fellow-laborers with the prisoner in the Gloucester Mills, were questioned as to the prisoner's state of mind before the murder. They all agree that he is perfectly sane, and that no man who was not so could have been employed in such work as the prisoner had to do in the mills. His own account of the manner and object of the murder all bear evidence of the sanity of the man. It is perfectly established then that, *at the time he committed the murder*, he was in his right mind and responsible for his actions. The question left then to be decided is,—is he *now* mad ? If he is mad, the trial, as regards him, is a nullity ; and, if he is not mad, he has been tried and found guilty. The Civil Surgeon, who has been watching him for some days, has given a most vacillating and equivocating opinion in regard to the prisoner's sanity or otherwise.* By his own account, he thinks him sane ; and yet says he is in doubt about it. It is plain, from his deposition, that Dr. ——— could never make up his mind whether what he describes as the indications of madness are, in the case of the prisoner, assumed or not. That they are assumed is, I think, palpable. Mr. Floyd, the Alipore Jailor, describes, with great clearness, the *sudden* transition of the prisoner from perfect sanity to a state which, if real, could be nothing short of downright madness. His own impression, after very careful and close watching, is that the man is pretending to be a fool. That opinion I have every reason to coincide in. The confessions of the prisoner show him to have been quite in his proper mind when he gave them ; his own conduct, as described by himself, is evidence of the same. He was not mad, nor did he show the slightest symptom of madness, for three days after his lodgment in the Alipore Jail.† It is not in the least probable that madness would commence in the sudden way that the prisoner's assumed appearance of madness did. I watched him with great care during the trial ; his conduct before me gives me reason to believe that he is as much in his right senses as he ever was. He pretends to understand nothing, and he speaks in monosyllables ; but I feel convinced that he both understands, and that he would speak clearly and intelligibly, if he dare make any better defence than pretend-

---

* The late Dr. ——— had been an officer of considerable talent, but was now very aged, and was upon the point of retiring.

† The two last sentences, I believe, convey the learned Judge's meaning which, in the original, is obscured by typographical errors.

ing madness. I am led to think that he understands what is said from the increased attention with which he watched and heard such parts of the evidence as concerned the part he took in the murder, and his own state of mind. When the doctor had given his deposition, I read it out to him ; he unconsciously evinced, in his countenance, the interest he took in it ; when I explained Mr. Floyd's deposition, he could not conceal the effect it had upon him." Sentence—Death.*

A very important case of feigned insanity occurred at Ahmednugger, in 1836. Hoozoorshah, having entered into an engagement to marry, and to defray the marriage expenses, advanced some money to the girl's father on this account, but was unable, from want of means, to meet his engagement ; consequently the marriage was broken off, and it only remained that the money should be repaid, when Hoozoorshah, seeing the girl and her mother entering a house, seized the former by the hand, and asked her what her intentions were. She referred him to her father, upon which he stabbed her four times with his dagger. These wounds proved fatal. He was tried ; and, nothing being elicited to show that he was suffering from mental derangement, he was sentenced to death, as it clearly appeared that, under the impulse of jealousy and revenge, he had fully resolved to marry or murder the girl. After the order for his execution was issued, the Civil Surgeon sent in a certificate to the effect that he was in hospital undergoing medical treatment for insanity. Consequently, the Sessions Judge stayed the Court's warrant. Upon this the superior Court directed the Sessions Judge to make inquiries as to the prisoner's state of mind about the time at which he committed the murder, and to report whether there was any reason to suppose that *the prisoner was insane at the time he perpetrated the murder*. In compliance, the Sessions Judge certified the depositions of eight witnesses who had been long and intimately acquainted with the prisoner, and some of whom were constantly living with him up to the day of the murder. From these depositions it appeared that the prisoner had never shown any indication of insanity. The Sessions Judge further stated that the prisoner's conduct on his trial did not indicate any aberration of intellect, and that he was therefore led to conclude that the prisoner's incoherent behaviour, since the sentence, was feigned and assumed. The Sessions Judge was then desired by the Court to inform them whenever the Civil Surgeon could certify that the prisoner had become sane, and to suspend execution of the warrant until further instructions. Two months later, it was duly reported that the prisoner was no longer in a deranged state of mind, and that, while in hospital, he was detected at night in an attempt to escape by making a hole in the mud wall of his cell. He was executed under a new warrant. When on the scaffold, he confessed

---

* Nizamut Adawlut Reports, February 2nd, 1856, p. 331.

that he had feigned madness in the hope that his capital sentence would be remitted.*

For a remarkable trial in which there was conflict of medical opinion as to whether a criminal was insane or simulated madness, see the case of Bissun Chunder Baboo, Nizamut Adawlut Reports, February 18, 1858, p. 57.

The above cases are cited, not on account of any very striking features of medico-legal interest which they present, but as affording a fair idea of the kind and amount of feigning which is likely to come under investigation in the criminal Courts of India.

The most difficult class of cases met with in this country is probably that in which individuals, of decidedly and conspicuously weak intellect, but gifted with a degree of cunning almost compensatory to the higher faculties in which they are deficient, having been made tools of by dangerous persons in effecting their nefarious designs, fall into the hands of the authorities, who demand reports upon the state of their minds as accountable beings. Here, however, the contest between the intellect of the Surgeon and that of the idiot should, of course, terminate in favor of the former, especially as these impostors, if watched sufficiently long, rarely fail to neglect or over-act their parts.

The chief modes of judging of the insanity or sanity of natives is, by observing whether they adhere to their rules of caste, or the customs laid down in their religion ; by having surveillance maintained upon them by the Native Doctors and by their fellow-prisoners (an unsafe practice) ; by watching them when they are unconscious of observation ; by noticing whether they are sleepless at night ; and also by employing most of the other plans of investigation which we have recourse to in England. Dr. Kenneth McLeod has recently told me of a case in which a prisoner, feigning insanity and dumbness, was detected by the administration of chloroform.

Law.

For the Indian laws as affecting the Insane, see Indian Penal Code, Section 84; Mayne's Commentaries, 5th Ed., pp. 52 to 55; Cowell and Woodman, p. 350 ; Code of Criminal Procedure, Sections 388 to 397.

* Bellasis' Reports, p. 111.

APPENDIX.

A.—Page 107.

LIST OF POISONS PROCURABLE IN INDIAN BAZARS.

Compiled from the Works of O'Shaughnessy, Royle, Fleming, Piddington, Honigberger, Burton Brown, Waring, Kanny Lall Dey, &c., and from the Chemical Examiners' Reports.

Vernacular Names.		Botanical or English Names.
————————	...	Actea Acuminata.
Afarbiyun, Farfiyun	...	Euphorbia Officiuarum.
Afeem (Duk.), Ufyoon (Arab.), Sheer-i-kush-kush (Pers.), Apaynum (Sans.)	...	Concrete juice of the Papaver Somniferum.
Ajwain, Khorasani or Banj	...	Hyoscyamus Niger.
Akundar Attaha	...	Juice of the Calotropis Hamiltonii.
Arrub-al-Salib	...	Solanum Nigrum.
Bag-Barendee (Beng.), Napatain (Tel.)	...	Jatropha Curcas.
Beheyra	...	Bellerie Myrobalon.
Belaschora Toombee	...	Lagenaria Vulgaris.
Belawine or Bhela (Duk.), Belader (Arab.)	...	Semecarpus Anacardium.
Bichattee	...	Tragia Involucrata.
Bijoyah, or Set Oprajeeta	...	Cannabis Indica.
————————	...	Bryonia Dioica.
————————	...	Cerasus Laurocerasus.
————————	...	Clematis Gouriana.
Bish	...	Aconitum Ferox.
Bish Cuchoo	...	?
Bernee Zumal	...	Saxus Baccata.
Bouran	...	Rhododendron Arboreum.
Cheena Kurrubæ	...	Thevetia Neriifolia.
Dadmaree, Bunmurich (Beng.)	...	Ammannia Vesicatoria.
Dakra	...	Aconitum Ferox.
Dampel (Beng. and Hind.)	...	Garcinia Pictoria.
Darmooz	...	Preparation of Arsenic?
Dhatoora (Kala)	...	Datura Fastuosa.
——— (Sada)	...	——— Alba.
Ghet-kol, Ghet-kuchoo (Beng.)	...	Arum Orixense.

Vernacular Names.		Botanical or English Names.
Gokatu or Kana-goraka (Cing.)	...	Hebradendron Cambogioides.
Goonch	...	Abrus Precatorius.
Gundhera	...	Daphne.
Gunduck-ke-tesab (atr)	...	Sulphuric Acid.
Gungla, Shulghum	...	Ranunculus Acris.
Gunjah	...	Cannabis Indica.
Hartal	...	Orpiment.
Heera kasis	...	Sulphate of Iron.
Hidgelee Badam (Hind. and Beng.)	...	Cashew.
Hoormaigatta	...	?
Hooroou (Beng.)	...	Sapium Indicum.
Hulla Hull	...	?
Hurreeana or Hurinah	...	Root of the Aconite or of the Gloriosa Superba ?
Hutteah	...	?
Indrain (Hind.), Vishala (Sans.), Hunzil, Irsa. (Pers. and Arab.)	...	Cucumis Colocynthis.
Indrayun and Bisloombhee	...	——— Pseudo Colocynthis.
Indrain Puharee	...	Hardwickii.
Ishlonga	...	?
Jamalghota (Hind.), Jayapœla (Sans.), Dund (Pers. Arab.)	...	Croton Tiglium.
———————	...	Janipha Manihot, Tapioca Plant.
Kadishen	...	Cluytia Collina.
Kahoo (Hind.)	...	Lactuca Sativa.
Kakmari (Sans.), Kakmari-ke-Beenje (the seeds)	...	Anamirta Cocculus (or Cocculus Indicus.)
Kalikootkie	...	Helleborus Niger (also Cobra Poison and Aconite Root.)
Kanapa-tiga (Tel.) Kusar (Hind.)	...	Vitis Carnosa.
Kerula (Hind.)	...	Cucumis Indicus (wild species.)
Kiwach	...	Mucuna Pruriens.
Kokibung	...	Hyoscyamas Insanus.
Koytasaper Bish	...	A Snake Poison ?
Kuchila-ke-Melung	...	Viscum of the Nux Vomica.
Kuchila, &c., &c.	...	Strychnos Nux Vomica.
Kunnar, Kanar	...	Nerium Odorum.
Kuphoor, Kusar (Hind.)	...	Camphora Officinarum.
Kurreearee-ka-jer	...	Root of Gloriosa Superba.
Kurrubee (Hind.)	...	Nerium Odorum.
Kurwr-Badam (Beng.)	...	Bitter Almond.
Lal-Chitra	...	Plumbago Rosea,
Lunka Sij (Beng.)	...	Euphorbia Tirucalli.
Makal (Beng.)	...	Trichosanthes Palmata.
Mansil	...	Realgar.
———	...	Meconopsis Aculeata.
Meeta Bish	...	Aconitum Ferox.
Mishmee Bish	...	Aconitum Ferox ?
Mohoora	...	Root of Aconitum, Ferox or Gloriosa Superba ?
Moordar Sung	...	Litharge.

VERNACULAR NAMES.		BOTANICAL OR ENGLISH NAMES.
Mudar	...	Calotropis Hamiltonii.
Munsa Sij	...	Euphorbia Ligularia.
Naga Musada (Tel.)	...	Strychnos Colubrina.
Nimuk-ke-tesab	...	Hydrochloric Acid.
Nunguinlceah or Nooangooleah	...	Gloriosa Superba.
Papita	...	Strychnos Ignatia.
Puharee Indrayun	...	Cucumis Hardwickii.
Pulball, Potole	...	Trichosanthes Dioica.
Raskapur	...	Calomel, with 10 per cent. of Corrosive Sublimate.
Sendur	...	Red Lead.
Seorinjan (two varieties)	...	Hermodactyl (Colchicum.)
Shial-kanta (Beng.)	...	Argemone Mexicana.
Shingurf	...	Vermillion.
Shora-ke-tesab	...	Nitric Acid.
Shwet Keerooi (Beng.)	...	Euphorbia Thymifolia.
Suffaid Shumbal	...	White Arsenic.
Suranjan Shirin	...	Colchicum Autumnale.
Soorujhal	...	Ranunculas Sceleratus.
Sunkhya Suffaid	...	Arsenious Acid, opaque.
——— Bilourie	...	——— Vitreous.
——— Golabi	...	——— with Orpiment.
——— Kala	...	——— with Realgar.
——— Pili	...	——— with Orpiment.
Sumbulkar	...	Arsenious Acid.
Tambaca	...	Nicotiana Tabacum.
Telini	...	Meloe, Milabris Cichorei (Blistering Fly.)
Toombee	...	Lagenaria Vulgaris.
Tutiya, Neel-Tutiya	...	Sulphate of Copper.
Ugooroo	...	Excæcaria Agallocha.
Usgund, Caknaj (Hind)	...	Physalis Somnifera.
Wallursi (Teling.), Walsura (Tamul.)	...	Walsura Piscidia.
Zangar Pitrai	...	Acetate of Copper.

It will be observed that the above List is evidently incomplete. It probably also contains some errors. Additions and corrections will be received, with many thanks, by the author.

A. 1.—PAGE 127.

Poisoning by Arsenuretted Hydrogen.

Dr. Mouat has published, in No. VIII. of the *Indian Annals of Medical Science for April* 1867, p. 657, the case of Mr. Andrew Robertson, Professor of Chemistry in the Calcutta Medical College, *ætat* fifty-seven. While exhibiting to his class the mode of applying Marsh's test to the detection of arsenic, and while the disengagement of Arsenuretted Hydrogen was rapid and abundant, a window was incautiously opened by a pupil; and, as it was directly in front of the Professor who lectured with his back to an open door, the want of air caused the gas to be carried directly to him:—he did not at first perceive it. He soon, however, became aware of it from the sense of burning and constriction in the throat, which compelled him immediately to close the lecture.

On the following morning, Dr. Mouat found that he had been laboring for several hours under excessive irritability of stomach, with an intense acrid burning sensation from the pharynx to the lower extremity of the alimentary canal. The vomited matters consisted, at first, of the food contained in the stomach, and then of bile and coffee-ground looking matter. The bowels had been obstinately constipated, and there had been severe pains in the loins, accompanied with the discharge of between three and four pints of bloody urine. This he had locked up for chemical examination after his recovery. He was afterwards quite satisfied that he discovered minute traces of arsenic. There was considerable fever, with a full, hard, frequent, and incompressible pulse; a dry, hot, unperspiring skin; deep-seated pain in the lumbar region, intense restlessness, anxiety, and general uneasiness, with a pale, anxious countenance, and considerable vital prostration.

On the third day, there was still constipation, the bowels not having been moved since the accident. There was a good deal of tenderness in the left iliac fossa, with a sense of weight and dragging in the fundament. A dose of castor-oil with laudanum produced a tolerably copious clay-colored evacuation, with a tubular slough somewhat ragged in appearance, and about four inches in length; it was found to consist of a portion of the lining membrane of the rectum, with a large quantity of fibrinous exudation. On the seventh day, there were symptoms of hepatitis; and, eighteen hours later, he was jaundiced. On the twenty-second day, he was free from all distressing symptoms. He died about three years subsequently from uremic coma in an attack of remittent fever.

B.—Page 134.

CATTLE POISONING.

Letter by Capt. Hedayet Ally, to Col. J. Emerson, Cantonment Magistrate, Dinapore.

Sir,—I beg to acknowledge the receipt of a pamphlet regarding the diseases of cattle, and the medicines discovered by Dr. McLeod for them, which you kindly favored me with. As a cursory view of the treatise seemed to interest me, I carefully perused it, and am persuaded to believe that the diseases therein laid down, breaking out among cattle, carry off thousands of them, and the treatment specified would prove efficacious in arresting the progress of their baneful effects. I have therefore sent the work to the tehsildar in my zemindary, with injunctions to try the remedies recommended therein, in case of such maladies breaking out.

2nd.—Since the attention of Government has been attracted to the disease, which annually breaks out, and of a sudden destroys thousands of cattle, inasmuch as, in the first place, the husbandmen are the sufferers; and in the next, the decrease of those useful animals in every place enhances their price ten-fold. In this country the loss of cattle, the only beasts employed for tillage (and quite unlike in most parts of Europe, where horses are used for that purpose), in one year is severely felt; in the next, by causing decline of crops, and the poor, not getting a sufficiency of corn, experience great hardship; consequently I set myself diligently to trace out, to the best of my ability, the real cause, besides death by the visitation of God, to which these creatures fell victims, and am happy to find my researches have not proved altogether fruitless. From conversation held with those in the hide trade, and others familiar with the subject, I have succeeded in ascertaining the following facts, which I shall fully undertake to detail.

3rd.—Should a retrospective view of the hide trade, as far back as the year 1841, be taken, and enquiry made as to the number and description of people who were then engaged in it, it will be found that they have increased ten-fold. Formerly the trade was confined to a few, *viz.*, Chamars and Butchers : the former dealt in hides obtained from cattle dying of natural death ; and the latter of those slaughtered for consumption. Now-a-days many carry on this trade, who, having only one object in view,—*viz.*, the greater the receipt of hides, the more profitable the trade,—have established warehouses, both in towns and districts, especially in the latter, and have appointed gomashtahs in different villages, for collecting this commodity. A very limited number of dealers in this article engaged gomashtahs on fixed salaries, the greater number do so on the percentage system, giving them half the profits accruing from sales of hides procured through their agency, reserving the other to themselves. Such lucrative inducements, without any risk, being held out to the gomashtahs, they continually watch the opportunity of effecting large purchases of good hides by every means within their reach.

4th.—By "good hides" is meant such as are heavy, uninjured, and the hair not spoiled, because they meet with ready and profitable sale ; whereas those of the dead animals have bad hair on them, and are less in weight, owing to the effects of the disease, and are consequently sold at a cheaper rate ; hence all traders study to purchase good hides, and for that purpose advance large sums to the Chamars in the interior without security.

5th.—It appears that Chamars in the districts have peculiar modes of poisoning cattle ; they contrive in some instances to poison the pasture where cattle are wont to graze, or mix it up with fodder when not taken out to graze ; and the poor creatures taking their food so poisoned, either drop down instantaneously, or die in a day or two afterwards, but never survive its effects ; their skins are ranked as "good hides," inasmuch as neither its weight diminishes, nor the hair gets spoiled. Impelled by the love of gain alone, they feel not the stings of conscience in carrying on this cruel and nefarious practice, to obtain good hides within a shorter space of time than that required for collecting slaughtered ones. These are facts well known, and reason suggests the same ; for it is customary in Hindustan for Chamars to have the privilege of removing the carcases of cattle dying in towns, villages, and parishes, situated within the limits assigned to them ; and by way of remuneration for their trouble in removing the carcases, they are allowed the enjoyment of the horns, hides, and fat of the dead cattle. This tempts them to bring about the death of more cattle than would die of themselves at the places within their respective jurisdictions.

6th.—During the rains and cold weather, cattle are poisoned in excess ; and it is also said that the Chamars mix up poison with *suttoo* (pulverised parched gram used by the common people as food), and sprinkle the mixture on the pasture, or where grass is found in abundance, and the cattle feeding thereon die. It has also come to my knowledge that they have a kind of awl or needle tipped with poison, with which they wound the animal's tender part so as to draw blood, and the poison coming in contact with the blood pervades the whole system in circulation, and brings on the poor beast's death. This cruel method of killing, the Chamars have designated in their professional technicality *thokeea* (by a poke), and that by poisoning grass or fodder, *beeroo* (medicines). The former mode is less in vogue than the latter, as it is more easily detected than the other. For instance, one of the fraternity asking another of the quantity and description of hides he has, is answered by the other in their own slang, such a quantity of slaughtered, and such of dead, as also so many *thokeea* and so many *beeroo*—the two last-mentioned kinds are ranked as slaughtered ones. This mode is more extensively practised in the country than in towns.

7th.—Tradesmen advance large sums of money to Chamars in the country for the supply of hides, which practice, in my opinion, is objectionable ; for to clear the advance received, they are induced to compass the destruction of cattle in such large numbers. It is also said that, if the Chamars be not able to clear the advances received from the hide dealers within a reasonable time, they are sent for by the latter, warned to clear their prescribed number of hides without delay, and the former promise to do so in a week or two, which they actually fulfil, when further advances are made to them, and they continue to compass the death of such numbers as would enable them to clear the advance money received afresh.

8th.—In Hindustan, trade in hides is carried on mostly by the lower class, and by very few of the respectable circle. Among the latter only those do it who observe that others engaged in it become rich within a short time, [and] naturally feel the same desire to become so also; very few of the lower class, who follow any trade or profession, care about good or evil, provided it is a source of profit, whilst the respectable part of the people think of making their fortune by their own honest exertions only, and thereby add to their respectability.

9th.—I am of opinion that, if enquiry be made into this matter, the number of cattle destroyed by poison will be easily ascertained ; especially if notice be taken of the number of hide godowns in towns and the country, the number of hides annually exported from each, and the proportion of slaughtered and dead ones,—the proportion of these two descriptions will be apparent. By slaughtered hides is meant those of animals killed for food, and by dead those that die by natural death. On enquiry at the godowns, it will undoubtedly be discovered that such quantities of hides were sent thence as never could have come from the number of cattle killed for actual consumption, which plainly proves the description of hides mentioned in para. 5.

10th.—Since 1857-58, when the mutiny broke out, a larger number of European Regiments are, of course, kept up, which necessarily causes a proportionately greater number of cattle to be killed for their use ; yet not to the extent which the books of hide merchants will show to have been exported from Bengal and other parts of India.

11th.—Should the books of consignees and brokers of Calcutta, through whom all the hides of Bengal are sold, as also those of the dealers in other towns who carry on this trade, be examined as to the quantity of hides lodged in their respective warehouses by dealers from 1865 to the current year, and the proportion of slaughtered and dead hides in them, the aggregate will show an excess of the latter over the former ; and the quantity of buffalo hides would also be ascertained. Moreover, the proportion of hides speciously denominated as slaughtered, will far exceed the actual number of cattle annually slaughtered in Bengal, from which the poisoning of cattle will fully be proved. The hides of those quadrupeds that are killed by poison are made to resemble those of the slaughtered, as neither the weight diminishes, nor the hair thereon gets spoiled. From the merchants' books, it will be apparent that so many heads of buffalo were never brought under the butcher's knife in Bengal, as the hides sold would indicate, for buffalo meat is seldom used as food : hence a very limited number are killed for that purpose. From the above facts, their natural death and that by poison will fairly be brought to light.

12th.—The Police should keep a vigilant eye over them, and take notice of the number of cattle dying of natural death, besides by the sickness which Dr. McLeod treats of ; for which purpose books should be kept at the Police Stations and outposts, in which causes of the death of cattle ought to be entered, and chowkeydars ordered to report to the next Police Station or outpost, the nature of disease which brought on the death of the animals ; the Police on suspecting any unfairness should make investigations, and this will lead to the detection of poisoning or otherwise. Should the Police be active, it is not improbable that, in some districts, those having a hand in supplying the poison will be detected and apprehended. Moreover, when it is known that the Police are on the alert, the nefarious practice in question will cease, inasmuch as it will deter the perpetrators from doing so in future, and the sufferers will be relieved. Should the Police enter the causes of death in their books, the number of cattle annually carried off by different diseases, as well as the prevalence of murrain in any particular district, will be brought to the knowledge of Government.

13*th*.—Should the above measures be adopted, and the books of the consignees and brokers of Calcutta and other towns be examined, the excess or diminution of exports of one year and those of the one before will be known ; in all probability, it will show a great falling off, as, in consequence of the short receipts, the dealers will likewise decrease ; for, owing to the suppression of the practice of poisoning, it will be difficult to procure hides, which will considerably discourage dealings in that commodity, and bring it down to the scale as in time gone by, and will leave the trade confined to hides of animals actually slaughtered for consumption, or which die from natural causes. In addition to what is above detailed, there are persons who can fairly detect hides produced by poisoning ; should such persons be engaged to examine the different descriptions of hides in the several godowns, it will deter both the merchants from purchasing such hides, and the Chamars from poisoning for that purpose.

14*th*.—I have thought it proper to bring to light whatever has come to my knowledge, so that by some suitable and wise enactment, the poisoners may be detected, and others warned from practising similar acts of cruelty in future, which will thus prove beneficial to the poor.

In submitting the above for your perusal and consideration, I entertain the hope that you will be pleased, if you deem it necessary, to forward it to higher authority.

I have, &c.,

(Sd.) HEDAYUT ALLY, *Capt.*,

A. D. C. to His Excellency the Commander-in-Chief.

DINAPORE, 11*th June* 1869.

B. 1.—PAGE 171.

Road-Poisoning in the Upper Provinces in 1869.

The *Englishman* gives an extract from the Report of the Chemical Examiner for the N. W. P., which shows that, in 1869, that officer had cognizance of *twenty-two* deaths from Datura-poisoning. He gives the following case :—

"Three men and a boy were travelling, last May, from Bombay, towards the North-West Provinces. They were joined at Hurdah by a man, who ingratiated himself by pleasant companionship, and every day as they travelled evinced his good-fellowship by making sherbet for the whole party during their mid-day rest. At length, at a solitary spot on the banks of a stream near Bansa, in the Dumoh District, they drank his sherbet for the last time. The three men were found dead, and the boy roaming about close to their bodies in the restless delirium caused by datura. A man said to have been the poisoner was apprehended soon after in the Hoshungabad District, and on him was found a carefully-made powder of datura seeds, mixed with a little flour and sugar. I detected datura in the stomachs of all the three victims."

C.—Page 212.

ON THE SYMPTOMS OF POISONING BY THE INDIAN SPECIES OF DATURA—BY DR. H. GIRAUD.

From the 1st January 1848 to the present date (20th January 1849), fifty-one cases of poisoning by datura have been treated in the Jamsetjee Jeejeebhoy Hospital; the general character of their symptoms have closely resembled those induced by *Datura stramonium*, in several instances exhibiting the three distinct stages: 1st, of primary delirium; 2nd, of sopor or even coma; and 3rd, of final delirium,—which have been observed to mark the action of henbane, belladonna, and other solanaceous plants, as well as that of the stramonium. It is seldom, however, that patients are brought to hospital before the second stage (that of sopor) has commenced; and very frequently not until the third stage (that of secondary delirium) has supervened; and, in the great majority of cases, either from the small quantity of the poison, from the large amount of food ingested with it, or from peculiarity of constitution, one single stage of delirium is alone observed.

The following is the general course of those cases in which the full effects of the poison are manifested:—The patient, in the primary stage of delirium, is found in a state of extreme restlessness, usually attempting to wander about as if in search of something, but frequently from giddiness and extreme muscular weakness he is unable to walk or even to stand; he either vociferates loudly or is garrulous, and talks incoherently; sometimes he is mirthful and laughs wildly, or is sad and moans as if in great distress; most generally he is observed to be very timid, and when most troublesome and unruly, can always be cowed by an angry word, frequently putting up his hands in a supplicating posture. When approached, he suddenly shrinks back, as if apprehensive of being struck, and frequently he moves about, as if to avoid spectra. But the most invariable accompaniment of this, and of the final stage of delirium, and frequently also of that of sopor, is the incessant picking at real and imaginary objects. At one time the patient seizes hold of parts of his clothes or bedding, pulls at his fingers and toes, takes up dirt and stones from the ground, or as often catches at imaginary objects in the air, on his body, or on anything near him;—very frequently he appears as if amusing himself by drawing out imaginary threads from the ends of his fingers; and occasionally his antics are so varied and ridiculous that I have seen his near relatives, although apprehensive of danger, unable to restrain their laughter. Many of these singular movements appear to originate in a curiously impared or disordered state of vision, in which distant objects seem to the patient as if very close to him, and those that are near as if highly magnified; for frequently, after gazing for some time at a distant object, he will attempt to grasp it as if it were close at hand; and he starts back, when approached, as if he thought the person approaching would the next moment touch him. This state of vision may, in part, depend upon the widely-dilated pupil, which, as in poisoning by other solanaceous plants, is an invariable symptom in all cases, and is persistent through each stage, and even continues for some time after complete recovery. With the foregoing symptoms, great diversity in the state of the circulation is met with in different individuals, and even in the same individual at different periods. In the greater number of cases, the temperature of the surface and the strength of the pulse are natural—although the rate of the latter is usually somewhat accelerated (90 or 100). In other instances the pulse is much quicker than natural (112 or 120), full, firm, or even sharp; the temples throb; the respiration is hurried; and the surface of the body is hot. Whilst, as a third and less frequent condition, the pulse is quick, small, and feeble, the respiration slow, and the surface cold.

The second stage, that of sopor, is the state in which a great number of cases are first brought under notice. They are then found either in a state of profound sopor, or in one of excessive drowsiness, from which they may be partially and momentarily aroused to some degree of consciousness ; there is low muttering delirium, tremor, subsultus tendinum, and most usually the characteristic catching at objects, although the patient's eyes may be closed at the time. In four cases only have I met with deep coma, utter insensibility and stertorous breathing, and in two of these there was a remarkable tympanitic state of the abdomen.

These all appeared to be in great danger ; but, like the milder cases, ultimately recovered after passing through the final stage of delirium.

As great a diversity in the state of the circulation has been observed in this second as in the preceding stage of the operation of the poison, the pulse being frequently quick, full, and firm, with throbbing temples, and heat of surface ; whilst, in other cases, a cold damp skin has accompanied a small feeble pulse, scarcely perceptible at the wrist ; and this without any corresponding difference in the nature of the other symptoms.

The third stage of final delirium has not been observed to differ, in any respect, either in regard to the nature of the delirium or to the condition of the circulation, from the primary stage.

The most numerous cases are those in which neither sopor nor coma is observed, but only the symptoms common to both stages of delirium.

The following is a statement of the condition of the patients at the time of their admission into the Jamsetjee Jeejeebhoy Hospital :—

In a state of excitement—afterwards comatose	2
In a comatose state	2
In a state of sopor	18
In a delirious state, without sopor or coma	29
Total ...	51

The patients, on recovery, usually state that they have little or no recollection of anything that occurred subsequent to their last meal, which may be supposed to have contained the poison ; so quickly does it appear to take effect. In one instance, however, I ascertained that a coachman drove his horses very steadily two hours after taking a meal which had been drugged; but, at the expiration of the third hour, active delirium came on, and continued for about eight hours. It would be interesting to discover the general duration of each of the stages above indicated; but this is rendered extremely difficult from the varied periods that elapse before the patients come under treatment; and the final stage of delirium is that only in which I have been able to arrive at even an approximate conclusion on this point. When the patient revives from the state of sopor, he recovers through that of final delirium usually in from six to ten hours; and this appears to be the general duration of the delirium of those milder cases in which neither coma nor sopor occur; doubtless the action of the poison is prolonged in some cases by the quantity of food ingested with it.

The treatment of these cases of poisoning by Datura must, of course, be guided both by the nature of the general symptoms, and by the particular state of circulation, which, as before mentioned, may be very varied under the same train of general symptoms. If the patient be seen soon after the poison has been taken, a promptly acting emetic, as sulphate of zinc, may be administered; and, where sopor with cold clammy skin and feeble pulse has supervened, an emetic of ipecacuanha and sesquicarbonate of ammonia seldom fails thoroughly to evacuate the stomach. In the stage of coma, or even of sopor, attended with heat of skin, throbbing temples, and full, firm pulse, emetics, I think, should not be employed; both because their operation might favour cerebral congestion, and because, when the case has advanced to this stage, the poison has probably left the stomach. In the stages of delirium where this is of an active kind and attended with much excitement of the circulation, great relief is usually obtained by the application of a few leeches (one to two dozen) to the temples; the exhibition of the cold affusion once or twice, and the use of small doses of tartar emetic and opium. This combination, in doses of from half a grain of tartar emetic with twenty or thirty minims of laudanum, repeated every two or three hours, generally proves as efficacious as in the analogous state of excitement that occurs in delirium tremens. On the other hand, when either the delirium or the sopor is accompanied by coldness of the surface of the body and a small feeble pulse, the use of the stimulants, as ammonia and ether, will be indicated. As it probably occurs in many cases that the action of the poison is prolonged by its being taken with large quantities of food, and that being only gradually absorbed in its passage through the intestinal canal, the early administration of an aperient as castor oil, is obvious.

[About two months ago, my own coachman ate, late at night, a considerable quantity of *Datura leaves* in a mess with brinjal, which some one had recommended for rheumatism. He was caught in a delirious state, and immediately dosed with sulphate of zinc. He was quite well in the morning, and *the pupils were not diluted.* I attribute this to early emesis.—N. C.]

C. 1.—Page 279.

The following very important case of Poisoning by Camphor has been given me by Baboo Kanny Lall Dey, who saw the case about a year ago in consultation with Baboo Juggernauth Sen :—

"Baboo ————————, aged twenty-two years, a patient of Baboo Juggernath Sen, was advised to take small doses of camphor for gonorrhœa. About 8 P.M. on the evening of ————, he took about a scruple of the drug. Feeling a pleasant and exhilarating effect therefrom, and considering camphor to be a homely and consequently not a very active remedy, he shortly after consumed about 1½ tola (*thirteen and-a-half* scruples) with a bottle of lemonade. There was nothing worthy of notice till three quarters of an hour afterwards, when he began to feel a slight warmth in the pit of the stomach, and shortly after a severe burning sensation in that organ, as also in the throat. This was soon followed by giddiness, dimness of sight, ringing in the ears, and numbness all over the body. His body became covered with a cold clammy perspiration, and he felt an icy coldness all over. There was a sense of impending suffocation, the respiration was hurried, and the breath surcharged with camphorous smell. He lost all control over the limbs, and, when raised up, reeled like a man under the influence of liquor. The tongue was felt as if it were too large for the cavity of the mouth, although there was no perceptible redness or swelling of the organ. Gradually the patient became quite delirious, and began to get convulsions at 11½ P.M., or two hours and-a-half from the commencement. He continued in this state till the morning, when, after profuse emesis from the treatment adopted, the symptoms began to subside. After ten hours, the patient became relieved from all the urgent symptoms ; but the secondary effects continued for a much longer period, and it was not until three days had elapsed that the patient was restored to perfect health.

"The treatment adopted was plenty of warm water to drink, in order to excite vomiting, and small doses of tincture of opium."

This case, I believe, represents the largest dose of Camphor but one that has ever been taken. Dr. Taylor (on Poisons, p. 727) has given one which occurred to Wendt of

Breslaw. *Eight scruples* were swallowed by a drunkard dissolved in spirit. The symptoms were vertigo, dimness of sight, delirium, and burning pain in the stomach. There was *no vomiting*. The man recovered. Dr. Taylor adds that this case shows that Camphor cannot be regarded as a very active poison.

My House Physician, Baboo Taruknauth Gangooly, tells me of a case in which a lad of fifteen was killed in a few hours by a dose of two tolas, or *eighteen scruples*, of Camphor.

C. 2.—Page 313.

Poisoning by Darnel.

The *Englishman* quotes the Report of the Chemical Examiner for the North-Western Provinces, Oudh, and the Central Provinces, for 1869, to the effect that the document contains a remarkable instance of wholesale poisoning by the use of flour mixed with *Darnel Seeds*. The soldiers of a Goorkah regiment having suffered severely from vomiting, headache, and vertigo, a searching investigation was made, whence it appeared that the seed of the *Darnel* had not been sifted with sufficient care from the wheat. The two plants grow side by side, and the bad grains can only be separated from the wholesome grain by both being thrown into a sieve, when the one will pass through and the other be retained.

C. 3.—Page 314.

White Arsenic and the Poison-Fang of a Cobra made up with Pan.

Baboo Kanny Lall Dey has kindly shown me a *Betle* sent to his office on the 31st August 1870, by the Assistant Commissioner, Sonthal Pergunnahs, it having been "given for chewing to some person in that district." This diabolical peace-offering contains two lumps of Arsenic and the Poison-Fang of a Cobra, identified as such by Dr. Fayrer. It is distinctly grooved, and was concealed by a coating of some adhesive filth.

C. 4.—Page 331.

Andromeda.

In Vol. XIV., Journal of the Agricultural and Horticultural Society of India, Dr. Cleghorn has written upon the poisonous properties of certain species of *Andromeda*, more especially *A. Ovalifolia*, so common in our Himalayan Stations. Royle mentions, p. 259, that *Andromeda Ovalifolia* is said to be fatal to goats in the Himalayas.

C. 5.—Page 380.

SNAKE-BITE—MORBID CHANGES IN THE BITTEN PART.

On the 8th of August 1870, Dr. Woodford was so obliging as to show me, in the police dead-house, in the body of a Brahmin, who had died in fifteen minutes after having been bitten by a snake, a condition of parts which he has long considered to be characteristic of this form of poisoning. For about a hand's-breadth around the puncture there was a dusky livid, somewhat lead-colored appearance of the integument not amounting to ecchymosis. Below this the cellular tissue was infiltrated with a glairy exudation like that which would appear at the first onset of hard œdema : no serum escaped from the divided areolar tissue. Dr. Woodford regards these appearances as certainly pathognomonic of snake-poisoning.

C. 6.—Page 386.

HORNET STINGS.

Dr. Ormerod refers to the fate of a party of engineers who, while surveying on the banks of the Jumna, were attacked by hornets. Two were stung to death, and several were severely injured.

D.—Page 396.

HUMAN SACRIFICE.

The following statement of a crime resembling Human Sacrifice appeared in the Calcutta *Englishman* for August 4th, 1870. The facts are asserted to have been established at the Sessions trial. I have not been able to obtain any further information regarding this case.

"There was, in a certain large town, in the Upper Doab, a carcass butcher of good position and extensive dealings, whose wife bore him none but still-born children. After bearing these disappointments for several years, the unfortunate couple resolved to practice the rites of *Karee,* or magical incantation, one of which was no less than the disgusting ceremony of eating human flesh. Accordingly the butcher spoke to a neighbour, who said that he was acquainted with a wizard—*Syana* or 'cunning man,' being the vernacular expression used,—and it was resolved to sacrifice *a fine lad of about nine years of age,* the son of a highly respectable widow, who kept a school for girls in the place. The auspicious day arriving, the boy was induced to play with the son of one of the conspirators whose house was near that of the schoolmistress. Presently the butcher, who was watching the children, persuaded the intended victim to take a walk with him, on the pretence of giving him some sweetmeats. Shortly after the party was observed walking along towards the butcher's house ; the wizard and the go-between being behind, while the butcher went in advance, holding by the hand the poor little boy, who trotted by his side—said one of the witnesses—'as if going with his father.'

"Scarcely had the door of the house closed upon the three ogres and their victim, when the rites began. The party was joined by the butcher's wife, the boy sate among them awaiting the promised treat of sweetmeats, and the wizard began to mutter spells out of a book. What followed is almost too sickening for description. Arriving at a certain point of his incantation, the wizard said, 'Now to your work.' On this the butcher advanced to the boy, threw him down, and kneeling upon him ripped him open, cut out the liver and the tongue, and making them into a mess, gave them to his wife to eat! Other parts of the body, likely to be usful as spells in other cases, were removed, and the trunk and legs separated, and disposed of in a neighbouring thicket just outside the town, in conformity with the rules of the horrible art.

"But public opinion was, for once, fairly roused. The position of the widowed mother, and the tender age of the victim, excited the interest of relatives and friends, who happened to be men of local influence. The carriers of the body had dropped a pair of shoes, which were recognised by the artizan who had made them for the dead boy. Search was made in the wood toward which they had been seen going, and the scattered fragments recovered and identified. One of those who had been present at the bloody rites turned Queen's evidence, and two of the prisoners, arrested on these indications, confessed to the charge. They have all been sentenced to transportation for life,—the Judge, as we understand, having been of opinion, with the assessors, that it was in ignorance rather than in bad faith that the accused had acted in committing the offence."

E.—Page 621.

OPINION UPON A QUESTION WHETHER DEATH WAS CAUSED BY SUFFOCATION OR STRANGULATION.

I have carefully and fully weighed the whole of the medico-legal questions involved in the case of ——.

I shall take the 1st, 3rd, and 5th Questions proposed by the counsel for the defence together.

1st.—"Whether, from the *post-mortem* appearances described, Strangulation was not more likely to have been the cause of death than Suffocation?"

3rd.—"Is the story told by Ram Tohal—*viz.*, the deceased died of Suffocation within a few moments, because Bocha stopped the boy's mouth—a probable one?"

5th.—"Is it likely that the marks of ecchymosis round the neck and the wrists of the deceased were produced after death?"

The leading statements of the Medical Officer, explanatory of the causes of death, are as follow:—

A sheet, twisted into a rope, was tied or fastened tightly round the neck. The hands were tied with a cloth behind the back. There were two slight marks corresponding to the cloth-rope round the wrists. The boy's hands were tied behind his back with a *dhooty*, but not in the same degree (of tightness) as the sheet. It (the *dhooty*) was soft. Ecchymosis was caused by the tightness of the *dhooty*. Certainly the *dhooty* was not very tight round the wrists. Apparently the wrists were not swollen; but virtually they might have been, as the whole body may have been swollen.

Putrefaction was just commencing, features swollen and of a reddish color. There was a clot of blood that had issued from the nostrils. The eyes congested, tongue not protruded, the teeth were closed; on undoing the cloth-rope that was round the neck, a mark of ecchymosis was found round the neck; no injury to the wind-pipe. Blood extravasated under scalp; brain congested. There were some spots of extravasation of blood on the membrane surrounding the brain. The veins in the chest and right side of the heart full of liquid blood. Lungs almost healthy. There was no blood in the lungs. Expulsion of hard fœces.

The medical witness first stated that death was caused by Strangulation. He afterwards changed his opinion and held that death resulted from Suffocation, that the sheet was tied round the neck immediately after life was extinct, or "probably with the last moments," and that the hands were tied after death. The medical witness's explanation of the fact that, latterly, he changed his opinion and maintained that death was caused by Suffocation and not by Strangulation, is as follows:—

"The signs I have described in the dead body might arise from Strangulation, with exception of extravasation of blood on the brain. This was not the only reason why I thought death was caused by Suffocation. There were no other signs except extravasation of blood. From the manner in which the cloth was tied I inferred it was not Strangulation, and also from the tongue not protruding, the eyes not being opened to my satisfaction, blood issuing from nostrils. As far as I know, in Strangulation the eyes ought to be wide open. In cases of Strangulation, if pressure be made above the larynx, the tongue does not protrude."

Not one of the above reasons can be regarded as positive proof that death was due to Suffocation and not to Strangling—neither can their aggregate be so regarded.

First.—Strangling is sometimes attended with extravasation of blood on the brain. It is a rare appearance, but, when present, as it was in this case, it is very significant equally of death from Suffocation and Strangling.

Dr. Taylor says (edition of 1865, p. 655) that, in Strangulation by Hanging, "the vessels of the brain are commonly found congested; and in some rare instances, it is said, extravasation of blood has been met with on the membranes or in the substance of the organ. Effusion of blood is, however, so rare that Romer found this appearance described only once in a hundred and one cases; and, in one hundred and six cases described by Casper, it was only found in a single instance. Sir Benjamin Brodie found a large effusion of blood in the substance of the brain, and he refers to another case in which there was considerable effusion between the membranes."

In a large number of cases of asphyxia the brain is congested; effusion of blood is the result of such congestion (however caused) in a rather extreme degree.

Second.—The medical witness inferred from the manner in which the cloth was tied round the neck, that it was not the cause of Strangulation.

As he did not further explain the grounds upon which he formed this opinion, it is impossible to argue upon his reasons for arriving at it. We, however, read that "A sheet twisted like a rope was tied or fastened tightly round the neck." That there was a mark of ecchymosis all round the neck about an inch long (broad?) The depression round the neck was circular. The witness adds—"I found no other violent marks on neck of deceased save depression around the neck. I do not think it true in every case that it is scarcely possible that a murderer in the strangling of a living person by a cord should avoid producing on the neck marks of violent injury. Perhaps one of the causes that led me to suppose that Strangulation was not the cause of Prosunno's death was this. This was one of the causes of my belief in this case. I formed my opinion in this before the trial."

It is thus evident that the medical witness considered that the marks of injury about the neck were not so severe as they would have been had the boy been strangled. This is a debateable question. In my Medical Jurisprudence (published in 1856, p. 382) I have written—"It would not appear, from the records, that those very severe injuries to the neck, such as laceration of the muscles of the throat, rupture of the tracheal rings, &c., &c., occasionally observed in European cases of strangling, are frequent in similar cases in India. I have more than once found traces of very severe contusion of the muscles of the throat." . . "Still, whether to the employment of several accessories in these cases, or to the use of long soft cloths, which form a part of nearly every native's dress, or to a theoretical acquaintance with the practices of the Phansigars, which must exist among all classes in India—it is certain that the rule which maintains that 'in strangling, a much greater degree of violence is commonly employed than is necessary to cause asphyxia' (Taylor), will be found to have very numerous exceptions in this country." In his last edition Dr. Taylor says: "In the strangling of a living person with a cord it is scarcely possible that the murderer can avoid producing on the neck marks of severe injury; and, in the existence of these, we have evidence of the violent manner in which death has taken place. On the other hand, a person may be strangled, and yet the ligature, in consequence of its being soft and of a yielding nature, will not cause a perceptible depression or ecchymosis—scarcely anything more than a slight depression of the skin. If we except cases of suicide, such a condition must be rare, because assailants usually produce a much more violent constriction of the neck than is necessary to ensure the death of a person."

I consider that the death of Prosunno was such as might be expected upon the supposition of his having been held down and strangled by a twisted *dhooty* tied round his neck.

Third.—The medical witness holds that death was probably not caused by Strangulation, because the tongue was not protruding. He adds—"In cases of Strangulation, if pressure is made above the larynx, the tongue does not protrude."

He is supported in the first part of his opinion by Taylor, who remarks (p. 675) that swelling and protrusion of the 'tongue are more marked in Strangulation than in Hanging. On the other hand, Casper says (New Sydenham Society's Edition, Vol. II., p. 162): "In regard to the protrusion of the tongue or the clenching of it between the teeth, I have already pointed out the inconstancy and consequent untrustworthiness of this symptom, which is just as often absent as present in persons strangled, whether they have died from apoplexy, suffocation, or neuroparalysis."

Fourth.—The medical witness inferred that the case was not one of Strangulation, because "the eyes were not open to his satisfaction." Here Dr. Taylor is with him, observing that the "eyes are wide open, prominent and congested" (p. 674). Casper, on the other hand, says (p. 162, Vol. II.): "Most of those strangled have a pale, peaceful, and not a turgid countenance. Precisely the same may be said of the protrusion of the eyes, which is seldom observed, and only when the countenance is very turgid."

Dr. Taylor says (p. 655) that the protrusion or non-protrusion of the tongue depends "simply upon congestion." The protrusion of the eyes, when present after Strangulation, results wholly from the same cause—turgesense of blood. If then Casper, an authority second to none, found that the majority of strangulated Europeans "have a pale, peaceful, and not a turgid countenance," without protrusion of the eyes and tongue, it is not needful that we should demand, as proof of Strangulation these almost extreme evidences of congestion in a rice-fed Hindu boy of twelve, "of an average constitution." Casper has shown that an ecchymosed appearance may result in the part compressed by the cord where a body is suspended by the neck shortly after death, and he maintains that this condition of the structures is often not to be distinguished from that produced in death by hanging. The medical witness says that, on undoing the cloth-rope that was round the neck, a mark of ecchymosis was found round the neck. He adds, on cross-examination, that "the rope may have been tied at the last moment or a minute after death" "I cannot assert that it was not tied an hour after death. It is my opinion it was tied within a minute." He is by no means minutely particular in describing the appearance of this ecchymosis, but, judging by the last expression quoted above, I infer that there was positively effusion of blood into the structures, such as is produced during life by the pressure of the ligature in some cases of death by Strangulation and Hanging.

Taking this and all the other circumstances of the case together, and especially remembering that the extravasation of blood upon the surface of the brain *certainly occurred during life*, I consider that the aggregate of the facts stated in the medical evidence is perfectly compatible with the opinion that the deceased was strangled and killed by a twisted cloth tied round his neck.

The arguments of the medical witness in favor of Suffocation and against Strangling are founded upon authority, but I consider that, when a large view of the question is taken, the correctness of his conclusions is highly questionable.

All the physical conditions of the case being absolutely compatible with the opinion that the deceased was strangled by the cloth tied round his neck, why should we depart from the conclusion that his death was so caused? Only, I believe, because it appears in the evidence that a witness, Ram Tohal, asserts that he saw a man in the act of endeavouring to suffocate the deceased by compressing his mouth and nostrils with one hand.

The remaining evidences of Suffocation as distinguished from Strangulation rest wholly upon the statements of Ram Tohal, to the effect that, "when the boy began to cry, Bocha stopped his mouth with his right hand. He placed his open hand on the face and nose of the lad. Bocha stopped both the boy's nostrils and mouth. There was only a slight sound. When the boy's mouth was stopped, he screamed out. I did not see any struggle. I only heard a scream after boy's mouth was stopped. Bocha's other hand was by his side. The room was light. Bocha was standing erect while he stopped the boy's mouth."

Ram Tohal testifies at one time that he saw the felonious act, during which he asserts the Suffocation took place, from beginning to end; on another occasion he declares that the act was not completed when he left.

He is consistent in stating that he left and went to the Golaghur, either before or after the felonious act was completed; and then, on his return, Bocha placed a *chadar* over the body of the boy, that the body was lying motionless, and that no sound was heard.

If Ram Tohal's statement is believed to be true, it must be considered as proved that Bocha was seen to compress the mouth and nostrils of one who certainly died from asphyxia or suspended respiration. If Ram Tohal is believed to have left the room at this crisis, it cannot be known what further violence, possibly ending in Suffocation or Strangulation, was had recourse to during his absence; but it is quite impossible to accept Ram Tohal's statement as fully descriptive of the manner in which a boy of twelve, of average health, was suffocated. No man, however powerful, could suffocate such a lad by holding one hand over his mouth and nostrils while the other hand was by his side. The struggle in such a case would be furious, and, no serious injury being inflicted upon the windpipe (there was no such injury here), the violent conflict for life would be protracted for at least two minutes.

F.—Page 709.

OPINION UPON A QUESTION OF UNNATURAL CRIME.

(Continuation of the above Case.)

The remaining questions put by the Counsel are—

2. "Whether it is possible, or at all probable, that an unnatural offence should be committed by force upon a boy of twelve, and yet no marks of injury should be found in the anus."

4. "Is it probable, from the circumstances of the case, that the substance which the Doctor says he found round the fœces was semen, or is it not more likely that rather the substance itself was an invention of the Doctor,* or that it was mucus from the intestines?"

* I do not think this.—N. C.

I distinctly consider that the evidence of an unnatural crime in this case is wholly Ram Tohal's.

In a boy of that age, accustomed to such crime, there would probably be no injury to the parts. In one upon whom such an outrage was *completed* for the first time, there would probably be some laceration of the mucus membrane within the anus, with more or less effusion of blood.

The medical witness does not appear to have made any close examination of those parts, and he certainly did not observe any signs of injury or traces of bleeding.

I do not coincide with the medical witness in the opinion that the appearance presented by the fœces was due to the presence of semen. I differ from him on the ground that, when mucus is present in the rectum, in certain cases of rectal dysentery, when hard fœces are passed, the mucus *invariably passes separately* from the fœces which are not at all coated by it. Physically, the two cases are parallel.

My belief in this case consequently is that—

First—Death was probably caused by Strangulation by a twisted cloth tied round the neck.

Second.—That what Ram Tohal says that he saw Bocha do, could not possibly have caused death by Suffocation.

Third.—That there is no evidence of the commission of an unnatural offence, except that offered by Ram Tohal.

Fourth.—There is nothing in the medical evidence in favor of the belief that the deceased had been the subject of an unnatural offence.

Fifth.—That, as it has not been even hinted in the case that the deceased child was accustomed to unnatural practices, the fact that no blood was noticed in the evacuation from the bowel affords strong reason for the belief that the outrage in question was at least not completed.

Sixth.—There remains another point which may be regarded as rather one of opinion than of fact. If we are to accept the idea of the medical witness that the matter seen on the fœces was seminal fluid, we must consider that an unnatural crime was *completed*, that *penetration* was effected. Is it probable that such an act could be effected by a man of sixty upon a boy unhabituated to the crime? I believe it to be almost in the last degree improbable.

Seventh.—That, should it ever be decided that Ram Tohal's testimony is untrustworthy, there remains nothing in the evidence of the medical witness to criminate the accused. There would then, as I have before suggested, be strong reason for believing that an unnatural outrage was not perpetrated, while there would be nothing to show by whom or in what place the murder, by Strangulation, was committed.

(Sd.) NORMAN CHEVERS, M.D.

MEDICAL COLLEGE, CALCUTTA,
12*th October* 1869.

G.—PAGE 807.

OINOMANIA.

The following observations on *Oinomania* deserve careful attention :—

" Another form of drunkenness remains to be described,—namely, the *paroxysmal.* This is the form which has been mentioned by writers (first by Hufeland, who termed it *Dipsomania*) as a true mania, and which is recognised to be such by all practically acquainted with Insanity. Erdmann first observed this affection in Russia, where it is termed *sapoi* (sauf-sucht, drinking disease, or mania). Bruhl-Kramer, Erdmann, Friedreich, Henke, Guislain, and others have also treated of it. Broussais and Rayer adopted the term *Oinomania.* Many writers have, however, treated of the affection as if it were a form of delirium tremens, to which it is undoubtedly generically allied, but from which, nevertheless, it is specially distinct. Persons affected with the *paroxysmal* form are, for the most part, of temperate or even abstinent habits, and are only attacked at intervals with the disorder, which consists in the gratification of an impulse to swallow stimulants in enormous doses for a period of definite duration, when the paroxysm ceases and the individual resumes his temperate or abstinent mode of life. Dr. Hutcheson, of the Glasgow Lunatic Asylum (Report for 1842), has given the best detailed account of the disease in the English language. He notes three forms—the acute, the periodic, and the chronic. The acute is the rarest of the three, and occurs as a sequel of exhausting causes, as fevers, puerperal or uterine hæmorrhage, excessive venereal indulgence, &c., or in certain forms of dyspepsia ; in the latter case it is very apt to become chronic. The periodic form is met with *in persons who have experienced injury of the head,* or who have overworked the brain, or who are the offspring, directly or collaterally, of drunkards or lunatics. Women are apt to become the subjects of it during pregnancy. The *chronic* is simply the paroxysmal form changed into *continuous* drunkenness.

When a person is about to have a paroxysm of *Oinomania,* and it is not induced by any manifest excitant, as alcohol, fatigue, &c., he feels listless, uneasy, restless, and depressed, and is incapable of steady application. These feelings are accompanied by a gradually increasing craving for stimulants, which at last is yielded to. The individual perhaps then disappears from his home or usual place of business, and spends his days and nights in alternate sleep and intoxication, haunting the lowest dram-shops, and associating with depraved persons. Or perhaps he shuts himself up in his room, never leaving it for any purpose, and rapidly gulps down glass after glass of liquor he has procured, reckless of all consequences to himself, his family, or his affairs. The paroxysm being exhausted, a stage of apathy and depression succeeds, in which bitter regrets for his folly, and resolutions never again to yield to temptation, are prominent. This period of temperance may continue for some months, when, after an apparently trivial circumstance, the morbid cerebral condition which constitutes the paroxysm is again developed.

Friedreich notes five stages of the affection, as follows : 1.—The *premonitory* stage. After a period of apparent health, and moderate use of stimulants, the eyes present a wild expression, there is spasmodic action of the muscles of the orbit, a winking of the eyelids, photophobia, flushing of the face, headache, disturbed sleep, loss of appetite, indigestion, flatulence, anxiety, and dread. This stage continues for from a few hours to a few days. 2.—The *commencement* of the attack. Increased desire for spirituous drinks, which relieve the restlessness for a short time, and to this end the patient takes them, but always more and more rapidly. 3.—Stage of *developement.* The desire for spirits is now more than ever urgent, and the relief given by them less in time and extent ; if the attempts to take them be forcibly resisted, so that, if the supply is cut off, the want is immediately followed by great distress, and feelings of anguish, fainting, and suffocation; indeed, not unfrequently, persons thus deprived of the desired stimulants become actually insane or maniacal. 4.—*The crisis* occurs in 3, 5, 7, 9, 11, 13, or 21 days. It is characterized by feelings of intense distress, so that the patient loudly bewails his state, or groans deeply, until at last urgent vomiting supervenes, when either " corrupted " bile, or in many cases a watery fluid, is thrown up. To this succeeds the greatest disgust for spirituous drinks, so that the person who but a short time before urgently demanded brandy now shudders at the bare idea of it. 5.—The stage of *convalescence* is marked by the *sequelæ* of the affection, amongst which an excited condition of the entire system is the principal. There are also sleeplessness, frightful or disagreeable spectral illusions and depressing and distressing sensations,—the phenomena more or less, in short, of *delirium tremens.*

The leading symptoms, in the typical form of the disease, are those which show themselves in the thoracic viscera in connection with the appetite for stimulants,—namely, the feelings of anguish, restlessness, and impending death by suffocation, and those which are more purely mental, and in which the insatiable appetite is the most prominent. To these may be added the direct results of the alcoholic poisoning. In discussing the pathology of paroxysmal drunkenness, it is necessary to determine carefully the order of causation. Now, it is undeniably certain that, in every case, whether it be acute or periodic, there is a special condition of the cerebrum which predisposes the individual to the paroxysm. This may be termed the *predisposing* cause. Without this, those circumstances upon which the outbreak immediately supervenes, or, in other words, the *exciting* causes, could never take effect. The *proximate* cause is that condition of the cerebrum which is developed by the exciting causes in a person duly predisposed, which condition is necessary to the manifestation of the paroxysm. The operation of these causes is best illustrated by cases. A member of a liberal profession is subject to paroxysms of *Oinomania.* He is fully aware of his infirmity, and is a water-drinker on principle, for, so long as he abstains from alcoholic stimuli, he is safe. If, however, he yields to temptation ever so little,—if he takes but a single glass of wine,—he is lost. The irresistible appetite is excited, and all the misery and disgrace of a paroxysm of drunken madness follows. This individual has a near blood-relative, a man of superior talents, who is equally predisposed to *Oinomania,* and who, when attacked by a paroxysm, disappears from his family and home, and is found in the lowest haunts of vice and depravity, drinking with the most depraved. Both these examples are members of a family in which Insanity is hereditary. In another similar case of an individual—a member of an artistic profession—there is great natural talent and aptitude for business, so that he gives the highest satisfaction to his employers ; but, at varying intervals of time—from a few weeks to several months—the *oinomaniac* is absent from his office for several days on a drunken "spree." When he returns, great is his remorse, bitter his self-condemnation, loud and resolutely expressed his promises to resist temptation. For a while all goes on well ; but, sooner or later, the temptation comes, the alcoholic stimulant is presented, is irresistible, and a paroxysm is the result, to end as before. Now the *brother* of this impulsive *oinomaniac* is the victim of continuous drunkenness ; the *father* of both was a continuous drunkard, who believed himself to be a tea-pot, to be made of glass, &c., and who, in a paroxysm of inebriate fury, burnt a cat alive ; and the *grandmother's* brother was also an impulsive and finally a continuous *oinomaniac.* It is related of this grand-uncle, that his friends having taken away his clothes on a Sunday morning, hoping to confine him to the house by the want of clothing, he went into his warehouse, and donning a funeral-cloak made his way to the dram-shop! These cases illustrate the *hereditary* transmission of the predisposition from generation to generation.

Like insanity, epilepsy, and other analogous affections of the cerebrum, *Oinomania* may be *periodic.* Bruhl-Kramer mentions a case in which the paroxysm occurred regularly every four weeks, at the new moon ; and Most remarks that he thinks he has observed, in several instances, that the impulse to drink was the most urgent about the same time. In Henke's "Zeitschrift fur Staatsarzneikunde" (vol. 34), a case is related of monthly periodic drunkenness prolonged for seven years ; each attack occupied eight days. The patient was a mechanic ; orderly, industrious, and moral, until he was thirty-four, when he became subject to paroxysms of *oinomania,* during which his whole character underwent a change. After being for three weeks most industrious and steady, he would return home of an evening in apparently his usual health; but, on going to bed, he could not sleep on account of great depression and a peculiar sensation in the head. About one o'clock he would leap out of bed, run about the house, rush into the street, in nothing more than his shirt, and shout and rave so violently for spirit at the dram-shops, that the people were compelled to supply him; this he would drink greedily and in large quantities, until he lost the use of his limbs. Towards morning, he would be taken home unconscious, where he would be confined and bound. After lying in that state, with half-closed eyes, for a length of time, he would raise himself up, look round with a wild, melancholy look, the veins of the forehead starting, his face bathed in perspiration, his pulse quick and full, his hair dishevelled, his body almost naked; he would first be abusive, twist about, and make violent efforts to free himself from restraint, and then would piteously beg and implore for spirits, his voice gradually becoming weaker. He rejected all food and drink, except coffee, demanding brandy only, for without it he felt he must perish. He was usually given to drink, for the purpose of quieting him, brandy-and-water, in the proportion of one of brandy to three of water, which he would drink off with the utmost eagerness, and immediately ask for more. In this way he would go on without resting or sleeping for one moment for eight days, having brandy-and-water given to him two or three times a day, and taking hardly anything else. During this time, he became gradually weaker, and his voice more and more feeble, and at last he would fall asleep, exhausted. On awaking, he had no recollection of what had happened, felt weak, and trembled a good deal. The appetite for food then returned; he would drink water only, abhorred brandy, went back to his employment, and was an industrious, steady, temperate man until the next paroxysm. This would return at the regular period, whether he took brandy or not, and continued whether his desire for brandy was gratified or not. As years went on, the duration of the paroxysms became gradually shortened to six, or five, and four days. There was no very striking decay of the intellect, although, at last, the termination of the case in imbecility began to threaten. He died unexpectedly during a paroxysm on the third day, appearing as if he had fallen asleep. During the paroxysms his room was more like that of an insane person than of a rational being, had a very offensive smell, and was very filthy. The patient himself, also, looked like a maniac. The father of this man was a confirmed drunkard, and committed suicide by hanging; two of his brothers were drunkards,—only a sister and himself of the family remained free from the vice; and he showed no symptoms of *oinomania* until he was thirty-four.

This case illustrates the disease in the acute form described by Friedreich, and is specially interesting, inasmuch as, by the character of regular periodicity which it presented, it brings *Oinomania* into the general category of cerebral and cerebro-spinal affections, the majority of which are thus periodic. It will occur at longer intervals, however, than the month, just as mania, epilepsy, somnambulism, &c., will. Cases continuing for one week, and recurring at intervals of twelve weeks, have been observed.* In the first case which Guislain saw, the paroxysm occurred at still longer intervals; it was that of a music-master, who every year, or every two years, suddenly ceased to practise his profession, and for about three months would be continually intoxicated. The paroxysm would then suddenly cease, and the patient become scrupulously temperate, drinking nothing but water, and avoiding all chances of temptation. Feeling during one of these lucid intervals, the premonitory symptoms of

* Most's "Ausfuhrliche Encyclopadie der gesammten Staatsarzneikunde," Vol. II., p. 995.

a paroxysm, he committed suicide. In another case (a woman) mentioned by Guislain the paroxysms came on after lucid intervals of from three to four years.

H.—Page 829.

LEGAL DEFINITIONS OF SOUNDNESS AND UNSOUNDNESS OF MIND.*

"A *Sound Mind*," says Shelford, "is wholly free from delusion" [all *popular* delusions of course being excepted]; "all the intellectual faculties existing in a certain degree of vigour and harmony, the propensities, affections, and passions being under the subordination of the judgment and will, the former being the controlling power with a just perception of the natural connection or repugnancy of ideas. Weak minds, again, differ from strong in the extent and power of their faculties; but, unless they betray symptoms of a total loss of understanding, and of idiotcy, or of delusions, they cannot be considered unsound. An *Unsound Mind*, on the contrary, *is marked by delusions*" [which are not popularly entertained], "mingles ideas of imagination with those of reality, those of reflection with those of sensation, and mistakes the one for the other; and such delusion is often accompanied with an apparent insensibility to or perversion of those feelings which are peculiarly characteristic of our nature. Some lunatics, for instance, are callous to a just sense of affection, decency, or honor; they hate those, without cause, who were formerly most dear to them; others take delight in cruelty; many are more or less affected at not receiving that attention to which their delusions persuade them they are entitled. Retention of memory, display of talents, enjoyment of amusing games, and an appearance of rationality on various subjects, are not inconsistent with unsoundness of mind; hence sometimes arises the difficulty of distinguishing between sanity and insanity. The man of insane mind, from disease, having been once *non compos mentis*, pertinaciously adheres to some *delusive idea*, in opposition to the plainest evidence of its falsity, and endeavors by the most ingenious arguments, however fallacious they may be, to support his opinions."—*On the Law of Lunacy*, 1847.

---

* See Med. Chir. Rev., July 1855, p. 272.

INDEX.